FEMALE GENITAL CANCER

S. B. Gusberg, M.D., D.Sc.

Distinguished Service Professor and Chairman Emeritus
Department of Obstetrics – Gynecology and Reproductive Science
Mount Sinai School of Medicine of the City University of New York
New York, New York

Hugh M. Shingleton, M.D.

J. Marion Sims Professor and Chairman,
Department of Obstetrics and Gynecology
Professor, Department of Pathology
University of Alabama School of Medicine
Birmingham, Alabama

Gunter Deppe, M.D.

Professor, Department of Obstetrics and Gynecology
Wayne State University School of Medicine
Director, Department of Gynecologic Oncology
Hutzel Hospital
Detroit, Michigan

CHURCHILL LIVINGSTONE
New York, Edinburgh, London, Melbourne   1988

Library of Congress Cataloging in Publication Data

Female genital cancer / edited by S.B. Gusberg, Hugh M. Shingleton,
   Gunter Deppe.
        p.   cm.
   Includes bibliographies and index.
   ISBN 0-443-08525-0
   1. Generative organs, Female — Cancer.   I. Gusberg, Saul B. (Saul
Bernard), date.   II. Shingleton, Hugh M.   III. Deppe, Gunter.
   [DNLM: 1. Genital Neoplasms, Female.   WP 145 F329]
RC280.G5F38   1988
616.99′465 — dc19
DNLM/DLC
for Library of Congress   88-2593
                                                                              CIP

© **Churchill Livingstone Inc. 1988**

Distributed in the United Kingdom by Churchill Livingstone, Robert Stevenson House, 1–3
Baxter's Place, Leith Walk, Edinburgh EH1 3AF, and by associated companies, branches, and
representatives throughout the world.

Accurate indications, adverse reactions, and dosage schedules for drugs are provided in this
book, but it is possible that they may change. The reader is urged to review the package
information data of the manufacturers of the medications mentioned.

Acquisitions Editor: *Toni M. Tracy*
Assistant Editor: *Nancy Terry*
Copy Editor: *Ann Ruzycka*
Production Designer: *Melanie Haber*
Production Supervisor: *Sharon Tuder*

Printed in the United States of America

First published in 1988

Contributors

Hervy E. Averette, M.D.
Professor and Director, Division of Gynecologic Oncology, Department of Obstetrics and Gynecology, University of Miami School of Medicine, Miami, Florida

Vicki V. Baker, M.D.
Assistant Professor, Department of Obstetrics and Gynecology, Division of Gynecologic Oncology, University of Alabama School of Medicine, Birmingham, Alabama

Hugh R. K. Barber, M.D.
Director, Department of Obstetrics and Gynecology, Lenox Hill Hospital, New York, New York

Arthur F. Battista, M.D., M.Sc., M.A.
Professor, Department of Neurosurgery, New York University School of Medicine, New York University Medical Center, New York, New York

Suzanne Bergen, M.D.
Clinical Instructor, Department of Obstetrics and Gynecology, Division of Gynecologic Oncology, University of California, Irvine, California College of Medicine, Irvine, California

John A. Blessing, Ph.D.
Director of Statistics, Gynecologic Oncology Group, Roswell Park Memorial Institute, Buffalo, New York

Marcia C. Bowling, M.D.
Assistant Professor, Department of Obstetrics and Gynecology, Division of Gynecologic Oncology, University of Cincinnati College of Medicine; Department of Clinical Obstetrics and Gynecology, The Christ Hospital, Cincinnati, Ohio

Gunter Deppe, M.D., F.A.C.O.G., F.A.C.S.
Professor, Department of Obstetrics and Gynecology, Wayne State University School of Medicine; Director, Department of Gynecologic Oncology, Hutzel Hospital, Detroit, Michigan

Philip J. DiSaia, M.D.
Professor and Chairman, Department of Obstetrics and Gynecology, University of California, Irvine, California College of Medicine, Irvine, California

Daniel M. Donato, M.D.
Assistant Professor, Department of Obstetrics and Gynecology, Division of Gynecologic Oncology, University of Miami School of Medicine, Miami, Florida

Joseph F. Fraumeni, Jr., M.D.
Associate Director, Epidemiology and Biostatistics Program, Division of Cancer Etiology, National Institutes of Health, National Cancer Institute, Bethesda, Maryland

Martin S. Goldstein, M.D.
Associate Clinical Professor, Department of Obstetrics – Gynecology and Reproductive Science, Mount Sinai School of Medicine of the City University of New York, New York, New York

Alan N. Gordon, M.D.
Assistant Professor, Department of Obstetrics and Gynecology, Division of Gynecologic Oncology, Vanderbilt University School of Medicine, Vanderbilt University Medical Center, Nashville, Tennessee

Hazel Gore, M.B., B.S.
Professor, Departments of Obstetrics and Gynecology and Pathology, University of Alabama School of Medicine, Birmingham, Alabama

Erlio Gurpide, Ph.D.
Professor, Departments of Biochemistry and Obstetrics – Gynecology and Reproductive Science, Mount Sinai School of Medicine of the City University of New York, New York, New York

S. B. Gusberg, M.D., D.Sc., F.A.C.S., F.A.C.O.G., F.R.C.O.G. (A.E.), D.Sc.(Hon.)
Distinguished Service Professor and Chairman Emeritus, Department of Obstetrics – Gynecology and Reproductive Science, Mount Sinai School of Medicine of the City University of New York, New York, New York

John V. Hagen, M.S., A.M.I.
Medical Illustrator, Section of Medical Graphics, Mayo Clinic and Foundation, Rochester, Minnesota

Charles B. Hammond, M.D.
Professor and Chairman, Department of Obstetrics and Gynecology, Duke University School of Medicine, Duke University Medical Center, Durham, North Carolina

Kenneth D. Hatch, M.D.
Professor and Director, Division of Gynecologic Oncology, Department of Obstetrics and Gynecology, University of Alabama School of Medicine, Birmingham, Alabama

Marc J. Homer, M.D.
Professor, Department of Radiology, Tufts University School of Medicine; Chief, Mammography Section, New England Medical Center Hospital, Boston, Massachusetts

Robert N. Hoover, M.D.
Chief, Environmental Epidemiology Branch, Epidemiology and Biostatistics Program, Division of Cancer Etiology, National Institutes of Health, National Cancer Institute, Bethesda, Maryland

Mary K. Howett, Ph.D.
Associate Professor, Department of Microbiology, Pennsylvania State University College of Medicine, Hershey, Pennsylvania

Raymond H. Kaufman, M.D.
Professor and Chairman, Department of Obstetrics and Gynecology, Baylor College of Medicine, Houston, Texas

Robert Y. Kim, M.D.
Associate Professor, Department of Radiation Oncology, University of Alabama School of Medicine, Birmingham, Alabama

Julie Johnson Knox, M.D.
Assistant Professor, Department of Psychiatry and Behavioral Sciences, University of Arkansas for Medical Sciences, Little Rock, Arkansas

W. Dwayne Lawrence, M.D.
Assistant Professor, Department of Pathology, Wayne State University School of Medicine; Chief, Department of Anatomic Pathology, Hutzel Hospital, Detroit, Michigan

John L. Lovecchio, M.D.
Director, Division of Gynecologic Oncology, Department of Obstetrics–Gynecology, North Shore University Hospital, Manhasset, New York

John M. Malone, Jr., M.D.
Assistant Professor, Department of Obstetrics and Gynecology, Wayne State University School of Medicine; Division of Gynecologic Oncology, Hutzel Hospital, Detroit, Michigan

Vinay K. Malviya, M.D.
Assistant Professor, Department of Obstetrics and Gynecology, Wayne State University School of Medicine; Vice Chief, Department of Gynecologic Oncology, Hutzel Hospital, Detroit, Michigan

Douglas J. Marchant, M.D.
Professor, Departments of Obstetrics and Gynecology and Surgery, Tufts University School of Medicine, Boston, Massachusetts

Cheryl F. McCartney, M.D.
Associate Professor, Department of Psychiatry, Adjunct Associate Professor, Department of Obstetrics and Gynecology, Associate Dean of Student Affairs, and Former Director, Psychiatric Consultation — Liaison Service, University of North Carolina at Chapel Hill School of Medicine, Chapel Hill, North Carolina

George W. Mitchell, M.D.
Professor, Department of Obstetrics and Gynecology, Division of Gynecology, University of Texas Medical School at San Antonio, University of Texas Health Science Center, San Antonio, Texas

James H. Nelson, Jr., M.D.
Professor, Department of Obstetrics and Gynecology, University of Cincinnati College of Medicine; Director, Division of Gynecologic Oncology, University of Cincinnati Hospital and The Christ Hospital, Cincinnati, Ohio; Joe V. Meigs Professor of Gynecology Emeritus, Harvard Medical School, Boston, Massachusetts

James W. Orr, Jr., M.D.
Director, Gynecologic Oncology, The Watson Clinic, Lakeland, Florida

Karl C. Podratz, M.D., Ph.D.
Associate Professor, Department of Obstetrics and Gynecology, Mayo Medical School; Chairman, Department of Obstetrics and Gynecology, Mayo Clinic and Foundation, Rochester, Minnesota

Joseph Ransohoff, M.D.
Professor and Chairman, Department of Neurosurgery, New York University School of Medicine, New York University Medical Center, New York, New York

Fred Rapp, Ph.D
Professor and Chairman, Department of Microbiology, Pennsylvania State University College of Medicine, Hershey, Pennsylvania

Frank J. Rauscher, Jr., Ph.D.
Senior Vice President for Research, The American Cancer Society, Inc., New York, New York

Peter E. Schwartz, M.D.
Professor, Department of Obstetrics and Gynecology, Director, Division of Gynecologic Oncology, Yale University School of Medicine, New Haven, Connecticut

Bernd-Uwe Sevin, M.D., Ph.D.
Associate Professor, Department of Obstetrics and Gynecology, Division of Gynecologic Oncology, University of Miami School of Medicine, Miami, Florida

Hugh M. Shingleton, M.D., F.A.C.S., F.A.C.O.G.
Professor and Chairman, Department of Obstetrics and Gynecology, Professor, Department of Pathology, University of Alabama School of Medicine, Birmingham, Alabama

John T. Soper, M.D.
Assistant Professor, Department of Obstetrics and Gynecology, Division of Gynecologic Oncology, Duke University School of Medicine, Duke University Medical Center, Durham, North Carolina

Richard E. Symmonds, M.D.
Emeritus Professor, Department of Obstetrics and Gynecology, Mayo Medical School; Emeritus Member, Mayo Clinic and Foundation, Rochester, Minnesota

C. C. Wang, M.D.
Professor, Department of Radiation Therapy, Harvard Medical School; Clinical Head, Department of Radiation Medicine, Massachusetts General Hospital, Boston, Massachusetts

Preface

The increase in the literature of gynecologic cancer and the multiplication of monographs concerning tumors of the female genital tract speak to the increasing knowledge and sophisticated, specialized technology that have led to the formalization of the discipline of gynecologic oncology. Though gynecologists have long shown an interest in the prevention and treatment of cancer, the demand for specialists who understand radical pelvic surgery, radiotherapy, chemotherapy, and pathology and who have mastered one of these disciplines has fostered an increasing concentration that has resulted in expanding scholarship in this field.

Female Genital Cancer is comprehensive but not encyclopedic. Certain infrequently encountered lesions will require a special search of the literature by the clinician requiring special information. Yet the reader will find in this book a presentation of the principal bases upon which our discipline is built. Section one concerns the oncologic sciences upon which clinical care depends and advances, section two the clinical science of the disease sites, section three the surgical treatment of genital cancer, and section four deals with special problems. To make each of these sections valuable, the editors have gathered a distinguished group of clinicians and scientists to contribute their knowledge and their teaching authority, as well as scholarship, in their respective fields of interest. No one person can encompass this whole field with maximum authority any longer.

An analysis of the development of gynecologic oncology reveals that early diagnosis has contributed more to its advance than innovative treatment, although the advent of modern chemotherapy has offered the possibility of curative treatment of advanced disease. The supremacy of diagnostic advance is based partly on the accessibility of many of the tumors that we treat, which has enabled us to study and define meticulously the histogenesis of these tumors, prevent progression to the invasive stage in some, and cure those established cancers in the earlier stages of advancement. The precursor stages of gynecologic tumors have been studied so well that they are regarded as prototypes for those of tumors in other less accessible organ systems.

As we have learned to surgically excise greater volumes of cancer, the increasing insights of tumor cell biology have led us to two modifying hypotheses: Surgery and radiation, no matter how radical, are essentially local or regional treatments while cancer is frequently a general disease that requires, in some situations, general treatment; and so we have begun to incorporate chemotherapy. With this increased knowledge of the biology of tumors, especially of their developmental nature, we have found that we can cure some precursors and tumors of low virulence with less intervention, reserving the more aggressive treatments for the more virulent diseases. This concept of individualization has decreased morbidity and enhanced the quality of life of these subjects without sacrificing longevity.

At the same time the astonishing advances in molecular biology in the past two decades, sometimes referred to in the lay press as the "biologic revolution," and the developing bridge from the laboratory to the bedside have forced us to consider our increasing need for surgical scholars, clinician scientists who have the capacity to scan the scientific horizon as it broadens and deepens. We must seek advances that can be translated into therapeutic gain in patient care if we are to swim with this scientific tide rather than allow it to drown us and deprive our patients of this accelerating knowledge of cell growth and cell death.

As the complexity of technology increases, we must also maintain our physicianly role by attending to the humanistic considerations of cancer treatment. The psychosocial aspects of cancer involving the problems of mutilations and diminished self image, of sexuality and reconstruction, and even of environment and lifestyle and risk factors with their concomitant behavioral problems must remain important issues.

We hope that the tri-generational experience among the authors and editors of *Female Genital Cancer* has allowed us to recognize the advances made by those who came before us while keeping ourselves sensitive and receptive to new evidence as it evolves.

To those who have collaborated with us in this labor of love, we offer our profound gratitude. We believe their efforts will be rewarded by grateful readers, who will respect their scholarship and authority, and by grateful patients, who will benefit from increasingly expert care.

We also acknowledge the devoted assistance of Mrs. Margaret Masler and Mrs. Shirley Waldemar, who helped in the preparation of this volume at The Mount Sinai School of Medicine. In addition, the responsibility for reference work, manuscript typing, preparation of photomicrographs and drawings, and editing of the chapters from the University of Alabama at Birmingham was assumed by Jean Elliot and Josephine Taylor. At Wayne State University, we acknowledge the assistance of Jane Wittersheim and Karen Wojotowicz.

Finally, to our publisher, Churchill Livingstone, and its sophisticated editors, Toni Tracy, Nancy Terry, and Ann Ruzycka, must go our gratitude for their devotion to this project.

S. B. Gusberg
Hugh M. Shingleton
Gunter Deppe

Contents

Section III.   SURGICAL PROCEDURES

Section IV.   SPECIAL PROBLEMS

1
Introduction: Cancer Control

S. B. Gusberg

The subject of cancer control is important to gynecologists, for we are entrusted with the health care of women, and much of our effort relates to the sector of that care previously called preventive medicine. This is as true in prenatal care as it is in cancer screening. There are special reasons for the study of gynecologic oncology and the interest in prevention, early diagnosis, and treatment of female genital cancer by all gynecologists and obstetricians:

1. Cancer of the female genital tract is frequent (Tables 1-1 and 1-2; Figs. 1-1 and 1-2).
2. Cancers of the uterus and of the lower genital tract are accessible.
3. The histogenesis of those tumors is well known, perhaps better known than malignant tumors elsewhere in the body.
4. These factors increase our opportunities for prevention by early detection and prompt eradication of precancerous lesions.
5. In addition, gynecologists have the opportunity to care for large groups of healthy asymptomatic women for whom cancer screening and counseling is appropriate and important.
6. In fact, most malignant tumors of the female genital tract are not only preventable but highly curable. Unfortunately, cancer of the ovary is an exception.

Indeed, if a female genital cancer is less than 1 cm in diameter, the cure rate will be 90 percent or better. Even if the tumor is more advanced but still confined to the organ of its origin, we may cure approximately 80 percent. The contrast of this figure with the 50 percent cure rate now obtainable if one includes all cases diagnosed suggests the importance of early diagnosis and screening. One can carry this thesis one step further with the knowledge that precancerous lesions and noninvasive cancers are curable in virtually 100 percent of cases. This goal is attainable when both patients and physicians play their appropriate responsible roles.

THE NATIONAL EFFORT

It is now 73 years since the founding of the American Cancer Society (ACS), 49 years since the inception of the National Cancer Institute (NCI), and 15 years since the passage of the National Cancer Act that transformed that institution into the major cancer research facility in the world. Thousands of hours of creative thinking, millions of person-hours of scientific work, and billions of dollars have been expended in this effort. It seems appropriate that an accounting is in order, and that we should set down where we have been in cancer control and where we are going (Fig. 1-3).

Table 1-1 Estimated New Cancer Cases by Sex for All Sites: United States, 1986[a,b]

Site	Total	Male	Female
All sites	930,000[d]	465,000[d]	465,000[d]
Buccal cavity and pharynx (oral)[c]	29,500	19,800	9,700
Lip	4,600	4,000	600
Tongue	5,300	3,300	2,000
Mouth	10,700	6,300	4,400
Pharynx	8,900	6,200	2,700
Digestive organs	217,800	110,700	107,100
Esophagus	9,300	6,600	2,700
Stomach	24,700	15,000	9,700
Small intestine	2,200	1,100	1,100
Large intestine (colon[c])	98,000	45,000	53,000
Rectum[c]	42,000	22,000	20,000
Liver and biliary passages	13,600	6,800	6,800
Pancreas	25,500	13,000	12,500
Other and unspecified digestive	2,500	1,200	1,300
Respiratory system	164,500	112,300	52,200
Larynx	11,700	9,600	2,100
Lung[c]	149,000	100,000	49,000
Other and unspecified respiratory	3,800	2,700	1,100
Bone	2,000	1,100	900
Connective tissue	5,100	2,700	2,400
Skin[c]	23,000[e]	12,000[e]	11,000[e]
Breast[c]	123,900[f]	900[f]	123,000[f]
Genital organs	169,800	96,400	73,400
Cervix, uterus[c]	14,000[f]	—	14,000[f]
Corpus, endometrium	36,000	—	36,000
Ovary	19,000	—	19,000
Other and unspecified genital, female	4,400	—	4,400
Prostate	90,000	90,000	—
Testis	5,100	5,100	—
Other and unspecified genital, male	1,300	1,300	—

Continued

Table 1-1 Estimated New Cancer Cases by Sex for All Sites: United States, 1986[a,b] *Continued*

Site	Total	Male	Female
Urinary organs	60,500	41,700	18,800
Bladder	40,500	29,000	11,500
Kidney and other urinary	20,000	12,700	7,300
Eye	1,800	900	900
Brain and central nervous system	13,800	7,700	6,100
Endocrine glands	11,700	3,500	8,200
Thyroid	10,600	2,900	7,700
Other endocrine	1,100	600	500
Leukemias	25,600	14,000	11,600
Lymphocytic leukemia	12,300	6,900	5,400
Granulocytic leukemia	12,600	6,700	5,900
Monocytic leukemia	700	400	300
Other blood and lymph tissues	44,500	22,800	21,700
Hodgkin's disease	6,900	3,900	3,000
Multiple myeloma	10,400	5,200	5,200
Other lymphomas	27,200	13,700	13,500
All other and unspecified sites	36,500	18,500	18,000

[a] The estimates of new cancer cases are offered as a rough guide and should not be regarded as definitive. Especially note that year-to-year changes may only represent improvements in the basic data.

[b] Incidence estimates are based on rates from NCI SEER program 1977 to 1981.

[c] One of six major sites designated by the American Cancer Society (colon and rectum constitute one site).

[d] Carcinoma in situ and nonmelanoma skin cancers are not included in totals. Carcinoma in situ of the uterine cervix accounts for more than 45,000 new cases annually, and carcinoma in situ of the female breast accounts for more than 5,000 new cases annually. Nonmelanoma skin cancer accounts for more than 400,000 new cases annually.

[e] Melanoma only.

[f] Invasive cancer only.

(Silverberg E, Lubera J: Cancer statistics. CA: 36:16, 1986.)

Table 1-2 Estimated Cancer Deaths by Sex for All Sites:
United States, 1986

Site	Total	Male	Female
All sites	472,000	253,500	218,500
Buccal cavity and pharynx (oral[a])	9,400	6,350	3,050
Lip	175	150	25
Tongue	2,100	1,400	700
Mouth	2,825	1,800	1,025
Pharynx	4,300	3,000	1,300
Digestive organs	119,700	62,500	57,200
Esophagus	8,800	6,400	2,400
Stomach	14,300	8,400	5,900
Small intestine	800	400	400
Large intestine colon[a]	51,800	24,800	27,000
Rectum[a]	8,200	4,300	3,900
Liver and biliary passages	10,600	5,300	5,300
Pancreas	24,000	12,300	11,700
Other and unspecified digestive	1,200	600	600
Respiratory system	135,350	93,000	42,350
Larynx	3,800	3,100	700
Lung[a]	130,100	89,000	41,100
Other and unspecified respiratory	1,450	900	550
Bone	1,400	800	600
Connective tissue	2,800	1,300	1,500
Skin[a]	7,500[b]	4,500	3,000
Breast[a]	40,200	300	39,900
Genital organs	49,400	27,000	22,400
Cervix, uterus[a]	6,800	—	6,800
Corpus, endometrium	2,900	—	2,900
Ovary	11,600	—	11,600
Other and unspecified genital, female	1,100	—	1,100
Prostate	26,100	26,100	—
Testis	500	500	—
Other and unspecified genital, male	400	400	—
Urinary organs	19,800	12,800	7,000
Bladder	10,600	7,200	3,400
Kidney and other urinary	9,200	5,600	3,600
Eye	400	200	200
Brain and central nervous system	10,200	5,500	4,700
Endocrine glands	1,750	750	1,000
Thyroid	1,100	400	700
Other endocrine	650	350	300
Leukemias	17,400	9,600	7,800
Lymphocytic leukemia	6,600	3,800	2,800
Granulocytic leukemia	10,400	5,600	4,800
Monocytic leukemia	400	200	200

Continued

Table 1-2 Estimated Cancer Deaths by Sex for All Sites: United States, 1986 *Continued*

Site	Total	Male	Female
Other blood and lymph tissues	23,700	12,300	11,400
Hodgkin's disease	1,500	900	600
Multiple myeloma	7,600	3,900	3,700
Other lymphomas	14,600	7,500	7,100
All other and unspecified sites	33,000	16,600	16,400

[a] One of six major sites designated by the American Cancer Society (colon and rectum constitute one site).

[b] Melanoma 5,600; other skin 1,900.

(Silverberg E, Lubera J: Cancer statistics. CA: 36:17, 1986.)

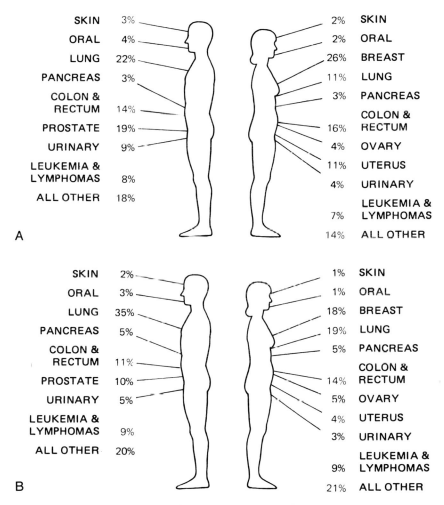

Fig. 1-1 1986 estimated cancer incidence **(A)** and cancer deaths **(B)** by site and sex. The estimates of the incidence of cancer are based on data from the National Cancer Institute's Surveillance, Epidemiology and End Results (SEER) program (1977–1981). Nonmelanoma skin cancer and carcinoma in situ have not been included in the statistics. The incidence of nonmelanoma skin cancer is estimated to be more than 400,000. (Prepared by Edwin Silverberg, supervisor of Epidemiology and Statistics, American Cancer Society, New York.) (Modified from Silverberg E, Lubera J: Cancer statistics. CA 36:9, 1986.)

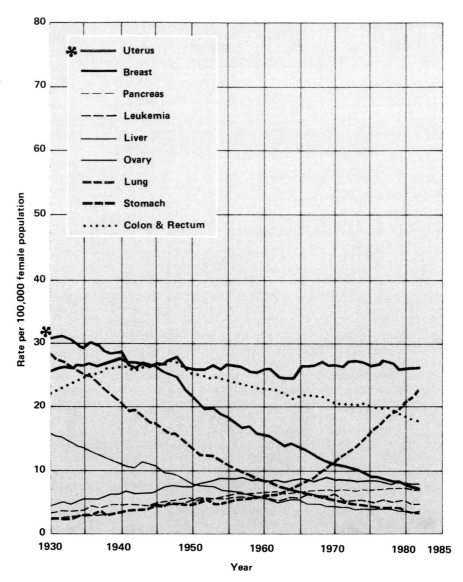

Fig. 1-2 Age-adjusted cancer death rates for selected sites in females in the United States, 1930–1982. (Rates adjusted to the age distribution of the 1970 U.S. Census population. Data from the U.S. National Center for Health Statistics and U.S. Bureau of the Census.) (Modified from Silverberg E, Lubera J: Cancer statistics. CA 36:9, 1986.)

No one who is informed about the progress in cancer control can doubt the wisdom of this effort. We have established cancer centers in most regions of the country; we have an increasing pool of trained oncologists in gynecology surgery, radiation, and medicine; we have speeded the technology transfer of the latest advances in diagnosis and treatment from the austerity of the research facility to the front-line community physician; and we have witnessed a tremendous growth in the body of knowledge about malignant cell growth and death (Tables 1-3 and 1-4).

That we have problems remaining must be acknowledged, for our gains have been somewhat muted by an aging population susceptible to cancer, common cancers like those of the breast, colon, and lung that have been slow to yield to treatment, and a

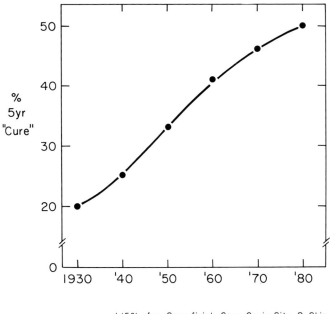

+15% for Superficial Ca:— Ca-in-Situ & Skin

Fig. 1-3 Cancer cure by decade.

Table 1-3 Cancer Incidence in Five Continents: Age Standardized

Site	Columbia (Calif.)	United Kingdom (S.W.)	Japan	United States (Conn.)	Israel Born in Europe	Born in Africa or Asia
Cervix	75.6	13.6	20.6	10.3	4.2	6.7
Corpus	6.8	10.2	1.3	15.3	10.7	4.5
Breast	27.3	50.6	11.0	62.3	55.5	22.2
Prostate	23.2	21.7	3.2	33.0	11.4	13.2
Stomach (F)	24.8	11.2	44.7	6.8	11.1	17.9

(Modified from Doll R, Muir G, Waterhouse J (eds): Cancer Incidence in Five Continents, Vol. 2, Springer-Verlag, Berlin, 1970.)

Table 1-4 Cancer Risk Change for Japanese Females Migrant to the United States[a]

Site	Japanese	Japanese Migrants to United States	U.S.-Born Japanese	U.S. White
Stomach	100	55	48	18
Colon	100	218	209	483
Breast	100	166	136	591
Ovary	100	337	—	535
Cervix	100	52	33	48
Corpus[b]	100	209	—	330

[a] Standardized mortality rates; Japan = 100.
[b]Japanese figures include chorioca; U.S. figures do not.
(Haenszel W, Kurihara M: Studies of Japanese migrants. J Natl Cancer Inst 40:43, 1968.)

Table 1-5 Mortality for the Five Leading Cancer Sites for Females by Age Group: United States, 1983

All Ages All Cancer (204,603)	Under 15 All Cancer (915)	15–34 All Cancer (3,548)	35–54 All Cancer (26,497)	55–74 All Cancer (102,382)	75+ All Cancer (71,233)
Breast (37,979)	Leukemia (332)	Breast (676)	Breast (7,770)	Lung (21,764)	Colon and rectum (13,496)
Lung (34,685)	Brain and CNS (201)	Leukemia (473)	Lung (4,973)	Breast (19,432)	Breast (10,091)
Colon and rectum (27,811)	Connective tissue (47)	Uterus (337)	Colon and rectum (1,927)	Colon and rectum (12,211)	Lung (7,827)
Ovary (11,375)	Bone (45)	Brain and CNS (304)	Ovary (1,728)	Ovary (6,319)	Pancreas (5,028)
Pancreas (11,292)	Kidney (43)	Hodgkin's disease (217)	Uterus (1,724)	Pancreas (5,439)	Uterus (3,287)

(Vital Statistics of the United States, 1983.)
(Silverberg E, Lubera J: Cancer statistics. CA 36:11, 1986.)

major, self-imposed environmental factor related to the latter, cigarette smoking (Table 1-5). Cigarette smoking is responsible for more than 80 percent of lung cancer, not readily curable as yet, and also appears to play a role in pharyngeal, laryngeal, esophageal, bladder, and cervix cancer (Fig. 1-4). Doll, a British epidemiologist, estimates that 50 to 60 percent of cancers in British males and a somewhat smaller percentage in females is attributable to cigarette smoking.

The frequency of malignant tumors of the female genital tract is significant (Table 1-6).

EARLY DIAGNOSIS AND CURE

The importance of gynecologic cancer has, in modern medicine, attracted the study and training of some gynecologists in this field and in recent years this has resulted in formalizing this training is preparation for certification in the subspecialty of gynecologic oncology. Almost parallel to this development, the era of Papanicolaou (Pap) screening has resulted in a steady decline in mortality from cervix cancer in the United States, while early diagnosis has resulted in increasing cure due to earlier-stage disease and even the detection of easily cured precursors by this method. That this decline in mortality is related to screening may be deduced from the Canadian experience presented in the Walton Report. While there are doubters who emphasize lead-time bias as responsible for the increasing longevity of some cancer patients, especially since we pragmatically and conveniently refer to "cure" as living and well for 5 years free of disease, mature physicians have witnessed the increasing survival of patients who formerly uniformly died of their disease, mostly within 3 years. Indeed, the rate of cure for invasive cancer generally, has risen from less than 20 percent in 1920 to approximately 50 percent in 1985. If we were to include superficial and in situ cancers, this cure rate would rise to 65 percent.

The working definition of cure as that of a person living and well and free of disease at 5 years from diagnosis has served us well, for most patients with persistent or recurrent disease present with this failure before 5 years and most afflicted with female genital cancer who survive 5 years are well forever (Table 1-7). The alternate definition of cure states that a

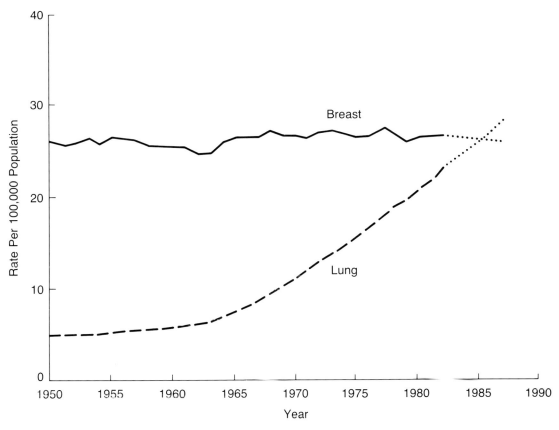

Fig. 1-4 Death rates of lung and breast cancers among women in the United States, 1950–1982. (Data from U.S. National Center for Health Statistics and U.S. Bureau of the Census. Death rates have been adjusted to the age distribution of the 1970 U.S. Census Population.)

Table 1-6 Frequency of Malignant Tumors of the Female Genital Tract: American Cancer Statistics for 1986

Organ	New Cases	Deaths
	73,400	22,400
Breast	123,000	39,900
Lung	49,000	41,100
Colon	53,000	27,000

Pap cytologic smear: may be considered a prototype for screening measures; has resulted in a greater than 50 percent reduction in mortality from cervix cancer in American women

Definition of uterine cancer precursors: dysplasia and cancer in situ for the cervix and adenomatous hy-

Table 1-7 Cancer Control: The Cure

Type of Cancer	%
Choriocarcinoma	0 → 90
Childhood leukemia	0 → >50
Hodgkin's disease	0 → >50
Wilm's tumor	0 → >50
Osteogenic sarcoma	0 → >70
Testicular cancer	>60
Cervical cancer	>60

treated woman can be considered cured when she arrives at a life expectancy equal to that of an age matched control never treated for cancer. Computers may render such complex terms clinically useful.

We can readily illustrate diagnostic advances during the modern biomedical era that have broadened our diagnostic scope:

perplasia for endometrium and similar lesions elsewhere in the body

Mammography: enables us to detect breast lesions not palpable to examination in asymptomatic women

Ultrasonography: permits discrimination between deep bodily masses

Computed tomography (CT) scan: offers a total view of body cross sections for the discovery of tumor masses and extension

Laparoscopy: permits direct vision and even biopsy of abdominal viscera without open surgery

Gastroscopy, colonoscopy, colposcopy, hysteroscopy: permit visualization of internal organs with direct access (also include other endoscopic techniques)

Magnetic imaging: a very recent diagnostic addition that offers not only internal body images without radiation but has the capacity for analyzing chemical body composition as well

Antigen tumor markers: enable us to follow the course of disease after treatment in some tumors

Although a long list, it becomes incomplete each year.

While early diagnosis permitted most of the advance until recent decades, therapeutic gains have increased survival in some malignant tumors formerly almost uniformly fatal, especially, those of childhood and early adulthood:

1. Childhood leukemia survival has increased from near zero to more than 50 percent.
2. Hodgkin's disease survival is now greater than 50 percent and in early stage disease 65 percent, whereas formerly it was almost invariably fatal
3. Choriocarcinoma, always fatal earlier, is now cured in 90 percent of cases.
4. Osteogenic sarcoma has been improved from zero percent to greater than 50 percent survival, recently, without limb amputation in appropriate individuals.
5. Kidney tumors of childhood now show greater than 50 percent survival.
6. Testicular cancer, even in advanced state, is now cured in more than 70 percent of cases, and ovarian cancer is beginning to yield to surgery and intensive chemotherapy.

Many of these therapeutic advances are based on combinations of surgery or radiation followed by chemotherapy. It seems important to remind gynecologic oncologists that cancer can be a general, rather than a local or regional, disease; surgery and radiation therapy, no matter how radical, are essentially local treatments. Only chemotherapy constitutes general bodily treatment with the capacity to seek out the cancer cell and destroy it. This does not diminish the important role of surgery or irradiation; it only recognizes our need to respect the enlargement of our scope with modern chemotherapy.

In fact, advances in the control of female genital cancer have come from several areas of technology. One may inspect this in the following examples, a list that is extensive but not exhaustive:

1. Definition of uterine cancer precursors
   a. Dysplasia and carcinoma in situ of the cervix
   b. Adenomatous hyperplasia of the endometrium
   c. Dysplasia and carcinoma in situ of the vulva
2. Pap cytologic smear
   a. Decline in mortality
   b. Monitoring high-risk patients
   c. Viruses as etiologic agents
3. Colposcopy and directed biopsy
   a. Ambulatory diagnosis
   b. Ambulatory treatment with cryotherapy or laser
4. Aspiration curettage of endometrium
   a. Histologic sample
   b. Ambulatory surveillance
5. Ultrasonography and laparoscopy
   a. Diagnosis and monitoring ovarian tumors
   b. Measurement
   c. Solid versus cystic
6. Hysteroscopy and hysterography
   a. Extent and localization of endometrial tumors
   b. Involvement of cervix
7. Mammography
   a. Breast screening
   b. Breast diagnosis
8. Rediscovery of radical hysterectomy; pelvic exenteration
   a. Roles defined
9. Pretreatment surgical staging
   a. Geographic extension of disease
   b. Planning treatment

10. Hormone dependence of endometrial cancer
    a. Steroid receptors
    b. Hormone treatment
    c. Progestins as estrogen antagonists
11. Individualization of treatment for endometrial cancer
    a. Virulence factors
    b. Primary surgery
    c. Adjuvant irradiation
    d. Selective lymphadenectomy
12. Treatment of advanced ovarian cancer
    a. Cytoreduction or debulking
    b. Intensive chemotherapy
    c. Post-treatment surgical staging—the second look

SCREENING FOR CANCER

The concept of screening asymptomatic individuals for preclinical disease or early clinical change for secondary prevention, with public education and counseling against carcinogens for primary prevention, has improved our strategic goal for cancer control (Fig. 1-5; Tables 1-8 and 1-9).

In general, screening efficiency rests on a benefit/risk ratio. The criteria frequently used are as follows:

The test should be effectual to decrease morbidity and mortality.
The benefit should exceed the risk.
The benefit should justify the cost.
The test should be technically acceptable to both patient and physician.

Most effective screening tests will depend on an interval between exposure and clinical establishment of cancer, with an interval of exfoliation of cells that permits detection of preclinical precancerous activity. The prototype of such tests is the Pap smear. It may be difficult to imagine risks related to any screening, but on analysis, one can understand a few:

Induction of anxiety or cancerphobia
Overtreatment
False security
Induction of cancer

The American Cancer Society decided to put its screening advice for asymptomatic persons on a more scientific basis in 1978 to 1979 and presented guidelines in 1980 based on an analysis of the literature by David Eddy and his group then at Stanford University, and subsequently reviewed by several of the expert committees of the ACS (Table 1-10).

These guidelines were based on rather conservative assumptions with respect to carcinoma of the cervix:

1. The Pap smear can detect precursor lesions
2. A 50 percent accuracy rate only was assigned
3. An 8-year transit time was allowed (i.e., from precursor to invasive cancer)
4. It offset the assumption that 5 percent would progress to invasion within 2 years
5. No case of dysplasia would regress spontaneously

In spite of this supple framework, physicians generally, especially gynecologists, while accepting the premise of most of these guidelines, objected strongly to the "at least every 3 years" phrase for the Pap

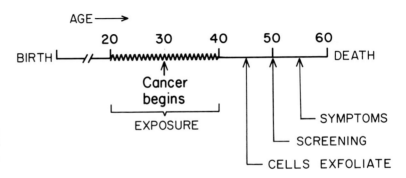

Fig. 1-5 Basis for screening. (Cole P, Morrison AS: p. 7. In Basic Issues in Cancer Screening. U.I.C.C. Report, Vol. 40. Geneva, 1978.)

Table 1-8 Summary of ACS Recommendations for the Early Detection of Cancer in Asymptomatic Persons

Test or Procedure	Population		
	Sex	Age	Frequency
Sigmoidoscopy	M, F	>50	Every 3–5 years; after 2 negative exams 1 year apart
Stool guaiac slide test	M, F	>50	Every year
Digital rectal examination	M, F	>40	Every year
Pap test	F	At 18 or earlier, if sexually active	At the physician's discretion after 3 consecutive negative Pap smears 1 year apart
Pelvic examination	F	20–40 >40	Every 3 years Every year
Endometrial tissue sample	F	At menopause women at high risk[a]	At menopause
Breast self-examination	F	>20	Every month
Breast physical examination	F	20–40 >40	Every 3 years Every year
Mammography	F	35–39 40–49 >50	Baseline Consult personal physician Every 1–2 years
Chest radiography		Not recommended	
Sputum cytology		Not recommended	
Health counseling and cancer checkup[b]	M, F M, F	>20 >40	Every 3 years Every year

[a] History of infertility, obesity, failure of ovulation, abnormal uterine bleeding, or estrogen therapy.
[b] To include examination for cancers of the thyroid, testicles, prostate, overies, lymph nodes, oral region, and skin.
(Silverberg E: Cancer statistics. CA 30:231, 1980.)

Table 1-9 Use of Cancer-Detection Tests in Asymptomatic Patients[a]

Study/ Examination	All Physicians (N = 1,035) %	General/ Family Practitioner (N = 532) %	Internist (N = 211) %	Obstetrician/ Gynecologist (N = 292) %	Age When Testing Usually Begins (Median Years)
Digital rectal	96	97	95	94	40.0
Stool blood	75	83	86	40	42.3
Proctoscopic	35	43	41	8	46.5
Breast physical	97	99	93	99	18.9
Mammogram	49	45	44	68	44.9
Pap test	94	96	86	100	18.7
Prostate[c]	90	90	89	NA	42.7
Chest radiography	42	44	57	14	NA

[a] "When you are examining a patient who has no personal history of cancer and who is asymptomatic, do you ever do. . . ?"
[b] Weighted to represent physicians in each group in their correct proportion in this and subsequent tables.
[c] Not asked of obstetricians/gynecologists. Total describes general/family practitioners and internists.
(Silverberg E: Cancer statistics. CA 35:201, 1985.)

Table 1-10 Recommendations for the Screening of Cancer
in Asymptomatic Persons, American Cancer Society, 1980

Test	Sex	Age	Frequency
Sigmoidoscopy	M&F	>50	q 3–5 years after two negative annual examinations
Stool Guiac	M&F	>50	Every year
Digital rectal	M&F	>40	Every year
Pap test	F	20–65	At least every 3 years
		<20 if sexually active	After two negative examinations
Pelvic examination	F	20–40	
		>40	Every 3 years
			Every year
Endometrial sample	F	Women at high risk	At menopause
Breast self-examination	F	>20	Every month
Breast examination	F	20–40	
		>40	Every 3 years
			Every year
Mammography	F	40–50	
		>50	Every 2 years
			Every year
Chest radiography			Not recommended
Sputum cytology			Not recommended

smear. Their concerns were expressed mainly with respect to several problems:

Loss of "anniversary" date interval

A high-risk population with an allegedly faster transit time

Loss of Pap entry into the health system

Some inadequate commercial Pap laboratories

The low cost of the Pap test, making cost an irrelevant factor

In fact, some of these concerns seem only theoretical and out of focus.

1. The low cost of the Pap test becomes larger when the physician's fee for examination and possible colposcopy are included.
2. There are cytology laboratories with poor quality control, but physicians should be aware of this by experience; in addition, they should exert great care in taking the cytologic sample.
3. Women between 20 and 40 years of age will usually consult a physician for contraception, pregnancy, or menstrual disorders, at which time they can be advised about preventive measures at whatever interval the physician deems appropriate to their needs.
4. There is no convincing evidence at present that high-risk women have a faster transit time than others, though it is clear from epidemiologic studies that their prevalence rate of precursors will be higher.

It would appear that the high-risk woman is frequently hard to reach with preventive measures and that we should concentrate on this problem. In addition, it is the opinion of some that a start to screening could be made with three or four annual Pap smears to offer the lesser laboratories more opportunities to detect abnormalities before going on to a 2–3-year interval.

PREVENTION AND DETECTION

While primary prevention, avoidance, or neutralization of all carcinogens is our theoretical ideal, early detection of preclinical or very early clinical disease is frequently all that we can attain in the present state of the art. The seven warning signals cited by the ACS, all possible symptoms of early cancer, have been widely publicized to caution the public against neglect.

ACS WARNING SIGNALS

1. Change in bowel or bladder habit
2. A sore that does not heal
3. Unusual bleeding or discharge
4. Thickening or lump in breast or elsewhere
5. Indigestion or difficulty swallowing
6. Obvious change in wart or mole
7. Nagging cough or hoarseness

This advice to consult a physician concerning those warning symptoms might well be accompanied and eventually superseded by prevention advice in this era of increased understanding of environmental causes of cancer.

SAFEGUARDS FOR WOMEN

1. Stop smoking to prevent lung cancer.
2. Practice breast self-examination.
3. Have periodic examination; some precancerous lesions can be detected.
4. Undergo periodic mammography.
5. Eat a prudent diet.
6. Limit sunlight exposure.
7. Limit alcohol intake.

As can be seen, some aspects of cancer care are no longer strictly biomedical in the narrow sense, for they relate to behavioral and psychosocial factors. In fact, in the traditional role, the physician's office can be a significant place in which to conduct a complete cancer examination for women. The 10-point screen can be quickly and effectively managed during the course of the regular periodic consultation visit.

THE CANCER EXAMINATION

1. Oral region
2. Thyroid and neck
3. Lymph nodes
4. Breasts
5. Skin
6. Abdomen
7. Pelvis
8. Rectum
9. Testes
10. Prostate

COUNSELING

We will fail in our role in preventive health care if we do not act as health counselors. If, in fact, we regard this as a distraction from the diagnosis and treatment of life-threatening disease, we should instruct the allied health personnel in our office or clinic in this sector of care whether they be nurses or technical assistants. They are capable of carrying out the educational and technical aspects of preventive care with great efficiency, frequently with a missionary zeal.

First, with respect to breast disease, the patient should be carefully instructed in the techniques of breast self-examination and advised to carry this out each month after the menses, when the breast is least congested. We know that most breast lumps are first detected by women rather than their physicians; it seems wise to practice this on a regular basis. For women over the age of 40, the detection of nonpalpable disease by mammography now appears to be a safe and efficient method of screening. The irradiation involved is insignificant in mature women screened by modern radiographic equipment; the efficiency of interpretation may be judged by the result of a recent national collaborative breast screening effort mounted as a demonstration project. In this project, women were screened by traditional examination and by mammography (Table 1-11).

This result has convinced most experts of the value of this screening effort.

Second, clear and formal instruction should be given to individual women as to the danger of smoking. There is increasing restriction of cigarette smoking in the U.S. adult population, more restriction in men than in women, but adolescents, who have not

Table 1-11 Breast Cancer Detection Demonstration Project[a]

Findings	%
Detected by mammography alone	41.6
Detected by physical examination alone	8.7
Mammography Alone Detected	
Noninfiltrating cancer	59.0
Infiltrating cancer < 1 cm	52.6

[a] Of 276,593 women screened, 4,443 cancers were found, 80 percent with negative nodes.

yet faced their mortality, have continued this habit at a great rate — especially young women. The result of this relative increase in smoking in the female population is now evident in the dramatic rise in lung cancer in women. Death from this disease has risen so precipitously that it will exceed death from breast cancer, itself high in the United States, this year.

Perhaps we can alter the adolescent's views of the smoking habit, not by the specter of disease in middle age, a time of life dimly perceived, but by pointing to the dangers of smoking in pregnancy, wherein pregnancy wastage by miscarriage and prematurity can occur, as well retarded growth of the infant in the uterus, because of nicotine and CO_2 that may result in developmental problems in small-for-date babies. In addition, they must be informed that the infrequent blood clotting problems of the oral contraceptive pill, so commonly used by young women, are increased by cigarette smoking.

Advice about diet and overexposure to the sun can be given readily by the physician or his assistants, but for the approximately 50 percent of women in the workforce, knowledge of toxic industrial chemicals must be imparted by more specialized persons.

THE DEVELOPMENT OF CANCER CONTROL

The decades of cancer control might be characterized in the following sequence:

1940s	Saw the sharpening of therapeutic technology both in surgery and radiotherapy, wherein radical surgery advanced due to the support system afforded by the emergence of scientific anesthesiology, antibiotics, blood banks, and the ability of surgeons to restore their patient's physiologic balance; radiotherapy acquired new machinery devised by the ingenious strategies of physicists and engineers
1950s	Could be called the decade of early diagnosis, wherein the concept of precancerous preclinical lesions and preinvasive cancer or carcinoma in situ was clearly defined and widely adopted
1960s	Saw the emergence of chemotherapy as a whole body treatment of cancer that could not only be palliative but actually curative
1970s – 1980s	Were marked by the so-called biologic revolution, for there was an explosion of scientific information, especially at the molecular level, concerning cell growth, cell metabolism — cell life and cell death
Late 1980s – 1990s	Could be called the era of therapeutic translation, for the basic sciences of the cancer cell and its host environment are ready to be taken up by the prepared scientific clinician into the improvement of diagnosis and treatment of clinical cancer.

CANCER CONTROL: THE FUTURE THRUST

1. High risk defined by site
2. Nutrition
3. Interferon and biologic modifiers
4. Chemoprevention
5. Environmental cancer and prevention
6. Screening by antibodies and enzymes
7. Combined treatment

Examples can be offered as evidence for this view of therapeutic translation already occurring from the basic oncologic sciences. Some of these options have been satisfactorily fulfilled; others are important already, but require significant further development.

Cell Biology

The insights of the cell biologists have freed us from the pharmaceutical era of chemotherapy, which was totally empirical. They have fostered the development of cytotoxic agents, reconoitering to seek out cancer cells remote from the primary site, with increased capability for discriminating destruction of these abnormal cells. These insights have also been programmed to intrude into the operative cell organelles and thus frustrate further cell division. In addition, the hope for chemoprevention has resulted from the development of substances that appear to restore cell maturation and therefore abort the inexorable transit of precancerous lesions to invasive cancer. Certain analogues of vitamin A (e.g., retinoic acid) appear to have this property, among others.

Radiobiology

Radiobiology has given us radiosensitizers to enhance the healing effect of therapeutic irradiation. It has shown that high-energy beams can make irradiation more efficient by nullifying the oxygen effect.

Immunology

Tumor immunology offers the prospect of bolstering host resistance to cancer cells and has developed some antigen and antibody markers for earlier diagnosis and even therapy. Monoclonal antibodies are already in clinical use.

Virology

Virology has taught us the transmissible nature of some malignant diseases, for viruses have been implicated in an etiologic mode in several human cancers: Epstein-Barr virus in Burkitt's lymphoma and nasopharyngeal cancer, hepatitis B virus in liver cancer, human papillomavirus in cancer of the cervix, and HTLV-1 in a certain type of lymphoma-leukemia.

These observations open the prospect of vaccines against such infections.

Genetics

Genetic studies have started to give us certain biologic markers, such as those in certain leukemias, and some familial breast and colon cancers, so that the possibility of prevention or earliest treatment becomes more feasible.

Endocrinology

Endocrinology by defining hormone sensitive tumors, especially in the breast, prostate, and uterus, has made hormonal antagonists important in the treatment spectrum.

Epidemiology

The science of epidemiology enables us to define high-risk groups for certain tumors, increasing our possibility for surveillance. The increased risk may be genetic, metabolic, or environmental.

EVALUATIONS OF QUALITY CANCER CONTROL

One can construct a scoring strategy for evaluation of oncologic care for female genital cancer, assigning 10 points for each heading, five for each subset, so that a score approaching 50 points indicates excellence if not perfection, in the following scheme:

1. Screening
   a. Technique
   b. Quality control
2. Diagnosis
   a. Technique
   b. Review of pathology
3. Treatment
   a. Surgical expertise
   b. Radiotherapeutic and chemotherapeutic knowledge
4. Rehabilitation
   a. Follow-up
   b. Quality of life

5. Communication
  a. Patient
  b. Public

We have made important strides in cancer control, but we surely have not reached our goal with 50 percent of patients afflicted with significant cancer still succumbing to their disease. The accelerated pace of discovery in the oncologic sciences and concurrent clinical advance would seem to give us cause for optimism about the future.

SELECTED READINGS

Cancer Facts and Figures. American Cancer Society, New York, 1985

Christopherson WM, Kurikara M: Studies of Japanese migrants. J Natl Cancer Inst 40:43, 1968

Collen M: Multiphasic Health Testing Services. Wiley, New York, 1978

Doll R: Strategy for detection of cancer hazards to man. Nature (Lond) 265:589, 1977

Doll R, Peto R: Mortality in relation to smoking. Br Med J 2:1525, 1976

Eddy DM: ACS report on the cancer related health checkup. CA 40:194, 1980

Fidler HK, Boyes DA, Worth AJ: Cervical cancer detection in British Columbia. J Obstet Gynecol Br Commonw 75:392, 1968

Gusberg SB, Deppe G: Role of Guidelines for Cancer Screening: Issues in Cancer Screening and Communications. Alan R. Liss, New York, 1982

Gusberg SB, Deppe G: The earliest diagnosis of cervical cancer and its precursors. Semin Oncol 9, No. 3, 1982

Haenszel W, Kurihara M: Studies of Japanese migrants. J Natl Cancer Inst 40:43, 1968

Miller AB, Lindsey J, Hill GB: Mortality from cancer of the uterus in Canada and its relation to screening for cancer of the cervix. Int J Cancer 17:602, 1976

National Cancer Institute: Consensus Development Meeting on Breast Cancer Screening: Issues and Recommendations. J Natl Cancer Inst 60:1519, 1978

Screening in Cancer: UICC Report of the International Workshop, Toronto, Canada. UICC Tech Rep Ser 40, 1978

Seidman H, Silverberg E, Bodden A: Probability of developing and dying of cancer. CA 28:33, 1978

Shapiro LJ, Associates: Survey of physicians' attitudes and practices in early cancer detection. CA 40:197, 1985

Silverberg E: Cancer statistics. 35:201, 1985

Silverberg E: Cancer statistics. CA 30:235, 1980

Walton Report: Cervical cancer screening programs. Can Med Assoc J 114: 1003, 1976

Winauer SJ, Leidner SD, Miller DG: Result of screening program for early colon cancer and polyps using fecal occult blood testing. Gastroenterology 127:1150, 1977 (abst 72)

Zdeb MS: The probability of developing cancer. Am J Epidemiol 106:6, 1977

Section I

ONCOLOGIC SCIENCES

2

The Epidemiologic Method of Research

Robert N. Hoover
Joseph F. Fraumeni, Jr.

The study of human populations in an attempt to identify the causes of disease has been a fascination of physicians and laypersons alike for some time. It was raised by Hippocrates in his treatise, On Airs, Waters, and Places[1]:

> Whoever wishes to investigate medicine properly should proceed thus: in the first place to consider the seasons of the year . . . then the winds, the hot and the cold, . . . one should consider most attentively the waters which the inhabitants use . . . and the ground . . . and the mode in the which the inhabitants live, and what are their pursuits, whether they are fond of drinking and eating to excess, and given to indolence, or are fond of exercise and labor.

However, most of the meaningful work in this area has only occurred during the last 150 to 200 years. For most of this more recent time, the fascination with study of diseases in human populations had focused primarily on the epidemics of the major scourges of infectious disease that had plagued mankind for centuries. With the elucidation of the causes of these diseases, and the opportunities for prevention that have flowed from these investigations, both the quantity and quality of life have improved to the point where the chronic diseases have become the major scourges that attract the interest and concern of the clinician and layperson. Thus, it has only been very recently, primarily the past 40 years, that studies of disease in human populations have focused on malignancy. While important etiologic insights have come from these investigations for a variety of cancer sites (e.g., cigarette smoking and lung cancer), the organ system that has received the most attention, and for which the number and variety of risk factors identified had been most numerous, is the female reproductive tract.

From the earliest observations of the rarity of cancer of the uterine cervix among nuns,[2] interest in risk factors for this organ has focused on sexual practices and related suspect infectious agents. Current enthusiasm over such agents, particularly papillomaviruses, keep this a hot topic for both research and debate in gynecology.[3] For endometrial cancer, early observations concerning the role of obesity, polycystic ovarian disease, and other risk factors, raised the likelihood of an estrogenic etiology.[4] The subsequent epidemic of exogenous estrogen-induced endometrial cancer, controversies over the indications for such treatment, the influence of added progestins, and risk-benefit questions, have all brought the epidemiology of this disease into the everyday discussions of gynecologists. Longstanding anxiety over possible carcinogenic effects of the oral contraceptive, supported by studies suggesting such a role for cancers of the cervix,[5] and muted by the observations of protection for endometrial and ovarian cancer,[6] has also become a part of the daily practice of obstetrics and gynecology. This same clinical community has also had to deal with suggestions that things as personal as the patient's use of body talc, and the surgeon's use of talc on his gloves may in some way relate to the risk of subsequent ovarian cancer.[7]

In the face of these observations and many others, the gynecologist, and particularly the gynecologist interested in malignancy, is confronted with the frequent task of interpretation of epidemiologic findings, with opportunities for scientific collaboration with epidemiologists, and with prospects for making etiologic observations at the bedside himself. For these reasons, it is probably more important for this specialty to understand the principles and methods of epidemiologic investigation than it is for any other clinical specialty.

DEFINITION

The root of the word *epidemiology* is *epidemic*. This is entirely appropriate, since the methods of the discipline are primarily those developed for the investigation of classic epidemics. On a practical level, also, the concept of excessive frequency of disease that is implied by the word epidemic is central to all epidemiologic investigations. Clearly, the goal of an epidemiologic investigation is to establish why, or if, a particular disease is excessive in a specific population group. However, since the word in its general usage seems to engender very subjective and differing opinions of how excessive the frequency must be to qualify as epidemic, thinking about epidemiology in these terms can often distract from an understanding of the principles involved. For example, in utero exposure to diethylstilbestrol (DES) would be unlikely to be considered responsible for an epidemic of gynecological malignancies when it has been responsible for less than one-tenth of 1 percent of all gynecologic malignancies diagnosed in the United States over the past 20 years. However, in terms of vaginal adenocarcinoma among young women, the epidemic nature of

the same observed number of cases is undeniable. Likewise, the marked decline in invasive cancers of the uterine cervix over the past 30 years would seem to be the antithesis of an epidemic. Using the same data, however, the rate of this disease among women aged 45 to 49 would be considered to be clearly epidemic compared with the rate among women aged 15 to 19.

Because of these semantic nuances, it is probably more useful not to think of epidemiology in terms of epidemics but rather in terms of its most popular textbook definition, that is, "the study of the distribution and determinants of disease frequency in human populations."[8] Although brief, this definition uses a number of key words:

1. *Epidemiology* refers to humans, a feature distinguishing it from a variety of other disciplines in cancer research.
2. It entails the study of populations. This distinguishes it from other disciplines, such as clinical research, which also study disease processes in human beings, but at the individual or case-series level. By contrast, epidemiology is the study of groups of people, groups definable in a variety of different ways that would permit them to be characterized as a population.
3. The term *frequency* denotes the quantitative orientation of the discipline. Epidemiology is a numerate science, based on the principle that if you can't count it, you don't understand it. Thus, rather than seeking solely qualitative differences, the epidemiologic method attempts to quantify the risks of disease attributable to various causes.
4. The terms *distribution* and *determinants* describe the two major approaches of the epidemiologic method. Descriptive studies examine the distribution of disease and are usually employed to generate etiologic hypotheses, while analytic studies are used mainly to test hypotheses and identify the determinants of disease. A primary objective of epidemiology is to identify and quantify relationships between exposure to environmental agents and deleterious health effects. These associations may lead to causal inferences, which in turn provide the basis for instituting preventive measures for various diseases.

EPIDEMIOLOGIC INVESTIGATIONS

Descriptive and Correlational Studies

Descriptive (or demographic) studies are concerned with identifying the distribution or patterns of disease in populations.[8] It is a basic tenet of epidemiology that diseases, including cancer, do not occur randomly, but fluctuate according to factors such as age, sex, race, time, and geographic location. The use of rates as measures of disease frequency is fundamental in describing patterns of cancer among these population groups. Prevalence, incidence, and mortality rates of cancer define the levels of risk prevailing in different populations and permit comparisons between groups. Descriptive surveys of cancer occurrence have been valuable in stimulating etiologic hypotheses and in providing direction for analytical studies, which are then necessary to establish whether risks are associated with particular exposures.[9] Thus, important leads to etiology have come from population-based cancer surveys, which have demonstrated substantial international variations in cancer incidence, shifts in risk among migrant populations, changes in risk over time, and geographic peculiarities from mapping cancer mortality at the county level.[10]

Descriptive studies may use the correlational (or ecological) approach, in which the rate of disease in a population is compared with the spatial or temporal distribution of suspected risk factors.[9] This type of study may be particularly helpful in developing or refining hypotheses about carcinogenic risks but falls short of establishing causal relationships.

Correlational studies have the advantage of being much less expensive and time consuming than analytic investigations because they often use mass statistics previously collected for another purpose.[11] The primary weakness of such studies, as with descriptive studies generally, is that data are collected on populations rather than individuals. In other words, the rate of disease and the prevalence of exposures to variables of interest are known for various population groups, but information on the exposure status of persons who have the disease and those who do not within each population is lacking.

Thus, one cannot infer from the correlations at the population level that the exposure of concern is associated with the risk of developing disease within each population.[11] For example, in early surveys of lung cancer, the international variation in mortality rates and temporal increases among males appeared consistent with the reported patterns of cigarette smoking, but these correlations by themselves may have been circumstantial rather than causal, since a variety of other exposures (e.g., occupational hazards, air pollution) also varied concomitantly with the patterns of lung cancer. It took the analytic studies that pursued these leads to establish the cause-and-effect relationships between smoking and lung cancer.

Correlational studies may also provide supporting evidence in evaluating relationships detected by analytic studies or laboratory data. This is illustrated by the more recent temporal increase in lung cancer among females, who have lagged about 20 years behind males in their adoption of smoking habits. Because correlational studies deal with aggregate exposures and disease occurrence at the population level, they are often also seriously limited by the imprecise measurements of exposure and the many potentially confounding variables. A relevant example in regard to these points concerns the relationship between menopausal estrogen use and the risk of endometrial cancer. One study evaluating the time trends in endometrial cancer from the late 1940s to the early 1970s noted a lack of any appreciable increase over this period,[12] leading some workers to conclude that this exonerated any recently introduced risk factors, including the use of menopausal estrogens. A subsequent evaluation of time trends during the 1970s reached the opposite conclusion.[13] Certainly the analytic studies of these issues have solidly supported the conclusions of the latter investigation.

Many reasons have been suggested for the failure of the first descriptive study to note a trend that could have pointed to newly introduced risk factors, the most prominent being the relatively small proportion of women exposed in the period covered and, perhaps more importantly, the rising rates of hysterectomy over this same time period, which tended to reduce the real number of women at risk of developing this tumor. Whatever the explanation, the dangers of the shift to causal interpretations on the basis of descriptive studies should be clear.

Analytical Studies

In order to test etiologic hypotheses and to identify and quantify carcinogenic risks to humans, it is necessary to conduct analytic epidemiologic studies.[8,9,11] These studies are the principal means of determining the human health hazards of specific environmental exposures and agents. In contrast to descriptive surveys, data are obtained on disease occurrence and putative risk factors for specific individuals, using mainly the case-control or cohort method. Thus, by grouping exposed individuals and comparing them to those unexposed, after controlling for all other relevant variables, the risk of disease associated with exposure can be estimated. While it is important to avoid imposing unnecessary constraints on epidemiologic investigation, some methodologic guidelines should be considered in designing a study. In particular, the study groups should be sufficiently large, and the time intervals between initial exposure and tumor onset sufficiently long, to identify the lowest excess risk considered important to detect. Reliable and valid estimates of exposure should be sought, with quantitative measurements to permit dose-response evaluations. Studies should be designed in a manner that minimizes potential sources of bias, and permits detection and control of confounding variables.

CASE-CONTROL STUDIES

Case-control studies start by identifying persons with a particular disease (cases) and a group of similar persons without the disease (controls). Information on past exposure to known or suspected risk factors is then collected from interviews, questionnaires, medical records, occupational logs, or other sources. The frequency of a particular exposure among the cases is compared with that in the control group, after making appropriate adjustments for other relevant differences between the two groups. If the proportion of cases with a certain exposure is significantly greater than that of the controls, an association between exposure and disease may be indicated. The case-control approach is especially well suited in studying relatively rare conditions, such as most cancers, in which the putative exposure is common in the general population (e.g., menopausal estrogens and endometrial cancer), or when the exposure is rare but accounts for a large portion of a particular cancer (e.g., DES and vaginal adenocarcinoma).[14]

COHORT STUDIES

Cohort studies begin by identifying a group of individuals with a particular exposure and a similar group of unexposed persons and following both groups over time to determine subsequent health outcomes. The rates of disease in the exposed and unexposed groups are then compared. Information on disease frequency and other factors may be identified from medical records, occupational records, physical examinations, interviews, questionnaires, or death certificates. An association between exposure and disease may be indicated if the rates of disease are greater in the exposed group than in the unexposed group. These investigations may be based on current exposure and future health outcomes (prospective cohort study), but more commonly they use past exposure information and disease occurrence (retrospective cohort study). Instead of an unexposed comparison group, general population mortality or incidence rates (specific for age, sex, race, and calendar time) are often used to determine the expected number of cases of disease. This method assumes that in the absence of specific exposure the study group would have had the same probability of developing the disease as the general population, but differences in ethnic, socioeconomic, and other variables must be considered in evaluating the validity of this assumption. The cohort approach is used mainly when it is possible to evaluate heavy exposures in clearly defined subgroups of the population. Thus, it has been especially helpful in assessing the carcinogenic risk from occupational hazards or medical exposures, including radiation and certain drugs (e.g., the risk of leukemia following treatment of ovarian cancer patients with alkylating agents).

Both the case-control and cohort methods are characterized as having certain strengths and weaknesses, although they complement each other in testing specific etiologic hypotheses. Case-control studies provide (1) a more efficient means of studying rare diseases, with fewer individuals needed for study as compared with the cohort approach; (2) a shorter time period for study completion and generally lower costs as compared with the cohort method; an opportunity to evaluate simultaneously several causal hypotheses as well as interactions (the extent and manner in which two or more risk factors modify the strength of one another); and (3) a capacity to evaluate the effects of common exposures as well as those rare exposures that may account for a large proportion of the cases. By contrast, the case-control approach has some problems in (1) directly estimating the risk associated with a particular exposure; (2) reducing certain biases (e.g., selection, historical recall) that affect the comparability of cases and controls; and (3) providing detailed and precise information on exposures occurring in the past.[8] By definition, such investigations can only evaluate one disease or outcome at a time.

The advantages of cohort studies are their capacity (1) to estimate directly the risks attributed to a particular exposure, since incidence or mortality from disease is actually being measured; to reduce subjective biases by obtaining information before the disease develops; (2) to determine associations between a particular exposure and multiple health outcomes; and (3) to evaluate temporal relationships such as latency period and duration of effect.

The most obvious temporal relationship that can be established by the cohort method, and in some circumstances established only by this method, is the timing between the exposure of interest and the development of the disease in question. From the first observations of excesses of indices of herpes virus infection among patients with cervical cancer, concerns were raised that such infection might have actually followed the development of the disease, and that the uterine cervix in the first stages of malignancy might, in fact be in some way particularly vulnerable to infection by these viruses.

Virtually the only way to assess these critical questions was to draw bloods from a large population of women for the evaluation of antibodies and then follow them over time to determine the frequency of cervical cancer development in those with and without evidence of prior infection. The first such major investigations designed to address this issue have failed to produce support for the hypothesis that there is a relationship between prior infection and the development of this malignancy.[15] However, cohort studies are usually expensive and complex undertakings. They require (1) large numbers of exposed individuals, particularly when relatively rare events as in the case of most cancers are being investigated; (2)

long periods of follow-up to accommodate the latency period for chronic diseases such as cancer; and (3) special handling of problems associated with persons lost to follow-up and with biased estimates of risk as from the healthy worker effect of occupational studies.[8]

INTERVENTION STUDIES

Also referred to as experimental studies,[16] intervention studies represent a third strategy of analytic epidemiology that is especially useful in confirming causal relationships suggested by case-control or cohort studies. This approach may be applied in programs designed, for example, to reduce cigarette smoking and alcohol intake, modify diet, control occupational pollutants, or evaluate candidate preventatives (e.g., vitamin A supplements, the addition of progestins to treatment regimens for menopausal symptoms). Ethical considerations are obviously critical when developing this approach and, after intervention, the statistical procedures resemble those employed for cohort studies.

EPIDEMIOLOGICAL MEASURES

Rates

If epidemiology is a numerate science, the measurement of frequency of disease should be a central feature of the discipline. The basic measure of frequency that has epidemiologic value is the rate. Within this context, this refers to an enumeration of the number of diseased persons expressed per unit size of the population in which these cases were observed. The addition of the element of time to this expression (e.g., time at which cases were observed, or period of time during which they developed) is a key feature, making any rate epidemiologically useful. A typical example in the area of cancer is that the overall incidence rate of cancer in the entire population is estimated to be approximately 325 cases per 100,000 population per year.[17] As can be seen, the expression of disease in this manner permits comparison of the rate of disease in one population with that in another, taking into account the likely prospect that the populations were of different size or were observed over differing periods of time. A variety of mechanisms also exist to adjust these rates for a variety of factors, including age, race, and social class.[18] Such adjustments remove the influence on disease rate of differences among the populations being compared with respect to these variables.

A variety of different types of rates can be developed for measurement of different disease states. For malignancy, the most common rates used are prevalence rates (numbers of cases in existence at a particular point in time divided by the number of people in the population in which they exist), mortality rates (number of deaths due to a particular malignancy over a specified period of time divided by the population under surveillance for these deaths over the same period of time), and incidence rates (number of new cases of a malignancy occurring over a specified period of time divided by the population under surveillance for such cases over the same period of time). Each type of rate has its own particular uses and its own particular drawbacks. For purposes of doing etiologic research, incidence rates are generally preferable. Both prevalence rates and mortality rates reflect the influence of prognosis as well as factors that lead to the occurrence of a disease. Prevalent cases (all those alive in the population at a particular point in time) tend to be heavily weighted with long-term survivors. By contrast, mortality rates clearly reflect the experience of those cases with the poorest prognosis. Incidence rates, reflecting as they do all of the cases of the disease that occur, are representative of the true spectrum of disease. In addition, incidence rates generally measure the frequency of disease at a point much closer in time to etiologic influences than do the other measures.

Measures of Association

The key ingredient in the epidemiologic method is the comparison of attributes between different populations. The question then arises as to how these attributes are to be compared. Considerable interest on the part of clinical and laboratory investigators is focused on tests of the statistical significance of differences between groups. While this assessment of the likely role of chance in producing any differences observed is important, it does not measure the magnitude of the differences and thus the strength of any observed relationship between an exposure and a disease. The main

measures of differences between populations utilized by epidemiologists are based on rates of disease. Specifically, two measures are most prominently used. The relative risk RR is the disease rate in the exposed divided by the disease rate in the referent (usually nonexposed) population. This measure gives an estimate of the relative difference in disease risk between the two populations. Thus, a RR value of 2.0 would indicate that the exposed group has twice the risk of the unexposed group (or a 100 percent increase in risk). The other measure of association is the risk difference. As implied, this estimate results from the subtraction of the rate among the unexposed from that among the exposed. This difference in risk is also frequently referred to as the attributable risk, AR. The implication of this terminology is that if the relationship observed is causal, then the difference between the risks is the amount of disease produced among the exposed that is attributable to that exposure.[8]

These two measures have somewhat different uses. The measure of relative risk is usually assumed to be an indicator of how strongly, and thus how likely, an exposure is related to a disease. Thus, the magnitude of the RR value is used as an indicator of how likely the relationship is to be causal. The difference between risks is also influenced by the magnitude of the difference between the exposed and unexposed but is also influenced by the rate of the disease in the absence of exposure. Thus, for a very rare condition, the relative difference between the rates in the exposed and the unexposed can be substantial, but the actual number of cases produced among the exposed could be quite small, owing to the rarity of the disease itself.

A recent follow-up study of 1-year survivors of ovarian cancer from five different randomized trials measured the incidence rate of acute non-lymphocytic leukemia and preleukemia among women treated with no chemotherapy, those treated with cyclophosphamide, and those treated with melphalan.[19] The incidence rates were 0.18, 3.21, and 11.46 cases per 1,000 women per year, respectively. The RR of these conditions compared with those receiving no chemotherapy was 18-fold for women taking cyclophosphamide and 64-fold for those taking melphalan. The RR value for women taking melphalan versus those taking cyclophosphamide was 3.6. The size of the relative excesses for women taking chemotherapy versus those receiving none makes it extremely unlikely that the excess risks are due to anything other than the drugs themselves. On the other hand, while the RR value of 3.6 for melphalan versus cyclophosphamide suggests that there may be a differential leukemogenicity for one drug versus another, the strength of the association is much less than for any chemotherapy versus none and thus requires a more cautious interpretation.

While the RR values are very high for these two alkylating agents as compared with no chemotherapy, the differences between the absolute risks are not very great. Thus, the attributable risk for these conditions among those treated with cyclophosphamide is approximately 3 per 1,000 per year and for melphalan is approximately 11 per 1,000 per year. Given all the other problems confronting ovarian cancer patients, including competing causes of mortality, these excesses probably do not represent a major public health problem. This also explains how it could be difficult for an individual clinician or even a large group practice to notice important etiologic observations, such as these differences in risks. If one were following as many as 100 patients who had been treated with one drug and 100 patients who had been treated with the other, even this 3.5-fold excess risk would result in a differential of only approximately one case of leukemia per year.

One other measure that is sometimes used in epidemiologic investigations is an estimate of the amount of disease attributable to a particular exposure not just among the exposed but in a population that has both exposed and unexposed individuals. This measure would thus reflect the amount of disease that would exist in some definable population if the exposure were removed. This measure is referred to as the population attributable risk or, when expressed as a proportion of the total disease in the population, as the etiologic fraction. This measure is calculated by subtracting the rate among the unexposed from the rate that exists in the total population of interest. It can be seen that the magnitude of this particular estimate relates not only to the magnitude of the relative difference between the exposed and unexposed, and to the level of the disease among the unexposed but to the prevalence of the exposure of interest in the particular population being addressed as well.

Using the example outlined above, even though the relative risk for alkylating agents versus none is very large, if exposure to all alkylating agents were removed, it would have very little impact on the total leukemia rate in the general population, since very few persons in the general population are being exposed to these drugs. By contrast, among the clinical population investigated in this particular study, the overall rate of these leukemic conditions was 2.35 per 1,000 patients per year. Subtracting the rate among those not treated with chemotherapy (0.18 per 1,000 per year) from this yields a population attributable risk of 2.17 cases per 1,000 women per year or, expressed as an proportion of the total observed rate, an etiologic fraction of 92 percent. This high proportion of leukemic disorders among ovarian cancer patients attributable to the use of alkylating agents is a result not only of the high relative risk associated with the use of alkylating agents but of a high prevalence of exposure to these agents in this population of patients.

All these measures have been illustrated in the context of a cohort investigation, within which these rates and risks can be directly measured. In case-control investigations, there are no exposed and unexposed populations per se, and, thus, no ability to calculate rates of disease and relative and attributable risks directly. However, over the years, reliable and reasonable procedures for estimating these parameters within the context of a case-control study have been developed and have become the preferred measures of association in these studies. Relative risks is estimated by the odds ratio, also referred to as the relative odds. By making some assumptions about the representativeness of the exposure among cases and controls with respect to a population to which inferences are to be made, estimates of the differences in risks can be attempted as well.

BIAS AND CONFOUNDING

Epidemiology is primarily an observational rather than an experimental science. Thus, many of the concerns mitigated by a randomization process and a controlled experimental environment have to be addressed specifically by the epidemiologist in the development of the protocol and study procedures, as well as in the analyses and interpretation of data. The major concern is over sources of bias or differential handling of the groups being compared. The result could be the acquisition of groups that are not comparable to each other, and/or the acquisition of data from these groups in a noncomparable manner. These circumstances can arise as a result of actions by the investigator, by the study participants, or by other persons or forces.

Covering all the possibilities for bias is beyond the scope of this review. However, some examples may be illustrative. Two of the more common ways of achieving noncomparable groups are through selection bias and response bias. For example, all the cases of a disease hospitalized at a specialized referral center could be selected for comparison with a random sample of the general population of the area. In this circumstance, any characteristics of the cases that differed from the controls might have nothing to do with the disease but rather could reflect characteristics that would lead to referral to this one institution. Likewise, a differential response rate to a questionnaire (e.g., 90 percent for cases and 60 percent for the controls) could lead to subsets (respondents) of cases and controls that are different from each other, while a comparison of the entire targeted series of cases and controls might yield no such differences.

Bias in the acquisition of data can also come about by a variety of means. One of the most discussed is recall bias or the tendency of cases to recall past exposures more completely because they have been searching their memories for possible reasons for their illness. The tendency of mothers of children with congenital heart defects to report taking virtually every type of medication more frequently during pregnancy than mothers of children without congenital defects is thought to reflect this phenomenon.[20] Similar bias in collection of information concerning cases versus controls can be introduced by others as well. The widely recognized practice of clinicians to record their patients' prior use of exogenous estrogens in a chart only if it would have relevance to a specific problem being worked up leads to a much more complete reporting of such exposure for endometrial cancer patients if chart information from the diagnostic workup is included. To avoid this bias, chart abstraction studies of this issue have had to exclude information recorded in the chart for some arbitrary period of time just prior to diagnosis for the cases and the date of case-matched diagnosis for the controls. This approach undoubtedly results in a failure to identify some cases and controls has having had prior exposure, but this procedure ensures that this will be just as likely for the cases as it will for the controls, these eliminating a biased recording of exposures.

An issue that has received considerable attention in epidemiology, and that will consider to do so, is that of confounding. Confounding of an association between a factor and a disease potentially exists when some other risk factor for the disease (in the context of the study) is also related to the factor under study. This correlation of a another variable with both the exposure and the disease under study can act to produce false associations between the exposure and the disease or to obscure a relationship when one actually exists. A common example is the confounding influence of age. Age is related quite strongly and directly with most malignancies. If this is not accommodated in the design of a case-control study, and a simple random sample of controls is chosen, they will almost always be, as a group, much younger than the cases. If this disparity is also ignored in the analysis, and the crude characteristics of the case group are compared directly with those of the controls, any variable associated with older age will falsely appear to be related to the risk of cancer.

While some confounding relationships are easily recognizable, others can be quite subtle. In a recent study of invasive cervical cancer,[5] the crude estimate of the RR value between this disease and prior long-term use of oral contraceptives was 0.9. However, there was concern that this relationship could be confounded by the time interval between inclusion in the study (diagnosis for the cases) and a prior Papanicolaou (Pap) smear. Since this was invasive cancer, as one might expect, the cases had a much longer time interval between their diagnostic workup and their last previous Pap smear than did the controls. In addition, this same time interval was also related to oral contraceptive use. Oral contraceptive users tended to participate in more regular Pap smear practices and thereby had a much shorter interval between study inclusion and previous Pap smear than did nonusers. Thus, it was believed that a biologic relationship between oral contraceptive use and invasive cervical cancer risk could be obscured by the tendency for oral contraceptive users to be screened more frequently. Indeed, this appeared to be the case. When the relationship was controlled for interval since last Pap smear, the RR value for long-term oral contraceptive use was noted to be 1.8.

STRENGTHS AND LIMITATIONS OF EPIDEMIOLOGY

Strengths

In contrast to studies in other biologic systems, epidemiology directly evaluates the experience of human populations and their response (risk of disease) to various environmental exposures and host factors. Thus, it is often possible to evaluate the consequences of an environmental exposure in the precise manner in which it occurs and will continue to occur in human populations. This includes such important considerations as dose, route of exposure, and concomitant exposures to other exogenous and endogenous factors. Through epidemiologic studies, human cancer has been linked to a number of lifestyle and other environmental hazards, including tobacco products and alcohol, ultraviolet (UV) and ionizing radiation, certain occupational and medicinal chemicals, dietary factors, and some infectious agents.[10,21,22] Epidemiology has played a central role in determining carcinogenic exposures, and it has complemented studies in laboratory animals in clarifying the carcinogenic potential of specific agents.[23] Another strength of the epidemiologic approach is its ability to provide insights into the mechanisms of human carcinogenesis. Thus, epidemiologic observations have complemented experimental evidence that carcinogenesis is a multistage process and that many cancers may result from the cumulative effect of environmental factors and host susceptibility states that accelerate or retard the transition rates at various stages of carcinogenesis.

Limitations

Although epidemiology is the only means of directly assessing the carcinogenic risks of environmental agents in humans, the method has several limitations that are difficult to overcome.[8] One problem is that evidence of an environmental hazard is usually obtained from persons with high or intermediate levels of exposure. Just as for studies in laboratory animals, detecting causal relationships at low exposure levels is difficult, since the observed associations with disease are usually less pronounced and may have alternative explanations, including those related to

chance, errors, biases, or confounding variables. To provide a valid basis for risk estimates, large numbers of human subjects are often needed, especially if the exposure is low or rare or if the excess risk is small compared with that of the baseline incidence rate.

Another obstacle to epidemiology is the long latency period between exposure and the development of cancer. This complicates the detection of relationships and makes it impossible to identify the carcinogenic risks to humans of agents newly introduced into the environment. Another common problem in epidemiology is that of exposure assessment. Often the specific exposure of interest cannot be measured directly, so that surrogate measures must be used (e.g., occupation, place of residence).Since exposure data are usually derived from historical records generated for other purposes or from the recollections of subjects, opportunities for either random or biased misclassification of exposure are frequently encountered. In addition, appropriate study groups are often simply unavailable or inaccessible. Furthermore, it may be difficult to implicate specific carcinogens when the environmental hazards involve complex exposures to a variety of agents, the effects of which are difficult to disentangle. Still another difficulty is the inability of epidemiologic studies to adjust for unknown risk factors, since control can be introduced only when the risk factors are already recognized.

Thus, when a particular factor is related to exposure and disease outcome, it may be confounded and give the appearance of an association when in fact none exists, or it may inflate or decrease the magnitude of an association. In view of these difficulties, it is not surprising that epidemiologic data exist for only a small proportion of the many chemicals that have been shown to be carcinogenic in laboratory animals.

BIOCHEMICAL EPIDEMIOLOGY

It seems likely that some limitations of cancer epidemiology may be overcome by incorporating laboratory methods in analytic investigations. This has been a valuable routine practice in infectious disease epidemiology for the past century. This approach, sometimes called biochemical or molecular epidemiology,[15,24] has only recently been developed in cancer epidemiology. There is current enthusiasm for these kinds of investigations, since they merge the strengths of observational human studies with newly developed experimental probes to derive information that could not be developed by epidemiology or laboratory study alone. The laboratory aspect may make it possible to define past exposures and subclinical or preclinical response to initiators, promoters, and inhibitors of carcinogenesis, or to evaluate host-environmental interactions. There is special interest in using this technique to clarify carcinogenic risks associated with nutritional influences or specific environmental agents that can be detected in tissues or body fluids.

Opportunities are also available to assess specific host factors that influence susceptibility to carcinogenesis, including endocrine parameters, immunocompetence, and genetic markers. Techniques are being refined to detect and quantify particular carcinogens or their metabolites in tissues or body fluids through chemical analyses, mutagenesis assays, or immunologic detection techniques. It is already possible to measure the interaction of specific agents with cellular target molecules, for example, through adduct formation with proteins and nucleic acids, excretion levels of excised adducts, or markers of altered gene expression.[24] the task of identifying the effects of lifestyle and other environmental and host factors is obviously formidable. Biochemical epidemiology represents an innovative approach that may help elucidate further the causes of cancer and the actual mechanisms of carcinogenesis.

DETERMINING CAUSALITY

In interpreting epidemiologic findings, one is guided by the magnitude of the risk estimates, their statistical significance (likelihood of being due to chance), and the rigor of the study design to avoid various kinds of bias, including those related to selection, confounding, classification, and measurement. A determination of causality in epidemiology is bolstered by dose-response relationships, the consistency and reproducibility of results, the strength and specificity of the association, its biological pausibility, and other considerations. Thus, inferences from epidemiology, as from other methods of inquiry, are not made in isolation but should take into account all relevant biologic information. Although epidemiologic and other observations can accumulate to the point that a causal hypothesis is likely, it is not possible to ever prove causality (in the strict sense, a hypothesis can only be disproved). Nevertheless, a causal hypothesis can be sufficiently probable, as in the case of menopausal estrogens and endometrial cancer and DES and vaginal adenocarcinoma, to provide a reasonable and even compelling basis for preventive and public health action.

REFERENCES

1. Hippocrates: On Airs, Waters, and Places. (Transl.) Classics 3:19, 1938
2. Rigoni-Stern D: Fatti statistici alle mallattie cancerose che servirono di base alle poche cose dette dal dott. G Progr Patol Terap 2nd Ser. 2:499, 1842; see also (transl) Scotto J, Bailar JC III: Rigoni-Stern and Medical Statistics: A nineteenth-century approach to cancer research. J Hist Med 65, 1969
3. Annonymous: Human papillomaviruses and cervical cancer. A fresh look at the evidence. Lancet 1:725, 1987
4. Gusberg SB: Precursors of corpus carcinoma, estrogens and adenomatous hyperplasia. Am J Obstet Gynecol 54:905, 1947
5. Brinton LA, Huggins GR, Lehman HF, et al: Long-term use of oral contraceptives and risk of invasive cervical cancer. Int. J Cancer 38:339, 1986
6. Hoover RN: Sex hormones and human carcinogenesis: Epidemiology. In Becker KL (ed): Principles and Practice of Endocrinology and Metabolism. JB Lippincott, Philadelphia, 1987
7. Hartge P, Hoover R, Lesher LP, et al: Talc and ovarian cancer. JAMA 250:1844, 1983
8. MacMahon B, Pugh TF: Epidemiology: Principles and Methods. Little, Brown, Boston, 1970
9. Doll R: The epidemiology of cancer. Cancer 45:2475, 1980
10. Fraumeni JF, Jr: Epidemiological approaches to cancer etiology. Annu Rev Public Health 3:85, 1982
11. Lilienfeld A, Pederson E, Dowd JE: Cancer Epidemiology: Methods of Study. Johns Hopkins Press, Baltimore, 1967
12. Cramer DW, Cutler SJ, Christine B: Trends in the incidence of endometrial cancer in the United States. Gynecol Oncol 2:130, 1974
13. Austin DF, Roe KM: The decreasing incidence of endometrial cancer: Public health implications. Am J Public Health 72:65, 1982
14. Cole P: Introduction: The analysis of case-control studies. p. 14. In Breslow NE, Day NE (eds): Statistical

Methods in Cancer Research. Vol. 1. International Agency for Research on Cancer, Lyons, 1980

15. Hoover RN: Hormonal, infectious and nutritional aspects of cancer of the female reproductive tract. p. 313. In Harris CC (ed): Biochemical and Molecular Epidemiology of Cancer. Alan R. Liss, New York, 1986

16. Hutchison GB: The epidemiologic method. p. 3. In Schottenfeld D, Fraumeni JF Jr (eds): Cancer Epidemiology and Prevention. WB Saunders, Philadelphia, 1982

17. Young JL Jr, Percy CL, Asire AJ (eds): Surveillance, Epidemiology, and End Results. National Cancer Institute Monograph 57. National Institutes of Health, US Department of Health and Human Services, Bethesda, MD, 1981

18. Hill AB: Principles of Medical Statistics. Oxford University Press, New York, 1966

19. Greene MH, Harris EL, Gershenson DM, et al: Mel-phalan may be a more potent leukemogen than cyclophosphamide. Ann Intern Med 105:360, 1986

20. Rothman KJ, Fyler DC, Goldblatt A, et al: Exogenous hormones and other drug exposures of children with congenital heart disease. Am J Epidemiol 109:433, 1979

21. Doll R̄, Peto R: The causes of cancer. J Natl Cancer Inst 66:1191, 1981

22. MacLure RM, MacMahon B: An epidemiologic perspective of environmental carcinogenesis. Epidemiol Rev 2:19, 1980

23. Tomatis L, Breslow NE, Bartsch H: Experimental studies in the assessment of cancer risk. p. 44. In Schottenfeld D, Fraumeni JF Jr (eds): Cancer Epidemiology and Prevention. WB Saunders, Philadelphia, 1982

24. Perera FP, Weinstein IB: Molecular epidemiology and carcinogen-DNA adduct detection: New approaches to studies of human cancer causation. J Chron Dis 35:581, 1982

3

Immunology

Philip J. DiSaia
Suzanne Bergen

Immunity means freedom from burden; according to the original application, burden implies invasion by microorganisms. In modern times, the burden upon the body is much larger, encompassing the reaction of the body to foreign tissue, such as an organ transplant, or to altered tissue, such as neoplastic growth.

Imagine a child opening a carefully wrapped, oversized birthday package and finding in it thousands of the bits and pieces of many games (checkers, chess pieces, jacks, tinker toys)—some familiar, some never seen before—all thoroughly mixed together. Before the child and playmates can begin to enjoy this jumbled birthday gift, they face the monumental task of sorting and organizing the pieces and figuring out the rules of the games.

Immunologists have faced much the same task in studying the body's defense mechanisms, its complex system for withstanding infections and combatting diseases including cancer. During the past decade, scientists have been figuratively shaking out the bits and pieces of the body's immune system for closer scrutiny. Having found an enormous array of highly sophisticated pieces, scientists have persistently been putting them together, trying to establish the basic rules of the game. Although scientists are generally excited with the progress made, they are also awed at the task that lies before them.

The immune system is without doubt one of the most complicated organizations within the body. The body itself is a citadel under constant siege. Its billions of cells are subject to frequent attack from outside invaders, such as viruses, bacteria, and other microbes. There is also the paramount threat that normal healthy cells may somehow be converted into uncontrollable cancer cells, trying to push their way into healthy tissues to destroy normal functions. Some immunologists believe that the same system that helps withstand foreign invaders also stands vigilant to prevent and combat cancer. The rules for fighting those different battles are not the same, however, nor are the parts of the immune system that must wage those battles quite the same. This growing realization has gradually changed the strategy of the immunologists' assault on cancer for reasons that now seem inevitable.

Perhaps the most current compelling evidence of an association between immune incompetence and cancer is the high incidence of Kaposi's sarcoma in homosexual men with acquired immunodeficiency syndrome (AIDS). Older clinical evidence is found in the reports of spontaneous regression of malignant neoplasms. While spontaneous regression of cancer is rare, it is an unpredictable phenomenon that has drawn the attention of physicians for many years. An important review was carried out by Everson and Cole,[1] who studied and carefully reported cases between 1900 and 1966 from the literature and experience of their colleagues.

A brief overview of our knowledge of the fundamentals of the human immune system as it is operational against human tumors follows. This field is in a constant state of flux, and our knowledge of the details changes almost daily. A student of this field must have an open mind and a propensity for diligent review of current literature.

ANATOMY OF TUMOR IMMUNITY

Antigens

Tumor cells express most of the same cell-surface antigens (e.g., transplantation or HLA antigens) as do normal cells (Table 3-1). In addition, most tumor cells also express specific antigens not found in similar normal cells. These antigens are termed tumor-specific antigens in animal studies and tumor-associated antigens in human malignancies. Experiments designed to demonstrate tumor-specific antigens involve a demonstration that pretreatment with a syngeneic tumor will influence the growth of a subsequent challenge with the same tumor. Foley[2] produced the first such evidence in 1953, shortly after the introduction of syngeneic inbred mouse strains. This finding was later confirmed by the studies of Prehn and Main.[3] Such studies are not possible in humans; however, there are in vitro techniques for detecting tumor antigens, and these have been liberally applied to human tumors. Tumors vary widely in their immunogenicity. In general, those neoplasms induced experimentally in vivo with chemical or viral agents are highly immunogenic, whereas tumors arising spontaneously in vivo are poorly immunogenic. Human tumor antigens tend to behave like weak histocompatibility antigens with less specificity and unfortunately are not as distinct as many found in lower animals. An example of such a human tumor antigen (CA 125) has been described by Bast et al.[4] to be common to most non-

mucinous epithelial ovarian carcinomas. Thirty years after the publication of the classic experiments by Prehn and Main, it has not been established with certainty that spontaneous human malignancies bear antigenic determinants not found on their nonmalignant counterparts. Perhaps the presence of a unique antigen on a tumor cell surface is not a requirement for its immunologic rejection, and the presence of an unusual protein or antigen may be sufficient. Monoclonal antibody studies have identified several unusual proteins that are candidates for the designation of tumor antigen, if immunogenicity can be demonstrated. The isolation of these proteins, as well as efforts to abrogate suppressor T-cell function, seem to be promising approaches for transforming these tumor-associated proteins to functionally specific human tumor-associated antigens.

Oncofetal antigens have also been described. These antigens are found in both fetal and malignant tissue. These normal antigens in the fetus are repressed as the process of intrauterine development proceeds toward birth and are then de-repressed during the malignant transformation process. Their existence supports the concept that cancer represents a dedifferentiation to a more primitive cell type. The most specific oncofetal antigens in gynecologic cancer are carcinoembryonic antigen (CEA) and α-fetoprotein (AFP). The apparent importance of these antigens is not in their possible protective value but rather in their ability to serve as tumor markers for various cancers. AFP is detectable immunologically in serum from human fetuses. In the adult, it is found in patients with malignancies of endodermal origin, such as liver tumors, and with gonadal tumors, such as endodermal sinus tumor of the ovary. Like CEA, there does not appear to be a clear correlation between the level of the protein and the prognosis for the patient. Also, like CEA, AFP is not disease specific.

Table 3-1 Transplantation Immunology

Genetic Relationship	Antibody	Transplant	
		Old Term	New Term
Identical, same individual	Auto	Auto	Syngeneic (autochthonous)
Identical twin	Iso	Iso	Syngeneic
Different individual, same species	Iso	Homo	Allogeneic
Different species	Hetero	Hetereo	Xenogeneic

Macrophages

Cells of the macrophage-histiocyte series are important components of the host system responsible for the maintenance of homeostasis. A primary function of macrophages in the body is the phagocytosis and disposal of effete cells, such as aged red blood cells (RBCs), cellular debris, and serum proteins. The removal of effete RBCs is a continuous process requiring that macrophages distinguish old from young cells as well as damaged from healthy cells. In addition to phagocytosis, macrophages are involved in the controlled metabolism of lipids and iron, in host response to injury (inflammation), and in the defense against microbial and parasitic infestations. Macrophages are also an important component of both the afferent and efferent arms of the immune system. Finally, these cells are important in the defense against neoplasms.

Lymphocytes

The lymphocyte was a poorly respected member of the family of circulating cells until the recent recognition of its key role in immunity. It is the principal cell involved in the recognition of an antigen as foreign and then initiating mechanisms to rid the host of the invader. The lymphocyte's recognition of self from nonself provides the host's key mechanism of homeostasis and is the starting point for all immune reactivity. These small cells, with a very large nucleus, circulate into every tissue of the body; when a processed antigen comes in contact with a lymphocyte, a series of events is triggered. The lymphocyte increases dramatically in size and undergoes lymphoblastogenesis, resulting in an immunoblast. The immunoblast proceeds toward development of humoral or cell-mediated immunologic effectors.

Humoral Factors

Some of the immunoblasts differentiate into plasma cells, which are largely responsible for humoral immunity. Antibodies are secreted by plasma cells into the vicinity of the antigenic stimulus; there, binding takes place with the inciting antigen. The basic unit of all antibodies is composed of four polypeptides: two light chains and two heavy chains linked by several disulfide bridges. There are five classes of antibodies or immunoglobulins: IgG, IgM, IgA, IgE, and IgD. It is estimated that 100,000 different antibodies can be produced by humans; specificity is a basic property of this system. An antibody directed toward a particular antigen will not confer protection against other antigens. This concept is termed the clonal selection theory, which states that each antibody-producing cell is committed to one particular antibody in production.

MECHANISMS OF IMMUNITY

The immune mechanism consists basically of initial recognition and processing of foreign matter, an afferent mechanism leading to activation of the central immune system, and an efferent mechanism leading to the elimination of the offending material. The basic study of immunology concerns the reactions of the body to certain foreign materials, both living and nonliving, presented to it. The immune reaction can be defined as an interaction between the invading process and its antigenic information and conveyance of it to the central immune mechanisms capable of reacting specifically to this information. The cells of the central mechanism, termed immunologically competent, are of the lymphoid series. This lymphoid tissue is present in peripheral lymph nodes, bone marrow, spleen, thymus, Peyer's patches of the intestine, the thoracic duct, and the bloodstream itself. All antigens are recognized as either self or nonself. When recognition occurs, it is very specific and precisely directed against certain molecular configurations on the antigen. In addition, antigen and immunocompetent cells apparently must have physical contact to evoke a response.

Specific immune responses are mediated by two major categories of effectors, with considerable interaction between the two. One category of response can be transferred from one individual to another only by transferring living, immunologically competent cells, or cultured products of these cells. This type of response is termed cell-mediated immunity. The second type of response can be transferred by cell-free serum and is therefore called humoral immunity. The key to both responses is the small lymphocyte, which until recently was relegated to a position of relative obscurity in textbooks of physiology and hematology. The small lymphocyte is formed in the bone marrow from precursor stem cells and then released into the circulation, eventually coming to rest in the lymphoid organs. The small lymphocyte specializes early in its life by either passing through the thymus gland or differentiating into a cell that will mediate humoral immunity. Despite the crucial differences between these two types of cells, they are morphologically indistinguishable under the light microscope.

Cell-Mediated Immunity

Cell-mediated immunity is produced by the lymphocyte that has passed through the thymus in its development. The precise mechanism of the thymic influence is ill understood in the human organism but is suspected of being hormonal. Once through the thymus, the lymphocyte remains under the influence of the thymus and is variously termed the thymic-dependent lymphocyte, T lymphocyte, or simply T cell. These cells may also be involved in the pathogenesis of the more common autoimmune disorders. Cell-mediated immunity is commonly influenced by drugs (e.g., anesthetic agents and corticosteroids), deficiencies in nutrition, major injury, and aging.

In recent years, techniques have been introduced that permit cellular migration to be followed. The techniques use isotopic labeling of cells for short-term studies of chromosomal markers for long-term investigations. These experiments have demonstrated that the lymphocytes of the thymus arise by differentiation of cells that enter the thymic primordium from without, namely, from the bloodstream. In the adult, these cells are derived from the bone marrow. When these migrant stem cells enter the epithelial primordium of the thymus, they proliferate and mature into small lymphocytes. Some investigators have postulated the presence of a diffusible substance or a thymic hormone; others have postulated that cell contact and interaction within the thymic environment are the crucial factor. Another complex issue for which we have little information is whether T-cell subpopulations represent separate lines of T-cell development or whether they are stages in a single differentiation pathway.

The thymus manufactures a large number of T lymphocytes (Fig. 3-1). These T cells leave the thymus to enter the bloodstream, where they make up about 60 percent of the peripheral blood lymphocytes. The T lymphocytes then enter a unique pattern of recirculation, with many moving from blood to lymph node to thoracic duct, then returning to the blood. In the lymph node, most T cells reside in the deep cortex in and between germinal centers. This pool of mature T lymphocytes is often called the recirculating pool of long-lived T lymphocytes, some of which are undoubtedly memory cells. A portion of these resting cells have been shown to live more than 20 years without dividing. It is important to note that the path of recirculation does not involve the thymus; for unknown reasons, once a T cell leaves the thymus, it does not appear to return to it.

Subpopulations of T Cells

Several subpopulations of T cells (Fig. 3-2) have been observed, each having different functions. There is substantial evidence for separate categories of functional T lymphocytes, such as the helper cell and suppressor cells, but it is unclear whether these categories represent different functional states in a common differentiation pathway or separate pathways of maturation. Normal T cells do not produce conventional immunoglobulins as is characteristic of B cells. However, T cells do have a crucial role in the regulation of immune responses by acting as potentiators or inhibitors of the B-cell transition into immunoglobulin-secreting plasma cells. The cells that potentiate this B-cell transition are classified as helper cells, whereas those that inhibit it are classified as suppressor cells. Suppressor cells have been identified in human beings through a variety of circumstances. There is compelling evidence in mice, and corroborating evidence in human beings, that potentiation and suppression are mediated by distinct subsets of T cells, each with a genetic calling committed to mediate only one of these two functions. In mice, helper T-cell and suppressor T-cell subsets can be readily distinguished by their surface membrane antigen. Other evidence suggests that immunoregulatory T cells may have an interim existence as inactive precursors. These might be referred to as pro-helper cells and pro-suppressor cells which in turn must react with a different set of activated T cells before maturing into fully functional helper effector cells or suppressor effector cells. Physiologically, suppressor cells may terminate excessive immune responses after antigenic exposure, and they probably provide a safeguard against autoimmune reactions. It is not surprising that recent evidence from a number of animal models of autoimmunity suggests that impaired suppressor T-cell function can lead to overt autoimmune disease.

An understanding of suppressor cell function in human neoplasia may alter the perspective and direction of oncologic researchers and clinicians. There is a real possibility that chemotherapy, radiation, and surgery might, in certain cases, benefit cancer patients by an indirect effect on suppressor cells as well as the obvious effect on the neoplasm itself. New immunotherapeutic strategies that incorporate recent insight regarding the suppressor cell network are nullifying suppressor cell systems that oppose tumoricidal im-

mune effector mechanisms. In addition to switching off antibody production by B cells, suppressor T cells apparently are capable of preventing lymphokine production by other T cells.

Natural killer (NK) cells are a more recently discovered subpopulation of lymphoid cells present in most normal persons. NK cells exhibit spontaneous cytolytic activity against a variety of tumor cells and some normal cells, and their reactivity can be rapidly augmented by interferon. They have characteristics distinct from other types of lymphoid cells are are closely associated with large granulated lymphocytes, making up about 5 percent of blood or splenic leuko-

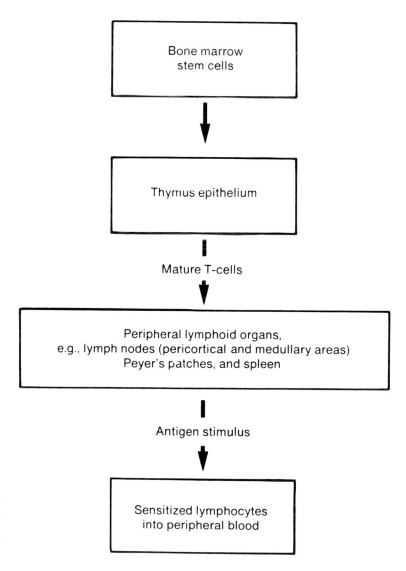

Fig. 3.1 Progress of T-cell lymphocyte maturation. (DiSaia PJ, Creasman WT: Tumor immunology. p. 475. In Clinical Gynecology Oncology. CV Mosby, 1984.)

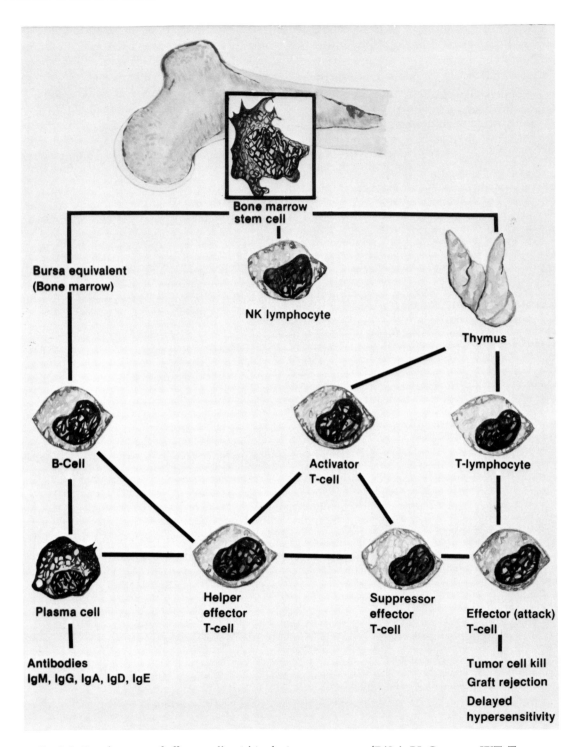

Fig. 3-2 Development of effector cells within the immune system. (DiSaia PJ, Creasman WT: Tumor immunology. p. 474. In Clinical Gynecologic Oncology. CV Mosby, 1984.)

cytes. There is increasing evidence that NK cells, with the ability to mediate natural resistance against tumors in vivo, may play an important role in immune surveillance. By contrast, T cells have virtually no detectable spontaneous cytotoxic activity; rather, they must be activated usually by being exposed to specific antigens on accessory cells, such as macrophages. There may be a considerable latent period, usually 7 to 10 days or more, before T cells develop their initial or primary activity. This is not so with NK cells, which appear to be able to react immediately and without prior sensitization.

Macrophage Immunity

Hibbs[5] suggested that macrophages may provide a surveillance system for the detection and destruction of nascent transformed neoplastic cells. Treating mice with a macrophage stimulant prolongs the latent period of tumor development when the mice are exposed to ultraviolet (UV) radiation and are protected against the carcinogenesis of other toxins. There are two major pathways whereby macrophage activation can be achieved in vivo. Frequently, macrophages are activated as a consequence of their interaction with microorganisms and their products, for example, endotoxins, the bacterial cell wall skeleton, and certain small components of the bacterial cell wall. In vivo activation of macrophages can also take place after their interaction with soluble mediators released by antigen- or mitogen-sensitized lymphocytes. The soluble lymphokine that induces macrophage activation is referred to as macrophage-activating factor (MAF); it first binds to a macrophage surface receptor and is then internalized to elicit tumoricidal properties in the macrophages.

Regardless of the method of their activation, rodent and human tumoricidal macrophages acquire the ability to recognize and destroy neoplastic cells both in vitro and in vivo, while leaving nonneoplastic cells unharmed. The mechanism for this is unknown but appears to be nonimmunologic in nature and to require intimate cell-to-cell contact. The ability of tumoricidal macrophages to distinguish tumorigenic from normal cells presents an attractive possibility for the treatment of disseminated cancer. The data generated in rodent and human systems indicate that, at least in vitro, tumoricidal macrophages can discriminate between neoplastic and nonneoplastic cells by a

process independent of transplantation antigens, species-specific antigens, tumor-specific antigens, and cell-cycle time. Although the precise mechanisms by which macrophages recognize and lyse tumor cells is unclear, it is probably regulated by a tumor cell characteristic that is linked with the tumorigenic capacity of tumor cells.

Humoral Immunity

As the term suggests, humoral immunity is mediated by factors present in and transferrable by serum; these factors include the classic antibody globulins. The cell responsible for the production of these antibodies is the second type of small lymphocyte, or the B cell. In the chicken, these lymphocytes are aggregated in a small organ called the bursa of Fabricius. Removal of the bursa was noted to render the chicken unable to produce antibodies; the B cells have thus come to be known as bursa-dependent cells. In humans, there was a great deal of controversy as to the origin of these cells, but recent evidence has made it quite clear that these cells originate in the bone marrow and that they do not undergo maturation in the thymus.

In humans (in whom there is no bursa of Fabricius) no one organ appears to have control of the B-cell production. Rather, B cells are distributed in all areas of lymphoid tissue, including the spleen, lymph nodes, appendix, and Peyer's patches of the small intestine. With suitable stimulation, B cells become metabolically active and begin to synthesize antibodies with great facility. The antibodies soon become detectable in the cytoplasm and are then secreted into the surrounding medium. It is at this point that the B cell has undergone transformation into a plasma cell, which is the actual antibody producer. In a typical peripheral lymph node, B cells occupy the germinal centers, and T cells populate the cortical areas; these areas are referred to, respectively, as the bursa- and thymus-dependent areas of the node. Although the bone marrow appears to be the source of cells destined to make antibodies, the bone marrow itself is not the focus of large-scale antibody formation. Rather, it is the site of intense lymphocyte proliferation leading to the production of mature B lymphocytes that quickly leave the marrow and travel to peripheral lymphoid tissues. These cells may then meet the appropriate antigen, become stimulated to divide and differentiate into large lymphocytes and plasma cells, and actively manufacture antibodies.

Escape from Surveillance

Several mechanisms have been postulated (Fig. 3-3) by which mutant cells might avoid an interaction with a potentially damaging immune system. A commonly held concept in the past was that the patient in whom a clinical malignancy developed had a paralyzed or otherwise depressed system. More recent evidence would strongly suggest that most patients with a clinical neoplasm have a competent immune system (at least in the early stages of malignancy) and the emergence of the neoplasm is due to an escape mechanism against the homeostatic principle of immune surveillance. Immunologic surveillance has been defined as the continuous monitoring of body cells by the immunologic system in order to destroy aberrant cells not specified by the genetic blueprint. This was first suggested by the great investigator Burnet[6] as a natural control mechanism to destroy incipient tumor cells.

Factors that seem to be at least partly responsible for the escape of neoplasms from host surveillance are as follows:

1. *Lowered tumor antigenicity:* Neoplasms that arise spontaneously are noted to be considerably less antigenic than those induced experimentally. Many human tumors may be weak or nonantigenic.
2. *Sneaking through:* Old and others have reported neoplastic systems in which large inocula of immunogenic tumor cells fail to grow in a synegeneic recipient, but smaller doses will grow and eventually overwhelm the host. The mechanism of "sneaking through" is unknown, but it may be related to the time of vascularization of the neoplasm.
3. *Immunoresistance:* Diminished sensitivity to rejection may develop in the same way that bacteria develop resistance to antibodies after repeated exposure. The cells may develop a decrease in cell-surface antigenic sites (antigenic modulation) or relevant antibody-binding sites. Another mechanism that is easy to conceive calls for antigenic

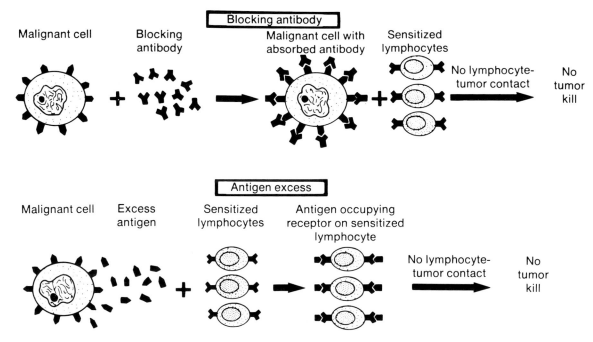

Fig. 3-3 Two methods of escape from surveillance: (1) blocking antibody absorbed onto antigen sites on tumor cell surface, and (2) excess antigen flooding the tumor cell environment, preventing lymphocyte attack.

molecules on the surface of the tumor cell to be shed in large amounts into the surrounding extracellular fluid. The cell surface will then be rendered relatively immunoresistant as its locality becomes flooded with excess antigens. This may be classified then as a blocking factor. Some have suggested that tumors that shed antigen rapidly are those of low immunogenicity that metastasize most rapidly.

4. *Vascularization:* Tumors probably reach 1 to 2 mm in diameter before vascularization takes place. Folkman and Hochberg's[7] studies suggest that the vessels result from ingrowth of host cells; instead of rejection of the endothelium of the tumor vessels it may be misrecognized as self. Thus, some neoplasms may proliferate with their antigens locked away behind a wall of normal endothelial cells unpenetrated by attack lymphocytes.

5. *Immunosuppression:* It has been well established that the presence of a cancer can significantly reduce the capacity to mount a response to a great variety of antigens. Immunosuppressive factors have been described in the serum of cancer patients and confirmed in vitro. The mechanism by which these factors cause immunosuppression is not understood, but some authorities have suggested that they suppress macrophage function. Some degree of immunosuppression has been found in almost all cancer patients studied. DNCB, DNFB, and a variety of skin test antigens have been used in patients with gynecologic malignancies. An increase in tumor burden is associated with a decreased percentage of patients responding to these tests, and both are associated with a poorer prognosis.

6. *Blocking factors:* Neoplasms may escape the immune mechanism by the development of systemic factors that abrogate the usual interaction with host-defense capabilities. A number of serum factors have been identified in vitro: blocking antibodies, antigen-antibody complexes, and soluble antigen excess. When these blocking factors are operational, the state of the tumor-host relationship is one of tumor enhancement. The mechanisms involved may be similar to those described for immunoresistance. Excess free antigen may paralyze lymphocyte activity. In addition, recent studies suggest that the cellular factors of the immune system may be capable of causing tumor enhancement. In some animal and in vivo systems, small numbers of sensitized (tumor-specific) lymphocytes can enhance tumor growth, whereas larger numbers of the same cells will retard growth. This phenomenon has been referred to as immunostimulation; if valid, it will help explain the emergence of neoplasms beyond the subclinical stage at which tumor cell numbers are small and vulnerable. The puzzle is made more difficult by the fact that deblocking factors have also been described in the serum of cancer patients undergoing remission or following surgical debulking procedures. The mechanism involved in deblocking is unknown.

GENERAL PRINCIPLES OF IMMUNOTHERAPY

It is obvious that the ultimate goal of immunotherapy or of any manipulation of the host-defense mechanisms is the complete destruction of all neoplastic cells. Short of that, the suppression of growth of tumor cells is desired. An expression of this therapeutic effect would be the prolongation of remission and the prevention of the appearance of metastatic disease. More often than not, the immunotherapist must be satisfied with evidence that the approach has achieved at least a reduction in the mass of tumor cells. Before the institution of immunotherapy, it is crucial to reduce tumor mass to a minimum, preferably less than 10^8 cells, by whatever means is at hand—radical surgical procedures, chemotherapy, or irradiation therapy. It has been shown that immunotherapy by itself appears to be relatively ineffectual. It is currently used in conjunction with other cancericidal modalities, which are depended on to significantly reduce the tumor burden. As one would expect, immunotherapy has shown more effectiveness in neoplasms that are highly antigenic, such as Burkitt's lymphoma, malignant melanoma, and neuroblastoma. Most important, the reader should fully comprehend the embryonic nature of immunotherapy, and an attidude of cautious optimism must be maintained as this fetal area of research is brought to full term.

Nonspecific Immunotherapy

A substance that increases response to an antigen is an adjuvant. Adjuvants may be effective by altering either the antigen itself or the immunologic reaction to the antigen. In the former instance, a mechanism can be postulated whereby the adjuvant would increase the release of antigen. Nonspecific immunotherapy directed toward the reaction to the antigen has focused on the cellular response. A long list of studies suggests at least two cellular cytotoxic mechanisms. One involves independent cytotoxic lymphocytes, such as NK cells or thymus-processed cytotoxic cells (T cells) which recognize the target antigens; the other is controlled by a thymus-independent effector cell system, which is independent of the target antigen. The latter system is triggered to kill by recognition of antibody bound to the target, refuting our previously held simplistic view that stimulation of the cellular mechanism is beneficial, whereas humoral immunity is of no aid. Present knowledge suggests four methods of stimulation of the host-response mechanism: (1) increased or improved localization of cytotoxic antibody, (2) suppression of blocking factors, (3) more effective use of macrophage activity, and (4) heightened CMI. The most widely used nonspecific immunotherapy has employed adjuvants such as bacillus Calmette-Guérin (BCG), *Corynebacterium parvum,* levamisole, and methanol-extruded residue (MER). BCG is a live attenuated strain of *Mycobacterium bovis. Corynebacterium parvum* is a gram-negative anaerobe given in a nonviable form. Levamisole is a synthetic antihelminthic drug that has been found to have significant effects on tumor immunity. MER is a methanol extraction of killed tuberculin bacilli.

Interferons

A new category of substances that may have therapeutic value is the interferons. Interferons are inducible secretory glycoproteins produced both in vivo and in vitro by eukaryotic cells in response to viral infection and other stimuli. They induce broad-spectrum resistance to viral infection. Interferon preparations have effects on tumor cells in vitro and antitumor activity in vivo by mechanisms that have not yet been identified but appear to be mediated in part through effects on several components of the immune response. These substances can be extracted from many cell types, but the leukocyte and lymphoblast appear to hold the most promise for therapeutic quality. Type I interferons (classic) are divided into α-interferon (IFN$_\alpha$) (virus-activated leukocytes) and β-interferon (IFN$_\beta$ (virus-activated fibroblasts). Type II in-

terferons (immune) are produced in response to mitogens or antibody-activated lymphocytes and are referred to as γ-interferon (IFN$_\gamma$). The mechanism of interferon activity is not totally clear but at least in part involves the recruitment and augmentation of NK cells. Interferons also prolong and inhibit cell division, having this effect on almost every cell system studied, whether transformed or normal. In addition, interferons stimulate the induction of several intracellular enzyme systems with a resultant profound effect on macromolecular therapeutics.

It is unclear whether the interferons work primarily by their antiproliferative activity or through alterations of immune responses. What is clear from both preclinical and clinical studies is that the interferons do exhibit antitumor activity. Methods of production and purification are becoming less expensive, and therapeutic trials are under way.

Lymphokines and Cytokines

Many of the biologic agents being tested as response modifiers are cell products (cytokines) of lymphocytes (lymphokines) or direct cytotoxic factors of activated lymphocytes (lymphotoxins) or macrophages (cytotoxins). The lymphokines have a specific ability to regulate certain components of the immune response, which may be useful in altering the growth and metastasis of cancer in man. For example, it is possible that certain lymphokines may augment the ability of T cells to respond to tumor-associated antigens, and others may induce higher responsiveness with respect to B-cell activity in cancer patients.

Interleukin-1 (IL-1), originally known as lymphocyte activating factor, is a macrophage-derived cytokine originally identified as a result of its nonspecific enhancing effect on murine thymocyte proliferation. Both IL-1 and viable macrophages are necessary for the initial step in activation of specific T cells and the process of further in vivo production of T cells. IL-1 in its purest form stimulates the production of IL-2, also known as T-cell growth factor. The assistance of macrophages is also required in this step. Human lymphotoxin has been produced from peripheral blood lymphocytes or tonsillar lymphocytes by stimulation with mitogens, such as phytohemagglutinins (PHA). Lymphotoxin may be the principal effector of delayed hypersensitivity. Depending on the type of tumor cell involved, the in vitro effect of lymphotoxin may be either cytolytic or cytostatic. Isolation of human lymphotoxin for in vivo studies is complicated by the occurrence of at least five major species and several subspecies that result from the association with other components and subsequent spontaneous degradation to lower-molecular-weight forms.

It has been estimated that more than 100 molecules have already been described as lymphokines. Several lymphokines, such as lymphotoxins, macrophage-activating factor, IL-2, and possibly tumornecrosis factor, merit evaluation as antitumor agents, since each may contribute to tumor control through its own distinct mechanisms. Such studies require quantities of material sufficiently pure to exclude contributions by other factors to permit definitive evaluation of each lymphokine-cytokine. Large-scale studies will require standardized preparations in quantities best ordained through genetic engineering with the use of sensitive and rapid assay procedures suitable to monitor production, purification, and bioavailability.

Thymic Factors

Other factors (thymosins) have been identified that exhibit thymic hormonelike activity. In general, these hormones can be expected to specifically increase host resistance through stimulation of the maturation of T cells from precursor cells. This would represent an immunoaugmenting effect that should be helpful to patients with cancer, particularly those with T-cell deficiencies. Thymosin fraction 5 is an extract containing a variety of thymic polypeptides and thymosin-α_1 is a synthetic polypeptide component that is also present in many thymic extracts. Similar to interferons, thymic extracts represent a family of compounds. Studies are in progress with thymic fraction 5 and with thymosin-α_1 to determine their efficacy in preclinical models and in patients with cancer.[8,9]

Specific Immunotherapy

Tumor immunotherapy has been under study with extensive clinical trials, but less has been attempted using specific immunotherapy than with nonspecific modes. Specific immunotherapy can be active, passive, or adoptive.

Active specific immunotherapy calls for administration to the cancer patient of tumor cells, or their equivalent, bearing antigens that will cross-react with the neoplasm. Tumor antigens are usually weakly antigenic, so that often immunostimulants (e.g., BCG) are administered jointly. Other attempts to heighten the immunogenicity of the tumor cells have been studied, such as surface changes by enzymes, viral incorporation, physical treatments, and chemical modifications. Although this remains an exciting field for future research, trials to date in humans have been disappointing.

A major limitation of active specific immunotherapy is the source and availability of the tumor antigens. As presently established, the necessity of adhering to a strict protocol for vaccine whole-cell preparation (which may differ among different tumors) constitutes a major limitation of this procedure for the clinician. While the present vaccine preparations must contain viable nontumorigenic cells prepared from individual tumors, it is possible that in the future nonclonal antibody defined purified tumor antigens would be available for large-scale immunizations. With these, a procedure can be visualized that would include antigen purification and characterization, followed by genetic engineering of the antigen for vaccine production. All these technologies are at hand and specific tumor antigen preparations will soon be available for clinical evaluation.

Passive Immunotherapy

Passive immunotherapy is the production of immunity resulting not from an active immune response but from a passive transfer of antibody of sensitized lymphocytes from another individual (for the latter transfer, the term adoptive immunity is favored). This mechanism will not be discussed at length in this chapter because this has not been a fruitful concept in human immunotherapy trials published to date. However, promising trials are under way using in vitro IL-2 stimulated lymphocytes borrowed from the patient and later returned to that patient. These preliminary studies may renew interest in this method of immunotherapy.

TUMOR MARKERS

A large body of work has been reported in the literature in the last two decades in the field of gynecologic oncology suggesting that the anatomy and physiology alluded to above does exist and is operational in the gynecologic system of cancer. The following is a brief description of the highlights of this body of work, beginning with evidence for the existence of tumor-associated antigens (Fig. 3-4) and cell-mediated immunity and ending with a description of immunotherapeutic trials.

Tumor-Associated Antigens

Kato and Torigoe[10] reported that a heterologous antiserum for human cervical squamous cell carcinoma had been prepared and specifically determined by Ouchterlony immunodiffusion and immunofluoresence studies. With this antiserum, a tumor antigen (TA-4) was purified from human cervical squamous cell carcinoma tissue. The specificities of the antigen and the antiserum were then reexamined by a RIA method using ^{125}I-labeled purified antigen. Although normal cervical tissue extract showed moderate cross-reactivity in the RIA, the circulating antigen activity could not be detected in normal women or in several patients with other carcinomas, whereas 27 or 35 patients with cervical squamous cell carcinoma showed detectable serum antigen activity. All patients with advanced stages of cervical squamous cell carcinoma showed detectable antigen levels. These results indicate that there is a quantitative abnormality of this

tumor antigen in patients with cervical squamous cell carcinoma. In 1979, Kato et al.[11] reported on further work with this tumor antigen. TA-4 purified from cervical squamous cell carcinoma was discovered to be a glycoprotein with a molecular weight of approximately 48,000. Once again, these workers reported that although TA-4 activity was found in normal squamous proteins of the female genital tract, clinical studies using RIA demonstrated that the appearance of TA-4 in the circulation was highly suggestive of the presence of squamous cell carcinoma; there was also a correlation between the progress of the disease and the change in the serum TA-4 levels; 55.2 percent of patients with cervical squamous cell carcinoma were reported as being positive. Also in 1979, Kato et al.[12] reported a double-antibody RIA for serial determinations of TA-4. The correlation of serum antigen levels with disease progress was investigated in 23 patients with cervical squamous cell carcinoma. Ten cases with widespread metastases received either radiotherapy or chemotherapy, or both. The nine patients who showed progression of their disease had a corresponding increase in serum antigen levels, while the one case with regression of its disease showed a corresponding decrease in serum antigen levels. Thirteen patients received radical surgery, and in all of these, high pretreatment antigen levels declined to undetectable levels 1 or 2 weeks after surgery. A panel

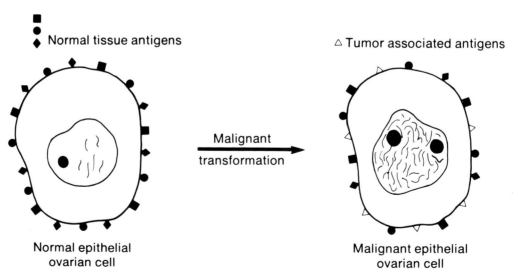

Fig. 3-4 Tumor-associated antigens (TAAs) are also expressed on tumor cell surface. (DiSaia PJ, Creasman WT: Tumor immunology. p. 468. In Clinical Gynecologic Oncology. CV Mosby, 1984.)

of coded sera from the National Cancer Institute (NCI)-Mayo Clinic Serum Bank was also studied to evaluate the specificity of the assay. Thirteen of 25 patients (52 percent) with cervical squamous cell carcinoma showed positive serum antigen levels, while only 1 of 58 controls (1.7 percent) showed false-positive results. These results suggest that serial TA-4 determinations may provide a useful method for evaluating regression or progression of the disease. This assay is now available commercially, and larger studies are under way studying its clinical value.

Nadkarni et al.[13] reported an in vitro demonstration of cell-mediated immune responses to tumor-associated antigen observed with autologous tumor extracts from patients with cervical cancer. Seventy-six percent of their patients exhibited an inhibitory effect with autologous antigens, while 59 percent reacted with homologous antigens. A progressive rise in percentage inhibitory activity was associated with increasing stage of disease. The physiochemical and immunochemical characterization of the tumor-associated antigen found on the membrane of cervical tumor cells suggested that it may be a lipid-protein complex containing an enzyme with immunologic determinants such as those of term-placental alkaline phosphatase enzyme.

CA 125

Bast et al.[4] reported CA 125 as an antigenic determinant expressed by greater than 80 percent of nonmucinous epithelial ovarian carcinomas. An immunoradiometric assay has been developed using a murine monoclonal antibody (OC 125) to quantitate CA 125 in human serum. Studies indicate that elevation of CA 125 serum levels above values normally found in healthy people can be detected in patients with serous, endometroid, clear cell, and undifferentiated ovarian carcinoma. adenocarcinoma of the endometrium or fallopian tube, as well as some nongynecologic malignancies and certain nonmalignant conditions. Elevated CA 125 levels also have been observed in pregnant women, most often during the first trimester. RIA testing of CA 125 may have significant value in the monitoring of subjects with diagnosed ovarian carcinoma. A persistently rising CA 125 value may be associated with progressive malignant disease and poor therapeutic response. A declining CA 125 value appears to be indicative of a favorable prognosis and

good response to treatment. A value greater than 35 U/ml is considered positive in most laboratories.

The status of tumor markers for ovarian carcinoma was well summarized by Bhattacharya and Barlow[14] in 1979. Two common tumor-associated antigens, or antigenic determinants in serous and mucinous cystadenocarcinoma of the ovary (OCAA and OCAA-l), were described and partially characterized. These antigens seemed to have potential for immunodiagnosis of ovarian cancer. Other well-defined embryonic proteins that have been examined in ovarian cancer included CEA, AFP, β-oncofetal antigen, Regan and Nagoa isoenzymes, and human chorionic gonadotropin (hCG). The presence of pregnancy-zone protein has also been reported in ovarian cancer. Enzymes, especially those involved in glycoprotein biosynthesis (e.g., glycoprotein : glycosyltransferases and glycosidases) have been explored as possible early biochemical indicators of ovarian neoplasia. A serum-specific deficiency of α-l-fucosidase has been found in patients with ovarian cancers. Of all the glycoprotein : glycosyltransferases studied, galactosyltransferase has been found to be the best enzyme marker for ovarian carcinoma. The determination of serum levels of this enzyme reflected the clinical status of the patient with respect to tumor progression as well as tumor burden. An assay of phosphodiesterase, which specifically hydrolyzes cytidine 5′-monophospho-N-acetylneuraminic acid, has been found promising in the detection and management of patients with ovarian cancer. Many of these markers have the requisite specificity to be useful in the diagnosis of ovarian cancer with further refinement. The use of several assays may provide more highly discriminatory data than can be obtained by a single assay.

Carcinoembryonic Antigen

Many investigators have studied CEA in gynecologic cancers.[15-25] Van Nagell et al.[26] reported in 1978 on a series of plasma CEA determinations attained prior to therapy in 300 patients with invasive carcinoma of the uterine cervix followed at the University of Kentucky Medical Center from 1971 to 1976. CEA levels were elevated (greater than 2.5 ng/m) in 48 percent of cervical cancer patients. The level of CEA varied directly with the stage of disease and histologic differentiation of the tumor. Plasma CEA levels were more commonly elevated in patients with endocervical adenocarcinoma than in those with squamous cell carcinoma but were unrelated to vascular invasion in the specimen or regional lymph node morphology. Two hundred and four patients had 2 to 15 (mean = 5) follow-up plasma CEA determinations after treatment. Thirty patients had progressively increasing plasma CEA levels following therapy; 29 of these patients developed recurrent cervical cancer. A progressive rise of serum CEA preceded the clinical diagnosis of recurrence by 1 to 23 months (mean: 6 months) in 13 of these patients and occurred at the same time as or after the clinical diagnosis of recurrence in 16 cases. It was concluded that patients with progressively rising plasma CEA levels following therapy for cervical cancer should be vigorously evaluated to rule out the presence of occult recurrence. In a similar study on ovarian carcinoma. Van Nagell et al.[27] reported that immunoperoxidase staining for CEA was performed on the tumors of 88 patients with epithelial ovarian cystadenocarcinomas treated at their medical center between 1962 and 1975. Pretreatment plasma CEA determinations were obtained in 45 of these patients, and 40 had serial plasma CEA measurements following therapy. Cyst-fluid CEA concentrations were measured in 14 patients. Immunoperoxidase staining indicative of a tissue CEA concentration of at least 3 ng/m was detected in 75 percent of mucinous cystadenocarcinomas but in no serous tumors. Plasma CEA levels were related both to tissue and cyst-fluid CEA concentrations and to the extent or stage of disease. Plasma CEA was highest in poorly differentiated mucinous tumors. All patients with progressively increasing plasma CEA levels showed the development of recurrent ovarian cancer and later died of their disease. In nine patients recurrent cancer developed despite normal plasma CEA values, but none of the tumors in these patients contained measurable concentrations of CEA. Serial plasma CEA determinations most accurately reflected the clinical status of disease in those patients whose tumors contained high levels of antigen. It was concluded that pretherapy plasma and tumor levels of CEA should be measured in order to identify those patients in whom serial plasma CEA determinations following therapy will be useful to monitor the effects of therapy.

Rutanen et al.[22] reported on a series of patients with gynecologic tumors, using RIA and immunoperoxidase techniques to determine the CEA level in the serum and tissues of patients. Among 328 patients with gynecologic cancer, the serum CEA concentration was elevated over the normal background level of 5 ng/ml in 32 cases (9.8 percent), and the frequency of elevated CEA levels increased with advancing clinical stage. Among 84 patients with benign tumors, CEA was elevated in 5 cases (6 percent). Elevated levels were most commonly seen in patients with ovarian cancer (20 percent). In squamous cell carcinoma of the uterine cervix, elevated levels occurred in 10 percent, and in cervical adenocarcinoma CEA elevation took place in 19 percent of the cases. In endometrial cancer, CEA was less frequently elevated (7 percent). After radical surgery, the CEA concentration decreased, remaining low in 20 of 24 cancer patients (83 percent). Fifteen of these patients remained clinically tumor free during the follow-up period of 4 to 24 months. Three of four patients whose CEA concentration did not significantly decrease after operation were found to have residual tumor. Radiotherapy resulted in an increased CEA concentration in three of five patients with advanced cancer.

DiSaia et al.[16] also found that in patients with elevated plasma CEA values, radical surgery, such as radical vulvectomy[15] (Fig. 3-5), would result in an abrupt return to negative levels during the postoperative period. This was demonstrated not only in patients with advanced vulvar carcinoma but in patients with recurrent cervical carcinoma who were undergoing exenteration.

Khoo et al.[19] reported on the predicative value of serial levels of CEA in tumor monitoring as examined in 213 patients with ovarian cancer; each patient had follow-up evaluation at monthly intervals for at least 12 months. CEA was not detectable throughout the period of observation in 35 percent of patients. In general, patterns showing a disappearance of CEA or persistently low levels were associated with a good prognosis, whereas those showing a reappearance or highly elevated and rising levels were associated with a poor prognosis. A transient reappearance of CEA was observed in 10 patients; this did not appear to be associated with tumor recurrence or progression. False-positive results were obtained in six patients in whom no tumor has been clinically detectable to date. False-negative results were obtained in four patients with obvious tumor progression. In terms of a good or poor prognosis, the use of CEA levels was highly accurate in patients with minimal residual disease (97

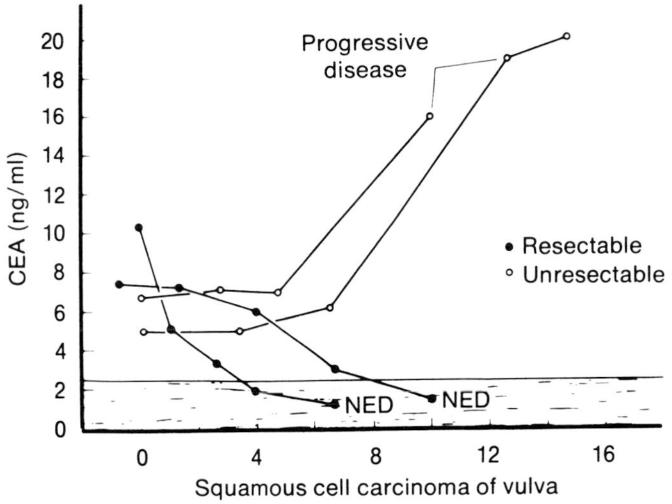

Fig. 3-5 Four patients with positive plasma (CEA) value before therapy are followed up subsequent to treatment. Progressive disease results in rising titers. (Reprinted with permission from the American College of Obstetricians and Gynecologists. DiSaia PJ, Morrow C, Haverback B, Dyce B: Carcinoembryonic antigen in cervical and vulvar cancer patients: Serum levels and disease progress. Obstet Gynecol 47:95, 1976.)

percent and 89 percent, respectively); the rate fell to 62 percent in patients with extensive disease. It was concluded that as the clinical significance and limitations become better known, serial CEA levels should contribute substantially to the monitoring of patients with ovarian cancer.

In conclusion, CEA can be found in many gynecologic malignancies. Its presence in measurable amounts is more obvious in the advanced stages of these malignancies. If present in measurable amounts in the plasma of the patient, the potential exists for utilization of this marker in the subsequent surveillance of the patient's status following therapy. However, when one looks at the number of patients with detectable amounts of CEA in the plasma versus the number of patients in whom various gynecologic malignancies develop when a positive titer is potentially in existence, one can only conclude that the yield would be small and the cost high if one were to recommend routine CEA determinations for all patients with gynecologic cancer. A more practical approach would be to seek a routine determination for all patients with advanced disease for whom a positive value is obtained on initial examination; periodic assays in the post-therapy period may then be helpful in detecting recurrent disease. The frequency of these subsequent determinations has not been specifically prescribed in the literature, and no credible analysis of the cost effectiveness of such a program has ever been determined. Clinicians must analyze the facts presented herein and reach their own conclusions concerning CEA determinations in patients with gynecologic malignancies.

Other Oncofetal Antigens

Goldenberg et al.[28] reported in 1978 on the identification of β-oncofetal antigen in cervical squamous cell cancer and its demonstration in neoplastic and normal tissues. An extract of human cervical squamous carcinoma was used to produce rabbit antiserum with immunoreactivity against an antigen in several types of normal and neoplastic tissues. This antigen was abundant in cervical cancer as well as in normal adult and fetal kidney and liver. The antigen had a β-mobility in immunoelectrophoresis and a molecular weight range of 74,000 to 90,000 as determined by gel chromatography. Since some of its properties were similar to those of the β-oncofetal antigen described in Fritsche and Mach, a comparison was undertaken that indeed revealed identical immunoreactivity of the anti-β-oncofetal antigen and anticervical cancer antisera when reacted in immunodiffusion against a cervical cancer extract. Their results did not support the designation of this antigen as an oncofetal antigen.

Tatarinov and Kalashikov[29] used nonspecific antisera to identify a new embryonic antigen in human fetal sera and in some adenocarcinoma extracts. The newly discovered antigen migrated with α-globulin and prealbumin in immunoelectrophoresis. Immunodiffusion analysis revealed analogous antigen in sera of newborns (20/20 positive) as well as in some individual extracts of ovarian (13/26 positive) and colonic (7/17 positive) adenocarcinomas, but not in adult sera or in other normal and malignant tissues. Comparative immunodiffusion showed that the reported embryonic antigen was not identical to AFP, CEA, bovine fetuin, or pregnancy-specific β_1-globulin.

Talerman et al.[30] studied AFP in germ cell neoplasms. Levels were measured serially whenever possible in 70 patients attending their institute with testicular or ovarian germ cell neoplasms. In 15 patients, the disease was active; in the others it was in remission. Patients with active disease had elevated serum AFP levels that correlated well with disease activity; no patient without evidence of active disease had elevated serum AFP levels. There was no correleation between serum AFP and CEA levels in patients with germ cell neoplasms, but there was good correlation between serum AFP levels and disease activity. As serum CEA levels did not correlate with disease activity, serial determinations would not be useful in monitoring progress in this group of diseases.

Talerman et al.[31] later reported on the use of AFP in diagnosis and management of endodermal sinus (yolk sac) tumor and mixed germ cell tumor of the ovary. There were four patients with pure dysgerminoma, one with pure endodermal sinus tumor, and eight with mixed germ cell tumors, all containing elements of endodermal sinus tumor. Patients with dysgerminoma and gonadoblastoma had normal serum AFP at all times. All patients with tumors containing endodermal sinus components had elevated serum AFP levels. In most cases, the level was first determined between 1 and 3 weeks postoperatively, and there was no evidence of metastasis. Serum AFP returned to normal 5 to 7 weeks postoperatively and began to rise again when disease recurred. Serum AFP determinations detected the presence of recurrent disease long before it became detectable by other means. Serum CEA was determined serially by RIA in eight of these patients, including two who died with metastases, and was normal on all occasions.

Donaldson et al.[32] reported in 1979 on AFP as a biochemical marker in patients with gynecologic cancer. AFP was measured by RIA in the sera of 348 patients with gynecologic malignancies and in 385 patients with benign gynecologic disease. Serum AFP was elevated (greater than 20 ng/ml) in 50 percent of patients with invasive cervical, endometrial, and ovarian cancers and in 20 percent of the control population ($P < 0.001$). However, there was no statistical evidence in the incidence of AFP elevation in patients with cervical intraepithelial neoplasia and in those with benign gynecologic disease. Serum AFP levels returned to normal within 2 months following complete tumor excision or radiation therapy in patients without clinical evidence of persistent disease.

In summary, the clinical usefulness of AFP and hCG assays is limited to patients with germ cell tumors of the ovary (primarily embryonal carcinoma and endodermal sinus tumor), and the more traditional use of hCG titers in patients with gestational and nongestational choriocarcinoma. Further studies in this area may prove that other oncofetal antigens are present in gynecologic cancers and that serial determination may be of value, but sufficient data are wanting.

Monoclonal Antibodies

On October 15, 1984, the Nobel Prize for medicine was awarded to Kohler and Milstein,[33] who in 1975 first described the Hybridome technique for producing stable long-lived clones of specific antibody producing cells (Fig. 3-6). Antibodies can now be produced in large quantities with such high intrinsic specificity that only one or two antigenic determinants are recognized. Their revolutionary findings and technique will certainly have a profound impact on the entire field of oncology. The potential for using monoclonal antibodies in diagnosis is obvious and probably will materialize sooner than those procedures with therapeutic implications.

The use of monoclonal antibody and its conjugates in the treatment and radioimaging of cancer is in a very early stage. While it is clear that much needs to be done to clarify many of the issues surrounding the use of antibody alone or of conjugates of the antibody with other toxic substances, it has already been demonstrated in both animal tumor models and in human subjects that antibody alone and antibody conjugated with drugs, toxins, and radioisotopes can have therapeutic effects. The potential for monoclonal antibodies in cancer therapeutics is enormous, given the specificity that is inherent to the antibody-antigen reaction. The use of isotope-labeled antibody has enormous potential for the detection and treatment of cancer. There are still significant problems with these conjugates in terms of potential toxicity for the organs

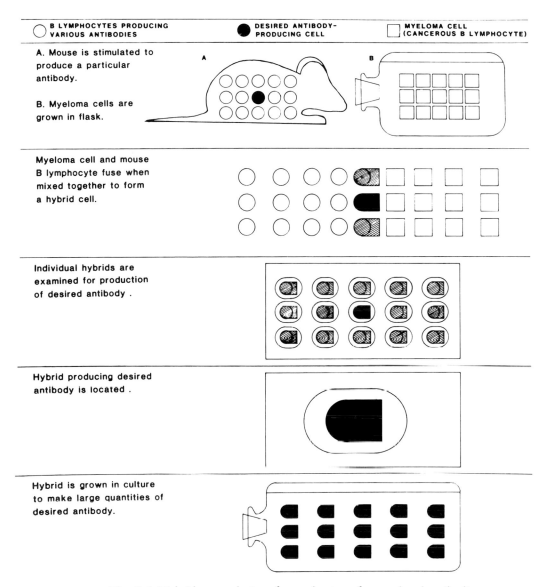

B LYMPHOCYTES PRODUCING VARIOUS ANTIBODIES   **DESIRED ANTIBODY-PRODUCING CELL**   **MYELOMA CELL (CANCEROUS B LYMPHOCYTE)**

A. Mouse is stimulated to produce a particular antibody.

B. Myeloma cells are grown in flask.

Myeloma cell and mouse B lymphocyte fuse when mixed together to form a hybrid cell.

Individual hybrids are examined for production of desired antibody.

Hybrid producing desired antibody is located.

Hybrid is grown in culture to make large quantities of desired antibody.

Fig. 3-6 Hybridoma technique for production of monoclonal antibodies.

nonspecifically accumulating radioactivity from the conjugate or its products, and any nonspecific binding of isotope-labeled conjugates will represent a significant and clinical problem for the use of these conjugates in therapy. The hypothesis that lower levels of drug toxicity and greater antitumor activity may be seen by virtue of increased specificity of the drug-antibody conjugate remains to be demonstrated in humans.[34,35]

Although large numbers of monoclonal antibody trials are initiated, only a few trials have been under

way for a sufficient period of time to have reported any results. Certain conclusions can be drawn on the basis of these preliminary studies. A major difficulty with antibody alone appears to be that of antigenic modulation. Thus far, antigenic modulation has been observed more with the antigens on hematopoietic cells than with those on solid tumors.

A central question, as yet unanswered, is whether monoclonal antibodies will identify antigens expressed on tumor cells that are not shared with normal tissues and furthermore, whether such neoantigens, if they exist, are really tumor specific or only tumor associated. In the field of gynecologic oncology, several antibodies that are supposed to recognize such tumor associated antigens have been reported, such as CA 125 raised against ovarian cancer cells. CA 125 is detected on the cell surface in more than 80 percent of nonmucinous ovarian cancers, while only traces of the antigen are expressed in some normal adult tissues.[4]

CELLULAR IMMUNE RESPONSE

Cellular immunity in gynecologic malignancies has been studied by many investigators. Activity has been documented primarily in cervical and ovarian cancer. Rivera et al.[36] used the leukocyte migration inhibition assay to demonstrate this activity in patients with cervical squamous cell carcinoma. The leukocyte migration inhibition test was used to study specific tumor immunity in carcinoma of the cervix. The test was done by the capillary tube method using Sykes Moore chambers. Test antigen was extracted from the ME-180 cervical squamous cell carcinoma cell line (either uninfected or infected with herpes simplex virus II) by the hypotonic lysis, low-frequency sonication method. Control antigen preparations from nonsquamous cell carcinoma tissues were used as well. Thirty patients with invasive cervical carcinoma, 16 patients with cervical dysplasia or in situ carcinoma, 19 normal controls, and 40 patients with other malignancies were studied. A significantly greater degree of leukocyte migration inhibition by the cervical cancer antigen was observed among the leukocytes of patients with invasive cervical carcinoma than in the other four groups. Significant migration inhibition (defined as a migration index under 0.70) was not frequently seen among the leukocytes of patients with in situ carcinoma or cervical dysplasia. Significant migration inhibition was not seen in any group with the control antigens. In patients with invasive carcinoma there was no relationship of the degree of migration inhibition to the stage of the disease. The data indicated that (1) there is specific tumor immunity in cervical carcinoma, (2) there may be a common antigen expressed on the ME-180 cell line, and (3) the tumor burden may have to reach either a critical size or level of invasiveness before it can elicit a host reaction detectable by these methods.

Murray[37] used the leukocyte migration inhibition test as an index of cell-mediated immune response to material derived from carcinoma of the cervix and normal cervical epithelium, in groups of patients and control donors. These control donors comprised preoperative patients with benign gynecologic lesions and a normal cervical smear. Higher reactivity to tumor-derived antigen was found in more patients with invasive carcinoma of the cervix than in control donors. Reactivity with the same tumor extract in patients with preinvasive lesions of the cervix (carcinoma in situ and dysplasia) was less than that found in the benign control women. The diagnosis was established in each of the former by colposcopy and selective punch biopsy after collection of the blood for examination. In four cases with microinvasive lesions of the cervix, no reactivity was found.

Levy et al.[38] reported on thymus-dependent immunity of 42 patients with squamous cell carcinoma of the cervix evaluated by delayed cutaneous reactions to ubiquitous antigens, dinitrochlorobenzene sensitization, and lymphocyte response to PHA. In addition, T and B lymphocytes were detected in peripheral blood and in tumor sections, by adherence to sheep RBC (E) and human RBC, antibody-complement sensitized (HEAC). Depressed cell-mediated immunity was more intense in patients with disseminated disease, although premature impairment was observed in some patients with initial-stage tumors. The absolute number of peripheral T lymphocytes showed association with both cutaneous reactions and PHA response. However, there appeared to be no significant correlation between the stage of the tumor and the pattern of adherence of E or HEAC to the biopsies.

Mashiba et al.[39] studied the cytotoxic activity of peripheral blood lymphocytes from patients with carcinoma of the uterine cervix examined by the microcytotoxicity assay using a cervical cancer line (QG-K). Lymphocytes from healthy persons and myoma patients were not cytotoxic for the cultured uterine cancer cells, but lymphocytes from uterine cancer patients were cytotoxic: those from patients with stage 0 disease showed cytotoxicity ranging from 22.0 to 56.2 percent. In stage IV and recurrent cases, cytotoxic activity was markedly reduced. In stages I, II, and III, the cytotoxic activity of lymphocytes and PHA reactivity were not correlated, and there were cases showing decreased PHA response with a high degree of cytotoxic activity.

DiSaia et al.[40] reported on the relationship between peripheral blood lymphocyte count and survival of patients with primary stage IIIB cancer of the cervix, investigated in a follow-up study of 30 patients (24 to 49 years old; mean age 42 years) (Fig. 3-7). All patients had peripheral blood lymphocyte counts measured immediately prior to treatment and were followed up for at least 23 months. All patients received as initial therapy 5,000 to 6,000 rads whole-pelvis irradiation, followed by brachytherapy in doses of 3,000 to 5,000 rads in one to two applications. Most deaths (13 of 18) occurred in the first 17 months after the start of therapy, and all but two of these deaths occurred in patients who had an initial total lymphocyte count of less than 2,000. All of the 12 patients alive at 23 months had initial peripheral lymphocyte counts of greater than 1,000. Division of the patients into three groups according to their initial total lymphocyte counts (I < 1,000; II < 1,999 and > 1,000; and III ≥ 2,000) showed that duration of survival increased steadily from group I to group III ($P = 0.005$). The data suggest that simple peripheral lymphocyte counts can give a comparatively accurate assay of immune competence as measured by survival duration.

Stratton et al.[41] reported on the number and functional abilities of lymphocytes from patients with either breast cancer or cervical cancer assessed before, during, and after radiation therapy given to treat the disease, and during several years of follow-up management. Radiation therapy depleted both T and B cells and depressed the responses to PHA and concanavalin A (Con-A) in all patient groups. The responses to mitogens in the weeks immediately following radiation therapy were greater in patients whose disease did recur and were depressed for a much longer time in patients whose disease recurred in the next 2 years. This difference was most clearly reflected in the ratio of mitogen response to the number of T cells. The relationship of response to nonresponsive or suppressive leukocytes in the weeks following radiation therapy was suggested as a possible clue to future prognosis.

Cell-mediated immunity is also being studied in ovarian carcinoma. Mandell et al.[42] reported on the immunologic assays of B and T-lymphocyte function performed on 21 patients with epithelial ovarian cancer prior to either chemotherapy or radiotherapy. The results were compared with similar studies in 12 age-matched normal women. The total peripheral blood lymphocyte counts, proportion of erythrocyte (E) rosette-positive cells, stimulation of T cells by PHA and Con-A, recall skin tests, and the ability to mount a primary delayed hypersensitivity response to

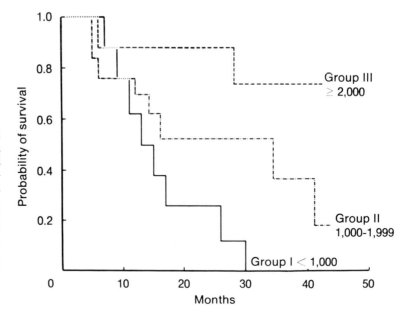

Fig. 3-7 Patients with stage III cervical cancer who received optimal radiation therapy. Survival (months) is correlated with initial peripheral blood lymphocyte counts. (Reprinted with permission from DiSaia PJ, Morrow CP, Hill A, Mittelstaedt L: Immune competence and survival in patients with advanced cervical cancer; peripheral lymphocyte counts. J Radiat Oncol 4:449, 1978. Copyright 1978, Pergamon Press, Ltd.)

keyhole limpet hemocyanin did not differ between patients and controls. However, patients with ovarian cancer had statistically significant reduction in surface immunoglobulin-positive cells; proliferative response to pokeweed mitogen and primary antibody response to keyhole limpet hemocyanin did not differ between patients and controls. Finally, patients with ovarian cancer had a statistically significant reduction in surface immunoglobulin-positive cells, proliferative response to pokeweed mitogen, and primary antibody response to keyhole limpet hemocyanin. In contrast to results in patients with other solid tumors, these data indicate that untreated patients with ovarian cancer have evidence of normal immune function but abnormal B-cell function.

Toyokawa[43] studied the early diagnosis of ovarian cancer by cell-mediated immunologic techniques. Lymphocyte response/50 μl peripheral blood to PHA was tested to elucidate nonspecific aspects of the immune state by testing the immunosuppressive effect of serum on the response of normal lymphocytes to PHA stimulation (serum effect), as done by a modification of the Park and Good method. The procedure to elucidate the specific immune state was determined by the leukocyte adherence inhibition test. The serum effect differed significantly between patients with ovarian carcinoma and benign ovarian tumors and was found to increase significantly even when the cancer mass was large (approximately 5 × 5 × 5 cm in diameter) in size. Serum immunosuppressive effects in venous blood at the vicinity of cancer mass were greater than in peripheral blood. In the leukocyte adherence inhibition test, white blood cells (WBC's) obtained from patients with cystadenocarcinoma adhered to a significantly lesser extent (adherence ratio was less than 70 percent) to a glass surface; in the control group, this ratio was more than 75 percent when tested with cystadenocarcinoma extract (antigen). WBCs from patients with cystadenocarcinoma did not react with extract from any other histologically different tumor, such as epidermoid cancer of the cervix. The measurement of the serum effect of peripheral blood on the normal lymphocyte response to PHA may be useful in the early detection of ovarian carcinoma. Application of the leukocyte adherence inhibition test made it almost possible to determine the histologic type of the ovarian carcinoma prior to laparotomy.

The effect of radiation on cell-mediated cytotoxicity in lymphocyte subpopulations has been a subject of great interest. Kohorn et al.[44] reported on lymphocyte subpopulations and cell-mediated cytotoxicity during and after radiotherapy in 16 patients with ovarian carcinoma. Tumor resection was performed in 9 of 16 patients with stage I and II disease. The tests were repeated for up to 77 days after the beginning of radiotherapy. All patients showed a reduced total lymphocyte count during radiotherapy (especially on days 7 to 35), with recovery after radiotherapy. Total T and B-cell counts decreased, but only the T cells showed a proportionate change. This selective reduction of T cells was associated with a decline in mononuclear cell cytotoxicity in vitro (lymphocyte kill of ovarian carcinoma target cells) in patients with stage I and II disease. Only one of seven patients with stage III disease showed this change in cell-mediated immunity. The surviving mononuclear cells in patients with stage III disease may have been sensitized to the tumor antigen and more resistant to radiotherapy, or radiotherapy may have induced a selective depression of T-suppressor cells. Lymphocytes from patients with tumors other than ovarian carcinoma were less cytotoxic to ovarian cancer cells than were lymphocytes from women with ovarian cancer (including 44 untreated patients). Cross-reactivity with lymphocytes from patients with nonovarian tumors (especially carcinoma of the endometrium and cervix) was noted in the cell-mediated immunity test. However, lymphocytes from patients with ovarian cancer were usually not cytotoxic to nonovarian tumor cells.

There has been similar interest in this aspect with regard to cervical carcinoma. Savage et al.[45] reported on the effect of radiotherapy on patients with carcinoma of the cervix at different stages assessed by lymphocyte transformation with PHA, T and B rosettes, and analysis of peripheral blood studies. Blood samples were taken before and after radiotherapy treatment and at the first follow-up clinic. A normal range of values was obtained from healthy donors for comparison. Preliminary results indicate that there is a difference in T and B rosetting between normals and patients with cancer of the cervix. Radiotherapy appears to diminish the percentage of T cells and cell yields. Comparison between stages shows a tendency for T cells to be depleted in the later stages. PHA transformation has not shown any significant differences between the groups.

A similar study by Hancock et al.[46] reported in

1979 involved the immune status of 15 women given radiotherapy (7,500 rad to point A and 5,000 rad to point B; ^{137}Cs insertion and external megavoltage radiotherapy) for stage I to II carcinoma of the cervix. All patients showed good tumor regression. Three months after the end of radiotherapy, 14 patients had minimal or no evidence of disease. A recurrence developed in one patient after 6 months. At the time of the report, 7 of 14 patients had been in remission for 1 year. Neutrophil function was essentially unaffected by radiotherapy, but absolute neutrophil and lymphocyte counts declined after radiotherapy and remained depressed 3 to 12 months later. The proportions of T and B cells declined and then returned almost to the pretreatment level during the follow-up period, although absolute counts remained depressed. Cellular immunity in vitro was reduced by radiotherapy and remained depressed during the follow-up period. There was no change in cutaneous immunity at any time. Four pretreatment plasmas inhibited PHA transformation of lymphocytes; this activity was not observed after radiotherapy. The variable immunologic response observed in patients in remission after radiotherapy for localized cervical cancer stresses the importance of assessing several aspects of immune function. Persistent depression of certain indices does not adversely affect the host-tumor response. In two patients who relapsed after an apparently good initial response, all aspects of immune function deteriorated except for serum immunoglobulin levels and neutrophil function.

Check et al.[47] reported that patients with advanced gynecologic cancer have a depressed immunologic function. These workers performed a battery of tests on peripheral blood samples from 42 patients with gynecologic cancer in an effort to determine the extent to which this depression was due to abnormal lymphocyte function, as compared with changes in the number of lymphoid cells in the peripheral blood or in the efficiency of purification of cells in Ficoll:Hypaque gradients in preparation for testing. The percentage of lymphocytes in the gradient-derived cell suspension (percent LG) and the absolute lymphocyte counts were more informative than mitogen stimulation, mixed leukocyte culture, and T- and B-cell measurements. Both values decreased significantly with the advancing stage of disease. The percent LG correlated with survival better than did any other test when multivariate analyses of all test combinations were performed. Low values of percent LG reflected both the depressed lymphocyte counts and the altered buoyant density of the leukocytes of many patients with advanced cancer. A large portion of the depression in other immune function tests was statistically attributed to changes in percent LG and the lymphocyte counts. It was concluded that these two simple measurements provide valuable information about patients with gynecologic cancer.

In summary, it is abundantly evident that the lymphocyte plays a major role in the drama of host versus tumor. This role has been repeatedly modified as our knowledge of mechanism of action and subpopulations of lymphocytes has grown over the past two decades. The interplay of certain populations (e.g., helper T cells, suppressor T cells, NK cells) appears to be quite intricate, and a better understanding of the overall effect has been hampered by inadequate methodologies available for monitoring the status of the immune system, both in health and disease. It would appear that the elements of cell-mediated immunity are multifactorial, carefully orchestrated to produce the integrity of the immune system in any patient at any particular point in time. The studies quoted herein only suggest a correlation between the cell-mediated immune status and the host's defenses against a particular clinical neoplasm. Further refinement or quantitation of this immune status must await better understanding of the methods of orchestration between elements and methods of truly evaluating this complex interplay.

STATUS OF IMMUNOTHERAPY OF GYNECOLOGIC CANCER

One of the predominant concepts in modern-day cancer research is that malignant tissues are foreign to the host and therefore subject to control and prevention by manipulation of the host immune system. As a first principle in attempting to develop immunotherapy, one would hope that tumors might have defined tumor antigens that could be extracted, studied, characterized, and used as immunogens to generate specific cytotoxic antibody and specifically sensitized lymphocytes that could kill tumor cells bearing this antigen. In several animal systems, the antigenic makeup of tumors is distinctive; indeed, the antigenic character of tumors induced by carcinogens is different from that produced by oncogenic viruses. Irrespective of the inducing agent, tumors induced in one strain of animals are usually rejected by normal members of an unrelated strain. Within the same strain of host animal, however, tumors often grow without interference, suggesting that tumor-specific antigens are not recognized by normal members of the same strain.

Among human malignancies, the evidence for tumor-specific antigens is suggestive but controversial, although there is reasonable evidence to suggest that at least some tumors do carry such antigens. On the assumption that such tumor-specific antigens do exist, the body's immune response against them would likely be dependent on several factors, similar to those that affect homograph rejection: (1) the immunologic competence of the host; (2) the immunogenicity of the tumor-associated antigens; and (3) the ability of these antigens to induce cell-mediated immunity, as opposed to humoral immunity, which tends to block protective responses against tumors.

The normal immune system is a complex myriad of interactions among lymphoid cells, soluble substance generated by these cells, and humoral factors, including antibodies. Suffice it to say that it is generally held that the principal way in which the body reacts against tumors is through the action of cells that have become sensitized either by active intrinsic sensitization or by passive acquisition of tumor-specific antibodies on their surfaces. In animal systems, specific immunity can be clearly demonstrated by a variety of procedures. First, tumors can be transplanted without restriction between genetically identical animals but are rejected by genetically unrelated hosts. Second, administration of tumor cells that have been killed by irradiation will often confer immunity when the animal is later challenged with live tumor cells. Such protection is tumor specific: growth of an unrelated tumor is not affected. Nevertheless, the original animal host does not destroy its own tumor. Third, immunity may be passively transferred to normal animals by lymphoid cells taken from an animal that has been exposed to the particular tumor in question. Human tumor interaction has not been as clearly defined.

There is little question that serious alteration of the immune function may accompany human cancer and that such disturbances are less pronounced early in the course of the disease or in patients having tumors that grow slowly. In general, alterations of cell-mediated immunity are the most evident and are usually first seen when depression of humoral immunities become manifest in later stages of the disease. An impressive example of loss of cell-mediated immune function is the state of anergy seen in patients with advanced gynecologic cancer.[48,49] Attempts to alter this derangement of immune function have been addressed with trials of immunotherapy.

Nonspecific Immunotherapy

Nonspecific immunotherapy implies stimulation of the reticuloendothelial system by injection of various substances unrelated to the malignancy under therapy. In recent years, BCG and *C. Parvum* have been in vogue as nonspecific reticuloendothelial stimulants. Various trials using nonspecific immunotherapy in gynecologic malignancies have been conducted with equivocal results.

Melchert et al.[50] reported on influencing the immune system of carcinoma patients with oral BCG treatment. Individual doses of 120 mg were administered with fruit juice weekly during the first month, every 14 days during the second and third months, and finally on a monthly basis. The group of patients treated had either breast or cervical cancer. Although there was some evidence of augmentation of the immune system in the patients with breast cancer, studies in patients with radium-telecobalt-treated cervical carcinoma indicated that the ability of the immune system to be stimulated was suppressed by immunotherapy.[50]

Olkowski et al.[51] reported on the effects of combined immunotherapy with levamisole and BCG on immunocompetence of patients with squamous cell carcinoma of the cervix. Immunologic tests were performed before and immediately after a full course of radiotherapy in 25 patients with squamous cell carcinoma of the cervix, stages IB through III. Patients were randomized to immunotherapy with oral levamisol and intradermal BCG or no immunotherapy. Lymphocyte responses to PHA and pokeweed mitogen were subnormal before radiotherapy and declined still further afterward. Both treatment groups showed a gradual recovery from immunosuppression (T- and B-lymphocyte counts and mitogenic responses) during follow-up, but the immunotherapy group showed a tendency (not significant in the preliminary data) to slower recovery. Lymphocyte cytotoxicity to allogeneic tumor cells was variably affected by radiotherapy but was generally higher 8 weeks after radiotherapy than in preceding tests. At the time of the report, follow-up had been too short to evaluate the effects of immunotherapy on recurrence or survival rates.

DiSaia et al.[52] reported the results of a Gynecologic Oncology Group study on the treatment of women with advanced carcinoma of the uterine cervix with radiotherapy alone versus radiotherapy plus immunotherapy with intravenous *C. parvum.* One hundred and sixty-seven patients in the preliminary report and 295 patients in the final unpublished study were considered evaluable at the time of analysis. The conclusion reached was that *C. parvum* did not add any therapeutical effect as an adjuvant to radiotherapy in the patient population study. Further analysis of this data is under way.

Mangan et al.[53] studied intralymphatic BCG in the treatment of gynecologic malignancies. An intralymphatic infusion of BCG (2 to 4 ml) was used to treat 13 women with advanced gynecologic malignancies including squamous cell carcinoma of the cervix (three patients) or vagina (one patient), adenocarcinoma of the endometrium (two patients) or fallopian tube (one patient), ovarian adenocarcinoma or cystadenocarcinoma (five patients), or pelvic metastases from melanoma of the eye (one patient). After BCG infusion, 10 of 13 patients were treated with radiotherapy (three patients) or chemotherapy (seven patients) with semustine, cyclophosphamide plus methotrexate or Alkeran. All patients developed inflammatory reactions to BCG, including fever and lymphangitis with adenitis along the lymphatic pathways of the infused legs. No correlation was noted between reactions to a standard anergy panel and either survival or inflammatory responses to intralymphatic BCG, but there was a positive correlation between inflammatory responses to BCG and survival. Inflammatory responses were slight in 4 of 13 patients who survived 1.5 to 8 months (mean 3.5 months). Grade 2+ or 3+ responses were noted in 4 of 13 patients who survived 2 to 6 months (mean: 5 months). Severe reactions were noted in 5 of 13 patients who survived 7 to 25 months (mean: 16.4 months). Whether the inflammatory reaction to intralymphatic BCG was prognostic or therapeutic could not be determined.

Kalpaktsoglou et al.[54] studied immunochemotherapy in adenocarcinoma of the ovary. Immunochemotherapy combined with total hysterectomy was used in the treatment of 21 cases of adenocarcinoma of the ovary, of which 7 were stages IC to IIB, 8 in stage III, and 6 in stage IV. Another six cases had irradiation with or without hysterectomy or various other schemes of treatment prior to immunochemotherapy. The immunotherapy depended on stimulation of the humoral and cellular immunity by a battery of antigens (tetanus, diphtheria-tetanus, influenza, mumps). Chemotherapy consisted of administration of cyclophosphamide 3 days after each course of immunotherapy. Each course of immunochemotherapy was followed by a period of 10 days free from any medication. The stimulation of the immune mechanism with BCG started 10 days after the fourth course of immunochemotherapy. This last course of treatment was repeated up to the end of the first year of immunochemotherapy. The same annual scheme of treatment was continually repeated. The patients were under constant clinical and laboratory follow-up. The cyclophosphamide was discontinued whenever the WBC fell below 4,500 to 4,000 per mm^3. All patients received vitamins A, E, C, and B complex. All the patients with stages IC to IIB and III, with total hysterectomy and without any prior treatment, showed a progressive recovery and are living normal lives. The lymphocytes, immunoglobulins, and RBC rosettes returned, in most cases, to normal levels. The favorable results in the survival rate obtained in cases of cancer without distant metastasis may be attributed to the reduction of the tumor masses by surgery, to the administration of antigens prior to chemotherapy, which seems to diminish the side effects of cyclophosphamide, to the administration of cyclophosphamide in small daily doses to avoid leukopenia, and finally, to the fact that patients are under continuous protective immunochemotherapy.

Gall et al.[55] reported on the effectiveness of immunotherapy (melphalan plus *C. parvum*) in 45 evaluable patients with untreated stage III ovarian cancer; these results were compared with a melphalan-alone series in similarly staged patients. Their response rate, progression-free interval, and survival were considerably better in the chemoimmunotherapy group than in either of the two melphalan-alone comparison groups studied. This study led to a prospective randomized trial conducted by the Gynecologic Oncology Group and is as yet unreported. Two hundred and one patients were randomized between melphalan (7 mg/

m²/day × 5 days every 28 days) versus melphalan plus *C. parvum* (4 mg/m² on day 7 of each treatment cycle). As compared with the nonrandomized trial by Gall's group, patients with minimal residual disease were selected for this trial. Preliminary data suggest that there is no difference in the duration of progression-free interval and survival in the two treatment arms.

Alberts[56] has one of the more exciting reports in the literature concerning nonspecific immunotherapy of ovarian carcinoma. He studied the effect of adding BCG to Adriamycin and cyclophosphamide (Cytoxan) for the treatment of stage III and IV or recurrent epithelial-type ovarian carcinoma. One hundred and thirty-one patients with no prior chemotherapy and measurable disease were randomly assigned to receive A-C or A-C + BCG. Adriamycin, 40 mg/m² on day 1, and cyclophosphamide, 200 mg/m² on days 3 to 6, were given every 3 to 4 weeks for a total Adriamycin dose of 500 mg/m². BCG was administered by scarification to alternating upper and lower extremity sites on days 8 and 15. There was a similar distribution between the two study arms of patients with stage IV disease, bulky tumor masses, types of surgical procedures, performance status, prior radiation therapy exposure, and type and grade of tumor histology. The complete remission (CR) + partial remission (PR) rate for A-C + BCG-treated patients of 52 percent was significantly different (*P* less than 0.05) from the 30 percent CR + PR rate observed in the A-C-treated group. The median duration of responses of 13+ months for the A-C + BCG-treated groups was not statistically better than the 7.2 months for the A-C-treated patients. Median survival duration of the A-C + BCG-treated patients (21 months) was statistically better than that of patients receiving only A-C (13.5 months) (*P* less than 0.005). Therapy was well tolerated. There were no drug-related deaths and no serious systemic BCG toxicities. The addition of BCG to the standard A-C treatment for far advanced ovarian carcinoma appears to have increased response rate and overall survival duration without markedly adding to drug toxicity (Table 3-2).

The Gynecologic Oncology Group has initiated a prospective randomized trial to test the efficacy of BCG by scarification in patients with advanced ovarian adenocarcinoma. Several optimal patients with bulk disease stages III and IV are now being randomized between chemotherapy with cisplatin, Adriamycin, and cyclophosphamide versus this three-drug

Table 3-2 Chemoimmunotherapy—Epithelial Ovarian Cancer: Stages III–IV

	A-C + BCG	A-C
Evaluable	53	56
Complete response	5(9%)	0
Partial response	23(43%)	22(40%)
Median duration of response	21	13.5
Stable disease	21	28
Increasing disease	4	6
Dead	16	28

A, Adriamycin, 40 mg/m², day 1; C, cyclophosphamide, 200 mg/m², days 3–6 repeat every 4 weeks; BCG bacillus Calmette-Guérin days 8 + 15.

regimen plus BCG given in a manner identical to that reported by Alberts. Although the chemotherapy given in this study by the Gynecologic Oncology Group is at variance with that used by Alberts, the methodology is otherwise identical.

Wanebo et al.[57] reported on a randomized chemoimmunotherapy trial of cisplatin–Adriamycin–5-fluorouracil (5-FU) and intravenous *C. parvum* for resistant ovarian carcinoma. A pilot study showed apparent benefit of immune stimulation with intravenous *C. parvum* and combination therapy with Cytoxan–Adriamycin–5-FU in advanced ovarian cancer resistant to alkylating agents. A randomized study was done to compare cisplatin–Adriamycin–5-FU and IV *C. parvum* versus cisplatin–Adriamycin–5-FU alone in 38 patients with progressive disease (stage II and IV) after prior chemotherapy (single agent in 26, combination in 12) and with radiation in 12. Reductive surgery was attempted in 10. Most patients had immune depression: 70 percent were DNCB-negative, 95 percent had depressed lymphocytes, and 50 percent had depressed PHA responses. Twenty patients were randomized to receive cisplatin–Adriamycin–5-FU and IV cyclophosphamide and 18 patients cisplatin–Adriamycin–5-FU alone. Intraveous cyclophosphamide was given in escalating doses (0.5 to 10 mg/day × 14). Cyclic administration was then begun: oral cyclophosphamide 60 mg/m²/day × 15; Adriamycin 30 mg/m² IV, and 5-FU 400 mg/m² IV on days 1 and 8; subcutaneous cyclophosphamide 0.5 to 4 mg was given weekly. Only 3 of 38 patients responded. One patient had a complete response (CR) to cisplatin–Adriamycin–5-FU + cyclophosphamide for 53 weeks. After the three-drug regimen alone, there was one CR for 47 weeks and two partial responses (PR) for 28 and 33 weeks. After cisplatin–Adriamycin–5-FU and cyclophosphamide, 10 patients were alive 20 weeks (median) compared with 9 patients (median 24 weeks) after cisplatin–Adriamycin–5-FU alone. Nine patients died in each group (median: 8 and 11 weeks, respectively). The addition of IV cyclophosphamide to the three-drug regimen has not improved response rate, duration of remission, or short-term survival in advanced ovarian cancer.

A similar study was reported by Rao et al.[58] in 1977 dealing with intravenous C. parvum as an adjuvant to chemotherapy for resistant ovarian carcinoma. Preliminary results were provided on the treatment of 39 women (28 to 74 years old; median age: 57 years) with advanced stage III and IV ovarian cancer who had progressive disease despite prior surgery, chemotherapy, and/or radiotherapy by a program of reductive surgery, intensive immune stimulation, and combination chemotherapy. Exploratory laparotomy was done in 16 patients either for alleviation of obstruction or in an effort to remove tumor; reductive surgery (removal of 50% of tumor) was accomplished in 8. The course of IV C. parvum was given in escalating doses as tolerated over 10 to 14 days, infused over 30 min. Cyclic chemotherapy was started on day 15: daily oral Cytoxan (60 mg/m² on days 1 to 14), Adriamycin (30 mg/m² on days 1 and 8), and 5-FU (400 mg/m² on days 1 and 8). The cycle was repeated after a 2-week rest; after the initial course of C. parvum, 4 mg was given subcutaneously at intervals as maintenance therapy. Pretreatment immune tests showed marked immune depression in most patients; two-thirds had depressed PHA responses and were negative to 2,4-dinitrochlorobenzene (DNCB). All but two had markedly depressed lymphocyte counts. Pretreatment immune function correlated with clinical response to therapy, with patients showing a favorable response having better pretreatment immune response than those with poor responses (10 of 12 of the former patients were DNCB positive versus 4 of 12 of the latter). However, there were no consistent patterns of change in immune tests during administration of IV C. parvum or during cisplatin–Adriamycin–5-FU plus SC C. parvum. Of the 11 patients receiving only IV C. parvum, none had a measurable response and none survived for 1 month after the start of therapy. Of four patients receiving IV C. parvum and fewer than three cycles of cytoxan–

Adriamycin–5-FU, two survived 6 weeks and two survived 8 weeks after starting therapy, but none had a response to therapy. Patients receiving C. parvum and more than three cycles of cytoxan–Adriamycin–5-FU had clinical response; four had a complete regression and were free of disease 9 to 12 months after starting therapy; eight had a 50 percent regression for 3 months and five of these were living with disease 5 to 11 months after starting therapy; five had a 25 to 50 percent response and three were living from 4 to 8 months; seven had no response, four were alive 2 to 4 months after therapy. Of these responders, eight had reductive surgery, with three free of disease for a median of 10 months and five having a partial response living with disease for a median of 9 months.

Corynebacterium-parvum in escalating doses and as subcutaneous maintenance was generally well tolerated; individual doses ranged from 0.5 to 23 mg with total doses from 10 to 177 mg. Common side effects were fever, headache, chills, transient rise in blood pressure and respiratory rate, and, in 50 percent of patients, drop in platelet or WBC counts.

Active Specific Immunotherapy

Active specific immunotherapy is accomplished by the injection of tumor vaccine made primarily from irradiated tumor cells and given in the hope that they will create an efficient antitumor action in the host. Active specific immunotherapy in ovarian cancer was reported by Crowther and co-workers.[59,60] Active specific immunotherapy of patients with ovarian cancer consisted of the monthly administration of allogeneic irradiated tumor cells and BCG. In a Planar freezer, two out of 10 viable tumor cells from surface epithelial ovarian carcinomas were cryopreserved in medium and 10 percent dimethylsulfoxide, and the ampules were stored in liquid nitrogen. Before the cells were used, the donor patients were tested for Austriala antigen; and each bath of cells was subjected to bacterial culture. Prior to immunotherapy, one ampule per patient was rapidly thawed at 37°C, washed twice, and made up to 0.4 m in medium without antibiotic for immediate irradiation with 10,000 rad. Glaxo strain BCG was reconstituted to 1 m, and 0.1 m of a 1:40 dilution containing approximately 2×10^5 live organisms was added to the reconstituted tumor cells for final IV injection in four sites in either the deltoid region or the thigh. Chemotherapy was given, usually as a bolus, midway in the immunotherapy regimen. Most patients received cyclophosphamide, (1 g PO during 3 days); however, patients in relapse were changed over to IV chemotherapy with Adriamycin (40 mg/m²); cyclophosphamide, 500 mg/m²; and cisdichloradiamineplatin II, 20 mg/m². Side effects were minimal; no BCG granulomata, systemic infection or tumor deposits at the site of immunization were seen. Actuarial survival curve calculations for 17 patients receiving chemoimmunotherapy (15 of whom were followed greater than 2 years, or until death) showed that the median survival shifted from 12 months for a control group to 24 months for patients receiving the active specific immunotherapy. A downward trend was observed, however, and at 48 months the survival for the immunotherapy group was 19 percent compared with 4 percent for the control group. Immunotherapy also appeared to facilitate responses to changes in chemotherapy for patients in relapse and appeared to offer some measure of protection from the immunosuppressive effects of chemotherapy.

Hudson et al.[61] reported a similar study of active specific immunotherapy in advanced ovarian cancer. Cryopreserved, disaggregated, and irradiated allogeneic tumor cells admixed with BCG were given (2×10^7 cells $1 \times$/day and 2×10^5 live BCG cells $1 \times$/month) to 10 postoperative patients with advanced ovarian cancer. When immunotherapy was begun, the patients had shown no clinical evidence of tumor progression for 3 months. The follow-up period was 2 years. At the time of the report, the median survival time was 23 months. Four patients were alive with no evidence of disease after 20 to 24 months. Three of these patients had never relapsed; one had relapsed at 12 months but responded to further treatment (unspecified). One patient relapsed after about 8 months and died after 1 year. Four patients relapsed (one twice) but responded well to further treatment; one was alive with disease at 2 years, and the others died of disease after 20 to 22 months. One patient remained alive with no evidence of disease for nearly 20 months, then relapsed and died within a short time. In a historical control group, 15 of 25 patients died after 6 to 12 months, 6 of 25 died after 12 to 18 months, and 4 of 25 survived 2 years (1 of 4 alive with no evidence of disease). After nearly 200 cycles of immunotherapy, there were no major side effects. Two patients apparently became hyperimmunized to

BCG. Serial studies of lymphocyte blastogenesis disclosed an increase in activity in several patients after immunization with tumor cells (alone or plus BCG) and in a patient who was not receiving alternating immunosuppressive chemotherapy (no further details). Immunotherapy is indicated only after a certain amount of tumor control has been obtained by conventional treatment. It should be regarded as an adjuvant to cytoreductive therapy, effective only when the tumor burden is minimal.

Juillard et al.[18] reported a phase I study of active specific intralymphatic immunotherapy. A total of 21 patients (17 women, 4 men) with advanced malignancies were immunized with 1×10^7 to 1.2×10^8 autochthonous (auto) tumor cells (7 patients) or allogenic (allo) tumor cells (14 patients) monthly. The patients received no other cancer treatment. There were no side effects involving temperature, blood pressure, complete blood count, electrolytes, SMA-12, or creatinine levels; however, there was one case of bacterial lymphangitis. Nine patients had failed to respond to recall antigens in the skin before active specific intralymphatic immunotherapy; of these, seven regained hypersensitivity to two or more antigens after treatment. Two patients died early in the study. Of the remaining 19 patients, five showed an objective regression (a 50 percent or greater reduction in tumor mass); these included patients with ovarian carcinoma (one auto, one allo), epidermoid carcinoma of the maxilla (one allo) and tongue (one allo), and leiomyosarcoma (one auto). Six patients showed stabilization of tumor growth and eight patients had progressive disease. The results indicate that active specific intralymphatic immunotherapy is a relatively safe treatment method that can induce regression.

Other Immunotherapy Trials

Freedman[62] reported on his experiences with transfer factor in advanced gynecologic cancer. Leukocytes used in the preparation of transfer factor were obtained from various donors, including spouses, and two long-term cures from trophoblastic disease. Transfer factor was prepared according to the method of Lawrence with minor modifications. The transfer factor was administered to three patients with recurrent uterine cervical carcinoma and two with metastatic choriocarcinoma unresponsive to chemotherapy. All patients were monitored with delayed hypersensitivity reaction to recall antigens, E-rosettes, and microcytotoxicity in the cervix group. In patients with trophoblastic disease, human chorionic gonadotropin titers were plotted against hematologic values, E-rosettes, and delayed hypersensitivity reaction, and the administration of chemotherapy and transfer factor. There was one partial responder among the cervix patients. All patients demonstrated either heightened or increased immune responses after transfer factor.

Ikic et al.[63] studied interferon treatment of uterine cervical precancerous lesions. Human leukocyte interferon was applied topically on the uterine cervix in 10 patients with persistent cytologic findings of nondysplastic atypia and dysplastic atypia. Patients were treated 14 to 21 days at a daily dose of 1×10^6 units. Cytologic findings after treatment consisted of minor inflammations, that is, normalized cytologic findings (IIA according to Papanicolaou's nomenclature) in all 10 patients. No relapses were found in the 6 months after treatment control examinations. A follow-up report in 1981 by Ikic et al.[64] studied groups of patients with cervical intraepithelial neoplasia randomly selected for treatment with human leukocyte interferon (13 patients with cervical intraepithelial neoplasia, grades 1 and 2) or placebo (18 patients with cervical intraepithelial neoplasia, grades 1 to 3). Follow-up studies at 2 years showed significant differences between the treatment in the placebo groups with regard to cytologic findings and pathohistological diagnoses. In the controls, the pathologically changed epithelium was persistent in 7 of 18 cases and there were 7 of 18 progressions. Among the controls, no regressions were observed. In the patients treated with human leukocyte interferon, abnormal epithelium persisted in 4 of 13 cases, progressed in 1 of 13, and regressed in 8 of 13. In the control and human leukocyte interferon-treated groups, significant progressions and regressions respectively, were observed in relation to morphogenesis of cervical carcinoma. The differences were greater when the groups were compared. The results indicated that human leukocyte interferon has an impact on the regression of cervical intrepithelial neoplasia. Therapy with human leukocyte interferon is particularly indicated in women in the reproductive age in whom fertility is to be preserved since it may obviate the need for surgery.

Krusic et al.[65] reported on the application of human leukocyte interferon in patients with invasive cervical carcinoma. Fifteen patients with invasive squamous cell carcinoma of the uterine cervix were treated with crude human leukocyte interferon for 3 weeks before surgical removal of the tumor. Nine patients were given human leukocyte interferon topically and intramuscularly, and 6 received it topically only. In three patients the surgical material was free from tumor cells, in three it showed a lower grade of carcinoma, and in nine the findings remained unchanged. In only one patient did the tumor metastasize to the lymph nodes. Typically a tumor regressed to about one-third its original size. There was a sharp distinction between the tumor mass and the healthy tissue manifested in the formation of a fibrous wall. On the basis of the scores, that is, stromal response, relationship between tumor-cell and macrophage activity and reactivity, and reactivity of the original lymph nodes, the overall appraisal of the response caused by human leukocyte interferon therapy was as follows: in six patients excellent, in five very good, in one moderate, in two poor, and in one no response. It is suggested that human leukocyte interferon is suitable for administration both before and after surgery in patients with cervical cancer of grades 1 or 2. If stroma cannot be induced to respond with 21 days of treatment, application of human leukocyte interferon should be discontinued.

Einhorn et al.[66] reported on a series of patients treated with human leukocyte interferon for advanced ovarian carcinoma. Daily intramuscular injections of 3×10^6 IU of human leukocyte interferon were given to five patients with advanced ovarian carcinoma, all of whom previously received other forms of treatment. Ascitic fluid production ceased in two of two patients. According to the criteria specified by Young and DeVita,[66a] a partial response was observed in one patients and in two other patients the disease was stable for more than 1 year. Side effects of the interferon therapy were relatively mild.

Freeman et al.[67] reported on the administration of human leukocyte interferon to 15 patients with epithelial ovarian carcinoma after previous chemotherapy or therapeutic irradiation. One objective response was observed. Three patients had stable disease for up to 6 months.

Abdulhay et al.[68] reported on 36 patients with measurable epithelial ovarian cancer who had failed conventional chemotherapy treated with lymphoblastoid interferon alone. Twenty-eight patients were evaluable for response: two with complete response (7.1 percent), three with partial response (10.8 percent), 14 with stable disease (50.0 percent), and nine with increasing disease (32.2 percent). It was concluded that interferon therapy may have cytostatic and possible cytotoxic effects. A logical next study would be to use interferon with conventional chemotherapy as first-time therapy if the combination is tolerable in pilot studies.

The introduction of interferon therapy was followed by an increase in the NK cell activity of peripheral blood lymphocytes in all three patients examined. NK cell activity decreased after cessation of interferon therapy in the one patient in whom this was tested.

CONCLUSIONS

Immunotherapy has recently been approached by most scientists with skepticism. However, the term immunotherapy has been much abused and is not infrequently applied to a host of procedures that lack a clear scientific rationale and involve ill-defined products of natural origin. There are several not mutually exclusive explanations for the lack of success within the past decade to translate immunotherapy successes in rodents to the human species. An optimistic view is that conditions for success for immunotherapy are highly critical and that they are achieved by serendipity in the rat experiments and still remain to be determined for human cancer. Some support for this interpretation comes from animal investigations in which it was shown that the antitumor effect obtained by auto-immunizing with irradiated tumor cells depends critically on the number of cells innoculated.[69,70]

In a classic article on this subject, Alexander[71] dismissed failure to optimize treatment procedures that are effective in some animal experimental systems and useful in clinical practice. Alexander suggested that the most plausible reason why immunotherapy has not been successfully translated from the experimental to clinical situation is that the animal models on which they were based were not realistic. The core problem of the clinical class of human cancer is disseminated disease. Control of primary and local spread can, in most cases, be achieved by surgery and radiotherapy and treatment failure due to local recurrences is a relatively rare situation. The challenge of

cancer is to eliminate distant metastases. It appears that the more immunogeneic a tumor is, the less likely it is to metastasize. Tumors that are highly immunogeneic respond to immunotherapy, but these are the very tumors that are curable by local treatment such as surgery and radiotherapy. The tumors that present the clinical problem of distant dissemination may be tumors that are not very immunogeneic and that do not respond to the immunotherapeutic procedures so far in experimental systems. Indeed, Alexander suggested that we could go further and claim that surgery or local radiotherapy is the best type of immunotherapy we know. Because tumors invariably shed malignant cells and dissemination therefore always occurs, such disseminated cells are destroyed by the host's immune reaction when the tumor is immunogeneic. Thus, the tumor is cured by the surgery, since the surgeon enables the host's response to deal with the disseminated tumor cells by removing the bulk of the tumor mass. In other words, immunotherapy works in a situation in which surgery or radiotherapy is simpler and more effective but fails in situations in which surgery or radiotherapy does not cure because of the presence of metastatic disease. One can take this rationale one step further and assume that all tumors have disseminated and those tumors that are cured by local therapy are the highly immunogeneic type which are then ultimately cured by the host's immune defenses operating against a minimally disseminated tumor burden.

Another theoretical explanation is suggested by current data consistent with the view that a contributing factor to metastatic spread is that tumor cells that are shed have developed the capacity to bypass host reactions directed against tumor-associated antigens on their surface, in much the same way that many bacterial infections persist in the presence of an active immune response. If efficient escape is associated with the capacity to metastasize, immunotherapeutic procedures that rely on increasing the magnitude of the reactions against the tumor either by specifically stimulating the host or by passively administering effective instruments, such as cytotoxic cells or antibodies, are unlikely to be useful for the control of metastasis.

New procedures of immunotherapy need to be developed that concentrate on devising ways of bypassing the escape mechanism rather than boosting an already developed and paralyzed host-defense response. The emphasis in immunotherapy must change from an approach predicated on increasing the magnitude of the host's response to an attempt to render ineffective the escape mechanisms developed by tumors that metastasize. The clinical application of such concepts lies in the future.

REFERENCES

1. Everson TC, Cole WH: Spontaneous Regression of Cancer. WB Saunders, Philadelphia, 1966
2. Foley EJ: Antigenic properties of methylcholanthrene-induced tumours in mice of the strain of origin. Cancer Res 13:835, 1953
3. Prehn RT, Main J: Immunity to methylcholanthrene induced sarcomas. J Natl Cancer Inst 18:769, 1957
4. Bast RC, Feeney M, Lazarus H, et al: Reactivity of a monoclonal antibody with ovarian carcinoma. J Clin Invest 68:1331, 1981
5. Hibbs JB Jr: Heterocytolysis by macrophages activated by BCG. Science 184:468, 1974
6. Burnet FM: Cellular Immunology. Cambridge University Press, Melbourne, 1969
7. Folkman J, Hochberg M: Self-regulation of growth in three dimensions. J Exp Med 138:745, 1973
8. Dillman RO, Beauregard JC, Mendelson J, et al: Phase I trials of thymosin fraction 5 and thymosin L-1. J Biol Response Mod 1:35, 1982
9. Smalley RV, Talmadge TA, Oldham RK, et al: The biological response modifiers program: Preclinical and clinical studies with thymosin preparations. In Byrom WA, Hobbs JR (eds): Thymic Factor Therapy. Academic Press, London, 1983
10. Kato H, Torigoe T: Radioimmunoassay for tumor antigen of human cervical squamous cell carcinoma. Cancer 40:1621, 1977
11. Kato H, Moioka H, Aramaki S, Torigoe T: Radioimmunoassay for tumor antigen of human cervical squamous cell carcinoma. J Cell Mol 25:51, 1979
12. Kato H, Miyauchi F, Morioka H, et al: Tumor antigen of human cervical squamous cell carcinoma: Correlation of circulating levels with disease progress. Cancer 43:585, 1979
13. Nadkarni JJ, Satam MN, Damle SR, et al: Characterization of tumor-associated antigen from human carcinoma of the uterine cervix. Gynecol Oncol 13:175, 1982
14. Bhattacharya M, Barlow J: Tumor markers for ovarian cancer. Int Adv Surg Oncol 2:155, 1979
15. DiSaia PJ, Morrow C, Haverback B, Dyce B: Carcinoembryonic antigen in cervical and vulvar cancer patients: Serum levels and disease progress. Obstet Gynecol 47:95, 1976
16. DiSaia PJ, Morrow C, Haverback B, Dyce B: Carcinoembryonic antigen in cancer of the female reproductive system: Serial plasma values correlated with disease state. Cancer 39:2365, 1977
17. Ito H, Kurihara S, Nishimura C: Serum carcinoembryonic antigens in patients with carcinoma of the cervix. Obstet Gynecol 51:468,1978
18. Juillard GJ, Boyer PJ, Yamashiro CH: A phase I study of active specific intralymphatic immunotherapy (ASILI). Cancer 41:2215, 1978
19. Khoo S, Whitaker S, Jones I, MacKay E: Predictive value of serial carcinoembryonic antigen levels in long-term followup of ovarian cancer. Cancer 43:2471, 1979
20. Kjorstad K, Orjaster H: Studies on carcinoembryonic antigen levels in patients with adenocarcinoma of the uterus. Cancer 40:2953, 1977
21. Magnin G, Rudigoz R, Kassier J, et al:Level of carcinoembryonic antigen and other polypeptides in the diagnosis and surveillance of breast cancer and cancers of the female genital tract. Rev Fr Gynecol Obstet 74:119, 1979
22. Rutanen E, Lindgren J, Sipponen P, et al: Carcinoembryonic antigen in malignant and nonmalignant gynecologic tumors. Cancer 42:581, 1978
23. TeVelde E, Zegers B, Ballieux R, et al: Carcinoembryonic Antigen (CEA), alpha-fetoprotein (AFP), beta-human chorionic gonadotrophin (BETA HCG) and alpha-2-pregnancy-associated glycoprotein (alpha(2)-PAG) in patients with invasive cervical cancer. Presented at the Sixth Meeting of the International Research Group for Carcinoembryonic proteins, Marburg/Lahn, West Germany, Sept. 17–21, 1978
24. Van Nagell J, Donaldson E, Gay E, et al: Carcinoembryonic antigen in ovarian epithelial cystadenocarcinomas. Cancer 41:2335, 1978
25. Wahlstrom T, Lindgren J, Seppala M: Presence of carcinoembryonic antigen in tumor cells lacks prognostic significance in epidermoid carcinoma of the uterine cervix. Vol. II Elsevier/North-Holland Biomedical Press, New York, 1979
26. Van Nagell J, Donaldson E, Gay E, et al: Carcinoembryonic antigen in carcinoma of the uterine cervix. Cancer 42:2428, 1978
27. Van Nagell J, Donaldson E, Gay E, et al: Carcinoembryonic antigen in carcinoma of the uterine cervix 2. Tissue localization and correlation with plasma antigen concentration. Cancer Res 44:944, 1979
28. Goldenberg D, Garner T, Pant K, Van Nagell J: Identification of beta-oncofetal antigen in cervical squamous cancer and its demonstration in neoplastic and normal tissues. Cancer Res 38:1246, 1978
29. Tartarinov Y, Kalashikov V: New human embryonic

antigen and its presence in some adenocarcionomas. Nature (Lond) 265:638, 1977

30. Talerman A, Van der Pompe W, Haije W, et al: Alpha-Fetoprotein and carcinoembryonic antigen in germ cell neoplasms. Br J Cancer 35:288, 1977

31. Talerman A, Haije W, Baggerman L: Serum alpha-fetoprotein (AFP) in diagnosis and management of endodermal sinus (yolk sac) tumor and mixed germ cell tumor of the ovary. Cancer 41:272, 1978

32. Donaldson ES, Van Nagell JR, Gay EC, et al: Alpha-fetoprotein as a biochemical marker in patients with gynecologic malignancy. Gynecol Oncol 7:18, 1979

33. Kohler G, Milstein C: Continuous cultures of fused cells secreting of predefined specificity. Nature (Lond) 256:495, 1975

34. Foon KA, Bernard M, Oldham RK: Monoclonal antibody therapy. J Biol Response Mod 1:277, 1982

35. Oldham, RK: Monoclonal antibodies in cancer therapy. J Clin Oncol 1:582, 1983

36. Rivera E, Hersh E, Bowen J et al: Leukocyte migration inhibition assay of tumor immunity in patients with cervical squamous cell carcinoma. Cancer 43:2297, 1979

37. Old LJ, Boyse EA, Clarke DA, Carswell EA: Antigenic qualities of chemically induced tumors. Ann NY Acad Sci 101:80, 1962

38. Levy S, Kopersztych S, Musatti CC, et al: Cellular immunity in squamous cell carcinoma of the uterine cervix. Am J Obstet Gynecol 13:160, 1978

39. Mashiba H, Matsunaga K, Ueno M, Jimi S: Cell-mediated cytotoxicity *in vitro* of human lymphocyte against a cervical cancer cell line. Gann 68:53, 1977

40. DiSaia PJ, Morrow C, Hill A, Mittelstaedt L: Immune competence and survival in patients with advanced cervical cancer: Peripheral lymphocyte counts. Int J Radiat Oncol Biol Phys 4:449, 1978

41. Stratton JA, Fast PE, Weintraub I: Recovery of lymphocyte function after radiation therapy for cancer in relationship to prognosis. J Clin Lab Immunol 7:147, 1982

42. Mandell G, Fisher R, Bostick F, Young R: Ovarian cancer: A solid tumor with evidence of normal cellular immune function but abnormal B cell function. Am J Med 66:621, 1979

43. Toyokawa M: Immunological diagnosis of ovarian carcinoma. Adv Obstet Gynecol 29:267, 1977

44. Kohorn E, Mitchell M Dwyer J, et al: Effect of radiation on cell mediated cytotoxicity and lymphocyte subpopulations in patients with ovarian carcinoma. Cancer 41:1040, 1978

45. Savage A, Pritchard J, James K: Immunological status of patients with carcinoma of the cervix. Br J Cancer 37:474, 1978

46. Hancock B, Bruce L, Heath J, et al: The effects of radiotherapy on immunity in patients with localized carcinoma of the cervix uteri. Cancer 43:118, 1979

47. Check IJ, Hunter RL, Rosenberg KD, et al: Preduction of survival in gynecologic cancer based on immunological test. Cancer Res 40:4612, 1980

48. Nalick RH, DiSaia PJ, Roth TH, Morrow MH: Immunologic response in gynecologic malignancy as demonstrated by the delayed hypersensitivity reaction; clinical correlations. Am J Obstet Gynecol 118:393, 1974

49. Nalick RH, DiSaia PJ, Rea TH Morrow CP: Immunocompetence and prognosis in patients with gynecologic cancer. Gynecol Oncol 2:81, 1972

50. Melchert F, Goldhofer W, Kreienberg R, Lemmel EM: Influencing the immune system of carcinoma patients with oral BCG treatment. Arch Gynaekol 224:476, 1977

51. Olkowski ZL, McLaren JR, Skeen MJ: Effects of combined immunotherapy with levamisole and bacillus Calmette-Guerin on immunocompetence of patients with squamous cell carcinoma of the cervix, head and neck and lung undergoing radiation therapy. Cancer Treatm Rep 62:1651, 1978

52. DiSaia PJ, Gall S, Levy D, et al: Preliminary report on the treatment of women with cervical cancer, stages IIB, IIIB, and IVA (confined to the pelvis and/or periaortic nodes), with radiotherapy plus immunotherapy with intravenous *Corynebacterium parvum,* phase II. p. 331. In Terry WD, Rosenberg SA (eds): Immunotherapy of Human Cancer. Elsevier/North-Holland, New York, 1982

53. Mangan C, Jeglum KA, Sedlacek TV, et al: Intralymphatic BCG in the treatment of gynecologic malignancies: A phase I study. Cancer 40:2933, 1977

54. Kalpaktsoglou PK, Ioannidou GB, Kondyli AP, et al: Immunochemotherapy in adenocarcinoma of the ovary. Acta Obstet Gynecol Scand 57:85, 1978

55. Gall SA, Creasman WT, Blessing JA, et al: Chemoimmunotherapy in primary stage III ovarian epithelial cancer. p. 337. In Terry, WD, Rosenberg SA (eds): Immunotherapy of Human Cancer. Elsevier/North-Holland, New York, 1982

56. Alberts D: BCG as an adjuvant to adriamycin-cytoxan for advanced ovarian cancer: A Southwest Oncology Group Study. Program and Abstracts of the Second International Conference on the Adjuvant Therapy of Cancer, Tucson University of Arizona Cancer Center, March 28–31, 1979, abst 38

57. Wanebo HJ, Ochoa M, Gunther U, et al: Randomized chemoimmunotherapy trial of CAF and intravenous *C. parvum* for resistant ovarian cancer—Preliminary results. Proc Am Assoc Cancer Res 18:225, 1977 (abst)

58. Rao B, Wannebo HJ, Ochoa M, et al: Intravenous *Cor-*

ynebacterium parvum: An adjunct to chemotherapy for resistant advanced ovarian cancer. Cancer 39:514, 1977

59. Crowther ME, Levin L, Poulton TA, et al: Active specific immunotherapy in ovarian cancer. Recent Results Cancer Res 68:166, 1979

60. Crowther ME, Hudson C: Experience with a pilot study of active specific immunotherapy in advanced ovarian cancer. Clin Oncol 3:397, 1977 (abst)

61. Hudson CN, Crowther ME, Poulton T, et al: Experience of a pilot study of active specific immunotherapy in advanced ovarian cancer. Characterization and treatment of human tumors. p. 332. In Harrap DW (ed): Advances in Tumor Prevention, Detection, and Characterization. Proceedings of the Seventh International Symposium on the biological characterization of human tumors, Budapest, April 13–15, 1977. Excerpta Medica, Amsterdam, 1978

62. Freedman RS: Experiences with transfer factor (TFD) in advanced gynecologic cancer. J Clin Hematol Oncol 8:130, 1978 (abst)

63. Ikic D, Singer Z, Sips D, et al: Interferon treatment of uterine cervical precancerosis. J Clin Hematol Oncol 9(4):299, 1979 (abst)

64. Ikic D, Singer A, Sips D, et al: Interferon treatment of uterine cervical precancerosis. J Cancer Res Clin Oncol 101:303, 1981

65. Krusic J, Kirmajer V, Knezevic M, et al: Influence of

human leukocyte interferon on squamous cell carcinoma of uterine cervix: Clinical, histological, and histochemical observations. III. Communication. J Cancer Res Clin Oncol 101:309, 1981

66. Einhorn N, Cantell K, Einhorn S, Strander H: Human leukocyte interferon therapy for advanced ovarian carcinoma. Am J Clin Oncol 5:167, 1982

66a. Young RC, Knapp RC, Fuks Z et al: Cancer of the ovary. p. 1083. In DeVita VT, Hellman S, Rosenberg SA (eds): Cancer: Principles and Practice of Oncology. JB Lippincott, London, 1985

67. Freeman RS, Gutherman TO, Wharton JT, Rutledge FN: Leukocyte interferon in patients with epithelial ovarian carcinoma. J Biol Response Mod 2:133, 1983

68. Abdulhay G, DiSaia PJ, Blessing J, Creasman WT: Human lymphoblastoid interferon in the treatment of advanced epithelial ovarian malignancies: A Gynecologic Oncology Group Study. Am J Obstet Gynecol 152:418, 1985

69. Vaage J: Specific de-sensitization of resistance against a syngeneic methylcholanthrene-induced sarcoma in C3HF Mice. Cancer Res 32:193, 1972

70. Vanwijik RR, Godrick EA, Smith HG, et al: Stimulation or suppression of metastases with graded doses of tumour cells. Cancer Res 31:1559, 1971

71. Alexander P: Back to the drawing board—The need for more realistic model systems for immunotherapy. Cancer 40:467, 1977

4

Endocrinology

Erlio Gurpide

HORMONE ENVIRONMENT AND GYNECOLOGIC CANCER

Epidemiologic studies of uterine cancer have demonstrated hormonal influences in tumorigenesis: a higher risk is noted under conditions characterized by the chronic presence of estrogens in the absence of progesterone,[1] such as menopause, presence of estrogen-secreting ovarian tumors, polycystic ovarian disease, and obesity. In polycystic ovarian disease the ovaries secrete estrogens and androgens but no progesterone; obesity is marked by increased production of circulating estrogens, formed by extraglandular aromatization of adrenal androgens and decreased blood levels of sex steroid binding globulin.[2] Further evidence for the existence of a correlation between chronic exposure to estrogenic compounds and endometrial cancer has been provided by studies on women who were using estrogens for climacteric problems: the risk for development of endometrial cancer was estimated to be four to eight times higher in estrogen users than in nonusers.[3-5]

The preceding considerations point to the importance of evaluating biochemical factors responsible for a hormonal environment that may favor the development of gynecologic cancer. Knowledge of these factors could be used for preventive as well as therapeutic purposes.

DETERMINANTS OF THE HORMONAL AVAILABILITY TO THE TARGET CELL

In order to identify factors affecting hormonal availability at the site of action, several parameters must be considered:

1. Rate of production of the hormone
2. Level of the circulating hormone and binding to plasma proteins
3. Metabolic rate clearance of the hormone in blood
4. Metabolism and concentration of the hormone in target cells

The steroid hormones most commonly considered to influence gynecologic cancer are the estrogens, progestins, and androgens.

Hormone Production

ESTROGENS AND PROGESTERONE

Figure 4-1 depicts sources of estradiol and estrone, the hormones most directly involved in the promotion and maintenance of gynecologic neoplasms. The main source of estrogens in cycling women is the active ovary. In an idealized menstrual cycle, the se-

65

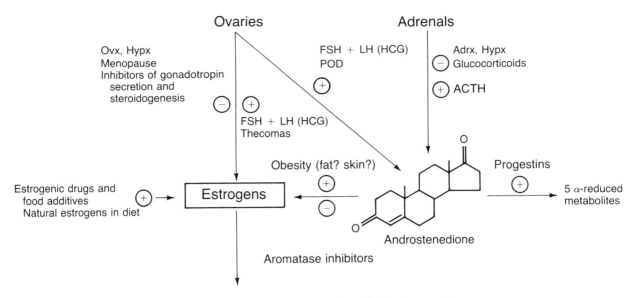

Fig. 4-1 Sources of estrogens (estradiol and estrone).

cretion rate of estradiol begins to rise significantly at about day 6 after the onset of menstruation, increasing in almost logarithmic fashion until day 14, the time of ovulation. At this time, the secretion of estradiol practically stops and significant secretion of progesterone by the corpus luteum begins. Secretion of estradiol is reinitiated, reaching a second wide maximum, coincidental with a high plateau of progesterone secretion between cycle days 19 and 25; the rates of secretion of both hormones then decline and reach baseline levels at the time of menstruation. Mean values of ovarian secretion rates of estradiol and progesterone during the menstrual cycle are shown in Table 4-1.

After the menopause, the circulating estrogens do not originate in the ovaries, as is evident from the observation that oophorectomy performed after the menopause does not reduce the blood levels of estradiol or estrone.[6,7] Postmenopausal estrogens are formed exclusively by extraglandular metabolism of androgens, mainly of adrenal origin (Table 4-1). Specifically, androstenedione, produced by the adrenals at a rate of about 1.4 mg/day is aromatized to estrone, which is then partially converted to estradiol. About 40 µg/day of estrogens is produced by this route, an amount that is small as compared with the average rate of secretion of estrogens by the premenopausal

normal ovary but large enough to provide a significant level of estrogenic stimulation of the genital tract after the menopause. It should be noted that peripheral aromatization of androgens (formation of the benzene ring in the steroid molecule) produces mostly estrone and little estradiol, whereas the estrogen secretion by the ovaries during the fertile years is practically all estradiol and little estrone.

The quantitive importance of the peripheral conversion of androgens to estrogens and the significance of this process in postmenopausal women, as well as in men, was demonstrated by the studies of Siiteri and MacDonald.[8] These investigators and others have described several interesting characteristics of these conversions, for example, that the extent of aromatization of intravenously administered radioactive androstenedione is directly related to weight and body surface area. This finding may explain why obesity is a risk factor in the development of endometrial cancer. Conversion of androgens to estrogens can occur in adipose tissue[9] and skin.[10] It is not possible, however, to evaluate from in vitro results the extent of conversion that may occur in these tissues in vivo. Metabolic characteristics of obesity, such as a reduced hepatic extraction of the androgens, may contribute to the increased conversion of androstenedione to estrone, which is also elevated in patients with liver disease.

Table 4-1 Sources of Steroical Sex Hormones in Normal Women

Steroid	Ovary	Metabolic Clearance Rate (MCR) Peripheral Plasma	Concn. in Plasma	Production Rate (PR) of Circulating Steroid (All Sources)	Sources of Circulating Steroid		
					Ovarian Secretion (%)	Adrenal Secretion (%)	Extraglandular Formation (%)
		liter/d	*pg/ml*	*µg/d*			
Estradiol (E_2)	Early follicular	1350	40	50	85	Nil	5(A); 10(E_1)
	Late follicular		300	400	>90	Nil	<10(A, E_1)
	Mid-luteal		150	200	>90	Nil	<10(A, E_1)
	Postmenopause	901	15	14	Nil	Nil	>90(A)
Estrone (E_1)	Early follicular	2210	50	110	70	Nil	20(A); 10(E_2)
	Late follicular		150	330	70	Nil	7(A); 25(E_2)
	Mid-luteal		80	180	60	Nil	13(A); 23(E_2)
	Postmenopause	1610	25	40	Nil	Nil	>90(A)
			ng/ml	*mg/day*			
Androstenedione (A)	Premenopause	2010	1.6	3.2	30–70	30–70	15(D)
	Postmenopause		0.7	1.4	<30	70–100	15(D)
Testosterone (T)	Premenopause	440	0.4	0.18	<30	20–40	50(A)
	Postmenopause		0.2	0.09	15–35	25–45	40(A)
Dehydroisoandrosterone (D)	Premenopause	1640	5	8	<30	>30	<60(DS)
	Postmenopause		2	3.3	<30	>30	<60(DS)
Progesterone (P)	Follicular	2400	0.4	1.0	10–70	5–65	25(Δ^5P)*
	Luteal		15	36	>90	—	1(Δ^5P)
	Postmenopause		0.2	0.5	Nil	>90	5(Δ^5P)
17-Hydroxyprogesterone (17HOP)	Early follicular	2000	0.5	1	20–80	—	20–80(17HOΔ^5P)*
	Late follicular		1.5	3	>90	—	—
	Mid-luteal		2	4	>90	—	—
	Postmenopause		0.3	0.6	Nil	—	—

Δ^5P, pregnenotone; 17HOΔ^5P, 17 hydroxypregnenolone
(Adapted from Gurpide E: Secretion of steroids from normal ovaries. In Scholler R (ed): Endocrinology of the Ovary. Editions Seppe, Paris, 1978.)

Postmenopausal women show an increased peripheral aromatization in comparison to premenopausal subjects. A slower metabolism of estrone after the menopause[11] contributes to the augmented effectiveness of secreted androstenedione in building plasma levels of estrogens.

Excessive estrogen production may also result from elevated rates of secretion of androstenedione, as noted in postmenopausal women with ovarian tumors and in young anovulatory women with polycystic ovarian disease. Abnormally high production rates of androstenedione or elevated fractional conversion of this androgen to estrone have been observed in patients with postmenopausal uterine bleeding.

The secretion of ovarian estrogen is controlled by pituitary gonadotropins. In addition to estradiol, androgens and progestins are capable of inhibiting gonadotropin secretion, mainly by reducing the output of hypothalamic luteinizing hormone–follicle-stimulating hormone (LH-FSH) releasing factors and their actions on the pituitary.[12] Lowering of the endogenous production of estrogens can also be achieved by the use of drugs that inhibit ovarian or adrenal steroidogenesis, such as aminogluthetimide[13] or ketoconazole.[14] More recently, administration of LH releasing hormone (LHRH) analogues, as well as LHRH antagonists that compete for binding of the hypothalamic factors to their pituitary receptors, has been shown to suppress gonadotropin secretion.[15,16]

After the menopause, production of endogenous estrogens can also be effectively reduced by the administration of glucocorticoids to suppress the production of adrenocorticotropin (ACTH), or by treatment with compounds capable of inhibiting aromatization, such as aminogluthetimide or 4-hydroxyandrostenedione.[17,18]

ANDROGENS

Androgens may have a direct influence on tumors, either by themselves or through their conversion to estrogens. Among the main four C_{19} steroids secreted by the endocrine glands in humans, that is, dehydroepiandrosterone sulfate, dehydroepiandrosterone, testosterone, and androstenedione (precursors of the classic urinary 17-ketosteroids), only the latter is of quantitative importance as a precursor of estrogens in normal postmenopausal women. Conversion of dehydroepiandrosterone and its sulfate to blood-borne androstenedione, testosterone, or estrogens is negligi-

ble in nonpregnant women. Most of the testosterone in female plasma is derived by metabolic conversion of secreted androstenedione.[19] Although testosterone can be aromatized directly to estradiol, this conversion is less efficient than that of androstenedione to estrone. Androstenedione is secreted by both the adrenals and the ovaries. It has been estimated that in premenopausal women 30 to 70 percent of the circulating androstenedione is secreted by the ovaries. Secretion of androgens by the ovaries after the menopause was demonstrated from measurements of concentrations of testosterone and androstenedione in arterial blood and in ovarian venous effluent; this finding contrasts with the absence of estrogen secretion. Postmenopausal ovariectomy resulted in significant reduction of levels of testosterone and androstenedione in plasma.

In addition to extraglandular aromatization, C_{19} steroids may act as estrogens by interacting with the estrogen receptor. These effects are noted at concentrations higher than those necessary to elicit androgen effects and can be antagonized by antiestrogens. In particular, dehydroepiandrosterone sulfate can stimulate in vitro prostaglandin production by endometrial tissue at concentrations found in plasma of normal subjects and this effect is suppressed by hydroxytamoxifene (Markiewicz L, Gurpide E, unpublished).

Metabolism and Blood Levels of Hormones

The plasma level of a hormone (c_p) is determined both by the rate at which it is supplied to the circulation (its production rate, PR) and by metabolic factors, as expressed by the relation

$$C_p = PR/MCR$$

where MCR denotes the metabolic clearance rate.[20] Average values of these parameters in normal pre- and postmenopausal women are listed in Table 4-1.

Special emphasis has been placed on studies of metabolism of estradiol, the hormone most directly related to the stimulation of tumor growth. The normal pattern of metabolism of either estradiol or estrone released into the systemic circulation is practically identical in men and in pregnant or nonpregnant women. These hormones are excreted in urine as estrone, estradiol, 16α-hydroxyestradiol (estriol), 2-hydroxyestrone, 16-epiestriol, and other minor metabolites.[21] Pregnancy results in a disproportionate increase in the levels of estriol, which in this case is mainly formed by aromatization in the placenta of 16α-hydroxylated C_{19} steroids produced by the fetus.[22]

Most of the estradiol is metabolized by conversion to estrone followed by either 2- or 16α-hydroxylations. the biologic effects of the 16α- and 2-hydroxylated metabolites are quite distinct: estriol has been shown to be capable of stimulating uterine growth when repetitively injected into rats,[23] whereas 2-hydroxyestrone displays no uterotropic activity in the rat.[24]

The metabolism of the estrogens can vary under various physiologic conditions and can be modified by drugs. Fishman and collaborators have shown that thyroxine and 7β, 17α-dimethyltestosterone, a drug that has produced remissions of breast tumors, reduce the conversion of estradiol and estrone to estriol and increases their metabolism to 2-hydroxyestrone.[25,26] The metabolism of estrogens is different in lean and obese women, the latter producing less 2-hydroxyestrone and more estriol, the estrogenic metabolite.

The fraction of estradiol undergoing 16α-hydroxylation is significantly higher in patients with breast or endometrial cancer than in normal women, whereas 2-hydroxylation is not significantly different in these two groups. The increase in 16α-hydroxylation, estimated by measuring the specific activity of tritiated water in blood after administration of 17α-^{3}H-estradiol, involves an increase in the production of 16α-hydroxyestrone, the intermediate in the conversion of estradiol and estrone to estriol. This metabolite can act as an estrogen and has the unique property of forming covalent bonds with amino groups of biologic macromolecules.[27] On the basis of these and other relevent observations, Fishman and co-workers suggested that metabolic characteristics of individual subjects or families can result in an increased production of 16α-hydroxyestrone and elevate the risk of development of cancer in estrogen target tissues through its interaction with nuclear DNA and proteins.

In spite of its estrogenic activity, estriol has been postulated to exert a protective effect against stimulation of tissues by estradiol, particularly in relationship to the development of breast tumors,[28] with a possible extension of this concept to uterine cancer. This suggestion has been based mainly on the antiuterotropic effect of estriol observed when a single dose of a mixture of estradiol and estriol is administered to immature or oophorectomized rats,[29] and on the failure of implantation noted when estriol is administered to rats at a critical period after mating,[30] a finding that can be interpreted to indicate neutralization by estriol of the estradiol surge necessary for nidation. However, these effects may be related to the short nuclear retention of estriol[23] and only relevant to the experimental condition used since this compound can produce estrogenic effects as complete as those achieved with estradiol when administered in repeated doses or when added to cultures of endometrial tissue or isolated glandular epithelial cells to stimulate $PGF_{2\alpha}$ productions.[31] Since physiologic conditions are characterized by sustained levels of estriol derived from estradiol, this metabolite can hardly be considered antiestrogenic.

Estrone is a compound of particular interest in relationship to gynecologic cancer because of its preponderance after the menopause. The relative increase in the ratio of rates of production of estrone to estradiol after the fifth decade of life has been related to the high incidence of endometrial cancer after the menopause.[32] The implication of this suggestion is that estrone and estradiol may differ qualitatively in their effects on endometrium. In vitro experiments have shown, however, that the competition of estrone for the binding of estradiol actually occurs after its conversion to estradiol in the tissue; estradiol, and not estrone, shows the binding to the nuclear chromatin required for the hormone to exert its mitogenic action.[33] These results indicate that estrone may not be estrogenic per se. Endogenously produced or exogenously administered estrone or estrone conjugates may exert their estrogenic action after conversion to estradiol, both peripherally and in the target tissue.

Estrogen metabolism by the intestinal flora, which can be influenced by diet and drugs, is another potentially important determinant of the availability of estradiol and its metabolites to tissues, since extensive enterohepatic circulation of the estrogens has been demonstrated.[34,35]

Metabolic Regulation of Hormonal Levels within Target Cells

Although the hormonal environment of neoplasia is generally evaluated on the basis of the concentration of the hormones in peripheral blood, many factors influence the tissue uptake of the circulating hor-

Table 4-2 Some Determinants of the Intracellular Concentration of a Hormone in Target Cells

$$c_{intracell} = \frac{\text{intracellular production rate (entry + synthesis)}}{\text{intracellular clearance}}$$

Parameter	Process	Regulatory Factors
Intracellular production rate $\left(\dfrac{nmole}{g \times hr}\right)$	Entry	Plasma concentration
		Binding to plasma proteins
		Capillary permeability
		Diffusibility (transport?) across cell membranes
	Synthesis	Intracellular conversion of circulating precursors
Intracellular clearance (hour^{-1})	Metabolism	Activity and localization of enzymes
		Levels and localization of cofactors
		Binding
	Exit	Diffusibility (transport?) across cell membranes
		Binding
	Binding	Specific (including receptors)
		Nonspecific (high capacity)

mone. In vivo and in vitro measurements have demonstrated a wide range of tissue/plasma or tissue/medium concentration ratios for various hormones at steady state. Several physiologic or pathologic conditions, as well as pharmacologic agents, influence these ratios mainly by modifying intracellular enzymatic activities acting on the hormones. Table 4-2 lists some of the factors that determine the intracellular concentrtion of a hormone in a target cell.

By analogy to the concept of metabolic clearance of a hormone in blood, the rapidity of the overall metabolism of the hormone in a cell can be represented by intracellular clearance (IC), defined as the quotient of the rate at which the hormone appears de novo in the cell (its production rate, PR) and the resulting intracellular concentration (c), as measured by isotopic methods.[33]

The rate at which the hormone is supplied to the cell can be resolved into two components: the transfer of hormone from circulation to the cell, and the intracellular formation of the hormone from blood-borne precursors. The rate of entry depends on the concentration of the unbound hormone in plasma and its diffusibility across capillaries and cell membranes. Steroids apparently enter cells by diffusion, although

the possible existence of saturable carrier systems for steroid hormones in plasma membranes of target tissues has not been ruled out.

ESTRADIOL IN HUMAN ENDOMETRIAL CELLS

The regulation of the intracellular concentration of a hormone can be illustrated with results from detailed studies of estradiol in human endometrium. Measurements of endogenous concentrations of estradiol in endometrium and in plasma showed a ratio of 10 and 3.8 in the follicular and luteal phase, respectively.[36] Superfusions of tissue with ^{3}H-estradiol in buffer solutions have shown that the steady-state intracellular concentration of the hormone was nine times higher in proliferative endometrium than in the medium but only twice as high when secretory tissue was used.[37] Results from both in vivo and in vitro experiments clearly indicate tissue factors affecting the intracellular concentration of the hormone.

Figure 4-2 shows some of the possible circulating contributors to the intracellular estradiol pool (e.g., estradiol itself, estrone, estrone sulfate, and androstenedione). Estrone sulfate is the estrogen in highest

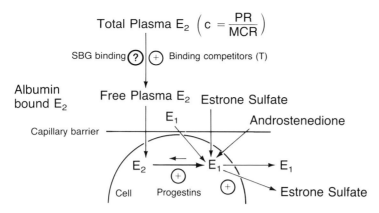

Fig. 4-2 Factors influencing intracellular concentration of estradiol in human endometrium.

concentration in plasma and can be converted in the tissue to estradiol[38]; although its utilization as a source of estradiol may be limited by the permeability of the blood capillaries to the ionized compound.[39,40] Perfusions of excised human uteri have suggested, however, that permeability of endometrial capillaries to estrone sulfate relative to that of estrone, is much larger in the endometrium than in the myometrium.[41] Evidence for aromatization of C_{19} steroids in endometrium was recently demonstrated in vitro.[42] It should be noted that even a very small conversion to estradiol would be significant in view of the high levels of androstenedione in plasma.

An important route of metabolism of estradiol in endometrium is its oxidation to estrone, promoted by a 17β-hydroxysteroid dehydrogenase. Estrone leaves the tissue, although a small fraction can be converted back to estradiol. In the presence of this metabolic pattern, it can be predicted that an increase of dehydrogenase activity will result in a higher clearance of estradiol, and a lower intracellular concentration of the hormone.[43] Since estrone appears not to be estrogenic per se, an augmentation of the estradiol dehydrogenase activity reduces the total estrogenic activity in the tissue. The levels of this regulatory enzyme change during the menstrual cycle: its activity in mid-secretory endometrium is about 10-fold higher than in proliferative endometrium.[44] Both in vitro and in vivo experiments have indicated that progesterone is responsible for the increase in enzymatic activity observed during the luteal phase. Induction of the enzyme in cultures of proliferative endometrium in noted when progestins are added to the medium[45];

in vivo, the activity of the endometrial estradiol dehydrogenase is augmented when medroxyprogesterone acetate is administered to women at the follicular phase of their cycles.[45] Furthermore, intrauterine devices (IUDs) releasing progesterone can increase the level of estradiol dehydrogenase[45,46] and can lower the levels of endogenous estradiol in endometrium.[47]

Another enzyme of physiologic importance in the intracellular regulation of estradiol levels in human endometrium is the sulfotransferase that catalyzes the sulfation of estrone and estradiol. This enzyme has been found to have an unusually low Michaelis constant (approximately 1 nM), a characteristic that makes it of particular relevance to the metabolism of estrogens in the endometrium, where the concentration of the substrate is very low.[48] Furthermore, the activity of the endometrial enzyme, found mainly in cytosol of the glandular epithelium, can be increased by progesterone in vitro.[49] Studies with cells from the Ishikawa endometrial adenocarcinoma cell line have also revealed an extensive conversion of estradiol (10^{-8}M) to estradiol 3-sulfate which is drastically reduced at higher substrate concentrations.[50]

The hormonal control of enzymatic activities affecting the levels of estradiol in the glandular epithelium of the human endometrium points to the potential importance of intracellular metabolism in the regulation of the hormonal concentrations and actions in target cells. It also reveals a mechanism that contributes to the well-known antiestrogenic effect of progesterone against continuous stimulation of target tissues by estradiol secreted by the ovaries throughout the menstrual cycle.

ACTIONS OF HORMONES AND ANTIHORMONES

Stated in general terms, estrogens promote proliferation and progestins induce differentiated functions in cells of the human genital tract. These hormonal actions, clearly evident in endometrial tissue during the menstrual cycle, are mediated by specific receptor molecules that, after binding the corresponding hormone, undergo structural changes that make possible their interaction with chromosomal acceptor sites located in specific protein-DNA complexes or in regulatory elements of inducible genes.[51-53] As a result of such interactions, expression of these genes is either initiated, suppressed, or quantitatively modified. Changes in the rates of transcription of a limited number of genes, with the corresponding formation of messenger RNA (mRNA) coding for the synthesis of specific proteins, can have a remarkable influence in target cells, since some of the proteins whose synthesis is affected by the ovarian hormones exhibit enzymatic activity controlling key cellular processes. For example, estrogens and progestins affect the activity of DNA polymerases and the synthesis of DNA, as well as the production of specific products, such as glycogen, mucins, and prostaglandins in epithelial cells of the endometrium that may be essential for implantation and survival of the embryo. In endometrial stroma, these hormones promote changes that result in the appearance of predecidual cells capable of producing prolactin. The estradiol-induced synthesis of progesterone receptor affects actions controlled by progestins; conversely, the inhibitory effect of progesterone on the estrogen receptor levels are as important as hormonal levels in the expression of hormonal effects.

Specific effects of estrogens, progestins, and glucocorticoids on human endometrium have been demonstrated in vitro, using tissue fragments, isolated epithelial and stromal cells, or endometrial adenocarcinoma cell lines. Results obtained in several laboratories, including ours, have shown direct actions of these hormones on cell proliferation, on glycogen accumulation, on activities of DNA polymerase α, 17β-hydroxysteroid dehydrogenase, steroid sulfotransferases, peroxidase, alkaline phosphatase, isocitric dehydrogenase, aromatase, plasminogen activator and creatine kinase, and on the production of prostaglandins, lipocortin, IgA secretory component, prolactin, and a variety of proteins characterized by their molecular weight, electrophoretic behavior, and, in some cases, their primary structure. These inducible secreted proteins, such as progestagen-associated protein (PEP),[54] are valuable markers of still undefined physiologic roles. In vitro studies have also served to confirm that the hormonal actions are direct and not mediated by circulating compounds formed in other tissues when the hormones are administered in vivo, a possibility that receives deserving attention. Furthermore, in vitro experiments have demonstrated endometrial responses to agonists other than steroid hormone, e.g. prolactin, oxytocin, epidermal growth factor, and cholinergic agents. A summary of in vitro hormonal responses of human endometrium and endometrial cells has been published elsewhere.[55,55a]

Of particular relevance to gynecologic cancer are in vitro studies of hormonal effects on endometrial neoplasms or endometrial cancer cell lines aimed to identify biochemical differences with normal tissue and cells.

Studies on the human breast cancer cell line MCF-7, summarized by Dickson and Lippman,[55b] have revealed that estrogens and antiestrogens can affect cell proliferation by regulating rates of production of growth stimulatory and inhibitory factors. These effects were observed in MCF-7 cells growing in culture dishes or forming tumors in nude mice.

Endometrial adenocarcinoma cells of the Ishikawa line were found to respond to estrogens by markedly but transiently elevating DNA polymerase α activity[55c] and by increasing rates of proliferation after several days in culture,[55d,55e] as well as by enhancing progesterone receptor level[55d] and alkaline phosphatase activity.[55f] These results could also been obtained in the absence of serum, an indication of direct action of the hormone on the cancer cell.

RATIONALE FOR HORMONE-RELATED THERAPY

Hormone-related methods of therapy fall within three large groups: treatment aiming at the elimination of endogenous hormones that may stimulate tumor growth, administration of drugs that interfere with the action of the endogenous hormones, and the use of pharmacologic doses of hormones or antihormones as specific cytotoxic or cytostatic agents for cancer cells. These therapeutic approaches are listed in Table 4-3.

Table 4-3 Hormone-Related Gynecologic Cancer Therapy

I. Elimination of endogenous hormones
   A. Ablation of endocrine gland
      1. Oophorectomy before menopause
      2. Adrenalectomy after menopause
      3. Hypophysectomy
   B. Suppression of hormone production
      1. By inhibition of hypophyseal secretions
         a. Of gonadotropins (hence of estrogens) with progestins, LHRH agonists, and antagonists
         b. Of ACTH (and hence of adrenal androgens) with dexamethasone or other glucocorticoids
      2. By inhibition of steroidogenesis with aminoglutethimide, ketoconazole or other inhibitors
      3. By inhibition of extraglandular aromatization with 4-hydroxyandrostanedione or other inhibitors
II. Interference with hormonal action at the target tissue
   A. By reduction of levels of estradiol receptors in endometrium with progestins
   B. By competition for binding to receptors with antiestrogens, e.g., Tamoxifen, or other triphenylethylene derivatives
   C. By enhancement of metabolism of estradiol in endometrium with progestins
III. Cytotoxic action on tumors
   A. By coupling ligand to hormone receptor with cytotoxic drugs
   B. By pharmacologic doses of estrogens or progestins

Oophorectomy is the obvious means of eliminating the sources of estrogens and reduces the production of androgens in premenopausal women. Adrenalectomy further eliminates endogenous steroids; in postmenopausal women, the adrenals are the main source of androgens and, indirectly, of estrogens. Removal or destruction of the hypophysis not only suppresses trophic hormones necessary for steroidogenesis but eliminates the source of other peptide hormones whose effects on tumor growth have not been clearly defined.

Pharmacologic control of endocrine function can be achieved by suppressing the secretion of pituitary hormones (e.g., gonadotropins with progestins, ACTH with dexamethasone) or by interfering with either steroidogenesis in the endocrine glands or the extraglandular formation of estrogens.

The available information on the mechanism of action of steroid hormones has led to the design of new forms of therapy. Drugs that inactivate the hormonal receptor in a target tissue would actually suppress the action of the hormone. Progestins, for instance, have been found to lower the levels of estradiol receptors in human endometrium.[56] Many compounds can compete with estradiol for binding to the estrogen receptor. Some of them are capable of promoting the activation of the receptor, its transfer to the nucleus, and the expression of the receptor-mediated estrogenic activity. Compounds in this category, such as ethynylestradiol, diethystilbestrol (DES), hexestrol, estriol, and many others, are therefore active estrogens. Others, however, once bound to the receptor, cannot exert full estrogenic effects, because they are unable to promote its activation or its binding to proper acceptor sites with kinetic characteristics compatible with sustained hormonal action. Drugs in this category would interfere with the action of the endogenous hormone. Among other triphenylethylene antiestrogens, tamoxifen is widely used, alone or in combination with cytotoxic agents, as adjuvant therapy for breast and endometrial cancer.[57-59]

The therapeutic effect of progestins on endometrial cancer was first described by Kelley and Baker[60] and was further documented by the studies of Bonte et al.,[61] Reifenstein,[62] and others. Remissions of metastatic endometrial adenocarcinoma were noted in about 30 percent of patients treated with either medroxyprogesterone acetate (Provera) or 17-hydroxyprogesterone caproate (Delalutin). Two effects of progestins on endometrium that can be related to their antiestrogenic and therapeutic action have already been described: (1) reduction of the levels of estradiol receptor, and (2) induction of the 17β-hydroxysteroid dehydrogenase, the enzyme that metabolizes estradiol. Estradiol dehydrogenase activity is low in endometrial adenocarcinoma of postmenopausal women, as could be expected from the absence of progesterone; administration of medroxyprogesterone acetate for 1 week to postmenopausal patients with endometrial carcinoma produced an increase in the activity of the enzyme in some but not all cases.[55,63]

Another application of the receptor concept has been the design of drugs combining a chemotherapeutic moiety (e.g., a nitrogen mustard) with a phenolic steroid that provides specificity for estrogen-responsive tumors.[64,65]

The mechanisms by which steroids given in pharmacologic doses are effective in provoking remission in patients with breast cancer are unknown. Some of the effects of progestins on endometrial tumors, obtained at concentrations beyond those necessary to saturate their receptors, are also unclear and may involve interference with cell membrane function.

PREDICTION OF RESPONSE TO HORMONE-RELATED THERAPY

Only about one-third of patients with metastatic breast cancer in a general population will respond to ablation of endocrine glands or treatment with steroids.[66] Also, only one-third of patients with endometrial adenocarcinoma respond to progestin therapy.[60] Tests for the prediction of responsiveness of individual patients to hormone-related therapy have proved helpful in the identification of those who are likely to benefit from this kind of treatment.

Hormone Receptor Content

Current knowledge of the processes involved in hormonal action provided a rationale for developing predictive tests. As originally proposed by Folca et al.[67] and Jensen et al.,[68] the absence of receptor for a hormone in tumor samples would invalidate therapeutic approaches based on the reduction of levels of endogenous hormone or on the interference with its action. The results shown in Tables 4-4 and 4-5 support this concept. A low incidence of response is found among breast cancer patients with tumors lacking estrogen receptors (ER$^-$) (Table 4-4). Among ER$^+$ patients, the percentage of positive responses to hormone-related therapy is twice that observed in the

Table 4-4 Objective Breast Tumor Regressions According to Estradiol Receptor Assay and Type of Therapy as Judged by Extramural Review

Therapy	ER$^+$	ER$^-$	ER$^\pm$	All Patients
Adrenalectomy	32/66	4/33	3/8	39/107
Castration	25/33	4/53	0/2	29/88
Hypophysectomy	2/8	0/8	—	2/16
Total	59/107 (55%)	8/94 (8%)	3/10 (30%)	70/211 (33%)
Androgen	12/26	2/24	0/1	14/51
Estrogen	37/57	5/58	0/2	42/117
Glucocorticoid	2/2	—	—	2/2
Total	51/85 (60%)	7/82 (8%)	0/3 (0%)	58/170 (34%)
Antiestrogens	8/20	5/27	—	13/47
Other	2/3	0/5	—	2/8
Total	10/23 (43%)	5/32 (16%)	—	15/55 (27%)

ER, estradiol receptor.
(Adapted from McGuire WL, Carbone PP, Sears, Escher GC: Estrogen receptors in human breast cancer; an overview. p. 1. In McGuire WL, Carbone PP, Vollmer EP (eds): Estrogen Receptors in Human Breast Cancer. Raven Press, New York, 1975.)

Table 4-5 Relationship Between Response of Recurrent or
Advanced Endometrial Adenocarcinoma to Progestins

Series	Responders		Nonresponders	
	PR(+)	PR(−)	PR(+)	PR(−)
McCarty et al.(1979)[69]	4	0	1	8
Martin et al. (1979)[70]	13	1	0	6
Benraad et al. (1980)[71]	6	2	0	5
Ehrlich et al. (1981)[72]	7	1	1	15
Total	30 (88%)	4 (12%)	2 (6%)	34 (94%)

(Adapted from Ehrlich CE, Young PCM, Cleary RE: Cytoplasmic
progesterone and estradiol receptors in normal, hyperplastic, and
carcinomatous endometria; therapeutic implications. Am J Obstet
Gynecol 141:539, 1981.)

general population. In patients with endometrial cancer, an average of 94 percent of those with tumors containing progesterone receptors (PR$^+$) responded to progestin treatment, whereas only 11 percent of PR$^-$ patients responded to the same treatment (Table 4-5).

Estrogen and progesterone receptors have been found in some specimens of ovarian cancer,[73-77] but their presence has not been demonstrated to be of value for the prediction of responses to treatment with progestins, antiestrogens or cytostactic drugs, in vivo or in vitro.[78,79]

Two different methodologies are commonly used in the routine evaluation of receptor content in tumors: (1) biochemical procedures, in which high-affinity specific binding of the ^{3}H-labeled hormone is measured in cytosol fractions from tissue homogenates,[80] and (2) immunocytochemical methods, based on colorimetric or fluorometric visualization of complexes formed by interaction of estrogen and progesterone receptors with the corresponding monoclonal antibodies that are commercially available.[81-83] These antibodies can also be used to measure receptors in immunoassays performed in tissue homogenates.

The results obtained using biochemical procedures are greatly affected by the heterogeneity of the tumor samples, which often include noncancerous and necrotic tissue. Furthermore, an undetermined fraction of the total intracellular receptor can remain associated to nuclei and thereby be excluded from the cytosol sample. The size of this fraction is influenced by the levels of the hormone in plasma, since the receptor activated by binding to the hormone is more tightly held by nuclear acceptors. Results from bio-

chemical tests may also depend on the ligand concentration, as several specific binders with different affinity for the hormone may be present in the sample. To obviate this problem and characterize the type of binder present in the sample, measurements are often conducted at various concentrations of the labeled hormone and affinity constants calculated using Scatchard plots or suitable computer programs.[84] Results are also influenced by the temperature at which the assays are performed: at 0 to 4°C, only unoccupied receptors are able to bind the labeled ligand during short incubations, whereas at higher temperatures exchange of the ^{3}H-ligand with the receptor-bound endogenous hormone may occur.

Regarding the interpretation of results from receptor measurements by biochemical methods, it is important to note that above the limit of sensitivity of the assay there is no clear information about the minimal level of receptor necessary to obtain hormonal responses. Concentrations of progesterone receptor at least as high as 300 fmoles/mg protein seemed necessary to obtain glycogen accumulation in endometrial adenocarcinoma under the influence of progestins, both in vivo and in vitro.[85] Furthermore, detection of receptors does not exclude the existence in the sample of cancer cells lacking receptors likely to be unresponsive to hormonal therapy. Immunocytochemical methods have the advantage of allowing the evaluation of tissue heterogeneity and a direct documentation of the presence of cancer cells with or without receptors, both nuclear and cytoplasmic.

In addition to the measurement of hormone receptors, assays for binding of tamoxifen or its 4-hydroxylated metabolite to antiestrogen receptors which do not bind estradiol may be relevant to the evaluation of responsiveness to tamoxifen therapy. The actions of triphenylethylene and diphenylmethane antiestrogens may be complex and these compounds can exert specific effects by mechanisms other than competition for the estrogen receptor.

Responses to Hormones and Antihormones

Binding to the receptor is only one of the steps in a series of events leading to the expression of hormonal action. It can therefore be expected that some tumors could be unresponsive to a hormone even in the presence of the corresponding receptor. Therefore, evaluation of in vivo and in vitro responses to hormones and antihormones may provide a more direct approach to determine responsiveness of the tumor to a particular therapy.

End points for the evaluation of progestin actions on endometrial adenocarcinoma have already been described, viz., stimulation of 17β-hydroxysteroid oxidoreductase activity,[55,63] promotion of glycogen accumulation,[85] and lowering of prostaglandin production,[86] of estrogen receptor levels[55,87] and of plasminogen activator activity.[87] More recently, the proportion of cells undergoing DNA synthesis in a tumor sample, estimated by flow cytometry (fraction in S phase), has been proposed to serve as a prognostic marker[88]; this interesting approach may also be useful in the evaluation of responses to hormones. The presence of progesterone receptors in a tumor sample may itself indicate the presence of functional estrogen receptors, since estrogens are necessary for the formation of the progesterone receptors in many tissues.[89] There are, however, examples of cancer cells containing progesterone binders independent of estrogen stimulation.[90]

Responsiveness to tamoxifen can be tested by measuring its effects on progesterone receptor levels, since they are also elevated by this antiestrogen. This effect of tamoxifen provides the basis for therapeutic approaches based on combinations of antiestrogens and progestins.[87] Further evaluation of this modality of treatment is necessary, however, since its advantages have not been confirmed.[58]

Another approach to the prediction of responsiveness of endometrial tumors is offered by the possibility of transplanting tissue fragments into nude mice, where they can form tumors. The rate of growth of such tumors provides an objective end point to evaluate the effects of test compounds.[91,92] One limitation of this approach is that only about one-third of the transplanted specimens yield measurable tumors.

Studies on cells from human gynecologic tumors in culture or in host animals may eventually serve to clarify current uncertainties related to several factors: (1) the regulation of cell proliferation by production of autocrine growth stimulatory or inhibitory factors; (2) the synthesis and effects of cellular oncogene products; (3) the secretion of proteolytic enzymes or their activators, which may permit cancer cells to break through basal membranes; and (4) the mechanisms of cytostatic or cytotoxic effects of some hormones and antihormones, which are only seen at high concentrations, well above those necessary for receptor saturation, but only in receptor-rich cells.

REFERENCES

1. Gusberg SB: Precursors of corpus carcinoma: Estrogens and adenomatous hyperplasia. Am J Obstet Gynecol 54:905, 1947
2. Enriori CL, Orsini W, Cremona MC et al: Decrease of circulating levels of SHBG in postmenopausal obese women. Gynecol Oncol 23:77, 1986
3. Ziel HK, Finkle WD: Increased risk of endometrial carcinoma among users of conjugated estrogens. N Engl J Med 293:1167, 1975
4. Smith DC, Prentice R, Thompson DJ, Hermann WL: Association of exogenous estrogen and endometrial carcinoma. N Engl J Med 293:1164, 1975
5. Mack TM, Pike MC, Henderson BE, et al: Estrogens and endometrial cancer in a retirement community. N Engl J Med 294:1262, 1976
6. Vermeulen A: Hormonal activity of the postmenopausal ovary. J Clin Endocrinol Metab 42:247, 1976
7. Judd HL, Lucas WE, Yen SSC: Serum 17β-estradiol and estrone levels in postmenopausal women with and without endometrial cancer. J Clin Endocrinol Metab 43:272, 1976
8. Siiteri PK, MacDonald PC: The role of extraglandular estrogens in human endocrinology. p. 615. In Greep RO (ed): Handbook of Physiology, Sec. 7, Vol. II, Part 1. American Physiology Society, Washington, DC, 1973
9. Schindler AE, Ebert A, Friedrich E: Conversion of androstenedione to estrone by human fat tissue. J Clin Endocrinol Metab 35:627, 1972

10. Schweikert H, Milewich L, Wilson JD: Aromatization of androstenedione by cultured human fibroblasts. J Clin Endocrinol Metab 43:785, 1976

11. Longcope C: Metabolic clearance and blood production rates of estrogens in postmenopausal women. Am J Obstet Gynecol 111:778, 1971

12. Speroff L, Glass RH, Kase NG: Clinical Gynecologic Endocrinology. Williams & Wilkins, Baltimore, 1983

13. Salhanick HA, McIntosh EN, Uzgiris VI, et al: Mitochondrial systems of pregnenolone synthesis and its inhibition. p. 525. In Crozier R, Corfman PA, Condliffe PG (eds): The Regulation of Mammalian Reproduction. Charles C Thomas, Springfield, IL, 1973

14. Pont A, Williams PL, Loose DS, et al: Ketoconazole blocks adrenal steroid synthesis. Ann Intern Med 97:370, 1982

15. Manni A, Santen R, Harvey H, et al: Treatment of breast cancer with gonadotropin-releasing hormone. Endocr Rev 7:39, 1986

16. Vickery BH: Comparison of the potential for therapeutic utilities with gonadotropin-releasing hormone agonists and antagonists. Endocr Rev 7:115, 1986

17. Santen RJ, Worgul TJ, Samojlik E, et al: Randomized trial comparing surgical adrenalectomy with aminoglutethimide plus hydrocortisone in women with advanced breast carcinoma. N Engl J Med 305:545, 1981

18. Brodie AMH, Wing L-Y, Goss P, et al: Aromatase inhibitors and the treatment of breast cancer. J Steroid Biochem 24:91, 1986

19. Lipsett MB, Migeon CJ, Kirschner MA, Bardin CW: Physiologic basis of disorders of androgen metabolism. Ann Intern Med 68:1327, 1968

20. Tait JF: Review: The use of isotopic steroids for the measurement of production rates in vivo. J Clin Endocrinol Metab 23:1285, 1963

21. Slaunwhite WR, Kirdani RY, Sandberg AA: Metabolic aspects of estrogens in man. p. 485. In Greep RO (ed):Handbook of Physiology, Sec. 7, Vol. II, Part 1. American Physiologic Society, Washington, DC, 1973

22. Beling CG: Estrogens. p. 32. In Fuchs F, Klopper A (eds): Harper & Row, New York, 1971

23. Anderson HN, Peck EJ Jr, Clark JH: Estrogen-induced uterine responses and growth. Relationship to receptor estrogen binding by uterine nuclei. Endocrinology 96:160, 1975

24. Fishman J, Martucci C: Differential biologic activity of estradiol metabolites. Pediatrics 62:1128, 1978

25. Fishman J, Hellman L, Zumoff B, Gallagher TF: Effect of thyroid on hydroxylation of estrogen in man. J Clin Endocrinol Metab 25:365, 1965

26. Fishman J, Hellman L: 7β, 17α-Dimethyltestosterone (Calusterone)-induced changes in the metabolism, pro-

duction rate and excretion of estrogens in women with breast cancer; a possible mechanism of action. J Clin Endocrinol Metab 42:365, 1976

27. Fishman J, Schneider J, Hershcopf RJ, Bradlow L: Increased estrogen 16α-hydroxylase activity in women with breast and endometrial cancer. J Steroid Biochem 20:1077, 1984

28. Lemon HM, Miller DM, Foley JF: Competition between steroids for hormonal receptor. Natl Cancer Inst Monogr 34:77, 1971

29. Brecher PI, Wotiz HH: Competition between estradiol and estriol for end organ receptor proteins. Steroids 9:431, 1967

30. Wotiz HH, Scublinsky A: The contraception action of impeding oestrogens. II. Post-coital effects of oestriol. J Reprod Fertil 26:363, 1971

31. Schatz F, Markiewicz L, Gurpide E: Effect of estriol on $PGF_{2\alpha}$ output by cultures of human endometrium and endometrial cells. J Steroid Biochem 20:999, 1984

32. Siiteri, PK, Schwarz BE, MacDonald PC: Estrogen receptors and the estrone hypothesis in relation to endometrial and breast cancer. Gynecol Oncol 2:228, 1974

33. Gurpide E: Enzymatic modulation of hormonal action at the target tissue. J Toxicol Environ Health 4:249, 1978

34. Adlercreutz H, Martin F, Pulkinen M, et al: Intestinal metabolism of estrogens. J Clin Endocrinol Metab 43:497, 1976

35. Papaioannou AN: The Etiology of Human Breast Cancer, Springer-Verlag, New York, 1974

36. Guerrero R, Landgren BM, Montiel R, et al: Unconjugated steroids in the human endometrium. Contraception 11:169, 1975

37. Tseng L, Gurpide E: Changes in the in vitro metabolism of estradiol during the menstrual cycle. Am J Obstet Gynecol 114:1002, 1972

38. Tseng L, Stolee A, Gurpide E: Quantitative studies on the uptake and metabolism of estrogens and progesterone by human endometrium. Endocrinology 90:390, 1972

39. Holinka CF, Gurpide E: *In vivo* uptake of estrone sulfate by rabbit uterus. Endocrinology 106:1193, 1980

40. Verheugen C, Pardridge WH, Judd HL, Chaudhuri G: Differential permeability of uterine and liver vascular beds to estrogens and estrogen conjugates. J Clin Endocrinol Metab 59:1128, 1984

41. Bulletti C, Jasonni V, Lubicz L, et al: Extracorporeal perfusion of the human uterus. Am J Obstet Gynecol 154:683, 1986

42. Tseng L: Estrogen synthesis in human endometrial epithelial glands and stromal cells. J Steroid Biochem 20:877, 1984

43. Gurpide E, Tseng L: Factors controlling intracellular

levels of estrogens in human endometrium. Gynecol Oncol 2:221, 1974

44. Tseng L, Gurpide E: Estradiol and 20α-dihydroprogesterone dehydrogenase activities in human endometrium during the menstrual cycle. Endocrinology 94:419, 1974

45. Tseng L, Gurpide E: Induction of human endometrial estradiol dehydrogenase by progestins. Endocrinology 97:825, 1975

46. Janne O, Ylostalo P: Endometrial estrogen and progestin receptors in women bearing a progesterone-releasing intrauterine device. Contraception 22:19, 1980

47. Hagenfeldt K, Landgren BM: Contraception by intrauterine release of progesterone. Effects on endometrial trace elements, enzymes, and steroids. J Steroid Biochem 6:895, 1975

48. Tseng L, Mazella J: Cyclic changes of estradiol metabolic enzymes in human endometrium during the menstrual cycle. p. 211. In Kimbal FA (ed): The Endometrium. Spectrum, New York, 1980

49. Tseng L, Liu HC: Stimulation of estrogen sulfurylation and arylsulfotransferase activity in human endometrium *in vitro*. J Clin Endocrinol Metab 53:418, 1981

50. Hata H, Holinka CF, Pahuja SL, et al: Estradiol metabolism in Ishikawa endometrial cancer cells. J Steroid Biochem 26:699, 1987

51. Spelsberg T, Littlefield B, Seelke R, et al: Role of specific chromosomal proteins and DNA sequences in the nuclear binding sites for steroid receptors. Recent Prog Horm Res 39:463, 1983

52. Comptom J, Schrader W, O'Malley B: Selective binding of chicken progesterone receptor A subunit to a DNA fragment containing ovalbumin gene sequences. Biochem Biophys Res Commun 105:96, 1982

53. Payvar F, Wrange O, Carlstedt-Duke J, et al: Purified glucocorticoid receptors bind selectively in vitro to a cloned DNA fragment whose transcription is regulated by glucocorticoids in vivo. Proc Natl Acad Sci USA 78:6628, 1981

54. Joshi SG: A progestagen-associated protein of the human endometrium; basic studies and potential clinical applications. J Steroid Biochem 19:751, 1983

55. Gurpide E, Tseng L, Gusberg SB: Estrogen metabolism in normal and neoplastic endometrium. Am J Obstet Gynecol 129:809, 1977

55a. Gurpide E: In vitro effects of steroids on human endometrium. p. 569. In Genazzani AR, Volpe A, Facchinetti F, (eds), Gynecological Endocrinology. Parthenon, Lancs, UK, 1987

55b. Dickson RB, Lippman ME: Estrogenic regulation of growth and polypeptide growth factor secretion in human breast carcinoma. Endocr Rev 8:29, 1987

55c. Gravanis A, Gurpide E: Effects of estradiol on DNA

polymerase α activity in the Ishikawa human endometrial adenocarcinoma cell line. J Clin Endocrinol Metab. 63:356, 1986

55d. Holinka CF, Hata H, Kuramoto H, Gurpide E: Responses to estradiol in a human endometrial adenocarcinoma cells line (Ishikawa). J Steroid Biochem 24:85, 1986

55e. Holinka CF, Hata H, Gravanis A et al: Effects of estradiol on proliferation of endometrial adenocarcinoma cells (Ishikawa line). J Steroid Biochem 25:781, 1986

55f. Holinka CF, Hata H, Kuramoto H, Gurpide E: Effects of steroid hormones and antisteroids on alkaline phosphatase activity in human endometrial cancer cells (Ishikawa line). Cancer Res 46:2771, 1986

56. Tseng L, Gurpide E: Effects of progestins on estradiol receptor levels in human endometrium. J Clin Endocrinol Metab 41:402, 1975

57. Kauppila A: Progestin therapy of endometrial breast and ovarian carcinoma. Acta Obstet Gynecol Scand 63:441, 1984

58. Carlson JA, Allegra JC, Day TG, Wittliff JL: Tamoxifen and endometrial carcinoma: Alterations in estrogen and progesterone receptors in untreated patients and combination hormonal therapy in advanced neoplasia. Am J Obstet Gynecol 149:149, 1984

59. Jordan VC, Fritz NF, Tormey CT: Endocrine effects of adjuvant chemotherapy and long-term tamoxifen administration on node-positive patients with breast cancer. Cancer Res 47:624, 1987

60. Kelley RM, Baker WH: The role of progesterone in human endometrial cancer. Cancer Res 25:1190, 1965

61. Bonte J, Decoster JM, Ide P, et al: Progesterone in endometrial cancer. p.285. In Persianinov LS, Chervakova TV, Presl J (eds): Recent Progress in Obstetrics and Gynaecology. Proceedings of the Seventh World Congress of Obstetrics and Gynaecology, Moscow, August 12–18, 1973. Excerpta Medica, Amsterdam, 1974

62. Reifenstein EC: The treatment of advanced endometrial cancer with hydroxyprogesterone caproate. Gynecol Oncol 2:377, 1974

63. Pollow K, Boquoi E, Lubbert H, Pollow B: Effect of gestagen therapy upon 17β-hydroxysteroid dehydrogenase in human endometrial adenocarcinoma. J Endocrinol 67:131, 1975

64. Kirdani RY, Mittleman A, Murphy GP, Sandberg AA: Studies on phenolic steroids in human subjects. XIV. Fate of nitrogen mustard of estradiol-17β. J Clin Endocrinol Metab 41:305, 1975

65. Terenius L: Antiestrogens and their role in mammary cancer. p. 82. In Stoll BA (ed): Mammary Cancer and Neuroendocrine Therapy. Butterworth, London, 1974

66. McGuire WL, Carbone PP, Sears ME, Escher GC: Es-

trogen receptors in human breast cancer; an overview. p. 1. In McGuire WL, Carbone PP, Vollmer EP (eds): Estrogen Receptors in Human Breast Cancer. Raven Press, New York, 1975

67. Folca PJ, Clascock RF, Irvine WT: Studies with tritium labeled hexoestriol in advanced breast cancer. Lancet 2:796, 1961

68. Jensen EV, DeSombre ER, Jungblut PW: Estrogen receptors in hormone-responsive tissues and tumors. p. 15. In Wissler RW, Dao TL, Wood S (eds): Endogenous Factors Influencing Host-Tumor Balance. University of Chicago Press, Chicago, 1967

69. McCarthy KS Jr, Barton TK, Fettler, B.F., Creasman, W.T., and McCarty K.S., Sr.: Correlation of estrogen and progesterone receptors with histologic differentiation in endometrial adencarcinoma. Am J Pathol 96:171, 1979

70. Martin PM, Rolland PH, Gammere M, et al: Estradiol and progesterone in normal and neoplastic endometrium. Correlations between receptor, histopathologic examinations and clinical responses under progestin therapy. Int J Cancer 23:321, 1979

71. Benraad TJ, Friberg LG, Koenders AJM, Kullander S: Do estrogens and progesterone receptors (E_2R and PR) in metastasizing endometrial cancer predict the response to gestagen therapy? Acta Obstet Gynecol Scand 59:155, 1980

72. Ehrlich CE, Young, PCM, Cleary RE: Cytoplasmic progesterone and estradiol receptors in normal, hyperplastic, and carcinomatous endometria; therapeutic implications. Am J Obstet Gynecol 141:539, 1981

73. Janne O, Kauppila A, Syrjala O, Vihko R: Comparison of cytosol estrogen and progestin receptor status in malignant and benign tumors and tumor-like lesions of human ovary. Int J Cancer 25:175, 1980

74. Schwartz PE, Keating G, Maclusky N, et al: Tamoxifen therapy for advanced ovarian cancer. Obstet Gynecol 59:583, 1982

75. Willcocks D, Toppila M, Hudson CN, et al: Estrogen and progesterone receptors in human ovarian tumor. Gynecol Oncol 16:246, 1983

76. Hochberg RB, Maclusky NJ, Chambers J, et al: Concentration of [16α-^{125}I] iodoestradiol in human ovarian tumors in vivo and correlation with estrogen receptor content. Steroids 46:775, 1985

77. Spona J, Gitsch E, Kubista E, et al: Enzyme immunoassay and Scatchard plot estimation of estrogen receptor in gynecological tumors. Cancer Res. 46(suppl.):4310, 1986

78. Gronroos M, Kangas L, Maenpaa J, et al: Steroid receptors and response of ovarian cancer to hormones in vitro. Br J Obstet Gynecol 91:472, 1984

79. Gronroos M, Kangas L, Maenpaa J, et al: Steroid receptors and response of ovarian cancer to cytostatic drugs in vitro. Br J Obstet Gynecol 91:479, 1984

80. Clark JH, Peck EJ Jr: Monographs on Endocrinology. Vol. 14. Springer-Verlag, New York, 1979

81. King WJ, DeSombre ER, Jensen EV, Greene GL: Comparison of cytochemical and steroid-binding assays for estrogen receptor in human breast cancer. Cancer Res 45:293, 1985

82. DeSombre ER, Thorpe SM, Rose C, et al: Prognostic usefulness of estrogen receptor immunocytochemical assays for human breast cancer. Cancer Res 46 (suppl):4256, 1986

83. Perrot-Applanat M, Logeat F, Groyer-Picard MT, Milgrom E: Immunocytochemical study of mammalian progesterone receptor using monoclonal antibodies. Endocrinology 116:1473, 1985

84. Mechanick JI, Peskin CS: Resolution of steroid binding heterogeneity by Fourier-derived affinity spectrum analysis (FASA). Anal Biochem 157:221, 1986

85. Holinka CF, Deligdisch L, Gurpide E: Histological evaluation of in vitro responses of endometrial adenocarcinoma to progestins and their relation to progesterone levels. Cancer Res 44:293, 1984

86. Markiewicz L, Gravanis A, Schatz F, Holinka CF, Deligdisch L, Gurpide E: Prostaglandin production by human endometrial adenocarcinoma in vitro. p. 420. In Baulieu EE, Iacobelli S, McGuire WL (eds): Endocrinology and Malignancy. Parthenon, Lancs, U.K., 1986

87. Robel P, Gravanis A, Roger-Jallais L, et al: Female sex steroid receptors i postmenopausal endometrial carcinoma. Biochemical responses to antiestrogen and progestin. p. 167. In Gurpide E, Calandra R, Levy C, Soto RJ (eds): Hormones and Cancer. Alan R. Liss, New York, 1984

88. McGuire WL, Dressler LG: Emerging impact flow cytometry in predicting recurrence and survival in breast cancer patients. J Natl Cancer Inst 75:405, 1985

89. Horwitz KB, McGuire WL, Pearson OH, Segaloff A: Predicting response to endocrine therapy in human breast cancer. A hypothesis. Science 189:726, 1975

90. Horwitz KB, Mockus MB, Lessey BA: Variant T47D human breast cancer cells with high progesterone receptor levels despite estrogen and antiestrogen resistance. Cell 28:633, 1982

91. Merenda C, Sordat B, Mach JP, Carrel S: Human endometrial carcinomas serially transplanted in nude mice and established in continuous cell lines. Int J Cancer 16:559, 1975

92. Satyaswaroop PG, Zaino RJ, Mortel R: Human endometrial adenocarcinoma transplanted into nude mice: growth regulation by estradiol. Science 219:58, 1983

5

Biostatistics

John A. Blessing

This chapter provides the clinician with a basic understanding of statistical concepts as they relate to scientific investigations in gynecologic cancer. It is not intended to eliminate the need for collaboration with a trained biostatistician but rather to foster meaningful dialogue when this interaction occurs. To that end, statistical issues such as probability distributions, confidence intervals, estimation, hypothesis testing, and P values are introduced and discussed in a fashion deliberately devoid of sophisticated mathematics.

Each of these topics is discussed in relationship to the primary vehicle for clinical investigation of gynecologic cancer, the clinical trial. Phase II and III trials will be introduced. Discussion of sample size requirements and false-positive and false-negative errors are featured in a presentation of study design. Following the completion of a study, the nuances of appropriate analysis and interpretation of results should be appreciated.

STATISTICAL CONCEPTS

Biostatistics may be visualized as an application of statistical methodology to biologic research. In order to discuss topics in biostatistics, it is necessary to introduce several basic statistical concepts. This presentation features a descriptive approach rather than a rigorous mathematical development.

Probability Distribution

In all scientific investigation, the outcome is typified by some degree of variability or uncertainty. The outcome of interest in the experiment is therefore called a *random variable*. Every random variable is governed by a *probability distribution*, which catalogs all possible outcomes and the associated probability of their occurrence. A random variable is termed *discrete* if the number of possible outcomes is finite. If the number of possible outcomes is not countable, the random variable is said to be *continuous*. In the clinical setting, tumor response is seen to be an example of a discrete random variable, while response duration and survival time are examples of continuous random variables. While the current topic does not necessitate an examination of each individual probability distribution, there are many distinct distributions. Determination of which probability distribution applies to a given experimental situation is essential if analyses are to be relevant.

Each probability distribution is actually a family of distributions. A given distribution is characterized by one or more *parameters,* which are constant for an individual application but which vary from application to application. In addition, the value of at least one parameter will usually be unknown.

As an example, suppose n independent binary trials (having only two possible outcomes) are conducted; the outcomes may be heads/tails, success/failure, response/nonresponse, and so forth. In clinical investigations, response/nonresponse is most frequently encountered. It is assumed that each trial has identical probability of success, P. The probability distribution that pertains to this experiment is called the *binomial distribution;* it has two parameters, n and P. Different binomial probability distributions are noted as the values of the parameters change. Generally, n is known, while the true value of P is unknown.

In conducting clinical research, it is seldom possible to test or treat all the subjects in a population. It is desirable to obtain a subset of the population, called a *sample,* and to use the accumulated information to make inferences regarding true, but unknown, population parameters. To do so, the investigator relies on the data gathered from the individual observations and employs a *statistic,* a function of the observations that does not depend on any unknown parameters.

Confidence Intervals and Estimation

One common practice employed to glean information from the sample or experiment is the construction of *confidence intervals.* Using properties of the relevant probability distribution, the appropriate statistic obtained from the sample, and statistical methodology, it is often possible to determine the points, l and u, such that it can be stated that the unknown parameter lies between l and u with a specified degree of confidence. The length of the confidence interval, l-u, can be predetermined, as can the degree of confidence; the required number of patients can then be determined.

Often it is preferable to develop an actual estimate of a parameter, rather than constructing an interval estimate. The statistic employed to do so is called an *estimator;* the actual realized value of the estimator is called an *estimate.* Intuitively, it would seem logical to employ sample means, variances, and proportions in order to estimate their population counterparts. Scientifically, these choices are warranted, as they possess the statistical properties sought in estimation.

Hypothesis Testing

In many situations, we will seek to test some hypothesis regarding the unknown parameter, rather than estimate it. In designing such an investigation, a *null hypothesis,* H_0, is determined and precisely stated. Often the null hypothesis implies no positive finding and the investigator hopes to be able to reject it. The null hypothesis must be tested against some *alternative hypothesis,* denoted by H_A. If H_0 implies no positive finding, H_A generally does imply one. It is essential that these hypotheses be formulated before the data are collected; that is, the data must not be employed to determine the research objectives.

Once the experiment has been conducted, the null hypothesis will either be accepted or rejected on the basis of the relevant test statistic. Table 5-1 shows that two types of error are possible. If the test statistic leads to rejection of H_0 when H_0 is actually true, the resulting error is known as a type I error. The erroneous rejection of H_0 (with its implied acceptance of H_A) is essentially a false endorsement of a positive result. Consequently, a type I error is often referred to as a *false-positive error.* Conversely, if H_0 is accepted and H_A is true, the result error is known as a *type II error,* or a *false-negative* error.

For a fixed sample it is not possible to minimize both types of error simultaneously. The probability of committing a type I error is fixed at some level α, called the *level* of *significance.* The probability of committing a type II error is denoted by β. The *power* of the test refers to the probability that a declared positive finding is really true (i.e., the probability of rejecting H_0 when it is false). It is readily seen to be equal to $1 - \beta$. In the clinical setting, common choices for α and β are 0.05 and 0.20, respectively. However, the actual values for a given situation should be determined through a consideration of the consequences of each type of error by medical and statistical collaborators. For example, a false-negative error rate of 0.20 might be intolerable if a potentially efficacious treat-

Table 5-1 Four Outcomes in a Test of Hypothesis

Reality	Decision	
	Accept H_0	Reject H_0
H_0 true	Correct decision	Type I error (false-positive)
H_0 false	Type II error (false-negative)	Correct decision

ment regimen could be erroneously abandoned and never investigated again.

Alternative hypotheses may be either one-sided or two-sided, depending on the current status of the disease entity being investigated. If a study is designed to compare the proportion of observed responses noted with two distinct chemotherapy regimens, A and B, the respective proportions would be denoted P_A and P_B. If there is no reason to believe that regimen A would be superior to regimen B, the appropriate test of hypothesis would be

$$H_0: \quad P_A = P_B$$

versus

$$H_A: \quad P_B > P_A \quad \text{one-sided alternative}$$

Figure 5-1 depicts the schema of the Gynecologic

Oncology Group (GOG) Protocol 60. The two treatments differed only by the presence of bacillus Calmette-Guérin (BCG) in one regimen. It did not seem likely that the addition of BCG would diminish the response rate. Consequently, a one-sided alternative was used.

If it appears likely that either regimen could prove superior to the other, the appropriate test of hypothesis would be

$$H_0: \quad P_A = P_B$$

versus

$$H_A: \quad P_A \neq P_B \quad \text{two-sided alternative}$$

Figure 5-2 displays the schema of GOG protocol 77. This study featured a comparison of two platinum analogues. At the time of study design, there was no

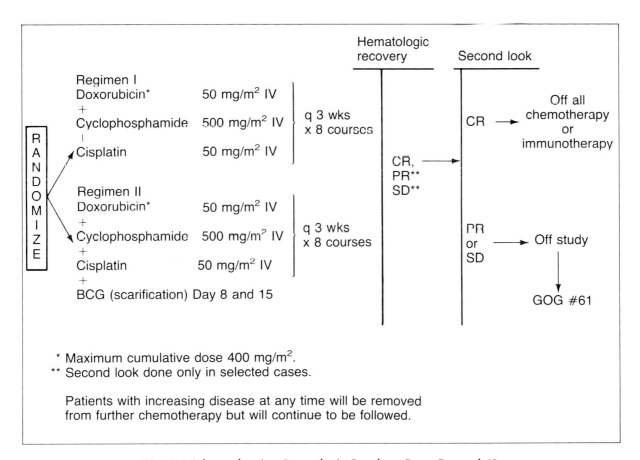

Fig. 5-1 Schema showing Gynecologic Oncology Group Protocol 60.

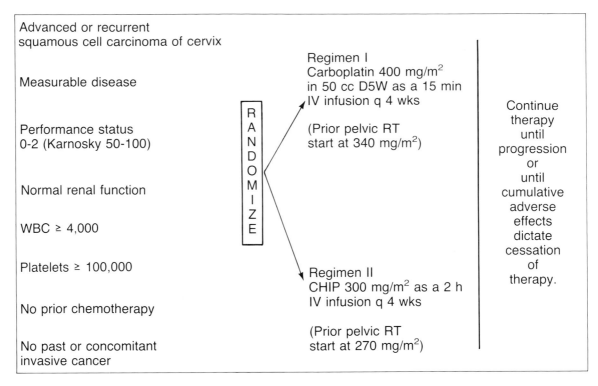

Fig. 5-2 Schema showing Gynecologic Oncology Group Protocol 77.

reason to speculate that one particular agent was superior to the other. Thus, a two-sided alternative was employed.

Having specified null and alternative hypotheses, specified appropriate values of α and β, and determined required sample size, the study is then conducted. At the conclusion, the appropriate test statistic is calculated. If the data are not consistent with H_0, it will be rejected; otherwise, H_0 will be accepted.

P Values

It has been determined that H_0 will be rejected if the data are not consistent with this hypothesis. How is it determined whether the data are consistent with H_0? We recall that a test statistic will be calculated. This statistic is some mathematical function of the observed data and is therefore a random variable itself. As such, probabilities regarding its outcome may be calculated. Of specific interest is the probability of observing data at least as inconsistent with the null

hypothesis as that which was observed, if the null hypothesis is actually true. This is the so-called *P* value familiar to most clinician-researchers. The smaller the *P* value is, the stronger the evidence is that the data are not compatible with H_0. It has become customary to present "significant" results with accompanying *P* values. In reality, a null hypothesis of no difference has been rejected because the experimental data do not support this conjecture; the *P* value depicts how likely it is that one could observe such data (or data more discrepant from H_0) if there is, in fact, no real difference.

CLINICAL TRIALS

It is not particularly uncommon for a clinician involved in the treatment of gynecologic malignancies to develop research interests and begin to collect patient data. Medical literature is saturated with case studies and small series of patients. The difficult task lies in conducting research in such a fashion that the applicability of the results extends beyond those who were treated. For example, if a small number of patients with recurrent squamous cell carcinoma of the cervix are treated with a new chemotherapeutic agent, the value of this research hinges on the ability to make appropriate inferences regarding the efficacy of this therapy for the population of patients suffering from this disease. Thus, merely collecting and summarizing patient data will not suffice; rigorous precise scientific investigation is necessary.

If one wishes to generate clinical data to ascertain the therapeutic efficacy of a particular mode of therapy on a given population, the *clinical trial* is the appropriate vehicle. Before the study is undertaken, a background of the disease entity must be summarized, a rationale for the current approach provided, objectives clearly stated, the treatment plan unambiguously detailed, data to be collected noted, and the number of patients to be treated specified. It is this latter facet that will ensure that the study will generate more than anecdotal information.

Several types of clinical trials are employed in therapeutic investigation. If trials in human subjects are warranted, an initial study, called phase I, will be initiated to determine the optimal dose and schedule of administration. Once an appropriate dose and schedule are determined, a phase II study is developed to examine tumor response and associated adverse effects. Such a study must be well conceived and soundly designed, as the results will dictate whether further study is warranted. If it appears that the response rate of the new agent is potentially higher than that of the standard therapy, or that the frequency of observed adverse effects may be reduced via the new agent, a definitive comparative study should be performed. A phase III study is a controlled clinical trial that compares a new potentially efficacious treatment regimen with the current standard mode of therapy. Treatment allocation should be random to promote comparable patient composition in each regimen and avoid bias (whether intentional or unintentional). This will help guarantee that any detected difference can only be ascribed to the agents themselves. Further descriptions of the various types of clinical trials are found in the reports by Gehan and Schneiderman[1] and Blessing.[2] The Phase II and phase III studies will be examined in more detail.

Phase II Trials

In attempting to evaluate new chemotherapeutic agents the primary outcome variable is objective response. Since this is a binary random variable (one having only two possible outcomes — response or nonresponse) and since the treatment of individual patients constitutes independent trials, we are sampling from a binomial distribution, characterized by two parameters: the number of trials, n, and the true probability of getting a response, P. Typically n is predetermined, while P is unknown. The purpose of the investigation is to obtain information regarding P. The accuracy of the resulting information is dependent on n. Thus a key concept in any phase II study is sample size determination, that is, the number of patients that will be treated.

One method of procedure involves determining a *confidence interval* about the observed response rate. Using basic statistical properties of the binomial distribution, it can be determined that to have 90 percent confidence that the observed probability of response is within $\pm$ 10 percent of the true population, probability of response requires 68 patients. If it is sufficient to be within $\pm$ 15 percent of the true value of P, only 30 patients are required. Similarly, the sample size will increase if the degree of confidence is increased from 90 percent. These are but a few of many possibilities. They serve to underscore two important points. First, there is a definite need for statistical-medical interaction before undertaking a phase II study. The degree of precision must be determined on the basis of the medical realities of the disease entity being investigated and available patient resources. Second, the required number of patients in these examples emphasizes the lack of credibility of journal publications featuring small numbers of cases.

Although the investigator should avoid directing research toward a collection of anecdotes, it is also wise to avoid the temptation to strive for excessive precision. The need for accuracy must be balanced with the ability to test new agents both promptly and efficiently. Consequently, it is advisable to strive for 90 percent confidence of being within $\pm$ 15 percent of the true probability. The required 30 patients facilitates a reasonable estimation of efficacy, yet permits the desired timeliness of the evaluation process.

It has become customary to build early stopping rules into the design of phase II studies. If an agent is found to be ineffective early in the study, valuable patient resources will not be wasted by continuing to the original accrual goal. The intention is laudable and the necessity of this consideration is also noted from an ethical viewpoint. However, it is essential that a thorough understanding of the use and consequence of early stopping be imparted by a trained statistician. The use of stopping rules generally requires a test of hypothesis approach, rather than a confidence interval scheme.

One such mechanism was developed by Gehan.[3] However, it is generally misunderstood, with most clinicians believing that observing 0 responses among the first 14 patients treated is always an indication for early stopping. Based on properties of the binomial distribution, Gehan stated if an agent "were 20 percent effective or more, there would be more than a 95 percent chance that one or more successes would be obtained in 14 consecutive cases." Thus, this criterion is reasonable if the response rate hypothesized is 20 percent. Other situations require different stopping rules.

Another phase II design currently in vogue is the so-called multiple testing procedure described in Flemming.[4] One determines P_o the largest responsibility, which if true implies that the agent does not warrant further study and P_A the smallest response probability which if true implies therapeutic efficacy. The hypotheses being tested are as follows:

$$H_0: \quad P \leq P_o$$

versus

$$H_A: \quad P \geq P_A$$

An initial number of patients are treated and followed. If the observed response rate is negligible, H_0 is accepted; no further cases are entered and the therapy abandoned. If the observed response rate is particularly high, no additional patients are required to demonstrate efficacy. However, if the observed response rate falls within a predetermined gray area, additional patients are then treated to obtain additional information, and the test of hypothesis is repeated. Here again, the input of the statistician will enable the appropriate study to be designed.

When dealing with gynecologic malignancies, care must be taken to address homogenous populations in phase II studies. It is not appropriate to lump many distinct populations into one group. For purposes of conducting phase II trials, each of the following cancers should be treated as a separate population and investigated in separate studies: epithelial tumors of the ovary, squamous cell carcinoma of the cervix, nonsquamous cell carcinoma of the cervix, mixed mesodermal sarcoma, leiomyosarcoma, carcinoma of the uterus, vulvar malignancies, and carcinoma of the vagina.

Phase III Studies

The cornerstone on which phase III studies must be built is feasibility. A blend of mathematical practicality and medical relevance must be sought. Seeking very large treatment differences may yield statistically feasible studies, but there must be sufficient medical rationale to indicate some hope that such a difference exists. Conversely, seeking to establish extremely small differences will require a very large number of patients to the extent that sufficient patients are not available. Even if the patient supply is abundant, one must consider whether such a difference would constitute a significant clinical finding; in addition to having sufficient patients to conduct a study, there must be sufficient reason to carry it out. Detection of 15 to 20 percent differences is most commonly sought. Sample size determination is another critical area in which interaction between clinician and statistician is essential.

If the primary outcome variable is objective tumor response, we may consider this variable to be binary; in gynecologic investigations, it is preferable to examine complete response. However, this discussion pertains equally well to examinations of responders (complete and partial combined). Sample size determination depends on four factors:

1. The magnitude of the difference considered clinically significant to detect: Verification of the existence of smaller differences requires a larger number of patients than detection of larger differences.
2. The baseline response rate of the standard therapy: Detection of the same magnitude of difference, requires more patients if the baseline is close to 50 percent than if it is at one extreme.
3. Values chosen for the probabilities of false-positive and false-negative errors: To decrease both simultaneously requires increased sample size.
4. The type of alternative hypothesis: If all other fac-

tors are held constant, two-sided alternatives require more patients than one-sided alternatives.

To depict how these four factors interact, Table 5-2 presents the number of patients requires in each regimen to demonstrate a 15 percent treatment difference for various levels of combination of factors 2 through 4. These figures are based on the methodology of Cochran and Cox.[5] It is readily seen that the number of patients required to document the existence of a 15 percent difference (if one exists) varies substantially as different constraints are imposed. Nonetheless, even the most lenient criterion depicted requires 76 patients per treatment regimen. This should provide a clear indication of the triviality of many published comparisons of small numbers of patients.

Time variables, such as survival, progression-free interval, and response duration, are continuous random variables. In addition, longer periods of patient follow-up are required to document the outcome of this variable. Thus, at any moment in time, many observations may be censored (alive, disease-free, or in response). Studies designed to compare therapeutic efficacy in terms of time variables therefore differ dramatically from those based on response comparisons. Nonetheless, there are parallels; the size of the difference in median survival and α and β must be specified. The statistical methodology is cumbersome and not at all intuitive. George and Desu[6] defined the number of observed failures (not entries) required in each regimen to observe a significant difference in

Table 5-2 Number of Patients Required in Each Regimen to Detect a 15 Percent Treatment Difference[a]

Difference (%)	β	Number of Patients	
		One-Sided	Two-Sided
10–25	0.20	76	96
	0.10	105	130
	0.05	195	220
25–40	0.20	120	150
	0.10	165	200
	0.05	300	340
40–55	0.20	135	175
	0.10	190	230
	0.05	350	390

[a] $\alpha = 0.05$.

Table 5-3 Number of Failures Required in Each Regimen to Detect a 50 Percent Improvement in Median Survival

α	β		
	0.20	0.10	0.05
0.05	76	105	132
0.01	123	159	193

two survival distributions. An increase in the median survival of the standard therapy by 50 percent in the experimental group requires 76 to 193 failures (and a larger number of entries) per regimen, depending on choices of α and β (Table 5-3). Publications making dramatic conclusions (or any conclusion) based upon a small number of patients, must be viewed with considerable skepticism.

Designing a Clinical Trial

Having decided to embark on clinical research, how does the investigator proceed? In preparation for designing a scientific study, a literature search should be undertaken to verify the state-of-the art of treatment in the disease category of interest. Objectives of the study can then be set forth. In designing a trial to address these goals, early interaction with a statistician trained in clinical trials is crucial. This will enhance the likelihood of sound design, meaningful data to analyze, and unambiguous results.

One of the first issues to resolve is the nature of the study. That is, are the study objectives best addressed in a phase II or phase III setting? In almost all instances, phase II testing of new agents is accomplished prior to use in phase III trials.

If a phase II study is indicated, it must be determined whether a confidence interval, parameter estimation, or hypothesis testing approach will be taken. If a confidence interval is employed, a degree of confidence and the desired width of the interval must be specified. Likewise, a degree of precision should be specified in estimating parameters. If hypothesis testing is used, the null and alternative hypothesis must be explicitly defined as well as the desired values of α and β. Sample size can then be calculated and a determination made regarding the feasibility of the study.

In phase II trials the intent is generally to determine whether sufficient activity is observed to warrant further study. Precise estimation of the true response rate is therefore usually not the primary goal. Rather, there is interest in determining whether the true response rate exceeds some minimal value associated with the response rate of standard therapy. It must be stressed, however, that the phase II trial is not a vehicle with which to conduct a formal comparison between a new agent and the standard therapy; it is merely a method of screening new agents for potential efficacy.) Thus, the common phase II approach employs hypothesis testing to screen new agents expeditiously but uses estimation if more detailed information is required.

An example will help clarify why the phase II study is best suited for screening, rather than estimation. The Gynecologic Oncology Group (GOG) conducted a phase II trial of cisplatin at 50 mg/m^2 given every 3 weeks in patients with recurrent squamous cell carcinoma of the cervix. Thigpen et al.[7] reported the results of this study, which had produced 11 responses in 25 patients. The observed 44 percent re-

sponse rate was considered a definite sign of therapeutic efficacy and a clear indication for further study. However, the observed response rate was based only on 25 patients; consequently, a 90 percent confidence interval for the true response rate was defined by the interval from 25 percent to 61 percent.

In summary, this trial unambiguously demonstrated activity, which was the intent of the study, but did little to estimate precisely the true response rate. As a result of this trial, the GOG initiated Protocol 43 to compare three different regimens of cisplatin. The schema for this study is shown in Figure 5-3. One of the three regimens was the previously studied regimen of 50 mg/m^2 every 3 weeks. The observed response rate in 150 patients evaluated on this regimen was 21 percent. Reporting for the GOG, Bonomi et al.[8] states:

The 21 percent response rate observed in 150 patients treated with Regimen I confirms the fact that cisplatin is

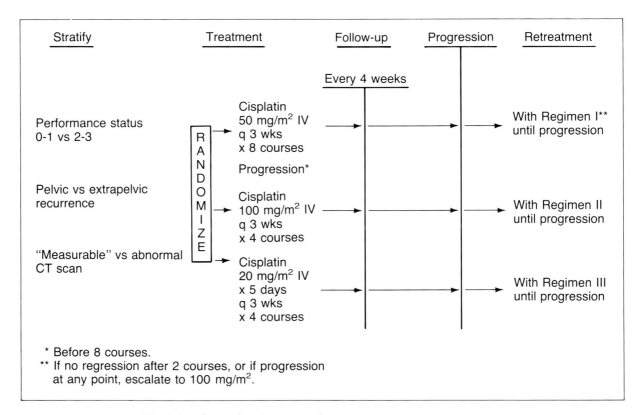

Fig. 5-3 Schema showing Gynecologic Oncology Group Protocol 43.

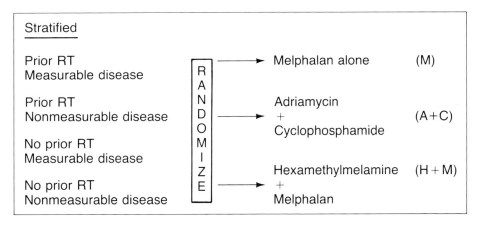

Stratified

Prior RT
Measurable disease

Prior RT
Nonmeasurable disease

No prior RT
Measurable disease

No prior RT
Nonmeasurable disease

R A N D O M I Z E

Melphalan alone   (M)

Adriamycin
+   (A+C)
Cyclophosphamide

Hexamethylmelamine   (H + M)
+
Melphalan

Fig. 5-4 Schema showing Gynecologic Oncology Group Protocol 22.

one of the most active drugs in squamous cell cervical cancer. The difference between the response rates observed in the two studies emphasizes the importance of the evaluation of new regimens in a large-scale trial.

If a phase III comparative study is indicated, the primary outcome variable must be determined, and suitable null and alternative hypotheses must be specified. Response or other discrete random variables are vastly different from survival or other continuous random variables. Nonetheless, in either instance, the probability of false-positive and false-negative errors, the baseline response or survival data, and the magnitude of the difference being sought must be specified. At this time, careful consideration must be given to the suitability of a one-sided or a two-sided alternative hypothesis. The sample size necessary to address the question can then be determined, and a decision can be reached regarding study feasibility. In instances in which more than one study objective is addressed, the sample size required to address the individual objectives will need to be determined. The larger number of patients will be required if each goal is to be addressed.

One last example will depict the logic of study design and the interrelationship of phase II and phase III studies. During the early 1970s, the GOG initiated Protocol 3, which compared melphalan with three combination chemotherapy regimens in advanced ovarian cancer. Park et al.[9] reported no advantage for the combinations, but less toxicity with melphalan, which therefore became the standard therapy. At that

time, Parker et al.[10] reported an 83 percent response rate using Adriamycin plus cyclophosphamide for previously untreated patients in an uncontrolled study. In a pilot study, Omura saw indications of possible activity using a combination of hexamethylmelamine and melphalan (GA Omura, unpublished data). Thus, the GOG designed Protocol 22 (Fig. 5-4). After statistically adjusting for the distribution of cell type and grade, the clinical response rate for Adriamycin plus cyclophosphamide was significantly ($P = 0.04$) higher (32 percent) than for melphalan (20 percent). However, survival was not appreciably improved.[11] Nonetheless, the improved complete response rate led to Adriamycin + cyclophosphamide as the standard therapy. At this time, Thigpen et al.[12] reported the results of a GOG phase II trial of cisplatin in patients with advanced ovarian carcinoma. This agent was found to be active. Also, Ehrlich et al.[13] indicated in a preliminary report that the addition of cisplatin to Adriamycin + cyclophosphamide constituted an active three-drug treatment regimen. Thus, the GOG developed Protocol 47 (schema shown in Fig. 5-5) to compare the two-drug regimen with cisplatin–Adriamycin–cyclophosphamide. As noted by Omura et al.[14] the overall complete response rate for the three-drug regimen was significantly ($P < 0.0001$) higher than for the two-drug approach (26 percent). Consequently, cisplatin–Adriamycin–cyclophosphamide became the standard therapy. Following an indication that the addition of bacillus Calmette-Guérin (BCG) to the standard regimen might enhance the

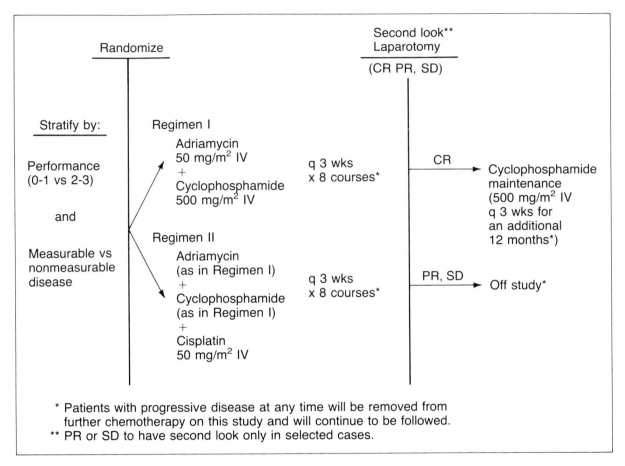

Fig. 5-5 Schema showing Gynecologic Oncology Group Protocol 47.

results, the GOG designed Protocol 60 in an attempt to compare cisplatin–Adriamycin–cyclophosphamide with the same three agents plus BCG (see Fig. 5-1). The study is not yet complete. Through careful planning the results of institutional pilot studies, cooperative group phase II and phase III studies have meshed together in a scientific fashion.

Once the study design is established, several other aspects must be addressed:

1. Precise eligibility criteria must be explicitly stated. In gynecologic investigations, particular attention should be paid to histology and stage. For example, stage III optimal and stage III suboptimal are two different ovarian populations that should generally not be lumped together. Likewise, squamous cell carcinoma of the cervix should be examined separately from other cervical lesions, as is the case with mixed mesodermal sarcomas and leiomyosarcomas.

2. The treatment plan must be well described. This includes not just dose and schedule but the nature of modifications and when they will occur as well.

3. Precise definitions of evaluation criteria must be given. If the study is to have any relevance, the measurement of results must be consistent with, as well as comparable to, those employed by other scientists.

4. The tests to be performed and measurements to be obtained must be clearly stated to foster comparable data for all patients.

5. Any other relevant information must be clarified prior to initiation of the study, including definition of surgical procedures, toxicity criteria, and other relevant factors.

Analysis of a Clinical Trial

It is by no means possible to introduce and describe all statistical methods of analysis that pertain to clinical trials. However, it is necessary to document the existence of several to emphasize the complexity of this issue. In this era of computerization, many scientists have access to computer software which features statistical programs. The results are extremely error prone if the user is not well versed in the underlying assumptions that determine whether specific types of analysis are appropriate. The clinician will often consider the program close enough to use, much like putting a screw in with a hammer. A more realistic analogy would often be putting a pane of glass in with a hammer.

ANALYSIS OF TUMOR RESPONSE DATA

Suppose an investigator has conducted a well-designed phase III study to compare the response rate of two chemotherapeutic regimens. The true response rates for the two regimens are denoted by P_1 and P_2. If a two-sided alternative is warranted, the appropriate hypotheses are

$$H_0: \quad P_1 = P_2$$

versus

$$H_A: \quad P_1 \neq P_2$$

In consultation with a biostatistician, it was determined that the study was feasible and that n patients would be required in each regimen. Probabilities of type I and II error were set at α and β, respectively.

The data from such a study are frequently presented in a *contingency table,* a cross-classification of the observations with respect to two variables, in this case treatment and response. A typical example is displayed in Table 5-4.

A test statistic is employed that has a chi-square probability distribution. H_0 can be readily tested. This situation is common; it would not be difficult to find computer software to conduct this elementary analysis, if it is appropriate. In practice, the situation is often much more complex. Information will also be available on other variables that may have some bearing on outcome. Examples include stage, histology, prior therapy, performance status, and age, to name a few. These are known as *prognostic factors.* It is hoped that randomization will permit both treatment regimens to have a similar patient composition with regard to these prognostic variables, but this is never guaranteed. If it appears that there are prognostic variables that must be considered, analysis becomes quite complex. To be sure, there are statistical techniques to employ, but can the casual user distinguish among regression, linear regression, multiple regression, and the multiple logistic model? In the situation described earlier, the multiple logistic model applies. An example of the need for this type of analysis is seen in the GOG Protocol 22. The complete response rate for the melphalan and Adriamycin plus Cytoxan regimens are shown in Table 5-5.

Omura et al.[11] stated:

> These results are not in themselves significantly different. However, there was some variation (not significant) in response by grade of tumor and by cell type. Moreover, there was some variation (also not significant) in the distribution of these features by treatment arm.

Thus, the role of prognostic factors cell type, grade, stage, prior radiotherapy, and age was examined. Only cell type and grade were of significance. Omura and co-workers further stated:

> When the results were simultaneously adjusted for distribution of grade and cell type (Cox's method), there was a significant advantage in complete response rate of A + C ($P = .04$) compared with M.

Table 5-4 Example of a Contingency Table

Response Classification	Treatment		Total
	Regimen 1	Regimen 2	
Responders	r_1	r_2	$r_1 + r_2$
Nonresponders	$17_1 - r_1$	$n_2 - r_2$	$(n_1 + n_2) - (r_1 + r_2)$
Total	n_1	n_2	$N_1 + n_2$

Table 5-5 Response by Regimen for M and A + C Arms of Gynecologic Oncology Group Protocol 22

Response Category	Regimen		Total
	M	A + C	
Complete Response	13	23	36
Other	51	49	100
Total	64	72	136

A, Adriamycin; C, cyclophosphamide.
M, melphalan.

In summary, a statistically significant therapeutic gain in complete response rate would have gone undetected if mere elementary analysis was used.

How complex are the multivariate techniques employed and how well are they understood? Omura's paper, when submitted for publication, was criticized by reviewers who interpreted the results as statistical manipulation. It was accepted after a response to this critique was written, which attempted to educate the journal reviewers. The methodology did not create the difference artificially; it removed a camouflage that would have otherwise obscured a true difference.

ANALYSIS OF SURVIVAL DATA

As was the case with tumor response, analysis of survival time can be accomplished via many available computer programs. However, different programs feature different test statistics with different probability distributions. It is therefore possible to find a significant difference via one method that is not considered significant via different methodology. It is essential to determine the appropriate methodology and inappropriate to "shop for significance" by employing various methods. In addition, it is quite possible for prognostic factors to influence the results. This must be examined in the analysis.

In GOG Protocol 47, Omura et al.[14] employed a Cox model

> to analyze the effect of treatment . . . adjusting for the influence of possible prognostic variables: stage, age, GOG performance status, grade and histology. Relation of this original set of variables was accomplished using a standard step-down technique. This resulted in three statistically significant prognostic variables: age, GOG performance status, and histology.

In this instance, the significant results which were found with simplistic analysis were reinforced by the multivariate techniques.

TIMING OF CLINICAL TRIAL ANALYSIS

As stated by Blessing and Anderson,[15] "When and how often a clinical trial is analyzed is as important as the use of appropriate methodology." We have seen that a substantial number of patients are necessary to obtain meaningful results in a clinical trial. Consequently, it is only logical that premature analysis can produce results that will vary greatly from the final analysis. Blessing and Anderson displayed the incidence of grade 4 leukopenia at various time points for patients with advanced endometrial carcinoma treatment with Adriamycin and cyclophosphamide according to GOG Protocol 48 (schema shown in Fig. 5-6). Eighteen months after activation, a premature analysis would have indicated no incidence of this adverse effect. However, examined yearly thereafter, the percentage of such cases continually rose, until final analysis demonstrated 11 patients of 108 (10 percent) experiencing grade 4 leukopenia. Thus, the true incidence would have been underestimated if results were disseminated early.

Another, example of the possible pitfalls of early analysis is exhibited by the GOG Protocol 43. This study was designed to seek a 15 percent difference in response rates among the three cisplatin regimens. One year after activation, a nonsignificant difference in response rates of 21.7 percent was present. This result was based upon a small number of patients. Four years later, the appropriate analysis demonstrated an actual difference of only 11.1 percent. In this instance, premature analysis would have proclaimed apparent dramatic findings that were subsequently not verified.

Survival curves are heavily weighted by early deaths until both substantial entries and reasonable follow-up are obtained. Moreover, a longer period of time is required to observe the outcomes than is necessary for tumor response and documentation of adverse effects. Premature analysis of survival can easily lead to an erroneous conclusion of treatment equivalence, which may preclude a subsequent appropriate analysis demonstrating some therapeutic effect.

Early presentation of results is a likely source of

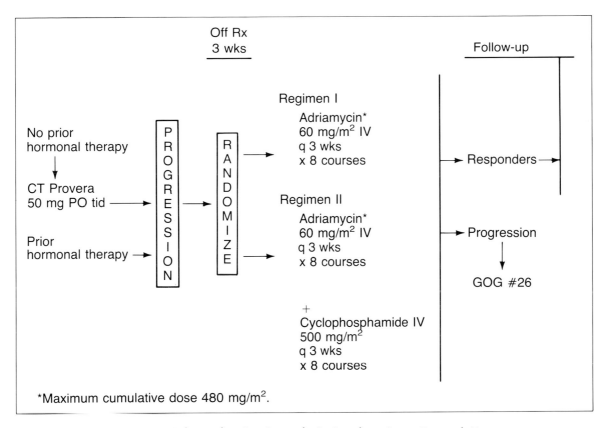

Off Rx
3 wks

Follow-up

No prior
hormonal therapy

CT Provera
50 mg PO tid

Prior
hormonal therapy

P R O G R E S S I O N

R A N D O M I Z E

Regimen I
Adriamycin*
60 mg/m² IV
q 3 wks
x 8 courses

Regimen II
Adriamycin*
60 mg/m² IV
q 3 wks
x 8 courses

+
Cyclophosphamide IV
500 mg/m²
q 3 wks
x 8 courses

Responders

Progression

GOG #26

*Maximum cumulative dose 480 mg/m².

Fig. 5-6 Schema showing Gynecologic Oncology Group Protocol 48.

investigator bias, which can jeopardize the study or taint the results. Perceived, but unfounded, differences may easily dampen enthusiasm for investigations leading to insufficient accrual and decreasing the likelihood of completion. In this fashion, unproved differences may be proclaimed, thereby misdirecting future areas of investigation.

While the data must not be analyzed or presented prematurely, ethical considerations require that ongoing results be monitored. This should be done to the extent required to ensure therapeutic efficacy and safety; conclusions should neither be drawn nor presented on the basis of study monitoring.

Repeated analyses are also of concern. If therapeutic comparisons are repeatedly done and statistical significance is eventually obtained, the true merit of this finding would have to be questioned. When testing a hypothesis, the probability of committing a false-positive error on any one of these is α; the probability of

committing a false-positive error on at least one comparison is greater than α. Peto et al.[16] noted that if α were fixed at 0.05 and a comparison were made on five occasions, "the chance that you will publish a 'significant ($P < .05$) difference' in a trial comparing two regimens which are, in fact, identical is probably more like 15% than the 5% which was claimed." If repeated analyses have been conducted, it would be advisable to require smaller P values before proclaiming significant differences.

Interpretation of Clinical Trials

Following the proper design, conduct, and analysis of a clinical trial, it is time to interpret the results and disseminate this information through publication. The principles espoused for the interpretation of one's own data can be equally well applied to the understanding of other journal articles.

THE PHASE II STUDY

It is alarming how frequently dramatic results with new agents are not reproducible. It has been stated many times that perhaps it does not matter what therapy a patient receives as long as he or she is one of the first 20 patients treated with a new drug. Although this statement is facetious, it does underscore the fact that there is growing concern over the inconsistency of initial trials with subsequent results.

A partial explanation is the penchant investigators have for excluding patients who did not receive a minimum number of courses, whose therapy was reduced because of therapy-related adverse effects, who died within a certain period of time from the onset of therapy, and so forth. To ensure comparable evaluation of all agents, it is recommended that any patient who received at least one course of therapy and for whom follow-up is available be considered evaluable. Excluding from analysis any patients who received therapy leads to inflated estimates of efficacy.

Another possible source of error is investigator bias. In an overzealous effort to confirm suspected positive findings, it is easy for investigators to rationalize not treating certain eligible patients they consider poor candidates. It is essential that all eligible patients seen be entered on study and treated, if data are to be representative of the population.

Finally, criteria for response determination must be explicitly stated and adhered to. The use of standard response definitions is essential in interpreting observed response rates. Typical responses may be classified as follows:

1. *Complete response:* disappearance of all gross evidence of disease for at least 4 weeks
2. *Partial response:* a 50 percent or greater reduction in the product of the largest diameter and its perpendicular of each lesion for at least 4 weeks

3. *Increasing disease:* a 50 percent or greater increase in the product of the largest diameter and its perpendicular of any lesion documented within 8 weeks of study entry or the appearance of any new lesion within 8 weeks of entry into study
4. *Stable disease:* disease not meeting any of the above three criteria

The use of such classifications as minimal response or stable disease as indications of efficacy is unwarranted and leads to overestimation of response rates.

THE NEGATIVE STUDY

The basic premise on which clinical research conducted is the hope of finding some positive result that will enhance patient care. Unfortunately, designing and conducting a study capable of detecting a positive result does not guarantee that one exists. Studies in which a significant finding is not proclaimed are often termed negative studies. In truth, the negative finding is much more limited in scope than is generally appreciated. It certainly does not state that no therapeutic difference exists. Rather, a difference of at least the magnitude considered clinically significant to detect when the study was designed does not exist. The possibility that a smaller difference might exist cannot be ruled out. The study was not designed to detect such differences and realistically should not address the issue. The negative finding should be presented within the context of the original study design.

Gynecologic Oncology Group Protocol 48 was designed to investigate whether the addition of cyclophosphamide to Adriamycin would improve the response rate over that noted for Adriamycin alone in patients with advanced carcinoma of the endometrium. Recent analysis by Thigpen et al.[17] yielded the response findings summarized in Table 5-6.

Table 5-6 Gynecologic Oncology Group Protocol 48 Response by Treatment

Response Category	Treatment		Total
	A	A + C	
Responders (%)	22 (22%)	34 (32%)	56
Nonresponders (%)	75	71	146
Total	97	105	202

A, Adriamycin; A + C, Adriamycin + cyclophosphamide.

It was determined that a 20 percent difference in response rates did not exist. The existence of a true 10 percent treatment difference cannot be determined from this study since it was not designed to detect differences smaller than 20 percent. (Had the study sought a 10 percent or greater difference, sample size requirements would have been 249 patients per regimen.) Thus, it is not possible to comment on the significance of the observed difference. By contrast, it is erroneous to state that "no therapeutic difference exists." It can only be concluded that a 20 percent difference does not exist.

Results must always be interpreted in the context of the study objectives. Under no circumstances should the objectives be altered to fit the findings. An interesting example is seen by returning to GOG Protocol 43. It was designed to detect a 15 percent or greater difference in response rates. When final analysis of the study was conducted a difference of 10.7 percent in overall response rates was noted between two of the treatment regimens. Because the number of evaluable patients in the study was larger than originally intended, this observed difference was statistically significant. Nonetheless, in designing the study, 15 percent was determined to be the minimum difference considered clinically significant to be detected. It would have been inappropriate to disregard this fact and proclaim a significant finding. Bonomi et al.[8] presented the results within the proper context: "The difference in response rates for regimens 1 and 2 is statistically significant ($P = 0.015$) but less than the magnitude originally considered clinically significant)."

It must also be repeated that if a significant result is not proclaimed, there is an inherent possibility of committing a false-negative error. It is currently popular to choose $\beta = 0.20$. This is an appropriate choice in most instances. Nonetheless, it should be understood that in such a design, proclamation of no significant difference stands a 1 in 5 chance of being wrong.

Perhaps the most grievous error with regard to negative studies is found in poorly designed studies in which no formal hypothesis is stated, no sample size determined, and no specification of α and β made. Often data are collected and comparisons made, with treatment equivalence proclaimed on the basis of such studies. The likelihood of error is high. Yet such studies are readily accepted and published by medical journals typically lacking in statistical review to complement medical peer review. It is again emphasized that lack of a significant finding, even in a well-designed study, does not endorse treatment equivalence.

THE POSITIVE STUDY

If the results of the study indicate a positive finding, it is customary to accompany the results with the appropriate P value. Recall that this value gives the probability of observing data as disparate from H_0 as was observed, if there is in fact no such difference. This is reiterated, as many investigators operate under the false assumption that the P value gives the probability that the stated difference does not exist. Also, if repeated analyses have occurred, the P value is a misrepresentation. In reading other articles, one should view P values between 0.03 and 0.05 somewhat skeptically, if it seems likely that multiple analyses have been used.

Finally, although clinical investigators tend to worship at the altar of 0.05, it is important to guard against too great a dependence on P values. Mathematical significance without clinical significance is of little significance!

An example documenting the unreliability of early analysis of time variable data is appropriate. The GOG recently completed a phase III study comparing two treatment regimens. The study was an appropriately designed randomized comparison of two chemotherapeutic agents. It was conducted to completion, and adequate follow-up was obtained and thoroughly analyzed. To facilitate a presentation of misleading interim results, the study is not identified. The appropriate final results did not demonstrate a significant advantage of one regimen over the other.

During the course of the study, results were monitored, but therapeutic comparisons were not undertaken. Copies of chronologic data files were preserved. To illustrate the present topic, graphs of progression-free interval have been constructed at various time points following activation. Figure 5-7 displays the duration of progression-free interval approximately 18 months following activation of the study. The curves are based on only 25 and 33 patients, respectively; they *appear* to indicate a potential superiority of regimen II over regimen I, with median durations of 3.4 and 7.6 months, respectively. Six months later, the difference between the regimens is less pronounced, but still noted (Fig. 5-8). This analy-

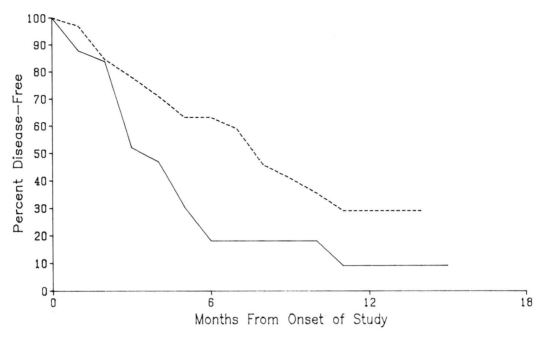

Fig. 5-7 Duration of progression-free interval by treatment. Premature analysis at 18 months. (——) Regimen I: free, 7; failures, 18; total, 25; median, 3.4 (----) Regimen II: free, 15; failures, 18; total, 33; median, 7.6.

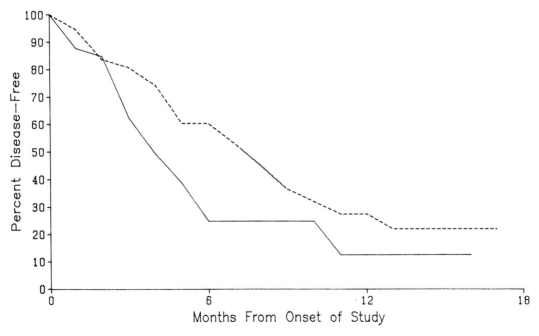

Fig. 5-8 Duration of progression-free interval by treatment. Premature analysis at 24 months. (——) Regimen I: free, 10; failures, 23; total, 33; median 3.9. (----) Regimen II: free, 15; failures, 22; total, 37; median 7.3.

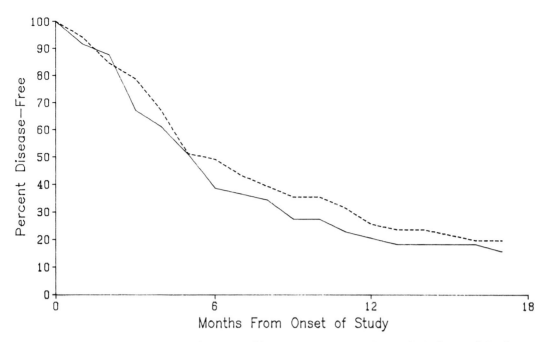

Fig. 5-9 Duration of progression-free interval by treatment. Appropriate analysis. (———) Regimen I: free, 7; failures, 45; total, 52; median, 4.9. (----) Regimen II: free, 9; failures, 46; total, 55; median 5.0.

sis is based on 33 and 37 patients and median durations now at 3.9 and 7.3 months, respectively. Figure 5-9 shows the same comparison with yet another 6-month patient accrual and follow-up. This analysis is based on 52 and 55 patients in the two respective regimens. Note that the previously observed differences have disappeared. Median duration of progression-free interval for the two regimens is 4.9 and 5.0 months, respectively. It is emphasized that Figures 5-7 and 5-8 do not reflect appropriate analyses and were presented merely to illustrate the problems that can arise from premature analysis.

TIME-VARIABLE CURVES

It has been demonstrated that graphs of time variables can prove very misleading if the analysis is premature. It is also true that appropriate analyses of time variables are frequently misunderstood because of the tails of the curves. Time-variable curves are commonly superimposed for several years and then separate. Investigators frequently believe that this represents some delayed therapeutic advantage. In truth, the tails of the curves usually represent few patients,

hence are subject to considerable fluctuation. Subsequent individual failures may change this portion of the curve dramatically. Emphasis must be given to the early part of the curve, which is based on most of the patients.

As an example, Figure 5-10 presents actual unpublished data depicting a treatment comparison of survival for two treatment regimens. Although the curves appear to diverge beyond 18 months, the difference is not significant ($P > 0.40$). Moreover, of 70 patients involved in this analysis, only 32 were observed longer than 18 months. Only 18 were observed beyond 30 months.

The format of the curves can play a vital role in proper interpretation. Figure 5-11 presents the same data contained in Figure 5-10; the only difference is that the data are only displayed to 18 months. This presentation would offer no hint of a therapeutic difference. Form should be determined in a manner that will present the results in the most accurate fashion.

It is also common for graphs depicting significant differences to cross in the tails. This does not negate the impact of the observed difference. Survival comparisons must not be viewed as comparing any one

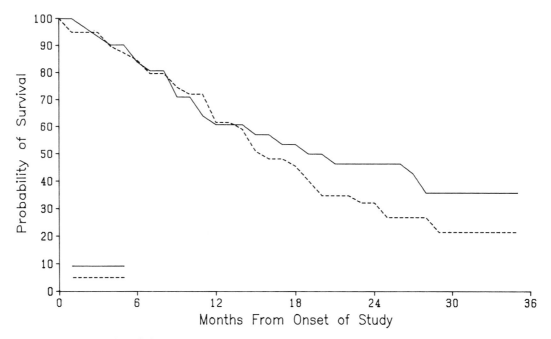

Fig. 5-10 Survival probability by treatment, displayed to 36 months. (———) Regimen I: alive, 6; dead, 25; total, 31; median, 19.0 (----) Regimen II: alive, 3; dead, 36; total, 39; median, 15.0.

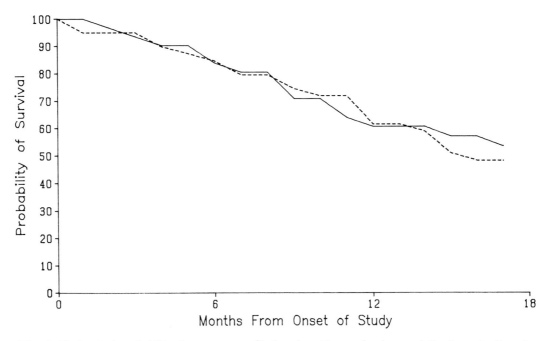

Fig. 5-11 Survival probability by treatment, displayed to 18 months. (———) Regimen I: alive, 6; dead, 25; total, 31; median 19.0. (----) Regimen II: alive, 3; dead, 36; total, 39; median, 15.0.

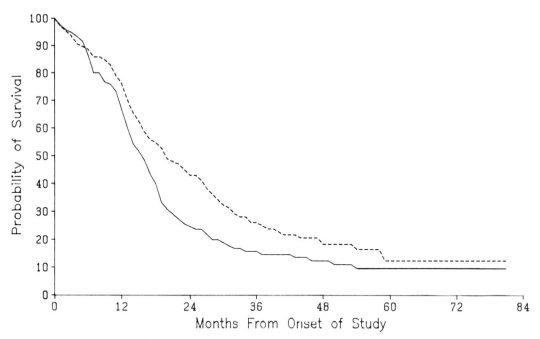

Fig. 5-12 Survival probability by treatment, showing actual data. (———) Regimen I: alive 17; dead, 104; total 121, median, 15.5. (----) Regimen II: alive, 22; dead, 85; total, 107; median, 19.7.

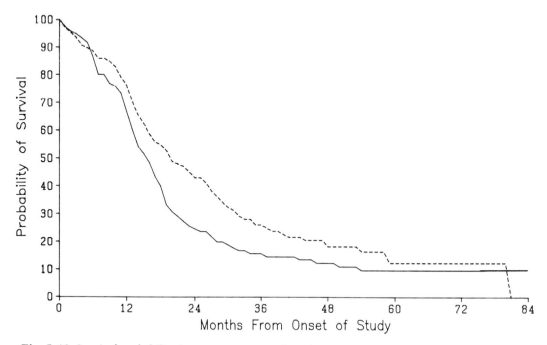

Fig. 5-13 Survival probability by treatment. Asterisks indicate one case altered.* (———) Regimen I: alive, 17; dead, 104; total, 121; median, 15.5. (----) Regimen II: alive 21; dead, 86*; total, 107*; median, 19.7

point (median, tail, or other); the true impact is best appreciated by examining the overall area between the curves.

To illustrate this principle, Figure 5-12 presents an unpublished comparison of two treatment regimens. Regimen II has significantly ($P < 0.02$) longer survival than those in regimen I. However, note that in Figure 5-13 the curves have been altered and now cross. The only difference in the two analyses reflected in Figures 5-12 and 5-13 is that the status of the last observed case in regimen II has been artificially changed from alive to dead. Thus, one late-occurring failure has caused the curve for regimen II to cross to zero. This is no reason to discount the significant finding illustrated in the entire survival comparison, graphically pointing out the ability of tails to fluctuate.

STATISTICAL-CLINICAL INTERACTION

One common theme has arisen throughout this chapter: the key to well-designed, appropriately analyzed, properly interpreted studies is continual interaction of clinical and statistical investigators. The aim of this chapter has been to establish an elementary understanding of relevant topics in order to enable this collaboration to take place in a more productive fashion. This will prove far more beneficial than any formal statistical presentation.

REFERENCES

1. Gehan EA, Schneiderman MA: Experimental design of clinical trials. p. 531. In Holland JF, Frei E (eds): Cancer Medicine. 2nd Ed. Lea & Febiger, Philadelphia, 1982
2. Blessing JA: Design, analysis, and interpretation of chemotherapy trials in gynecologic cancer. p. 49. In Deppe G (ed): Chemotherapy of Gynecology Cancer. Alan R Liss, New York, 1984
3. Gehan EA: The determination of the number of patients required in a preliminary and a follow-up trial of a new chemotherapeutic agent. J Chron Dis 13:346, 1961
4. Flemming TR: One-sample multiple testing procedure for phase II clinical trials. Biometrics 38:143, 1982
5. Cochran WG, Cox GM: Experimental Designs. 2nd Ed. John Wiley & Sons, New York, 1957
6. George SL, Desu MM: Planning the size and duration of a clinical trial studying the time to some critical event. J Chron Dis 27:15, 1974
7. Thigpen T, Shingleton H, Homesley H, et al: Cis-Platinum in treatment of advanced or recurrent squamous cell carcinoma of the cervix: A phase II study of the Gynecologic Oncology Group. Cancer 48:899, 1981
8. Bonomi P, Blessing JA, Stehman FB, et al: Randomized trial of three cisplatin dose schedules in squamous cell carcinoma of the cervix. (A Gynecologic Oncology Group Study.) J Clin Oncol 3:1079, 1985
9. Park RC, Blom J, DiSaia PJ, et al: Treatment for women with disseminated or recurrent advanced ovarian cancer with melphalan alone in combination with 5-fluorouracil and dactinomycin or with the combination of cytoxan, 5-fluorouracil and dactinomycin. (From the Gynecologic Oncology Group.) Cancer 45:2529, 1980
10. Parker LM, Griffiths CT, Yankee RA, et al: Combination chemotherapy with adriamycin-cyclophosphamide for advanced ovarian carcinoma. Cancer 46:669, 1980
11. Omura GA, Morrow CP, Blessing JA, et al: A randomized comparison of melphalan versus melphalan plus hexamethylmelamine versus adriamycin plus cyclophosphamide in ovarian carcinoma. Cancer 51:783, 1983
12. Thigpen JT, Lagasse L, Homesley H, et al: Cis-platinum in the treatment of advanced or recurrent adenocarcinoma of the ovary: A phase II study of the Gynecology Oncology Group. Am J Clin Oncol CCT 6:431, 1983
13. Ehrlich CE, Einhorn L, Williams SD, et al: Chemotherapy for stage III-IV epithelial ovarian cancer with cis-dichlorodiammine-platinum (II), adriamycin, and cyclosphosphamide: A preliminary report. Cancer Treatm Rep 63:281, 1979
14. Omura G, Blessing, JA, Ehrlich CE, et al: A randomized trial of cyclophosphamide and adriamycin with or without cisplatin in advanced ovarian carcinoma. A Gynecologic Oncology Group study. Cancer 57:1725, 1986
15. Blessing JA, Anderson, B: Analysis of clinical trials in gynecologic cancer—Timing and interpretation. Gynecol Oncol 23:275, 1986
16. Peto R, Pike MC, Armitage P, et al: Design and analysis of randomized clinical trials requiring prolonged observation of each patient. I. Introduction and design. Br J Cancer 34:585, 1976
17. Thigpen T, Blessing J, DiSaia P, et al: A randomized comparison of adriamycin with or without cyclophosphamide in the treatment of advanced or recurrent endometrial carcinoma. Proc Am Soc Cancer Oncol 4:115, 1985

6

Principles of Radiotherapy

C. C. Wang

Female genital cancer is one of the most common types of malignancy. Together with colorectal cancer, it ranks second in incidence and fourth in mortality. In 1985, approximately 75,000 new cases were diagnosed and 22,400 died, with a mortality rate of approximately 30 percent.[1] These malignant tumors have diverse epidemiologic and etiologic features, clinical courses, patterns of spread of disease, and prognoses. Their management is therefore vastly different and should be highly individualized. Surgery, radiation therapy, and chemotherapy are the three principal modalities available for the treatment of gynecologic malignant disease. It has been demonstrated that the best therapeutic results ensue when the treatment policy decisions are made by a multidisciplinary team rather than by individual specialists. It is also to be noted that some cancers that were considered incurable by previous standards have been found curable by a combination of either radiotherapy and surgery or chemotherapy, or both approaches. These specialists therefore must participate in the decision making for therapy from the very onset. It is the complementary effort of this team that offers most to the patient.

MODALITIES OF RADIATION THERAPY

Undue emphasis is often placed on the equipment of radiation therapy but, as in all medicine, the knowledge and skill of the radiation therapist are the determinants of success of a given treatment rather than the hardware. Nevertheless, the armamentarium of modern radiation therapy does make possible techniques previously unavailable with improvement in cure rates and reduction of undesirable local side effects and complications.

The tools of radiation therapy may be x-rays, γ-rays, or energetic particles such as electrons, protons, α-particles or neutrons. x-Rays result from rapid deceleration of fast-moving electrons through a vacuum tube. γ-Rays result from variation in the energy state of an atom. These changes occur at a characteristic rate in atoms, such as radium-226, cobalt-60, cesium-137, iridium-192, and other radioactive isotopes. Both x-rays and γ-rays are physically identical to similar biologic action and are part of the electromagnetic wave spectrum, sometimes called a photon beam.[2] According to the power of penetration and source of radiation, radiotherapeutic modalities can be divided roughly into four categories:

1. *Low-voltage x-ray:* operating in the range of 50 or 120 kV and used for superficially placed lesions, primarily cancer of the skin
2. *Kilovoltage x-ray:* operating from 200 to 400 kV
3. *Megavoltage x-ray:* operating over a range of several million volts to 25 or more million volts
4. *γ-ray sources of teletherapy:* principally cobalt-60 units

Megavoltage irradiation possesses certain inherent physical advantages, such as (1) a skin-sparing effect, reflected by the fact that often a full course of curative radiation therapy can be given without causing significant radiation dermatitis; (2) sharper beam and increase in depth dose, making it possible to deliver maximal homogeneous irradiation to tailor-fit the individual lesions, thus minimizing unnecessary damage to the adjacent normal tissues and organs; (3) a bone-sparing effect, due to decreased differential absorption between soft tissue and bone, resulting in a lower incidence of osteoradionecrosis as compared with kilovoltage irradiation; and (4) a substantial reduction in integral dose, hence less radiation sickness and better tolerance of treatment on the part of the patient.

Megavoltage Irradiation or Photon Beam

Present-day means of generating x- or γ-irradiation (or photon beam) in the megavoltage range is usually via one of several following devices.

TELECOBALT-60 MACHINE

Although technically not an x-ray machine, the telecobalt-60 machine is used in the same manner as, and for all practical purposes is, a megavoltage x-ray machine. The source of ionizing rays, in this case γ-rays having energies of 1.17 and 1.33 MeV, is several thousand curies of radioactive cobalt-60, housed in a shielded head with collimating devices. This is a common, practical machine for clinical radiation therapy available at most medical centers. Except for its relatively short half-life of 5.25 years, which may require frequent change of sources in a busy depart-

ment, it offers certain technical advantages, such as freedom from breakdown.

LINEAR ACCELERATOR

The linear accelerator, commonly known as a Linac or Clinac, provides a compact source of x-rays in a range of 4 to 25 million volts. Either x-rays or electron beams can be produced. Linear accelerators have the advantage of high output, (i.e., 200 to 1,000 cGy)* per minute at isocenter. They are also compact and have been found very popular at the major cancer centers.

BETATRON

The betatron is capable of accelerating electrons to very high speeds; it can generate highly penetrating, relatively homogeneous x-ray beams with energies up to 40 million volts. Although larger, the betatron is relatively compact for the energy level of radiation developed. However, it has the disadvantage of relatively low output and limited portal size for large-field radiation therapy.

Kilovoltage Irradiation

Radiation generated by the 100- to 250-kV x-ray machine may be used in the treatment of superficial cancers. It has no place in the primary management of deep-seated cancers. Most superficial lesions previously suitably treated by kilovoltage machines can now be satisfactorily managed by electron-beam therapy.

Particulate Irradiation

ELECTRON BEAM

Energetic electrons can be generated by either a linear accelerator or a betatron. According to the depth of the lesions, various energies ranging from 6 to 18 MeV or above can be selected for optimum irradiation. The characteristics of electron beam are rapid dose buildup and sharp falloff beyond the speci-

---

* 1 Gy (gray) = 100 rad = 100 cGy; centigray is a unit of energy absorbed.

fied energy applied; thus, the structures or organs further deep to the treatment target receive relatively less radiations. The principal areas of application suitable for electron-beam therapy include lesions of the skin and lip, primary lesions of the head and neck located at 2- to 5-cm depth, and metastatic disease in the superiorly placed nodes (e.g., inguinal adenopathy). Frequently, electron-beam therapy is given in conjunction with photon-beam irradiation.

HEAVY PARTICLES

Proton and α-particles have been used for radiation therapy during the past decade. These heavy particles are generated from a cyclotron and can penetrate deep into soft tissue. Because of minimal side scattering, these particles can be sharply focused deep into the body for specific high-dose irradiation. When the heavy particles are slowed down in the tissues, they release their maximum ionization shortly after stoppage, known as the Bragg peak. Using various thicknesses of absorbers, these Bragg peaks can be spread within the desired width of volume for wide-field irradiation, forming a so-called modulated beam. The idea of this form of radiotherapy is to improve physical dose distribution to the target volume in the hope of increasing local tumor control and decreasing radiation complications. This mode has been used for clinical radiation therapy particularly by radiation therapists at Massachusetts General Hospital, with the 160-MV protons from the Harvard cyclotron. In the gynecologic area, it has been used to irradiate paraaortic lymph node metastases with improved therapeutic results.

Radioactive Isotopes

Radium-226 was an important γ-ray source of radiation therapy. Because of its inherent hazard of unnecessary radiation exposure to the therapy staff, radium-226 has been replaced by other isotopes, such as cesium-137 or iridium-192 in clinical practice. Interstitial and intracavitary afterloading devices are available for the treatment of cancer of the uterus and cervix and metastatic cervical nodes. Radon is a gaseous daughter product of radium that is no longer available commercially; it has likewise been replaced by other isotopes, such as gold-198 and iodine-125 for permanent interstitial implant.

BASIC CONCEPTS OF RADIATION BIOLOGY

Developments in the fields of radiobiology have been received with great interest and understanding by clinical radiotherapists for the past decade. Ideas originating in the laboratory have begun to influence the choice of new treatment modalities, dose fractionation schemes, and radiotherapeutic techniques. The progress in this basic science, although slow, will probably continue to dominate the practice of future radiation therapy. In order to keep abreast of what is going on in present-day radiobiologic research, some basic knowledge would be desirable. For detailed study in this field, the reader is advised to consult Hall's text.[3]

When ionizing radiations traverse tissues and cells, certain radiation-induced changes result. Many of these events occur primarily in the water molecules of living matter—an indirect effect that results in generating a number of free radicals. These highly reactive free radicals may recombine swiftly without causing biologic effects, or they may combine in fractions of a microsecond with other atoms and molecules to produce biochemical effects in irradiated cells. In contrast to the indirect effect, the interaction of ionizing radiations with atoms or organic molecules in the cell results in inactivation without intervention of aqueous free radicals—a direct effect. This physical and biochemical phenomenon, although brief and yet extremely complex, may lead to a variety of nuclear and cytoplastic molecular changes, resulting in radiation damage to the cells.[3]

These radiation effects are expressed in a variety of ways, notably (1) loss of reproductive ability, (2) metabolic changes, (3) cell transformation, (4) acceleration of the cellular aging process, and (5) mutation.

When a cell is damaged by irradiation, various kinds of radiation injuries may take place[4-7]:

1. *Lethal damage*—loss of the ability of the cell to reproduce indefinitely. Daughter cells, if produced, are reproductively sterile.
2. *Potentially lethal damage*—slightly less severe impairment of the proliferative ability from which it might recover. Any modification in its environment, however, will interfere with repair and cause the cell to die.
3. *Sublethal damage*—the capacity of cells to sustain a

certain number or quantity of radiation lesions or events without cell death. These lesions may be repaired.

Radiobiologically, it is known that an approximately exponential relationship exists between the dose of ionizing radiation administered to a cell population and the survival fraction of these cells.[8-12] A survival curve describes the probability of cell kill plotted on a logarithmic scale by various doses of radiation plotted on a linear scale[12,13] (Fig. 6-1).

The slope of this curve varies with the radiosensitivity of the particular cell line, its environment during irradiation, the presence or absence of oxygen,[14] the type and method of administration of radiation, and the biologic state of the cells. The curve has a characteristic shoulder followed by a straight line. The sensitivity of the cells is expressed by the slope of the curve and the extrapolation number. D_0 is the single dose of radiation required to kill 63 percent of the cells in an exponential straight line portion of the curve resulting in 37 percent or $1/e$ survival fraction and is an expression of the radiosensitivity of the cells. The shoulder represents the accumulated sublethal injuries or the amount of waste radiations and is always present in x- or γ-radiation and is extremely small or almost absent in high linear energy transfer (LET) radiation, such as neutrons or α-particles. The projection of the straight exponential portion of the curve to the point of intersection with the ordinate represents the extrapolation number, which can be interpreted as a measure of the number of sensitive targets in the cell that must be hit to cause cessation of reproduction. D_q (quasithreshold dose) is the dose at which the extrapolated exponential portion of the curve intercepts the abscissa through the 100 percent survival level and is a measure of the width of the initial shoulder. D_{37} is the dose required to reduce the cell population to 37 percent in the initial portion of the survival curve and is equal to $D_q + D_0$. When the exponential curve is strictly exponential (single-hit kinetics), D_0 and D_{37} are the same. In most instances, however, such as x-ray and γ-ray survival curves, D_{37} is larger than D_0 because of the initial shoulder.

Although experimental studies show similar dose-survival curves in various normal and malignant mammalian cell lines with D_0 ranging between 100 and 250 cGy in an oxygenated environment,[3,8,9] the information thus far is not readily applicable to the clinical situation. Clinically, radiosensitivity refers to the rate of gross tumor shrinkage and anatomic and functional changes following a given dose-time-volume relationship. Tumor shrinkage, a common denominator of radiosensitivity, is determined by many factors, such as cell type, origin, rate of cellular proliferation, cell death and absorption, degree of oxygenation, and amount of vasculoconnective tissue in or about the tumor. Human tumors are extremely complex. An aggregate of cancerous growth represents an enormous biologic disorder. Various cells will grow differently, intermingled with various amounts of connective vascular tissue. A wide range of biologic factors affect the radiation response in different histopathologic types of malignancies. In spite of this complicated tumor biology and composition, clinically some tumors respond to radiotherapy better than others, and some respond with much lower or greater radiation doses.

An arbitrary classification of malignant gynecologic tumors according to radiosensitivity.

CLASSIFICATION OF MALIGNANT GYNECOLOGIC TUMORS

1. Very radiosensitive
   a. Lymphoma
   b. Dysgerminoma
   c. Granulosa cell tumor
2. Moderately radiosensitive
   a. Squamous cell carcinoma
   b. Adenocarcinoma
   c. Endometrioid carcinoma
   d. Epithelial ovarian tumor
   e. Stilbestrol-induced clear cell carcinoma
3. Relatively radioinsensitive
   a. Fibrosarcoma
   b. Leiomyosarcoma
   c. Carcinosarcoma
   d. Melanoma
   e. Malignant teratoma
   f. Sarcoma botryoides

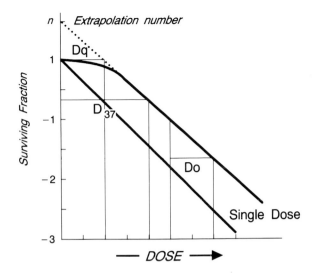

Fig. 6-1 Example of cell survival curves showing D_0, D_{37}, and D_q and extrapolated number.

FACTORS AFFECTING THE BIOLOGIC RESPONSE TO IONIZING RADIATION

Cell and Tissue Sensitivity to Ionizing Radiation

Over the years, cell differentiation and reproductive rate have been considered the basis of radiosensitivity.[15] The Bergonie-Tribondeau law states that the effect of radiation on living cells is more intense (1) the greater the reproductive activity, (2) the longer the mitotic phase, and (3) the lesser the morphology and function differentiated. It has been observed in general that embryologic immature tissues are more easily injured by radiations than are aged well-differentiated tissues. Tissues with rapid renewal capacity and active proliferation, such as the reproductive organs, bone marrow, and small bowel mucosa, are generally susceptible to radiation injury.

Oxygen Enhancement Ratio

In most biologic systems, under both normal and malignant conditions, the radiation effect of x-rays and γ-rays is considerably greater when the cells are irradiated in the oxygenated than in the hypoxic con-

dition.[16] The difference in radiosensitivity is in the neighborhood of two- to threefold and is called high oxygen-enhancement ratio (OER)[17] (Fig. 6-2).

The enhancement occurs only when the dissolved oxygen is present in the cells during irradiation. The mechanism of oxygen-enhancement radiosensitivity is not fully understood. It is believed that the dissolved oxygen molecules react and combine with the highly reactive radiation-induced free radicals, preventing recombination of these free radicals and resulting in irreversible radiation injuries. The oxygen may therefore be thought of as a fixer of radiation effects. Since the biologic damage by dense ionizing radiations, such as neutrons and α-particles, is primarily due to direct effect without the intervention of water molecules, the OER is observed to be considerably less marked than the sparsely ionizing radiations, such as x-rays. Neutron radiations are therefore less oxygen dependent or have a low OER.

All cells in the tumor are not benefited to the same extent by increased oxygenation. Increasing radiosensitivity associated with increasing intracellular oxygen occurs markedly when the cells are hypoxic, but such enhancement of radiosensitivity is much less if

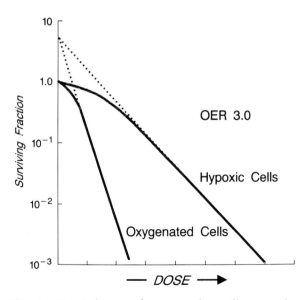

Fig. 6-2 Survival curves for mammalian cells exposed to x-rays under oxygenated and hypoxic environment. The difference in radiation sensitivity is threefold (i.e., OER = 3).

the cells are already full oxygenated. Under clinico-pathologic conditions, a tumor core greater than 150 to 180 μm distant from the functional capillaries often contains hypoxic cells that are insensitive to radiation therapy. By contrast, the cells at the periphery of the tumor mass or near capillaries are well oxygenated, hence radiosensitive and controllable by radiation. The availability of oxygen to the tumor can be altered by a variety of changes inside the body, such as impaired circulation from previous radical surgery, fibrosis from previous irradiation, and anemia secondary to hemorrhage.

Because of the recognition of the presence of the radioresistance of hypoxic cells in large rapid-growing tumors, radiation therapy has been given under hyperbaric oxygen,[9-11] or in conjunction with hyposic cell sensitizers. This is given in the hope that the hypoxic portion of the tumor masses will become more oxygenated or sensitized, hence more radiosensitive; thus, the overall radiosensitivity of the entire tumor would increase. The results of such approach are disappointing at the present time, however.

Time-Dose-Fraction Relationship

The radiation effects produced by a single dose of x-rays or γ-rays are more pronounced than those produced by the same amount delivered in divided daily fractionated doses over a period of time. This decreased response with daily fractionation appears to be related to cell recovery from sublethal damage occurring between doses and is less pronounced in densely ionizing radiations, such as neutrons. With fractionated radiation therapy given in daily increments, sublethal damage is repaired daily in less than 4 to 6 hours; the shoulder of the survival curve is therefore duplicated with each daily fraction (Fig. 6-3). This type of recovery accounts for most of the increased dose necessary with conventional clinical fractionation. This daily duplication of the "shoulder" is obviously not an efficient use of energy as far as inactivation of the reproductive capacity of a single cell type is concerned. Yet, in clinical radiation therapy of malignant tumors, the superiority of fractionated irradiation is thought to be partly attributed to the four Rs of radiobiology: repair of sublethal damage, redistribution of cells within the cell cycles, repopulation, and reoxygenation.[18]

Normal cells would repair and repopulate following sublethal damage during and after a course of fractionated irradiation. This includes the resumption of mitotic activity of the normal cell and repopulation from the stem cells. Radiation-induced cell death initiates a feedback mechanism that activates a reparative process. This has been called the homeostatic stimulus to normal tissue repair. Malignant cells also repopu-

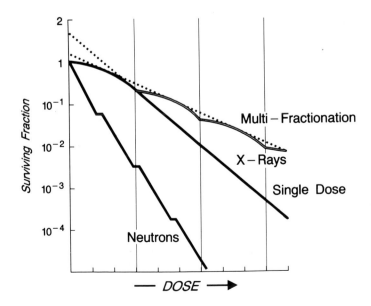

Fig. 6-3 Cell survival curves showing repair and duplication of initial shoulders after fractionated irradiation. The phenomenon of repair of sublethal damage is marked in x-rays and practically absent after neutron therapy.

late to a lesser extent and later after initial radiation exposure than do normal cells. Thus, after accumulated radiation dosages, the complete demise of the entire tumor eventually results.

Fractionated radiation therapy results in more damage to tumor cell population[18,19] because the process of reoxygenation of hypoxic cells and redistribution of radiosensitive cell cycle occurs between the dose fractions. During fractionation and protraction of treatment, radiosensitive oxygenated cells are destroyed, with subsequent reduction of tumor size; radioresistant hypoxic cells distant from functional vasculature are then close to the blood supply and become reoxygenated. Thus, the overall radiosensitivity and radiocurability of the entire tumor is enhanced. This concept is applied routinely in clinical radiation therapy.

Linear Energy Transfer and Relative Biologic Effectiveness

Linear energy transfer is the average energy deposited in each linear unit of track of secondary electron (or other charged particles) and is measured in electron volts per micron, or more practically, in keV/μm. Particle radiations such as neutrons and α-particles have dense ionization and high LET, whereas x-rays and γ-rays have sparse ionization and low LET. Biologic damage to cells is related to LET. Generally, particle radiations with high LET are more likely to produce substantial damage in a given volume of living matter, because the ionization is produced close together compared with low LET radiations, the ionization of which is produced relatively far apart. The increase in biologic damage or increased relative biologic effectiveness (RBE) does not continue indefinitely, however. With irradiation of extremely high LET, more energy is deposited to the targets than is needed to produce even the maximum biologic effect. Such irradiation deposits more energy in cell than is required and the excessive energies, resulting in overkill are therefore wasted. This phenomenon generally occurs in irradiation with LET above 100 keVμm.

Relative biologic effectiveness is used to compare the biologic effectiveness of different radiations relative to 200-kV x-rays as the standard. For low LET radiations, such as cobalt-60 γ-rays or low-megavoltage x-rays or electrons, the RBE is slightly less than unity (or 1), while higher LET radiations have greater RBE, ranging between >1 to 3.5, depending on the biologic system and end point tested.

Other Factors

Other factors capable of altering radiosensitivity include hypoxic cell sensitizers and hyperthermia. In pathologic conditions in which carcinomas invade cartilage, bone, and muscle, the radiosensitivity changes considerably.

CONCEPTS OF COMBINED RADIATION THERAPY AND SURGERY

Surgery and radiotherapy are equally effective in eradicating small limited human cancers. Each of these modalities has its own merits, indications, and limitations. Radiation therapy has the advantage of being able to control the disease in situ, thereby avoiding the removal of a useful and necessary part as well as preserving bodily function. Radiotherapy should therefore be considered the best "tissue- and organ-sparing procedure" available. On the other hand, for certain early lesions situated in less strategic locations, surgery can be carried out expediently and effectively without functional and cosmetic mutilation and is therefore preferred.

In the management of advanced carcinomas, surgical failures are often due to an inability to remove microscopic tumor extension at the periphery, resulting in marginal recurrence. Failure from radiation therapy is an inability to control the hypoxic cells commonly present in a large tumor and is therefore central rather than marginal in nature as in surgery. Tumor seeding in the wound after surgery and metastases via lymphatic and hematogenous routes are additional means to account for radiotherapeutic and surgical failures.

On the basis of the presently available radiobiologic knowledge and the mechanism of treatment failures, the major strength of radiation therapy is therefore to eradicate the radiosensitive, actively growing, well-oxygenated cells in the periphery of the tumor. The strength of surgery on the other hand is to remove the centrally situated, radioresistant hypoxic tumor cells. For extensive tumors, which are rarely curable by either method alone, the logical approach is combination radiation therapy and surgery. Two conceptual approaches to combined radiation therapy and surgery have emerged, that is, pre- and postoperative radiation therapy.

Preoperative Radiation Therapy

The aims of preoperative radiation therapy are to prevent marginal recurrences, to control subclinical disease at the primary site or in the lymph nodes or to convert technically inoperable tumors into operable ones. This form of combined approach has been found to decrease iatrogenic scar implant, local recurrence, and the incidence of distant metastases. The disadvantages of preoperative radiation therapy are (1) precise tumor extent is obscured due to shrinkage of the lesion prior to surgery; (2) delaying of surgery, thus creating a great deal of anxiety on the part of some patients; (3) increase in postoperative complications.[20]

The most common form of preoperative radiation therapy employs a modest dosage consisting of 4,500 cGy in 1 month. This is followed in 1 month by radical surgery according to the original extent of the disease, as though radiation therapy had not been given. The program is applicable mostly to medium-size or advanced tumors for which radical surgery can be satisfactorily carried out and is not associated with significant postoperative morbidity or mortality.

High-dose preoperative radiation therapy, that is, 6,000 to 6,500 cGy in 7 weeks to be followed by surgery, or so-called postirradiation resection, has been used for cancer of the uterus. Following the high dose of radiation, the magnitude of surgery must be decreased in that only the residual disease should be removed, that is, extrafascial hysterectomy for stage IB barrel-shaped cervix, stage II carcinoma of the endometrium.

Low-dose short-course preoperative radiation therapy, that is, 1,000 cGy divided into four or five daily fractions to be followed immediately by radical surgery, has been used in stage I high-grade carcinoma of the endometrium at the MGH for the past 10 years and found effective in preventing scar implant with satisfactory local control and survival. The detailed studies were published elsewhere.

Postoperative Radiation Therapy

The aims of postoperative radiation therapy are to eradicate residual disease transected at the tumor margins, to control subclinical disease implanted in the wound or in the lymph nodes. The procedure is usually carried out approximately three or four weeks after surgery when the wound is healed. Generally a dose of 4,500 to 5,500 cGy in 5 to 6 weeks is planned to the whole pelvis if surgery is radical in extent. On the other hand, if surgery is primarily a debulking procedure with gross residual disease remaining, high dose radiotherapy must be given, i.e. 6,500 cGy in 7 weeks through shrinking field technique to the area of known disease. This may be accompanied by increased incidence of complications.

TREATMENT PLANNING AND PREPARATION OF PATIENT FOR RADIATION THERAPY

After radiation therapy is elected, treatment should be carefully planned and executed. In the modern practice of radiation therapy, the treatment planning is based on the nature, size, and location of the tumor; the volume of tissue to be encompassed; the normal organ to be spared; and the intent of treatment (curative or palliative), and is carried out with the aid of a simulator and dedicated computer prior to actual treatment. This procedural preparation for radiotherapy must be as thorough as the preparation of a patient who is to undergo surgery. All workups should be complete, including evaluation of the extent of the primary lesion by inspection, palpation, and various diagnostic means such as radiographs (IVP, contract studies) and, when indicated, lymphangrography, ultrasonography, and computed tomography (CT) scans. This is mandatory in order to determine the exact tumor volume for optimum direction of the treatment beam.

In certain gynecologic tumor sites, adequate evaluation can only be carried out with the patient under general anesthesia. Also, the distant soft and bony parts must be examined for metastases, these include chest radiographs and bone scans.

Histologic confirmation of malignancy should be obtained before treatment. This is necessary for an understanding of the disease and the appropriate treatment planning. A complete physical examination, including blood and urine studies and a liver profile for appraisal of the patient's physical status, is highly desirable. Anemia, which may affect tumor control, should be corrected.[21,22]

The total dose to be given is determined by the total treatment time (protraction), number and dose of daily fractions (fractionation), cell type, the tolerance of the tumor bed, and, most importantly, the response of the tumor and the patient to treatment. In general, the radiosensitive tumors treated with intent to cure require a dose of between 4,500 and 5,500 cGy in about 1.5 month's time. For squamous cell carcinoma and adenocarcinoma, a dose for cure ranges between 6,500 and 7,000 cGy during a period of 7 to 8 weeks. For a large bulky tumor, a dose of 8,000 cGy is required; this often can only be achieved by combination of external high-energy beam therapy and brachytherapy, either intracavitary or interstitial.

INTENT OF RADIATION THERAPY

The intent of radiation therapy can be divided into three categories: (1) curative, (2) palliative, and (3) adjunct to surgery. Radical radiation therapy with the intent of cure is not without morbidity and should be performed with both care and justification. In curative radiation therapy, the treatment course is usually prolonged and physically taxing. Radiation reactions, both local and systemic, may be severe but should be accepted as an inevitable price for the possibility of cure. As a matter of fact, the discomfort suffered by patients from curative radiation therapy is not less and is sometimes more than that from radical surgery. When the patient is physically unfit for radical curative surgery because of severe anemia, cachexia, and rapid deterioration of physical condition, she is equally unfit for curative radiation therapy.

With incurable tumors due to extensive disease or distant metastases, or both, palliative radiation therapy for symptomatic relief should be the aim. Pain, foul discharge, obstruction, and ulceration can be alleviated by a modest dose of radiation. A shorter treatment course than used in curative radiation therapy is undertaken, without much additional discomfort to the patient, in the hope of prolonging a useful and comfortable life. The mere adding of days of existence and pain hardly justifies the word palliation. Palliative radiation therapy is not indicated in patients whose incurable cancer remains asymptomatic. For the debilitated patients in the terminal stage of their advanced malignant disease beyond palliative radiotherapy, the best treatment is human kindness, morphine, and good nursing care.

For moderately advanced cancers, there has been a tendency to combined radiation therapy and surgery with improvement in results. The concepts and rationale of combined modalities have been previously discussed.

RADIATION MANAGEMENT OF GYNECOLOGIC MALIGNANCIES

A considerable body of experience as to what can and cannot be accomplished by either irradiation or surgery for various types of gynecologic malignant diseases has been accumulated. The general principles of radiation therapy for various major gynecologic cancers are discussed.

Carcinoma of the Cervix

Squamous cell carcinoma of the cervix is the most common cancer of the female genital tract. It is a moderately radiosensitive cancer and in its early stage is radiocurable. Its control requires a high dose of local irradiation. Fortunately, the cervix and the corpus of the uterus have an unusually high tolerance to radiation. In general, these structures can withstand a much higher dose of irradiation than any comparable volume of tissues in other portions of the body. A dose of 20,000 to 30,000 cGy in 2 weeks is routinely well tolerated. Because of the relatively high radiation tolerance, a high dose of tumor-control radiation, that is, 7,000 to 8,000 cGy can often be delivered locally by intracavitary cesium implant to the cervix, uterus, and paracervical tissues without significant radiation complications. The success of intracavitary brachytherapy in the treatment of cancer of the cervix is due almost entirely to this high tolerance, that is, an extremely favorable therapeutic ratio. A tumor-control dose, however, cannot be delivered with safety beyond 3 to 4 cm laterally from the os to include the entire parametria and the pelvic walls. Therefore, for the treatment of advanced lesions, such as stages IIB and III, there is a gradual shift in emphasis in making external beam therapy the principal mode of radiation therapy with intracavitary cesium implant of reduced amount as a supplementary procedure. In general, a dose of approximately 5,500 to 6,000 cGy can be delivered to the lateral parametria and pelvic nodes by combination of cesium implant and external beam irradiation. Treatment of the paraaortic nodal metastases depends solely on external beam irradiation. A dose of 5,000 cGy in 6 weeks should not be exceeded if serious small bowel complications are to be avoided.

PRINCIPLES OF INTRACAVITARY BRACHYTHERAPY AND TECHNIQUES

Brachytherapy has proved the most effective single agent in controlling early carcinoma of the cervix. The development of technique to give an optimal dose to the cervix, vaginal vault, paracervical tissues, and corpus has utilized two routes of cesium placement, that is, uterine and vaginal sources. Many different techniques and applicators have been developed, but these are far less important than adherence to principles that have shown their merits by favorable results over many years:

1. Pelvic infection and trauma are avoided or minimized.
2. Radioactive sources are placed to obtain maximum irradiation of the uterus, cervix, and paracervical tissues and vaginal vault with the least irradiation of the rectum and bladder.
3. Each patient is handled individually and meticulously with respect to dosage distribution, protraction, individual anatomy, pathology, and complications. The limited radiation tolerance of the bladder, rectum, and rectovaginal septum should be respected. The distribution and calculation of doses from cesium and external beam therapy to various pelvic structures must be taken into consideration in the overall treatment of the patient. Such dosimetric factors can be accurately assessed with the aid of the dedicated computer.
4. The optimum dose for carcinoma of the cervix is determined by the tolerance of the rectum, recto-

vaginal septum, bladder, and small bowel. The total dosage must be reduced in the patients with poor protoplasm, pelvic inflammatory disease, or previous multiple pelvic or abdominal surgical procedures and in patients over 70 years of age or in physically debilitated condition.

METHODS OF RADIATION THERAPY

Brachytherapy

Intracavitary. Over the years, two principal methods of brachytherapy have been developed. These are two distinctly different techniques both in physical properties of the applicators and treatment philosophy[23] (Fig. 6-4).

1. *Paris Method.* The Paris method uses a small amount of radium over a long period of treatment. Typically, 33.3 mg is distributed in the uterus in a single line source and 13.3 mg in each of two corks in the vaginal fornices joined by a metal spring to form a colpostat. A third cork which contains 6.66 mg radium is interposed between the two if anatomic condition permits. The entire assembly is left in place continuously for 5 days. The principle is to employ low-intensity, continuous, low-dose rate radiation therapy. The dose to the paracervical triangle is approximately 70 to 80 Gy.

2. *Stockholm Method.* The Stockholm method uses a large amount of radium in short, intense, and sharp high-dose rate treatment. In the uterus, a line source containing 50 to 60 mg, and in the vagina, 80 to 100 mg radium is distributed in a flat or curved box closely apposed to the vaginal vault and cervix. Two treatments, each lasting 20 to 24 hours with 3-week intervals, are given. Although the dose to the cervix, lower uterine segment, vaginal vault, and the paracervical triangle is relatively high, approximately 70 Gy, laterally the dose to the pelvic nodes is relatively low with this technique. Individualization of each patient's treatment plays an important part in this scheme.

3. *Manchester Technique.* The Manchester technique[24] is a modification of the Paris method. This method employs a precalculated dosage system so that a predetermined dose of approximately 70 Gy is given to so-called point A, which is in the medial edge of the broad ligament where the uterine vessels cross under

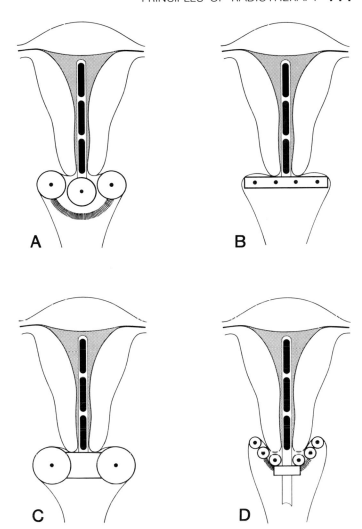

Fig. 6-4 Diagram showing varying basic brachytherapy methods used for treatment of carcinoma of the cervix **(A)** Paris method. **(B)** Stockholm method. **(C)** Manchester technique. **(D)** Ernst applicator.

the ureter. Physically, this point is located 2 cm laterally out from the uterine canal, 2 cm superior to the fornix. The dose to point B, which is 3 cm lateral to point A, is approximately 20 Gy. Each of the two treatments, staged about 1 week apart, extends for about 3 days. So-called vaginal ovoids and uterine tandem of various sizes and lengths are used. In this method, the radium loading in the vagina and uterus varies according to the size of the ovoids and the length of the tandem and is designed to keep the dose rate at point A relatively constant, approximately 50 cGy ±10 percent per hour. A practical loading combination for the tandem and ovoid system is illustrated as follows:

	Long	Medium	Short
1. Intrauterine tandem Loading from fundus down (mg of Ra eq slug)	15-10-10	15-10	20
	Large	Medium	Small
2. Vaginal ovoid (3 cm, 2.5 cm, 2 cm in diameter) Loading (mg of Ra equivalent in each of the pair ovoids)	25	20	15

The loading of the tandem may be altered for various conditions. If the bulk of the disease is in the lower uterine segment, the loading may be changed to

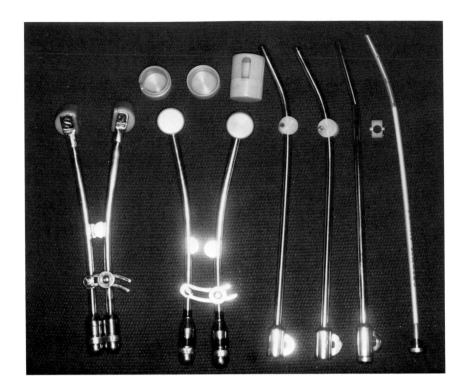

Fig. 6-5 Afterloading Fletcher-Suit applicator, ovoids, tandems, jackets, and cesium dummy source.

15-10-15 mg. The Manchester technique is more easily reproducible and is conveniently afterloaded; it has attracted a large number of followers in this country and abroad (Fig. 6-5).

Basic Physics of Intracavitary Brachytherapy

1. In the modern practice of radiation therapy, the expression of radiation dosage both from x-rays and radium is the amount of energy absorbed by the tumor in terms of cGy.[25] For intracavitary cesium therapy, unless there is a qualified statement as to the size of the applicators, geographic arrangement of the cesium sources, distance from the tumor and the adjacent organs, and the volume of tissue irradiated, the term milligram-hour is meaningless and cannot be used as an accurate expression of radiation dose in clinical radiation therapy.

2. Regardless of what techniques are used, the box, ovoids, or colpostats should be as large as possible to extend over the widest possible region to give maximum lateral dose, as well as fit snugly by packing so that they do not slip into the lower vagina; thus avoiding inadequate irradiation of the cervix and paracervical tissues. These vaginal sources are primarily responsible for radiation damage to the rectum and bladder and therefore should be placed away from these radiosensitive organs by careful packing. For a given dose to point A, the larger the box, ovoids, or colpostats, the higher the dose to point A, with the dose to the vaginal mucosa being constant (Fig. 6-6). Likewise, the larger the ovoid, the more of the vaginal walls are treated (Fig. 6-7).

3. The intrauterine tandem is the major contributor of the dose to the pelvic nodes and should be as long as possible. The longer the tandem, the greater the dose to point B, or pelvic nodes, with the dose to the mucosa of the uterus constant (Fig. 6-8).

4. In order to avoid unnecessary radiation exposure of the staff, most of the present-day intracavitary techniques employ some form of afterloading device. The Fletcher-Suit applicator using the tandem-ovoid Manchester technique is one of the representatives. Although cesium-137 has largely

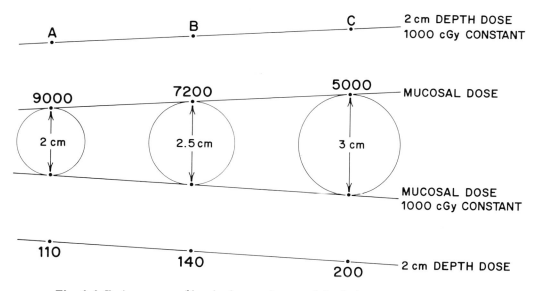

Fig. 6-6 Basic concept of brachytherapy. Increased depth dose versus size of ovoids.

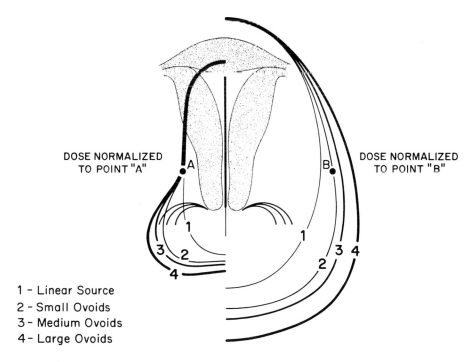

1 – Linear Source
2 – Small Ovoids
3 – Medium Ovoids
4 – Large Ovoids

Fig. 6-7 Graphic comparison of various sizes of ovoids versus dose distribution. The larger the ovoids the more coverage of the upper vagina and further lateral throw of radiation.

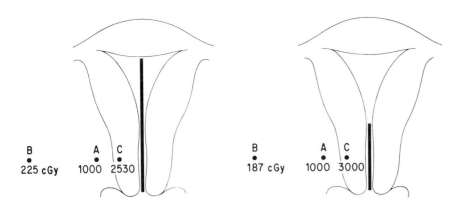

B
225 cGy

A
1000

C
2530

B
187 cGy

A
1000

C
3000

Fig. 6-8 Basic concept of brachytherapy. Increased depth dose versus length of tandem.

replaced radium-225 for most of the intracavitary work, the principles of radium therapy have been unchanged.

Interstitial. Interstitial implantation of the cervical tumor and broad ligaments is used to deliver additional radiation to the bulk of the tumor and/or when intracavitary implant is technically impossible. The procedure, however, is difficult to perform properly and runs the risk of overdosing with resultant local necrosis and underdosing with tumor recurrences. In experienced hands, the procedure is worthwhile and achieves higher local tumor control. For cervical stump carcinoma, this technique is used often when the remnant of either the cervical canal or the cervical os cannot be found.

Teletherapy

External beam therapy is primarily used for treatment of advanced tumors as a preparatory prior to intracavitary implant because the disease has spread beyond the effective range of brachytherapy. It is also used when the tumors are large with exophytic growth or when the cervical os cannot be identified because of extensive local lesion, or for pelvic recurrences following a surgical procedure. It should not be used as a substitute for an intracavitary implant as a primary treatment for early carcinoma of the cervix. The large irradiated volume and the limited radiation tolerance of the rectum, bladder, and rectovaginal septum prevents the delivery of high-dose irradiation and yields a lower cure rate and greater complication rate in potentially curable early lesions.

RADIATION THERAPY TECHNIQUE

Prior to treatment planning and simulation, a small bowel series is needed to ascertain the position and mobility of the bowel with bladder fully distended or emptied. If the small bowel can be pushed away from a fully distended urinary bladder, radiation therapy should be given with a full bladder. This may reduce greatly small bowel sequelae from whole-pelvis irradiation. Figure 6-9 shows the shift of small bowel position away from the pelvis with full and emptied bladder.

In order to identify the location of various anatomic structures, the primary tumor in the cervix is marked by a dura clip or a gold seed marker, the anterior rectal wall by barium and the base of the bladder by contrast substance in the balloon of the catheter prior to simulation (Fig. 6-10).

For most external beam therapy, a four-field box technique is used. The standard portal size for anterior-posterior fields is 15 × 15 cm or 16 × 16 cm. The upper border lies at the mid-sacroiliac joint and should not include the entire common iliac chain if small bowel complications are to be avoided. The inferior border includes the inferior margin of the obturator foramen or at least the upper two-thirds of the vagina. For the lateral portals, the anterior border includes the symphysis pubis and posteriorly the sacral prominence with a field size of 15 × 12 cm² (Fig. 6-11). High-energy photons, that is 10 MeV or above, are preferred. For a patient with anterior-posterior diameter greater than 25 cm, cobalt-60 radiation is not the optimum modality for the treatment of carcinoma of the cervix due to excessively high peripheral

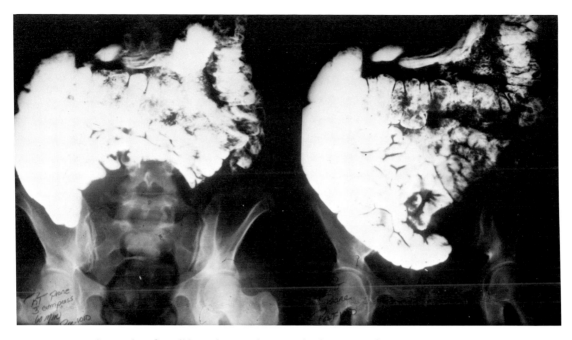

Fig. 6-9 Radiographs of small bowel series showing displacement of small bowel position away from the pelvis with full and empty bladder.

dose and inferior treatment results as compared with high-energy radiation.

RADIOTHERAPEUTIC MANAGEMENT OF CARCINOMA OF THE CERVIX

Owing to the high incidence of pelvic lymph node metastases in carcinoma of the cervix, that is, approximately 15 percent in stage I, 30 percent in Stage II and 45 percent in stage III lesions, the radiotherapeutic management of this disease, therefore must include the treatment of the primary lesion as well as the metastatic pelvic nodes according to the stage of the disease.

Generally, for the small, early, stage I and IIA lesions, treatment is primarily by intracavitary cesium implant first followed by external beam therapy to the pelvic nodes. For most other lesions having a great deal of exophytic component, or extensive tumors with poor identification of the cervical os, such as stage IIB and III disease, the radiotherapeutic program consists of initial whole pelvic irradiation to include the primary lesion and the nodes for maxi-

mum shrinkage of the tumor and irradiation of the metastases, followed by intracavitary implant with reduced amounts.

The following is a general scheme of treatment policy for cancer of the cervix in various stages and conditions as practiced at the Massachusetts General Hospital using Fletcher-Suit applicator and cesium-137 sources and 25 MV external beam from Clinac 35 linear accelerator:

Stage I and early IIA: Two implants (70 hours – 2 weeks – 70 hours) delivering 70 to 80 Gy to point A, 20 Gy to point B, to be followed by 40 Gy external beam therapy to the pelvic nodes.

Bulky stage I and extensive IIA: 40-Gy whole-pelvis radiation therapy first followed by two implants with reduced amount (40 hours – 2 weeks – 40 hours) or one implant of 60 to 65 hours, and 10 Gy to the pelvic nodes via external beam therapy.

Stage IIB and III: 45 Gy whole-pelvis irradiation first, followed by one implant of 60 hours or two implants of 30 hours each deliver 30 to 35 Gy to point A, and ? 500 cGy "boost" to the bulk of the lesion.

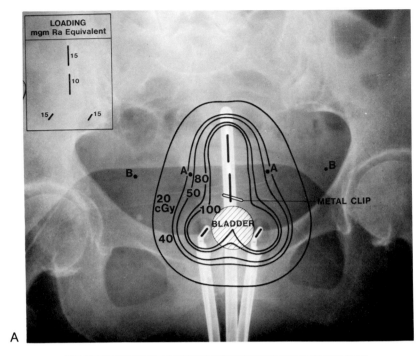

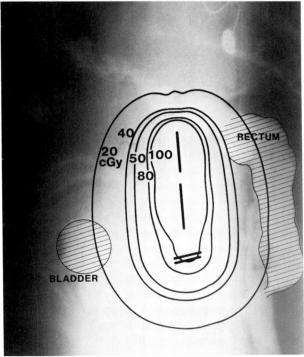

Fig. 6-10 Isodose distribution of intracavitary tandem-ovoid implant for carcinoma of the cervix. **(A)** AP projection. **(B)** Lateral projection.

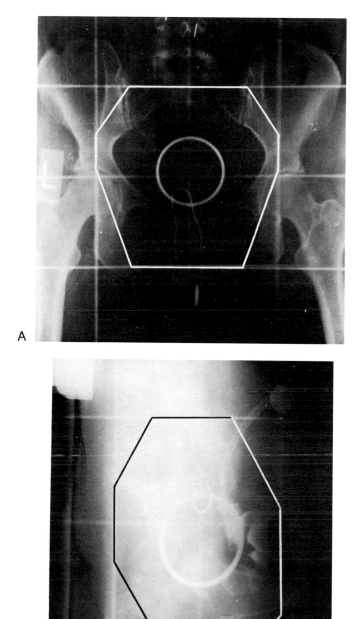

Fig. 6-11 Standard portal for external beam radiation therapy of carcinoma of the cervix. **(A)** AP view. **(B)** Lateral view.

Stage IV: 60-Gy whole-pelvis radiotherapy with ? short implant (40 to 45 hours), delivering 20 to 25 Gy to point A or an additional 10 Gy by external beam throughout reduced portals.

The duration of implant is based on 50 cGy ±10 percent/h with the Manchester system.

THE ROLE OF SURGERY IN THE MANAGEMENT OF STAGE I AND IIA CARCINOMA OF THE CERVIX

Although radiation therapy is applicable to most patients with carcinoma of the cervix, there are certain circumstances in which radical hysterectomy (Wertheim hysterectomy) for stage I and IIA carcinoma of the cervix may be preferred. These conditions may vary, depending on various individual institutions and the availability of the skills of the surgeon and radiation therapist:[25]

1. Relatively young, healthy, and thin individual (i.e., 50 years or younger)
2. Tumor associated with large uterine fibroid
3. Tumor extends to the fundus of the uterus
4. Funnel-shaped or distorted vaginal apex preventing effective use of vaginal cesium
5. Tumor associated with pelvic inflammatory disease, ulcerative colitis and diverticulitis
6. Unsatisfactory positioning of the radioactive sources after repeated attempts
7. Inability to identify uterine canal after 40 Gy whole-pelvis irradiation.

The misconception was often heard that metastatic nodes from carcinoma of the cervix cannot be sterilized by radiation therapy, indicating lymphadenectomy. Studies in which lymphadenectomy is done following a full course of radiation therapy showed greater than 50 percent decrease in positive nodes. As a corollary of this type of study, it developed that radical surgery after radiation therapy does not improve the survival rate and instead produces a fearfully high rate of complications, such as fistulas and necrosis, probably because both methods cause major impairment of vascular supply.

SPECIAL SITUATIONS

1. *Barrel-shaped cervix:* In the presence of stage I bulky endocervical tumor, the lower uterine segment and the cervix are much enlarged, forming a barrel-shaped mass. This special condition is defined when the mass is equal to or over 6 cm across, felt by rectal examination. Such lesions are associated with high central pelvic recurrence, approximately 15 percent. The management of barrel-shaped cervical cancer is external beam whole-pelvic radiation therapy of approximately 40 Gy, and an attenuated intracavitary implant of approximately 25 Gy to point A to be followed by an extrafascial hysterectomy.

2. *Carcinoma of the cervical stump:* If a supracervical hysterectomy has been performed for a benign condition at least 2 years prior to the onset of symptoms leading to the diagnosis of carcinoma of the cervix, it is presumed that the surgery was not performed in the presence of cervical cancer. Without an adequate intrauterine canal, radiation therapy of carcinoma of the cervical stump consists primarily of external beam whole-pelvis irradiation first, followed by an intracavitary or interstitial implant of reduced amount. The amount of external radiation therapy is usually one stage higher as compared with carcinoma of the intact uterus.

3. *Adenocarcinoma of the cervix:* Adenocarcinoma comprises approximately 10 percent of cancer of the cervix. It is a moderately radiosensitive neoplasm. Management is the same.

4. *Patients with paraaortic node metastases but with negative scalene nodes:* In the recent past, attempts have been made to irradiate paraaortic metastases in patients whose pelvic tumors have been controlled by either surgery or radiation therapy. Unfortunately for those patients treated with cobalt-60 unit using opposing AP-PA portals, an unacceptably high incidence of serious complications was reported after a dose of 50 Gy in 6 weeks.[27,28] Radiation therapy must therefore be meticulously carried out and requires high-energy photon technique from a linear accelerator preferably 25-MeV four-field box portals carefully shaped to individual circumstances. If metastatic nodes are localized and yet unresectable, intraoperative electron beam

radiation therapy may be considered in addition to external photon irradiation. At Massachusetts General Hospital, experimental use of the 160-MeV proton beam from the Harvard cyclotron has been used for paraaortic lymph node metastases. With precision technique, high-dose irradiation apparently is well tolerated.

5. *Recurrent or persistent carcinoma:* The conditions are defined as the presence of active malignant disease which appears more than or within 6 months after the completion of therapy, respectively. At times, the distinction between recurrent and persistent disease may be vague. The treatment of this group of patients is similar and must be highly individualized. When the situation occurs following radiation therapy, early surgical exploration is performed and if the lesion is still localized to the pelvis without extension to the pelvic wall or positive nodes, a pelvic exenteration is performed. The exenterative procedure can be anterior, posterior or total depending on the anatomic extent of the disease. In cases of recurrence following radical hysterectomy, either exenterative procedure or radiotherapy would be employed depending on the findings of the tumor survey, physical examination and, in some instances, surgical exploration.

6. *Reirradiation:* Reirradiation has little place in the management of recurrent carcinoma of the cervix because of the severe complications which may occur in the already heavily irradiated normal tissues. Small local recurrences however may be treated with interstitial implant, iodine-125 seeds or iridium-192 if the lesion is outside the previous portals, but in most instances the value of this procedure is limited. If the lesion is operable, pelvic exenteration may be considered with the understanding that postoperative complications may be frequent, particularly if the pelvis received a radiation dose greater than 60 Gy.

7. *Postoperative radiation therapy:* Information regarding the value of postoperative radiation therapy is limited. Patients with early carcinoma of the cervix whose specimens of the primary lesion show deep stromal penetration or tumor with lymph or blood vessel invasion or tumor in the parametria or resection margins after Wertheim hysterectomy or lymph node involvement should undergo a course of postoperative radiation therapy, although its beneficial effects are difficult to confirm without a randomized trial. The patients who underwent total hysterectomy for a benign condition but were inadvertently found to have occult invasive carcinoma of the cervix by histologic examination likewise should not be denied postoperative radiation therapy. Generally, external wholepelvis irradiation is the treatment of choice, and the dose is limited to 50 to 55 Gy in 6 to 7 weeks with or without supplementary vaginal vault brachytherapy.

RESULTS OF RADIATION THERAPY

The overall results of treatment of stage I carcinoma of the cervix by radiation therapy are comparable to those following Wertheim hysterectomy, i.e. 80 to 90 percent 5-year cure.[29,30] For stage II disease, the 5-year no-evidence-of-disease rates are approximately 50 to 60 percent. For stage III disease, the survival rate ranges between 25 to 40 percent. For stage IV disease, the rates are poor by radiation therapy alone, approximately 10 to 15 percent. For advanced lesions, most patients succumb to uncontrolled pelvic disease as well as to distant metastases.

Several groups have described their results of radiation therapy in treating cervical carcinoma, among the largest being M.D. Anderson Hospital and Mallinckrodt Institute,[29] including more than 2,500 patients. For patients with stage IB invasive cervical carcinoma, 5-year survival rates approximate 85 to 90 percent. For stage IIA and IIB carcinoma, 5-year survivals approximate 70 to 85 percent and 65 to 70 percent, respectively. In stage III carcinoma, 5-year survival is approximately 35 to 45 percent. In stage IV carcinoma, the survival obtained clearly depends on selection as well as radiation technique, but reported 5-year survival is in the range of 10 to 15 percent.

The Massachusetts General Hospital experience, including a period from 1976 to 1978, was published in the FIGO Nineteenth Annual Report.[31] The 5-year survival rate for stages I to IV was 52 percent. For stages I and II, the rates were 81 percent and 51 percent respectively. For the stage III disease, the 5-year survival rate was 11 percent, and there was no survival with stage IV disease. Most of the early lesions were treated by surgery with or without postoperative radiation therapy and the late stage lesions by radiation therapy only as reflected by our treatment policies as discussed. These results are quite comparable to most cancer centers in other parts of the country. In a selected group, however, the results are superior.

For barrel-shaped cervical carcinomas, the central recurrence rates are reduced from 15 percent to approximately 3 percent with a moderate increase in disease-free survival after planned combined radiation therapy and surgery as outlined earlier.[32,33] For patients with adenocarcinoma of the cervix treated with radiation therapy, the cure rates are nearly the same as those with squamous cell carcinoma for a given stage of the disease.[34] At the University of Maryland, 5-year survivals for 62 patients with stages I to III cervical adenocarcinoma were 85 percent, 77 percent, and 33 percent, respectively, similar to those quoted earlier for squamous cell carcinoma.[35]

In patients with carcinoma of the cervical stump, with modern radiotherapeutic techniques, the 5-year survival rate is about as good as for cervical carcinoma of the intact uterus. The M.D. Anderson Hospital series reported 263 patients treated with this condition with 5-year survivals of 91 percent, 77 percent, 46 percent, and 38 percent for patients with stages I to IV cancer, respectively.[36]

Results of postoperative irradiation have been variable. In patients who have undergone simple hysterectomy inadvertently in the presence of invasive cervical carcinoma, 5-year disease-free survivals following postoperative pelvic and vaginal irradiation were comparable to those seen in patients treated conventionally with radical surgery or irradiation, provided there was no gross residual tumor and irradiation commenced within 6 months after surgery.[37] The Massachusetts General Hospital series consisted of 10 patients. The 5-year no-evidence-of-disease rate was 90 percent for stages I and II lesions.

The use of irradiation in patients with positive pelvic lymph nodes has been especially vexing, hampered by the lack of properly randomized clinical trials and thus by questions regarding the comparability of treated and control groups. Major studies, including the Society of Gynecologic Oncologists' Presidential Panel with 49 treated patients and 146 controls, and the Memorial Hospital Study with 32 treated patients and 39 controls fail to support the use of postoperative irradiation in the presence of positive

nodes, with comparable survival and pelvic control for treated and control groups, although in the SGO Panel Report, there was a suggestion that postoperative radiation therapy improved survival in patients with more than five positive nodes, although the difference in survival, 85 percent versus 37 percent at 5 years, failed to reach statistical significance.[38] It should be pointed out that other reports with fewer patients dispute these results.[39] In general, the reported collected results suggest that postoperative irradiation may improve disease-free survival by approximately 20 percent.[40-44]

Results of radiation therapy in cervical cancer recurrent after surgery indicate that a fraction of such patients can be salvaged. Among patients with disease confined to the pelvis, those with central recurrence have the best prognosis, while those with pelvic sidewall recurrence do worst.[45] Using external beam irradiation, salvage rates as high as 80 percent for central disease have been claimed, although 40 to 60 percent is a more realistic figure. Irradiation of recurrent cancer with interstitial sources, generally in patients with prior irradiation, has yielded 2-year disease-free survivals of approximately 15 to 25 percent.[46-48]

Results of paraaortic irradiation in patients with cervical cancer must be reviewed with care, as radiation techniques and circumstances prompting irradiation affect morbidity and survival. In selected populations, however, irradiation of small amount of paraaortic nodal disease with modest doses can lead to survival rates of approximately 20 to 40 percent with minimal morbidity.[27,49] The experimental use of proton beam from the cyclotron at the Massachusetts General Hospital has resulted in a few long-term survivors without significant complaints.

Carcinoma of the Corpus Uteri

Adenocarcinoma is the most common primary malignant tumor of the corpus and shows a wide variety of cell types which can be classified according to the degree of differentiation. This tumor occurs predominantly in postmenopausal patients and often is associated with obesity, diabetes, and hypertension. It usually grows and spreads from its mucosal origin, infiltrating the myometrium and eventually reaching the peritoneal surface and breaking through and invading adjacent organs. Extension and metastases can

Table 6-1 Incidence of Pelvic Nodal Metastases for Stage I
Carcinoma of the Endometrium

	Endometrium	Inner Third	Middle Third	Outer Third	Total
Boronow et al.[50]					
Grade I	0	0	0	25	5.5
Grade II	0	2.7	33	20	10
Grade III	0	25	25	42	26
Lewis et al.[51]					
All Grades	0	0	14	36	11.2

occur along the lymphatics with secondary growth appearing in the ovaries, vagina, parametria, and pelvic and paraaortic lymph nodes.

Prognosis of this disease depends on three factors:

1. Cell type and degree of cellular differentiation
2. Degree of myometrial invasion
3. Presence or absence of endocervical involvement

The lymphatics of the body of the uterus drain via the infundibulo-pelvic ligament to the common iliac and paraaortic nodes. When the tumor extends to involve the cervix, the spread of the tumor is via the paracervical lymphatic to the pelvic, obturator, common iliac, and paraaortic nodes. The incidence of pelvic nodal metastases for stage I carcinoma of the endometrium depends on tumor grade and the degree of myometrial invasion (Table 6-1).

Irradiation and surgery are both effective methods of therapy. Primary surgery consists of total abdominal hysterectomy and bilateral salpino-oophorectomy and is preferred in cases in which the operative risk is low and in which growth is limited to the uterus and the cell type is well-differentiated adenocarcinoma. Wertheim hysterectomy with preoperative radiation therapy is reserved only for selected patients with endocervical involvement (i.e., stage II).

Radiation therapy for inoperable cases consists of whole-pelvis irradiation of 45 to 50 Gy in 5 to 6 weeks followed by intracavitary cesium implant. The cure rate following radiation treatment alone is not so high as with surgery, partly because it is often used in the poor-risk group and in patients with more extensive disease.

SELECTION OF THERAPY

Management of carcinoma of the endometrium is complex and controversial. For a preoperative procedure, some recommend high-dose external beam whole-pelvis radiation, that is, 45 Gy in 5-weeks, and some favor intracavitary implant while others favor combination of these two. There are pros and cons related to such approach. At Massachusetts General Hospital, we have not employed preoperative intracavitary brachytherapy for almost 25 years or high-dose whole-pelvis radiation therapy for over 10 years. The reasons are as follows:

1. For Stage IA well-differentiated adenocarcinoma, many patients can be cured without adjuvant radiation therapy.
2. For the patients with high grade tumors, the incidence of pelvic and paraaortic nodal metastases is not negligible. Without staging laparotomy, the extent and location of the involved nodes cannot be determined; therefore, these nodes are often not irradiated with the traditional portals if high-dose preoperative radiation therapy is given.
3. Some patients with extrauterine spread of the tumors or positive peritoneal washings cannot be adequately assessed preoperatively and high-dose radiation therapy to the pelvis would destroy recognition of their presence which may well represent the tip of the iceberg of extensive disease and offer the physician a false sense of security; thus, the patient may well be undertreated.
4. If the depth of myometrial invasion is marked, which cannot be determined preoperatively, the

high-dose radiation therapy would destroy the primary lesion and the propensity for nodal metastases would not be appreciated in such irradiated uteri.

5. Based on the foregoing arguments, high-dose external radiation therapy and/or brachytherapy may undertreat a sizable group of patients with high incidence of nodal metastases, and overtreat the patients with good prognosis without nodal metastases or with superficial lesions.

Because of these facts, a program of low-dose preoperative radiation therapy was initiated 10 years ago, consisting of 10 Gy in 5 days, only for stage I high-grade lesions. There are several advantages:

1. On the basis of study of carcinoma of the bladder,[52] low-dose preoperative radiation therapy can decrease the incidence of wound implant as well as distant metastases effectively. Since carcinoma of the endometrium is a highly implantable lesion, such a program appears to be attractive.

2. Low-dose preoperative radiation therapy permits immediate surgery without wound healing problems.

3. Low-dose preoperative radiation therapy permits the benefits of stage laparotomy without affecting the true stage of the disease, nodal status, peritoneal washing cytology, extrauterine spread, and so forth.

4. Low-dose preoperative radiation therapy does not distort the precise histopathologic nature of the disease; the degree of depth of myometrial invasion, thus allowing immediate postoperative adjuvant therapy to be given (i.e., radiation therapy or chemotherapy); and so forth.

5. During the past 10 years, such a program has been found effective with satisfactory results. The results are reported in another section of this chapter.

The treatment policy for carcinoma of the corpus uteri as practiced at the Massachusetts General Hospital can be briefly summarized as follows:

1. For stage I undifferentiated adenocarcinoma, and/ or lesion associated with enlarged uterus (more than 8-cm-long canal), a course of low-dose preoperative radiation therapy is planned. This is given in the form of external whole-pelvis irradiation of 1,000 cGy in five daily fractions to be followed immediately by total abdominal hysterectomy and bilateral salpingo-oophorectomy.

2. Stage I well-differentiated superficial carcinoma is treated by total abdominal hysterectomy and bilateral salpingo-oophorectomy without preoperative radiation therapy. Postoperatively, either intracavitary vaginal cesium implant to reduce the incidence of vaginal recurrences or whole-pelvis external radiation therapy is given.

3. For patients whose resected specimens show deep myometrial invasion by tumor (one half or more of its entire thickness) and/or the cell type is undifferentiated in nature, postoperative whole pelvis irradiation of 40 to 45 Gy in 5 weeks including the vagina is given in lieu of intracavitary vaginal cesium implant. From the standpoint of risk of nodal metastases, patients with stage I carcinoma of the endometrium can be divided into two groups (i.e., high and low risk); the recommendations for postoperative radiation therapy are shown in Figure 6-12.

4. For patients with carcinoma of the corpus with involvement of the endocervix (stage II), preoperative whole-pelvis irradiation of 10 Gy in five daily fractions is planned, to be followed by Wertheim hysterectomy. An alternative approach is to deliver external whole-pelvis irradiation of 40 Gy and one intracavitary cesium implant, tandem-ovoid combination, with 25 Gy to point A, to be followed by extrafascial abdominal hysterectomy. Either method is effective and is determined by the physical status of the patient and the availability of the skills of the surgeon or the radiation therapist. Most of the failures from either approach are due to distant metastatic disease.

5. Stage III carcinoma (tumor outside the uterus but within the pelvis), is infrequent and may involve the ovary, peritoneum, and paracervical tissues or may spread laterally to the pelvic sidewall or inferiorly to the vagina. Some cases may be resectable, that is, adnexal mass not fixed to the pelvic sidewall. Patients deemed to be resectable should be explored if the medical condition of the patient permits. Therapy in these cases must be individualized according to the findings at surgery, consisting of irradiation, chemotherapy, or both.

6. Stage IV carcinoma is infrequent. Its treatment is primarily palliative and must be individualized ac-

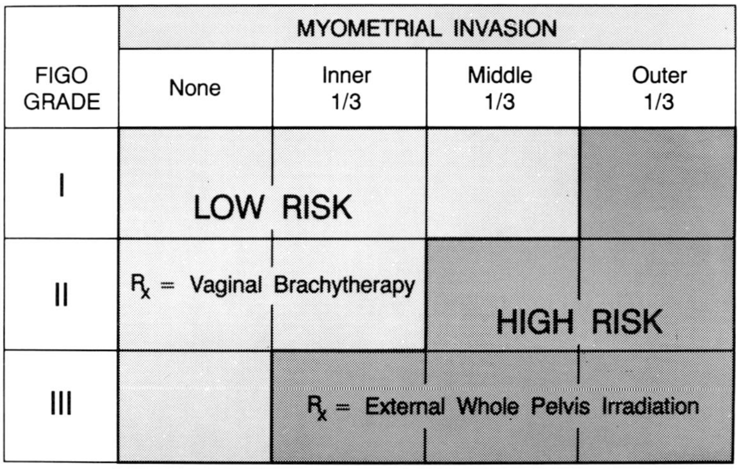

FIGO GRADE	MYOMETRIAL INVASION			
	None	Inner 1/3	Middle 1/3	Outer 1/3
I	LOW RISK			
II	R_x = Vaginal Brachytherapy		HIGH RISK	
III			R_x = External Whole Pelvis Irradiation	

Fig. 6-12 Diagram showing relative risk of pelvic lymph node involvement versus FIGO grade and extent of myometrial involvement by carcinoma of the endometrium. The recommended radiation procedure is shown in the graph that is, external beam whole-pelvis radiation therapy and intracavitary vaginal brachytherapy.

cording to the findings in each case. Irradiation, surgery, or combination of both or hormonal therapy or chemotherapy may be considered.

7. Recurrent carcinoma therapy is individualized depending on the site(s) of recurrent carcinoma and may include surgery, irradiation, or chemotherapy. If the recurrence is demonstrated by laparotomy to be limited to the vagina or pelvis, in previously unirradiated patients high-dose radiation therapy with external beam and/or implant may be considered with a fair degree of local control.

8. The reported incidence of vaginal recurrence after total abdominal hysterectomy alone varies from 10 to 15 percent.[53,54] Its incidence is directly related to the tumor grade and depth of myometrial invasion. The most common region involved by a well-differentiated carcinoma is at the vaginal vault. For a small local recurrence, intracavitary or interstitial implant may eradicate the disease. For large vaginal vault lesions, however, combined external whole-pelvis irradiation and isotope implant is the procedure of choice. Vaginal recurrences from undifferentiated adenocarcinomas tend to develop more rapidly and extensively and involve the anterior vaginal wall and suburethral area and are frequently associated with tumor spread outside the vaginal vault and into the pelvis as well as with distant metastases. Such lesions are treated primarily by external whole-pelvis irradiation with a dose of 55 to 60 Gy in 6 to 7 weeks, to be followed by an implant delivering 20 Gy to bulk disease, if lasting local controls are to be expected.

INTRACAVITARY BRACHYTHERAPY TECHNIQUES FOR CARCINOMA OF THE CORPUS

Single Linear Cesium Source

If the uterus is small (i.e., the canal measures less than 8 cm), a single linear tandem source with heavy loading at the top such as 20 to 15 to 10 mg, can be used for intracavitary irradiation to deliver approximately 25 to 30 Gy 2 cm from the central sources. Figure 6-13 shows the isodose distributions with differential loading of sources suitable for intracavitary boost after external radiation therapy. This is used following high-dose external whole-pelvis radiation therapy of 45 to 50 Gy.

Heyman's Packing Technique

The aim of Heyman's packing technique is to insert eight or more irradiators in the form of capsules, each containing 10 mg radium tightly in the uterine cavity. In experienced hands, this technique may be used in lieu of hysterectomy as primary treatment of patients with medically inoperable carcinoma with an enlarged uterus. It is accompanied by the risk of uterine perforation, cervical laceration, and potential spread of cancer cells with the stretching and distention of the uterine cavity during the operation. Various sizes of Heyman's capsules, including afterloading Simon applicators, are available. Generally, two impants are

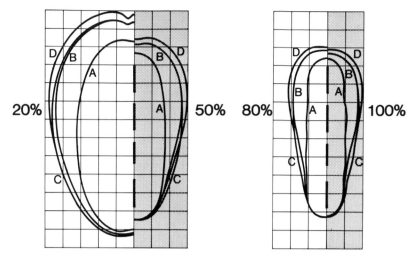

20%   50%   80%   100%

Loading Arrangement

mgm Radium Equivalent in Tandem	A	B	C	D
	10	25	25	35
	10	20	20	20
	10	10	15	10
	10	10	10	10

Fig. 6-13 Isodose distributions with various differential loadings for intracavitary boost by a line applicator for endometrial carcinoma.

given, each delivering approximately 25 to 30 Gy to 1.5 cm below the mucosal surface, staged 3 weeks apart. With the advent of high-energy whole-pelvis radiation therapy, this technique with Heyman's capsule packing is no longer used at our institution.

Intracavitary Vaginal Implant Therapy

A cylindrical applicator is used, available in varying diameters, ranging from 2 to 3.5 cm, and varying lengths of 4 to 7 cm (Fig. 6-14). The largest applicator that the vagina can accept is commonly chosen. The cylinder is generally loaded with 30 to 45 mg Ra eq^{137}Cs sources arranged either in tandem or in a T-shaped arrangement.[55] Figure 6-15 shows the T-source cylinder currently used at Massachusetts General Hospital. A dose of 40 to 45 Gy to the vaginal mucosa in 48 hours is given. The procedure is performed under local anesthesia in a departmental operating room, after the vaginal apex is healed, 4 to 6 weeks postsurgery.

RESULTS OF TREATMENT

For patients with FIGO stage I grades 2 and 3 endometrial adenocarcinoma, 5-year survival approximates 75 to 85 percent and 55 to 65 percent, respectively. When analysis is confined to patients with disease being confined to the corpus following surgery and pathologic evaluation, the corresponding figures are 90 to 95 percent and 75 to 80 percent.[56,57] Using these results as a benchmark, the program in using low dose preoperative radiation therapy at Massachusetts General Hospital has yielded 5-year survival of 97 percent and 94 percent for patients with grades 2 and 3 carcinoma, respectively, in 53 patients whose disease was surgically proven to be limited to the corpus, that is, postsurgical stage I.[58] While the results in grade 2 carcinoma appear no better, there does appear to be an improvement in prognosis in patients with grade 3 disease. This is in keeping with the results of others who described a beneficial response to irradiation in stage I carcinoma only in those patients with poor prognostic features.[59,60]

For medically inoperable cases of endometrial ade-

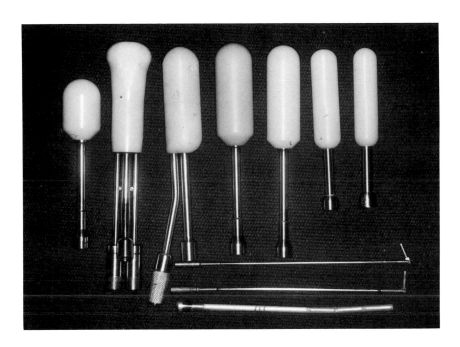

Fig. 6-14 Various vaginal applicators.

nocarcinoma, the use of radiation therapy alone offers a modest chance for cure; 285 patients treated with a variety of irradiation techniques at Roswell Park Memorial Institute[61] demonstrated a 63 percent corrected 5-year survival rate, with best results seen in patients treated with combined external beam and intracavitary therapy, while 85 patients treated at the M.D. Anderson Hospital, primarily with intracavitary radium alone, demonstrated a 5-year survival of 75 to 80 percent.[62]

Results in stage II carcinoma appear to vary with tumor grade and extent of the tumor within the endometrial cavity and the myometrium and cervix. Five-year survivals varied from 60 to 80 percent, with patients undergoing combined surgery and irradiation doing better than the patients treated with irradiation alone in most, but not all, series.[63-65]

Patients with clinically evident extrauterine tumor, FIGO stage III, have a poorer prognosis than do those found at surgery to have unsuspected extrauterine disease, with 5-year survivals of 16 percent and 40 percent, respectively.[66] Furthermore, the location of extrauterine disease is important, since in patients with surgically staged disease, those with metastases to the ovaries or fallopian tubes only demonstrated an 80 percent 5-year survival, versus 15 percent for those with disease involving other pelvic structures.[67]

The Massachusetts General Hospital experience of 1976 through 1978 was published in the FIGO Annual Report.[31] For the entire group of 157 patients stages I to IV, the 5-year survival rate was 71 percent (112 of 157 patients). For stages I and II, the corresponding rates were 80 percent and 65 percent, respectively. In stage III and IV lesions, the rates were poor, with only a few patients alive at 5 years.

The results of treatment of recurrent cancer vary with the location of the recurrence, characteristics of primary tumor and the interval following surgery. In patients treated with irradiation, and with combined irradiation plus surgery, 5-year survivals for postoperative recurrent cancer were 15 to 25 percent.[68,69] Vaginal recurrences represent a distinct variety of local recurrence, which is prevented by adjuvant irradiation. Vaginal recurrences appear to comprise two populations, those appearing soon after surgery and involving the distal vagina have only a few survivors. Those whose recurrence involves the apex at some time after surgery, may expect a 5-year survival in excess of 50 percent, however.[53,77]

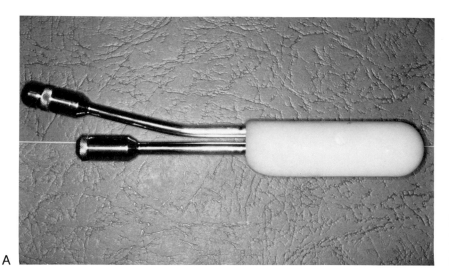

A

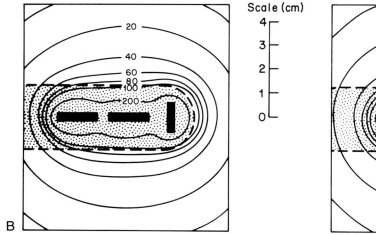

B

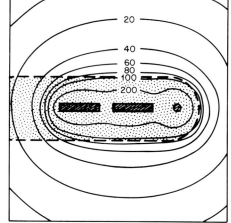

Fig. 6-15 T-source cylinder. **(A)** External appearance. **(B)** Isodose distribution along the applicator.

Carcinoma of the Ovary

Malignant ovarian tumors may arise from any of the component cells of the ovary. Although the laparoscope may be helpful in differentiating nonneoplastic from neoplastic tumors, laparotomy is essential in making a definitive diagnosis and evaluation of the extent of the tumor. The management of ovarian carcinomas is surgical excision, if the condition is operable.

Carcinoma of the ovary tends to spread rather early and extensively by three routes:

1. Seeding along the peritoneal surface and omentum
2. Invasion of the adjacent pelvic structures
3. Metastasis to the regional nodes and to right hemidiaphragm

Any of these conditions can render complete surgical removal impossible with low surgical survival rates and can thus dictate the use of postoperative adjuvant treatment.

SELECTION OF THERAPY

Stage I   For stage I disease, the treatment of choice is surgical resection, in the form of total abdominal hysterectomy and bilateral salpingo-oophorectomy and omentectomy, except in the well-explored young woman with a well-differentiated tumor strictly confined to one ovary in whom conservative surgery may preserve fertility.

Stage II   Every attempt should be made to perform a total abdominal hysterectomy, bilateral salpingo-oophorectomy, and omentectomy resecting as much tumor as possible to reduce residual nodules to less than 2 cm. Careful recording of the residual tumor nodules is important. Postoperative adjuvant irradiation may be given to residual disease, to areas of prior tumor fixation or adherence, or to the entire abdomen.

Stage III   If the lesions are resectable, total abdominal hysterectomy, bilateral salpingo-oophorectomy, and omentectomy with resection of gross tumor are performed and adjuvant postoperative therapy is indicated. For the nonresectable lesions, as much tumor as possible should be removed if the procedure does not endanger the life of the patient as both chemotherapy and radiotherapy are more effective when fewer cancer cells are present. Postoperatively, the patient is treated with chemotherapy or radiotherapy. The exact size and location of the residual nodules need to be clearly spelled out in the operative note.

Stage IV   Individualization must be carried out. Total abdominal hysterectomy, bilateral salpingo-oophorectomy, and omentectomy (when possible) are performed, to be followed by radiation therapy.

ADJUVANT THERAPY

Postoperatively, there are several choices. The first is chemotherapy, generally the treatment of choice. Radiation therapy may also be given, but requires large fields to encompass the entire abdomen with questionable effectiveness. A third alternative is intraperitoneal instillation of chromic ^{32}P.

RADIATION THERAPY MANAGEMENT OF OVARIAN CANCERS

Radiation therapy for ovarian carcinomas is primarily adjuvant in nature. For IA and IB low-grade carcinomas, the results following curative surgery are satisfactory, and therefore no postoperative radiation therapy is indicated. For the high-grade tumors, whole pelvis irradiation may be considered but its usefulness is unproven. For the Stage IC lesions, administration of chromic ^{32}P intraperitoneally is limited to (1) those situations in which all gross disease has been removed, (2) cases in which peritoneal miliary seeding is present, or (3) localized tumor that ruptured during surgical removal. The prime requisite for ^{32}P instillation is an adhesion-free peritoneal cavity demonstrated by radiographic studies. A dose of 15 mCi is usually given per injection.

For stage II lesions with residual disease limited to the pelvis, high-dose whole-pelvis radiation therapy is given. The irradiation portals should be adequate to include all the pelvic structures to the pelvic brim, for a tumor dose of approximately 50 Gy in 6 weeks. This dose can only be accomplished safely by using high-energy megavoltage modality with AP and PA portals.

For stage III disease, radiation therapy requires total abdominal irradiation. Such large radiation portals always compromise the radiation dose and therefore the effectiveness, and the dose is further compromised by the necessity for shielding the kidneys and liver after doses of approximately 25 to 30 Gy, respectively. Except for radiosensitive tumors, such as dysgerminoma, granulosa cell tumor, or lymphoma, and for some epithelial tumors having residual nodules less than 2 cm in diameter, whole-abdominal irradiation does not provide good palliation, and the amount of radiations tolerable by the radiosensitive abdominal organs will not eradicate the advanced epithelial tumors. Furthermore, bone marrow depression from whole abdominal irradiation prevents subsequent use of effective chemotherapeutic agents. In a group of patients where minimal disease has been left at surgery but which is too extensive to employ ^{32}P instillation, abdominopelvic irradiation, including the diaphragms, may be given instead of chemotherapy. Recent reports suggest this approach may be worthwhile.[71]

Total abdominal irradiation may be given using the moving strip technique[72,73] or by wide-field abdominopelvic irradiation, the so-called abdominal bath. The moving strip technique delivers 28 Gy in 13 days to each strip; a pelvic boost is generally added. Wide-field whole abdominal irradiation causes severe acute GI toxicity unless the fraction size is reduced to approximately 1 Gy, and the total abdominal dose is limited to approximately 25 Gy in 5 to 6 weeks. A pelvic boost field can bring the total dose to the pelvis to approximately 45 Gy. Moving strip irradiation has not been shown to be superior to "abdominal bath" as far as long-term cures are concerned,[74] and therefore is not commonly used.

The recent development of employing twice-daily radiation therapy for some human malignancies arising in the head and neck area[75] has extended such approach to treatment of gynecologic cancers.[76] For total abdominal irradiation, two fractions a day with 1 Gy per fraction, 4 hours between fractions, for a total of 30 Gy in 3 weeks, has been found to be well tolerated even in patients who failed multiagent chemotherapy, following second-look laparotomy. Additional pelvic boost of 15 Gy in 1 week can be completed without further difficulties. Most patients had a marked bone marrow depression yet recovered in a few months. GI symptoms were minimal. Whether multifraction a day radiation therapy can improve the local control for this unfortunate group of patients remains to be seen in the coming years. The short-term results thus far are encouraging.

Ovarian carcinomas of borderline malignant potential have a much better prognosis, stage by stage, than do the frankly invasive malignant ovarian carcinomas.[77,78] The beneficial effect of radiation therapy for these particular tumors is uncertain but, if the residual tumors are limited to the pelvis, one may consider postoperative radiation therapy to control the residual disease. The radiosensitive tumors, such as dysgerminoma, granulosa cell tumor, and lymphoma, may be benefited by postoperative radiation therapy even if the extent of the lesions calls for irradiation of the entire abdomen because of their high radiosensitivity and radiocurability

RESULTS OF TREATMENT

The results of treatment are closely related to the stage of the primary lesion, the degree of cellular differentiation and the presence or absence of gross residual tumors after surgical resection.[79,80] For stage I disease, the 5-year survival rates range from 80 to 90

percent following surgical resection.[81] Selected patients with favorable grades and histology may be treated by conservative surgery alone to preserve fertility.[82] The results of conventional once-daily radiation therapy for more advanced ovarian tumors, mainly stage II and III, are more difficult to interpret, since with more meticulous surgical staging, cases with microscopic evidence of extrapelvic disease are removed from stage II group, improving the results in that stage, and placed in stage III, improving results in that stage as well. Typical 5-year survivals in stage II carcinoma in multiple series treated with either postoperative pelvic irradiation or whole abdominal irradiation are in the range of 50 to 60 percent.[83] For patients with stage III carcinoma results vary from as low as 12 percent to 70 percent survival.[83,71] For serous cystadenocarcinomas, stage for stage, the low-grade lesions generally carry a better survival rate than do high-grade lesions. Likewise, those patients with residual tumors of small size, that is, 2 cm or less, were found to have somewhat better survival rates than those patients with large residual tumors following surgical removal.

The role of intraperitoneal chromic ^{32}P is unclear; most studies are uncontrolled evaluations of patients with relatively favorable tumors. Chemotherapy is thought to be beneficial in stage I disease with tumor present on the external surface of the ovary or tumor spillage into the peritoneal cavity during surgical removal and is clearly indicated for stage II and III lesions with expected objective responses in 40 to 50 percent of cases treated. For stage IV inoperable and unresectable lesions, chemotherapy and radiation therapy are, at times, effective in providing long-term palliation and growth restraint.

SEX CORD STROMAL TUMORS

The sex cord stromal tumors are rare and include granulosa and thecal cell tumors. These are benign. Granulosa cell tumors tend to recur many years after surgery and can produce excessive estrogen. The treatment of choice for these tumors is surgical resection. Radiation therapy is effective in an adjuvant setting or in controlling inoperable lesions with a dose of approximately 40 Gy in 4 weeks.

Dysgerminoma occurs in the young age group (i.e., 20 to 30 years) and is infrequent. Its management is surgical resection. Like seminoma in males, it is extremely radiosensitive and radiocurable. The tumor is frequently unilateral (less than 10 percent bilateral); thus, in younger women conservative surgical resection can be performed with preservation of fertility and endocrine function.[84] This tumor spreads by the lymphatic route to the paraaortic nodes and then to the mediastinum and supraclavicular nodes. For tumors more extensive than stage IA, postoperative radiation therapy is indicated at least to the lymphatic drainage area if not the whole abdomen with high survival rates. A dose of 30 Gy in 4 weeks should suffice.

For the dysgerminoma with mixed choriocarcinoma, endodermal sinus tumor, or teratoma, multidrug multicyle chemotherapy is indicated postoperatively. The cure rates for these malignant germ cell tumors are good.

RESULTS OF TREATMENT

The beneficial effects of radiation therapy for ovarian sex cord stromal tumors are well recognized. In one series[85] with granulosa cell tumor; of 13 patients who did not receive radiation therapy after surgery, of whom nine had stage I disease, eight (62 percent) died of their disease. By contrast, of 46 patients who were irradiated postoperatively, of whom 21 had stage I disease, only 17 (34 percent) died of their disease.

In the M.D. Anderson Hospital series of patients with dysgerminoma,[86] those with unilateral encapsulated tumors were treated conservatively, and the remainder were irradiated postoperatively, generally to the entire abdomen. All 16 patients with stage I and II disease survived, as did 75 percent of those with stages III and IV. Similar results were obtained at the Holt Radium Institute.[87]

MISCELLANEOUS OVARIAN TUMORS

Other ovarian tumors include primary malignant lymphoma and mesenchymal tumors, although they are rare. Management should be highly individualized with surgical resection first to be followed by adjuvant therapy, such as radiation therapy and/or chemotherapy. Unfortunately, these tumors tend to spread early and widely, and the prognosis is poor.

Metastatic tumors to the ovary are not uncommon and include Krukenberg's tumor of the GI tract, breast, or lung cancers. Treatment is primarily palliative and depends on the nature of the primary lesions. In general, chemotherapy with or without radiation therapy is preferred.

Carcinoma of the Vagina

Carcinoma of the vagina is an uncommon tumor, comprising approximately 1 to 2 percent of gynecologic malignancies. More than 90 percent of these tumors are squamous cell carcinoma, although adenocarcinoma, sarcoma, malignant melanoma, and diethylstilbestrol (DES)-induced clear cell carcinoma is occasionally seen. Sarcoma botryoides occurs in children and infants.

More than one-half of squamous cell carcinomas occur in the upper third of the vagina and about one-third in the lower third.[88] The lesion arising from the middle and upper third of the posterior vaginal wall at times is difficult, if not impossible, to differentiate from carcinoma of the cervix. Vaginal bleeding is a nonspecific symptom of the disease. Careful palpation and inspection of the lesion followed by biopsy are needed in order to establish the diagnosis.

The pattern of lymphatic spread varies with the location of the lesion. For the upper third of the vagina, the lymphatics follow those of the cervix and lymph node metastases occur in the external iliac and hypogastric nodes. For the lower third of the vagina, the lymphatics merge with those of the vulva and drain to the inguinal nodes. The middle third of the vagina possesses dual drainage of the upper and lower third, and the lymphatics drain to the external iliac and inguinal nodes.

The anterior vaginal wall is relatively fixed, so that tumors arising from this location may often invade the urethra and bladder base, although the lesions may be small. The posterior vaginal wall however is relatively pliable and the tumors although large may expand by direct extension without invading the rectal mucosa. Such pattern of spread has great therapeutic implications and may determine the extent of surgery and/or choice of radiotherapeutic procedures.

SELECTION OF THERAPY

The location and extent of the vaginal tumors determine the selection of therapy:

1. Carcinoma in situ or stage I carcinoma of the vagina can be treated either by local excision, partial vaginectomy, or local radiation therapy. For multifocal lesions, radiation therapy is the treatment of choice with good local control.

2. When the early lesion (stage I) is located in the upper third of the vagina, treatment is similar to

that for carcinoma of the cervix. If the patient is a good surgical risk, radical hysterectomy with wide vaginal cuff and pelvic lymphadenectomy is preferred.

3. For advanced stage I lesions involving the lower two-thirds of the vagina, radiation therapy is preferred, with surgery held in reserve.

4. For the extensive stage II lesions involving primarily the anterior or posterior vaginal wall, high-dose radiation therapy involves risks of radiation injury of the urethra, bladder or rectum respectively. Such lesions are preferably treated by excision either before or after external beam radiation therapy. The lesions arising from the lateral wall may be vigorously treated by combined external beam therapy and interstitial implant with good local control and yet without the high risks of bladder or bowel damage.

5. For stage III disease with tumor extending onto the pelvic wall, radiation therapy is the only reasonable therapeutic procedure. In some instances, pelvic exenteration may be possible for removal of residual nidus of the tumor after high-dose radiation therapy.

6. For stage IV disease with involvement of the bladder and/or rectum, combined radiation therapy and surgery in the form of anterior or posterior exenteration may be considered.

7. Clear cell carcinoma in a young adult, stage I or II disease, can be managed similarly by total vaginectomy with radical abdominal hysterectomy lymphadenectomy and vaginal vault reconstruction. The ovaries can be preserved. Radiation therapy can be added if pelvic nodes are positive and/or there is evidence of residual disease in the pelvis and/or positive resection margins. If radical surgery is done, the ovaries should be moved out of the pelvis, with blood intact, in case postoperative radiotherapy is necessary.

TECHNIQUE OF RADIATION THERAPY

Some of the vaginal applicators for treatment of carcinoma of the endometrium are available for irradiation of vaginal carcinoma. Commonly, a large vaginal cylinder is used to treat the superficial stage I lesions. Because of the rapid steep falloff of radiation by intracavitary technique, a dose of 60 to 70 Gy may be delivered to the vaginal mucosa and the tumor, yet the dose to the neighboring structures is low. Thus, the rectum and bladder can be spared from the high-dose effect. The procedure is relatively straightforward and can be done under local anesthesia and generally consists of two sittings of 30 to 35 Gy 2 weeks apart. For large stage I or II lesions, external beam whole-pelvis radiation therapy is given first for approximately 45 Gy, to be followed by interstitial implant or intracavitary vaginal cylinder irradiation for an additional 30 Gy.

Figure 6-16 shows an applicator developed at the Massachusetts General Hospital using template technique for carcinoma of the vagina. Essentially a two-plane interstitial implant, the inner plane lies along the vaginal mucosal surface intracavitarily and the outer plane interstitially below the base of the tumor. The two planes are separated for a distance of 1.5 cm. The dose prescribed is referenced at midpoint between the planes.

Most of the advanced lesions, stages III and IV, require high-dose external whole pelvis radiation therapy. The treatment techniques are similar but not identical to those for carcinoma of the cervix.

RESULTS OF TREATMENT

Prognosis in carcinoma of the vagina treated by irradiation depends most heavily on stage and nodal status, and somewhat less on tumor grade. Review of major series of patients treated with radiation therapy[54,89–91,93] indicates approximately 80 to 90 percent 5-year actuarial survival for stage I, 50 to 60 percent survival for stage II, 30 to 40 percent survival for stage III, and 5 percent for stage IV carcinomas. Approximately 40 percent of patients develop recurrences which are commonly in the pelvis. Unfortunately, the pelvic recurrence is often extensive with metastatic nodal disease, making surgical salvage often impossible or unsuccessful. For incurable and inoperable lesions, radiation therapy or combined multiagent chemotherapy is effective for palliation with alleviation of distressing symptoms and, remotely, for prolongation of comfortable and useful life.

Carcinoma of the Vulva

Cancer of the vulva constitutes approximately 5 percent of all gynecologic malignancies. Squamous cell carcinoma is by far the most common malignant

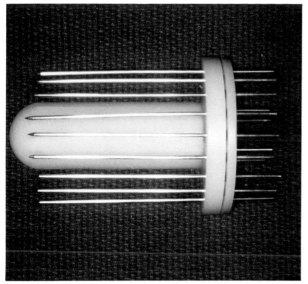

A

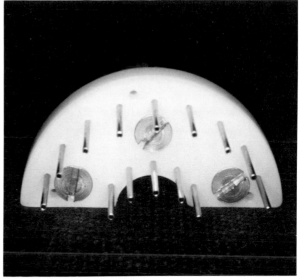

B

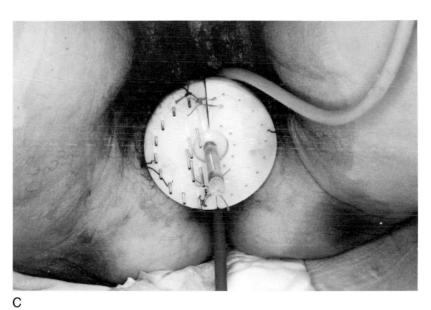

C

Fig. 6-16 Applicator for template implant for carcinoma of vagina. **(A)** Lateral view. **(B)** End view. **(C)** In a patient.

tumor although other tumors, including melanoma, carcinoma of the Bartholin gland, adenocarcinoma, and sarcoma are occasionally seen in this region. Pre-malignant lesions include in situ carcinoma, Paget's disease, and erythroplasia of Queyrat and others.

Squamous cell carcinoma is a disease of advanced age, although it has been seen with increasing fre-quency in young women in the third and fourth dec-ades of life. Because of the rich lymphatics of the vulva, careful palpation of the lymphatic areas is indi-cated as part of the complete physical examination. Most of the primary lymphatic drainage of the vulva is to the superficial femoral nodes, and then to the deep femoral nodes. There are many crossings between both vulvae, and bilateral metastases are not uncommon. The incidence is high.

Cloquet's node is located in the femoral canal beneath Poupart's ligament and represents the most proximal lymph node in the deep femoral chain. If Cloquet's node is negative for metastases, it is unlikely that the vulvar cancer has spread to involve the hypogastric or external iliac nodes within the pelvis. This peice of information has great radiotherapeutic implication. If Cloquet's node is not involved by the carcinoma, there is no indication that the pelvic nodes should be included within the postoperative radiation therapy portal.

SELECTION OF THERAPY

The preferred treatment for squamous cell carcinoma of the vulva is surgical resection, consisting of radical en bloc vulvectomy with bilateral inguinal lymph node dissection. Pelvic lymph node dissection is occasionally added, but the survival of patients with positive nodes is low. Older patients, even with many medical problems, have tolerated such radical surgery quite well.

Radiation therapy may be useful as primary management for patients who refuse surgery or for medically inoperable patients with small localized tumors. It can be used prior to inguinal dissection for fixed nodes and/or for palliation for widespread disease. Postoperative radiation therapy is indicated when the resection margins are close to, or involved by, tumor; for patients with multiple positive lymph nodes in the resected specimen; and for tumors with extracapsular extension.

RADIATION THERAPY TECHNIQUE

In patients of advancing age, the vulvar tissues tend to be atrophic and have low tolerance to radiation therapy. Any curative radiation therapy may result in brisk symptomatic radiation dermatitis and mucositis and is extremely uncomfortable to the patients. Radiation therapy must be carried out with great caution and care.

For the localized inoperable lesions, external beam radiation therapy consisting of 40 Gy to the primary site and inguinal and pelvic nodes is followed by an interstitial implant for an additional 30 to 35 Gy. For small superficial lesions, low-energy electron beam

plays an important role in treating this disease[94]—just like skin cancer for a dose of 60 Gy in 5 weeks. For the inguinal and pelvic nodal disease, high-energy external beam photon irradiation through anterior and posterior portals with or without electron beam boost to the superficial groin nodes is employed.

Likewise, because of constant moisture and folding of the skin, the groins generally tolerate high-dose radiation therapy poorly often with acute symptomatic sequelae.

RESULTS OF TREATMENT

The surgical results for carcinoma of the vulva are surprisingly good. The cure rates are related to the size of the primary lesions, the presence or absence of nodal metastases, and the histologic differentiation of the tumor.[95,96]

In general, patients with small primaries, absence of nodal metastases, and/or well-differentiated tumors have the highest survival. These factors are interrelatd however. For patients without nodes, a 5-year survival rate of 80 to 90 percent can be expected. For patients with positive nodes, the corresponding rate is decreased by a factor of 2, ranging from 30 to 50 percent. Likewise, the fewer the number of metastatic nodes, the better the survival.

Since most vulvar cancers are traditionally treated by surgery, the results of radiation therapy in the management of this disease are sparse. Three series have reported the use of preoperative external beam irradiation in 28 patients, using 36 to 55 Gy, in an attempt to debulk a tumor before surgery or to avoid inguinal lymphadenopathy.[97-99] Results are too preliminary to draw conclusions as to efficacy but the irradiation is well tolerated. Data on the use of postoperative irradiation are too sparse to summarize.

Prempree and Amornmarn[100] described the use of radiation therapy for recurrent vulvar carcinoma Prempree treated patients with recurrent vulvar carcinoma using combined pelvic irradiation and interstitial implant to doses in the neighborhood of 60 to 80 Gy. Twenty-one patients demonstrated a 38 percent 5-year survival with prognosis, depending on site and extent of recurrence.

Frischbier and Thomsen[94] report on 118 patients treated following biopsy, using an electron beam of 9 to 16 MeV to deliver 45 to 54 Gy to the vulva and inguinal areas. Of 33 patients with disease confined to the vulva, 70 percent survived 5 years; for patients with disease involving inguinal nodes or adjacent organs, 5-year survival was 39 percent. Eight percent of patients developed severe complications.

Miscellaneous Gynecologic Carcinomas

MALIGNANT TUMOR OF THE FALLOPIAN TUBE

Malignant tumor of the fallopian tube is a rare neoplasm and comprises fewer than 1 percent of gynecologic malignancies and is usually a papillary adenocarcinoma. Clinically it behaves and spreads in a manner similar to that of ovarian carcinoma with direct local extension and intraperitoneal implants. Therefore, early diagnosis of these tumors cannot be easily made.[101] An adnexal mass with intermittent pelvic pain is nonspecific but may herald the presence of this tumor. A positive Pap smear in the presence of a negative curettage should alert the clinician to this diagnosis. There is no official staging for this disease, but an attempt has been made using FIGO staging system as for ovarian cancer.

Selection of Therapy and Results

Although this tumor is quite radiosensitive, the cure rate by radiation therapy or surgery, is poor because of the frequent wide dissemination of the disease. Radiation therapy should be considered following total hysterectomy and bilateral salpingo-oophorectomy if residual disease remains or is suspected in the pelvis. A dose of 45 to 50 Gy to the whole pelvis in 5 to 6 weeks is sufficient for this condition. Like ovarian cancer, prognosis varies with stage and postoperative residual disease. The 5-year survival rates approximate 60 percent for stage I disease, 40 percent for stage II disease, and 10 to 20 percent for more advanced disease.[102,103] The roles of chemotherapy and whole-abdominal irradiation in this disease have not been systematically explored.

CARCINOMA OF THE URETHRA

Carcinoma of the urethra is a rare tumor. Most are squamous cell carcinomas, but adenocarcinoma and transitional cell carcinoma are occasionally seen. There is no official staging system for this disease.

Selection of Therapy

Surgery or radiation therapy can be used for this disease. When the lesion is small, radiation therapy is the treatment of choice. If radiation therapy is unsuccessful, the lesion may be dealt with by radical surgery including anterior pelvic exenteration and lymph node dissection. For the inoperable lesions, external beam therapy is useful for palliation.

Radiation Procedure

When the lesion is small and limited to the urethra, the radiotherapeutic procedure is a combination of approximately 45 Gy by external beam therapy to the primary to be followed by interstitial implant delivering 25 Gy by either a volume implant or two-plane implant. When the disease extends outside the urethra into the vulva, bladder neck, or periurethral tissue, the treatment of choice is external beam whole-pelvis radiation therapy of 55 to 60 Gy with or without supplementary interstitial implant. Anterior pelvic exenteration is reserved for radiation failure. Figure 6-17 shows a photograph of a template applicator for interstitial brachytherapy for carcinoma of the urethra developed at Massachusetts General Hospital.

Results of Treatment

Results of treatment are best for small anteriorly situated tumors that are limited to the urethra. Of 62 patients treated at the University of Vienna, the overall 5-year survival rate was 64 percent. For anterior lesions, the survival rate was 71 percent versus 50 percent for posterior lesions. In the series conducted at the University of Maryland, 77 percent of 14 patients treated for cure survived 5 years. The Massachusetts General Hospital experience consisted of 22 patients treated by radiation therapy; of these, 64 percent were free of disease at 5 years but, when the disease extended outside the urethra into the vulva, bladder neck, or periurethral tissue, the results were uniformly poor, with an overall 5-year disease free rate of 32 percent.[104,105]

SIDE EFFECTS AND COMPLICATIONS

A distinction must be made between radiation therapy side effects and complications. The former is the

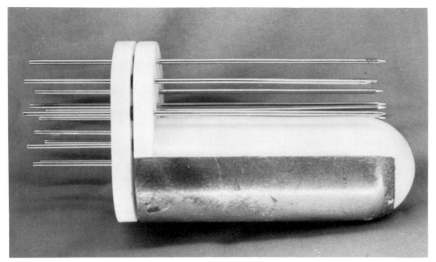

A

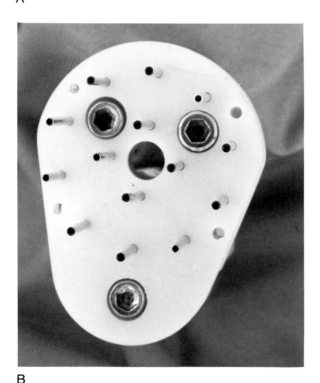

B

Fig. 6-17 Applicator for template implant for urethral carcinoma. **(A)** Lateral view, showing lead shield for protection of rectal wall. **(B)** End view.

Predisposing Factors

1. *Intrinsic:* These factors are related to the patient's medical condition,[106,107] including the advanced stage of the lesions, presence of adhesions after previous surgery or chronic pelvic inflammatory disease or endometriosis with fixation of loop of small bowel in the pelvis, diabetes, or hypertension.[108]

2. *Extrinsic:* These factors are related to the conduct of radiation therapy and the associated surgical procedures. In general, a large irradiated pelvic volume, high total dose or fraction size, a limited number of portals, (i.e., AP and PA versus four-field), or low-energy photon beam (cobalt-60 versus 25 MeV) all may increase radiation side effects and complications. Likewise, pretreatment transperitoneal staging laparotomy is often fraught with severe complications, especially if high-dose radiation therapy is given for pelvic and/or paraaortic lymph node metastases. Combined high-dose irradiation and radical hysterectomy often results in increased complications.

Acute Side Effects

The acute side effects include cystitis, proctitis, and enteritis, the necessary concomitants of curative radiation therapy, although various in extent in individual cases, and should not be considered complications and usually respond to conservative treatment or reduction in fraction size or total dose of radiation therapy.

by-product of radiation therapy, willfully produced and often unavoidable. The latter is the result of high-dose radiation and often unintentionally produced and requires corrective measures other than irradiation. At times, the distinction between these two may be vague and the common factors affecting their incidence are as follows:

Late Side Effects

Some of the more serious late effects become severely symptomatic; they require surgical or medical intervention and are therefore called radiation complications:

1. *Small bowel:* The mucosa of the small bowel is much more susceptible to radiation damage than is generally appreciated. A conventionally fractioned dose of 30 to 40 Gy may lead to hyperemia and edema with transient desquamation of glandular epithelium, clinically manifested as acute enteritis, with frequent watery diarrhea. Late radiation effects may manifest themselves in the form of intestinal necrosis, perforation, or progressive narrowing of the lumen of the intestine with or without ulceration and subsequently intestinal obstruction. These complications are generally seen at doses in excess of 45 to 50 Gy. Treatment of these chronic irreversible small bowel injuries, justifiably called complications, requires resection or bypass with careful surgical techniques. The irradiated bowel with thickened bowel walls does not heal well because of microvascular changes causing an impaired blood supply and should not be used for either bypass or anastomotic procedure.

2. *Rectosigmoid and rectum:* These structures are more susceptible to radiation injury than other pelvic organs. Acute radiation proctitis is clinically seen as frequent bowel movements, tenesmus, and minor bleeding. It usually responds within a few days to conservative treatment and medication with bismuth subcarbonate, Kaopectate or Lomotil, or a low-residue diet. In severe cases, reduction of the radiation dose or temporary interruption of the radiation treatment may be required. Late radiation injuries are infrequent and usually occur 6 months to 2 years after radiation therapy. Ulceration of the rectal wall occurs in the upper anterior rectum and rectosigmoid colon and usually is at the level corresponding to maximum dose from vaginal radium in patients with cervical cancer. The ulceration usually heals with conservative treatment. In severe instances, it may progress to perforation, fistulas, hemorrhage, or obstruction though these are unusual. Other less frequent late radiation changes consists of woody induration and thickening of the bowel wall, completely encompassing a segment of rectum and rectosigmoid, with diarrhea, tenesmus, and bleeding. The bowel lumen may be markedly narrowed with partial or complete intestinal obstruction requiring colostomy. This severe radiation complication is often called sigmoiditis and is frequently associated with high-dose external beam therapy (60 Gy or more) when a fixed loop of sigmoid lies within the treatment fields.[109] Treatment of this complication requires colostomy or resection of the involved loop of bowel with bypass of the affected segment.

3. *Bladder and ureter:* With high-dose external beam therapy and intracavity implant for cancer of the cervix or corpus, late complications may develop after doses in excess of 70 Gy. These are slow in making their appearance, generally after 1 to 4 years. In severe instances, the irradiated bladder may ulcerate; subsequently vesicovaginal fistulas may develop, requiring urinary diversion. In the ureter, late ureteral complications may occur[110] but are rare despite high-dose irradiation for carcinoma of the cervix.[111] Generally, any ureteral abnormality or obstruction following radical radiation therapy must be considered recurrent carcinoma until proved otherwise, and its management should be planned accordingly.

4. *Kidney:* The kidneys have erroneously been thought to be immune to the adverse effects of radiations and complications. Doses of the order of 25 to 30 Gy in 3 weeks may result in radiation nephritis with secondary contraction of the kidney and when this is bilateral, the result can be fatal.[112] During abdominal irradiation the dose to both kidneys should be kept under 25 Gy in 3 weeks to avoid fatal nephritis.

5. *Cervix and vagina:* Postirradiation ulcers of the cervix or vaginal vault necrosis occasionally develop 6 to 12 months after intracavitary radium implant. These are relatively asymptomatic and are treated conservatively. Months may be required for reepithelialization. Fortunately, this complication is relatively infrequent, 1 to 4 percent. Vaginal stenosis and foreshortening of varying degrees occurs in about 60 to 70 percent of patients undergoing radiation therapy and intracavitary implant. The condition is caused by adhesions formed between the raw surfaces of the anterior and posterior vaginal walls and can be avoided by frequent use of vaginal dilators during the healing phase of the vagina or encouraging vaginal use after treatment.

6. *Skeleton:* Femoral neck fractures and pubic bone osteoradionecrosis are most commonly seen following pelvic irradiation through lateral portals with orthovoltage equipment. These complications generally develop a year or more after radiation therapy after a dose of 50 to 60 Gy in 6 weeks to the femoral neck and pelvic bones.[113] Treatment of this complication requires internal fixation. In spite of previous irradiation, bone union occurs in most cases. Since megavoltage radiation spares the bone, these complications are less likely to occur with dosages within the therapeutic range.

7. *Hematopoietic system:* Radiation can suppress stem cell regeneration, affecting the blood elements. This depression is a radiation side effect and likely occurs when the entire abdomen and pelvis are irradiated. If the depression is unduly severe, radiation therapy will have to be suspended. Recovery usually is rapid.

8. *Liver:* Irradiation of the whole liver to doses in excess of 30 Gy can produce sufficient damage to liver parenchyma with biochemical changes that death due to liver failure may follow a dose of 40 Gy in 4 weeks.[114]

REFERENCES

1. Cancer statistics. Ca 36:1, 1986
2. Johns HE, Cunningham JR: The Physics of Radiology. 3rd Ed. Charles C Thomas, Springfield, IL, 1977
3. Hall EJ: Radiobiology for the Radiologist. 2nd Ed. Harper & Row, New York, 1978
4. Elkind MM, Sutton G, Moses WB, et al: Sublethal and lethal radiation damage. Nature (Lond) 214:1088, 1967
5. Suit HD, Urano M: Repair of sublethal radiation injury in hypoxic cells of C3H mouse mammary carcinoma. Radiat Res 37:422, 1969
6. Elkind MM, Whitmore GF: The Radiobiology of Cultured Mammalian Cells. Gordon and Breach, New York, 1967
7. Pizzarello DJ, Witcofski RL: Medical Radiation Biology. Lea & Febiger, Philadelphia, 1972
8. Fowler JF: Differences in survival curve shapes for formal multi-target and multi-hit models. Phys Med Biol 9:177, 1964
9. Glassburn JR, Brady LW, Plenk HP: Hyperbaric oxygen in radiation therapy. Cancer 39:751, 1977
10. Gray LH: Radiobiologic basis of oxygen as a modifying factor in radiation therapy. AJR 85:803, 1961
11. Gray LH, Conger AD, Ebert M, et al: The concubation of oxygen dissolved in tissues at the time of irradiation as a factor in radiotherapy. Br J Radiol 26:638, 1953
12. Puck TT, Marcus PU: Actions of x-rays on mammalian cells. J Exp Med 103:653, 1956
13. Hewitt HB, Wilson CW: Survival curve for mammalian leukemia cells irradiated in vivo. Br J Cancer 13:69, 1959
14. Thomlinson RH, Gray LH: The histological structure of some human lung cancers and the possible implication for radiotherapy. Br J Cancer 9:539, 1955
15. Fertil B, Malaise EP: Intrinsic radiosensitivity of human cell lines is correlated with radioresponsiveness of human tumors: Analysis of 101 published survival curves. Int J Radiat Oncol Biol Phys 11:1169, 1985
16. Wright EA, Howard-Flanders P: The influence of oxygen on the radiosensitivity of mammalian tissues. Acta Radiol [Oncol] (Stockh) 48:26, 1957
17. Gray LH, Conger AD, Ebert M, et al: The concentration of oxygen dissolved in tissues at time of irradiation as a factor in radiotherapy. Br J Radiol 26:638–648, 1953
18. Withers HR: The four "R's" of radiotherapy. In Lett JT, Adler H (eds): Advances in Radiation Biology. Vol. 5. Academic Press, New York, 1975
19. Withers HR: Biologic basis for altered fractionation scheme. Cancer 55:2086, 1985
20. Powers WE, Palmer LA: Biologic basis of preoperative radiation treatment. AJR 102:176, 1968
21. Bush RS, Jenkins RP, Allt WE, et al: Definitive evidence for hypoxic cells influencing cure in cancer therapy. Br J Cancer 37:302, 1978
22. Blitzer PH, Wang CC, Suit HD: Blood pressure and hemoglobin concentration: Multivariate analysis of local control after irradiation for head and neck cancer. Int J Radiat Oncol Biol Phys 10:8, 1984
23. Cantril ST: Radiation Therapy in the Management of Cancer of the Uterine Cervix. Charles C Thomas, Springfield, IL, 1950
24. Paterson, R: The Treatment of Malignant Disease by Radiotherapy. 2nd Ed. Williams & Wilkins, Baltimore, 1963
25. Wang CC: Principles of radiation therapy of gynecologic cancers. Cancer 134:219, 1981
26. Allt WEC: Supervoltage radiation treatment in advanced cander of the uterine cervix; preliminary report. Can Med J 100:792, 1969
27. Potish R, Adcock L, Jones T, et al: The morbidity and utility of periaortic radiotherapy in cervical carcinoma. Gynecol Oncol 15:1, 1983
28. Wharton JT, Jones HW, Day HT Jr, et al: Pre-irradiation celiotomy and extended field irradiation for

invasive carcinoma of the cervix. Obstet Gynecol 49:333, 1977

29. Perez C, Breaux S, Madoc-Jones H, et al: Radiation therapy alone in the treatment of carcinoma of the uterine cervix. I. Analysis of tumor recurrence. Cancer 51:1393, 1963

30. Fletcher GH: Cancer of the uterine cervix. Janeway Lecture, 1970. AJR 111:225, 1971

31. Annual Report on Gynecological Cancer. Vol. 16. FIGO, Stockholm, Sweden, 1976

32. Durrance FY, Fletcher GH, Rutledge FN: Analysis of central recurrent disease in Stage I and II squamous cell carcinoma of the cervix on intact uterus. AJR 106:831, 1969

33. Durrance FY: Radiotherapy following simple hysterectomy in patients with Stage I and II carcinoma of the cervix. AJR 102:165, 1976

34. Cuccia CA, Bloedorn FA, Onal M: Treatment of primary adenocarcinoma of the cervix. AJR 99:371, 1967

35. Weiner S, Wizenberg M: Treatment of primary adenocarcinoma of the cervix. Cancer 35:1514, 1975

36. Miller B, Copeland L, Hamberger A, et al: Carcinoma of the cervical stump. Gynecol Oncol 18:100, 1984

37. Andras E, Fletcher G, Rutledge F: Radiotherapy of carcinoma of the cervix following simple hysterectomy. Am J Obstet Gynecol 115:647, 1973

38. Society of Gynecologic Oncologists Presidential Panel Report: Is pelvic radiation beneficial in the postoperative management of Stage IB squamous cell carcinoma of the cervix with pelvic node metastasis treated by radical hysterectomy and pelvic lymphadenectomy? Gynecol Oncol 10:105, 1980

39. Fuller A, Elliot N, Kosloff C, Lewis J: Lymph node metastasses from carcinoma of the cervix, Stages IB and IIA: Implications for prognosis and treatment. Gynecol Oncol 13:165, 1982

40. Chung C, Nahhas W, Stryker J, et al: Analysis of factors contributing to treatment failures in Stage IB and IIA carcinoma of the cervix. Am J Obstet Gynecol 138:550, 1980

41. Shingleton H, Gore H, Soong S-J, et al: Tumor recurrence and survival in Stage IB cancer of the cervix. Am J Clin Oncol 6:265, 1983

42. Hogan W, Littman P, Griner L, et al: Results of radiation therapy given after hysterectomy. Cancer 49:1278, 1982

43. Hughes R, Brewington K, Hanjani P, et al: Extended field irradiation for cervical cancer based on surgical staging. Oncology 9:153, 1980

44. Piver MS, Barlow JJ: High dose irradiation to biopsy confirmed aortic node metastases from carcinoma of the uterine cervix. Cancer 39:1243, 1977

45. Ciatto S, Pirtoli L, Cionini L: Radiotherapy for post-operative failures of carcinoma of the cervix uteri. Surg Gynecol Obstet 151:621, 1980

46. Nori D, Hilaris B, Kim H, et al: Interstitial irradiation in recurrent gynecological cancer. Int J Radiat Oncol Biol Phys 7:1513, 1981

47. Puthawala A, Syed A, Fleming P, DiSaia P: Re-irradiation with interstitial implant for recurrent pelvic malignancies. Cancer 50:2810, 1982

48. Buchsbaum JJ: Para-aortic lymph node involvement in cervical carcinoma. Am J Obstet Gynecol 113:942, 1972

49. Brookland R, Rubin S, Danoff B: Extended field irradiation in the treatment of patients with cervical carcinoma involving biopsy proven para-aortic nodes. Int J Radiat Oncol Biol Phys 10:1875, 1984

50. Boronow RC, Morrow CP, Creasman WT, et al: Surgical staging in endometrial cancer: Clinical-pathologic findings of a prospective study. Obstet Gynecol 63:825, 1984

51. Lewis BV, Stallworthy JA, Cowdell R: Adenocarcinoma of the body of the uterus. J Obstet Gynaecol Br Commonw 77:343, 1970

52. Van de Werf-Messing B: Carcinoma of the bladder treated by suprapubic implants. The value of additional external beam irradiation. Int J Cancer 5:277, 1969

53. Ingersoll FM: Vaginal recurrence of carcinoma of the corpus: Management and prevention. Am J Surg 121:473, 1971

54. Gusberg SB: Indication for radiation therapy in the treatment of cancer of the endometrium. p.320 In Simon N (ed): Afterloading Radiotherapy. DHEW Publ 72-8024. Department of Health and Human Services, Washington, DC, 1971

55. Wang CC: An afterloading applicator for intracavitary vaginal irradiation. Radiology 117:225, 1975

56. DePalo G, Kenda R, Andreola S, et al: Endometrial carcinoma: Stage I. Obstet Gynecol 60:225, 1982

57. Hendrickson M, Ross J, Eifel P, et al: Adenocarcinoma of the endometrium: Analysis of 256 cases with carcinoma limited to the endometrium. Gynecol Oncol 13:373, 1982

58. Wang CC, Shimm DS, Dosoretz DE, et al: Low-dose preoperative radiation therapy for adenocarcinoma of the endometrium. A pilot study. Cancer 54:1002, 1984

59. Vongtama V, Karlen JR, Piver SM, et al: Treatment, results and prognostic factors in Stage I and II sarcomas of the corpus uteri. AJR 126:139, 1976

60. Onsrud M, Kolstad P, Normann T: Postoperative external pelvic irradiation in carcinoma of the corpus Stage I: A controlled clinical trial. Gynecol Oncol 4:222, 1976

61. Badib AO, Kurohara SS, Vongtama VY, Webster JH:

Evaluation of primary radiation therapy in Stage I, Group 2, endometrial carcinoma. Radiology 93:417, 1969

62. Landgren R, Fletcher G, Delclos L, Wharton J: Irradiation of endometrial cancer in patients with medical contraindications to surgery or with unresectable lesions. AJR 126:148, 1976

63. Wallin T, Malkasian G, Gaffey T, et al: Stage II cancer of the endometrium: A pathological and clinical study. Gynecol Oncol 18:1, 1984

64. Greenberg S, Glassburn J, Antonaides J, Brady L: Management of carcinoma of the uterus Stage II. Cancer Clin Trials 4:183, 1981

65. Tak W: Carcinoma of the endometrium with cervical involvement (Stage II). Cancer 43:2504, 1979

66. Aalders J, Abeler V, Kolstad P: Recurrent adenocarcinoma of the endometrium: A clinical and histopathological study of 379 patients. Gynecol Oncol 17:85, 1984

67. Bruckman J, Bloomer W, Marck A, et al: Stage III adenocarcinoma of the endometrium: Two prognostic groups. Gynecol Oncol 9:12, 1980

68. Badib A, Kurohara S, Beita A, Webster J: Recurrent carcinoma of the corpus uteri. AJR 105:596, 1969

69. Aalders J, Abeler V, Kolstad P: Clinical (Stage III) as compared to subclinical intrapelvic extrauterine tumor spread in endometrial carcinoma: A clinical and histopathological study of 175 patients. Gynecol Oncol 17:64, 1984

70. Reddy S, Lee M-S, Hendrickson F: Pattern of recurrences in endometrial carcinoma and their management. Radiology 133:737, 1979

71. Dembo A: Radiation therapy in the management of ovarian cancer. Clin Obstet Gynaecol 10:261, 1983

72. Delclos L, Quinlan EJ: Malignant tumors of the ovary managed with postoperative megavoltage irradiation. Radiology 170:369, 1969

73. Dembo AJ, van Dyk J, Japp B: Whole abdominal irradiation by a moving-strip technique for patients with ovarian cancer. Int J Radiat Oncol Biol Phys 5:1933, 1977

74. Fazekas JT, Maier JG: Irradiation of ovarian carcinomas: A prospective comparison of the open-field and moving-strip techniques. AJR 120:118, 1974

75. Million RR, Parsons JT, Cassisi NJ: Twice-a-day radiation therapy for cancer of the head and neck. Cancer 55:2100, 1985

76. Wang CC: Altered fractionation radiation therapy. Presented to the ACS National Conference on Gynecologic Cancer, Atlanta, Ga, 1986

77. Scully RE: Common epithelial tumors of borderline malignancy (carcinoma of low malignant potential). Bull Cancer 69(3):228, 1982

78. Richardson GS, Scully RE, Nikrui N, Nelson JH: Medical Progress: Common epithelial cancer of the ovary. N Engl J Med 312:415, 483, 1985

79. Kottmeier HL: Ovarian cancer with special regard to radiotherapy. In Deeley TJ (ed): Modern Radiotherapy. Gynecological Cancer. Appleton & Lange, E. Norwalk, CT, 1971

80. Long RT, Johnson RE, Sala JM: Variations in survival among patients with carcinoma of the ovary: Analysis of 253 cases according to histologic type anatomical stage and method of treatment. Cancer 20:1195, 1967

81. Smith J, Rutledge F, Delclos L: Postoperative treatment of early cancer of the ovary: A random trial between postoperative irradiation and chemotherapy. Natl Cancer Inst Monog 42:149, 1975

82. Munnell E: Is conservative surgery unjustified in Stage I (I A) carcinoma of the ovary? Am J Obstet Gynecol 103:641, 1969

83. Haas J, Mansfield C, Hartman G, et al: Results of radiation therapy in the treatment of epithelial carcinoma of the ovary. Cancer 46:1950, 1980

84. Asadourian LA, Taylor HB: Dysgerminoma: An analysis of 105 cases. Obstet Gynecol 33:370, 1969

85. Pankratz E, Boyes D, White G, et al: Granulosa cell tumors—A clinical review of 61 cases. Obstet Gynecol 52:718, 1978

86. Krepart G, Smith J, Rutledge F, Delclos L: The treatment for dysgerminoma of the ovary. Cancer 41:986, 1978

87. Lucraft H: A review of thirty-three cases of ovarian dysgerminoma emphasizing the role of radiotherapy. Clin Radiol 30:585, 1979

88. Frick HC, Jacox HW, Taylor HC Jr: Primary carcinoma of the vagina. Am J Obstet Gynecol 101:695, 1968

89. Chau PM: Radiotherapeutic management of malignant tumors of the vagina. AJR 89:502, 1963

90. Brown G, Fletcher G, Rutledge F: Irradiation of "in situ" and invasive squamous cell carcinoma of the vagina. Cancer 28:1278, 1971

91. Perez C, Camel H: Long term follow up in radiation therapy of carcinoma of the vagina. Cancer 49:1308, 1982

92. Prempree T: Role of radiation therapy in the management of primary carcinoma of the vagina. Acta Radiol [Oncol] (Stockh) 21:195, 1982

93. Weghaupt K, Gerstner G, Kucera H: Radiation therapy for primary carcinoma of the female urethra: A survey over 25 years. Gynecol Oncol 17:58, 1984

94. Frischbier H, Thomsen K: Treatment of cancer of the vulva with high energy electrons. Am J Obstet Gynecol 111:431, 1971

95. Green TH Jr: Radical vulvectomy. Clin Obstet Gynecol 8:642, 1965

96. Green TH Jr, Ulfelder H, Meigs JV: Epidermoid car-

cinoma of the vulva: An analysis of 238 cases. Am J Obstet Gynecol 75:834, 1958

97. Hacker N, Berek J, Juillard G, Lagass L: Preoperative radiation therapy for locally advanced vulvar carcinoma. Cancer 54:2056, 1984

98. Daly J, Million R: Radical vulvectomy combined with elective node irradiation for TxNo squamous carcinoma of the vulva. Cancer 34:161, 1971

99. Acosta A, Given F, Frazier A, et al: Preoperative radiation therapy in the management of squamous cell carcinoma of the vulva: Preliminary report. Am J Obstet Gynecol 132:198, 1978

100. Prempree T, Amornmarn R: Radiation treatment of recurrent carcinoma of the vulva. Cancer 54:1943, 1984

101. Green TH Jr, Scully RE: Tumors of the fallopian tube. Clin Obstet Gynecol 5:886, 1962

102. Denham J, Maclennan K: The management of primary carcinoma of the Fallopian tube. Cancer 53:166, 1984

103. Eddy G, Copeland L, Gershenson D, et al: Fallopian tube carcinoma. Obstet Gynecol 64:546, 1984

104. Chu AM: Female urethra carcinoma. Radiology 107:627, 1973

105. Chu AM, Beechinor R: Survival and recurrence patterns in the radiation treatment of carcinoma of the vagina. Gynecol Oncol 19:298, 1984

106. El Senoussi M, Fletcher G, Borlase B: Correlation of radiation and surgical parameters in complications in the extended field technique for carcinoma of the cervix. Int J Radiat Oncol Biol Phys 5:927, 1979

107. Lagasse L, Ballou S, Berman M, Watring W: Pretreatment lymphangiography and operative evaluation in carcinoma of the cervix. Am J Obstet Gynecol 134:219, 1979

108. Maruyama Y, Van Nagelel J, Utley J, et al: Radiation and small bowel complications in cervical carcinoma therapy. Radiology 112:669, 1974

109. DeCosse J, Rhodes R, Wente W, et al: The natural history and management of radiation induced injury of the gastrointestinal tract. Ann Surg 170:369, 1969

110. Slater JM, Fletcher GH: Ureteral strictures after radiation therapy for carcinoma of the uterine cervix. AJR 111:269, 1971

111. Goodman M, Dalton J: Ureteral strictures following radiotherapy: Incidence, etiology, and treatment guidelines. J Urol 128:21, 1982

112. Luxton R: Radiation nephritis. Am J Med 22:215, 1953

113. Bickel D: Post irradiation fracture of the femoral neck. JAMA 176:175, 1961

114. Lewin K, Millis R: Human radiation hepatitis: A morphologic study with emphasis on the late change. Arch Pathol Lab Med 96:21, 1973

7
Principles of Chemotherapy

Gunter Deppe
Vinay K. Malviya

The modern era of cancer chemotherapy began during World War I following the observation of reduction in lymph node volume in soldiers exposed to nitrogen mustard.[1] The first patient to be treated with nitrogen mustard had Hodgkin's disease. Following almost 20 years of research, the first complete and sustained remission was accomplished with the antifolate agent methotrexate in a patient with metastatic gestational choriocarcinoma.[2] Since then, there have been significant advances in the field of chemotherapy.

Several cancers, even at advanced stages, may be cured by chemotherapeutic agents. Gestational trophoblastic tumors, testicular tumors, acute lymphoblastic leukemia, and Hodgkin's disease can be controlled in more than 70 percent of patients.

Among gynecologic malignancies, ovarian, endometrial, and cervical cancers have shown significant response to systemic chemotherapy, but with uncertain prolongation of survival. Chemotherapy is now used in the treatment of all stages of gynecologic malignancies; it is no longer reserved exclusively for patients with relapse or when the tumor is already disseminated on initial presentation. Better control of gynecologic malignancies with chemotherapy will depend on resolution of such problems as host intolerance, tumor heterogeneity, and resistance. This chapter summarizes the established principles underlying the current use of chemotherapy in gynecologic malignancies.

THE CELL CYCLE

The cell cycle is the interval between the midpoint of mitosis and the midpoint of the subsequent mitosis in one or both daughter cells. This concept was recently widened to include cellular and biochemical aspects that regulate either normal or abnormal cell growth.[3]

The life cycle of a normal or neoplastic cell begins with mitosis or cell division. After the cell has completed its division, it enters G_1 phase or the first gap phase, considered a relatively quiescent phase. DNA and protein synthesis are known to be initiated during this phase. This is the longest phase of the mammalian cell cycle, highly variable in duration, and often related to the proliferative activity of the tissue. When proliferative activity is high, G_1 phase tends to be short. Occasionally, cells rest for prolonged periods and are then known to be in G_0 phase. During this phase, the cell is being primed for DNA synthesis.

Upon emerging from G_1 phase, the cell enters S

141

phase, during which synthesis is completed. During this period, which lasts 10 to 20 hours, the cell doubles its DNA content. Following the S phase, there is a short premitotic or G_2 phase lasting 2 to 10 hours when the spindle apparatus is being synthesized. Finally, mitosis occurs during M phase, which lasts 30 minutes to 1 hour. The cell proceeds through the four classic steps of mitosis, consisting of prophase, metaphase, anaphase, and telophase, resulting in cellular division and formation of daughter cells.

Growth of an abnormal cell involves the same kinetic factors observed in normal cells. Many biochemical events that are cell-cycle specific have been described. These events seem to occur only in proliferating cells and are undetectable in dormant cells. A number of enzymes that are strictly related to DNA synthesis increase in activity during S phase. These enzymes include thymidine kinase, DNA polymerase, dihydrofolate reductase, and ribonucleotide reductase.[4-7] A unique-copy gene transcription is a prerequisite for cellular entry from G_1 into S phase. The cells enter S phase at a permissive temperature at which RNA polymerase II is functionally active. For a malignant cell, however, there is no evidence for an identifiable biochemical event that precedes such a transformation.

Once S phase begins, the enzymes necessary for purine, pyrimidine, and DNA synthesis increase in activity. After the DNA content has doubled, the cell enters G_2 phase when RNA and protein synthesis must occur before the cell can construct a mitotic apparatus and begin division. The fraction of cells in S phase can be estimated by ^{3}H-thymidine labeling or autoradiography.[8] It can also be determined from measurements of cellular DNA content using flow cytometry. The fraction of cells in S phase reflects the relative rate of cell production in a population. The higher the S fraction, the greater the rate of cell proliferation.

The RNA component of the cell provides a reasonable estimate of cell mass. The increase in the amount of RNA throughout the cell cycle can be demonstrated with flow microfluorimetry of cells stained with acridine orange.[9]

These considerations appear to be critical to the action of some chemotherapeutic agents. The original concept of drugs being truly phase specific requires modification. For most agents, several phases may be

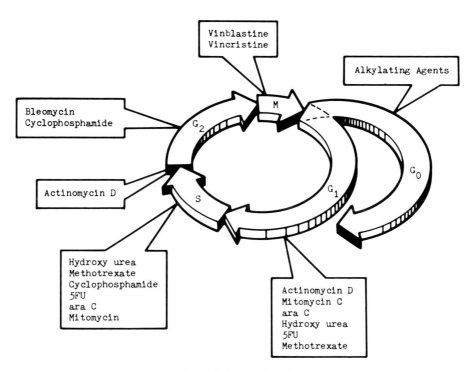

Fig. 7-1 The cell cycle.

susceptible to varying degrees. Agents that are effective only during a particular phase of the cell cycle, such as the S phase of cellular DNA synthesis, are phase specific. Those agents in which action is prolonged and independent of any specific cell cycle phase are phase nonspecific. Agents that are most effective in S phase are usually effective inhibitors of rapidly proliferating cell populations. Conversely, alkylating agents and other drugs that interact primarily with macromolecular DNA (e.g., Adriamycin) seem to be largely independent of the cell replication cycle and are effective against tumors displaying relatively low proliferative activity (Fig. 7-1).

TUMOR GROWTH

As recently as 1959, cancer was still believed to be a wild, unregulated growth subject to no control by the host.[10] However, the shorter cell cycle time of jejunal epithelial cells as compared with the fastest-growing mouse tumors supports the finding that tumor cells do not necessarily proliferate faster than normal cells; thus, therapy aimed at destroying rapidly proliferating cells may also result in destruction of normal cells.[11]

Since the cell-cycle time of tumor cells is not necessarily longer than that of normal cells, an explanation of why tumors grow while normal adult tissue does not depends on the growth fraction (fraction of cycling cells in the population) and the rate of cell loss. Growth of tissue is not just a function of the number of mitoses or the length of the cell cycle, but the real determinant is the excess of cells produced over cells that die per unit of tissue. It is therefore possible to calculate the growth of tumor experimentally by determining the cell-cycle time (T_c), the growth fraction, and the tumor doubling time. A tumor with a short cell-doubling time, a large growth fraction, and a low rate of cell loss will increase rapidly in size. Conversely, a tumor with a prolonged doubling time, a small growth fraction, and a high rate of cell loss may change minimally over a long period. These factors are responsible for the great variability in clinical behavior frequently observed even in histologically similar tumors.

Gompertz devised a mathematical formula for predicting the relationship between the size and growth rate of a fetus that fits the observed growth rates for most animal and some human tumors.[12] Both normal and neoplastic cells may be influenced by certain growth factors, and both populations appear to contain more dividing cells when the population size is small and fewer dividing cells when it is large.[13] The growth fraction is therefore inversely proportional to the size of the tumor.

An initial rapid growth phase (log phase) is followed by a slower phase (plateau) (Fig. 7-2). During the log phase of growth, the tumor is clinically nondetectable. As the tumor becomes clinically detectable, the growth slows, and it enters a plateau phase. It is likely that most, if not all, human tumors arise from a single abnormal cell that multiplies and eventually may kill the host when the body burden of tumor approaches or exceeds 1×10^{12} cells (one trillion cells: approximately 1 kg of tumor). The minimal detectable body burden of tumor in humans is considered 1×10^9 cells (1 g of tumor). At the time of clinical detection (1 cm^3), a malignant tumor has completed 75 percent of the doubling required to destroy the host (33 of approximately 40).

The growth rate of a solid tumor is also dependent on its subpopulation, which, being heterogeneous, has different growth characteristics, metastatic potential, and susceptibility to therapy.[14] Substantial reduction of the tumor volume (debulking) will render the tumor much more susceptible to chemotherapy or radiation therapy — the log-kill hypothesis proposed by Skipper and co-workers.[15] This concept was developed to account for the observation in mouse L1210 leukemia that multiple courses of treatment with cytotoxic drugs could be curative, although individual courses of treatment were not. Their data indicate that when the dose of an effective chemotherapeutic agent is administered, a constant fraction (percentage) of cells is destroyed and not a specific number of cells. This may vary from a small percentage to a maximum of 99.99 percent (Fig. 7-3). If the tumor burden in advanced malignancies is $>10^{12}$ cells and, since the best one can hope for with a single maximal exposure of tumor cells to a drug is between 2 and 5 logs of cell kill, it is apparent that the treatment must be repeated many times to achieve tumor control (10^6) cells. The tumor has the ability to regrow and ultimately destroy the host as long as even one viable cell is present. The tumor control is much better with a smaller initial tumor burden. There is evidence that immunologic

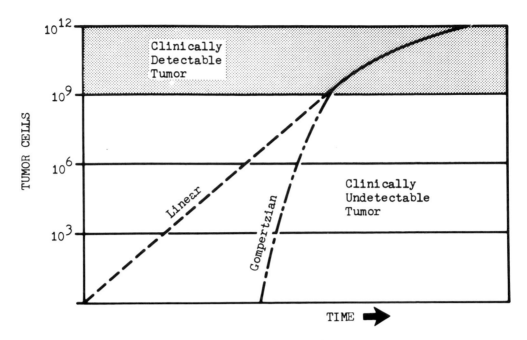

Fig. 7-2 Tumor growth.

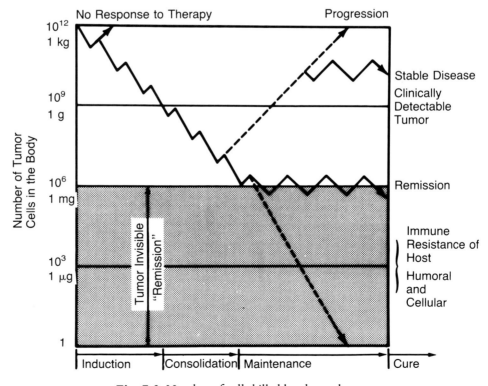

Fig. 7-3 Number of cells killed by chemotherapy.

approaches to therapy may be more effective than chemotherapy when the tumor mass is small. Log kills are small in relatively unresponsive tumors; even if clinical complete responses are observed, they will be of short duration.

DRUG INTERACTIONS

Drug interactions have been studied more completely in animals than in humans and may be synergistic, additive, or antagonistic. Combinations that improve therapy because of either increased antitumor activity or decreased toxicity are believed to be synergistic. Additive therapy produces enhanced antitumor activity, but in amounts roughly equal to the sum of both agents acting singly. Finally, antitumor agents may actually antagonize each other's actions, producing less therapeutic effect than when they are used singly.[16]

DRUG RESISTANCE

In mammalian systems, there is evidence that spontaneous and permanent mutation to phenotypic drug resistance could occur in genetically unstable, rapidly growing, malignant cell lines. This observation suggests that most mammalian cancer cells start with intrinsic sensitivity to anticancer drugs but simply develop spontaneous resistance at variable rates; thus, a tumor that is initially sensitive to chemotherapy may become progressively more resistant to treatment and may ultimately prove lethal. Marrow toxicity, however, always occurs with retreatment.

Goldie and Coldman[17] developed a mathematical model relating curability to the time of appearance of a singly or doubly resistant cell line. Assuming spontaneous mutation rate approximating natural frequency, there is a variation in the size of the resistant fraction in tumors. Because the proportion of these resistant cells within a tumor is small, they do not influence the initial response to treatment. This means that a complete clinical response may be obtained, however, relapse from complete remission is dependent upon the presence of these resistant cells.

This model also explains the unusual clinical observations of tumor heterogeneity and that phenotypic resistance may be associated with preferential site of metastasis. Fluctuations in drug sensitivity occur in different cell lines isolated from various tumor sites in the same patient. These data predict that metastases in different organs in the same patient may respond differently to various drugs. This theory leads one to believe that multiple effective drugs should be used early. To minimize the emergence of drug-resistant clones alternating rather than sequential cycles of chemotherapy may be used, since the latter would favor development of double drug-resistant mutants. Combination chemotherapy has several advantages; in some cases, however, the same drugs combined in different dosage and sequence may yield a spectrum of effects from antagonistic to synergistic. This sometimes is referred to as schedule dependency. Often, resistance to one specific drug can confer cross-resistance to structurally disimilar drugs that have different mechanisms of action—a phenomenon known as pleiotropic drug resistance.

CHEMOTHERAPY REGIMENS

Complete remission is a mandatory prerequisite to achieve cure and prolong survival significantly. Maximal drug dosages must be administered with the goal of achieving maximal tumor cell kill, since reduction to minimize toxicity may be ineffective and harmful to the patient.[18] Combination chemotherapy for most gynecologic cancers is considered superior to single-agent chemotherapy. Despite lethal effects produced in the bulk of the tumor by single agents, survival and eventual regrowth of a fraction of resistant neoplastic cells renders the single-drug therapy of questionable value. Spontaneous and pleiotropic drug resistance and toxicity limit the duration of therapy and the amount of drug that may be tolerated.

Drug combinations are designed with agents that produce different biochemical lesions that attack multiple sites in biosynthetic pathways or that inhibit several processes involved in the maintenance and function of essential macromolecules.[19,20] The specific sequence of administering multiple drugs in combination therapy regimens is usually determined by biochemical and cell kinetic effects of individual agents. The common goal is to decrease the production and availability of a specific end product vital for tumor cell growth and replication. Biochemical concepts of sequential concurrent blockage and that of complementary inhibition have been invaluable in selection of drug combinations.[20-22]

Thus, if one were to administer a cell cycle nonspecific agent that produced a two-log kill in a host bearing a tumor mass with 10^9 cells and no further therapy were given, the tumor would simply regrow. With simultaneous or sequential administration of cell-cycle-specific agents, however, one can consistently produce repetitive log kill in tumors. This may result in the magnitude of log kill required to induce a cure. Combination chemotherapy is now the standard, and often the regimens are complex and cyclical.

Drug toxicity can be minimized by certain therapeutic maneuvers that alter the pharmacokinetics or metabolism of drugs. Doxorubicin is much less cardiotoxic when infused over 96 hours as compared with bolus administration. Nephrotoxicity of cisplatin may be minimized with the simultaneous administration of hypertonic saline and sodium thiosulfate. Mesna (sodium 2-mercaptoethane sulfonate) has been used extensively to prevent hemorrhagic cystitis produced by cyclophosphamide.

PHARMACOKINETIC CONSIDERATIONS IN DRUG SCHEDULING

The route for drug administration is based primarily on the ability of the drug to reach its target site in an active form and the availability of an acceptable preparation for its administration. Oral administration is preferred for lipid-soluble drugs and drugs taken up by specific transport systems. The intramuscular (IM) route is not used for drugs that cause necrosis or in patients with high risk of bleeding. The intravenous (IV) route is preferred for water-soluble compounds, as complete absorption is guaranteed when the infusion is completed.

Bolus dosing provides maximal drug peak levels in plasma but a rapid decline thereafter as the drug is rapidly eliminated from the plasma compartment by metabolism or excretion. This form of dosing is optimal for cell-cycle phase-nonspecific drugs that do not have to be present during a specific phase of the cell cycle. For agents preferentially acting in a specific phase of the cell cycle, such as S-phase-specific drugs, prolonged intravenous infusion has advantages, particularly if the drug has a short plasma half-life ($t\frac{1}{2}$). Prolonged infusions provide a specific and constant plasma concentration and may serve to reduce drug toxicity. Tumor may be present in a body compartment, such as the central nervous system (CNS), which is not rapidly penetrated by systemically administered drugs.

INTRAPERITONEAL ADMINISTRATION

Regional chemotherapy has been designed to deliver high-dose chemotherapy to the tumor while protecting the patient from systemic toxicity due to a reduction of the drug going into the systemic circulation. The basic assumption is that higher drug concentration leads to greater tumor cell kill, leading to better tumor response. In recent years, intraperitoneal chemotherapy has been used extensively in ovarian cancer. The pharmacologic advantage of administering a drug into the peritoneum is related to the clearance of the drug through the peritoneum, total body clearance, and protein binding.

Ozols et al.[23] evaluated the intensity of intracellular fluorescence in mouse ovarian tumors treated both intraperitoneally and intravenously with doxorubicin. The top four to six cell layers in tumor masses and free-floating cells were intensely fluorescent, suggesting high drug concentrations with intraperitoneal administration. Drug diffusion into the tumor mass was minimal, however, and did not provide any advantage over intravenous administration. McVie et al. calculated platinum content on peritoneal surface tumors and found that the concentration in the first 3 mm of the tumor was higher than concentrations of the drug delivered intravenously.[24,25] On the basis of white blood cell (WBC) thickness, 3 mm is equivalent to approximately 50 cell layers. A marked variability of diffusion depths into tumor nodules exists among different neoplastic agents. All available data, including the initial work of Dedrick et al.,[26] suggests that intraperitoneal chemotherapy benefits patients with microscopic tumors or with very small gross nodules on the peritoneal surface. Table 7-1 lists the common chemotherapeutic agents that have been evaluated for intraperitoneal use. Patients with bulky intraperitoneal disease may be treated with concomitant administration of systemic and intraperitoneal chemotherapy. Furthermore, following initial debulking laparotomy, primary treatment with multi-agent intraperitoneal chemotherapy that ensures ade-

Table 7-1 Anticancer Drugs Evaluated Intraperitoneally with Pharmacokinetics

Drug[a]	IP Dose Range	Technique	Comments
Methotrexate[27]	15–50 μM 13.5–45 mg	Tenckhoff, 2-L 6-h dwells	Local toxicity
Methotrexate[28]	96 hr × 8, 30 mg/m²/day × 5	Tenckhoff	IV leucovorin protection
5-Fluorouracil[29]	1.3–2080 mg, q4h × 8	Tenckhoff, 2-L 4-h dwells × 2 weeks	Slight local toxicity, higher portal levels; systemic toxicity reaches 300 × plasma level
Doxorubicin[30]	9–54 μM (10–50 mg)	Tenckhoff, 2 L (one 4-hr dwell) × 2 weeks	Moderate to severe local toxicity; 10² differential in AUC of concentration × time IP over IV, dose limiting
Cisplatin[31]	100–270 mg/m²	Tenckhoff, 2 L (one 4-hr dwell)	Thiosulfate protection IV 12 AUC at highest dose
Cisplatin[32]	50 mg/m²	Thiosulfate infusion; infinite dwell	No protection, minimal residual disease
Cisplatin[33]	60 mg/m²	Ascites (20-min dwell)	No protection
Cisplatin[34]	120–180 mg	Ascites (20-min dwell)	No protection, 42–72 × plasma level
Cytosine arabinoside[35]	60 μM (30 mg) × 20 dwells	Tenckhoff, 2-L 5-h dwells	10²–10³ advantage
Mitomycin[36]	5–30 mg	Tenckhoff, 1.5 L	200 × advantage in AUC
Streptozocin[37]	1 g	Ascites	Local toxicity at high levels
Carboplatin[38]	200–300 mg/m²	Tenckhoff, 2 L (one 4-hr dwell)	Pharmacokinetic advantage being determined; no local toxicity
Cisplatin + ara-c + doxorubicin[39]	100–200 mg/m², 10³–10⁴ moles/L	4-h dwell with	Synergy, abdominal pain secondary to Doxorubicin
Cisplatin + ara-c[40]	100–200 mg/m² + 200 mg	4-h dwell with	Thiosulfate protection; hematologic toxicity at high ara-c levels
Cisplatin ara-c[41] Bleomycin	—	—	Ongoing

AUC, area under curve.
[a] Superscript numbers are references.

quate systemic exposure to cytotoxic agents remains a promising alternative.

Temporary access to the peritoneal cavity may be obtained by repeated punctures and drug instillation with acceptable morbidity.[42] Alternatively, a Tenckhoff catheter or surgically implanted infus-a-port may be used as a peritoneal portal permitting repeated access into the peritoneal cavity[43,44] (Fig. 7-4). Major complications and the risk of infection vary with the chemotherapeutic agent used and the frequency of administration. Septic complications occurred in 7.6 percent of patients with Tenckhoff catheters and in 6.6 percent of patients with implanted catheters. No septic complications were noted in patients with single-use intraperitoneal catheters.[45]

ADJUVANT CHEMOTHERAPY

Chemotherapy is rendered more effective with surgical reduction of tumor burden. To maximize the potential for cure by chemotherapy, treatment should

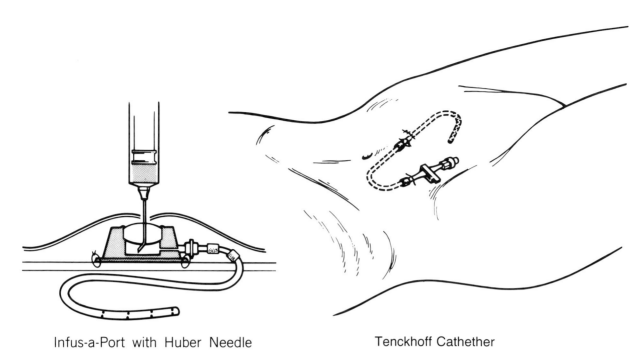

Infus-a-Port with Huber Needle   Tenckhoff Cathether

Fig. 7-4 Intraperitoneal chemotherapy.

be started as soon after surgery as possible. Combination, rather than single-agent, chemotherapy should be used in an adjuvant setting for maximal effectiveness. Patients should be treated as aggressively as those with clinically evident disease. Drugs that produce partial responses in patients with clinically evident disease should not necessarily be expected to produce better results in an adjuvant setting. Prolonged combination chemotherapy is no longer believed to be necessary. In fact, a lengthy period of adjuvant therapy could accelerate the growth of resistant population by enhancing its mutation rate.[46] Neoadjuvant, or induction, chemotherapy refers to the initial use of chemotherapy to reduce tumor bulk in an attempt to lower the stage of the tumor, making it surgically resectable.

RESPONSE CRITERIA

Cure in cancer as defined by Frei et al.[47] is the achievement of a plateau on disease free survival that extends without treatment, beyond the period of risk of relapse for a given disease. All tumor measurements should be recorded in centimeters and should consist of the longest diameter and the perpendicular diameter at the widest portion of the tumor. Liver-size measurements should be recorded at the xiphoid line and 8 cm lateral to xiphoid lines.

COMPLETE REMISSION

Complete remission is defined as a disappearance of all clinical evidence of active tumor for a minimum of 6 weeks. In addition, cytology performed on peritoneal washings must be consistently negative. A patient will be considered to have a pathologically complete response when no histologic or cytologic evidence of disease is found at laparotomy.

PARTIAL REMISSION

Partial remission is defined as 50 percent or greater decrease in the sum of the products of all diameters of measured lesions. In patients with liver metastases, there should be at least a 30 percent reduction in the sums of measurements below the costal margin. No simultaneous increase in size of any lesion or appearance of any new lesions should occur.

STABLE DISEASE

Stable disease refers to steady state or to a response less than partial remission or progression. There may be no appearance of new lesions and no worsening of symptoms.

PROGRESSION

Unequivocal increase of at least 25 percent in the size of any measurable lesion and appearance of new lesions is termed progression of disease.

RELAPSE

Relapse refers to the appearance of new lesions or the reappearance of old lesions in patients who have been in complete remission. For patients in partial remission, relapse is defined as an increase of 50 percent or more in the sum of the products of the diameters of all measured tumors over that which was obtained at the time of maximum tumor regression.

ADEQUATE TRIAL

An adequate trial is defined as two courses of treatment. Patients must be continually monitored for response, since the therapeutic index of chemotherapeutic agents is low. Most patients are evaluated clinically for response at monthly intervals; if progression or no response of disease is documented within three cycles, the patient is switched to an alternative therapy.

The response to treatment cannot be evaluated by a single set of criteria. Response criteria, both subjective and objective, are summarized below.

TYPES OF TUMOR RESPONSE: GYNECOLOGIC MALIGNANCIES

1. *Tumor size:* palpation, radiologic measurement, radioisotope scans
2. *Serum markers:* choriocarcinoma, endodermal sinus tumors, dysgerminoma, nonmucinous epithelial ovarian cancers

(Continues)

---

3. *Disappearance of effusions:* tumors involving pleural or peritoneal surfaces or obstructing lymphatics
4. *Organ function:* improved renal function after obstructive uropathy

---

CHEMOTHERAPEUTIC AGENTS

Continued success in the treatment of cancers is dependent on the development of new and more effective agents as well as the continued exploration of innovative approaches using established drugs. Each year, the National Cancer Institute (NCI) evaluates 15,000 new compounds and assesses their activity in P388 mouse leukemia cell lines. After initial screening, their activity is confirmed in mouse tumors and human tumor xenografts and most recently in human tumor stem cell assay. A brief outline of drug development and clinical trials to establish their clinical activity is outlined in Figure 7-5 and Table 7-2.

The rationale for use of a given drug requires a clear understanding of its mechanism of action as well as detailed knowledge of its clinical pharmacology. The chemotherapeutic agents most commonly used in gynecologic malignancies are listed in Table 7-3. The mechanism of action at the cellular level is represented in Figure 7-6. The dosages and toxicities shown are for traditional use as single agents. Certain agents may be used in experimental high-dose protocols or in combinations that require dose reductions.

ALKYLATING AGENTS

Alkylating compounds form covalent bonds with nucleophilic target molecules by proving reactive carbonium ion intermediates or their transitional complexes. Their primary mechanism is produced by the attachment of extremely unstable alkyl groups to DNA and interference with its function and replication as well as with transcription of RNA. Most alkylating agents have two or more unstable alkyl groups per molecule.

Their chemical variability explains their different

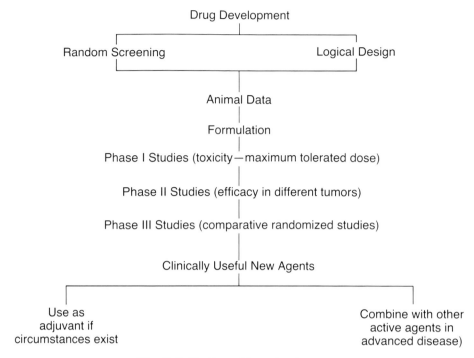

Fig. 7-5 Outline of drug development.

Table 7-2 Types of Clinical Trials

Phase	Goal	Comment
I	Determine the MTD for a given schedule of a drug in humans.	The mechanism of action, likely toxicities, and probable useful schedule are generally available from preclinical animal studies. Patients do not have to have measurable disease for study entry.
II	Define the spectrum of antitumor action of a drug.	The MTD of a drug is used in patients with different kinds of measurable cancer. The response rate is determined and rare side effects are looked for.
III	Compare two or more drugs, drug schedules, or drug combination to define the clinical value of a new therapy more precisely.	This is usually conducted as a randomized clinical trial with the control group receiving "standard" treatment. In some cases, this may include the use of a placebo or the use of supportive care without chemotherapy.

MTD, maximum (safely) tolerated dose.

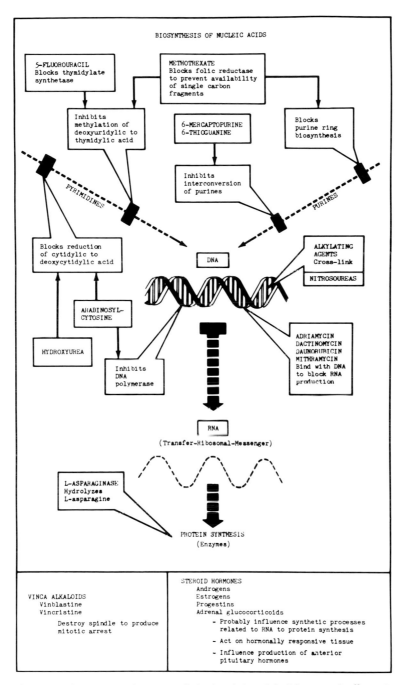

Fig. 7-6 Mechanisms of anticancer drugs at cellular level. (Modified from Krakoff IH: Cancer chemotherapeutic agents. CA 37:93, 1987.)

Table 7-3 Chemotherapeutic Agents

Compound	Route of Administration	Typical Treatment Schedule	Usual Toxicities
Alkylating agents			
Cyclophosphamide (Cytoxan)	PO, IV	PO: 100–250 mg/m² IV: 400–1,000 mg/m²	Myelosuppression, hemorrhagic cystitis plus bladder fibrosis, alopecia, hepatitis, amenorrhea and azoospermia
Chlorambucil (Leukeran)	PO	0.03–0.10 mg/kg/day	Myelosuppression, intestinal discomfort, dermatitis, hepatotoxicity
Melphalan (Alkeran, L-PAM)	PO	0.2 mg/kg/day × 5 days q4–6wk	Myelosuppression, nausea and vomiting (rare), mucosal ulceration (rare)
Cisplatin (cis-diamminodichloride) (Platinol)	IV	15–40 mg/m² IV × 3 wk 50–100 mg/m² IV × 3 wk 50–250 mg/m² IP × 3 wk	Nephrotoxicity, tinnitis and hearing loss, nausea and vomiting, thrombocytopenia
Dacarbazine (DTIC)	IV	80–160 mg/m²/day × 10 days	Myelosuppression, nausea and vomiting, flu-like syndrome, hepatotoxicity
CHIP	IV	270 mg/m²/day × 4 wk	Nausea and vomiting, myelosuppression, nephrotoxicity
Diamine (cyclobutane dicarboxylate platinum) (CBDCA)	IV	300 mg/m²/day × 4 wk	Thrombocytopenia, anemia, myelosuppression, nephrotoxicity, nausea, vomiting
Antitumor antibiotics			
Actinomycin D (Dactinomycin, Cosmegen)	IV	0.3–0.5 mg/m² IV × 5 days 2.5 mg/m² IV weekly	Nausea and vomiting, skin necrosis, mucosal ulceration, myelosuppression, hepatotoxicity, alopecia
Bleomycin (Blenoxane)	IV or IM	10–20 units/m² IV or IM: 1–2 ×/wk for a dose of 400 units For effusion: 60–120 units	Fever, dermatologic reactions, alopecia, anaphylactic reactions, myelosuppression, pneumonitis, and pulmonary fibrosis at cumulative doses over 400 units
Mitomycin C (Mutamycin)	IV	10–20 g/m² IV q6–8wk	Myelosuppression, local vesicant, nausea and vomiting, mucosal ulcerations, nephrotoxicity, hypercalcemia

Drug	Route	Dose	Toxicity
Vinca alkaloids			
Vincristine (Oncovin)	IV	1.4 mg/m²/weekly	Alopecia, mild myelosuppression, areflexia, muscular weakness, peripheral neuritis, paralytic ileus
Vinblastine (Velban)	IV	4–8 mg/m² q1–2wk	Myelosuppression, alopecia, nausea and vomiting, neurotoxicity, areflexia
Etoposide (VP-16)	IV	50–150 mg/m²/day × 5q3wk	Nausea and vomiting, alopecia, mild myelosuppression
Antimetabolites			
5-Fluorouracil (fluorouracil)	IV	500 mg/m²/day × 3 wks; 1,000 mg/m²/wk continuous infusion × 3 wk; 1,000 mg/m² continuous infusion × 5 days	Stomatitis, diarrhea, myelosuppression, nausea, vomiting, anorexia, cerebellar ataxis, hyperpigmentation of nail beds
Methotrexate (MTX amthopterin)	PO, IV	PO: 2.5–5 mg/day; IM/IV: 25–50 mg 1–2 wk; IM: 200 mg–10 g with leucovorin rescue; 1 mg/kg IM with leucovorin rescue with 1 g/m² IV wk; Intrathecal: 12–15 mg/m² 1–3 wk	Mucosal ulceration, myelosuppression, hepatotoxicity
Hydroxyurea (Hydrea)	PO, IV	PO: 1–2 g/m²/day; IV: 1–2 g/m²/day	Myelosuppression, nausea and vomiting, anorexia
Cytarabine (ara-c)	IV, IP	200 mg/m²/day × 5 by continuous infusion	Nausea, vomiting, bone marrow depression, megaloblastosis, leukopenia, thrombocytopenia
Progestins—Hydroxyprogesterone caproate (Delalutin)	IM	1 g/IM biweekly	Fluid retention, epithelial changes in genital tract, nausea, sterile injection, abscess
Medroxyprogesterone acetate (DepoProvera)	IM, PO	200–600 mg IM q1–2wk	
Megestrol acetate (Megace)	PO	20–40 mg PO qid	
Miscellaneous agents			
Hexamethylmelamine	PO	4–8 mg/kg/day	Nausea and vomiting, myelosuppression, neurotoxicity, skin rashes
Tamoxifen	PO	2–12 mg/m² bid	Gastrointestinal discomfort, hot flashes, flare reaction

distribution and site of action. The alkylating agents are not phase specific and have different toxicities and tumor spectrum. The most commonly used alkylating agents in gynecologic malignancies are cis-diammino-dichloroplatinum (cisplatin), dacarbazine (DTIC), cyclophosphamide (Cytoxan), chlorambucil (Leukeran), and melphalan (Alkeran) (Table 7-3).

ANTIMETABOLITES

The general mechanism of action of antimetabolites consists of interference with metabolic steps crucial to cell growth leading to inhibition of biosynthesis of DNA. These antitumor agents are structural variations of the normal purines and pyrimidines required for RNA and DNA synthesis. They specifically inhibit enzymatic processes necessary for nucleic acid biosynthesis. They may act as substitutes for a normal metabolite essential to a vital metabolic pathway or may bind to an enzyme forming an inactive drug enzyme complex. Other methods of their action may involve competition with a normal metabolite acting at an enzyme regulatory site to interfere with the catalytic rate of an essential enzyme or blocking a catalytic site of an enzyme.

Although many antimetabolites are employed in medical oncology, only a few are used in the therapy of gynecologic malignancies: 5-fluorouracil (5-FU) and cytosine arabinoside, both pyrimidine antagonists. Methotrexate is a folate antagonist that binds to the enzyme dihydrofolate reductase and hydroxyura, an inhibitor of ribonucleotide reductase. Their doses and usual toxicities are shown in Table 7-3.

ANTITUMOR ANTIBIOTICS

The antitumor antibiotics are anthracyclines that occur in nature. The mechanism of action of the anthracyclines appears to involve intercolation into the DNA structure, resulting in an inhibition of DNA replication and also of RNA sysnthesis. Cells in the S-phase of the cell cycle are found especially sensitive to anthracycline toxicity. Actinomycin D (dactinomycin), Blenoxane (bleomycin), Mutamycin (mitomycin C), and Adriamycin (doxorubicin) are most commonly used in gynecologic oncology (Table 7-3).

VINCA ALKALOIDS

The vinca alkaloids, vincristine and vinblastine, are structurally similar multiringed substances derived from the periwinkle plant *(Vinca rosea)*. These compounds have a different spectrum and vary in antitumor activity and toxicity. They bind to cellular microtubular protein and prevent the formation of the mitotic spindle structure resulting in metaphase arrest. At higher concentrations, they interfere with nucleic acid and protein synthesis. Their typical treatment schedule and toxicities are listed in Table 7-3.

EPIPODOPHYLLOTOXINS

The epipodophyllotoxins are a class of semisynthetic derivatives of podophyllotoxins (extract of mandrake plant). They have multiringed structures linked to glucopyranose sugar moiety. The epipodophyllotoxins exert an effect late in S or G_2 phase. Cytotoxicity is believed to be related to DNA damage. The member of this group used for treatment of gynecologic malignancies is etoposide (VP_{16}) whose pharmacologic and clinical features are shown in Table 7-3.

BIOLOGICAL RESPONSE MODIFIERS

Corynebacterium parvum, bacillus Calmette-Guérin (BCG), and β-interferon have been used in the treatment of gynecologic malignancies, both intravenously and intraperitoneally. They may be used singly or in combination with various chemotherapeutic agents. The precise mechanism of action with these agents has not been determined. It appears, however, they influence transcription of RNA to protein. The use of biologic response modifiers in gynecologic cancer needs further investigation.

TOXICITY

The usefulness of anti-cancer drugs is often limited by toxic reactions. Chemotherapeutic agents have a low therapeutic index, hence, the margin of safety of these agents is small. For this reason, one should be familiar with their spectrum.[49-51] Numerous complications may occur, and the physician must be alert to both the known complications of cancer chemotherapy and unrecognized complications of this emerging discipline. The toxicity grading of the Southwest Oncology Group (Table 7-4) is useful in dosage modification.

GASTROINTESTINAL TOXICITY

Anorexia, nausea and vomiting are the most common and distressing acute reactions to a wide variety of cancer chemotherapeutic agents.[52] Apart from the emesis induced by the stimulation of the chemoreceptor trigger zone (CTZ), there may be a considerable psychologic component manifested as anticipatory emesis.[53,54] Suppression with phenothiazines, given intravenously or as rectal suppositories, may be adequate; however, emesis induced by DTIC or cisplatin often requires intravenous antimetics. The best available agent is metoclopramide, 2 mg/kg/$\frac{1}{2}$ hour prior to chemotherapy, then every 2 hours for five doses, then every 3 to 4 hours on demand.[55] The toxicity includes mild sedation, diarrhea and reversible extrapyramidal reactions which are controlled with intravenous diphenhydramine.

Use of other adjuncts include lorazepam, 0.05 mg/kg (not to exceed 4 mg), which causes amnesia in addition to its antiemetic effects.[56] Lorazepam may be repeated every 4 to 6 hours. The use of high-dose steroids, tetrahydrocannabinol, and nabilone also remain as useful additives.[57,58]

Other toxicity includes mucositis (especially with 5-FU) with stomatitis, esophagitis, and diarrhea. These are usually self-limiting and are dose-related, and, therefore, can be controlled. Frequent gargles with dilute hydrogen peroxide (1 percent) or viscous Xylocaine are useful. Oral candidiasis should be aggressively treated with mycostatin or clotrimazole troches. Patients who have difficulty swallowing may require additional aggressive nutritional support.

BONE MARROW TOXICITY

Clinically, bone marrow toxicity is the most important form of toxicity for many of the antineoplastic drugs in clinical practice. These include leukopenia with resultant infection, thrombocytopenia with bleeding complications, and symptoms requiring blood transfusions. The approximate timing of myelosuppression with various agents is outlined in Table 7-5. Depending on the severity of myelosuppression, the chemotherapeutic dosages may require modifications (Table 7-6).

Patients with grade 4 bone marrow toxicity require hospitalization and frequently require aggressive support with antibiotics, infusion of blood and blood products.[70] Alkylating agents, mitomycin C, and nitrosoureas, may lead to pancytopenia.[71] Mitomycin C also is associated with microangiopathic hemolytic anemia.[72] Efforts to prevent leukopenia with lithium carbonate have not been widely accepted.[73] Experimental programs of autologous bone marrow transplantation may hold the key to managing chemotherapy-induced leukopenia.[74,75]

IMMUNOSUPPRESSION

Most of the commonly used antineoplastic agents suppress cellular and humoral immunity.[76] The immunologic parameters studied include delayed macrophage entry into inflammatory sites, and attenuated lymphocyte blastogenic response to phytohemagglutinen (PHA). There is a marked decrease in host defenses during treatment; however, in some patients, there may be immunologic overshoot during the recovery period. The true clinical significance of this remains to be determined.

SKIN REACTIONS

Skin reactions may include local necrosis from drug extravasation, alopecia, and allergic or hypersensitivity reactions.[77] Less serious skin reactions include changes in skin pigmentation, photosensitivity reactions, and oncholysis. Transverse banding of nails, folliculitis (Actinomycin D), and radiation recall the phenomenon (Adriamycin). The effect of chemotherapy on wound healing remains extremely controversial and is probably of no clinical significance.[78]

DRUG EXTRAVASATION

The severity of reaction is a function of drug doses extravasated and varies from erythema to extensive tissue necrosis requiring skin grafting (Fig. 7-7). Even

Table 7-4 Chemotherapy Toxicity Criteria (Southwest Oncology Group)

System	0	1	2	3	4
Hematopoietic (Hb g/dl)	>2 y ≧ 10.0	9.0–9.9	7.0–8.9	5.0–6.9	<50
WBC (granulocytes) μl	>4,000 (>1,500)	3,000–3,999	2,000–2,999	1,000–1,999	<1,000
Platelets/μl	≧100,000	75,000–99,999 (<1,500)	50,000–74,999 (<1,000)	25,000–49,999 (<500)	<25,000 (<250)
Genitourinary Renal Creatinine clearance	>50	40–50	30–39	20–29	<20
Bladder	Normal	Dysuria requiring therapy and/or microscopic hematuria	Dysuria requiring therapy and/or hematuria	Hematuria + drop in Hb: by 2 g/dl	
Hepatic SGOT	(normal 2 ×n) <40	(2–4.9 ×n) 41–60	(5–10 ×n) 61–200	200 (>10 ×n)	
SGPT	<30	30–35	51–100	100 (>10 ×n)	
Bilirubin	<1 mg/dl	1–2 mg/dl	2.1–5 mg/dl	5 mg/dl	
				5 mg/dl	
				Clinical evidence of liver failure	
Gastrointestinal Stomatitis	Normal	Erythema	Ulcers—able to eat	Unable to eat because of ulcerations	
Abdominal pain	None	No Rx needed	Rx needed — helpful	Rx needed — not helpful	
Constipation	Daily BM	No BM <2 of	No BM × 2–4 days	No BM >4 days	
Diarrhea	<3 BM daily	3–4 liquid stools / No dehydration	>4 liquid stools / Needs IV to hydrate	Blood diarrhea / Needs IV +/or blood	
Gastrointestinal Nausea and vomiting	Normal	Nausea; no vomiting	Vomiting can be prevented by Rx <6 × day	Vomiting >6 ×day in spite of antiemetics	
Pulmonary	Normal	No symptoms pulmonary function and parameter 10–25% <pre-Rx	Pulmonary symptoms requiring Rx without need for assisted ventilation	Assisted ventilation needed	

Cardiac	Normal in all	ECG changes only or sinus tachycardia not to exceed 110 at rest	Arrhythmias except ventricular tachycardia ± ECG charges	CHF, ventricular tachycardia, pericarditis and/or effusion
Neuromuscular Peripheral nerves	None	+DTRs +/or paresthesias	Absent DTRs weakness + peripheral nerve pain	Incapacity, weakness to bedridden state, paresis
CNS	Normal	Drowsiness and nervousness	Confusion, anxiety or depression requiring therapy	Convulsions Coma Psychosis
Skin				
Acute	Normal	Transient erythema	Vesiculation	Ulceration
Chronic	Normal	Pigmentation, atrophy, depilation	Subepidermal fibrosis	Ulceration + necrosis
Allergy	None	Drug fever <38°C Transient rash	Urthicaria fever >38°C, asthma	Anaphylactic reaction or anaphylactic shock
Hypertension	Normal	<10%+	10–25%+	>25%+
Fatigue	Stays at baseline	1-level deterioration in performance status	2-level deterioration in performance status	3-level deterioration in performance status

Performance Status Ranking

AJCC Scale	Rank	Karnofsky Scale
0	Fully active	90–100
1	Restricted but ambulatory, capable of light work	70–80
2	Up more then 50%, capable of self-care, unable to work	50–60
3	Limited self care, more than 50% confined to bed or chair	30–40
4	Completely bedridden	10–20
	Dead	0

Table 7-5 Granulocyte, Nadir, Recovery, and Plasma Half-Life of Chemotherapeutic Agents Useful in Gynecologic Oncology

Drug[a]	Nadir of Granulocytes (days)	Recovery (days)	$t\frac{1}{2}$ (min)
Melphalan[52]	10–12	—	40
Vinblastine[60]	5–9	14–21	4
Cyclophosphamide[61]	8–14	18–25	240–390
5-Fluorouracil[62]	7–14	20–30	10–20
Methotrexate[63]	7–14	14–21	45
Actinomycin D[64]	15	22–25	20
Doxorubicin[65]	6–13	21–24	198
Mitomycin C[66]	28–42	42–56	47
Vincristine[67]	4–5	7	1
Bleomycin[68]	—	—	16–45
Cisplatin[69]	—	—	25–49

[a] Superscript numbers are references.

with meticulous attention to the detail of drug administration, the incidence is 1 : 1000 venipunctures.[79] Strategies for management are outlined in Table 7-7. The treatment and management of intravascular chemotherapeutic drugs is controversial because there are no standard treatments that are well documented with regard to effectiveness. It is often difficult to determine that an infiltration has occurred. The intensity of intravascular reaction may vary and can occur hours after extravasation. In an attempt to identify and treat this problem, infusion should be discontinued if the patient complains of pain, burning, stinging, or swelling at the IV site, loss of blood return, and color changes at needle insertion site, mandates stopping the drug infusion. The needle should be left in place, approximately 5 ml blood drawn along with the residual drug, then 100 mg solucort-F should be injected intravenously and an appropriate antidote given. If, however, one is unable to inject or in the event of symptoms of extravasation after discontinuing intravenous infusion, inject the site with 100 mg solucort-F, subcutaneously. Topical 1 percent hydrocortisone cream, along with warm or cold compresses, should be applied. The timing and the drug that has extravasated should be documented carefully. Skin grafting is often necessary to cover the area of necrosed skin and to protect underlying vital structures (Table 7-7).

Table 7-6 Dose Adjustment of Therapy

WBC Before Starting New Course	Dose Adjustment
>4,000/mm³	100% of drugs
3,999–3,000/mm³	100% of nonmyelotoxic agent
	50% of each myelotoxic agent
	Wait an additional week
2,999–2,000/m³	100% of nonmyelotoxic agent
	25% of each myelotoxic agent
	Wait until count equals 3,000/m³
1,999–1,000/m³	50% of nonmyelotoxic agent

(Data from refs. 80 and 81.)

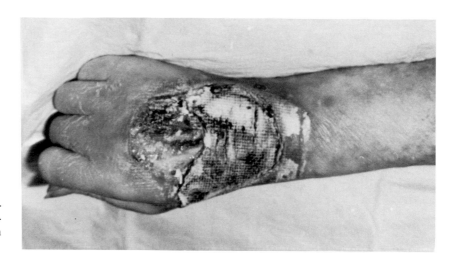

Fig. 7-7 Extravasation of mitomycin C with extensive necrosis. Patient required skin graft.

VASCULAR AND HYPERSENSITIVITY REACTIONS

The most catastrophic form of hypersensitivity is anaphylactic shock and commonly is seen with L-asparaginase, but rarely may be seen with cyclophosphamide, doxorubicin, cisplatin, and high-dose methotrexate.[77] Bleomycin can cause a unique hyperpyrexic reaction as well as Raynaud's phenomenon and a scleroderma-like reaction.[77,82] Cytabarine may rarely cause a distinctive syndrome of fever, conjunctival suffusion, and a maculopapular rash that can be prevented by corticosteroids.[83]

Table 7-7 Vesicant Drugs and Treatment of Drug Extravasation

Drug		Type of Compress
Dactinomycin (actinomycin D)	Sodium thiosulfate 10%, 4 ml	Cold
Dacarbazine	No specific antidote	Cold
Daunomycin or Daunorubicin (Cerubidine)	Sodium bicarbonate 8.4%, 4 ml	Cold
Doxorubicin (Adriamycin)	Sodium bicarbonate 8.4%, 5 ml	Cold
Mithramycin (mithracin)	Edetate disodium 150, mg/ml 1 ml	Hot
Mitomycin (Mutamycin)	Sodium thiosulfate 10%, 5 ml	Cold
Estramustine phosphate (Estracyte)	No specific antidote	Cold
Mechlorethamine (nitrogen mustard)	Sodium thiosulfate 10%, 4 ml	Cold
Vinblastine (Velban)	Hyaluronidase 150 units/ml, 1 ml	Hot
Vincristine (Oncovin)	Hyaluronidase 150 units/ml, 1 ml	Hot
Carmustine (BCNU) — an irritant	Sodium bicarbonate	Cold

HEPATOTOXICITY

The spectrum of toxicity ranges from transient elevations of transaminase enzymes with cytarabine, nitrosoureas, and doxorubicin, fibrosis and cirrhosis with methotrexate, cholestasis and possibly hepatic necrosis with 6-mercaptopurine, or mithramycin and fatty metamorphosis with L-asparaginase.[84] Rarely, severe hepatic veno-occlusive disease has been reported with mitomycin C, 6-thioguanine, or cytabarine alone or in combination with radiation therapy in preparation for bone marrow transplantation.[85,86]

PULMONARY TOXICITY

Pulmonary fibrosis caused by Bleomycin appears to be dose related, occurring in doses greater than 400 units.[87] Some degree of pulmonary dysfunction also is caused by methotrexate, procarbazine, and most alkylating agents.

CARDIOTOXICITY

Dose-limiting toxicity of doxorubicin, daunomycin, and high doses of cyclophosphamides resulting in cardiac dysfunction have been reported in the literature.[88] The usual dose of Adriamycin for cardiac dysfunction is 450 mg/m^2; these patients need to be carefully monitored by estimation of cardiac systolic ejection fraction.

NEUROTOXICITY

Many patients with advanced malignancies develop neurologic symptoms from either the cancer or its treatment at some point in the natural history of the disease. The neurotoxicity of chemotherapeutic agents have been elaborated by Kaplan and Wiernik.[89]

Ararchnoiditis, myelopathy, or encephalomyelopathy may result from intrathecal Methotrexate or Thiotepa. Chronic encephalopathies and the somnolence syndrome from cerebral irradiation and/or intrathecal Methotrexate or cytarabine have also been described. Acute encephalopathies (as with methotrexate, 5-FU, procarbazine, hexamethylmelamine,

cytarabine) have also been reported. Vincristine, cisplatin, hexamethylmelamine, VP$_{16}$, and procarbazine cause troublesome peripheral neuropathy. Cerebellar syndrome and ataxia have been reported with 5-FU, HMM, and procarbazine, Ototoxicity and optic nerve damage have been described with cisplatin. Autonomic dysfunction and cranial nerve paresis are known to occur from vinca alkaloids, cisplatin, and 5-FU.

True alterations of taste and smell are also known to occur with chemotherapy using doxorubicin and vincristine.[90] Epileptic seizures are also known to occur due to cisplatin toxicity.[91] Most recently, high dose cyclophosphamide has been reported to cause transient blindness in children.[92] Inappropriate antidiuretic hormone syndrome due to cyclophosphamide and cisplatin may lead to severe electrolyte imbalance.[93]

GENITOURINARY TOXICITY

Drug-induced nephrotoxicity due to cisplatin often alters the number of courses that can be administered.[94] Consequent forced hydration and the use of mannitol and 10 percent sodium thiosulfate have limited nephrotoxicity and permit the use of cisplatin in higher doses. Uric acid nephropathy may also be a problem preventable by the use of allopurinol and hydration. Hemorrhage cystitis appears in 10 percent of patients treated with cyclophosphamide.

SEXUAL AND GONADAL DYSFUNCTION

Alkylating agents may lead to amenorrhea and azoospermia.[95] Post-therapy gynecomastia and impotence may also result from Leydig cell dysfunction.[96] Recently, the use of luteinizing hormone releasing hormone (LHRH) in protecting patients undergoing chemotherapy for leukemia and other disorders is under investigation.

CONCLUSION

In summary, chemotherapy of gynecologic cancer has made major strides over the last decade. The gynecologic oncologists who know the underlying principles of chemotherapy will understand its effectiveness and relationship to surgery and irradiation. Such knowledge will enable the physician to critically evaluate current treatment schemes and to design effective future studies. The goal of therapy in gynecologic malignancies should be long-term disease-free survival. Additional progress may require more knowledge about the mechanics of cancer cell growth and death in order to develop new and more effective chemotherapeutic drugs and schedules.

REFERENCES

1. Goodman LS, Wintrobe MW, Dameshek W, et al: Nitrogen mustard therapy. JAMA 132:126, 1946
2. Li MC, Hertz R, Spencer DB: Effect of methotrexate therapy upon choriocarcinoma and chorioadenoma. Proc Soc Exp Biol Med, 93:361, 1956
3. Baserga R: The cell cycle. N Engl J Med, 304:453, 1981
4. Brent TP, Butler JAV, Crathorn AR: Variation in phosphokinase activities during the cell cycle in synchronous population of heLa cells. Nature (Lond) 207:176, 1965
5. Spadari S, Wiessbach A: The interrelation between DNA synthesis and various DNA polymerase activities in synchronal heLa cells. J Mol Biol 86:11, 1974
6. Johnson JF, Fuhrman CL, Wiedmann LM: Regulation of dihydrofolate reductase gene expression in mouse fibroblasts during the transition from the resting to growing state. J Cell Physiol 97:397, 1978
7. Larson A: Ribonucleotide reductase from regenerating rat liver. Eur J Biochem 11:113, 1969
8. Harriss EB, Hoelzer D: An evaluation of various double labeling and autoradiographic techniques for the measurement of DNA synthesis time in leukemic cells. J Microsc 96:205, 1972
9. Darzynkiewicz Z, Evenson DP, Staiano-Gico L, et al: Correlation between cell cycle duration and RNA content. J Cell Physiol 100:425, 1979
10. Quastle H, Sherman FG: Cell population kinetics in the intestinal epitheium of mouse. Exp Cell Res 17:420, 1959
11. Baserga R, Kisieleski WE: Comparative study of the kinetics of cellular proliferation of normal and tumorous tissue with the use of tatiated thymidine. J Natl Cancer Inst 28:331, 1962
12. Skipper HE, Perry S: Kinetics of normal and leukemic leukocyte populations and relevance to chemotherapy. Cancer Res 30:1883, 1970
13. Antoniades HN, Owen AJ: Growth factors and regulation of cell growth. Annu Rev Med 33:445, 1982
14. Tsuruo T, Fidler IJ: Differences in drug sensitivity among tumor cells from parental tumors, selected variants and spontaneous metastases. Cancer Res 41:3058, 1981
15. Skipper HE, Schabel FM JR, Wilcox WS: Experimental evaluation of potential anticancer agents on the criteria and kinetics associated with "curability" of experimental leukemia. Cancer Chemother Rep 35:1, 1964
16. Chabner BA (ed): Clinical pharmacokinetics and drug monitoring. p. 106. In Pharmacologic Principles of Cancer Treatment. WB Saunders, Philadelphia, 1982
17. Goldie JH, Coldman AJ: A mathematical model for relating the drug sensitivity of tumors to their spontaneous mutation rate. Cancer Treatm Rep 63:1727, 1979
18. Devita VT Jr: The Richard and Hinda Rosenthal Foundation Award Lecture. American Association for Cancer Research, Los Angeles, May 1986
19. Devita VT JR, Young RC, Canellos GP: Combination versus single agent chemotherapy. A review of the basis of selection of drug treatment of cancer. Cancer 35:98, 1975
20. Sartorelli AC: Approaches to the combination chemotherapy of transplantable neoplasms. Prog Exp Tumor Res 6:228, 1965
21. Potter VR: Sequential blocking of metabolic pathways in vivo. Proc Soc Exp Biol Med 76:41, 1951
22. Elion GB, Singer S, Hitchings GH: Antagonists of nucleic acid derivatives. VIII. Synergism in combinations of biochemically related antimetabolites. J Biol Chem, 208:477, 1954
23. Ozols RF, Locker GY, Goroshone JH, et al: Pharmacokinetics of Adriamycin and tissue penetration in murine ovarine cancer. Cancer Res, 39:3209, 1979
24. McVie JG, Dikhoff T, Van der Heide J, et al: Tissue concentration of platinum after intraperitoneal cisplatin administration in patients. Proc Am Assoc Cancer Res 26:162, 1985
25. Jenkins J, Sugarbarker P, Granola F, et al: Technical consideration in the use of intraperitoncal chemotherapy administration by Tenckhoff catheter. Surg Gynecol Obstet 154:858, 1982
26. Dedrick R, Myers C, Bungay P, et al: Pharmacokinetic rationale for peritoneal drug administration in the treatment of ovarian cancer. Cancer Treatm Rep 62:1, 1978
27. Jones RB, Myers CE, Guarina AM, et al.: High volume intraperitoneal chemotherapy ("belly bath") for ovarian carcinoma. Cancer Chemother Pharmacol 1:161, 1978
28. Howell SB, Chu BCF, Wung WE, et al: Long duration intracavitary infusion of Methotrexate with systemic leucovorin protection in patients with malignant effusions. J Clin Invest 67:1161, 1981

29. Speyer JL, Collins JM, Dedrick RL, et al: Phase I and pharmacological studies of 5-fluorouracil administered intraperitoneally. Cancer Res 40:657, 1980

30. Ozols RF, Young RC, Speyer JS, et al: Phase I and pharmacological studies of Adriamycin administered intraperitoneally to patients with ovarian cancer. Cancer Res 42:4265, 1982

31. Howell SB, Pfeifle CE, Wung WE, et al: Intraperitoneal cisplatin with systemic thiosulfate protection. Ann Intern Med 97:845, 1982

32. Cohen CJ: Surgical considerations in ovarian cancer. Semin Oncol 12(suppl 4):53, 1985

33. Casper ES, Kelsen DP, Alcock NW, et al: IP cisplatin in patients with malignant ascites pharmacokinetic evaluation and comparison with the IV route. Cancer Treatm Rep 67:235, 1983

34. Pretorius RG, Hacker NF, Berek JSM et al: Pharmacokinetics of IP cisplatin in refractory ovarian carcinoma. Cancer Treatm Rep 67:235, 1983

35. King ME, Pfeifle CE, Howell SB: Intraperitoneal cytosine arabinoside in ovarian carcinoma. J Clin Oncol 2:662, 1984

36. Gyves J, Ensminger W, Niederhuber J, et al: Phase I study of intraperitoneal 5-day continuous 5-FU infusion and bolus Mitomycin-C. Proc Am Soc Clin Oncol 1:15, 1982

37. Panasci LC, Skalski V, St Germain J, et al: Pharmacology and toxicity of IP streptozolocin in ovarian cancer: A case report. Cancer Treatm Rep 66:1595, 1982

38. McVie G: In Carter S, Rozencweig M (eds): Investigational New Drugs European Conference on Clinical Oncology Symposium, Stockholm, 1985

39. Markman M, Howell SB, Lucas WE: Combination intraperitoneal chemotherapy with cisplatin, cytarabine, and doxorubicin for refractory ovarian carcinoma and other malignancies principally confined to the peritoneal cavity. J Clin Oncol 2:1321, 1984

40. Markman M, Cleary S, Lucas WE, et al: Intraperitoneal chemotherapy with high dose cisplatin and cytosine arabinoside for refractory ovarian carcinoma and other malignancies principally involving the peritoneal cavity. J Clin Oncol 3:925, 1985

41. Markman M, Cleary S, Lucas WE, et al: Combination intraperitoneal chemotherapy with cisplatin, cytarabine and Bleomycin. Proc Am Soc Clin Oncol 4:112, 1985

42. Myers C: The use of intraperitoneal chemotherapy in the treatment of ovarian cancer. Semin Oncol 11:275, 1984

43. Pfeifle CE, Howell HB, Markman M, et al: Totally implantable system for peritoneal access. J Clin Oncol 2:1277, 1984

44. Piccart MJ, Speyer JL, Markman M, et al: Intraperitoneal chemotherapy: Technical experience at fine institutions. Semin Oncol 12:90, 1985

45. Runowicz CD, Dottino PR, Shafor MK: Catheter complications associated with intraperitoneal chemotherapy. Gynecol Oncol 24:41, 1986

46. Weiss RB, Devita VT: Multimodal primary cancer treatment (adjuvant chemotherapy): Current results and future prospects. Ann Intern Med 91:251, 1979

47. Frei E III: Curative cancer chemotherapy. Cancer Res 45:6523, 1985

48. Krakoff IH: Cancer chemotherapeutic agents. Ca 37:93, 1987

49. Chabner BA: The role of drugs in cancer treatment. p. 3. In Pharmacologic Principles of Cancer Treatment. WB Saunders, Philadelphia, 1982

50. Calabresi P, Parks RE: Chemotherapy of neoplastic diseases. p. 1240. In Goodman LS, Gilman RS (eds): The Pharmacological Basis of Therapeutics. Macmillan, New York, 1985

51. Cadman E, Becker FF: Toxicity of chemotherapeutic agents. A comprehensive treatise. Cancer 5:59, 1977

52. Siegel LJ, Longo DL: The control of chemotherapy induced emesis. Ann Intern Med 95:352, 1981

53. Wilcox PM, Fettony JH, Nettesheim KM: Anticipatory vomiting in women receiving cyclophosphamide, methotrexate and 5-FU (CMF) adjuvant chemotherapy for breast carcinoma. Cancer Treatm Rep 66:1601, 1982

54. Morrow GR, Morrell C: Behavioral treatment for the anticipating nausea and vomiting induced by cancer chemotherapy. N Engl J Med 307:1476, 1986

55. Gralla RJ: Metoclopramide — A review of antiemetic trials. Drugs 25:63, 1983

56. Laszlo J: Antiemetics and Cancer Chemotherapy. Williams & Wilkins, Baltimore, 1983

57. Cassileth PA, Lusk EJ, Torri S, et al: Antiemetic efficacy of dexamethasone therapy in patients receiving cancer chemotherapy. Arch Intern Med 143:1347, 1983

58. Carey MP, Burish TG, Brenner DE: Delta 9 tetrahydrocannabinol in cancer chemotherapy: Research problems and issues. Ann Intern Med 99:106, 1983

59. Albert DS, Chang SY, Chen H-SG, et al: Kinetics of intravenous Melphalan. Clin Pharmacol Ther 26:73, 1979

60. Nelson RL: The comparative clinical pharmacology and pharmacokinetics of vindesine, vincristine and vinblastine in human patients with cancer. Med Pediatr Oncol 10:115, 1982

61. Bagley CM, Bosteck FW, Denla VT: Clinical pharmacology of cyclophosphamide. Cancer Res 33:226, 1973

62. Colvin M, Hetton J: Pharmacology of cyclophosphamide and metabolites. Cancer Treatm Rep 65(suppl 3):89, 1981

63. Huffman DH, Wan SH, Azarnoff DL, et al: Pharmacokinetics of methotrexate. Clin Pharmacol Ther 14:572, 1973

64. Tattersal MHN, Sodergren JE, Dengupta SK, et al: Pharmacokinetics of Actinomycin-D in patients with malignant melanoma. Clin Pharmacol Ther 17:701, 1975

65. Benjamin RS, Riggs CE, Bachur NR: Plasma Pharmacokinetics of doxorubicin and its metabolism in humans with normal hepatic and renal function. Cancer Res 37:1416, 1977

66. Van Hazel GA, Kovach JS: Pharmacokinetics of Mitomycin-C in rabbits and humans. Cancer Chemother Pharmacol 8:189, 1982

67. Jackson DV, Sethi VS, Spurr CL, et al: Pharmacokinetics of vincristine infusion. Cancer Treatm Rep 65:1043, 1981

68. Ohnuma T, Holland JF, Masada H, et al: Microbiological assay of Bleomycin: Inactivation tissue distribution and clearance. Cancer 33:1230, 1975

69. Ribaud P, Gouveia J, Bonnay M, et al: Clinical pharmacology and pharmacokinetics of cisplatin and analogues. Cancer Treatm Rep 65(suppl 3):97, 1981

70. Henderson ES: The granulocytopenic effects of cancer chemotherapeutic agents. p. 207. In Dimitrov NV, Nodine JH (eds): Drugs and Hematologic Reactions. Grune & Stratton, Orlando, FL, 1974

71. Trainor KJ, Morley AA: Screening of cytotoxic drug for residual bone marrow damage. J Natl Cancer Inst 57:1236, 1976

72. Zimmerman SE, Smith FP, Phillips TM: Gastric carcinoma and thrombolic thrombocytopenia purpura: Association with plasma immunocomplex concentration. Br Med J 284, 1432, 1982

73. Rothstein G, Clarkson DR, Larson W: Effect of lithium on neutrophil mass and production. N Engl J Med 298:178, 1978

74. Lazarus HM, Herzig RH, Graham-Pole J, et al: Intensive melphalan chemotherapy and cryopreserved autologus bone marrow transplantation for the treatment of refractory cancer. J Clin Oncol 1:359, 1983

75. Barbasch A, Higby DJ, Brass C: High dose cytoreductive therapy with autologus bone marrow transplantation in advanced malignancy. Cancer Treatm Rep 76:143, 1983

76. Harns JE, Sinkovics JG: Suppression of human immune response in the Immunology of Malignant Disease. CV Mosby, St. Louis, 1976

77. Dunagin WG: Clinical toxicity of chemotherapeutic agents: Dermatologic toxicity. Semin Oncol 9:14, 1982

78. Ferguson MK: The effect of antineoplastic agent on wound healing. Surg Gynecol 154:421, 1982

79. Larson DL: Treatment of tissue extravasation by antitumor agents. Cancer 49:1796, 1982

80. Faehnich J: Extravasation. NITA 7:49, 1984

81. Cancer chemotherapy guidelines and recommendations for nursing education and practice. Oncol Nursing Soc 1984

82. Vogelzang NJ, Bosl GJ, Johnson K: Renaud's phenomenon: A common toxicity after combination for testicular cancer. Ann Intern Med 95:288, 1981

83. Shah SS: The cytarabine syndrome in an adult. Cancer Treatm Rep 67:405, 1983

84. Perry MC: Hepatotoxicity of chemotherapeutic agents. Semin Oncol 9:65, 1982

85. Woods WG, Dehner LP, Nesbit ME, et al: Fatal veno-occlusive disease of the liver following high dose chemotherapy, irradiation and bone marrow transplantation. Am J Med 68:285, 1980

86. Gill RA, Onstad GR, Cardamone JM, et al: Hepatic veno-occlusive disease caused by 6-thioquanine. Ann Intern Med 96:58, 1982

87. Ginsberg SJ, Comis RL: The pulmonary toxicity of antineoplastic agents. Semin Oncol 9:34, 1982

88. Cadman E: Toxicity of chemotherapeutic agents. p. 59. In Becker FF (eds): A Comprehensive Treatise. Cancer. Vol. 5. Plenum Publishing Corporation, New York, 1977

89. Kaplan RS, Wiemik PH: Neurotoxicity of antineoplastic drugs. Sem Oncol 1:103, 1982

90. Schiffman SS: Taste and smell in disease. N Engl J Med 308:1275, 1983

91. Mead GM, Arnold AM, Green JA, et al: Epileptic seizures associated with cisplatin administration. Cancer Treatm Rep 66:1719, 1982

92. Kende G, Sirkin SR, Thomas PR, et al: Blurring of vision — A previously undescribed complication of cyclophosphamide therapy. Cancer 44:69, 1979

93. Levin L, Sealy R, Barron J: Syndrome of inappropriate antidiuretic hormone secretion following dis-dichlorodiammineplatinum II in a patient with malignant thymoma. Cancer 50:2279, 1982

94. Riselbach RE, Garnick MD (eds): Cancer and the Kidney. Lea & Febiger, Philadelphia, 1982

95. Chapman RM: Effects of cytotoxic therapy on sexuality and gonadal function. Semin Oncol 9:84, 1982

96. Trump DL, Davy MD, Stall S: Gynecomastia in men following antineoplastic therapy. Arch Intern Med 142:511, 1982

8

Viruses and Cancer

Mary K. Howett
Fred Rapp

BACKGROUND

Studies in carcinogenesis during this century have followed two parallel but separate tracks of investigation. One large area of research has been the study of chemical and physical agents that cause altered cell properties in culture and/or tumors in animals. Although many agents have tested positive for such abilities, the mechanisms by which normal cells are altered remain unclear in most instances. The alternative path of study is carcinogenesis by viruses. The concept that infectious agents, especially viruses, can also modulate normal cells to cancer cells is an attractive one, in part, because viruses can be purified and their proteins and nucleic acids examined in molecular detail. While precise mechanisms also remain unclear, a major thrust has been to identify a single viral gene product required for carcinogenesis and to study the structure and function of such a product.

Demonstration of a viral association with malignancy was first noted by Ellermann and Bang,[1] who showed that filtrates of chicken leukemic cells, known to be free of bacteria, could transmit the disease when reinoculated into disease-free chickens. Because leukemia was not yet recognized by physicians as a true cancer, the importance of this finding was overshadowed by the demonstration by Rous[2] that a solid tumor (a transplantable sarcoma of chickens) could be transmitted in the same manner.

The technology with which to exploit these important early experiments remained to be developed decades later. The advent of modern virology and molecular biology produced inroads associating viruses with the etiology of cancer. Several major approaches include (1) the development of in vitro models to study virus replication and the ability of viruses to alter normal cellular growth regulation; (2) the development of in vivo models to study tumorigenesis by viruses; (3) the isolation of viruses from naturally occurring tumors; (4) the development of specific and sensitive methods with which to probe morphologically altered cells and tumors for virus nucleic acids and proteins; and (5) epidemiologic studies, especially in human populations, to associate viruses with certain tumor types. As a result of these efforts, both DNA and RNA viruses have been implicated in animal and human tumors. (For thorough and extensive reviews[3,4] of this subject, the reader is referred to the references at the end of the chapter.)

Virus groups with known tumorigenic activity include certain DNA viruses: adenoviruses; papovaviruses (both the papilloma and polyoma subgroups); herpesviruses; the hepadnavirus, hepatitis B virus; and one major group of RNA viruses, the retroviruses. Retroviruses have been associated extensively with tumors in animals and recently two human retroviruses have been linked with rare T-cell lymphomas. This chapter discusses the associations of these viruses with human tumors, with special emphasis on those associated with genital neoplasms.

PROPERTIES OF CANCER CELLS

Regardless of the agent for inducing carcinogenesis, many cancer cells share the same altered properties. With apology to the many outstanding scientists who have published a wealth of information on the cancer cell phenotype, we shall briefly discuss some of these properties and cite a few selected references.

Most of the properties found in cancer cells convey a selective growth advantage. The growth of cancer cells in an abnormal site can interfere with normal organ function. The term transformed cell is generally used to describe a cell that is altered during carcinogenesis. The term transformation can be best defined within this context as the acquisition of a new and heritable trait by a cell.[5,6] Cells from animal tumors possess many of the same traits as cells transformed in culture, thereby justifying the use of in vitro transformation as a model for in vivo tumorigenesis.

The infection of cells or a multicellular organism by a virus usually results in productive or lytic infection but occasionally, especially if the infected cell type does not fully support viral replication, leads to stable acquisition by the cell of the virus nucleic acid or a subset of the virus genome. In carcinogenesis, this heritable change results in the immortalization of the cell and it may become tumorigenic. The altered cell is now removed from normal growth regulation. The consequence in vitro is the establishment of a continuous cell line with new growth properties; in vivo, the cell may be capable of tumorigenesis. In many cases, continued expression of viral gene products is required for this immortalization but it is not known whether this is always true.

It is possible to think of transformed cells as more vigorous than their normal counterparts. This vigor is reflected in several characteristics. These altered characteristics reflect a genetic change in the cell. Heritable changes are listed below.

Attempts to describe and understand the cancer phenotype have involved growth of tumor cells in vitro as well as generation de novo of transformed cells by addition of viruses and/or carcinogens.

PROPERTIES OF CELLS TRANSFORMED BY VIRUS

Altered morphology

Decreased contact inhibition in culture

Increased saturation density in culture

Decreased length of cell cycle

Growth without attachment to a physical substrate

Chromosomal aberrations

Altered karyotype

Ability of cells to divide in low serum medium

Decreased actin filaments

Increased synthesis of the protease plasminogen activator

Acquisition of virus nucleic acids

Acquisition of new cell surface antigens and often, of intranuclear antigens

Decrease in the ratio of cytoplasmic to nuclear volume

Ability to form tumors in immunologically compromised or syngeneic hosts

---

Transformed cells are usually more rounded and refractile than their normal cell counterparts; while normal cells may grow in a recognizable oriented monolayer in culture, this pattern may also change as a consequence of transformation. Normal cells generally respect territorial boundaries much more strictly. The phenomenon, known as contact inhibition, controls growth. In cell culture, normal cells will grow until their membranes touch, but the cells usually will not grow on top of one another to a significant degree. The multilayered growth of transformed cells results in an increased number of cells per given area (saturation density) in a culture flask. When cell lines exhibiting different in vitro saturation densities were prepared from BALB/c inbred mouse embryos and tested for tumorigenicity, a strong correlation between saturation density in vitro and initiation of tumor formation was noted.[7] Transformation by viruses will also produce cell cultures with increased saturation densities. Growth without attachment to a solid substrate also will frequently take place. This latter quality allows one transformed cell to form a focus by growing, after suspension, in medium containing soft (sloppy) agar (3 percent) or 0.5 percent methylcellulose. Stoker et al.[8] termed this phenomenon anchorage dependence of multiplication on the part of normal cells. In addition, while most mammalian cells need serum for growth,[9,10] transformation results in decreased serum dependence.

Changes in cell morphology can be accompanied by an accelerated growth rate and a corresponding decrease in the ratio of cytoplasmic to nuclear volume. Certain cell structures are also altered in cells transformed by viruses or carcinogens or in cells that become otherwise transformed. Chromosomal aberrations and abnormal chromosome numbers are common,[3] and structural actin filaments (the cell cytoskeleton) are decreased in number. It is possible to demonstrate an abnormal but stable karyotype in cells transformed by certain herpesviruses. By using fluorescently labeled anti-actin antibody, it has been shown that transformation of rodent cells by papovaviruses leads to a disruption of the cell cytoskeleton.

Macromolecular changes in cells also accompany transformation. These include the acquisition of a variety of newly synthesized antigens, both virus specific and cell induced. Papovavirus- and retrovirus-transformed cells demonstrate about 50 new cell proteins in addition to antigens specific to the transforming virus. These new cell proteins include molecules involved in membrane changes and in mechanisms of proteolysis.

It can be concluded from these transformed cell properties that multicomponent mechanisms are involved in the establishment and maintenance of the transformed state. Regardless of the criterion selected by the investigator, the biologically significant characteristic of transformation is tumor formation. Thus, in vitro measurements of transformation merely indicate possible success for malignant transformation of cells. In modern tumor virology, transformed cell lines are usually derived after introduction of viral genetic information by focus formation of morphologically altered cells on monolayers of normal cells or alternatively by growth of colonies in soft agar. Lines derived by these approaches can be tested for the other parameters.

PAPOVAVIRUSES

The papovaviruses can be divided into the polyoma and the papillomavirus subgroups. The name *papova* is derived from three principal members of the group: *pa*pillomaviruses, *po*lyomavirus, and simian *va*cuolating virus [simian virus 40 (SV40)]. These viruses are unenveloped and contain a double-stranded, circular, covalently closed and supercoiled DNA.[11] Considerable evidence that members of this group affect cell proliferative control has been obtained.[3,4] The polyoma subgroup has been extensively researched, and SV40 DNA has been completely sequenced.[12,13] Work on SV40, originally isolated from monkey cell cultures used to prepare poliovirus vaccine, led to investigation of the possible role of this virus in human oncogenesis. Although a significant role in human tumor formation has not been established for SV40, this virus has become a model for the study of tumor viruses and transforming genes. SV40 is briefly discussed as a prototype virus of the polyoma subgroup, since polyomavirus has many properties similar to SV40. The virus, discovered in cultures of rhesus monkey kidney cells,[14] has the ability to lyse permissive (e.g., African green monkey kidney) cells and can transform a variety of nonpermissive (e.g., hamster or other rodent) cells in culture.[15-17] Injection of SV40 into some newborn hosts, (e.g., hamsters) will directly result in the formation of tumors.[18,19]

The DNA of the virus is a supercoiled, circular, double-stranded molecule with an approximate molecular weight of 3×10^6.[11] When permissive or nonpermissive cells are infected by SV40, the virus adsorbs to, and is engulfed by, the cell membrane (viropexis) and then traverses the cytoplasm within a vesicle formed by the cell membrane.[20] This vesicle coalesces with the nuclear membrane and virus is released into the nucleus, where uncoating and replication occur.[21] During lytic infection by SV40, the events that occur are generally divided into early and late events. Early refers to the period prior to replication of virus DNA. Immediately after uncoating, early virus messenger RNA (mRNA) is transcribed, stimulating cellular RNA and DNA synthesis.[22]

Prior to DNA synthesis, the induction of several distinct enzymes occurs in infected cells.[23-26] These enzymes include RNA polymerase, DNA ligase, thymidine kinase, dTMP kinase, dTDP kinase, cytidine kinase, dCMP deaminase, CDP reductase, dTMP synthetase, dehydrofolate reductase, and probably others. Following early RNA and antigen synthesis, cellular DNA synthesis is induced.[3,27] Histones and nuclear acidic proteins are induced at this time, as is the replication of mitochondrial DNA.[28,29] The mechanism of the induction is not fully understood, but it seems to depend, at least in part, on the early region of the virus genome. Tegtmeyer[30] in 1972 showed that induction is a gene A (early gene) function, since a functional gene A product is required for initiation of virus DNA synthesis. The gene A product is referred to as the tumor (T) antigen.

At the same time, or shortly after the induction of cellular DNA synthesis, the replication of virus DNA begins in the nuclei of permissive cells.[31] Concurrent with or shortly after viral DNA synthesis, the structural proteins of the virus are synthesized. After synthesis of SV40 progeny DNA and structural proteins,

assembly and maturation of new virions occur in the nuclei.

When nonpermissive cells (i.e., hamster or mouse) are infected by SV40, the virus is adsorbed to the cell and enters the nucleus just as in permissive cell-virus interactions. The viral infection is capable of transiently altering the growth pattern of the cells; thus, they behave like transformed cells. This transformation is abortive, however, since most of the cells regain their normal somatic cell properties after several mitoses. Viral DNA synthesis does not occur. Abortive transformation of 3T3 cells infected with SV40 was first observed by Smith and colleagues.[32] Abortively transformed cells have the ability to grow in low concentrations of serum; their altered growth patterns seem to depend on the expression of early viral genes because the altered appearance is blocked by interferon.[33,34] Abortive transformation induces the same spectrum of cellular enzymes (especially

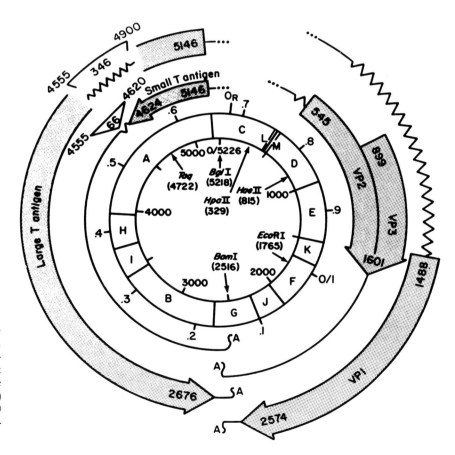

Fig. 8-1 Genomic organization of simian virus 40 (SV40). (Adapted from Fiers W, Contreras R, Haegman G, et al: Complete nucleotide sequence of SV40 DNA. Nature (Lond) 273:113, 1978. Copyright © 1978 Macmillan Journals Limited.)

those involved with DNA synthesis) seen in infected permissive cells, and cellular DNA synthesis also is induced. Attempts to demonstrate synthesis of viral DNA or structural antigens in infected nonpermissive cells have consistently failed.

A small percentage of abortively transformed cells becomes stably transformed. The fixation of transformation is dependent on at least one round of mitosis in infected cells.[35] In synchronized cells that are abortively transformed, the addition of interferon before the S period of the cell cycle prevents the fixation of transformation, implying that fixation occurs either in the S or G_2 phase of the cell cycle.[36] Stably transformed cells permanently possess all the properties described for abortive transformants; several techniques have demonstrated that these cells possess stably integrated viral DNA.

Many SV40-transformed lines contain the equivalent of one complete virus genome, as SV40 can be rescued by the formation of cell hybrids between these lines and permissive cells either by cocultivation[37] or by fusion of the two cells in the presence of inactivated Sendai virus.[38-41] Transformed cell lines from which viruses cannot be rescued by these techniques are presumed to contain SV40 DNA lacking complete viral genetic information.

The state of the viral DNA in the transformed cells was examined by Sambrook and co-workers.[42] Because the high-molecular-weight portion of cellular DNA contains SV40-specific gene sequences and because the association was alkali stable, these workers concluded that the SV40 DNA is covalently integrated into the DNA of the transformed host cell. These results were confirmed by several other investigators. SV40 DNA also has been detected in various transformed lines by measuring the nucleic acid hybridization between virus-specific RNA and the total DNA extracted from the cells.[42,43] Radioactively labeled viral RNA for use in hybridization experiments can be synthesized by transcription in vitro of SV40 DNA by *Escherichia coli* RNA polymerase. Similar measurements also have been performed by hybridizing small amounts of denatured labeled SV40 DNA, with the total DNA extracted from the transformed cells.[44,45] Transformed lines containing up to 60 integrated SV40 genomes have been examined.

Because of the limited coding capacity of SV40 DNA, a great deal of attention was paid to identification of the transforming genes and gene products. An antigen synthesized early after viral infection as well as in transformed cells was first identified using serum from tumor-bearing hamsters.[46-48] This was named the T antigen, which can be detected by immunofluorescence or complement-fixation assay. Accurate purification of the T antigen took a long time, with Del Villano and Defendi[49] reporting the first molecular-weight (M_r) estimate as 100,000 for this protein. Prives and colleagues[50] were able to show that in vitro synthesis of T antigen could be directed by the early 19S SV40 mRNA. Since that time, careful studies have clearly defined two proteins whose synthesis can be directed in vitro by the 19S early mRNA: a 94,000-M_r protein, now termed large T and a 17,000-M_r protein, referred to as small t.[51] Thus, in the 19S early mRNA, there are two species of mRNA. These mRNAs for T and t antigens have now been mapped. The coding sequences for the messages are shown in the SV40 genomic map (Fig. 8-1).

PROPERTIES OF LARGE T ANTIGEN

Binding to the SV40 origin
Initiation of viral DNA replication
Autoregulation of early transcription
Induction of late viral transcription
ATPase activity
Protein kinase
Adenovirus helper function
Tumor-specific transplantation antigen
Target for cytotoxic T cells
Binding to cellular DNA
Stimulation of cellular DNA synthesis
Binding to p53
Activation of rDNA transcription
Induction of cellular enzyme synthesis
Initiation of transformation
Maintenance of transformation

Considerable evidence has implicated both of these antigens in malignant cell transformation. T antigen has been shown to bind to DNA, and numerous investigators have shown specific binding to the origin of SV40 DNA replication. It is now known that T antigen (the viral gene A product) is required for SV40 DNA synthesis, controls transcription of the late region of the virus, and self-regulates transcription of the early strand. Those functions now ascribed to the T antigen are shown below, and this subject has been thoroughly reviewed.[51]

The question of the oncogenicity of a human polyoma subgroup of papovaviruses has become an issue due to the isolation of several papovaviruses from human subjects. One group, typified by the JC isolate, was obtained from biopsies of patients with progressive multifocal leukoencephalopathy (PML), a progressive degenerative disease of the central nervous system (CNS).[52] JC virus has a very limited host range in culture, growing only in fetal human glial cells; however, this virus causes transplantable brain tumors in hamsters.

A second human papovavirus, BK virus, was isolated from the urine of an immunosuppressed renal allograft patient.[53] BK virus is similar to SV40 and is capable of in vitro transformation.[3] BK virus has been the subject of intensive molecular studies; in fact, the entire genome of this virus has been sequenced,[54] as has SV40 DNA.

The human population has a high prevalence of antibodies to the human papovavirus isolates, but so far these viruses have not been associated with human cancer. Research is under way to try to establish an etiologic role for the JC virus in the pathogenesis of PML. Virtually every PML biopsy shows evidence of papovaviruses, and JC virus has been used to produce PML syndrome in macaques. It must be remembered that SV40 fails to cause any known disease in its natural host, the cynomolgus monkey. The possibility of a similar relationship between humans and the human papovavirus isolates must therefore be considered.

nents. One virus, hepatitis B virus (HBV) has been implicated in the development of primary hepatocellular carcinoma, a neoplasm derived from the parenchymal cells of the liver.

EVIDENCE FOR THE ASSOCIATION OF HEPATITIS B VIRUS INFECTION WITH PRIMARY HEPATOCELLULAR CARCINOMA

Correlation of PHC and HBV carrier rate

Correlation of PHC and HBV carrier state, both in high PHC and low PHC incidence areas

Superimposition of PHC on post-hepatic cirrhosis

HBsAG* and HBcAg in cells of PHC biopsies

Identification of integrated HBV DNA in hepatoma cell lines derived from PHC patients

Familial clustering of HBV carrier state, chronic liver disease, post-hepatic cirrhosis, and PHC

Maternal transmission of the HBV carrier state to newborns in areas where PHC rate is high

Evidence that a similar virus/disease complex leads to PHC development in the Pennsylvania woodchuck

HBsAG, hepatitis B surface antigen; HBcAG, hepatitis B core antigen; HBV, hepatitis B virus; PHC, primary hepatocellular carcinoma.

HEPATITIS B VIRUS

Hepatitis can be defined as inflammation of the liver. This inflammation can be caused by viral agents and by chemical agents that are toxic to liver compo-

It has long been suggested that damage due to chronic liver disease, such as that associated with HBV infection, may result in the development of primary hepatocellular carcinoma. Primary liver cancers represent a small percentage (1 to 2 percent) of all malignancies found in the Americas and Europe but may constitute 20 to 30 percent of African and Asian tumors.[55] The incidence of primary liver cancer in men is substantially higher (two- to fourfold) than in women, with a peak incidence between 50 and 70 years of age.[56] Clinical observations have associated about 75 percent of liver cell cancers (hepatomas) and about 20 to 50 percent of duct cell cancers (cholangiomas) with cirrhosis.[57] Hepatomas often occur (10 to 15 percent of cases) subsequent to postnecrotic cirrhosis and hemochromatosis but do not occur commonly in patients with Laennec's cirrhosis. Other factors in the environment besides viruses (aflatoxins, cycads, nitrosamines, and alcohol) may damage the liver. In addition, these agents may influence the rate of primary hepatocellular carcinoma in HBV-infected populations.[56]

Acute liver infections can be caused by at least three different viruses; the diseases are commonly referred to as hepatitis A (infectious hepatitis), hepatitis B (serum hepatitis) and hepatitis C (non-A, non-B hepatitis).[58,59] Hepatitis A infections are characterized by a short incubation period (about 30 days), and the virus is shed into the feces of infected individuals. The primary path of infection is the oral/fecal route. Such infections are acute and do not become chronic. Hepatitis A is presently thought to be transmitted by a small RNA-containing virus. The pathology of non-A-non-B hepatitis is similar to that of hepatitis B, but its etiology is not well understood.

Hepatitis B virus causes serum hepatitis, a disease characterized by a longer incubation than that of hepatitis A. The primary route of spread of this agent is via infected blood or blood components, but the virus also can be transmitted by other routes. During the 1960s, Krugman and co-workers[60] demonstrated that serum from patients with long-incubation hepatitis could transmit a similar disease to human volunteers, a hepatitis with an incubation period of about 60 days. If this serum was boiled prior to administration, it was capable of immunizing patients and no longer transmitted disease.

In screening thousands of blood samples to examine genetic variation of serum proteins, Blumberg et al.[61] in 1963 found an antigen in a serum from an Australian aborigine that reacted with antibodies in a serum of an American hemophilia patient. Further studies[62-64] demonstrated that this antigen was rare in North America and western Europe and more common in Africa and Asia. It is now known that this antigen is indicative of serum hepatitis, and the nature

of the Australia antigen as well as the structure of HBV have been worked out in detail. This antigen is currently designated hepatitis B surface antigen (HBsAg).

A large number of individuals infected with HBV develop the carrier state, (i.e., chronic infection that may or may not be accompanied by active liver disease[58]) and chronically infected women transmit the disease to newborn infants.[58] While blood or blood products represent the major mode of spread in low prevalence areas, Third World countries often have a dramatically increased chronic infection rate because of perinatal transmission.

Hepatitis B virus, as an infectious entity, appears to be composed of a virus particle (average diameter of 42 nm) and is commonly referred to as the Dane particle[65] (see Fig. 8-2). Essentially, it is an enveloped virus with an internal core structure containing a double-stranded circular DNA[66] (with a gap in one strand and a nick in the opposite strand) and a virus-specific DNA polymerase.[67] Dane particles are found in the blood of acutely and chronically infected persons and also in sections of infected liver.

The concentration of infectious particles in blood is low compared with the presence of circulating subunits of virus particles, HBsAg. This surface antigen is identical to the Australian antigen and is composed of spheres (22 nm) or filaments (22 nm wide, 100 to 700 nm long) in blood or other body fluids of infected persons.[68,69] These particles can be present in the blood of carriers at a concentration of 10^{12}/ml blood. Antibody to HBsAg will agglutinate these subunit structures and the Dane particles. Naked cores, however, can be prepared by treating Dane particles with lipid solvents. The core structure is not agglutinated by antibody to HBsAg but possesses its own specificity, the core antigen (HBcAg).[70]

In infected liver cells, HBsAg is found in the cytoplasm, whereas HBcAg is found only in the nucleus. The core contains a double-stranded DNA and a virus-specific DNA polymerase. The core contains about three proteins and the polymerase possesses its own antigenicity, commonly referred to as HBeAg.[71] Serologically, HBeAg is found only in patients with HBsAg[72] and is accompanied by increased numbers of Dane particles and increased HBV polymerase activity.[73,74] A carrier who is positive for HBeAg (HBeAg+) is more likely to have active liver disease. Transmission to newborn infants is more likely when

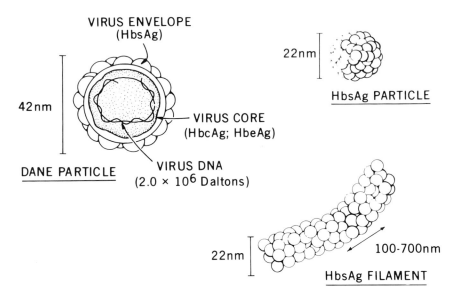

Fig. 8-2 The major structural elements found in the blood of patients with hepatitis B virus (HBV). The Dane particle represents the infectious virion and is an enveloped DNA virus containing a circular double-stranded DNA molecule with a large gap in one strand and a nick in the other. The nucleocapsid contains a core antigen (HBcAg), HBeAg, and a DNA polymerase. The relative frequency of Dane particles is low as compared with the presence of hepatitis B surface antigen (HBsAg) particles and filaments. HBsAg is present in large amounts in the blood of acutely infected persons and of HBV carriers. HBsAg-containing human blood serves as a source for preparation of a formalin-inactivated vaccine against HBV infection. (Rapp F, Howett MK: Tumor viruses — vectors of carcinogenesis at the molecular level. p 65. In Pilch YH (ed): Surgical Oncology. McGraw-Hill, New York, 1984. Reprinted with permission.)

the mother is HBeAg[+], and HBeAg[+] blood is more likely to transmit disease.

The development of the carrier state seems heavily implicated in the development of primary hepatocellular carcinoma.[67,75-81] High frequencies of primary hepatocellular carcinoma occur in areas with high frequencies of HBV carriers. Familial clustering of chronic liver disease, cirrhosis, and primary hepatocellular carcinoma has been noted in areas in which the HBV carrier rate is high. Since maternal virus transmission to offspring often occurs, these areas have large numbers of persons who are essentially lifelong carriers of HBV. In controlled studies in these areas, hepatocellular cancer has been associated with active HBV infection. It is interesting that primary hepatocellular carcinoma patients show a high incidence of HBV infection even in areas in which HBV and primary hepatocellular carcinoma rates are low. HBV structures, proteins, and viral DNA can frequently be demonstrated in primary hepatocellular carcinoma biopsies.

Several groups have identified HBV DNA inte-

grated into cell DNA from primary hepatocellular carcinoma biopsies.[82-84] Integrated virus DNA also can be detected, however, in chronic active hepatitis with or without cirrhosis.[85] Integration of HBV DNA therefore is a common event in the HBV life cycle. Its precise role in carcinogenesis requires definition.

A cell culture system for growing HBV is not yet available, hampering work aimed at detailing viral gene expression; the precise role of viral gene products in the transformation of liver cells is therefore unknown. The discovery of a woodchuck hepatitis virus will undoubtedly aid study of this disease complex since this virus (similar physically to HBV) can cause a spectrum of diseases including acute and chronic hepatitis, cirrhosis, and primary hepatocellular carcinoma in the Pennsylvania woodchuck.

Recent advances in the prevention of HBV infection may yield long-range information proving the relationship of this virus to carcinoma. Early studies showed antibody to HBsAg to be protective against serum hepatitis. A vaccine is now available to vaccinate humans with a surface antigen (free of nucleic acid) prepared from the blood of human HBV carriers.[56,86] If its use in Africa and Asia proves successful in preventing HBV infection, this vaccine may eventually reduce the endogenous incidence of chronic liver disease and of primary hepatocellular carcinoma and constitute the first effective human cancer vaccine.

HERPESVIRUSES

The herpesviruses are a large group of double-stranded DNA-containing viruses that can be identified morphologically by means of electron microscopy, sensitivity to ether, characteristic genome size, and antigenic constitution. Herpesviruses have been identified as common agents in a large number of species and all members of the group have essentially the same structure: an icosahedral nucleocapsid that contains the DNA and is surrounded by one or more lipid bilayer envelopes (Fig. 8-3). These agents have been reviewed in depth.[87]

These viruses are particularly well adapted to survival, since acute infection frequently results in establishment of latency. Virus persists in the infected host, commonly in nerve or blood cells in an unknown but apparently noninfectious state. Latent herpesviruses can be reactivated and repeatedly establish active infections that may or may not be similar in pathology to the primary infection. Primary and recurrent diseases are often accompanied by virus shedding, and

even latently infected hosts that lack overt disease can shed virus intermittently. Transmission and propagation of the herpesviruses are therefore highly efficient.

Herpesviruses are interesting because they have been implicated in a number of naturally occurring neoplastic diseases.[88-90] Limitations in the scope of this chapter do not permit a detailed discussion of all the animal models that have been established for oncogenesis by herpesviruses; we concentrate instead on the five human agents.

HERPES SIMPLEX VIRUSES

Although herpesviruses have also been shown to produce tumors in rabbits, cattle, guinea pigs, and monkeys, this discussion concentrates on the human herpesviruses and their suspected role in human neoplasia. Of the five known human herpesviruses, four are associated with various types of human tumors either by epidemiologic studies or by direct virologic techniques. In addition, the same four, herpes simplex virus (HSV) types 1 and 2 (HSV-1, HSV-2), Epstein-Barr virus (EBV), and human cytomegalovirus (HCMV), have been shown to transform normal cells in vitro to a malignant phenotype. These agents all cause primary, latent, and recurrent diseases (see Table 8-1). The fifth human herpesvirus, varicella-zoster virus (VZV), causes chickenpox as a primary infection and can recur as shingles later in life. To date

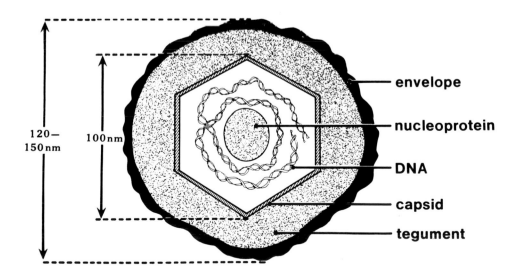

Fig. 8-3 Structure of a typical herpesvirus.

Table 8-1 Diseases Attributable to Human Herpesviruses

Virus	Disease/Condition
Herpes simplex virus type 1	Acute herpetic gingivostomatitis Recurrent herpes labialis Keratoconjunctivitis Herpes genitalis Neonatal encephalitis Neonatal herpetic septicemia Primary herpetic dermatitis Eczema varicelliform herpeticum Kaposi Traumatic herpes Herpetic encephalitis in adults Trigeminal neuralgia Carcinoma of lip?[a] Cervical carcinoma?
Herpes simplex virus type 2	Herpes genitalis Neonatal encephalitis Neonatal herpetic septicemia Acute herpetic gingivostomatitis Recurrent herpes labialis Keratoconjunctivitis Primary herpetic dermatitis Eczema varicelliform herpeticum Kaposi Traumatic herpes Herpetic encephalitis in adults Trigeminal neuralgia Cervical carcinoma?[a] Carcinoma of lip?[a]
Cytomegalovirus	Cytomegalic inclusion disease Mononucleosis-like syndrome Pneumonia in immunosuppressed patients Cancer of the prostate? Kaposi's sarcoma?
Epstein-Barr virus	Infectious mononucleosis Burkitt's lymphoma? Nasopharyngeal carcinoma?
Varicella-zoster virus	Chickenpox Shingles Ophthalmic zoster Varicella pneumonia Congenital abnormalities Hemorrhagic varicella Encephalitis

[a]Neoplastic diseases associated with viral agent.
(Rapp F, Howett MK: Tumor viruses—vectors of carcinogenesis at the molecular level. p. 65. In Pilch YH (ed): Surgical Oncology. McGraw-Hill, New York, 1984. Reprinted with permission.)

VZV has not been associated with malignancy in vivo; however, transformation in vitro has been demonstrated,[91] and its true oncogenic potential is unknown. It is suspected by analogy to the other members of this group.

HSV-1 and HSV-2 were originally distinguished by serologic procedures. These two herpesviruses are similar in composition, and both are capable of causing the same disease syndromes in humans, although HSV-1 generally is associated with oral or facial infections, whereas HSV-2 is found in sexually transmitted herpetic infections. The genomes of these two viruses vary in base composition by 2 percent, with HSV-1 (69 percent guanine + cytosine) sharing about 50 percent DNA homology with HSV-2 (71 percent guanine + cytosine). The DNA of HSV is large (100×10^6 daltons) and extremely complex in structure and function. The reader is referred to comprehensive reviews[92,93] for information concerning the molecular biology of HSV DNA.

In 1971, the observation was made that HSV-2 rendered nonlytic by ultraviolet (UV) irradiation is capable of transforming hamster embryo fibroblasts to tumorigenicity.[94] Subsequently, HSV-1 was also used to transform hamster cells; other investigators have demonstrated formation of morphologically transformed foci after HSV infection of mouse, rat, chicken, and human cells. In most cases, the lytic capacity of the transforming virus is hampered, often to enable transformation. Temperature-sensitive (*ts*) mutants of HSV also have been used for transformation. By infecting cells with ts mutants and holding cultures at a nonpermissive temperature, virus fails to replicate lytically, and transformed foci of cells can be established. In the absence of inactivation, most susceptible cells are killed by HSV and therefore no longer serve as targets for transformation. It is possible that in the body, defective or incapacitated HSV particles may initiate the transforming event. The possibility that host defenses dampen virus replication should also be considered. A general review[95] of transformation by HSV can be found at the end of this chapter.

Both serotypes of HSV are associated with human cancer. HSV-1 is implicated as a factor in squamous cell carcinoma of the lip. This tumor is rare, however, and additional studies are necessary before a strong etiologic role for HSV-1 can be established for this disease. More substantial evidence has linked HSV-2

with cervical carcinoma.[88] Data indicating a causal role for HSV-2 in cancer of the cervix are summarized below. Most data involve epidemiologic studies; direct biologic observations have been more difficult to obtain.

STATUS OF THE ASSOCIATION OF HERPES SIMPLEX VIRUS TYPE 2 WITH CERVICAL CANCER

Conflicting epidemiology of virus isolation and anti-HSV-2 antibodies

Failure to detect a specific set of virus antigens in cultured tumor cells

Failure to detect HSV-2 DNA in the majority of cervical carcinoma biopsies

Transformation in culture of normal cells to malignancy by HSV-2

Failure to detect HSV-2 mRNA in carcinoma in situ and in dysplasia of the cervix

Controversy over induction of cervical carcinoma in mice by intravaginal administration of inactivated HSV-2

It appears that the occurrence of cervical cancer is linked to sexual contact and depends at least in part on low socioeconomic status, sexual promiscuity, and early first intercourse. Rigoni-Stern[96] was the first to observe that cloistered nuns and unmarried women in Italy demonstrate a low incidence of cervical cancer. This observation has been confirmed in many other countries; the corollary observation, that prostitutes are at high risk for cervical cancer, also has also been reported. Other factors that positively correlate with cervical cancer rates include promiscuity by the male spouse, rates of penile cancer, young mean age of first coitus, and relatively large total number of coital partners. The original citations to these numerous works can be found in zur Hausen.[88]

Secondary factors relative to infectious agents may also be etiologic for cervical cancer. Most recent are reports that cigarette smoking may increase the risk by twofold.[97–100]

The patterns described above make an infectious

agent likely as a causal factor in cervical cancer. Two groups of viral agents have been investigated in this light during the past 15 years: the herpesviruses and the human papillomaviruses. (Both groups are discussed later in this chapter.)

A number of seroepidemiologic studies illustrate the possibility that women with cervical carcinoma have a higher incidence of HSV-2 infection.[101,102] Initial studies demonstrated a higher frequency and higher titer of antibodies to HSV antigens in women with cervical cancer as compared with matched case controls. Many follow-up studies throughout the world led to similar conclusions. Not all studies have been positive, however, and a major rebuttal of the hypothesis that HSV-2 causes cervical cancer was recently published by Vonka and co-workers.[103] These investigators published a prospective study encompassing thousands of women in Czechoslovakia that failed to correlate viral infection with cancer incidence.

Because of data from other tumor virus host systems, including EBV, workers expected to detect virus nucleic acids in tumor biopsies. Frenkel and colleagues[104] reported the presence of HSV-2 DNA in only one cervical carcinoma biopsy. These investigators used DNA-DNA hybridization to measure reassociation of cervical biopsy DNA with a radioactively labeled HSV-2 DNA probe. Attempts by others, including Frenkel's group, to repeat these findings have been largely unsuccessful, but several valid reasons may contribute to these failures. The few positive reports[88] are referenced. Data already discussed for the papovaviruses and adenoviruses indicate that as little as 1 to 1.5×10^6 daltons of DNA is sufficient for a transforming gene. This would only represent 1 to 1.5 percent of the HSV genome, and the DNA-DNA hybridization techniques previously used in the HSV system might not be sensitive enough to detect such a small piece of DNA, even if it were present in every cell. Frenkle's laboratory recently reported detection of subgenomic rearranged portions of HSV-2 in two additional biopsies.[105]

Because of these problems, studies have also turned to the detection of HSV-specific mRNA in biopsy material. The rationale for these experiments is based on the assumption that any biologically relevant HSV-2 DNA sequences would exert their control in the tumor cell by transcription into mRNA and subsequent translation into protein gene products. If more than one copy of mRNA is transcribed, the DNA sequence will be amplified. Using in situ hybridization of radioactively labeled HSV-2 DNA probe to mRNA in cryostat sections of biopsy material, Jones et al.[106] and McDougall et al.[107] reported a fairly high incidence (about 60 percent) of positive hybridization of the HSV-2 DNA probe to sections from dysplasia and carcinoma in situ of the cervix. Control cervical tissues only rarely hybridized to the HSV-2 probe. In addition, radioactively labeled λ bacteriophage and SV40 DNA probes failed to hybridize to the experimental sections. At that time, however, these investigators failed to detect HSV-2-specific sequences in invasive cervical carcinoma, although McDougall's group reported positive results with carcinomas in a later study.[108] The possibility of detection limitations may again be relevant — or it is possible that the continued presence of virus genetic information is not required.

Observations in a number of other laboratories have suggested that HSV-2 mRNA sequences can be detected in biopsies of invasive carcinoma of the cervix. Subsequent studies by additional research groups demonstrated a statistically increased number of grains on autoradiographs by in situ hybridizations[109,110]; however, these experiments evidenced very low levels of hybridization to radioactive probe compared with those reported in previous investigations.

In addition to work on tumor biopsies, attempts to define a subset of HSV sequences that might effect transformation in vitro have been under way. These experiments are based on the assumption that the same sequences will potentiate tumor formation in vivo.[111,112] Several investigators have shown that not only can inactivated viral preparations transform but that transfection with intact HSV DNA can potentiate transformation. Random and fairly extensive shearing of the viral DNA prior to transfection or treatment of the DNA with certain, but not all, restriction endonucleases abolishes the transforming potential. This last piece of information indicates that extensive shearing and certain restriction endonucleases can introduce cuts into essential transforming genes. Because certain restriction enzymes do not appear to cut essential transforming genes, the possibility arises that one can transform by transfection of cells with purified DNA fragments (i.e., subsets of the virus genome). HSV DNA has the capacity to code for

50 to 100 proteins, so that dealing with a subset of the virus DNA narrows the number of potentially transforming virus gene products.

By transfecting hamster cells with DNA fragments, Camacho and Spear[113] reported morphologic transformation using the XbaI-F restriction fragment of HSV-1. This fragment maps in the region between 0.30 and 0.45 from the left-hand side of the HSV DNA genome and corresponds to the region coding for two virus glycoproteins. No tumors have yet been obtained by inoculation of these cells into syngeneic newborn hamsters, however, and a search for HSV-1 glycoproteins in the cells has proved negative. Whether these cells represent true HSV-1 transformants remains to be determined. Hayward and colleagues[114] have also reported morphologic transformation of hamster cells by the BglI-N fragment of HSV-2 DNA, which maps between 0.582 and 0.682 on the HSV-2 DNA map. Continued experiments with smaller and smaller HSV-2 DNA fragments achieved transformation of rodent cells, but no unique subset of HSV DNA sequences could consistently be demonstrated in the transformed cells.[115] These data taken collectively have led to the suggestion that HSV-2 might be involved in a "hit-and-run" mechanism of transformation.[115-118] To date, the mechanism of the hit has not been well defined.

In addition to a lack of consensus on detection of HSV-2 information in tumor biopsies and/or transformed cells, controversy also exists concerning the ability of HSV-2 to cause tumors after intravaginal inoculation of mice. Wentz and co-workers[119,120] have described a model in which cervical carcinoma can be induced in vivo by repeated exposure of the cervix to inactivated HSV-1 or HSV-2. These observations have been supported by reports from mainland China.[121] A strong counter to these reports, however has been published recently.[122] In a double-blind study using 1,000 mice, correlation of HSV-2 or HSV-1 inoculation with the development of dysplasia was not observed. In cases in which dysplasia developed, correlation with insertion of vaginal tampons was noted regardless of whether the tampons were soaked with virus solutions or mock-infecting fluids. This study is difficult to refute because of the large number of animals employed and the double-blind nature of the study.

In summary, while HSV (especially HSV-2) initially seemed a good candidate as the causative agent of cervical carcinoma, recent data have not strongly supported that role. However, the ability of the virus to transform in vitro and the ubiquitous nature of these viruses, warrant continued investigation to determine whether they play a primary or secondary role in human neoplasia.

EPSTEIN-BARR VIRUS

In 1958, Denis Burkitt, an English surgeon in Uganda, reported the prevalence of a particular, connective tissue, jaw tumor in African children.[123] Malignant jaw lymphomas with a similar pathology are seen only rarely in other parts of the world. In addition to a high rate of Burkitt lymphoma in native Ugandan children, children of foreign missionaries stationed in equatorial Africa were also at increased risk for the disease. In his original report, Burkitt noted that clustering of the disease occurred in areas where climate and environment allow the occurrence of endemic malaria. Burkitt lymphoma is most often found in the lower jaw but also can arise in the upper jaw, the thyroid, the ovaries, the liver, and the kidneys.

Attempts to grow tumor tissue in culture yielded lymphoblastoid cell lines that could be grown indefinitely in suspension culture. A subsequent search for a virus etiology of the tumor resulted in the discovery of herpesvirus-like particles in the cells of the tumor.[124] In addition, some of the cell lines derived from the lymphomas released virus particles (EBV), and it was possible to show that cell-free supernatants from these cultures were capable of transforming normal human lymphocytes to immortalized lymphoblastoid lines.[125] It is now known that only a few of the cells in the culture shed virus.

To date, normal lymphocytes from human umbilical cord, human adults and infants, marmosets, gibbons and owl, squirrel and cebus monkeys have been transformed by EBV. In response to the association of Burkitt's lymphoma with EBV, a large research effort was mounted to examine the relationship of the virus to tumor formation.[126] As a serendipitous by-product of this effort, Gertrude and Werner Henle discovered that EBV is the causative agent of infectious mononucleosis. This association was made when a research technician in the Henle laboratory contracted infectious mononucleosis and simultaneously seroconverted with antibody specific to EBV.[127]

The epidemiology of EBV infection is now more clearly understood. The virus is ubiquitous, and children in lower socioeconomic areas are commonly infected before adolescence. In higher socioeconomic backgrounds, infection usually occurs during mid to late adolescence and results in the disease syndrome known as infectious mononucleosis. The occurrence of infectious mononucleosis results in a nonmalignant proliferative response in certain types of lymphocytes; the clinical course of disease can vary from subclinical to prolonged disease characterized by sporadic fever and fatigue. Peripheral blood smears from infectious mononucleosis patients sometimes contain white blood cells (WBCs) suggestive of acute lymphocytic leukemia, but this response is limited and disappears as the patient recovers. Infectious EBV is shed into the oropharyngeal secretions of infected individuals and infection is usually transmitted by salivary contact (i.e., kissing).[128]

Antisera from infectious mononucleosis and Burkitt's lymphoma patients demonstrates three antigens: early antigens (EA), corresponding to those proteins made soon after EBV infection; virus structural or capsid antigens (VCA); and a nuclear antigen (EBNA) associated with EBV infection and transformation. An analogy between EBNA and the papovavirus T antigen can be made, since all the cells in a lymphoblastoid culture will be EBNA+, but only a small number cells will be EA+ or VCA+. VCA+ cells seem to be associated with the ability to shed virus.[129] We now know that EBNA is a complex structure of several different proteins.

There are apparently two types of EBV. One variety, P3J-HR-1, isolated from a patient with Burkitt's lymphoma, can superinfect EBV lymphoblastoid cell lines and induce virus antigen synthesis but cannot transform cord blood leukocytes.[130,131] The other, strain B95-8, was isolated from marmoset lymphoblastoid cells transformed by an infectious mononucleosis isolate of EBV. This strain does not induce EA but readily transforms umbilical cord leukocytes. Kieff and co-workers[132] have identified a region of virus DNA (about 15 percent of the genome) that is present in P3J-HR-1 but missing in B95-8. The deletion affects a portion of the genome involved in coding for one of the EBNA proteins.

The link between EBV and human cancer has been considerably strengthed since the first association was made. Outlined below is the cumulative evidence pointing to an etiologic role for EBV in Burkitt's lymphoma. A second geographically restricted tumor, nasopharyngeal carcinoma, has also been strongly linked to EBV,[133] and evidence that has accumulated is similar to that listed. Nasopharyngeal carcinoma is concentrated in the Southern Chinese population and recent studies suggest that genetic factors may predispose an individual for development of the disease. Epidemiologic and direct biologic studies, however, have again strongly implicated EBV in the causation of this disease. Simons and co-workers[134] in 1974 found that the presence of two HLA-related antigens (A2 and B Sin2) increased the risk for the development of nasopharyngeal carcinoma. This correlation has only held up for the Southern Chinese population and not for nasopharyngeal carcinoma patients of non-Chinese heritage. The exact role of HLA antigens in determining nasopharyngeal carcinoma risk is not clear.

EVIDENCE FOR THE ETIOLOGIC ROLE OF EPSTEIN-BARR VIRUS IN BURKITT'S LYMPHOMA

Association of virus particles, antigens, and nucleic acids with tumor tissues

Presence of the virus in Burkitt's lymphoma-afflicted regions

Increased anti-EBV antibody in patients with Burkitt's lymphoma

Transformation in vitro to immortality of human lymphocytes by EBV shed from Burkitt's lymphoma tumor tissue

Proliferative response to infectious mononucleosis patient lymphocytes

Transformation in vitro to immortality of human B lymphocytes by EBV

Induction of malignant lymphoma in nonhuman New World primates by EBV infection

In addition to its association with infectious mononucleosis, Burkitt's lymphoma, and nasopharyngeal carcinoma, EBV can infect B lymphocytes. Following infection, lymphoblastoid lines can be derived that replicate perpetually in culture.[135,136] Uninfected B lymphocytes represent terminally differentiated cells incapable of cell division. Immortalized lines continue to express EBNA and contain EBV DNA. A small percentage of the cells may produce virus. These latently infected cells express a cell surface antigen that allows them to serve as targets for lysis by T lymphocytes taken from EBV-immune donors.[137] This antigen has been termed lymphocyte-derived membrane antigen (CYDMA); its precise nature awaits characterization.

Finally, the argument that EBV plays an etiologic role in B-cell lymphomas has been strengthened by the observation that some species of nonhuman primates can develop B-cell lymphomas after EBV infection.[138] These experiments have been most frequently attempted in New World primates, such as marmosets. Baboons and other Old World primates are naturally infected with agents that are biologically and genetically related to EBV.[139-141] One baboon colony in the Soviet Union has a high incidence of malignant B-cell lymphomas, which occur in animals latently infected with the baboon EBV-related agent, herpesvirus papio.[142]

HUMAN CYTOMEGALOVIRUS

Another human herpesvirus that transforms cells and may have oncogenic potential is human cytomegalovirus (HCMV). HCMV causes many human diseases including classic cytomegalic inclusion disease, intrauterine death, congenital defects, an infectious mononucleosis, postperfusion syndrome, and interstitial pneumonia.[143,144] The virus can cause both persistent and latent infections.

HCMV infection is very common with close to 90 percent of the human population infected at some time in life. Infection of a healthy adult is usually clinically inapparent, but serious problems arise when congenital HCMV infection occurs. Such infections occur in a significant number of pregnant women in the third trimester.[145-147] Infected infants can have persistent HCMV infection that can be asymptomatic or encompass a range of symptoms from mild to severe CNS involvement, with growth of the virus in

other organs. This herpesvirus is also a problem in immunosuppressed patients, in whom HCMV pneumonia may develop. Post-transfusion reactivation of HCMV has been reported by several investigators.[148,149] The virus is able to persist in circulating polymorphonuclear lymphocytes[150] and possibly in blood lymphocytes.[151-153]

HCMV possesses properties commonly associated with known oncogenic DNA viruses; that is, it can stimulate DNA and RNA synthesis of host cells infected in culture.[154,155] Albrecht and Rapp[156] were the first to establish a continuous line of hamster cells transformed to malignancy by HCMV. Indirect immunofluorescence tests detected virus antigens in the cytoplasm and membranes of cells from this line, and the line was tumorigenic when inoculated into newborn hamsters. Work by Geder and colleagues[157] demonstrated that infection of human embryo lung cells with a prostatic isolate of HCMV (Major strain) can lead to a long-term persistent infection and that occasional cell transformants can arise in the culture. These transformants do not shed infectious virus but contain virus-specific membrane and intracellular antigens. These human cell transformants share common antigens with the HCMV-transformed hamster cells and can induce nondifferentiated tumors when injected into athymic nude mice.

In addition to the ability of the virus to transform cells in culture, genital cancers, including cancer of the prostate, are linked to HCMV by virtue of the persistent presence of the virus in the genitourinary tract, by its sexual mode of transmission, and finally by epidemiologic and direct studies associating viruses and virus antigens with these cancers. While several investigations have tried to link HCMV to cervical carcinoma, other viruses are more highly implicated. The involvement of HCMV in other human neoplasias has been suggested but not extensively studied. The genitourinary tract supports HCMV infection and the virus can be found in cervical secretions and in semen.[146,158-160] This, in part, suggests that the virus can be transmitted venereally.

Cancer of the prostate is the fourth most prevalent cancer in the United States and is found at increased incidence, particularly in black males.[161] Data have linked HCMV infection to this cancer. A serologic study of 92 patients demonstrated a positive correlation between HCMV antibody titers and this tumor. Controls included patients with benign prostatic hyperplasia and nonurogenital cancers. This latter group demonstrated lower antibody titer to HCMV.[162] In addition, lymphocytes from patients with prostatic cancer are cytotoxic for cells transformed by a prostatic isolate of the virus.[163] Further investigation of this problem is necessary to define whether these relationships are causal or brought about by the mere presence of HCMV in the flora of prostate tissue.

In addition, HCMV has been implicated in the genesis of colon carcinoma. This virus can be isolated from the gastrointestinal (GI) tract,[164] and colon tumors have been examined for HCMV nucleic acids.[165] A small number of colon carcinoma tissues were positive for HCMV DNA; however, in one patient, normal colon tissue also contained the virus genome. A small number of tissue samples from patients with familial polyposis or ulcerative colitis tested positive for HCMV genetic material; however, samples from patients with Crohn's disease were negative. The detection of HCMV in adenocarcinoma of the colon was confirmed by a second group[166]; however, additional reports failed to uphold these observations.[167,168] The role of this virus in colon cancer remains unclear.

Finally, HCMV has been linked to Kaposi's sarcoma. Until recently, this was considered a disease with particularly high incidence in children of equatorial Africa. The disease in this population is aggressive and highly fatal, whereas Eurpean and American cases are more benign. Outside the African continent, the disease is limited to older men, particularly those of Mediterranean descent.[169-171] A newly affected population for Kaposi's sarcoma is acquired immunodeficiency syndrome (AIDS) patients. Disseminated Kaposi's sarcoma and other unusual opportunistic infections appeared in young homosexual males in 1981,[172,173] and this tumor is now recognized as a common complication of AIDS. The fatal course of Kaposi's sarcoma in such patients and the severity of the AIDS epidemic have increased interest in the etiology of this tumor.

Giraldo and co-workers[174] were the first to report isolation of HCMV from a Kaposi's sarcoma biopsy. Patients with Kaposi's sarcoma also exhibit increased antibody titers to this virus and not necessarily to other human herpesviruses.[171,175] Virus antigens, as well as virus nucleic acids, have been demonstrated in tumor biopsies and in cell lines of tumors.[176,177] These data taken collectively establish a strong association of this human tumor with HCMV infection.

RETROVIRUSES

The retroviruses represent a group of RNA-containing viruses that have been isolated over several decades from an enormous number of naturally occurring animal tumors as well as from tumors that have been experimentally induced by chemical carcinogens, radiation, or by genetic breeding of animal strains with high tumor incidence.[178,179] These viruses can be transmitted both vertically and horizontally. In the past, retroviruses have been called leukoviruses, C-type RNA viruses, oncornaviruses and RNA tumor viruses, but all these names have been put aside, since they describe characteristics that do not apply to every member of this group. For example, not every member has been shown to be oncogenic. The name "retrovirus" refers to their distinguishing characteristic: the fact that they carry in the virion (virus particle) the enzyme reverse transcriptase, an RNA-dependent DNA polymerase.[180,181] This enzyme permits the RNA genome of these viruses to replicate through a DNA intermediate.

The single-stranded RNA of retroviruses replicates through a double-stranded DNA intermediate (Fig. 8-4). Briefly, the genome RNA is copied into a double-stranded complementary DNA molecule (provirus DNA) that integrates into the cell DNA after host cell division. The provirus DNA serves as the template for synthesis of new virion RNA and virus mRNA by host cell RNA polymerase. During synthesis of new virus RNA, the virus mRNA directs concomitant synthesis of virus proteins in the cytoplasm of the cell. Subsequently, the nucleocapsid leaves the cell by budding through the cytoplasmic membrane. This sequence is usually carried out without cell destruction, making retroviruses ideal tumor viruses.

The first association of viruses with neoplasia was made at the beginning of the twentieth century for avian leukemias and sarcomas. It is now known that these tumors are caused by retroviruses, but progress was slow until the 1950s, when a retrovirus was linked to leukemias in certain high-incidence strains of mice.[182] This virus group is now known to cause a large variety of tumors in connective tissue and in tissues of the hematopoietic and reticuloendothelial systems. A certain subgroup of retroviruses also has been shown to be involved in mammary tumor formation. The discovery in 1936 by Bittner,[183] of

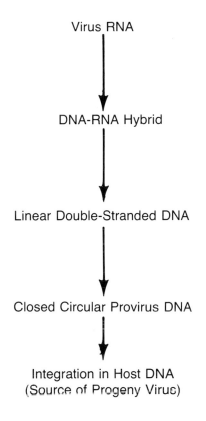

Virus RNA

↓

DNA-RNA Hybrid

↓

Linear Double-Stranded DNA

↓

Closed Circular Provirus DNA

↓

Integration in Host DNA
(Source of Progeny Virus)

Fig. 8-4 Scheme for retrovirus replication.

mouse mammary tumor virus in the milk of certain high-incidence mouse strains sparked a huge research effort based on the hope that retroviruses would be found in human tumors. This hope has been frustrated by the relative ease of detection of these agents in animal tissues coupled with the failure to readily isolate comparable viruses from human tissues. The evidence for the role of human retroviruses in human cancers is discussed later in this chapter.

In addition to neoplasia, the widespread appearance of these viruses in animal tissues led to hypotheses that retroviruses could be involved in normal biologic processes such as evolution, gene regulation, somatic cell mutation, and embryonic differentiation. These topics are outside the scope of this review but the reader should be aware of their existence.

The study of retroviruses converged with another area of scientific research, the study of oncogenes. Initial knowledge that gene products could convert normal cells to cancer cells came from the study of DNA and RNA tumor viruses. Many of these viruses contain transforming genes that can directly alter growth patterns of cells in culture and, in some cases, induce tumors after inoculation of animals.[184] As early as 1969, Huebner and Todaro[185,186] advanced the hypothesis that covert oncogenes might be present in normal cells. This hypothesis supposed that factors such as chemicals, radiation, or invading viruses might cause depression or alteration of oncogenes and result in carcinogenesis at the cellular level. This turns out to be true. We now know that the direct acting oncogenes of the retroviruses have cellular counterparts.[187,188]

In addition, experiments to demonstrate the transfer of cellular oncogenes from cancer cells into normal cells revealed that (1) such genes exist and can transfer the cancer phenotype, and (2) in some cases the genes correspond to identical or altered cellular genes that have been transduced into the transforming retroviruses.[189] The understanding that alteration and/or overexpression of cellular genes can result in an altered growth pattern and the knowledge that such genes can fall under control of virus gene regulation led to a hypothesis for the oncogenic mechanism of the leukemia viruses, retroviruses that lack directly transforming oncogenes but contain strong promoter regions that can influence transcription of cellular genes. In summary, normal cellular sequences "proto oncogenes" can be involved in tumorigenesis. In some cases, the genes can be mutated to change the function of the resulting protein and in other cases, chromosomal translocation, mutagenesis or gene amplification can alter the expression of the gene.[190,191]

Recently, a family of human retroviruses called the human T-lymphotropic viruses (HTLVs) has been isolated and shown to be associated with T-cell abnormalities.[192-195] Isolates known as HTLV-I are associated with an aggressive form of adult T-cell leukemia or lymphoma.[192-195] An infrequent isolate, HTLV-II was first identified in a T-cell varient of hairy cell leukemia.[196] In addition, it is now known that a third virus, HTLV-III (or HIV), is the causative agent of AIDS.[197-200]

HTLV-I and HTLV-II do not contain direct transforming oncogenes; nevertheless, these agents transform cells in culture. These retroviruses are suspected of transforming cells by production of a protein factor that transactivates transcription of genes from the virus genome and genes of the cell that may be involved in growth regulation.[201,202] HTLV-I and

HTLV-II represent important examples of retroviruses involved in rare human malignancies.

PAPILLOMAVIRUSES

Papillomaviruses of animals and humans can induce warts, benign tumors of the skin or other epithelial tissues. Most warts are benign and often regress; however, there is increasing interest in the role of papillomaviruses in malignancies. Lesions in humans attributable to these viruses include the well-known plantar, common, and flat warts of the skin, and genital warts (including condylomata acuminata and condylomata plana), and laryngeal papillomas of the mucosa. Only a few papillomaviruses are able to transform fibroblasts. The most well studied in this latter category are bovine papillomaviruses types 1 and 2.

The common human wart was first associated with a viral agent by Ciuffo[203] in 1907, who demonstrated that warts were transmissible by inoculation of cell-free filtrates of wart tissue. This experimentation was carried out at a time when it was considered ethical to inoculate human volunteers with potentially infectious material. The concept that warts could convert from benign lesions into carcinomas was described for the Shope[204] cottontail rabbit papillomavirus by the demonstration that a substantial percentage of these papillomas could progress to metastatic carcinomas[205-207] in infected wild rabbits. The fact that malignant conversion required 12 to 18 months pointed to secondary factors either in the host or in the environment that interacted with the infected tissue. Another condition in which secondary factors play a role in progression of warts to carcinomas is epidermodysplasia verruciformis,[208] a human familial disease characterized by large numbers of epidermal warts. These skin warts become cancerous at high frequency in areas exposed to sunlight. Juvenile laryngeal papillomas, thought to be caused by perinatal infection of children born to mothers with genital human papillomavirus infections also can progress to malignancy. Laryngeal papillomas were at one time ablated by x-irradiation. After long latent periods, it was found that many of these patients developed laryngeal cancers at the site of the former papilloma. Spontaneous progression was rare, so x-irradiation was a clear secondary factor.[209]

Although the cause of human warts has long been credited to human papillomaviruses, the nature of these viruses is not well understood because these agents have not yet been grown in cell culture. Recent advances in molecular biology have allowed extensive typing of papillomaviruses using cloned DNAs. This has revealed a number of previously obscured facts. First, the number of types of papillomaviruses greatly exceeds original expectations. Approximately 45 types have been described. These are detailed in Table 8-2. Since the known papillomavirus types numbered 16 in 1984, one can appreciate how rapidly this area of virology is growing. Many of these types may have overlapping or identical biologic targets in the host. Second, human papillomaviruses are found in a number of papillomatous lesions in a variety of human tissues. Third, while more than one type can cause a given lesion, the types may be grouped based on tissue tropism. For example, types 6, 11, 16, 18, 31, 33, and 35 are commonly found in genital warts. Finally, these viruses may play a significant biologic role in human tumors, as their presence was recently detected in both rare and common carcinomas, particularly in genital cancers. This concept is enhanced by the fact that papillomas are now recognized histologically as possible precursors to malignant lesions. This review describes the basic properties of this group and concentrates on the evidence that papillomaviruses are significant pathogens and cancer-causing agents in the human genital tract.

The papillomaviruses are a subgroup of the papovaviruses: small nonenveloped DNA viruses of icosahedral symmetry, containing a double-stranded circular genome that is covalently closed and supercoiled. The subgroup contains human papillomaviruses and a number of animal papillomaviruses, the most well studied of which include cottontail rabbit and bovine papillomaviruses. The biology and biochemistry of this virus group have been reviewed extensively by Pfister.[211] The molecular weight of papillomavirus DNA is approximately 5×10^6, denoting that it is a relatively small virus with a coding capacity for a small (probably less than a dozen) number of proteins. The size of the DNA is approximately 8 kilobase (kb) pairs. By analogy to the rest of the papovavirus group, the proteins can be divided into two types: early proteins that are made prior to the onset of viral DNA replication, and late proteins, the structural proteins for production of new progeny vi-

Table 8-2 Lesions Commonly Associated with Various Human
Papillomaviruses

HPV type	Lesion
1a–c	Plantar warts
2a–e	Common hand warts
3a,b	Flat warts/juvenile warts
4	Plantar warts
5a,b	Macules, epidermodysplasia verruciformis patients
6a–f	Condylomata acuminata
	CIN I, II, III
	VIN I, II, III
	Laryngeal papillomas
7	Butcher's warts
8	Macules, epidermodysplasia verruciformis patients
9	Warts and macules, epidermodysplasia verruciformis patients
10a,b	Flat warts
11a,b	Condylomata acuminata
	CIN I, II, III
	laryngeal papillomas
12	Warts and macules, epidermodysplasia verruciformis patients
13	Oral focal hyperplasia (Heck lesions)
14a,b	Skin lesions, epidermodysplasia verruciformis patients
15	Skin lesions, epidermodysplasia verruciformis patients
16	Condylomata acuminata
	CIN I, II, III
	VIN I, II, III
	Bowenoid papulosis
	Malignant carcinoma, cervix and penis
17a,b	Skin lesions, epidermodysplasia verruciformis patients
18	Malignant carcinoma, cervix and penis
19–29	Warts and hyperplastic lesions, epidermodysplasia verruciformis patients
30	Laryngeal carcinoma (rare)
31	CIN
	Malignant carcinoma, cervix
32	Oral focal hyperplasia (Heck lesions)
33	Bowenoid papulosis
	CIN
	Malignant carcinoma, cervix
34	Bowenoid papulosis
35	CIN
	Malignant carcinoma, cervix
36	Actinic keratosis
37	Keratoachanthoma
38	Melanoma
39	Cutaneous lesions
40	Laryngeal carcinoma
41	Flat warts

CIN, cervical intraepithelial neoplasia; VIN, vulvar intraepithelial neoplasia.
(Adapted from McCance DJ: Human papillomaviruses and cancer. Biochim Biophys
 Acta 823:195, 1986. Reprinted by permission from Elsevier Science Publishing Com-
 pany Inc.)

rions. Because of the great difficulty in obtaining purified populations of papillomaviruses in any quantity, not much work has been accomplished on protein characterization. Among the human papillomaviruses, the proteins of only a few types have been analyzed: these include types 1, 2, and 4.[212-214] Continued and detailed investigation of the proteins of the human papillomavirus types is necessary to understand fully the replication and structure of the viruses and their transmission. In addition, analysis of these proteins will uncover those serving as antigenic stimuli in the infected host and which proteins, if any, can elicit a protective immune response. This information will be essential to the eventual design of human papillomavirus vaccines.

Papillomaviruses are usually host-range restricted. Only the bovine papillomaviruses seem capable of infecting cells of different species. The host range of this group of viruses is usually limited to epithelial cells. In addition, certain types are found in given lesions. The molecular basis of the tissue specificity is not understood. Replication occurs in the nucleus of infected cells and virus DNA appears to exist as a stable episome present in high (50 to 200) copy numbers. It is a curious and not well understood fact that papillomavirus replication occurs in the maturing layers of keratinizing epithelium. It is presumed that the basal cells are infected and transformed by the virus, but the movement of the progeny of these cells into the keratinizing layers may be the signal for viral production. The initial event in the stratum basale results in increased proliferation. Friedmann and Fialkow[215] found this to be a polyclonal event; isoenzyme analysis of four condylomata acuminata demonstrated the multicellular origins of the lesions. In experimental infections in rabbit skin, cottontail rabbit papillomavirus-induced papillomas contained detectable levels of virus DNA in the stratum granulosum but not in less differentiated skin layers.[216] In addition, in situ hybridization of type 1-induced human warts showed that the viral DNA was first detectable in the stratum spinosum.[217] These and numerous subsequent studies indicate that the bulk of DNA replication occurs in the differentiating layers; however, they do not exclude the presence of DNA in the basal cells because low numbers of copies of virus DNA per cell would be very hard to detect. Evidence that replication in the differentiating layers involves the full virus replication cycle was provided by Almeida and co-workers,[218] who observed whole virus particles in the stratum spinosum. Aggregates of virus can be seen in keratinized stratum corneum. The conclusion then (summarized in Fig. 8-5) is that increased differentiation (keratinization) increases the permissiveness of infected cells. The molecular mechanism involved is not understood.

Attempts to propagate human papillomavirus in cell culture have failed. Rheinwald and Green[220] developed a method for long-term culture of human keratinocytes. In these cultures, human papillomavirus DNA persisted and replicated as a stable episome[221] with a high (50 to 200) genome copy number per cell. Mature virions, however, could not be detected. Attempts to duplicate in vivo conditions for wart development by inoculation of wart extracts into human skin grafted to hamsters or the backs of immunoincompetent mice also failed. This was somewhat surprising since rabbit skin grafted onto hamster cheek pouch or nude mice was successfully transformed with cottontail rabbit papillomavirus.[222-225] Recently, however, infection and papillomatous transformation have been accomplished in xenografted human tissues placed beneath the renal capsule of the nude mouse.[226-227] Human papillomavirus

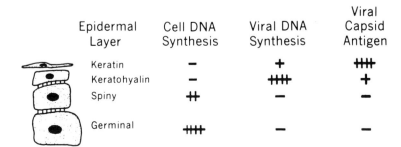

Epidermal Layer	Cell DNA Synthesis	Viral DNA Synthesis	Viral Capsid Antigen
Keratin	−	+	+++
Keratohyalin	−	+++	+
Spiny	++	−	−
Germinal	+++	−	−

Fig. 8-5 Differential localization of cell DNA, viral DNA, and viral capsid antigen synthesis in keratinizing epithelium. (With permission from Kreider JK, Bartlett GL: The Shope papilloma-carcinoma complex of rabbits: A model system of neoplastic progression and spontaneous regression. Adv Cancer Res 35:81, 1981.)

type 11-containing extracts successfully infected fragments of human uterine cervix, skin, and larynx. This experimental system offers a method of studying the basic process of human papillomavirus replication and the interaction of these viruses with host cells.

Only a small number of the human papillomaviruses have been examined biochemically at either the protein or nucleic acid level, due to the inability of virologists to obtain workable quantities of virus. The first studies performed on wart virus DNAs were conducted on tissue extracts of warts. The advent of molecular cloning, however, has advanced the field incredibly, particularly in the area of detection and characterization of new human papillomavirus types. By inserting the 8-kb virus DNA molecules into plasmid cloning vectors, many virus DNAs can now be propagated in bacterial hosts; mature virions are not made but a large amount of virus DNA can be obtained for study. A human papillomavirus is considered a new type if nucleic acid hybridization analyses indicate less than 50 percent homology with previous isolates.[228] Viruses sharing more than 50 percent homology but still differing from one another are considered subtypes within a given type.

Cloning of the genomes of these viruses also has permitted DNA sequence analyses, and we now know that animal and human papillomaviruses have a similar genetic organization. Some of the viruses have been studied in greater detail. Bovine papillomavirus 1 is one of the most amenable to study because of its ability to produce tumors in laboratory animals and to transform cells in culture.[229] Viral particles as well as cloned virus DNA have been used to transform cells,[230] and detailed studies have defined a subgenomic transforming fragment of this virus.[231] The virus DNA sequences are multiple and extrachromosomal,[232–233] and sequence analyses have detailed the RNA-coding regions of the virus.[234] This type of molecular biology has greatly advanced the understanding of how the viruses function.

Table 8-3 lists the common human papillomavirus types found in human genital lesions and references the first isolation of each type. Human papillomavirus type 6 was first identified and partially characterized in total nucleic acid of a human genital wart (condyloma acuminatum). In the initial report, six of six additional condylomata acuminata tested positive for human papillomavirus type 6, and subsequent screening of condylomata in several laboratories has demonstrated that this type is commonly found in such lesions. Human papillomavirus type 11 DNA was originally isolated and cloned from a laryngeal papilloma of a 15-year-old patient. In the initial report, four of nine laryngeal papillomas were positive for human papillomavirus type 11 DNA and human papillomavirus type 11 DNA also was detected in one patient with recurrent tracheal and pulmonary papillomatosis. Human papillomavirus type 11 also is found in condylomata acuminata. Human papillomavirus type 16 DNA, cloned from the DNA of a cervical cancer biopsy, shares some homology with human papillomavirus type 11. In the original report of this papillomavirus type, 61.1 percent (11 of 18) of cervical cancers from Germany were shown to contain human papillomavirus type 16. This was true for 34.8 percent (8 of 23) of cervical cancers from Brazil and for 28.6 percent (2 of 7) and 25 percent (1 of 4) of vulvar and penile carcinomas, respectively. Human papillomavirus type 16 was rarely present in condylomata acuminata (2 of 33) and when present, human papillomavirus type 6 or 11 was also present. Several detailed studies have subsequently confirmed that human papillomavirus type 16 is prominent in carcinomas of the uterine cervix; human papillomavirus

Table 8-3 Human Papillomavirus Types Involved in Genital Lesions

HPV Type	Tissue of Isolation	Investigators
6	Condyloma acuminatum	Gissmann and zur Hausen[235]
11	Laryngeal papilloma	Gissmann et al.[236]
16	Cervical carcinoma	Dürst et al.[237]
18	Cervical carcinoma	Boshart et al.[238]
31	Cervical dysplasia	Lorincz et al.[239]
33	Cervical carcinoma	Beaudenon et al.[240]

type 18 also has been cloned from a cervical cancer biopsy. In the initial report, 9 of 36 cervical carcinomas from Africa and Brazil, 2 of 13 cervical tumors from Germany, and 1 of 10 penile carcinomas contained this agent. However, human papillomavirus type 18 was not detected in 17 cervical dysplasias, 29 genital warts, 8 carcinomata in situ or 15 normal cervical biopsies. Several cervical cancer cell cultures that have been maintained in laboratories for many years also contain human papillomavirus type 16 and 18 DNA. In general, human papillomavirus type 6 or 11 infections are virus positive and contain koilocytotic cells; however, human papillomavirus type 16 or 18 lesions fail to demonstrate evidence of a high degree of koilocytosis and show atypia corresponding to cervical intraepithelial neoplasia II or III.[241] These latter lesions demonstrate aneuploid DNA patterns. Human papillomavirus type 31, a recent isolate cloned from a cervical dysplasia, has been detected in 20 percent of mild and moderate dysplasias, 6 percent of invasive cancers, but not in condylomata acuminata. An additional isolate, human papillomavirus type 33, has also been cloned from a cervical carcinoma and sequences of this type have been found in 4 to 8 percent of genital intraepithelial neoplasias and invasive cervical carcinomas. Since about 90 percent of all cervical carcinomas contain human papillomavirus-related sequences when examined under nonstringent hybridization conditions,[238] it seems likely that even additional human papillomavirus types will be associated with these tumors.

One of the most common cancers of the female genital tract is invasive squamous carcinoma of the cervix. The fact that the prevalence of this cancer correlates with promiscuity has led researchers to suggest that a transmissible agent is involved.[242] The prevalence of human papillomavirus in both the male and female genital tract and recent isolation of these viruses from papillomas, dysplasias, and cancers has convinced many scientists that papillomaviruses play an important etiologic role in genital malignancies. Infections with certain human papillomavirus types may be more likely to progress from papillomas to carcinomas and it is likely that secondary factors play a critical role in this progression. It is unlikely that human papillomavirus is sufficient for malignancy, since most human papillomavirus-induced lesions regress spontaneously. In addition, the latency for cancer development is long. A lesion diagnosed as cervical intraepithelial neoplasia type I may not progress to invasive cancer for 2 to 10 years. The identity of secondary cocarcinogenic or tumor-promoting factors that may influence neoplastic progression of warts awaits definition.

SUMMARY

Several groups of the viruses discussed are known to transform cells in culture and to cause tumor formation in animals. Some of these virus groups have been strongly associated with malignant tumors in humans, most notably human papillomavirus, EBV, and HBV. The case is overwhelming that EBV and HBV are involved in Burkitt's lymphoma and primary hepatocellular carcinoma, respectively. Even if the concession is made that the viruses fulfill only one of a number of causal roles, the evidence for involvement of these two viruses in human neoplasia has fulfilled all the necessary requirements short of showing that removal of the virus prevents the tumor. The ability to clone human papillomavirus sequences from human warts has permitted accumulation of strong evidence linking this agent with human cervical cancer. In many cases, this evidence could not be obtained for HSV-2 in relationship to this same tumor. The most recent evidence that human papillomavirus nucleic acids can be found in biopsies of dysplasia, carcinoma in situ, and invasive carcinoma of the cervix lends strong support to the accumulated evidence that this virus has oncogenic potential.

It has been difficult, however, to demonstrate an association for papovaviruses (other than human papillomavirus), adenoviruses, and retroviruses with neoplasia in the human population despite abundant examples of tumor formation by these agents in the animal kingdom. Especially disturbing is the paucity of data concerning the existence of naturally occurring human retroviruses. The ease with which the retroviruses can be obtained from animals would seem to indicate a fundamental oversight by biologists in their approach to isolation of retroviruses from human tissue. Isolation of HTLV-I and HTLV-III may herald a new age for isolation of these viruses from human tumors.

The failure to detect genomes of tumorigenic viruses in tumor samples can only be considered valid if the detection limit of the method used is sufficiently

EVIDENCE THAT HUMAN
PAPILLOMAVIRUS IS INVOLVED IN
CERVICAL CANCER

Knowledge that animal papillomas progress to carcinomas

Recognition that koilocytotic atypia of the cervix is human papillomavirus induced

Recognition that koilocytotic atypia can progress to carcinoma

Detection of human papillomavirus DNA in a large percentage of dysplasias and cervical carcinomas

Dysplastic transformation of human tissue after laboratory infection with human papillomavirus type 11

sensitive to pick up as little as one foreign gene per tumor cell. Even this approach is not proof positive, since persistence of virus genes in the tumor cell is not necessarily required, despite evidence in animal models.

The reader should also realize that association of an infectious agent with a tumor is not definite proof of a causal relationship. It is only by removing the infecting agent (e.g., by virus vaccination) and demonstrating concurrent cessation of tumor incidence that a precise etiologic role for a virus in neoplasia can be defined. Attempts in progress to obliterate hepatitis B virus infection in Third World countries by use of an HBsAg vaccine should yield data over the next 30 to 50 years that will definitely resolve whether this one putative tumor virus causes liver cancer. Preparation of vaccines against other viruses or eradication by immunotherapy or chemotherapy is a subject of ongoing research. Only effective prevention of virus infection will ultimately define their true role in oncogenic disease.

ACKNOWLEDGMENTS

The authors thank Elaine Neidigh for secretarial expertise and Melissa Clement for editorial assistance. New observations cited in this manuscript were supported in part by grants CA27503, CA25305, CA34479, and CA09124 awarded by the National Cancer Institute and by National Institutes of Health and Special Institutional grant SIG-11 awarded by the American Cancer Society.

REFERENCES

1. Ellermann V, Bang O: Experimentalle leukamie bei huhnern. Zentralbl Bakteriol Abt I 46:595, 1908
2. Rous P: Transmission of a malignant new growth by means of a cell-free filtrate. JAMA 56:198, 1911
3. Tooze J: Molecular Biology of Tumor Viruses. Parts 1, 2, and 3. Cold Spring Harbor Laboratory, Cold Spring Harbor, NY, 1980
4. Gross L (ed): Oncogenic Viruses. 3rd Ed. Pergamon Press, New York, 1983
5. Lindner D, Gartler SM: Glucose-6-phosphate dehydrogenase mosaicism: Utilization as a cell marker in the study of leiomyomas. Science 150:67, 1965
6. Fialkow PJ, Gartler SM, Yoshida A: Clonal origin of chronic myelocytic leukemia in man. Proc Natl Acad Sci USA 58:1468, 1967
7. Aaronson SA, Todaro GJ: Basis for the acquisition of malignant potential by mouse cells cultivated in vitro. Science 162:1024, 1968
8. Stoker M, O'Neill C, Berryman S, Waxman V: Anchorage and growth regulation in normal and virus-transformed cells. Int J Cancer 3:683, 1968
9. Rubin H: Growth regulation in cultures of chick embryo fibroblasts. p. 127. In Wolstenholm GEW, Knight J (eds): Growth Control in Cell Cultures. Ciba Foundation Symposium. Churchill Livingstone, London, 1971
10. Holley R, Kiernan J: "Contact-inhibition" of cell division in 3T3 cells. Proc Natl Acad Sci USA 60:300, 1968
11. Crawford LV, Black PH: The nucleic acid of simian virus 40. Virology 24:388, 1964
12. Reddy VB, Thimmappaya B, Dhar R, et al: The genome of simian virus 40. Science 200: 494, 1978
13. Fiers W, Contreras R, Haegeman G, et al: Complete nucleotide sequence of SV40 DNA. Nature (Lond) 273:113, 1978
14. Sweet BH, Hilleman MR: The vacuolating virus, SV40. Proc Soc Exp Biol Med 105:420, 1960
15. Rabson AS, Kirschstein RL: Induction of malignancy in vitro in newborn hamster kidney tissue infected with simian vacuolating virus (SV40). Proc Soc Exp Biol Med 111: 323, 1962
16. Black PH, Rowe WP: SV40-induced proliferation of

tissue culture cells of rabbit, mouse and porcine origin. Proc Soc Exp Biol Med 114:721, 1963

17. Shein HM, Enders JF, Levinthal JD, Burket AE: Transformation induced by simian virus 40 in newborn simian hamster renal cell cultures. Proc Natl Acad Sci USA 49:28, 1963

18. Rabson AS, O'Conor GT, Kirschstein RL, Branigan WT: Papillory ependymomas produced in Rattus (Mastomys) natalensis inoculated with vacuolating virus (SV40). J Natl Cancer Inst 29:765, 1962

19. Eddy BE, Grubbs GE, Young RD: Tumor immunity in hamsters infected with adenovirus type 12 or simian virus 40. Proc Soc Exp Biol Med. 117:575, 1964

20. Hummeler K, Tomassini N, Sokol F: Morphological aspects of the uptake of simian virus 40 by permissive cells. J Virol 6:87, 1970

21. Barbanti-Brodano G, Swetly P, Koprowski H: Early events in the infection of permissive cells with simian virus 40: Adsorption, penetration, and uncoating. J Virol 6:78, 1970

22. Weil R, Salomon C, May E, May P: A simplifying concept in tumor virology: Virus specific "pleiotropic effectors." Cold Spring Harbor Symp Quant Biol 39:381, 1974

23. Weil R, Petursson G, Kara J, Diggelman H: The interaction of polyoma virus with the genetic apparatus of host cells. p. 593. In Colter JS, Paranchych W (eds): The Molecular Biology of Viruses. Academic Press, New York, 1967

24. Kit S, Piekarski LJ, Dubbs DR, et al: Enzyme induction in green monkey kidney cultures infected with simian adenovirus. J Virol 1:10, 1967

25. Kit S: Viral induced enzymes and viral carcinogenesis. Adv Cancer Res 11:73, 1968

26. Eckhart W: Transformation of animal cells by oncogenic DNA viruses. Physiol Rev 48:513, 1968

27. Sambrook J, Sharp PA, Keller W: Transcription of SV40. I. Separation of the strands of SV40 DNA and hybridization of the separated strands to RNA extracted from lytically infected and transformed cells. J Mol Biol 70:57, 1972

28. Winocour E, Robbins E: Histone synthesis in polyoma and SV40-infected cells. Virology 40:307, 1970

29. Rovera G, Baserga R, Defendi V: Early increase in nuclear acidic protein synthesis after SV40 infection. Nature New Biol 237:240, 1972

30. Tegtmeyer P: SV40 DNA synthesis: The viral replicon. J Virol 10:591, 1972

31. Minowada J, Moore GE: DNA synthesis in X-irradiated cultures infected with polyoma virus. Exp Cell Res 29:31, 1963

32. Smith HS, Scher CD, Todaro GJ: Abortive transfor-

mation of Balb/3T3 cells by simian virus 40. Bacteriol Proc Abstr 217:187, 1970

33. Dulbecco R, Johnson T: Interferon-sensitivity of the enhanced incorporation of thymidine into cellular DNA induced by polyoma virus. Virology 42:368, 1970

34. Taylor-Papadimitriou J, Stoker MGP: Effect of interferon on some aspects of transformation by polyoma virus. Nature New Biol 230:114, 1971

35. Todaro GJ, Green H: High frequency of SV40 transformation of mouse cell line 3T3. Virology 28:756, 1966

36. Todaro GJ, Green H: Cell growth and the initiation of transformation by SV40. Proc Natl Acad Sci USA 55:302, 1966

37. Gerber P, Kirschstein RJ: SV40-induced ependymomas in newborn hamsters. I. Virus tumor relationships. Virology 18:582, 1962

38. Gerber P: Studies on the transfer of subviral infectivity from SV40-induced hamster tumor cells to indicator cells. Virology 28:501, 1966

39. Koprowski H, Jensen FC, Steplewski ZS: Activation of production of infectious tumor virus SV40 in heterokaryon cultures. Proc Natl Acad Sci USA 58:127, 1967

40. Watkins JF, Dulbecco R: Production of SV40 virus in heterokaryons of transformed and susceptible cells. Proc Natl Acad Sci USA 58:1396, 1967

41. Tournier P, Cassingena R, Wichert R, et al: Etude de mecanisme de l'induction chez des celluels de hamster Syrien transformees par le virus SV40. I. Proprietes d'une lignee cellulaire clonale. Int J Cancer 2:117, 1967

42. Sambrook J, Westphal H, Srinivasan PR, Dulbecco R: The integrated state of DNA in SV40-transformed cells. Proc Natl Acad Sci USA 60:1288, 1968

43. Westphal H, Dulbecco R: Viral DNA in polyoma and SV40-transformed cell lines. Proc Natl Acad Sci 59:1158, 1968

44. Gelb LD, Kohne DE, Martin MA: Quantitation of SV40 sequences in African green monkey, mouse, and virus-transformed cell genomes. J Mol Biol 57:129, 1971

45. Ozanne B, Vogel A, Sparp P, et al: Transcription of SV40 DNA sequences in different transformed cell lines. Lepetit Colloq Biol Med 4:176, 1973

46. Black PH, Rowe WP, Turner HC, Huebner RJ: A specific complement-fixing antigen present in SV40 tumor and transformed cells. Proc Natl Acad Sci USA 50:1148, 1963

47. Habel K: Specific complement-fixing antigens in polyoma tumors and transformed cells. Virology 25:55, 1965

48. Rapp F, Kitahara T, Butel JS, Melnick JL: Synthesis of SV40 tumor antigen during replication of simian papovavirus (SV40). Proc Natl Acad Sci USA 52:1138, 1964

49. Del Villano B, Defendi V: Preparation and use of an immunosorbent to study the molecular composition of the SV40 T-antigen from hamster tumor cells. Bacterial Proc Abst 222:118, 1970

50. Prives C, Aviv H, Gilboa E, et al: The cell-free translation of early and late classes of SV40 messenger RNA. INSERM Colloq 47:305, 1975

51. Rigby PWJ, Lane DP: Structure and function of simian virus 40 large T-antigen. p. 31. In Klein G (ed): Advances in Viral Oncology. Vol. 3. Raven Press, New York, 1983

52. Padgett BL, Walker DL: New human papovaviruses. Prog Med Virol 22:1, 1976

53. Gardner SD, Field AM, Coleman DV, Hulme B: New human papovavirus (BK) isolated from urine after renal transplantation. Lancet 1:1253, 1971

54. Seif I, Dhar R, Khoury G: The genome of human papovavirus BKV. Cell 18:963, 1979

55. London WT: Primary hepatocellular carcinoma. Hum Pathol 12:1085, 1981

56. London WT. Hepatitis B virus and primary hepatocellular carcinoma. p. 325. In Klein G (ed): Advances in Oncology. Vol 3. Raven Press, New York, 1983

57. Edmundson HA, Peters RL: Liver. p. 1321. In Anderson WAD, Kissane JM (eds): Pathology. 7th Ed. CV Mosby, St. Louis, 1977

58. WHO: Advances in viral hepatitis. Report of the WHO Expert Committee on Viral Hepatitis Tech Rep Ser 602, 1977

59. Joklik WK, Willett HP, Amos DB (eds): Zinsser Microbiology. 18th Ed. Appleton-Century-Crofts, E Norwalk, CT, 1984

60. Krugman S, Giles JP, Hammond J: Infectious hepatitis. Evidence for two distinctive clinical, epidemiological and immunological types of infection. JAMA 200:365, 1967

61. Blumberg BS, Alter HJ, Visnich S: A new antigen in leukemia sera. JAMA 191:541, 1965

62. Blumberg BS, Gerstley BJS, Hungerford DA, et al: A serum antigen (Australia antigen) in Downs syndrome leukemia and hepatitis. Ann Intern Med 66:924, 1967

63. Okachi K, Murakami S: Observations on Australia antigen in Japanese. Vox Sang 15:374, 1968

64. Prince AM: An antigen detected in blood during incubation period of serum hepatitis. Proc Natl Acad Sci USA 60:814, 1968

65. Dane DS, Cameron CH, Briggs M: Virus-like particles in serum of patients with Australia-antigen-associated hepatitis. Lancet 1:695, 1970

66. Summers J, O'Connell A, Millman I: Genome of hepatitis B virus: Restriction enzyme cleavage and structure of DNA extracted from DANE particles. Proc Natl Acad Sci USA 72:4597, 1975

67. Robinsin WS: The genome of hepatitis B virus. Annu Rev Microbiol 31:357, 1977

68. Robinson WS, Lutwick LI: Virus of hepatitis, type B. 1. N Engl J Med 295:1168, 1976

69. Robinson WS, Lutwick LI: Virus of hepatitis, type B. 2. N Engl J Med 295:1232, 1976

70. Hoofnagle JH, Gerety RJ, Barker LF: Antibody to hepatitis-B core antigen. Am J Med Sci 270:179, 1975

71. Magnius LO, Espmark JA: New specificities in Australia antigen sera distinct from Le Bouvier determinants. Immunology 109:1017, 1972

72. Magnius LO, Lindholm A, Lundin P, Iwarson S: New antigen-antibody system. Clinical significance in long-term carriers of hepatitis B surface antigen. JAMA 231:356, 1975

73. Alter HJ, Blumberg: Further studies on a "new" human isoprecipitin system (Australia antigen). Blood 27:297, 1966

74. Nielsen JO, Dietrichsin O, Juhl E: Incidence and meaning of E-determinant among hepatitis-B antigen positive patients with acute and chronic liver disease. Lancet 2:913, 1974

75. Szmuness W: Recent advances in the study of the epidemiology of hepatitis B. Am J Pathol 81:629, 1975

76. Vyas GN, Ibrahim AB, Rao KR, Schmid R: Tolerance to hepatitis-B antigen. Hypothesis for its termination with immune-RNA. Life Sci 15:261, 1974

77. Stevens CE, Beasley RP, Tsui J, Lee WC: Vertical transmission of hepatitis-B antigen in Taiwan. N Engl J Med 292:771, 1975

78. Chien DY, Vyas GN: Correlation of hepatitis-B surface and E-antigens. N Engl J Med 299:1253, 1978

79. Stevens CE, Neurath RA, Beasley RP, Szmuness W: HBeAg and anti-HBE detection by radioimmunoassay. Correlation with vertical transmission of hepatitis-B virus in Taiwan. J Med Virol 3:237, 1979

80. Krugman S, Overby LR, Mushahwar IK, et al: Viral hepatitis, type-B. Studies on natural history and prevention reexamined. N Engl J Med 300:101, 1979

81. Vyas GN, Cohen SN, Schmid R (eds): Viral Hepatitis. Franklin Institute Press, Philadelphia, 1978

82. Gerin JL, Shih JWK, Huyer BH: Biology and characterization of hepatitis B virus. p. 49. In Szmuness W, Alter HJ, Maynard JE (eds): Viral Hepatitis, 1981. Franklin Institute Press, Philadelphia, 1982

83. Brechot C, Pourcel C, Louise A, Rain B, Tiollais P:

Presence of integrated hepatitis B virus DNA sequences in cellular DNA of human hepatocellular carcinoma. Nature (Lond) 286:533, 1980

84. Shafritz DA, Kew MC: Identification of integrated hepatitis B virus DNA sequences in human hepatocellular carcinomas. Hepatology 1:1, 1981

85. Brechot C, Pourcel C, Hadchouel M, et al: State of hepatitis B virus DNA in liver diseases. Hepatology 2:27S, 1982

86. Blumberg BS, Millman I: Vaccine against viral hepatitis and process. Serial No. 864 filed 10/8/69; patent 36 36 191 issued 1/18/72, US Patent Office, 1972

87. Roizman B (ed): The Herpesviruses. Vols. 1, 2 and 3. Plenum Press, New York, 1982, 1983, 1985

88. zur Hausen H: Herpes simplex virus in human genital cancer. Int Rev Exp Pathol 25:307, 1983

89. Rapp F, Robbins D: Cytomegalovirus and Human Cancer. p. 175. In Plotkin SA, Michelson S, Pagano JS, Rapp F (eds): Birth Defects: Original Articles Series, March of Dimes Defects Foundation, Alan R Liss, New York, 1984

90. McDougall JK, Nelson JA, Myerson D, Beckmann AM, Galloway DA: HSV, CMV and HPV in human neoplasia. J Invest Dermatol 83:072S, 1984

91. Yamanishi K, Matsunaga Y, Ogino T, Lopetegui P: Biochemical transformation of mouse cells by varicella-zoster virus. J Gen Virol 56:421, 1981

92. Roizman B: The structure and isomerization of herpes simplex virus genomes. Cell 16:481, 1979

93. Roizman B, Jenkins FJ: Genetic engineering of novel genomes of large DNA viruses. Science 229:1208, 1985

94. Duff R, Rapp F: Oncogenic transformation of hamster cells after exposure to herpes simplex virus type 2. Nature New Biol 233:48, 1971

95. Jenkins FJ, Howett MK: Characterization of the mRNAs mapping in the BglII-N fragment of the herpes simplex virus type 2 genome. J Virol 52:99, 1984

96. Rigoni-Stern D: Fatti statistia relativi alle malatie cancerose. G Dervire Prog Pathol Terap 2:507, 1842

97. Winklestein W: Smoking and cancer of the uterine cervix: Hypothesis. Am J Epidemiol 106:257, 1977

98. Wright NH, Vessey MP, Kenward B, et al: Neoplasia and dysplasia of the cervix uteri and contraception: A possible protective effect of the diaphragm. Br J Cancer 38:273, 1978

99. Wigle DT, Mao Y, Grace M: Re: Smoking and cancer of the uterine cervix: Hypothesis. Am J Epidemiol 111:125, 1980

100. Clarke EA, Morgan RW, Newman AM: Smoking as a risk factor in cancer of the cervix: Additional evidence from a case-control study. Am J Epidemiol 115:59, 1982

101. Nahmias AJ, Josey WE, Naib ZM, et al: Antibodies to herpesvirus hominis types 1 and 2 in humans. II. Women with cervical cancer. Am J Epidemiol 91:547, 1970

102. Rawls WE, Tompkins WAF, Figueroa ME, Melnick JL: Herpesvirus type 2:Association with carcinoma of the cervix. Science 161:1255, 1968

103. Vonka V, Kanka J, Jellinek J, et al: Prospective study on the relationship between cervical neoplasia and herpes simplex type 2 virus. I. Epidemiological characteristics. Int J Cancer 33:49, 1984

104. Frenkel N, Roizman B, Cassai E, Nahmias A: A DNA fragment of herpes simplex 2 and its transcription in human cervical cancer tissue. Proc Natl Acad Sci USA 69:3784, 1972

105. Manservigi R, Cassai E, Deiss LP, et al: Sequences homologous to two separate transforming regions of herpes simplex virus DNA are linked in two human genital tumors. Virology 155:192, 1986

106. Jones KW, Fenoglio CM, Shevchuk-Chaban M, et al: Detection of herpesvirus 2 mRNA in human cervical biopsies by *in situ* cytological hybridization, IARC Sci Publ 24:917, 1979

107. McDougall JK, Galloway DA, Fenoglio CM: Cervical carcinoma: Detection of herpes simplex virus RNA in cells undergoing neoplastic change. Int J Cancer 25:1, 1980

108. McDougall JK, Crum CP, Fenoglio CM, et al: Herpesvirus-specific RNA and protein in carcinoma of the uterine cervix. Proc Natl Acad Sci USA 79:3853, 1982

109. Eglin RP, Sharp F, Maclean AB, et al: Detection of RNA complementary to herpes simplex virus DNA in human cervical squamous cell neoplasms. Cancer Res 41:3597, 1981

110. Eizuru Y, Hyman RW, Nahhas WA, Rapp F: Herpesvirus RNA in human urogenital tumors. Proc Soc Exp Biol Med 174:296, 1983

111. Tevethia MJ: Transforming potential of herpes simplex viruses and human cytomegalovirus. p. 257. In Roizman B (ed): The Herpesviruses. Vol. 3. Plenum Press, New York, 1985

112. Spear PG: Transformation of cultured cells by human herpesviruses. Int Rev Exp Pathol 25:327, 1983

113. Camacho A, Spear PG: Transformation of hamster embryo fibroblasts by a specific fragment of the herpes simplex virus genome. Cell 15:993, 1978

114. Reyes GR, LaFemina R, Hayward SD, Hayward GS: Morphological transformation by DNA fragments of human herpesviruses: Evidence for two distinct transforming regions in herpes simplex viruses types 1 and 2 and lack of correlation with biochemical transfer of the thymidine kinase gene. Cold Spring Harbor Symp Quant Biol 44:629, 1979

115. Galloway DA, McDougall JK: The oncogenic potential of herpes simplex viruses: Evidence for a "hit-and-run" mechanism. Nature (Lond) 302:21, 1983

116. Skinner GRB: Transformation of primary hamster embryo fibroblasts by type 2 simplex virus: Evidence for a "hit-and-run mechanism." Br J Exp Pathol 57:361, 1976

117. Hampar B, Aaronson SA, Derge JG, Chakrabarty M, Showalter SD, Dunn CY: Activation of an endogenous mouse type C virus by ultraviolet-irradiated herpes simplex virus types 1 and 2. Proc Natl Acad Sci USA 73:646, 1976

118. Hampar B, Boyd AL, Derg JG, et al: Comparison of properties of mouse cells transformed spontaneously by ultraviolet light-irradiated herpes simplex virus or by simian virus 40. Cancer Res 40:2213, 1980

119. Wentz WB, Reagan JW, Heggie AD: Cervical carcinogenesis with herpes simplex virus type 2. Obstet Gynecol 46:117, 1975

120. Wentz WB, Reagan JW, Heggie AD, et al: Induction of uterine cancer with inactivated herpes simplex virus types 1 and 2. Cancer 48:1783, 1981

121. Chen MH, Chang YD, Zhi-Hui L, et al: Prevention of type 2 herpes simplex virus induced cervical carcinoma in mice by prior immunization with a vaccine prepared from type 1 herpes simplex virus. Vaccine 1:13, 1983

122. Meignier B, Norrild B, Thuning C, et al: Failure to induce cervical cancer in mice by long-term frequent vaginal exposure to live or inactivated herpes simplex viruses. Int J Cancer 38:387, 1986

123. Burkitt DP: A tumour safari in east and central Africa. Br J Cancer 16:379, 1962

124. Epstein MA, Achong BG, Barr YM: Virus particles in cultured lymphoblasts from Burkitt's lymphoma. Lancet 1:702, 1964

125. Nadkarni JS, Nadkarni JJ, Clifford P, et al: Characteristics of new cell lines derived from Burkitt lymphomas. Cancer 23:64, 1969

126. Epstein MA, Achong BG (eds): The Epstein-Barr Virus. Springer-Verlag, New York, 1979

127. Henle W, Henle G: Seroepidemiology of the virus. p. 61. In Epstein M, Achong B (eds): The Epstein-Barr Virus. Springer-Verlag, New York, 1979

128. Henle G, Henle W: The virus as the etiologic agent of infectious mononucleosis. p. 297. In Epstein M, Achong B (eds): The Epstein-Barr Virus. Springer-Verlag, New York, 1979

129. Kieff E, Dambaugh T, Hummel M, Heller M: Epstein-Barr virus transformation and replication. p. 133. In Klein G (ed): Advances in Viral Oncology. Vol. 3. Raven Press, New York, 1983

130. Miller G, Robinson J, Heston L, Lipman M: Differences between laboratory strains of Epstein-Barr virus based on immortalization, abortive infection and interference. Proc Natl Acad Sci USA 71:4006, 1974

131. Ragona G, Ernberg I, Klein G: Induction and biological characterization of the Epstein-Barr virus (EBV) carried by the Jijoye lymphoma line. Virology 101:553, 1980

132. King W, Dambaugh T, Heller M, Dowling J, Kieff E: A variable region of the EBV genome is included in the P3HR1-deletion. J Virol 43:979, 1982

133. Klein G: The relationship of the virus to nasopharyngeal carcinoma. p. 340. In Epstein M, Achong B (eds): The Epstein-Barr Virus. Springer-Verlag, New York, 1979

134. Simons MJ, Wee GB, Day NE, et al: Immunologic aspects of nasopharyngeal carcinoma. I. Differences in HL-A antigen profiles between patients and control groups. Int J Cancer 13:122, 1974

135. Gerber P, Whang-Peng J, Monrol JH: Transformation and chromosome changes induced by Epstein-Barr virus in normal leukocyte cultures. Proc Natl Acad Sci USA 63:740, 1969

136. Henderon E, Miller G, Robinson J, Heston L: Efficiency of transformation of lymphocytes by Epstein-Barr virus. Virology 76:152, 1977

137. Svedmyr E, Jondal M: Cytotoxic effector cells specific for B cell lines transformed by Epstein-Barr virus are present in patients with infectious mononucleosis. Proc Natl Acad Sci USA 72:1622, 1975

138. Miller G: Experimental carcinogenicity by the virus *in vivo.* p. 352. In Epstein M, Achong B (eds): The Epstein-Barr Virus. Springer-Verlag, New York, 1979

139. Falk L, Deinhardt F, Nonoyama M, et al: Properties of a baboon lymphotropic herpesvirus related to Epstein-Barr virus. Int J Cancer 18:798, 1976

140. Gerber P, Pritchett R, Kieff E: Antigens and DNA of a chimpanzee agent related to Epstein-Barr virus. J Virol 19:1090, 1976

141. Gerber P, Nkrumah F, Pritchett R, Kieff E: Comparative studies of Epstein-Barr virus strains from Ghana and the United States. Int J Cancer 17:71, 1969

142. Rabin H, Neubauer RH, Hopkins RF, et al: Transforming activity and antigenicity of an Epstein-Barr like virus from lymphoblastoid cell lines of baboons with lymphoid disease. Intervirology 8:240, 1977

143. Weller TH: The cytomegaloviruses: Ubiquitous agents with protean clinical manifestations. N Engl J Med 285:203, 1971

144. Lang DJ: Cytomegalovirus infection in organ transplantation and post-perfusion: A hypothesis. Arch Ges Virusforsch 37,:365, 1972

145. Numazaki Y, Yano N, Morizaka T, et al: Primary infection with human cytomegalovirus: Virus isola-

tion from healthy infants and pregnant women. Am J Epidemiol 91:410, 1970

146. Montgomery R, Youngblood L, Medearis DN: Recovery of cytomegalovirus from the cervix in pregnancy. Pediatrics 49:524, 1972

147. Reynolds DW, Stagno S, Hosty TS, et al: Maternal cytomegalovirus excretion and perinatal infection. N Engl J Med 289:1, 1973

148. Feinstone SM, Kapikian AZ, Purcell RH, et al: Transfusion-associated hepatitis not due to viral hepatitis type A or B. N Engl J Med 292:767, 1973

149. Lerner PI, Sampliner JE: Transfusion-associated cytomegalovirus mononucleosis. Ann Surg 185:405, 1977

150. Huang ES, Pagano JS: Comparative diagnosis of cytomegalovirus. p. 241. In Kurstak E (ed): New Approaches in Comparative Diagnosis of Viral Diseases. Academic Press, New York, 1977

151. Caul EO, Clarke SKR, Matt MG, et al: Cytomegalovirus infections after open heart surgery. A prospective study. Lancet 1:777, 1971

152. St Jeor S, Weisser A: Persistence of cytomegalovirus in human lymphoblast and peripheral leukocyte cultures. Infect Immun 15:402, 1977

153. Rinaldo CR, Richter BS, Black PH, et al: Analysis of T lymphocyte subsets in cytomegalovirus mononucleosis. J Immunol 126:2114, 1981

154. St Jeor S, Albrecht TB, Funk FD, Rapp F: Stimulation of cell DNA synthesis by human cytomegalovirus. J Virol 13:353, 1974

155. Tanaka S, Furukawa T, Plotkin SA: Human cytomegalovirus stimulates host cell RNA synthesis. J Virol 15:297, 1975

156. Albrecht T, Rapp F: Malignant transformation of hamster embryo fibroblasts following exposure to ultraviolet-irradiated human cytomegalovirus. Virology 55:53, 1973

157. Geder L, Laychock A, Gorodecki J, Rapp F: Alteration in biological properties of different lines of cytomegalovirus-transformed human embryo lung cells following in vitro cultivation. IARC Sci Publ 24:561, 1978

158. Geder L: Oncogenic properties of human cytomegalovirus. p. 47. In Rapp F (ed): Oncogenic Herpesviruses. CRC Press, Boca Raton, FL 1980

159. Amstey MS, Lenin EB, Meyer MR: Herpesvirus infection in the newborn. Its treatment by exchange transfusion and adenosine arabinoside. Obstet Gynecol 47:33S, 1976

160. Lang DJ, Kummer JF: Demonstration of cytomegalovirus in semen. N Engl J Med 287:756, 1972

161. Cancer Facts and Figures. American Cancer Society, New York, 1986

162. Laychock AM, Geder L, Sanford EJ, Rapp F: Immune response of prostatic cancer patients to cytomegalovirus-infected and -transformed cells. Cancer 142:1766, 1978

163. Dagen JE, Sanford EJ, Rohner TJ, et al: Recognition of virally-transformed cells by lymphocytes from patients with prostatic cancer. Urology 12:532, 1978

164. Henson D: Cytomegalovirus inclusion bodies in the gastrointestinal tract. Arch Pathol Lab Med 93:477, 1972

165. Huang ES, Roche JK: Cytomegalovirus DNA and adenocarcinoma of the colon: Evidence for latent viral infection. Lancet 1:957, 1978

166. Hashiro GM, Horikami S, Loh PC: Cytomegalovirus isolations from cell cultures of human adenocarcinomas of the colon. Intervirology 12:84, 1979

167. Brichacek B, Hirsch I, Zavadova H, et al: Absence of cytomegalovirus DNA from adenocarcinoma of the colon. Intervirology 14:223, 1980

168. Hart H, Neill WA, Norval M: Lack of association of cytomegalovirus with adenocarcinoma of the colon. Gut 23:21, 1982

169. Oettle, AG: Geographical and racial differences of frequency of Kaposi's sarcoma as evidence of environmental or genetic causes. p. 330. In Ackermann LV, Murray JF (eds): Symposium on Kaposi's Sarcoma. Haefner Publishing Company, New York, 1963

170. Slavin G, Cameron HM, Singh H: Kaposi's sarcoma in mainland Tanzania: A report of 117 cases. Br J Cancer 23:349, 1969

171. Giraldo G, Beth E, Kourilsky FM, et al: Antibody patterns to herpes-viruses in Kaposi's sarcoma: Serological association of European Kaposi's sarcoma with cytomegalovirus. Int J Cancer 15:839, 1975

172. Gottlieb MS, Schroff R, Schanker HM, et al: *Pneumocystis carinii* pneumonia and mucosal candidiasis in previously healthy homosexual men. Evidence of a new acquired cellular immunodeficiency. N Engl J Med 305:1425, 1981

173. Hymes KB, Cheung T, Greene JB, et al: Kaposi's sarcoma in homosexual men—A report of eight cases. Lancet 2:598, 1981

174. Giraldo G, Beth E, Hagenau F: Herpes-type virus particles in tissue culture of Kaposi's sarcoma from different geographic regions. J Natl Cancer Inst 49:1509, 1972

175. Giraldo G, Beth E, Henle W, et al: Antibody patterns to herpesviruses in Kaposi's sarcoma. II. Serological association of American Kaposi's sarcoma with cytomegalovirus. Int J Cancer 22:126, 1978

176. Giraldo G, Beth E, Huang ES: Kaposi's sarcoma and its relationship to cytomegalovirus (CMV) III. CMV DNA and CMV early antigens in Kaposi's sarcomas. Int J Cancer 26:23, 1980

177. Boldogh I, Beth E, Huang ES, et al: Kaposi's sarcoma. IV. Detection of CMV DNA, CMV RNA and CMNA in tumor biopsies. Int J Cancer 28:469, 1981

178. Bishop JM: Retroviruses. Annu Rev Biochem 47:35, 1978

179. Coffin JM: Structure, replication and recombination of retrovirus genomes: Some unifying hypotheses. J Gen Virol 42:1, 1979

180. Temin H, Mitzutani S: RNA-dependent DNA polymerase in virions of Rous sarcoma virus. Nature (Lond) 226:1211, 1970

181. Baltimore D: Viral RNA-dependent DNA polymerase. Nature (Lond) 226:1209, 1970

182. Gross I: Viral etiology of cancer and leukemia: A look into the past, present and future. G. H. A. Clowes Memorial Lecture. Cancer Res 38:485, 1978

183. Bittner JJ: Some possible effects of nursing on the mammary gland tumor incidence in mice. Science 84:162, 1936

184. Tooze J (ed): DNA Tumor Viruses. Cold Spring Harbor Laboratory, New York, 1980

185. Huebner RJ, Todaro GJ: Oncogenes of RNA tumor viruses as determinants of cancer. Proc Natl Acad Sci USA 64:1087, 1969

186. Todaro GJ, Huebner RJ: The viral oncogene hypothesis. New evidence. Proc Natl Acad Sci USA 69:1009, 1972

187. Varmus HE: Viruses, genes and cancer. I. The discovery of cellular oncogenes and their role in neoplasia. Cancer 55:2324, 1985

188. Bishop JM: Viruses, genes and cancer. II. Retroviruses and cancer genes. Cancer 55:2329, 1985

189. Weinberg RA: The action of oncogenes in the cytoplasm and nucleus. Science 230:770, 1985

190. Bishop JM: Cellular oncogenes and retroviruses. Annu Rev Biochem 52:301, 1983

191. Klein G: The role of gene dosage and genetic transpositions in carcinogenesis. Nature (Lond) 294:313, 1981

192. Poiesz BJ, Ruscetti FW, Gazdar AF, et al: Detection and isolation of type C retrovirus particles from fresh and cultured lymphocytes of a patient with cutaneous T-cell lymphoma. Proc Natl Acad Sci USA 77:7415, 1980

193. Kalyanaraman VS, Sargadharan MG, Bunn PA, et al: Antibodies in human sera reactive against an internal structural protein of human T-cell lymphoma virus. Nature (Lond) 294:271, 1981

194. Posner LE, Robert-Guroff M, Kalyanaraman VS, et al: Natural antibodies to the human T cell lymphoma virus in patients with cutaneous T cell lymphoma. J Exp Med 154:333, 1981

195. Yoshida M, Miyoshi T, Hinuma Y: Isolation and characterization of retrovirus from cell lines of human adult T-cell leukemia and its implication in the disease. Proc Natl Acad Sci USA 79:2031, 1982

196. Kalyanaramon VS, Sarngadharen MG, Miyoshi I, et al: A new subtype of human T-cell leukemia virus (HTLV-II) associated with a T-cell variant of hairy cell leukemia. Science 218:571, 1982

197. Popovic M, Sarngadharan MG, Read E, Gallo RC: Detection, isolation, and continuous production of cytopathic retroviruses (HTLV-III) from patients with AIDS and pre-AIDS. Science 224:497, 1984

198. Gallo RC, Salahuddin SZ, Popovic M, et al: Frequent detection and isolation of cytopathic retroviruses (HTLV-III) from patients with AIDS and at risk from AIDS. Science 224:500, 1984

199. Schüpbach J, Popovic M, Gilden RV, et al: Serological analysis of a subgroup of human T-lymphotropic retroviruses. Science 224:503, 1984

200. Sarngadharan M, Popovic M, Bruch L, et al: Antibodies reactive with human T-lymphotropic retroviruses (HTLV-III) in the serum of patients with AIDS. Science 224:506, 1984

201. Sodroski JG, Rosen CA, Haseltine WA: *Trans*-acting transcriptional activation of the long terminal repeat of human T lymphotropic viruses in infected cells. Science 225:381, 1984

202. Haseltine WA, Sodroski JG, Patarca R, et al: Structure of 3'-terminal region of type II human T lymphotropic virus: Evidence for new coding region. Science 225:419, 1984

203. Ciuffo G: Innesto positivo con filtrato di verrucae volgare. Giorn Ital Mal Veneral 48:12, 1907

204. Shope RE: Infectious papillomatosis of rabbits. J Exp Med 58:607, 1933

205. Rous P, Beard JW: The progression to carcinoma of virus-induced rabbit papillomas (Shope). J Exp Med 65:523, 1935

206. Kidd JG, Rous P: Cancers deriving from the virus papillomas of wild rabbits under natural conditions. J Exp Med 71:469, 1940

207. Syverton JT: The pathogenesis of the rabbit papilloma-to-carcinoma sequence. Ann NY Acad Sci 54:1126, 1952

208. Lewandowsky F, Lutz W: Ein falleiner bisher nicht beschriebenen hauterkrankung (Epidermodysplasia verruciformis). Arch Dermatol Syph (Berl) 141:193, 1922

209. zur Hausen H: Human papillomaviruses and their possible role in squamous cell carcinomas. Curr Top Microbiol Immunol 78:1, 1977

210. McCance DJ: Human papillomaviruses and cancer. Biochim Biophys Acta 823:195, 1986

211. Pfister H: Biology and biochemistry of papillomaviruses. Rev Physiol Biochem Pharmacol 99:11, 1984

212. Favre M, Breitburd F, Croissant O, et al: Structural

polypeptides of rabbit, bovine and human papilloma viruses. J Virol 15:1239, 1975

213. Gissmann L, Pfister H, zur Hausen H: Human papilloma viruses (HPV): Characterization of 4 different isolates. Virology 76:569, 1977

214. Orth G, Favre M, Croissant O: Characterization of a new type of human papilloma virus that causes skin warts. J Virol 24:108, 1977

215. Friedmann JM, Fialkow PJ: Viral "tumorigenesis" in man: Cell markers in condylomata acuminata. Int J Cancer 17:57, 1976

216. Orth G, Jeánteur P, Croissant O: Evidence for localization of vegatative viral DNA replication by autoradiographic detection of RNA-DNA hybrids in sections of tumors induced by Shope papillomavirus. Proc Natl Acad Sci USA 68:1876, 1971

217. Grussendorf EI, zur Hausen H: Localization of viral DNA-replication in sections of human warts by nucleic acid hybridization with complementary RNA of human papilloma virus type 1. Arch Dermatol Res 264:55, 1979

218. Almeida JD, Howatson AF, Williams MG: Electron microscope study of human warts: Sites of virus production and nature of the inclusion bodies. J Invest Dermatol 38:337, 1962

219. Kreider JK, Bartlett GL: The Shope papilloma-carcinoma complex of rabbits: A model system of neoplastic progression and spontaneous regression. Adv Cancer Res 35:81, 1981

220. Rheinwald JG, Green H: Serial cultivation of strains of human epidermal keratinocytes: The formation of keratinizing colonies from single cells. Cell 6:331, 1975

221. La Porta RF, Taichman LB: Human papilloma viral DNA replicates as a stable episome in cultured epidermal keratinocytes. Proc Natl Acad Sci USA 79:3393, 1982

222. Kreider JW, Bartlett GL, Sharkey FE: Primary neoplastic transformation in vivo of xenogeneic skin grafts on nude mice. Cancer Res 39:272, 1979

223. Kreider JW, Haft HM, Roode PR: Growth of human skin on the hamster. J Invest Dermatol 57:66, 1971

224. Pass F, Niimura M, Kreider JW: Prolonged survival of human skin xenografts on antithymocyte serum-treated mice: Failure to produce verrucae by inoculation with extracts of human warts. J Invest Dermatol 61:371, 1973

225. Cubie HA: Failure to produce warts on human skin grafts on "nude" mice. Br J Dermatol 94:659, 1976

226. Kreider JK, Howett MK, Wolfe SA, et al: Morphological transformation in vivo of human uterine cervix with papillomavirus from condyloma acuminata. Nature (Lond) 317:639, 1985

227. Kreider JK, Howett MK, Lill NL, et al: In vivo transformation of human skin with human papillomavirus type II from condylomata acuminata. J Virol 59:369

228. Coggin JR, Jr, zur Hausen H: Workshop on papillomaviruses and cancer. Cancer Res 39:545, 1979

229. Lancaster WD, Olson C: Animal papillomaviruses. Microbiol Rev 46:191, 1982

230. Howley PM, Low MF, Heilman CA, et al: Molecular characterization of papillomavirus genomes. Cold Spring Harbor Conf Cell Prolif 7:233, 1980

231. Lowy DR, Dvoretzky I, Shober R, et al: In vitro tumorigenic transformation by a defined sub-genomic fragment of bovine papilloma virus DNA. Nature (Lond) 287:72, 1980

232. Lancaster W: Apparent lack of integration of bovine papilloma virus DNA in virus-induced equine and bovine tumor cells and virus-transformed mouse cells. Virology 108:251, 1981

233. Law MF, Byrne JC, Howley PM: A stable bovine papillomavirus hybrid plasmid that expresses a dominant selective trait. Mol Cell Biol 3:2110, 1983

234. Chen EY, Howley PM, Levinson HD, et al: The primary structure and genetic organization of the bovine papillomavirus type 1 genome. Nature (Lond) 299:529, 1982

235. Gissmann L, zur Hausen H: Partial characterization of viral DNA from human genital warts (condylomata acuminata). Int J Cancer 25:605, 1980

236. Gissmann L, Diehl V, Schultz-Coulon H, et al: Molecular cloning and characterization of human papillomavirus DNA derived from a laryngeal papilloma. J Virol 44:393, 1982

237. Dürst M, Gissmann L, Ikenberg H, et al: A papilloma DNA from a cervical carcinoma and its presence in cancer biopsy samples from different geographic regions. Proc Natl Acad Sci USA 80:3812, 1983

238. Boshart M, Gissmann L, Ikenberg H, et al: A new papillomavirus DNA, its presence in genital cancer biopsies and in cell lines derived from cervical cancer. EMBO J 3:1151, 1984

239. Lorincz AT, Lancaster WD, Temple GF: Cloning and characterization of the DNA of a new human papillomavirus from a woman with dysplasia of the uterine cervix. J Virol 58:225, 1986

240. Beaudenon S, Kremsdorf D, Croissant O, et al: A novel type of human papillomavirus associated with genital neoplasias. Nature (Lond) 321:246, 1986

241. Crum LP, Ikenberg H, Richart RM: Human papillomavirus type 16 and early cervical neoplasia. N Engl J Med 310:330, 1984

242. zur Hausen H: Herpes simplex virus in human genital cancer. Int Rev Exp Pathol 25:307, 1983

Section II

ORGAN SITES

9

Principles of Diagnosis

Hugh M. Shingleton
Hazel Gore

Breast and uterine cancer are two of the four most frequently occurring cancers in women; breast, ovarian, and uterine cancer are among the six leading causes of cancer death. For most female genital cancers, improved survival rates are reflections of greater efforts in early detection rather than of improved treatment modalities. Primary care physicians have the best opportunity to evaluate women for cancer and must avail themselves of every opportunity to inquire about risk factors and significant symptoms and to perform a comprehensive physical examination and pertinent diagnostic studies. In addition to a pelvic examination, a woman should also be evaluated for cancer of extragenital sites, since breast, colorectal, and lung cancers all exceed uterine and ovarian cancer in frequency. Early diagnosis and patient education must be emphasized if women in whom cancer develops are to have an opportunity to survive. As the female population ages, cancer will become an even greater health care problem. Figure 9-1 shows the probability at birth that white and black women in the United States will eventually develop cancer (listed by site); only the seven more common sites are listed. A woman can now expect to live more than 25 years beyond the menopause; it has been estimated that one-third of the total female population in Western societies is postmenopausal.

HISTORY AND PHYSICAL EXAMINATION

The diagnosis of cancer requires an able clinician, ever on the alert for signs or symptoms of cancer. Far too often, physicians, busy with the routine, contribute to delay in diagnosis of cancer and thus to tumor incurability. This problem is compounded by the patient's own tendency to deny symptoms and signs and to delay visits to physicians because of the fear of discovery of cancer. The young, slender, normotensive, nondiabetic woman can have endometrial cancer; the nulliparous, monogamous woman can have cervical cancer. Breast and gastrointestinal (GI) cancer, more common than any of the reproductive tract tumors in women, can occur in asymptomatic women or may present in atypical ways. Vaginal bleeding in pregnant women is not invariably due to pregnancy nor should rectal bleeding be dismissed as due to hemorrhoids. Failure to perform a rectal examination because it is uncomfortable for the patient or odious to the physician is no more excusable than the widespread failure of many physicians to perform routine pelvic examinations on women. Even captive audiences, such as women in hospitals for various reasons, seldom have pelvic examinations other than in obstetric or gynecologic wards. Since early detection

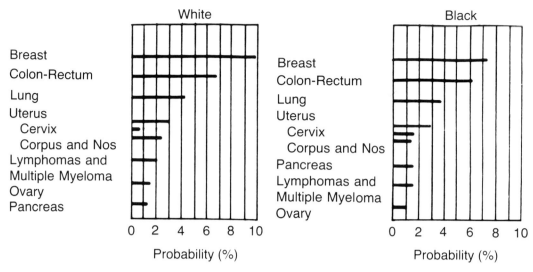

Fig. 9-1 Probability at birth of eventually developing cancer by site, females, United States, 1985. (American Cancer Society data.)

is generally associated with high curability, improvement in all these areas is mandatory, if women with cancer are to have the best possible chance for survival.

The Medical History

While the history and chief complaint are important parts of every physician's assessment, they are not as important as a comprehensive examination in the detection of cancer. However, cancer might be suspected from some historical details (Table 9-1). Breast, uterine, and colorectal cancers are familial; a family history of such malignant tumors should mandate close surveillance of other family members. A menstrual history suggesting anovulatory cycles or exposure to exogenous estrogen over a protracted period of time should raise the level of suspicion for endometrial cancer. Postmenopausal bleeding may suggest vulvar, vaginal, uterine, and cervical cancer, or even bladder or rectal cancer. Postcoital bleeding, at any age, bears investigation. Advancing age, in general, increases the risk for cancer. Unexplained major weight loss or a rapid increase in abdominal girth are ominous signs.

An association of obesity, hypertension, and diabetes with endometrial cancer was discussed in a recent textbook by Cavanagh et al.[1] In summary, while

it is true that large numbers of women with endometrial cancer are obese, it is not clear that screening the heavier women in the population would detect more than one-half of cases of endometrial cancer. Recent studies have shown the same rate of hypertension in women with endometrial cancer and women of similar age in the general population. The association of diabetes and endometrial cancer is unclear because of the tendency of investigators to in-

Table 9-1 Women at High Risk for Cancer

Cancer	Features
Breast	Family history of breast or gynecologic cancer
	Personal history of fibrocystic breast disease
	Late age at first pregnancy
Colorectal	Family history of polyposis or colon cancer
	Personal history of intestinal polyps
	Ulcerative colitis, other genital cancers
Lung	Personal history of cigarette smoking
Endometrial	Family history of cancer
	Personal history of obesity, nulliparity, late menopause, and/or unopposed estrogens
Cervical	Personal history of onset of sexual activity before age 20, multiple sex partners, and/or low socioeconomic status
Ovarian	Family history of ovarian, breast, or colon cancer

clude women with abnormal glucose tolerance as well as women with frank diabetes in their analyses; when the former are deleted from consideration, diabetes as such may not be a risk factor for endometrial cancer.

Ovarian cancer, although the deadliest of the major gynecologic cancers, is notoriously silent in presentation; in fact, such cancers are seldom detected on routine examination by physicians. More commonly they present as abdominal masses or ascites noted by the patients themselves. Ovarian cancer commonly presents in stage III with intraabdominal spread, making it difficult to cure. Only abdominal-pelvic examination at regular intervals by skilled physicians can identify earlier more curable lesions.

Signs and Symptoms of Pelvic Cancer

Many women present with self-discovered enlarged nodes in the neck or groin areas, abdominal masses or distention, breast lumps, or vulvar-vaginal lesions. In women without such findings, the most common symptoms are likely to be vaginal bleeding, abnormal vaginal discharge, vulvar irritation or itching, or rectal bleeding. Most women presenting with vaginal or rectal bleeding will not have cancer but will have other conditions causing the bleeding. There may be nothing specific about the bleeding to raise the suspicion of cancer, although either vaginal bleeding in elderly women or postcoital bleeding should lead to suspicion of cancer as the cause. It is not unusual for a woman to be unable at times to determine whether the bleeding is coming from the bladder, the vagina, or the rectum. Other women will complain of irritating or offensive vaginal discharges that may be associated with malignancy rather than infection. Finally, some women subsequently found to have cancer will present for routine examinations or for care of other conditions with no symptoms whatsoever. This is especially true of early cervical, ovarian, and vulvar cancer, including melanoma.

Cancer of the breast is a common disease. A woman faces a 7 to 10 percent chance of developing breast cancer in her lifetime. Certain high-risk factors are recognized: breast cancer is more common after age 40, increasing in incidence with advancing age. Women with a family history, particularly on the maternal side, and those who bear children late in

their reproductive life are more likely to have breast cancer. Those with other genital cancers, or with fibrocystic disease, also are at increased risk of developing breast cancer. Other factors associated with an increased risk are exogenous hormone intake, immunologic incompetence, high dietary fat intake, and previous exposure of the breast to significant amounts of radiation.

Rectal bleeding and changes in bowel habits are the most common complaints of patients with colorectal cancer. Persons at high risk are those with familial polyposis, a family history of polyps or colon cancer, as well as a personal history of female genital cancers of other types, intestinal polyps, or ulcerative colitis. Those in the high-risk group should be followed up regularly; the value of routine screening of asymptomatic women without risk factors for colorectal cancer remains open to question.

Office Equipment

The physician's office must be equipped to detect the major cancers affecting women. Comfortable examining tables are a necessity, as are vaginal specula of a variety of sizes and designs. The office should have adequate directable lights for use in the general examination as well as for the speculum evaluation. Cotton-tipped applicators moistened with saline, as well as wooden spatulas or other devices designed for cervical scraping, should be readily at hand. Spray fixatives have replaced the bottles of ether alcohol formerly used in office practice for fixing Papanicolaou (Pap) smears. Office equipment should include scalpels, forceps, a variety of sutures, and specially designed biopsy instruments for sampling the endometrium, cervix, vagina, and vulva. Suction devices for endometrial sampling are available, but the use of Novak, Duncan, or Kevorkian curettes for obtaining a simple endometrial biopsy is still popular, with adequate results. Kevorkian and other similar small punch-biopsy forceps have largely replaced alligator, Gaylor, and Gusberg punch-biopsy forceps in office practice[2] (Fig. 9-2). These forceps cause less discomfort and less bleeding than do the larger ones. A bottle of Lugol's solution is essential and enables the gynecologist to identify small vaginal or cervical lesions not otherwise visible other than through a colposcope. Iris hooks, Alis clamps, or long-toothed forceps may facilitate biopsy procedures of the vaginal walls.

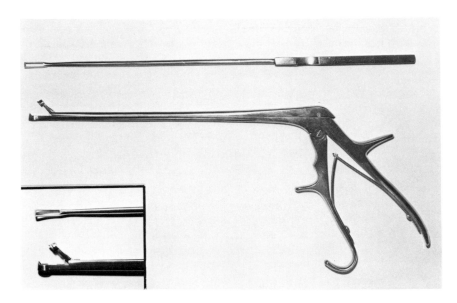

Fig. 9-2 Cervical biopsy instruments. Upper: Kevorkian-Younge endocervical curette. Lower: Burke biopsy forcep. (Shingleton HM, Orr JW Jr: Cancer of the Cervix: Diagnosis and Treatment. Churchill Livingstone, Edinburgh, 1987)

For vulvar biopsies, scalpels may be used. The cutaneous Keyes dermatologic biopsy instruments may be preferable, since they remove a small amount of tissue and rarely result in significant bleeding (Fig. 9-3). Monsel's solution (ferric subsulfate) is useful in controlling minor bleeding; interrupted sutures may be used if necessary to stop more brisk bleeding at the biopsy site.

Physical Examination

All women should have regular physical examinations. Comprehensive breast examination is recommended at 3-year intervals in women aged 20 to 40, and yearly thereafter. Palpation of nodes in the head and neck area, the axillae, and groins is not time consuming. An abdominal examination should include palpation of the liver, kidneys, and spleen and assessment for fluid, abnormal pulsations, or masses in all four quadrants. Pelvic examination should first focus on the vulva, then the vagina, and finally the cervix. Many busy clinicians ignore the vulva unless the patient draws attention to a symptomatic area or some abnormality. Lesions may be missed in the vagina by failure to look at all the epithelial areas; for instance, the anterior and posterior walls are covered by the bivalve speculum blades and may obscure a lesion. In elderly patients not taking exogenous hormones, an assessment of estrogen levels might be indicated, as an unusually youthful appearance of the vaginal epithelium might suggest an estrogen-producing ovarian tumor. Next, the cervix should be examined for general appearance, location, and consistency. Gross lesions, marked change in consistency (nodularity, hardening, asymmetric expansion), and friability require investigation. Colposcopic evaluation is not recommended routinely but is best applied in patients with atypical cervical cytologic findings. Involvement of the uterus in pelvic tumor masses may, however, displace the cervix, the first sign of which may be difficulty in locating the cervix with the speculum on routine examination. Deviation of the cervix from its normal position may also occur with benign conditions, however, as in simple retroversion of the uterus or in the case of large leiomyomata.

Pelvic masses not involving the epithelium of the vagina or cervix fall into two groups: those involving the uterus and those separate from the uterus. The group involving the uterus includes common benign conditions such as pelvic inflammatory disease, leiomyomata, or extensive endometriosis. Malignant conditions such as primary or metastatic ovarian tumors and cervical, endometrial, fallopian tube, and colorectal cancers may also involve, or apparently involve, the uterus. The group in which the mass is separate from the uterus includes pedunculated leiomyomata, some inflammatory ovarian or tubal masses, and certain benign or malignant ovarian tumors. Solid ovarian masses are more likely to be malignant than are cystic masses. Combined abdo-

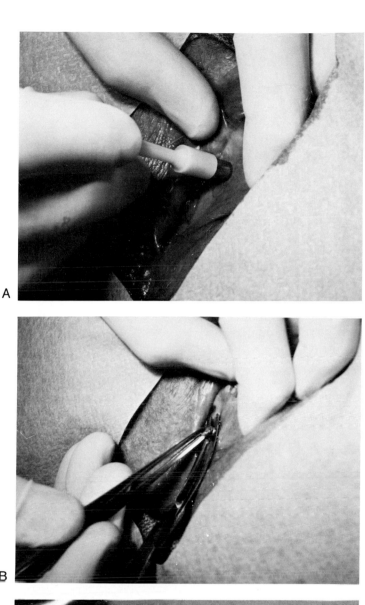

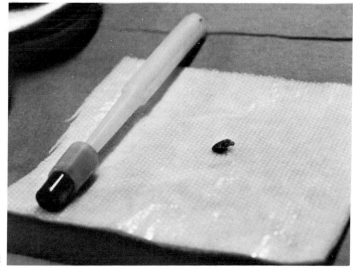

Fig. 9-3 (A) Disposable punch biopsy instrument of the Keyes type used to obtain a small plug (Baker and Cummins, Division of Keyes Pharmaceuticals Inc., Miami, FL). **(B)** The pellet-shaped specimen is grasped with forceps and cut with scissors. **(C)** The biopsy specimen is properly oriented on a piece of telfa and placed in formalin.

minopelvic examination and rectovaginal examination often provide unique information in regard to the location, size, mobility, and consistency of a mass as well as the probability of its being benign or malignant. In the presence of an abdominal or pelvic mass, it is essential to test for ascites.

All adult women should be encouraged to perform breast self-examination at monthly intervals. Even without universal compliance with this recommendation, most breast cancers are currently detected by the patient. Benign conditions of the breast, such as fibrocystic disease, fibroadenomas, intraductal papillomas, and ductal ectasia, are so common that, for some women, referral to experienced colleagues may be necessary and closer follow-up required.

Both cystic and solid masses of the breast can be evaluated using needle aspiration techniques. Some authorities believe that a cystic mass found to contain clear or cloudy fluid (nonbloody) need not be evaluated for malignant cells. Bloody fluid or perhaps any fluid in high-risk patients should be sent for cytologic study. Solid masses can be aspirated and a diagnosis of cancer made with a high degree of reliability (Fig. 9-4).

For detection of colorectal cancer, the American Cancer Society[3] recommends annual digital rectal examinations in persons aged 40 and above. Stool guaiac tests for occult blood should be added in women aged 50 and above. Sigmoidoscopy is recommended at age 50 and at 3- to 5-year intervals thereafter, if negative. For those at high risk, either barium enema or fiberoptic colonoscopy, or both, should be used to assess the entire colon and should be employed even before age 50. Fiberoptic colonoscopy is much more sensitive than an air-contrast barium enema in evaluating the colon and can ordinarily be performed on an outpatient basis.

Preconceived ideas on the part of the physician as to what the patient is likely to have may lead to mistakes in diagnosis. A common tendency in evaluating young women presenting with pelvic masses is to assign a diagnosis of pelvic inflammatory disease

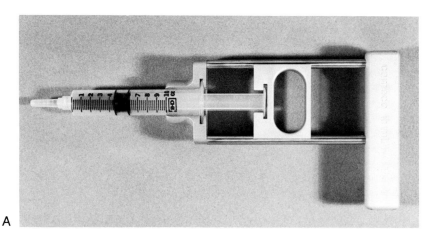

A

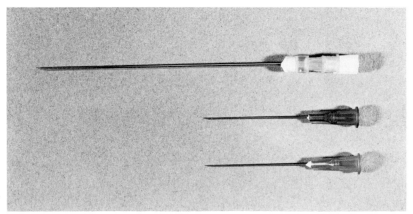

B

Fig. 9-4 Instruments for fine needle aspiration. **(A)** Syringe holder and syringe. **(B)** Types of needles. Longer needle of larger bore for deep aspirations and shorter needles for more superficial aspirations.

(PID) to those in the lower social classes and a diagnosis of endometriosis to those in higher classes. Rarely is cancer considered as part of the differential diagnosis. The inflamed cervix that bleeds on contact at the time of a Pap smear or digital examination is not always due to cervicitis nor are cervical lesions during pregnancy always related to the pregnancy. Rectal bleeding is not always due to hemorrhoids, even if the woman has hemorrhoids. Impartial observation and comprehensive physical assessment are the order of the day for the competent physician or health professions.

DIAGNOSTIC PROCEDURES

Before proceeding with more complex investigations, simple hematologic tests such as hemoglobin estimation and complete blood count (CBC) are important. The presence of anemia, although not a specific test, should always be investigated further.

Cytologic Evaluation

The Pap smear has been an important component of routine gynecologic examination for more than 30 years. Although initially applied to women over age 40, it became increasingly evident during the 1950s that the test should be used to detect early abnormalities in patients in their 20s and 30s. In her lectures and resident teaching, Johnson[4] advocated taking smears from pregnant women to pick up premalignant conditions, since this was a captive group, and to educate such women to return regularly for Pap smears after completion of their pregnancies. This approach followed her studies on obstetric patients with preinvasive lesions. Currently, regular Pap smears are thought to be indicated from the onset of sexual activity without considering the youth of the patient. How frequently smears should be repeated in the patient whose smears have always been negative is controversial. The American Cancer Society[5] considers smears taken at 3-year intervals, except in high-risk groups, adequate, but we advocate yearly testing as a general recommendation.

Although the clinician attempts to take an excellent sample, areas may be missed. The spray fixative may be imperfectly applied. Smears may be allowed to dry before fixation, or some areas may be missed by the spray, and these may be washed off in processing, giving a less than adequate smear. The drying and the inadequate quantity should be reported, but there is often pressure on the laboratories to give an answer. Under such circumstances, with the 3-year rule, there may be a 6-year gap between adequate smears. Quality of screening varies, and indeed even the most experienced cytotechnologist may have a bad day and miss atypicalities. Such atypicalities may be erroneously attributed to an inflammatory effect. Another factor is the occasional mislabeled specimen. All this is mentioned to make the clinician more sensitive to advocating yearly Pap smears for the asymptomatic previously negative patient. Certification of laboratories and education of physicians are needed.

Abnormal smears are an indication for further evaluation and as such are dealt with in individual chapters of this book. Frequency of repeat smears in pre-

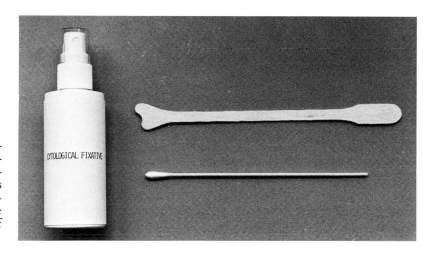

Fig. 9-5 Spatula and cotton-tipped applicator used for obtaining cervical scrape and endocervical swab specimens respectively. *Note:* Cotton-tipped applicator should be moistened with saline at time of use.

viously treated patients is dealt with in the discussion of patient management.

Originally Pap smears were vaginal and a true exfoliative cytologic examination. Gradually, cervical swabbing and then cervical scraping along with endocervical aspiration using a glass pipette with a thick rubber bulb were introduced. Endocervical aspiration was subsequently replaced by endocervical swabbing.

Between 1950 and 1960, physicians often took three routine smears from each patient, then two, cervical and endocervical. This practice has now been generally replaced by a single slide combining endocervical swabbing using a cotton-tipped applicator moistened with normal saline and cervical scraping (Fig. 9-5).

What can be learned from the Pap smear? Varying degrees of atypia and dysplasia may be recognized[2]

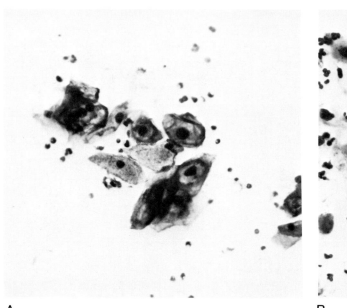

A

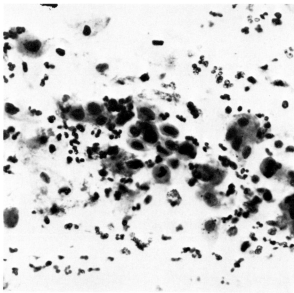

B

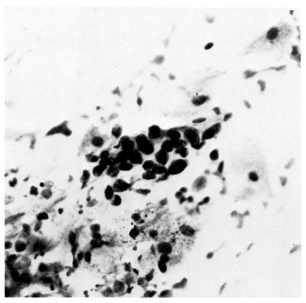

C

Fig. 9-6 Koilocytic atypia in a Papanicolaou smear. **(A)** Nuclei are minimally atypical and vary slightly in size. The large perinuclear vacuole, the classic cytoplasmic alteration of koilocytosis, is evident in several squamous epithelial cells of intermediate type and may be compared with an uninvolved cell in the center of the field. (×380.) **(B)** Moderate dysplasia in metaplastic epithelium with nuclear irregularity, variation in nuclear size, and increased nuclear to cytoplasmic ratio. (×380.) **(C)** Small hyperchromatic nuclei, with very little variation in size and scanty cytoplasm (often undetected by light microscopy), are found in smears from patients with carcinoma in situ. (×380.) (Shingleton HM, Orr JW Jr: Cancer of the Cervix: Diagnosis and Treatment. Churchill Livingstone, Edinburgh, 1987.)

(Fig. 9-6). Malignant squamous cells in a pattern suggesting carcinoma in situ or with a more bizarre pattern with inflammation and necrosis consistent with invasive squamous cell carcinoma may be detected. Atypical glandular cells may suggest adenocarcinoma of the cervix or adenocarcinoma of the endometrium[2] (Fig. 9-7). On rare occasions, malignant cells from tubal or ovarian carcinoma may be found, but such findings are exceedingly rare and are not of practical importance. The Pap smear should not be credited with picking up obvious vaginal or cervical carcinomas, but it is useful when the cervix appears only inflamed or when the carcinoma is entirely within the endocervical canal or endometrial cavity.

Candida and *Trichomonas* are reported, and such findings may be helpful if not detected on clinical examination. Involvement of cells by human papillomavirus, intracytoplasmic inclusions suggesting *Chlamydia,* and the classic changes associated with herpes may be noted.

Cervical smears are not suitable for the evaluation of estrogenic effect, although a mature squamous epithelial pattern in the postmenopausal patient must be noted and investigated further. Not always is it due to estrogen, but it may be related to inflammation. Lateral vaginal scrapings are better for evaluation of estrogen levels, although even from this site inflamed specimens or those with cytolysis are unsuitable.

The presence of endometrial cells beyond cycle days 10 to 12 should be explained. Any endometrial cells in the postmenopausal patient are abnormal, and the reason for their presence should be determined.

Vaginal and cervical smears have not been as useful in detecting endometrial carcinoma as they are for cervical carcinoma. During the 1950s, simple endometrial aspirations were attempted, followed by a variety of scraping and brushing techniques and various washings. Some of these methods have been successful in the hands of those who introduced them. Those physicians took the samples themselves with great care, and each clinician had a specific laboratory that took exceptional care in processing and reading. Such techniques employed in a routine manner have been less successful and are no longer generally employed.

In summary, Pap smears should be carefully taken, adequately fixed, and always labeled with the patient's name, using pencil on frosted ends, diamond marker on plain slides. Clinicians should select a reli-

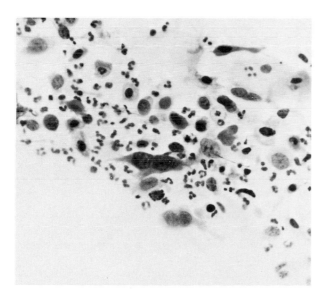
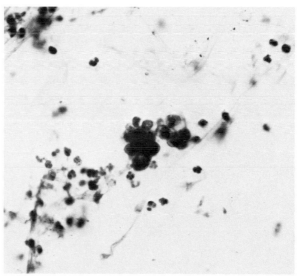

A   B

Fig. 9-7 Malignant squamous cells with nuclear variation, irregular chromatin distribution and varying amounts of cytoplasm. **(A)** There are numerous polymorphonuclear leucocytes, part of the commonly associated tumor diathesis. (×380.) **(B)** Tight clusters of malignant nuclei, some with prominent nucleoli. Vacuolated cytoplasm is evident in the group on the right and both clusters suggest an acinar formation consistent with adenocarcinoma. (×380.) (Shingleton HM, Orr JW Jr: Cancer of the Cervix: Diagnosis and Treatment. Churchill Livingstone, Edinburgh, 1987.)

able laboratory in their own area so that consultation is available with the pathologist; clinicians should not be influenced by the cheapest rate. Having made that decision, repeat smears should be sent to the same laboratory, so that all may be evaluated together if necessary. If a normal smear alters within a year to more than mild dysplasia, the concerned laboratory staff should review the former slide and search for even one dysplastic cell — not that a dysplasia report might have been made on a single cell, but to see whether anything was missed that should have been found. In short, quality control is essential. Flitting from laboratory to laboratory is not advisable because the form of report may differ and cause confusion. Any reservations about a given laboratory should be discussed with the pathologist; only if the clinician is still dissatisfied should another laboratory be employed. This same principle applies to biopsies, which should go to the same laboratory as the smears for correlation. This gives the pathologist the opportunity to tell the clinician when the atypical cells on the smears have not been explained.

Accuracy rates of cervical cytology vary widely from laboratory to laboratory and in some degree reflect quality control within the laboratory, numbers of slides screened per screener, and indeed the obsessional attention to detail of the screener, whether a pathologist or a cytotechnologist. The clinician tends to blame any discrepancy in regard to cytology on the pathologist or pathology laboratory. The fact is, however, that training of clinicians for obtaining proper cervical smears is slipshod, and the technique is not necessarily applied uniformly by the same clinician from day to day; as a result, numerous sampling errors and fixation artifacts contribute to the imperfection of the method. In a sense, this problem speaks for screening at more frequent rather than less frequent intervals, as advocated by some groups, such as the Walton Report[5a] and the American Cancer Society.

Those who do not understand the merits and limitations of cytology or who avail themselves of low-quality cytology services do not appreciate the great potential of the method under ideal circumstances. Squamous cell carcinoma can be differentiated from adenocarcinoma; endocervical cells can be distinguished from endometrial cells. Precursor lesions can be distinguished from invasive lesions. Inflammatory conditions can be detected, and hormonal evaluation is possible. Another common misconception is that modern genital cytology is as effective in detecting lesions of the upper genital tract as those of the cervix. Screening cytology is most inaccurate in detecting endometrial cancers. It cannot be relied on to rule out malignancy or premalignancy of the vulva or vagina. Only rarely does it identify cancer of the ovary or tube.

Colposcopic Examinations

For most women with atypical Pap smears, colposcopically directed biopsies are the preferred method for definitive diagnosis. By avoiding conization for

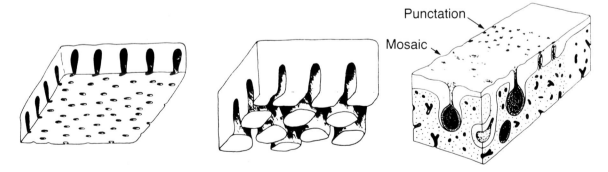

Fig. 9-8 Basis for colposcopic patterns. Left: Vertical penetration of vessels in neoplastic epithelium causes punctation pattern (modified from KA Bolten). Middle: Deep rete peg and surrounding vascular stroma cause mosaic pattern (modified from KA Bolten). Right: Diagram of normal and altered epithelium. (Modified from R Cartier). (Shingleton HM, Hatch KD, Orr JW Jr, et al: Diagnosis and treatment of preinvasive and microscopically invasive squamous cell carcinoma of the cervix. Cancer Bull 35(4):172, 1983.)

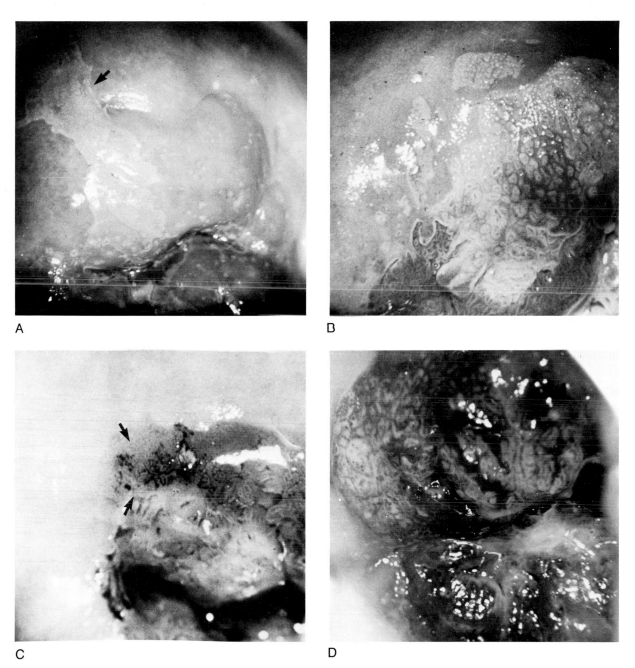

Fig. 9-9 (A) Demarcated acetowhite lesion in a large transformation zone. Area of fine mosaic is present (arrow), compatible with dysplasia in metaplasia. **(B)** Coarse mosaic and punctation patterns with acetowhite background, compatible with marked dysplasia–carcinoma in situ. **(C)** Abnormal blood vessels, suggesting microinvasive cancer. **(D)** Coarse mosaic, acetowhite epithelium, punctation, atypical vessels in cervix of pregnant woman. (Shingleton HM, Hatch K, Orr JW Jr: Diagnosis and treatment of preinvasive and microscopically invasive squamous cell carcinoma of the cervix. Cancer Bull 35(4):172, 1983.)

routine investigation of cytologic atypias, most women can avoid hospitalization. The colposcopic impression will often correlate as well as, or better than, the cytologic diagnosis with the final tissue diagnosis.

Basic patterns of colposcopy are acetowhite epithelium, punctation, and mosaic and atypical vessels[3] (Fig. 9-8). The basis for these patterns is well explained in the various atlases of colposcopy and will not be repeated here. The diagnosis of microscopically or deeply invasive cervical lesions by experienced colposcopists is possible, using visual criteria alone; however, biopsy confirmation of invasion is mandatory, and clinical decisions, based on colposcopic examinations alone, are inappropriate[3] (Fig. 9-9). Colposcopic evaluation of atypical smears in a background of severe cervical inflammation is difficult. Also, in lesions involving more than one cervical

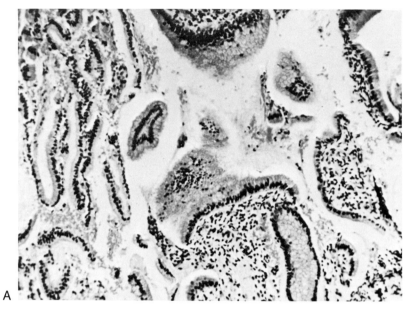

A

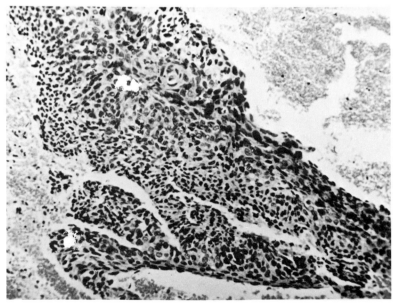

B

Fig. 9-10 Endocervical curettage specimens. **(A)** Normal columnar epithelium and bits of endocervix. **(B)** Fragment of poorly differentiated malignant squamous epithelium, whether carcinoma in situ or invasive carcinoma cannot be determined, therefore conization would be recommended unless invasive cancer had been found in a biopsy. (H&C, ×250.) (Shingleton HM, Orr JW Jr: Cancer of the Cervix: Diagnosis and Treatment. Churchill Livingstone, Edinburgh, 1987.)

quadrant, the inexperienced colposcopist may not appreciate the most appropriate area for biopsies and so the sampling problem may be the reason for underdiagnosis. Careful attention to the correlation of the cytologic, colposcopic, and biopsy findings is mandatory in order to succeed in making an accurate outpatient evaluation. The accuracy of the techniques is enhanced by liberal use of endocervical curettage to assess the status of the endocervical canal, which is not always accessible to direct view. Significant fragments of neoplastic epithelium, and especially those suggesting cervical intraepithelial neoplasia 3 (marked dysplasia – carcinoma in situ) or invasive carcinoma must be followed by conization of the cervix to ensure adequate tissue for proper diagnosis[2] (Fig. 9-10). With combined use of cervical cytology, colposcopy, cervical biopsies, and endocervical curettage for outpatient evaluation, serious error will be avoided in up to 99 percent of cases. A diagram is included to demonstrate steps in colposcopic evaluation (Fig. 9-11).

An experienced colposcopist should be able, in most cases, to distinguish preinvasive from invasive disease of the cervix, thus avoiding cervical biopsy in the pregnant patient (Fig. 9-12). The normal eversion of the cervix as the pregnancy progresses favors colposcopic evaluation and in most instances obviates the need for diagnostic conization during pregnancy. This is important, since conization may damage the cervix, risk abortion, or induce premature labor and is often associated with heavy bleeding.

Endometrial Cancer Detection and Screening

Endometrial cancer can be detected on an outpatient basis, both in symptomatic and in asymptomatic women. Endometrial biopsy may be performed with Novak, Duncan, or Kevorkian curettes. Endometrial tissue samples are preferred by most pathologists to cytologic samples for diagnosis of endometrial cancer.

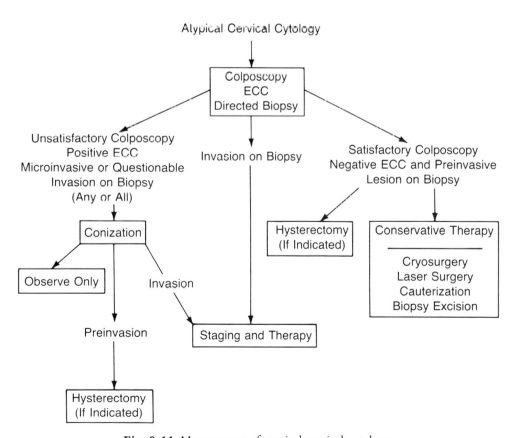

Fig. 9-11 Management of atypical cervical cytology.

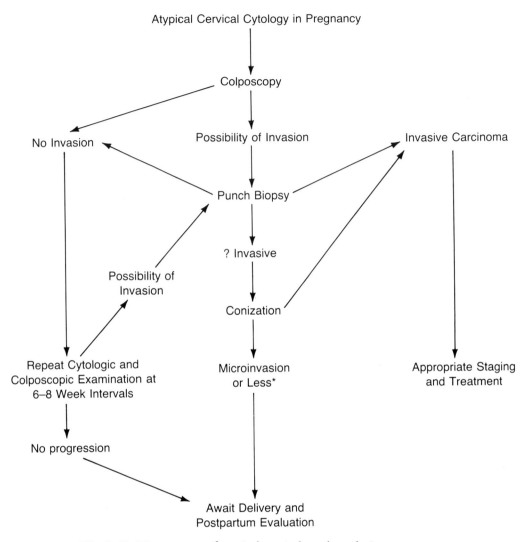

Fig. 9-12 Management of atypical cervical cytology during pregnancy.

Several commercial suction-aspiration biopsy instruments are available in addition to the above-mentioned curettes and provide superior samples, leading to high degrees of diagnostic accuracy[6] (Table 9-2). In the symptomatic patient, report of any cytologic or histologic abnormality short of a diagnosis of adenocarcinoma requires a fractional curettage to rule out focal invasive disease. For asymptomatic cases, detection of adenocarcinoma is more difficult, especially in postmenopausal women with stenotic endocervical canals. It is particularly important, however, to obtain periodic endometrial samples in women at high risk of endometrial cancer, especially those on exogenous estrogen therapy.

Specimen Handling

Visible lesions on the vulva may be evaluated by diagnostic biopsy or by excisional biopsy[3] (Fig. 9-3). A diagnostic biopsy should be taken from the area most suggestive of carcinoma. When a lesion is small, an excisional biopsy with a presumed clear skin margin may be indicated. The pathologist attempts to section such lesions in order to determine whether the

Table 9-2 Pooled Results in Diagnosis of Endometrial Cancer from a Number of Published Series Using Various Cytologic and Histologic Techniques of Endometrial Sampling

Technique	No. of Patients in Study	No. of Patients with Endometrial Cancer	Accuracy in Diagnosing Cancer (%)
Aspiration	12,480	331	88.5
Lavage	2,805	206	81.6
Endometrial brush	1,354	278	87.4
Jet wash			
Direct smear	2,258	90	86.7
Millipore filter	1,234	64	75.0
Cell block	4,701	184	87.5
Endometrial biopsy	1,679	445	87.4
Aspiration curettage	1,135	40	97.5

(Modified from Vuopala S: Diagnostic accuracy of the clinical application of cytological and histological methods for investigating endometrial carcinoma. II. Survey of the literature. Acta Obstet Gynaecol Scand 70(suppl):8, 1977.)

margins are histologically clear of tumor. In small lesions, this may be very difficult. Gross inspection may display what appears to be the closest margin, and this is given priority. With medium-size lesions removed within an ellipse of skin, a central cross section and blocks taken at right angles are used. Sometimes India ink is applied to margins, serving as a guide in the histologic sections to identify true surgical lines of excision.

Vaginal and cervical biopsies taken on the basis of grossly or colposcopically visible lesions should be labeled carefully as to site. An attempt should also be made for good orientation. The cucumber technique of Richart[7] is good if conscientiously applied, but it necessitates cooperation of pathologist and histotechnologist and a good understanding of what is being sought. Placing the biopsy flat on its deep surface on a piece of brown paper towel of the hard-surface type or on a square of Histowrap is another technique for making orientation easier after fixation (Fig. 9-13).

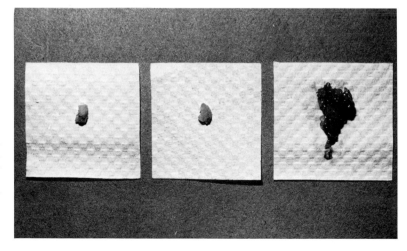

Fig. 9-13 Orientation of biopsy and curettage specimens. The tissue is placed on a 3 × 3-cm piece of paper towel or Telfa. Left: Cervical punch biopsy with deep surface on the paper towel. Middle: Cervical biopsy with cut edge on the paper towel. Right: Endocervical curettage.

Placing such a biopsy on its side is another technique, but it is less easy to orient consistently.

An endometrial biopsy is only a random sampling of the endometrium. When taken judiciously, it is useful for endometrial dating in infertility patients and may serve as a screening procedure to detect hyperplasia or carcinoma. As a screening method, the absence of hyperplasia or carcinoma on biopsy does not rule out such conditions. More extensive sampling of the endometrial cavity may be necessary. It should be realized that even endometrial curettage does not sample the entire endometrial surface. For practical purposes, it is accurate; a small adenocarcinoma within a hyperplastic endometrium that may be missed on curettage but found in a subsequent hysterectomy specimen has probably been adequately managed. Diagnostic curettings are always examined in their entirety and at several levels. Differential curettage, separating endometrial and endocervical curettings, is theoretically an excellent idea, but the findings should always be correlated with clinical observations. One must remember that endocervical tissue may be detached and included with endometrial curettings. Endometrial tumor may prolapse into the endocervical canal and be removed among endocervical curettings. The pathologist is well aware that isolated bits of adenocarcinoma not continuous with normal endometrium in an endometrial curettage may be a contaminant from the endocervix. On the other hand, to be sure that endocervix is involved when there is endometrial adenocarcinoma, it is necessary to find adenocarcinoma in recognizable endocervical tissue, not just lying detached among curetted bits of endocervix.

Endocervical curettings require careful handling. They should be applied carefully to a small paper towel square (about 3×3 cm) or to a piece of Histowrap or Telfa and lowered gently into a wide-mouthed container of fixative (Fig. 9-13). After fixation, they may be gently detached and pushed toward the center of this square, which is folded into an envelope and placed in the processing cassette. It is finally removed by the histotechnologist for embedding. The number of levels that should be made from such a block will depend on the concentration of material in the paraffin block. Whatever is found in the sections should be listed for evaluation of the adequacy of the endocervical curettings; for example, such curettings may appear abundant, but the tissue may be mostly endometrial with too little endocervical tissue in-

cluded for adequate evaluation. The pathologist can only report on what is seen. The clinician must determine whether the small fragments of atypical epithelium were really obtained from the endocervix or were perhaps a contaminant from the portio. This is an example of the importance of correlating colposcopic findings with histologic patterns.

Indications for Conization

Many believe that any patient with a positive endocervical curettage requires conization. When one gains experience, however, in evaluating endocervical curettage specimens and has the ability to examine the specimens or discuss them directly with an experienced pathologist, one can often avert conization in patients in whom only small fragments of mild or moderately dysplastic epithelium are contained in the curetted specimen. In order to avoid conization in this circumstance the colposcopist must have visualized the entire border of a colposcopic lesion; moreover, the cytologic diagnosis must agree — that is, not suggestive of invasive disease.

Colposcopists who do not have the ability to discuss each specimen directly with the pathologist should follow the general rule that positive endocervical curettings require conization for definitive diagnosis. Indications for conization of the cervix will vary with the experience of clinicians and their ability to correlate cytologic, colposcopic, and histologic findings. A cone may be diagnostic or both diagnostic and therapeutic. For this reason, the pathologist always treats a cone as potentially therapeutic and directs pathologic evaluation to include careful examination of lines of surgical excision[2] (Fig. 9-14).

Some patients have anatomic abnormalities of the cervix or upper vagina such that adequate examination of the cervix by colposcopy is prevented. Severe atrophy or infection at times may preclude adequate examination, and conization may be necessary. When there is a significant discrepancy among the cytologic report, colposcopic examination, and the biopsy diagnosis, a conization may be indicated, since the most important rule for a colposcopist is that there be no marked discrepancy in the three complementary techniques. The need for conization varies with the age of patients; at our colposcopy clinic, only about 2 percent of teenagers with atypical smears require conization while such a procedure is indicated in about one-

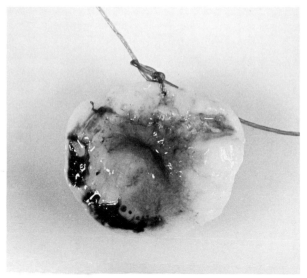

A

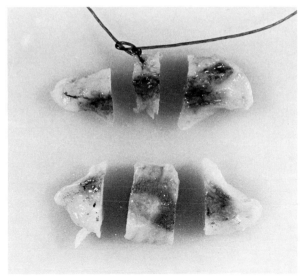

B

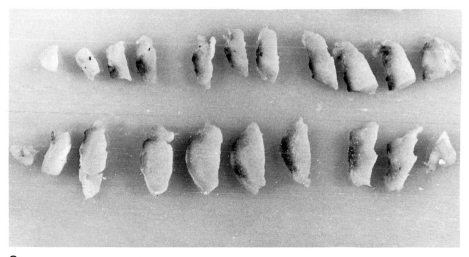

C

Fig. 9-14 Handling of conization specimen for optimal study. **(A)** The tie indicates the 12 o'clock position. **(B)** Cone is opened at the 3 and 9 o'clock positions. The central segment from each lip is complete from endocervix to portio margin. **(C)** Each of these segments is divided into blocks, taking care to preserve the lines of surgical excision. The lateral segments are also divided into blocks, realizing that only the portio margin is a line of surgical excision. (Technique of Hazel Gore.) (Shingleton HM, Orr JW Jr: Cancer of the Cervix: Diagnosis and Treatment. Churchill Livingstone, Edinburgh, 1987.)

third of women over the age of 50. This is explained by the tendency of neoplastic lesions to have endocervical locations in postmenopausal women with retraction of the squamocolumnar junction and the increased likelihood of higher-grade lesions of the cervix with advancing age.

Specialized Cytologic and Pathologic Techniques

In evaluating a pelvic mass, three pathologic techniques (short of examination of the excised mass) may be applied: fine-needle aspiration, needle biopsy, and

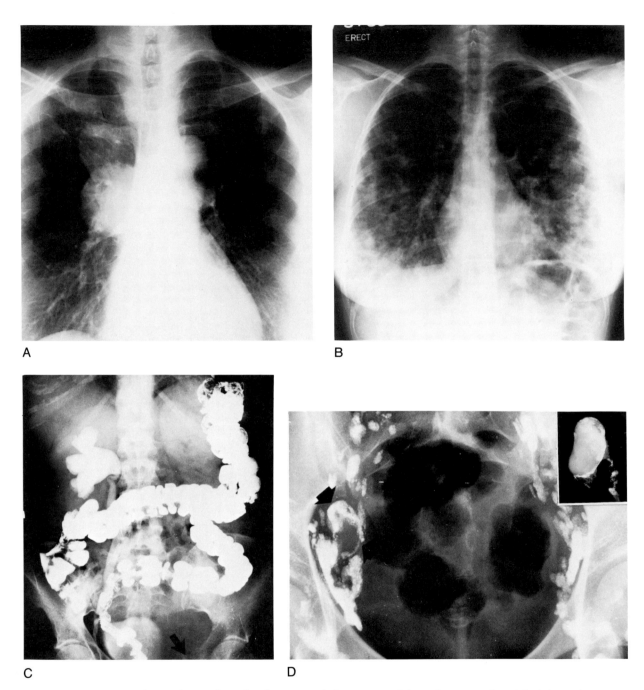

Fig. 9-15 Radiographic studies of malignancies. **(A)** PA view of chest, demonstrating right hilar and mediastinal involvement by metastatic cervical cancer. **(B)** Metastatic disease in chest of a woman with gestational trophoblastic disease. **(C)** Radiographic findings in a 44-year-old woman with advanced squamous cell cancer. The left kidney is nonvisualizing; note right hydronephrosis and hydroureter of a marked degree. A pelvic mass displaces the bladder and rectosigmoid to the right. In addition, bony invasion has occurred in the right pelvis (arrow). (Film courtesy of Dr. Larry Kilgore.) **(D)** Details of a lymphangiographic study of pelvic lymph nodes. A large right pelvic node (arrows) has a filling defect secondary to invasion by squamous cell carcinoma. The inset shows the same node after removal. **(A,C,D** from Shingleton HM, Orr JW Jr: Cancer of the Cervix: Diagnosis and Treatment. Churchill Livingstone, Edinburgh, 1987.)

scalpel biopsy. Fine-needle aspiration may be examined by smears stained by the Pap technique or by a cytospin technique similarly stained. Fine-needle aspiration is safe for evaluation of abdominal and pelvic masses, breast masses, and enlarged nodes. Fine-needle aspiration is a cost-effective, accurate, and safe procedure.[8] It can be performed on an outpatient procedure, yields results more rapidly than does surgical biopsy, and is particularly advantageous in view of diagnostic-related group reimbursement programs. The safety and accuracy of the technique have led to its use largely replacing surgical (scalpel) biopsies and needle biopsies. If indicated, other staining techniques may be applied for more specific identification. Should definite tissue be obtained during such a fine-needle aspiration, or if there is enough material to spin down for a cell block, such material may be examined by histologic techniques.

A needle biopsy of a mass may produce tissue for histologic evaluation. Fragments of tissue washed from the needle may be evaluated cytologically in conjunction with the histologic material. Biopsy by this technique may also be taken through a laparoscope or at laparotomy.

Peritoneal or pleural fluid or cyst contents may be aspirated and examined cytologically, as smears, as cytospin preparations, or as cell blocks. Such material should be delivered promptly to the laboratory, or a previous discussion with the pathologist should have produced instructions on how such material should be fixed (or when anticoagulants should be added to make such material suitable for processing in the laboratory). Such fluids produce a protein precipitate that makes processing difficult; therefore, most laboratories favor addition of anticoagulant if there is a delay in processing.

Radiographic Studies

The contribution of chest radiographs, intravenous pyelogram (IVP), and barium enema is apparent[2] (Fig. 9-15). While the diagnosis of any cancer requires tissue confirmation, pulmonary lesions consistent with metastases drastically change treatment planning. Such lesions also require cytologic or pathologic confirmation before treatment plans are determined or altered. An IVP showing obstruction or nonvisualization of the upper urinary tract constitutes a valid reason for upstaging cancer of the cervix and ureteral

obstruction is an ominous finding in any abdominopelvic malignancy. Barium enema is essential in the investigation of rectal bleeding and, together with such techniques as flexible colonoscopy or upper GI radiographic studies, is an integral part of the staging of abdominopelvic cancer of any type. Recently, computed tomography (CT) scans have contributed to diagnosis and staging, primarily in identifying abdominal masses, especially enlarged paraaortic and pelvic lymph nodes, and liver metastases (Fig. 9-16). Ultrasound scans, which are less expensive than CT scans, usually constitute confirmation of pelvic and abdominal masses and demonstrate whether such masses are cystic or solid. Cysts can be shown to be unilocular or multilocular (Fig. 9-17). Abdominopelvic CT scans and ultrasound scans are helpful when indicated but are requested excessively by clinicians. Physicians who prefer not to perform pelvic examinations (or who are not adept at performing them) often substitute abdominopelvic ultrasound scans or even CT scans for such examinations. While physical assessment in the form of pelvic examination is preferable and much cheaper, considerable numbers of abdominopelvic masses are detected on abdominal and pelvic ultrasound scans. Laparotomy may be necessary to evaluate women with such reported masses, although the techniques are not invariably accurate and the reports cannot always be accepted at face value.

Mammography is a safe and effective procedure that is recommended annually for women age 40 and over. A properly performed mammogram can detect at least 90 percent of breast cancers; occult tumors identified only by screening mammography are of low volume and have a low rate of axillary nodal metastases (Fig. 9-18). Thus, they have a better prognosis than do palpable breast cancers. The trend away from radical mastectomy as treatment of early tumors is a practical and important reason for women to avail themselves routinely of this diagnostic technique.

Magnetic resonance imaging (MRI) is being applied to abdominal and pelvic malignant disease. At this time, however, it has not been shown to be superior to CT or ultrasound scans and, since it is considerably more expensive, should be considered experimental. Ultimately, MRI may offer advantages over CT scans, since longitudinal as well as transverse cuts are possible with this technique. Identification of tumor within lymph nodes or its distinction from normal tissues within abdominal or pelvic organs by

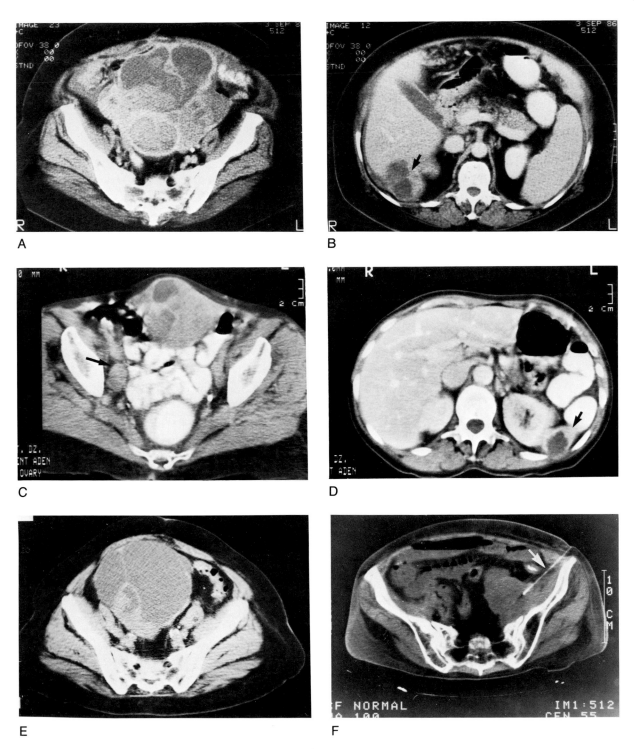

Fig. 9-16 Computed tomography (CT) scans of various malignancies. Advanced adenocarcinoma of endometrium **(A)** with extrauterine extention and **(B)** liver metastasis (arrow). **(C)** Clear cell ovarian adenocarcinoma involving abdominal wall and right pelvic nodes (arrow). **(D)** A parasplenic metastasis is present (arrow). **(E)** Retroperitoneal sarcoma presenting as a large solid/cystic pelvic mass. **(F)** Large pelvic nodal mass in advanced squamous cell carcinoma of the cervix. A long needle (arrow) is being used for aspiration cytology under CT scan guidance.

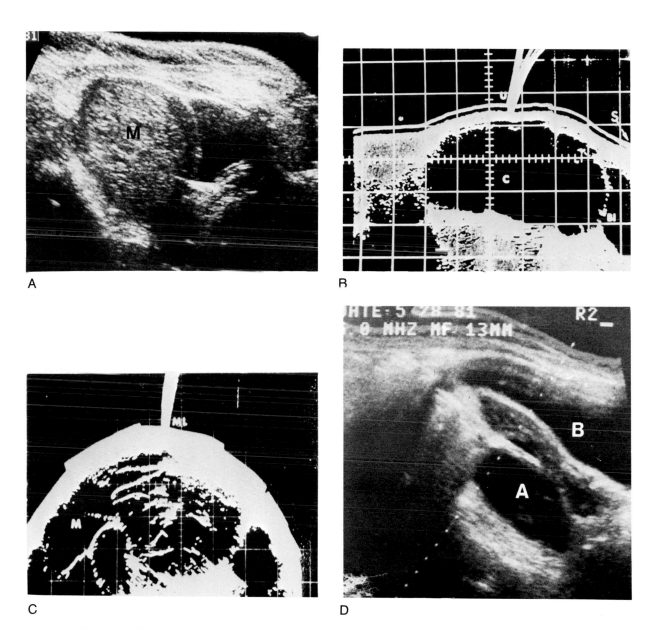

Fig. 9-17 Ultrasound scans of abdominopelvic masses. **(A)** Enlarged uterus containing the snowflake pattern of a molar pregnancy. M, mole. (Courtesy of Dr. Lincoln Berland.) **(B)** Longitudinal scan of a large mucinous cyst filling the abdomen. C, cyst; Bl, bladder; S, symphysis. **(C)** Transverse scan of a large multiloculated adenocarcinoma of the ovary. M, mass; M, midline. **(D)** Longitudinal midline ultrasound scan displaying a large abscess in the cul-de-sac in a patient with squamous cell carcinoma of the cervix. A, abscess; B, bladder.

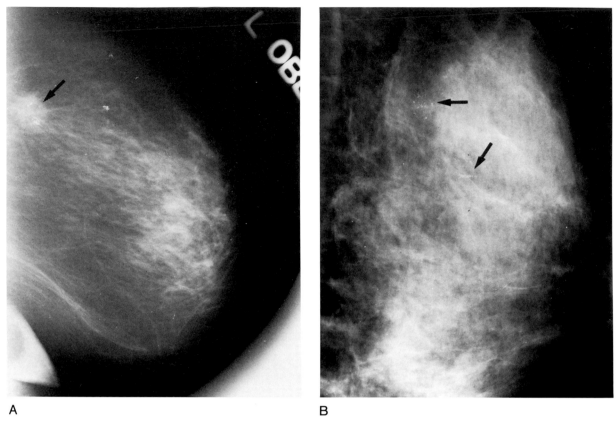

A   B

Fig. 9-18 (A) Mammogram demonstrating invasive duct cancer. A 16-m stellate tumor containing malignant calcification is seen (arrow). **(B)** Mammogram showing magnified view of two clusters of malignant microcalcification in tissue exhibiting in situ duct cancer. (Film courtesy of Dr. Eva Ruben.)

determining different densities of tissues was thought to be possible with this technique but is not yet established.

Serum and Tissue Markers

Among all the biochemical markers used for tumor diagnosis and monitoring of disease course in gynecologic cancers, the β-subunit of human chorionic gonadotrophin (β-hCG) in the management of gestational trophoblastic disease remains the best example. Following molar evacuation, women with hydatidiform moles are put under close surveillance with serum β-hCG determinations for 12 months. The titers of those undergoing spontaneous regression promptly fall to normal levels, whereas the titers of those whose disease persists either plateau at elevated levels or show serial elevation in β-hCG value. The use of the β-hCG serum assay, together with the availability of effective chemotherapeutic regimens, has made gestational trophoblastic tumors highly curable except in those patients in the high-risk metastatic categories. Khazaeli et al.[9] in 1986 reported a further development of the β-hCG serum assay; using a monoclonal antibody radioimmunassay (RIA) system that is only reactive with free β-hCG subunits dissociated from intact α-β-hCG molecules, these workers showed that the assay could accurately predict, at the time of uterine curettage, which women would undergo spontaneous regression and which would develop persistent disease. The significance of this work is that, subject to further confirmation of the preliminary findings, the free β-hCG assay could be used to identify the group who would benefit from prophylactic chemotherapy, using fewer courses of therapy than required if instituted once persistence has been established.

The continuous research and development of tumor markers for clinical applications have resulted in a number of new biochemical tests. In addition to the free β-hCG assay, the CA 125 and the squamous cell carcinoma (SCC) serum assays are two other techniques that have prompted field testings by gynecologic oncologists. Since 1983, reports by Bast,[10] Canney et al.,[11] Kerbs et al.,[12] and others have indicated that CA 125 is a sensitive and specific serum marker; serum CA 125 levels were found to correlate with disease progression and regression in most patients with epithelial nonmucinous ovarian malignancies. However, a subsequent report by Alvarez et al.[13] summarized our experience and showed that while rising CA 125 levels are a highly reliable indication of progressive disease, falling levels are not a reliable indication of tumor control. The study by Alvarez's group also showed that elevated CA 125 levels could be found in some mucinous as well as stromal and germ cell tumors. All published studies indicate that elevated CA 125 levels prior to second-look laporatomy are predictive of residual tumor and that rising CA 125 levels in follow-up is associated with, and predictive of, disease recurrence. A recent report by Bast[14] suggested that an elevated CA 125 level, in combination with an elevated level of either CA 15-3 or CA 72-3, is indicative of malignancy with a 98 percent specificity. This combined marker approach is also being tested for screening purposes.

The SCC antigen has been reported to be a serum marker for squamous cell carcinoma, especially that of the cervix. It is an antigenic subfraction of TA4, a tumor marker identified by a rabbit antiserum raised against purified tissue extract of cervical squamous cell carcinoma. Available data on the distribution of serum SCC antigen levels indicate that serum SCC levels are below 2.0 ng/ml in 95 percent of healthy subjects and in 94 percent of patients with benign diseases. In squamous cell carcinoma of the cervix, the frequency of elevation above 2.0 ng/ml increased with disease stage, being 16 percent in cervical dysplasia, 34 percent in stage I, 64 percent in stage II, 84 percent in stage III, 85 percent in stage IV, and 64 percent in recurrent disease. Holloway et al.,[15] at our laboratory, investigated the clinical value of serum SCC determinations in the management of patients with invasive squamous cell carcinoma of the cervix. In this pilot study, serum SCC levels were elevated in 67 percent of such patients (all stages included), and the levels were found to correlate with disease course.

The development of useful serum markers has been paralleled by research advances in tissue markers. In an immunohistochemical classification of germ cell tumors, Taylor et al.[16] showed that neither alphafetoprotein (AFP) nor hCG is present in pure germinoma or teratoma. Whereas both are present in embryonal carcinoma, AFP is present in endodermal sinus (yolk sac) tumor and hCG is present in choriocarcinoma. Immunohistochemical identification of these markers in tissue enables the use of the serum markers in follow-up management.

To et al.,[17] at our laboratory, reported in 1986 that the immunohistochemical expression of blood group ABH isoantigens on cervical tumor tissue is significantly related to patient survival. In cancer of the cervix, depth of stromal invasion, clinical lesion size, and lymph node involvement are three established clinicohistologic risk factors for tumor recurrence. Tumors with a depth of stromal invasion of more than 1.5 cm that are ABH negative were found to follow the most aggressive clinical course. The identification of potentially useful serum markers and clinicohistologic risk factors has opened up the possibility of applying closer surveillance to cervical cancer patients selectively identified at high risk of tumor recurrence.

Recommendations for Screening

General and specific recommendations for cancer detection evaluation of asymptomatic women are listed in Table 9-3. These recommendations are a composite of those of the American Cancer Society (ACS), the Division of Cancer Prevention of the National Cancer Institute (NCI), and our own ideas. The ACS recommendations (1980) met with considerable opposition from gyn-oncologists. The suggestion of smears every 3 years after two negative smears seems to de-emphasize the importance of yearly examination and was rejected by many physicians and groups such as the Society of Gynecologic Oncologists and the American College of Obstetricians and Gynecologists.

Our recommendations are related to women of various groups and apply to high-risk women as well as those at lesser risk. In regard to women at high risk of cervical and ovarian cancer, we believe that yearly pelvic examinations provide an opportunity for Pap smears as well as bimanual examinations, which may detect ovarian enlargements. Pelvic ultrasonography may be useful on an interval basis as well in screening

Table 9-3 Suggested Cancer Screening of Asymptomatic Women[a]

Recommendations	Age		
	20–40 Years	40–50 Years	≥50 Years
General			
Cancer-related checkup	3 years	Yearly	Yearly
Breast self-examination	Monthly	Monthly	Monthly
Specific			
Lymph nodes	3 years	Yearly	Yearly
Breast examination	3 years	Yearly	Yearly
Abdominal examination	3 years	Yearly	Yearly
Pelvic examination and Pap smear	Yearly[b]	Yearly	1–3 years
Digital rectal	—	Yearly	Yearly
Stool occult blood test	—	—	Yearly
Mammography	Baseline examination at age 35–50	1–3 years	Yearly
For high-risk women			
Pelvic examination and Pap smear (cervix/ovarian cancer)	Yearly[b]	Yearly	Yearly
Pelvic ultrasonography (ovarian cancer)	—	1–3 years	1–3 years
Proctoscopy, colonoscopy and/or barium enema (colorectal cancer)	—	2 or more evaluations	3–5 years after 2 neg. evaluations
CEA, CA 125 markers (colorectal/ovarian cancer)	—	Yearly	Yearly
Chest radiography (lung cancer)	—	Yearly	Yearly

CEA, carcinoembryonic antigen; Pap, Papanicolaou.
[a] These recommendations are a composite of those of the American Cancer Society, the Division of Cancer Prevention of the National Cancer Institute, and the present authors.
[b] Begin smears before age 20 if sexually active. The American Cancer Society recommends examination and Pap smears at 3-yearly intervals in this age group, except in high-risk women.

for ovarian lesions, particularly in obese women. At the time of the yearly examinations, CEA and CA 125 serum markers may be drawn and, if elevated, may lead to more intensive evaluation for colorectal or ovarian cancer, respectively. Yearly or interval chest radiographs are recommended for women over age 40 who are smokers, although the NCI makes no recommendation regarding screening for lung cancer. Primary prevention in the form of abstinence from tobacco use is the recommended policy position.

REFERENCES

1. Cavanagh D, Ruffolo EH, Marsden DE: Gynecologic Cancer: A Clinicopathologic Approach. Appleton-Century-Crofts, E. Norwalk, CT, 1969
2. Shingleton HM, Orr JW Jr: Cancer of the Cervix: Diagnosis and Treatment. Churchill Livingstone, Edinburgh, 1987
3. American Cancer Society: A Factbook for the Medical and Related Professions. Professional Education Publication. ACS, New York, 1986
4. Johnson LD: Dysplasia and carcinoma in situ in pregnancy. p. 382. In Norris HJ, Hertig AT, Abell MR (eds): The Uterus. Williams & Wilkins, Baltimore, 1973
5. Shingleton HM, Hatch KD, Orr JW Jr, et al: Diagnosis and treatment of preinvasive and microscopically invasive squamous cell carcinoma of the cervix. Cancer Bull 35(4):172, 1983
5a. Walton RJ: The task force on cervical cancer screening programmes. (Editorial.) Can Med Assoc J 143:981, 1976
6. Vuopala S: Diagnostic accuracy of the clinical application of cytological and histological methods for investigating endometrial carcinoma. II. Survey of the literature. Acta Obstet Gynaecol Scand 70(suppl):8, 1977
7. Richart RM: The handling of small tissue samples for pathologic examination. Bull Sloane Hosp Women 9:113, 1963
8. Bottles K, Miller TR, Cohen MB, Ljung B-M: Fine

needle aspiration biopsy: Has its time come? Am J Med 81:525, 1986

9. Khazaeli MB, Hedayat MM, Hatch KD, et al: Radioimmunoassay for free Beta HCG assay for early detection of persistent trophoblastic disease. Am J Obstet Gynecol 155:320, 1986

10. Bast RC Jr, Klug TL, St John E, et al: A radioimmunoassay using a monoclonal antibody to monitor the course of epithelial ovarian cancer. N Engl J Med 309:883, 1983

11. Canney PA, Moore M, Wilkinson PM, James RD: Ovarian cancer antigen CA125: A prospective clinical assessment of its role as a tumor marker. Br J Cancer 50:765, 1984

12. Krebs HB, Goplerud DR, Myers M, et al: The role of CA125 as tumor marker in ovarian carcinoma. Obstet Gynecol 67(4):473, 1986

13. Alvarez RD, To ACW, Boots LR, et al: CA125 as an indicator for poor prognosis in ovarian malignancies. Gynecol Oncol 26:284, 1987

14. Bast RC Jr: Pros and cons of tumor markers. National Conference on Gynecologic Cancer. American Cancer Society, New York, 1986

15. Holloway RW, To ACW, Boots LR, et al: The clinical utility of the serum SCC antigen radioimmunoassay in the management of patients with invasive squamous cell carcinoma of the cervix. Obstet Gynecol in press

16. Taylor CR, Kurman RJ, Warner NE: The potential value of immunohistologic techniques in the classification of ovarian and testicular tumors. Hum Pathol 9:417, 1978

17. To ACW, Gore H, Shingleton HM, et al: Lymph node metastases in cancer of the cervix: A preliminary report. Am J Obstet Gynecol 155:388, 1986

SUGGESTED READINGS

American Cancer Society: Mammography: Two statements of the American Cancer Society. Professional Education Publication. ACS, New York, 1986

Bibbo M, Rice AM, Wied GL, et al: Comparative specificity and sensitivity of routine cytologic examinations and the Gravlee jet wash technic for diagnosis of endometrial changes. Obstet Gynecol 43:352, 1974

Birnholz JC, Barnes AB: Early diagnosis of hydatidiform mole by ultrasound imaging. JAMA 225:1359, 1973

Bolten KA: p. 43. In Introduction to Colposcopy. Grune & Stratton, New York, 1960

Cartier R: p. 89. In Practical Colposcopy. S. Karger AG, Geneva, 1977

Casper S, van Nagell JR Jr, Powell DF, et al: Immunohistochemical localization of tumor markers in epithelial ovarian cancer. Am J Obstet Gynecol 149:154, 1984

Cohen CJ, Gusberg SB, Koffler D: Histologic screening for endometrial cancer. Gynecol Oncol 2:279, 1974

DiSaia P, Morrow CP, Haverback BJ, Dyce BJ: Carcinoembryonic antigen in cervical and vulvar cancer patients: Serum levels and disease progress. Obstet Gynecol 47:95, 1976

DiSaia P, Haverback BJ, Dyce BJ, Morrow CP: Carcinoembryonic antigen in patients with gynecologic malignancies. Am J Obstet Gynecol 121:159, 1975

DiSaia P, Haverback BJ, Dyce BJ, Morrow M: Carcinoembryonic antigen in patients with squamous cell carcinoma of the cervix uteri and vulva. Surg Gynecol Obstet 138:542, 1974

Goldenberg DM, Pletsch QA, Van Nagell JR Jr: Characterization and localization of carcinoembryonic antigen in squamous cell carcinoma of the cervix. Gynecol Oncol 4:204, 1976

Gusberg SB, Frick HC II (eds): Corscaden's Gynecologic Cancer. 5th Ed. Williams & Wilkins, Baltimore, 1978

Hacker NF: Breast disease: A gynecologic perspective. p. 350. In Hacker NH, Moore JG (eds): Essentials of Obstetrics and Gynecology. WB Saunders, Philadelphia, 1986

Hofmeister FJ: Endometrial biopsy, another look. Am J Obstet Gynecol 118:722, 1974

Jones KK: Feminization, virilization, and precocious sexual development that results from neoplastic processes. Ann NY Acad Sci 230:195, 1974

Jordan JA: Colposcopy in the diagnosis of cervical cancer and precancer. Clin Obstet Gynecol 12:67, 1985

Kato H, Tamai K, Magaya T, et al: Clinical value of SCC-antigen, a subfraction of tumor antigen TA-4, in the management of cervical cancer. Gann No Rinsho (Jpn) 31(suppl 6):594, 1985

Kerr-Wilson RHJ, Shingleton HM, Orr JW Jr, Hatch KD: The use of ultrasound and CT scanning in the management of gynecologic malignancies. Gynecol Oncol 18:54, 1984

Kobayashi M: Use of diagnostic ultrasound in trophoblastic neoplasms and ovarian tumors. Cancer 38:441, 1976

Kolstad P, Stafl A: Atlas of Colposcopy. University Park Press, Baltimore, 1972

National Cancer Institute: The cancer letter. J Natl Cancer Inst 12(37):3, 1986

Richart RM: Natural history of cervical intraepithelial neoplasia. Clin Obstet Gynecol 5:748, 1968

Silverberg E: Statistical and epidemiological information on gynecologic cancer. Statistical Information Service, Department of Epidemiology and Statistics, Department of Research. American Cancer Society, New York, 1986

10

Vulvar Dystrophy and Neoplasia

Gunter Deppe
W. Dwayne Lawrence

VULVAR DYSTROPHY

According to the International Society for the Study of Vulvar Disease (ISSVD), vulvar dystrophies are divided into three categories.[1]

CLASSIFICATION OF VULVAR DYSTROPHIES

1. Hyperplastic dystrophy
   A. Without atypia
   B. With atypia
      a. Mild
      b. Moderate
      c. Severe
2. Lichen sclerosus
3. Mixed dystrophy (lichen sclerosus with foci of epithelial hyperplasia)
   A. Without atypia
   B. With atypia
      a. Mild
      b. Moderate
      c. Severe

This classification groups the plethora of confusing and often overlapping conditions that exist in the literature into two types, hyperplastic dystrophy and lichen sclerosus; the third type consists of coexisting lesions of the first two varieties. On gross examination, the vulvar dystrophies often appear as thick white plaque(s). Clinically, such lesions are denoted as leukoplakia (literally "white patch"); the term is used properly to describe a gross condition only and defines no histologic entity. On microscopic examination, typical hyperplastic vulvar dystrophies show a variably thick superficial layer of parakeratotic or hyperkeratotic squamous epithelium, the histologic counterpart of leukoplakia. Hyperplastic and mixed dystrophies may exhibit no cytologic abnormalities, or they may show variable degrees of atypia graded as mild, moderate, or severe. In those without cellular atypia, the squamous epithelium has a hyperplastic appearance. The rete ridges are elongated, complex, and thickened; mitotic figures may be numerous in the lower levels of the epithelium. Nuclei appear bland. A chronic inflammatory infiltrate commonly is present (Fig. 10-1).

As with the hyperplastic varieties of vulvar dystrophy, lichen sclerosus often is accompanied by leukoplakia (Fig. 10-2). In addition, however, the lesions of lichen sclerosus are frequently associated with la-

223

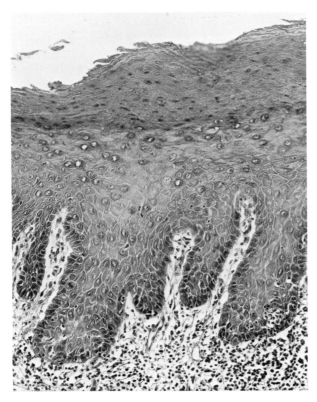

Fig. 10-1 Hyperplastic dystrophy without atypia. A thick layer of parakeratotic squamous cells overlies elongated and irregular rete ridges. Numerous chronic inflammatory cells are present in the dermis. (H&E, ×30.)

bial atrophy, particularly of the labia minora. Lichen sclerosus has a distinctive histologic appearance. The squamous epithelium is usually, but not invariably, thin, and rete ridges are flattened. The dermis has a highly characteristic bandlike zone of pale homogeneous tissue in which elastic fibers are scarce or absent. A dense lymphocytic infiltrate frequently borders the homogeneous zone. Hyperkeratosis may be a prominent feature (Fig. 10-3). Pigment, within both melanocytes and keratinocytes, is absent, contributing to the gray or white appearance of the vulvar skin on clinical examination.

Mixed dystrophy occurs when hyperplastic dystrophy and lichen sclerosus are present simultaneously on the vulva. This condition represents approximately one-fifth of vulvar dystrophies and may be more refractory to treatment than the pure forms.

Treatment

Inspection with magnification under bright light or colposcopy is helpful in the work-up.

VULVAR NEOPLASMS: DIAGNOSTIC METHODS

History

Inspection

Palpation

Colposcopy

Toluidine blue

Cytology

Biopsy

The toluidine blue test emphasizes for possible biopsy the suspicious ("blue") areas that may represent dystrophy.[2]

TOLUIDINE BLUE TEST

1. Clean vulva of lubricant or powder.
2. Paint vulva with 1 percent aqueous solution of toluidine blue.
3. After 3 minutes, rinse vulva with 1 percent acetic acid.

The toluidine blue test is not a cancer test; it merely confirms the presence of surface nuclei that bind the dye. A false-positive test may occur with any break in the continuity of the uppermost epithelial layers. The diagnosis depends on histologic examination of a representative biopsy specimen.

Vulvar biopsies are best done with a Reyes cutaneous punch, available in various sizes (Fig. 10-4). Following infiltration of the vulvar skin with a local anesthetic, 1 percent lidocaine (Xylocaine), the Reyes punch is pushed against the area to be biopsied and a circular area of skin is coned out. The skin plug is

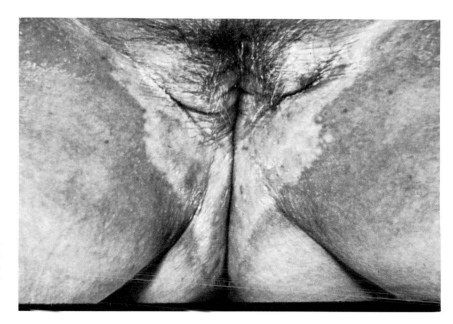

Fig. 10-2 Lichen sclerosus. The lesion shows leukoplakia and a symmetric distribution that extends to involve the inner thighs, perineum, and buttocks. The labia appear atrophic.

lifted with Adson forceps and cut out with a small scissors. The skin defect is closed either with a single figure-of-eight 3-0 Vicryl suture or left open. Monsel's solution or application of pressure usually controls bleeding.

The management of patients with vulvar dystrophies includes the elimination of contributing factors, such as vaginitis and excessive sweating and the use of deodorants, perfumes, douches, irritating soaps, detergents, powders, and nonabsorbtive underclothing.

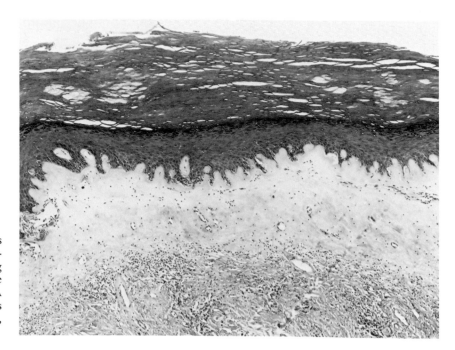

Fig. 10-3 The epidermis shows a thick layer of parakeratotic cells and an underlying pale homogeneous bandlike zone in the superficial dermis. A sprinkling of lymphocytes is seen below the latter. (H&E, ×12.)

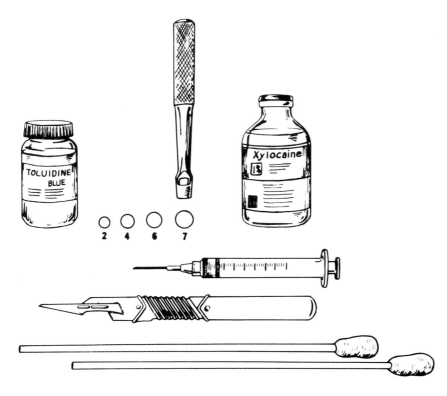

Fig. 10-4 Outpatient vulvar biopsy set.

Once the histopathologic diagnosis is established, treatment is as summarized below.

TOPICAL TREATMENT OF VULVAR DYSTROPHIES

Hyperplastic dystrophy	→ fluorinated hydrocortisone cream
Lichen sclerosus et atrophicus	→ 2% testosterone cream
Mixed dystrophy	→ Initial hydrocortisone/ long-term testosterone cream

---

Hyperplastic dystrophy without atypia is treated best with a twice-daily application of topical corticosteroid preparation (e.g., 0.5 percent hydrocortisone, Lidex ointment, Valisone).

For the prompt relief of pruritis, local twice-daily therapy with a cream consisting of seven parts fluorinated corticosteroid and three parts crotamiton is recommended. A 2 percent mixture of testosterone propionate in petrolatum jelly applied twice daily produces a 90 percent response rate in patients with lichen sclerosus. Control of symptoms may require applications for several months. Once pruritis abates and the disease appears to be controlled, applications of testosterone cream can be decreased initially to once daily, then to once weekly. The disease usually recurs if maintenance therapy is discontinued.

Progesterone in oil, 100 mg/ounce in a cream base, used twice daily, may be substituted when patients are unable to tolerate the side effects of testosterone (e.g., hirsutism, clitoral hypertrophy, voice change).

Mixed dystrophy may be treated by twice-daily applications of a hydrocortisone/testosterone mixture or by first treating with hydrocortisone cream for several weeks until cured, then substituting a maintenance testosterone treatment regimen for the hydrocortisone treatment. Vulvar dystrophies with variable degrees of atypia should be treated similarly.[3-7] Atypical areas should be sampled thoroughly and carefully watched on a regular 3-month basis to avoid over-looking the subsequent development of vulvar neoplasia.

VULVAR INTRAEPITHELIAL NEOPLASIA

Like the vulvar dystrophies, intraepithelial squamous cell carcinoma of the vulva has been designated by several terms. Perhaps the most common and widely used is Bowen's disease; others include erythroplasia of Queyrat and carcinoma simplex. More recently, in keeping with the widely accepted concept of cervical intraepithelial neoplasia, some investigators prefer the term vulvar intraepithelial neoplasia.[8,9] Using this classification, grades I and II represent mild and moderate dysplasia, respectively; the more severely dysplastic lesions and carcinoma in situ are combined under the designation grade III. The ISSVD has recommended, however, that previously popular eponyms be discarded and replaced simply by the term carcinoma in situ.

The most common symptom of vulvar carcinoma in situ is pruritis; nevertheless, one-third of patients may be asymptomatic. Carcinoma in situ frequently presents as a plaquelike lesion that may be white, red, or even darkly pigmented (Fig. 10-5). Some investigators have noted that approximately one-third of patients with vulvar carcinoma in situ have hyperpigmentation and that the latter are the second most common cause of vulvar pigmented lesions.[10]

In recent years, the incidence of carcinoma in situ of the vulva apparently has been increasing; furthermore, nearly 50 percent of such patients are in the 20- to 40-year age group, and approximately one-third of the affected patients have associated papillomavirus infection of the cervix, vagina, and vulva.

The precise potential of vulvar carcinoma in situ for invasion is unclear; however, important risk factors appear to be advanced age and immunosuppression. Older patients have a higher risk of developing invasive cancer. A literature review by Friedrich et al.[11] demonstrated that 30 percent of patients with carcinoma in situ of the vulva had antecedent or concomitant malignancies of other body sites; approximately 15 percent of patients had associated carcinoma in situ of the cervix.

In assessing the degree of severity of vulvar intraepithelial neoplasia, several histologic parameters are evaluated: the level (lower, middle, upper third) of involvement by atypical squamous cells, the degree of cellular crowding, nuclear atypicality, and mitotic activity, including both typical and atypical forms. In

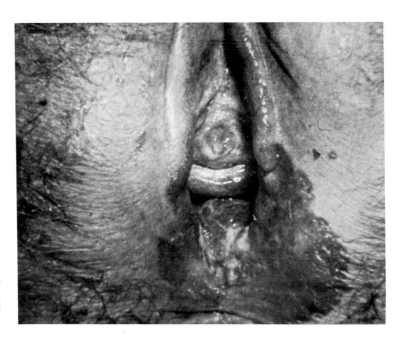

Fig. 10-5 Carcinoma in situ. A well-demarcated plaquelike erythematous lesion involves the labia and extends onto the fourchette.

carcinoma in situ (vulvar intraepithelial neoplasia type III), there is virtually full-thickness involvement of the squamous epithelium by densely crowded squamous cells showing loss of polarity, high nucleocytoplasmic ratios, enlarged nuclei containing coarsely clumped chromatin, and numerous, often atypical, mitotic figures involving the full epithelial thickness. Multinucleation, as well as giant cell formation, may be seen. These features are assessed in the squamous epithelium deep to the granular layer, above which is often a thick layer of hyperkeratotic or parakeratotic squamous cells (Fig. 10-6).

Treatment

A variety of treatments are available. Therapy of these lesions must be individualized, depending on the patient's age and extent of involvement. All therapeutic modalities have been successful in most patients and have similar recurrence rates regardless of treatment used. Wide local excision with at least 1 cm clear margins around the suspicious areas is acceptable treatment for individual lesions and permits histopathologic characterization of the specimen.[12,13]

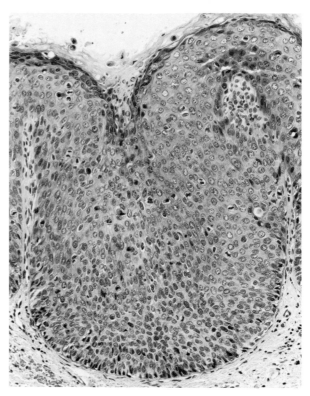

Fig. 10-6 Carcinoma in situ—vulvar intraepithelial neoplasia III. Virtually the entire epithelium is replaced by squamous cells with loss of polarity as well as crowding and mitotic activity in all levels of the epithelium. Superficially, a dark granular cell layer is immediately subjacent to a layer of hyperkeratotic cells. (H&E, ×30.)

TREATMENT MODALITIES FOR
VULVAR INTRAEPITHELIAL NEOPLASIA

Vulvectomy

Skinning vulvectomy

Local excision

Topical 5-fluorouracil cream

Cryosurgery

CO_2 laser

Patients with diffuse lesions may be managed with multiple wide local excision or a skinning vulvectomy with split-thickness skin graft.[14-16] A vulvectomy with loss of the clitoris is unnecessary, since that procedure has not decreased the recurrence rate of approximately 30 percent.

Local chemotherapy, consisting of 5 percent fluo-rouracil cream[17-19] or bleomycin,[20] and topical immunotherapy with dinitrochlorobenzene (DNCB), has been used.[21,22] The side effects of both these regimens include pronounced local irritation and painful ulcerations. Although the results have not met expectations, approximately 50 percent of patients demonstrate a complete response.

Cryosurgery may be used for small lesions, but the CO_2 laser is the method of choice for local tissue destruction. The CO_2 laser offers nonmutilating treatment with good cosmetic and functional results.[23-30] As with local chemotherapy, adequate biopsies of all suspicious areas are mandatory prior to laser therapy.

Laser evaporation should be performed to a depth of only 3 mm with 2.0-mm spot diameter and 20-W continuous time. Baggish[23] recommends Bioclusive

Table 10-1 Postoperative Regimen Following Laser Evaporation of Vulvar Intraepithelial Neoplasia

Therapy	Instruction	Frequency
Sitz baths	Ocean water (dissolved sea salts in tap water)	Four times/day
Betadine solution	Dilute 1 : 4 with water; squirt on perineum	After urination or defecation
Electric hair dryer	Dry vulva after sitz baths, showers, baths, or irrigation	As needed

(Modified from Baggish MS: Basic and Advanced Laser Surgery in Gynecology. Appleton-Century-Crofts, E. Norwalk, CT, 1985.)

(Johnson & Johnson) urethane dressing following laser evaporation. For undressed wounds, his recommendations are outlined on Table 10-1.

Whatever the choice of treatment modality, close follow-up is crucial. Because of the multifocal nature of this disease, the entire lower genital tract requires careful evaluation. Biopsies should be taken whenever a suspicious lesion is detected on follow-up examination.

VULVAR CONDYLOMA

Vulvar condyloma, or condyloma acuminata, commonly known as genital warts, is probably the most frequently encountered benign vulvar lesion, especially in females of reproductive age. Highly contagious and sexually transmitted, condyloma acuminata also frequently affects the vagina, perineum, perianal area, and cervix; in the latter, they more commonly take the form of flat lesions, hence the designation flat condyloma. The etiologic agent of condyloma acuminatum is the human papillomavirus, which has a predilection to involve stratified squamous epithelium, sparing neither epidermis nor moist squamous mucosa. In these areas, the lesions may grow as single, but usually multiple, small, soft, papillary excrescences; lesions tend to spread and coalesce to form larger verruciform masses (Fig. 10-7). With time, and especially under the influence of pregnancy, condyloma acuminata may grow to cover virtually the entire external genitalia. Large cauliflower-like condyloma must be differentiated from verrucous carcinoma of the vulva.

On microscopic examination, the typical condyloma acuminatum is shown to be composed of fronds of fibrous tissue thrown into fingerlike projections and covered by a thickened hyperplastic squamous epithelium (Fig. 10-8). The squamous cells forming the latter are well differentiated, and intercellular bridges are often prominent. Hyperkeratosis and parakeratosis are frequently seen, and mitotic figures may be numerous. Koilocytes, squamous cells with wrinkled convoluted nuclei and perinuclear clear zones (halos), are present in the mid- and superficial portions of the acanthotic epithelium. Koilocytes are virtually pathognomonic of human papillomavirus infection, although caution must be exercised in the diagnosis, since other conditions infrequently may result in perinuclear halos.

Special investigative techniques provide overwhelming confirmation of human papillomavirus within condyloma acuminata; ultrastructural studies have demonstrated virions, immunohistochemical studies have shown antibodies against human papillomavirus structural proteins, and DNA hybridization studies have found human papillomavirus DNA, all within the squamous cell nuclei of condylomas. Such investigations have virtually eliminated all doubt that human papillomavirus is the causative agent of condyloma acuminatum.

Given the well-known oncogenic potential of human papillomavirus, it is not surprising that much speculation has arisen over its role in the genesis of vulvar intraepithelial neoplasia as well as invasive squamous cell carcinoma and so-called verrucous carcinoma of the vulva. Recent research has provided ample evidence of an association between human papillomavirus and vulvar intraepithelial neoplasia;[8,9,32] more than two-thirds of vulvar intraepithelial

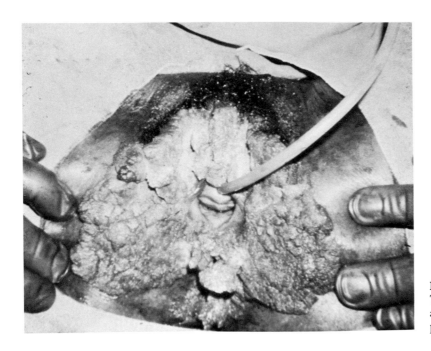

Fig. 10-7 Condyloma acuminata. The entire vulva, perineum, and perianal areas are covered by soft verrucous papillary lesions.

neoplasia lesions show cytologic features of human papillomavirus effect, and one-half to two-thirds can be shown by immunohistochemical means to stain positively for the structural proteins of human papillomavirus. In the report by Daling et al.,[33] epidemiologic studies strongly suggested a causal relationship between condyloma acuminatum and vulvar squamous cell carcinoma. Indeed, microspectrophotometrically proven aneuploid areas may occur within otherwise normal-appearing and polyploid condylomas; aneuploidy is generally associated with malignant epithelia, and its presence may represent foci of malignant transformation within otherwise benign condylomas.

BOWENOID PAPULOSIS

A relatively recently described entity that may affect the vulva is bowenoid papulosis.[34-36] Although the condition was first described in the skin of the penis,[37] lesions may involve the genital and perigenital skin of both sexes.

The vulvar and perivulvar skin involved by bowenoid papulosis usually exhibits multiple dome-shaped papules or plaques, measuring 1 to 10 mm in diameter (Fig. 10-9). Although the lesions of bowenoid papulosis have a characteristically violaceous hue, they also may vary from pink to red-brown to black; they are frequently grouped in linear or annular configurations.

On microscopic examination, the lesions of bowenoid papulosis are characterized by lack of full-thickness involvement by atypical squamous cells, vacuolated keratinocytes, numerous typical mitotic figures (often in metaphase), and hyperkeratosis or parakeratosis. Dark inclusion-like bodies surrounded by a clear halo may be seen in the stratum corneum and impart a salt-and-pepper appearance to the epithelium on low-power examination. A frequently cited diagnostic difference between bowenoid papulosis and carcinoma in situ is the lack of extension into pilosebaceous units in the former.[38]

Bowenoid papulosis currently is thought to represent a benign reactive disease that is self-limited and that may undergo spontaneous regression.[34] The etiology of bowenoid papulosis is unclear; however, some workers favor a viral etiology, as studies have found evidence of herpes simplex virus type 2 (HSV-2) in some and human papillomavirus in others.[35,38] In one recent study, human papillomavirus common antigens were demonstrated in almost three-fourths of cases examined.[35] Furthermore, re-

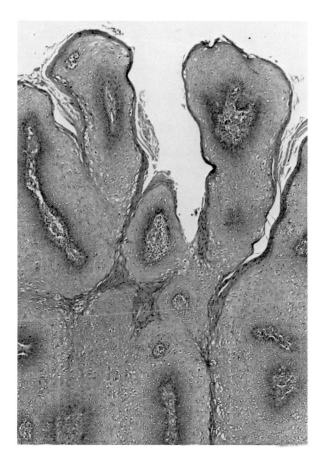

Fig. 10-8 Vulvar condyloma. The epidermis is thrown into fingerlike projections covered by hyperplastic squamous epithelium. Koilocytes with paranuclear halos can be seen in the upper layers of the epithelium. (H&E, ×12.)

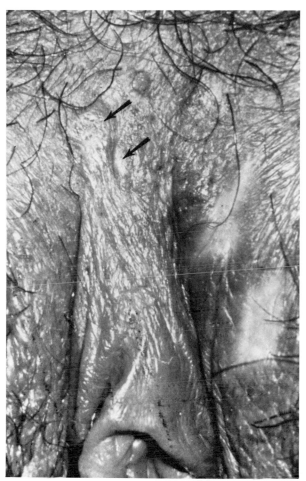

Fig. 10-9 Bowenoid papulosis. Slightly elevated ill-defined gray-blue plaques (arrows) are present near the clitoral hood. Gray-white areas on the left represent sites of previous biopsy for similar lesions.

cent studies have demonstrated human papillomavirus serotypes 16 and 18 in penile lesions of bowenoid papulosis;[36,39] such serotypes in the cervix have been designated high-risk serotypes due to their frequent association with invasive squamous cell carcinoma. More study is needed to determine whether an analogous situation exists in lesions of bowenoid papulosis occurring in the female genital tract.

The pathologist should be informed of the clinical presentation and gross appearance of the lesion(s), especially if there is clinical suspicion of bowenoid papulosis, to avoid both clinical and pathologic errors in diagnosis and consequent mismanagement of the patient. Surgical excision or local destructive methods appear to be adequate treatment for this condition.[38]

PAGET'S DISEASE

Paget's disease of the vulva, or extramammary Paget's disease, might be classified as a special form of vulvar intraepithelial neoplasia. It is essentially a dermatologic disorder, occurring most commonly in the nipple, but also in extramammary sites including the vulvar, perianal, and axillary skin.[40] Although mammary Paget's disease frequently is accompanied by an underlying carcinoma of the breast, extramammary forms are less often joined by an underlying carcinoma (20 percent). In addition, other carcinomas, such as breast, vaginal, cervical, and gastrointestinal

(GI) adenocarcinomas, may be concomitants of extramammary Paget's disease. The former occur with enough frequency that some physicians carry out appropriate exclusionary tests after the diagnosis of vulvar Paget's disease is made.

Typically, the gross lesions of vulvar Paget's disease are thickened, red, velvety, and soft with apparently well-demarcated borders (Fig. 10-10). Spots of excoriation and an eczematoid scaly appearance may be present. Although the disease generally involves the hair-bearing portions of the vulva first, it may extend to the perianal area and into the vagina. Pruritis, soreness, and burning are the most frequent symptoms, and extensive vulvar involvement may cause persistent tissue weeping. Patient- and physician-related

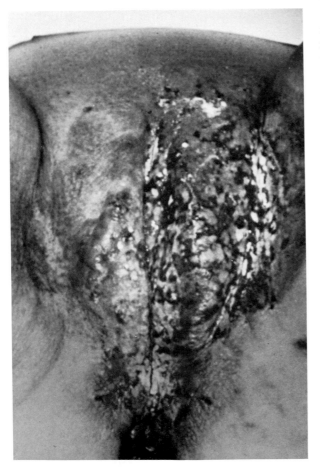

Fig. 10-10 Paget's disease. The vulvar, perineal, and perianal areas are thickened by red, velvety soft lesions with fairly well demarcated borders.

delay in establishing the diagnosis of Paget's disease is common. Clinically, the differential diagnosis of Paget's disease includes nonspecific dermatitis and candidiasis. Paget's disease may be suspected on the basis of gross inspection alone, but a vulvar biopsy is mandatory for accurate histologic diagnosis.

On microscopic examination, the squamous epithelium contains characteristic large, round to oval cells with abundant pale cytoplasm (Paget cells); nuclei may be vesicular or hyperchromatic and mitotic figures are usually rare to absent (Fig. 10-11). The Paget cells are found either singly or in nests within the epithelium and may extend deeply into hair shafts and accessory adnexal structures. Mucin stains differentiate Paget cells from those of amelanotic malignant melanoma; only the former stain positively for intracytoplasmic mucin.

Paget cells tend to infiltrate the epidermis laterally in a manner similar to the radial growth phase of malignant melanoma. Consequently, careful evaluation of the surgical margins of resection in a case of Paget's disease is of utmost importance. It must be remembered, however, that isolated nests or single Paget cells may be present in skin that appears grossly normal. Clear margins of resection are therefore no guarantee that Paget's disease will not recur, an occurrence that is not uncommon.

Treatment

The aim of surgical treatment is to remove the entire lesion with free margins and to exclude an occult underlying adenocarcinoma of the sweat glands. If the metastatic workup is negative, excision of the entire visible lesion is required; frequently, accomplishment of this goal necessitates a vulvectomy. The excision should extend at least 3 cm beyond the margins of the visible lesion and deep enough into the subcutaneous fat (down to the Colles fascia of the vulva) to include all adnexal structures.

Microscopic examination often demonstrates involvement of vulvar skin to be far greater than is apparent on gross examination of the lesion. Involved skin may appear unremarkable on gross examination, so that frozen sections are helpful in determining the free margins of resection. Since free surgical margins to not exclude the possibility of recurrence, patients should be followed closely and undergo careful examinations every 4 to 6 months.

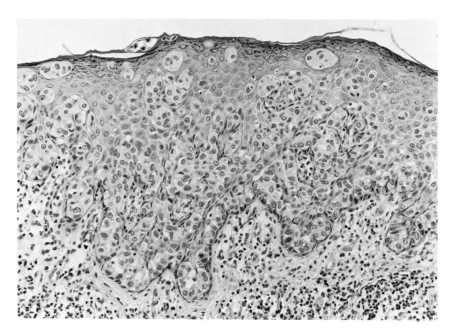

Fig. 10-11 Paget's disease. The squamous epithelium contains numerous large round to oval cells with pale cytoplasm (Paget cells). Cells invade the epidermis confluently, in small clusters, or as single cells. (H&E, ×30.)

Recurrent Paget's disease without underlying adenocarcinoma can be treated by repeat surgical excision, topical bleomycin, topical 5-fluorouracil (5-FU), or CO_2 laser vaporization.[4,41] If invasive adenocarcinoma of the sweat glands is present, a radical vulvectomy with bilateral inguinal-femoral lymphadenectomy should be performed. Pelvic lymphadenectomy or irradiation of the pelvic lymph nodes should be considered if metastatic tumor is found in the groin lymph nodes.

MICROINVASIVE SQUAMOUS CELL CARCINOMA

The rationale for recognizing such a category of squamous cell carcinoma is to define a specific population of women with small cancers that can be treated conservatively without significant risk of metastasis and death. Some observers believe that the incidence of vulvar intraepithelial neoplasia and invasive vulvar squamous cell carcinoma, including microinvasive forms, is increasing and is accompanied by a decrease in the average age at diagnosis.[42,43] Such figures offer ample justification for segregation of women, especially younger women, with tumors amenable to conservative surgery, sparing them the physical and psychological trauma of radical surgery. There is,

however, no currently accepted pathologic definition of vulvar microinvasive carcinoma. Attempts to compare survival of patients with microinvasive carcinoma in different series from the literature are hampered by several problems; among the histopathologic ones are (1) failure to state the reference point from which the measurement was taken, (2) confusion over the definition of vascular channels as well as failure to record presence or absence of vascular invasion, and (3) failure to denote the degree of tumor differentiation.

In order to arrive at a precise definition of microinvasive carcinoma that could be applied universally and engender meaningful and clinically relevant data, the ISSVD has proposed the following pathologic definition of microinvasive carcinoma of the vulva: a squamous carcinoma having a diameter of 2 cm or less, as measured in the fresh state, with a depth of invasion of 1 mm or less, measured from the epithelial-stromal junction of the most superficial adjacent dermal papilla to the deepest point of invasion. The presence of vascular space involvement by tumor would exclude the lesion from this definition.

The histologic parameters within the above definition (lesional diameter, depth of invasion, reference point of measured invasion, and presence or absence of vascular invasion) have been discussed exhaustively by numerous workers.[44-48] All these parameters are important for comparison with other series of microinvasive carcinoma and warrant inclusion in the pathology report.

The size of the lesion alone cannot be used as a criterion for metastatic prognostication, since tumors less than 1 cm in diameter with inguinal node metastases have been reported; however, there does appear to be a rough correlation between lesional size and metastatic potential. Donaldson et al.[49] indicated that 3 cm may be a reliable index of metastatic potential. In their study, tumors exceeding that figure were accompanied by lymph node metastasis nearly four times as frequently as those less than 3 cm in diameter.

The depth of stromal invasion appears to be the most important variable in the prediction of lymph node metastasis. Importantly, microinvasive carcinoma of the vulva appears to be a different disease from microinvasive carcinoma of the cervix, since comparable depths of invasion in the vulva are associated with higher and unacceptable rates of lymph node metastasis. For example, approximately 5 percent of vulvar squamous carcinomas invading to 3 mm or less are associated with lymph node metastases. By contrast, cervical microinvasive carcinoma with comparable depths of invasion (corresponding to the definition of cervical microinvasive carcinoma approved by the Society of Gynecologic Oncologists) are only rarely accompanied by lymph node metastasis. Vulvar squamous cell carcinomas invading to 5 mm or less have a 12 to 28 percent nodal metastasis rate as compared with a 1 to 3 percent nodal metastasis rate in cervical tumors of comparable invasive depth.[48,50] To the best of our knowledge, no lymph node metastases have been reported in squamous carcinomas of the vulva invasive to 1 mm or less.

The points of reference for measurement of invasion have been discussed extensively in the literature. Wilkinson et al.[48] suggested the most reliable reference point for standardization of measurement is the epidermal-stromal junction of the most superficial adjacent dermal papilla; the measured depth of invasion would then be from the latter to the deepest point of invasive tumor (Fig. 10-12).

In actual practice, precise histologic measurement using the previously described parameters frequently is difficult and sometimes impossible. Problems with orientation of the specimen, ulceration, and lack of dermal papillae in the section all contribute to confound the assessment of microinvasion.

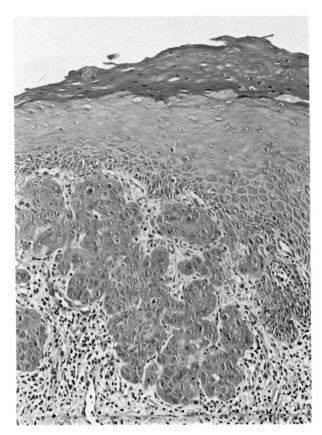

Fig. 10-12 Microinvasive squamous cell carcinoma. Small irregular nests of squamous cell carinoma invade the superficial dermis. The tumor appears to arise from atypical squamous cells in the lower portion of the epithelium. The middle and upper layers of the squamous epithelium have a dystrophic appearance. (H&E, ×30.)

The task of differentiating between true vascular invasion and tumor within artefactual spaces is a well-known histopathologic problem. Most workers agree that identification of true vascular invasion should exclude a tumor from the microinvasive category, although vascular involvement in vulvar squamous carcinomas invasive to 1 mm or less apparently is unusual.

Surgical approaches ranging from wide local excision to radical vulvectomy with bilateral groin dissection have been recommended for treatment of microinvasive carcinoma.[42,44,46,50-54] Each patient's case must be individualized.

The vulvar lesion should be excised and multiple sections should be examined for the previously mentioned histopathlologic parameters. The selection of wide local excision, hemivulvectomy or total vulvectomy depends on the clinical situation. It is perhaps prudent to sample groin lymph nodes if invasion is more than 1 mm. When the tumor is located in the midline, a bilateral groin lymphadenectomy is necessary. For unilateral lesions, an ipsilateral lymphadenectomy may be sufficient, since ipsilateral groin metastasis appears to be the rule.

SQUAMOUS CELL CARCINOMA

Squamous cell carcinoma is the most common primary tumor of the vulva, representing 90 to 95 percent of such cases, and is generally a disease of older women. Some investigators have noted a significantly higher incidence of concomitant primary tumors affecting other body sites;[55,56] this finding perhaps is related to the advanced age of the patient and may reflect a diminution in immunologic competence.

The great majority of invasive squamous cell carcinomas occur on the labia majora, favoring the medial aspect; conversely, the labia minora are involved primarily only one-third as often. Clitoral and periurethral areas are other favored sites. Small lesions may be present as raised nodules that are inconspicuous, escaping detection, especially in the absence of ulceration and bleeding (Table 10-2). Tumors less than 3 to 4 cm in diameter frequently do not ulcerate. At the time of diagnosis, squamous cell carcinoma of the

vulva is often large because of delay in treatment. Whether delay is secondary to psychosocial or other reasons, by the time of surgery most of these tumors are present as an exophytic fungating mass that has invaded the labia and urethra as well as the vagina and rectum (Fig. 10-13). Ulceration and friability may lead to bleeding and secondary infection. Induration may also arise from an inflammatory reaction to the tumor although actual fixation to underlying tumors may occur in more advanced cases. In contrast to the exophytic variety, some tumors grow as endophytic masses that may ulcerate centrally and form heaped-up ragged margins.

Often, hypopigmented gray to white skin, representing lesions of vulvar dystrophy, are seen adjacent

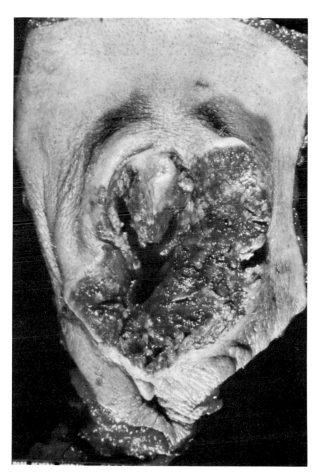

Fig. 10-13 Squamous cell carcinoma. The tumor grows as a large ulcerated nodular mass that has virtually destroyed the labia majora and minora.

Table 10-2 Presenting Symptoms of Invasive Vulvar Cancer[a]

Symptom	Frequency (%)
Pruritis	71
Vulvar lesion	58
Ulceration	28
Bleeding	26
Pain	23
Urinary tract symptoms	14
Vulvar or vaginal discharge	13

[a] N = 224 patients.
(Podratz KC, Symmonds RE, Taylor WF, et al: Carcinoma of the vulva: Analysis of treatment and survival. Obstet Gynecol 61:63, 1983.)

to the tumor. Carcinoma in situ, manifested grossly by leukoplakia or a red or pigmented plaque, may occur adjacent to the invasive squamous cell carcinoma; some workers have suggested that such tumors have a better prognosis.

On microscopic examination, most vulvar squamous cell carcinomas are either well or moderately differentiated; squamous pearl formation is common (Fig. 10-14). The tumor usually invades the underlying stroma in broad islands, nests and interconnecting strands of squamous cells with easily identifiable intercellular bridges. In many carcinomas, frequently at the advancing edge, there is invasion by single cells and small nests. The stroma is usually densely infiltrated by lymphocytes, and the ground substance is loose and edematous around foci of carcinoma. Mitotic activity generally parallels the degree of differentiation.

Invasive squamous cell carcinoma may be bordered by squamous cell carcinoma in situ or infrequently may arise from apparently normal mature squamous epithelium. Squamous cell carcinoma may arise directly from an epithelium showing vulvar dystrophy (Fig. 10-12); cases have been reported in which squamous cell carcinoma has arisen from lichen sclerosus and invaded the stroma. Approximately 3 percent of cases of lichen sclerosus are associated with an invasive squamous cell carcinoma.

Poorly differentiated vulvar squamous cell carcinomas occasionally are encountered; in these tumors, pearl formation may be sparse to entirely absent. Some varieties of poorly differentiated squamous carcinoma may have such a pronounced spindle cell appearance that they are mistaken for a sarcoma. Immunohistochemical studies, however, reveal such sarcomatoid tumors to stain strongly for epithelial cell markers such as cytokeratin.

Squamous cell carcinoma of the vulva may exhibit contiguous invasion of the vagina, urethra and anus or rarely may metastasize to distant sites by hematogenous routes. The predominant method of spread, however, occurs by lymphatic dissemination in an orderly fashion, proceeding first to the superficial inguinal lymph nodes, to the deep inguinal lymph nodes, and then through the femoral canal to the deep pelvic lymph nodes (obturator, external and internal iliac lymph nodes) and aortic lymph nodes[58-62] (Fig. 10-15).

The superficial inguinal lymph nodes function as the primary drainage sites for the vulva. The Cloquet

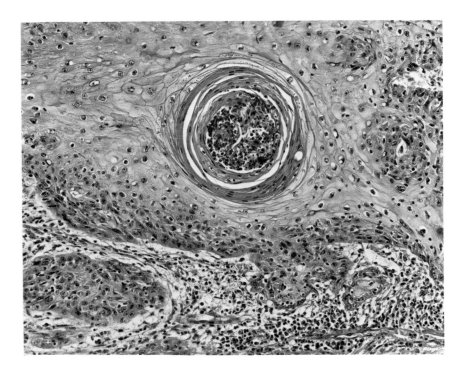

Fig. 10-14 Squamous cell carcinoma, well differentiated. The tumor invades as variable sized islands, the largest of which contains a squamous pearl with central necrosis. A dense lymphocytic infiltrate surrounds the tumor. (H&E, ×30.)

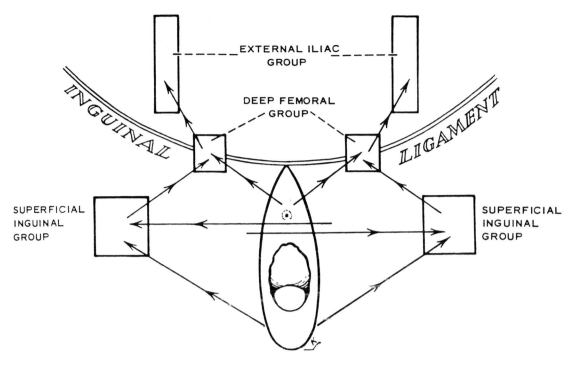

Fig. 10-15 Method of spread of squamous cell carcinoma of the vulva. (Modified after Way S: In Malignant Disease of the Vulva. Churchill Livingstone, Edinburgh, 1982.)

node is the most cephalad of the deep femoral group and is situated beneath the Poupart ligament; if this lymph node is negative for metastatic cancer, pelvic lymph node metastasis is uncommon. Lesions involving the clitoris, Bartholin gland, vagina, urethra, or rectum may spread through direct lymphatics to the pelvic and aortic lymph nodes; the practical importance of sampling these nodes appears to be limited, since no positive deep pelvic nodes in the absence of involved inguinal lymph nodes were found in 58 patients with clitoral cancer.[63]

Iverson[64] found metastases to the groin lymph nodes in 39 percent of 258 patients. Concomitant involvement of both groin and pelvic lymph nodes occurred in 6 percent of cases. Pelvic lymph node involvement in the absence of metastases to the groin lymph nodes was detected in 1 percent of patients.

Clinical Staging

The current staging classification of vulvar squamous cell carcinoma approved by the International Federation of Gynecology and Obstetrics (FIGO) is based on a clinical analysis of the primary tumor (T), regional lymph nodes (N), and distant metastases (M) (Table 10-3). Pretreatment workup may include cystoscopy, sigmoidoscopy, chest radiography, and, in advanced lesions, liver scan, bone scan, skeletal radiography, and computed tomography (CT) scan of the pelvis and abdomen, if clinically indicated.

Bassett,[65] in 1912, described an en bloc procedure for removal of the vulva and groin lymph nodes as treatment for vulvar carcinoma. Taussig,[66] in 1935, and Way,[61] in 1948, continued Bassett's work and demonstrated improved survival when radical vulvectomy and bilateral inguinal lymphadenectomy, with or without pelvic lymphadenectomy, are used for the treatment of invasive vulvar carcinoma.

The traditional butterfly incision (Way) with removal of wide areas of skin has been modified because of significant associated physical and psychological morbidity (Fig. 10-16). Many authorities recommend different approaches.[67-73] The question invariably arises as to how much "radicality" is necessary for optimal treatment.

The size of the tumor, location, and lymph node

Table 10-3 Clinical Stages of Invasive Carcinoma of the Vulva[a]

Stage	Tumor Classification			Description
				Invasive Carcinoma of the Vulva (FIGO Classification)
0				Carcinoma in situ
I	T1	N0	M0	All lesions confined to the vulva with a maximum diameter of
	T1	N1	M0	2 cm or less and no suspicious groin lymph nodes
II	T2	N0	M0	All lesions confined to the vulva with a diameter greater than
	T2	N1	M0	2 cm and no suspicious groin lymph nodes
III	T3	N0	M0	Lesions extending to the urethra, vagina, anus, or perineum,
	T3	N1	M0	but without grossly positive groin lymph nodes
	T3	N2	M0	
	T1	N2	M0	Lesions of any size confined to the vulva and having suspi-
	T2	N2	M0	cious lymph nodes
IV	T1	N3	M0	Lesions with grossly positive groin lymph nodes regardless of
	T2	N3	M0	extent of primary
	T3	N3	M0	
	T4	N3	M0	
	T4	N0	M0	Lesions involving mucosa of the rectum, bladder, urethra, or
	T4	N1	M0	involving bone
	T4	N2	M0	
	M1A			All cases with pelvic or distant metastases
	M1B			

Invasive Carcinoma of the Vulva (TNM Classification)

N	Regional Lymph Nodes	T	Primary Tumor
N0	No palpable lymph nodes	T1	Tumor confined to the vulva, 2 cm or less in larger diameter
N1	Palpable lymph nodes in either groin, not enlarged, mobile (not clinically suspicious for neoplasm)	T2	Tumor confined to the vulva, more than 2 cm in diameter
N2	Palpable lymph nodes in either one or both groins, enlarged, firm and mobile (clinically suspicious for neoplasm)	T3	Tumor of any size with adjacent tumor spread to the urethra and/or vagina, and/or anus
N3	Fixed or ulcerated lymph nodes	T4	Tumor of any size infiltrating the bladder mucosa and/or the rectal mucosa or both, including the upper part of the urethral mucosa and/or fixed to the bone
M	Distant Metastases		
M0	No clinical metastases		
M1A	Palpable deep pelvic lymph nodes		
M1B	Other distant metastases		

[a] If cytology or histology of lymph nodes reveals malignant cells, the symbol + (plus) should be added to N; if such examinations do not reveal malignant cells, the symbol − (minus) should be added to N.

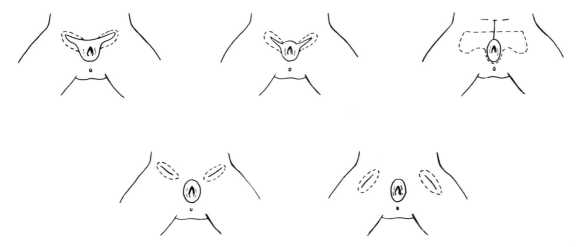

Fig. 10-16 Incisions used for radical vulvectomy and bilateral inguinal lymphadenectomy.

involvement must be considered prior to individualization of treatment. Optimal treatment should always assure ample free resection margins. To attain this goal, portions of urethra, vagina, and/or rectum must be resected in some patients.

Separate incisions for the inguinal-femoral lymphadenectomy might be considered in small lesions without clinically suspicious (N2) nodes and when the tumor is located in the posterior portion of the vulva. Laterally placed tumors generally spread to ipsilateral groin nodes; some workers therefore recommend initial ipsilateral removal of groin lymph nodes in patients with strictly unilateral tumors.[54,64] If positive groin lymph nodes are detected on frozen section, the corresponding contralateral nodes should be removed. It is impossible to predict with accuracy which lesions will spread to contralateral lymph nodes. Bilateral inguinal-femoral lymphadenectomy must be done in patients with midline vulvar lesions. Pelvic lymph node metastases in the absence of groin metastases are rare, even in tumors of the clitoris and Bartholin gland.

In a recent review of 82 patients with invasive vulvar cancer who underwent radical vulvectomy and bilateral inguinal lymphadenectomy, Iversen et al.[64] reported 5- and 10-year survival rates of 59 and 34 percent, respectively. Seventy-two patients managed with additional pelvic lymphadenectomy had respective 5- and 10-year survival rates of 53 percent and 38 percent. Further review of the literature studying patients with positive pelvic nodes shows 5-year sur-

Table 10-4 Carcinoma of the Vulva: Results of Radical Vulvectomy and Bilateral Groin and Pelvic Lymphadenectomy for Patients with Positive Pelvic Nodes

Investigators	5-Year Survival Rate (%)
Green et al. (1958)[74]	12.5
Collins et al. (1963)[75]	16.7
Morley (1976)[76]	16.7
Way (1982)[62]	21.2
Cavanagh et al. (1985)[77]	25.0
Shepherd and Monaghan (1985)[78]	18.0

vival rates that range from 12.5 to 25 percent (Table 10-4); with negative pelvic lymph nodes, the 5-year survival ranges from 69 to 100 percent (Table 10-5).

Most authorities agree that pelvic lymphadenectomy should only be considered if groin lymph nodes are positive. In a prospective randomized study carried out by the Gynecologic Oncology Group, patients with positive groin lymph nodes either underwent a pelvic node dissection or received bilateral groin and pelvic node irradiation following radical vulvectomy and inguinal lymphadenectomy.[82] The superiority and benefit of radiation were demonstrated in patients with suspicious or positive groin nodes or more than one positive groin node. Treatment recommendations for state I to IV squamous cell carcinoma of the vulva are summarized in Table 10-6.

Table 10-5 Carcinoma of the Vulva: Results of Radical Vulvectomy and Groin Dissection for Patients with Negative Lymph Nodes

Investigators	5-Year Survival (%)
Way (1960)[79]	77
Franklin and Rutledge (1971)[80]	100
Morley (1976)[76]	92
Krupp et al. (1973)[81]	91
Green (1978)[69]	87
Cavanagh et al. (1985)[77]	69
Shepherd and Monaghan (1985)[78]	88

Complications

Complications encountered with radical vulvectomy and groin dissection are divided into immediate and delayed types. The most frequent early complication is wound disruption and infection. Various investigators report some degree of wound breakdown in approximately one-half of cases.[74-81] In a review of the Mayo Clinic data, Podratz et al.[57] reported wound separation, infection, and necrosis in 85 percent of patients (Table 10-7). Thromboembolic disease was the most potentially serious postoperative complication, with an incidence of 9 percent. The overall postoperative mortality has been reduced to 1 to 4 percent,

Table 10-6 Treatment Options for Invasive Carcinoma of the Vulva

Stage	Description
I	Radical vulvectomy and groin lymph node dissection
	Radical local excision for lesions less than 1 mm in depth
II	Radical vulvectomy and groin lymph node dissection
III	Radical vulvectomy and groin lymph node dissection
	Deep pelvic lymph node dissection or groin and pelvic lymph node irradiation if inguinal lymph nodes are positive
IV	Radical vulvectomy and pelvic exenteration
	Surgery followed by radiation therapy
	Radiation of large primary lesion to improve resectability followed by radical surgery

Table 10-7 Complicatons Following Radical Vulvectomy and Groin Dissection (175 patients)

Complications	%
Early	
Wound separation, infection, necrosis	85
Urinary tract infections	18
Thromboembolic disease	9
Partial necrosis of symphysis	<1
Hemorrhage of femoral artery	<1
Delayed	
Leg edema	69
Lymphangitis, phlebitis, cellulitis	13
Vaginal stenosis	13
Pelvic relaxation	11
Urinary stress incontinence	11
Hernia	5
Urethral stenosis, prolapse	2
Fistula	2
Rectal incontinence, prolapse	1

(Modified from Podratz KC, Symmonds RE, Taylor WF, Williams TJ: Carcinoma of the vulva: Analysis of treatment and survival. Obstet Gynecol 61:63, 1983.)

despite the generally advanced age of the patients (Table 10-8), and the multiple associated medical disorders (Table 10-9).

Exenterative Surgery

Involvement of vagina, bladder, or rectum may require anterior, posterior, or total exenteration, together with vulvectomy and lymphadenectomy. Ex-

Table 10-8 Squamous Cell Carcinoma of the Vulva: Mean Age by Stage

Age (years)	Stage
65.5	I
69.6	II
69.4	III
68.4	IV

(Annual Report on the Results of Treatment in Gynecological Cancer. Vol 19. FIGO. Radiumhemmet, Stockholm, Sweden 1985.)

Table 10-9 Vulvar Carcinoma: Associated Medical Disorders[a]

Disease	Frequency (%)
Hypertension	42
Cardiac disease	35
Arthritis	18
Diabetes mellitus	14
Thyroid dysfunction	7

[a] N = 224 patients.
(Podratz KC, Symmonds RE, Taylor WF, et al: Carcinoma of the vulva: Analysis of treatment and survival. Obstet Gynecol 61:63, 1983.)

Table 10-10 Pelvic Exenteration for Invasive Vulvar Carcinoma[a]

Investigators	5-Year Survivors (%)
Thornton (1973)	57
Krupp (1975)	30
Kaplan (1975)	44
Morley (1976)[76]	6
Benedict (1979)	20
Cavanagh (1981)	50
Phillips (1981)	54

[a] N = 78 patients.
(Modified from Phillips B, Buchsbaum HJ, Lifshitz S: Pelvic exenteration for vulvovaginal carcinoma. Am J Obstet Gynecol 141:1038, 1981.)

enterative vulvectomy should be considered only after aortic lymph nodes have been sampled and found to be negative and a workup for distant metastases is negative.

A review of the literature by Phillips et al.[84] reveals that the 5-year survival rate in 78 patients who underwent radical vulvectomy and pelvic exenteration ranges from 6 to 57 percent (Table 10-10). Twelve patients were treated by anterior, 45 by posterior, and 21 by total pelvic exenteration.

Radiation Therapy

Historically, radiation therapy alone as the primary treatment of invasive vulvar carcinoma has been used infrequently in the United States; this could be attributed not only to the high incidence of associated radiation vulvitis but to the favorable results obtained with surgery as well. A favorable outcome, however, may be achieved with radiation therapy alone. One hundred and seventy-three patients with stage I and II vulvar squamous cell carcinoma have a 5-year survival of 52.6 percent. Of 212 such patients with stage III and IV cancer, 39.2 percent survived 5 years (Table 10-11). Generally, better results have been obtained with patients under the age of 60 (Table 10-12).

Radiation therapy may be used preoperatively to preserve either the bladder or rectum, or both, in treating patients with extensive vulvar carcinoma. Boronow[86] treated 33 such patients, achieving a 5-year survival rate of 75 percent and an associated operative and treatment-related mortality of 3 percent; two patients required removal of the bladder and rectum because of fistulas. For treatment of patients with positive groin nodes, postoperative irradiation to the groin and pelvic lymph nodes has replaced pelvic lymphadenectomy in many institutions. Prospective, randomized, multiinstitutional trials are necessary to define the precise role of irradiation in the treatment of patients with vulvar cancer.

Recurrence

Although the size of a tumor correlates well with patient survival, the number of lymph nodes involved by metastatic carcinoma is the major prognostic fac-

Table 10-11 Five-Year Survival with Radiation Therapy for Vulvar Carcinoma

N0-1		N2-3	
51.9%		39.3%	
T1-2	T3-4	T1-2	T3-4
52.6%	42.9%	43.6%	30.2%

T1		T2		T3	
57.9%		40.6%		34.7%	
N0-1	N2-3	N0-1	N2-3	N0-1	N2-3
59.1%	53.8%	44.3%	37.9%	42.9%	32.8%

(Modified from Frischbier HJ: Radiation therapy of vulvar carcinoma (Hamburg Method). p. 163. In Zander J, Baltzer J (eds): Erkrankungen der Vulva. Urban & Schwarzenberg, Baltimore, 1986.)

Table 10-12 Radiation Therapy for Vulvar Carcinoma: 5-Year Survival and Age

Age (years)	Stage I–IV (%)
<40	69.2
40–49	74.1
50–59	65.6
60–69	49.1
70–79	30.2
>80	16.0

(Modified from Frischbier HJ: Radiation therapy of vulvar carcinoma (Hamburg Method). p. 164. In Zander J, Baltzer J (eds): Erkrankungen der Vulva. Urban & Schwarzenberg, Baltimore, 1986.)

tor. Metastases usually occur within the first 2 years following treatment. Local metastases on the vulva can be surgically excised or irradiated. Small recurrent tumors in the groin are best treated with local irradiation.

Chemotherapy

The role of chemotherapy in the treatment of systemic and regional recurrences of squamous cell vulvar carcinoma, as primary treatment prior to surgery and radiation therapy, or as an adjuvant for high-risk patients, requires further investigation. No advantage in survival rates was noted in a randomized study of patients with vulvar cancer who received both bleomycin by infusion and surgical therapy.[87]

Mitomycin, 15 mg/m² on day 1, and a 5-day continuous infusion of 5-FU, 750 mg/m², followed by radiation therapy (3,000 rad) to the vulva prior to radical surgery, achieved a good response in two patients.[88]

Experience with systemic chemotherapy is limited because of the rarity of the disease and the relatively good results with surgery and radiation. The most successfully used agents and combinations are summarized in Table 10-13.

Prognosis

In the most recent Annual Report from the International Federation of Gynecology and Obstetrics (FIGO), 80 collaborators reported an overall 5-year survival rate of 46.3 percent in patients treated for squamous cell carcinoma of the vulva (Table 10-14).

Until the etiology of the disease is defined more accurately, improvement in results will be best accomplished through patient education (noting symptoms for earlier diagnosis), physician education (immediate biopsy of all vulvar lesions), and appropriate treatment planning. It is essential that the treating physician initiate immediate individual appropriate surgical and combined modality therapy.

Table 10-13 Single-Agent and Combination Chemotherapy in Squamous Vulvar Cancer

Agent	No. of Patients	Objective Response (%)
Single		
Adriamycin	6	67
Bleomycin	55	59
Cisplatin	2	50
Methotrexate	13	62
Combination		
Bleomycin/ mitomycin C	9	56
Cisplatin/ 5-fluorouracil	1	100

(Data from Deppe et al.,[89] Yordan et al.,[90] and Pfleiderer.[91])

Table 10-14 Carcinoma of the Vulva: 5-Year Survival by Stage

Stage	No. of Patients	5-Year Survival (%)
I	558	71.4
II	346	47.2
III	270	32.0
IV	23	10.5
No Stage	1	—
Total	1,198	46.3

(Annual Report on the Results of Treatment in Gynecological Cancer. Vol. 19. FIGO. Radiumhemmet, Stockholm, Sweden, 1985.)

VERRUCOUS CARCINOMA

Verrucous carcinoma is a rare type of squamous cell carcinoma that most often affects older women; cardinal features of verrucous carcinoma are slow and locally aggressive growth. Because of its gross and microscopic similarity to condyloma acuminatum, it may be confused with that entity and treated as such for an extended period of time before the true diagnosis is made.

Many investigators consider the so-called giant condyloma of Buschke-Lowenstein and verrucous carcinoma the same lesion, arising by malignant transformation of a previous, and probably longstanding, condyloma acuminatum.[92-98] Whatever its etiology, verrucous carcinoma warrants placement in a special category because its natural history is different from that of the usual squamous cell carcinoma of the vulva.

Grossly, the tumor grows in an exophytic papillary fashion (Fig. 10-17). On microscopic examination, verrucous carcinoma has such a deceptively bland histologic appearance that the lesion may be easily confused with condyloma or pseudoepitheliomatous (pseudocarcinomatous) hyperplasia; this is especially true if only the superficial portions of the tumor are biopsied. For proper microscopic evaluation of the neoplasm, a full-thickness biopsy is necessary, since histologic hallmarks of verrucous carcinoma include invasion of the stroma by broad bulbous pushing borders and cellular atypia at the bases of the rete pegs (Fig. 10-18). Distinction from ordinary condyloma is aided by the absence of fibrovascular cores within the proliferating papillary masses of tumor.

Both the clinician and pathologist must harbor a high index of suspicion for this tumor in order to arrive at a correct diagnosis. The occurrence of a lesion with the aforementioned gross and microscopic characteristics, especially in a woman at an age generally unassociated with condyloma, should raise the question of verrucous carcinoma.

Treatment

Depending on the size of the tumor, wide local excision, radical vulvectomy, or even an exenterative surgical procedure would be the choices for treatment of this condition. Lymphadenectomy is indicated

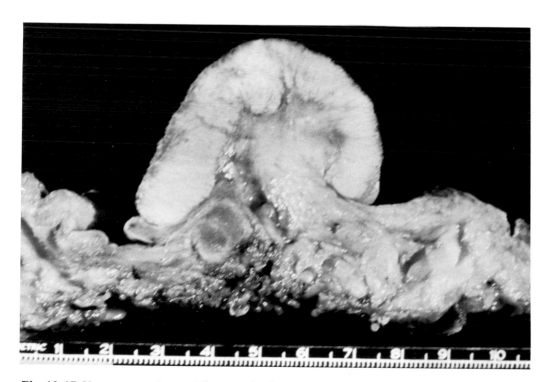

Fig. 10-17 Verrucous carcinoma. The tumor has been sectioned to show an exophytic growth pattern; invasion by bulbous pushing borders is evident even on gross examination.

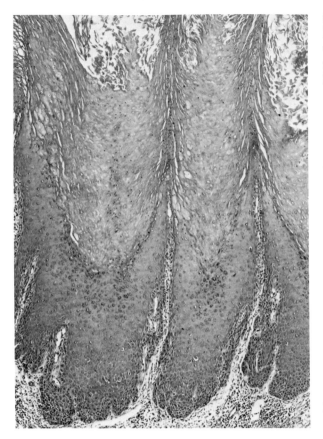

Fig. 10-18 Verrucous carcinoma. The tumor has bulbous rete pegs that invade the dermis in a pushing growth pattern. A thick layer of hyperkeratotic and parakeratotic epithelium is present; note the striking resemblance to condyloma. (H&E, ×12.)

when palpable suspicious lymph nodes are present. Radiation therapy has been implicated as an instigator of more aggressive biologic behavior, including transition to a more anaplastic tumor and even metastasis.[94,96,98]

MALIGNANT MELANOMA

Malignant melanoma of the vulva may occur at any age; however, women in the sixth and seventh decades of life are most commonly affected. In fact, the average age at the time of diagnosis is 55 years, with a range of 15 to 84 years. Chung[99,100] found approximately one-third of the patients in his study of vulvar melanoma to be premenopausal, but vulvar melanoma is extremely rare before puberty. Although malignant melanoma is an uncommon tumor of the vulva, it remains the second most common invasive neoplasm of that organ, occurring prodominantly in light-skinned and fair-haired persons.

The most common presenting symptoms in patients with vulvar melanoma are a vulvar mass or enlarging mole, pruritis, and bleeding. Melanoma can occur at any site on the vulva, but approximately 80 percent are situated on the labia minora or other mucosal surfaces. Pigmented nevi are common on the vulva (Fig. 10-19), and some malignant melanomas undoubtedly originate from such lesions. Because of their sometimes poorly accessible location and frequent covering by pubic hair, nevi exhibiting changes in size and pigmentation may not be noticed until they reach a large size, ulcerate, and bleed. In addition, psychosocial factors similar to those mentioned in the section on invasive squamous cell carcinoma may contribute to the delay of treatment.

As with other cutaneous sites in the body, the two most common types of vulvar melanomas are the superficial spreading and the nodular varieties. The former appears grossly as a slightly elevated irregularly shaped lesion; frequently, superficial spreading melanoma has a variegated color pattern, ranging from pink-tan to brown and black, but also containing shades of slate-gray to blue. Nodularity and ulceration within and around such a lesion may signal that dermal invasion has occurred. Nodular melanoma, in contrast, often begins as a more elevated lesion and rapidly assumes a nodular configuration; dark pigmentation within nodular melanoma is the rule (Figs. 10-19 and 10-20). On microscopic examination, both superficial spreading melanoma and nodular melanoma originate at the dermal-epidermal junction. The latter landmark often is completely obliterated, however, by the marked junctional activity of the malignant melanocytes. Tumor cells invade in both directions, extending into the lateral epidermis as well as into the dermis. Melanoma cells generally are large with copious cytoplasm and large nuclei, often containing huge eosinophilic nucleoli (Fig 10-21); however, spindle cells may form a minor or major component of the tumor, the latter instance occasionally contributing to confusion in the diagnosis. In nodular melanomas, the tumor cells stay relatively restricted to the nodular area of epidermis overlying the dermal component. By contrast, superficial spreading mela-

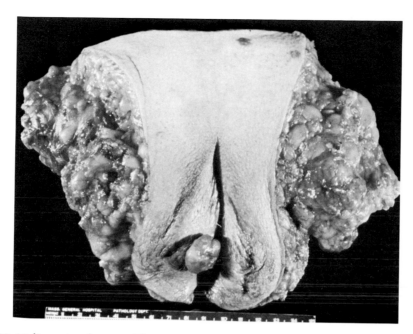

Fig. 10-19 Malignant melanoma. The tumor is present as a nodular growth arising from the right labium majus. Note two other macular pigmented lesions on the left mons pubis.

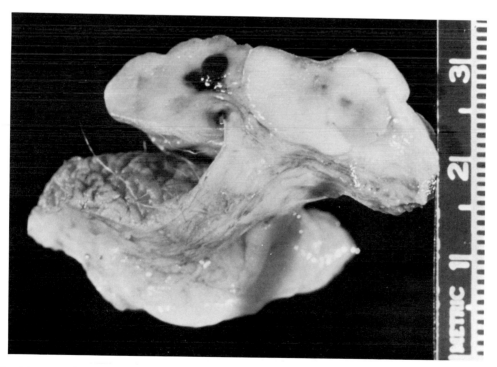

Fig. 10-20 Malignant melanoma. Enlargement of Figure 10-19, showing nodular sectioned surface of tumor. The melanoma is largely amelanotic, but a focus of dark pigmentation is present.

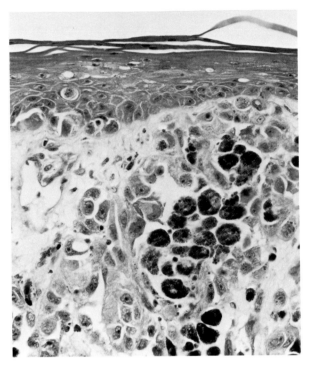

Fig. 10-21 Malignant melanoma. The superficial dermis contains large polygonal cells with enlarged nuclei and prominent nucleoli. The cytoplasm of some melanoma cells is full of dark-staining melanin pigment. A few melanoma cells are present at the dermal-epidermal junction and in the epidermis. (H&E, ×30.)

noma invade the stratified squamous eipthelium overlying and contiguous to the dermal component, if ulceration is not present. This behavior has engendered the terminology of pagetoid melanoma for superficial spreading melanoma; indeed, there may be a striking resemblance of superficial spreading melanoma to Paget's disease. Additional confusion may be created, since Paget's cells occasionally may engulf melanin granules in small quantities.

The most commonly used methods to judge prognosis in malignant melanoma involve assessment of tumor thickness. Clark et al.[101] first advocated reporting the depth of invasion by anatomic levels, which they designated I-V. Specific levels of invasion showed significant correlation with mortality. Using Clark's levels, Chung et al.[100] discovered few stage I vulvar melanomas, probably for reasons previously mentioned. In their study, no deaths occurred in patients with level II lesions; however, levels III and IV were associated with an approximately 60 percent mortality rate. The latter is higher than the 35 and 46 percent mortality rates originally reported by Clark for cutaneous melanoma. Level V had a dismal prognosis with an 80 percent mortality rate.

According to Breslow,[102] actual micrometer-aided measurement of melanomas affords more reliable prognostication than anatomic levels of invasion. Other workers have combined the Clark and Breslow[103] methods to identify low, moderate, and high risk groups in studies of cutaneous melanoma; however, to date, vulvar melanomas have not been studied using this approach.

Staging

Application to malignant melanoma of the staging system used for squamous cell carcinoma is less suitable because prognosis in the former depends more on the level, or depth, of skin involvement rather than on the size of the lesion. Furthermore, the widely used level system for cutaneous melanomas described by Clarkis less applicable to vulvar melanoma because of morphologic differences in vulvar skin and the skin of other body sites. Staging of vulvar malignant melanoma may be best accomplished using a modified level system defined by Chung (Table 10-15). The levels of invasion are measured from the granular layer or from the outermost epithelial layer in the squamous mucosa or its estimated position in the epidermis to the deepest point of invasion. Prognosis is related to the depth of skin involvement (Table 10-16).

Table 10-15 Staging System for Vulvar Melanoma

Level	Description
I	Tumor confined to the epithelium
II	Superficial penetration of the tumor into the dermis or lamina propria to a depth of 1 mm or less
III	Superficial penetration of tumor between 1 and 2 mm into the subepithelial tissues
IV	Invasion beyond 2 mm into the fibrous and fibromuscular tissue, but not into underlying fat
V	Extension of disease into underlying fat

(Chung AF, Woodruff JM, Lewis, JL: Malignant melanoma of the vulva. Obstet Gynecol 45:638, 1975.)

Table 10-16 Survival in Relationship to Level of Vulvar Melanoma

Level	No. of Patients	Dead of Disease (%)
II	8	0
III	5	60
IV	15	60
V	5	80

(Modified from Chung AF, Woodruff JM, Lewis JL: Malignant melanoma of the vulva. Obstet Gynecol 45:638, 1975.)

Treatment

The diagnosis of vulvar melanoma should be confirmed by histologic examination. Suspicious pigmented lesions require removal by total excision with wide margins. Partial excision or biopsy of melanoma is not recommended, but neither has been shown to affect the outcome adversely. Malignant melanoma of the vulva spreads predominantly by local extension and by both lymphatic and hematogenous routes.

The pretreatment workup should include a careful evaluation of the urethral meatus, vagina and all peripheral lymph nodes. To rule out distant metastases, chest radiography, liver scan, and CT scan of the pelvis and abdomen are necessary. Percutaneous needle biopsy of suspicious lesions identified by such studies or of enlarged lymph nodes should be done under CT-scan guidance prior to definitive treatment.

Patients with Chung's level I and level II lesions can be treated adequately with a wide local excision. Nodal metastases have not been reported in level II lesions. Radical vulvectomy with bilateral inguinal-femoral lymph node dissection appears to be justified for more deeply invasive lesions. Pelvic lymphadenectomy should be performed only if the inguinal lymph nodes contain metastatic melanoma. Lesions involving the urethra, vagina, or rectum may require total vaginectomy or exenteration to ensure adequate resection.

Patients with either advanced level disease (IV, V) or positive lymph nodes, or both, require individualized treatment. Radiation therapy alone appears to be less than effective in the primary treatment of malignant melanoma. The anecdotal use of adjuvant chemotherapy, immunotherapy, and radiation therapy to complement surgery has been reported[104]; prospective controlled cooperative group studies will be necessary to assess these modalities adequately and determine the extent of surgery required to cure malignant melanoma of the vulva.

Prognosis

Reported 5-year survival rates range from 14 to 50 percent with a mean of 30 percent; the 10-year survival rate is only slightly lower (27 percent).[99,105] Patients with involved lymph nodes have a 5-year survival rate of less than 7 percent compared with 40 percent with negative lymph nodes. Since earlier diagnosis obviously leads to better clinical outcome, suspicious lesions of the vulva should be promptly excised and further treatment, if required, begun with dispatch.

CARCINOMA OF THE BARTHOLIN GLAND

Carcinoma of the Bartholin gland is rare and represents approximately 1 to 3 percent of all vulvar neoplasms. Approximately 100 cases are reported in the literature. Leuchter et al.[106] identified adenocarcinoma and squamous cell carcinoma as the most common histologic types (Table 10-17). In this study, the median age of patients at diagnosis was 57 years with a range from 14 to 85 years. The most frequent presenting symptoms were a vulvar mass and pain. Diagnosis

Table 10-17 Histology of Carcinoma of the Bartholin Gland

Histology	No. of Patients
Squamous	34
Adenocarcinoma	29
Adenoid cystic carcinoma	14
Mixed	4
Transitional	3
Anaplastic	4

(Modified from Leuchter RS, Hacker NF, Voet RL, et al: Malignant melanoma of the vulva. Obstet Gynecol 66:361, 1982.)

was often delayed (mean time to diagnosis: 10 months) because cancers were misdiagnosed as a Bartholin gland cyst.

In this series reported by Leuchter, a high incidence of groin lymph node metastasis (37.3 percent) was found. When groin lymph nodes were negative, no positive pelvic lymph nodes were detected. The 5-year survival rate, even in the absence of positive inguinal lymph nodes, was approximately 50 percent.

Treatment

The recommended treatment for carcinoma of the Bartholin gland is a radical vulvectomy with bilateral inguinal-femoral lymphadenectomy. Deep pelvic lymph node dissection or irradiation to the groin and pelvic lymph nodes may be necessary only if four or more inguinal-femoral lymph nodes are positive.[63]

Thirty-seven reported cases of adenoid cystic carcinoma of the Bartholin gland were recently reviewed by Copeland et al.[107] in 1986; the age range of those patients was 25 to 70 years, and the median age was 42 years. On the basis of this review of clinical and pathologic characteristics, the recommended treatment for adenoid cystic carcinoma is radical wide local excision, obtaining clear surgical margins, and an ipsilateral inguinal lymphadenectomy.

BASAL CELL CARCINOMA

Basal cell carcinoma is rarely encountered on the vulva. The reported incidence ranges from 2 to 12 percent of all vulvar malignancies. The tumor predominantly affects Caucasian postmenopausal women; in a review by Breen[108] in 1975, the average age was 59 years. Commonly, the tumor was located on the labium majus and pruritis and a vulvar mass were the most common presenting symptoms. Basal cell carcinoma frequently was accompanied (20 percent) by other neoplasms.

The etiology of basal cell carcinoma is unknown. Since it is a locally invasive tumor that usually does not metastasize, recommended treatment is wide and deep local excision. The results are excellent if the margins are free of tumor. Basal cell carcinoma is relatively radiation resistant.

REFERENCES

1. International Society for the Study of Vulvar Disease. New nomenclature for vulvar disease. Obstet Gynecol 47:122, 1976
2. Brown EM, Ostergard DR: Toluidine blue and colposcopy for screening and delineating vulvar neoplasia. Obstet Gynecol 38:775, 1971
3. Friedrich EG: Vulvar dystrophy. Clin Obstet Gynecol 28:178, 1985
4. Friedrich EG: Vulvar Disease. WB Saunders, Philadelphia, 1983
5. Friedrich EG: Topical testosterone for benign vulvar dystrophy. Obstet Gynecol 37:677, 1971
6. Kaufman RH, Gardner HL, Brown D Jr, et al: Vulvar dystrophies: An evaluation. Am J Obstet Gynecol 120:363, 1974
7. Zelle K: Treatment of vulvar dystrophies with topical testosterone proprionate. Am J Obstet Gynecol 109:570, 1971
8. Crum CP, FU YS, Levine RU, et al: Intraepithelial squamous lesions of the vulva: Biologic and histologic criteria for the distinction of condylomas from vulvar intraepithelial neoplasia. Am J Obstet Gynecol 144:77, 1982
9. Crum CP, Liskow A, Petras P, et al: Vulvar intraepithelial neoplasia (severe atypia and carcinoma in situ). A clinicopathologic analysis of 41 cases. Cancer 54:1429, 1984
10. Friedrich EG, Kalra PS: Serum levels of sex hormones in vulvar lichen sclerosus and its effect of topical testosterone. N Engl J Med 310:488, 1984
11. Friedrich EG, Wilkinson EJ, Fu YS: Carcinoma in situ of the vulva: A continuing challenge. Am J Obstet Gynecol 36:830, 1981
12. Wolcott HD, Gallup DG: Wide local excision of vulvar carcinoma in situ: A reappraisal. Am J Obstet Gynecol 150:695, 1984
13. Woodruff JD: Carcinoma in situ of the vulva. Clin Obstet Gynecol 28:230, 1985
14. DiSaia PJ, Rich WM: Surgical approach to multifocal carcinoma in situ of the vulva. Am J Obstet Gynecol 140:136, 1981
15. Rettermain MA, Braly PS, Roberts WS, et al: Treatment of cutaneous vulvar lesions with skinning vulvectomy. J Reprod Med 30:478, 1985
16. Rutledge F, Sinclair M: Treatment of intraepithelial carcinoma of the vulva by skin excision and graft. Am J Obstet Gynecol 102:806, 1968
17. Carson TE, Hoskins WJ, Warzel JF: Topical 5-fluorouracil challenge of carcinoma in situ of the vulva. Obstet Gynecol 47(suppl):59S, 1976
18. Lifshitz S, Roberts JA: Treatment of carcinoma in situ

of the vulva with topical 5-fluorouracil. Obstet Gynecol 56:242, 1980

19. Krupp PJ, Bohn IW: 5-Fluorouracil topical treatment on in situ vulvar cancer: A preliminary report. Obstet Gynecol 51:702, 1978

20. Roberts JA, Watling WG, Lagasse LD: Treatment of vulvar intraepithelial neoplasia (VIN) with local bleomycin. Cancer Clin Trials 3:351, 1980

21. Foster DC, Woodruff JD: The use of dinitrochlorobenzene in the treatment of vulvar carcinoma in situ. Gynecol Oncol 11:330, 1981

22. Raaf JH, Krown SE, Pinsky CM: Treatment of Bowen's disease with topical DNCB and 5-fluorouracil. Cancer 37:1633, 1976

23. Baggish MS, Dorsey JH: CO$_2$ laser for the treatment of vulvar carcinoma in situ. Obstet Gynecol 57:371, 1981

24. Crum CP: Using lasers to treat condylomas and VIN. Contemp Ob/Gyn 20:57, 1982

25. Kaufman RH, Friedrich EG: The carbon dioxide laser in the treatment of vulvar disease. Clin Obstet Gynecol 28:220, 1985

26. Leuchter RS, Townsend DE, Hacker NF, et al: Treatment of vulvar carcinoma in situ with the CO$_2$ laser. Gynecol Oncol 19:314, 1984

27. Reid R, Elfont EA, Zirkim RM, et al: Superficial laser vulvectomy. II. The anatomic and biophysical principles permitting accurate control over the depth of dermal destruction with the carbon dioxide laser. Am J Obstet Gynecol 152:261, 1985

28. Reid R: Superficial laser vulvectomy. I. The efficacy of extended epidermal ablation for refractory and very extensive condylomas. Am J Obstet Gynecol 151:1047, 1985

29. Stein S: Co$_2$ laser surgery of the cervix, vagina and vulva. Surg Clin North Am 64:885, 1984

30. Townsend DE, Levin RU, Richart RM, et al: Management of vulvar intraepithelial neoplasia by carbon dioxide laser. Obstet Gynecol 60:49, 1982

31. Baggish MS: Basic and Advanced Laser Surgery in Gynecology. Appleton-Century-Crofts, E Norwalk, CT, 1985

32. Crum CP, Braun LA, Shah KV, et al: Vulvar intraepithelial neoplasia: Correlation of nuclear DNA content and the presence of a human papilloma virus (HPV) structural antigen. Cancer 49:468, 1982

33. Daling JR, Chu J, Weiss NS, et al: The association of condylomata acuminata and squamous carcinoma of the vulva. Br J Cancer 50:533, 1984

34. Berger BW, Hori Y: Multicentric Bowen's disease of the genitalia. Spontaneous regression of lesions. Arch Dermatol 114:1698, 1978

35. Penneys NS, Mogollon RJ, Nadji M, et al: Papilloma virus common antigens. Papillomavirus antigen in verruca, benign papillomatous lesions, trichilemmoma, and bowenoid papulosis: An immunoperoxidase study. Arch Dermatol 120:859, 1984

36. Ikenberg H, Gissman L, Gross G, et al: Human papillomavirus type 16-related DNA in genital Bowen's disease and in Bowenoid papulosis. Int J Cancer 32:563, 1983

37. Wade TR, Kopf AW, Ackerman AB: Bowenoid papulosis of the penis. Cancer 42:1890, 1978

38. Patterson JW, Kao GF, Graham JH, Helwig EB: Bowenoid papulosis: A clinicopathologic study with ultrastructural observations. Cancer 57:823, 1986

39. Gross G, Hagedorn M, Ikenberg H, et al: Bowenoid papulosis: Presence of human papillomavirus (HPV) structural antigens and of HPV 16-related DNA sequences. Arch Dermatol 121:858, 1985

40. Sitakalin C, Ackerman AB: Mammary and extramammary Paget's disease (groin, vulva, perianal). Am J Dermatopathol 07:335, 1985

41. Watring WG, Roberts JA, Lagasse LD, et al: Treatment of recurrent Paget's disease of the vulva with topical bleomycin. Cancer 41:10, 1978

42. Hacker NF, Nieberg RK, Berek JS, et al: Superficially invasive vulvar cancer with nodal metastases. Gynecol Oncol 15:65, 1983

43. Wilkinson EJ: Superficial invasive carcinoma of the vulva. Clin Obstet Gynecol 28:188, 1985

44. Buckley CH, Butler EB, Fox H: Vulvar intraepithelial neoplasia and microinvasive carcinoma of the vulva. J Clin Pathol 37:1201, 1984

45. Buscema K, Stern JL, Woodruff JD: Early invasive carcinoma of the vulva. Am J Obstet Gynecol 140:563, 1981

46. Guaschino S, Bagliani F, Pesando PC, et al: Microinvasive carcinoma of the vulva. Eur J Gynaecol Oncol 5:99, 1984

47. Hacker NF, Berek JS, Lagasse LD, et al: Management of regional lymph nodes and their prognostic influence in vulvar cancer. Obstet Gynecol 61:408, 1983

48. Wilkinson EJ, Rico MJ, Pierson KK: Microinvasive carcinoma of the vulva. Int J Gynecol Pathol 1:29, 1982

49. Donaldson ES, Powell DE, Hanson MB, et al: Prognostic parameters in invasive vulvar cancer. Gynecol Oncol 11:184, 1981

50. Zucker PK, Berkowitz RS: The issue of microinvasive squamous cell carcinoma of the vulva: An evaluation of the criteria of diagnosis and methods of therapy. Obstet Gynecol Surv 40:136, 1985

51. Boice CR, Seraj IM, Thrasher T, et al: Microinvasive squamous carcinoma of the vulva: Present status and reassessment. Gynecol Oncol 18:71, 1984

52. DiSaia PJ, Creasman WT, Rich WM: An alternate approach to early cancer of the vulva. Am J Obstet Gynecol 133:825, 1979

53. DiSaia P: Management of superficially invasive vulvar carcinoma. Clin Obstet Gynecol 28:196, 1985

54. Hacker NF, Berek JS, Lagasse LD, et al: Individualization of treatment for Stage I squamous cell vulvar carcinoma. Obstet Gynecol 63:155, 1984

55. Buchler DA: Multiple primaries and gynecologic malignancies. Am J Obstet Gynecol 123:376, 1975

56. Deppe G, Dolan TE, Zbella EA, et al: Synchronous multiple primary malignant neoplasms of the breast, colon and vulva. A case report. J Reprod Med 29:878, 1984

57. Podratz KC, Symmonds RE, Taylor WF, Williams TJ: Carcinoma of the vulva: Analysis of treatment and survival. Obstet Gynecol 61:63, 1983

58. Figge DC, Tamimi HK, Greer BE: Lymphatic spread in carcinomas of the vulva. Am J Obstet Gynecol 152:387, 1985

59. Iversen T, Aas M: Lymph drainage from the vulva. Gynecol Oncol 16:179, 1983

60. Plentl AA, Friedman EA: Lymphatic System of the Female Genitalia. WB Saunders, Philadelphia, 1971

61. Way S: The anatomy of the lymphatic drainage of the vulva and its influence on the radical operation for carcinoma. Am R Coll Surg Engl 3:187, 1948

62. Way S: Malignant Disease of the Vulva. Churchill Livingstone, Edinburgh, 1982

63. Curry SL, Wharton JT, Rutledge FN: Positive lymph nodes in vulvar squamous carcinoma. Gynecol Oncol 9:63, 1980

64. Iversen T: New approaches to treatment of squamous cell carcinoma of the vulva. Clin Obstet Gynecol 28:204, 1985

65. Bassett A: Traitement chirurgical operatoire de l'epithelioma primitif du clitoris. Rev Chir Paris 46:546, 1912

66. Taussig FJ: Cancer of the vulva: An analysis of 155 cases (1911–1940). Am J Obstet Gynecol 40:764, 1940

67. Choo YC: Invasive squamous carcinoma of the vulva in young patients. Gynecol Oncol 13:158, 1982

68. Christopherson W, Buchsbaum HJ, Voet R, et al: Radical vulvectomy and bilateral groin lymphadenectomy utlizing separate groin incisions: Report of a case with recurrence in the intervening skin bridge. Gynecol Oncol 21:247, 1985

69. Green TH: Carcinoma of the vulva. A reassessment. Obstet Gynecol 52:462, 1978

70. Hacker NF, Leuchter RS, Berek JS, et al: Radical vulvectomy and bilateral inguinal lymphadenectomy through separate groin incisions. Obstet Gynecol 58:574, 1981

71. Iversen T: New approaches to treatment of squamous cell carcinoma of the vulva. Clin Obstet Gynecol 28:204, 1985

72. Green TH, Ulfelder H, Meigs JV: Epidermoid carcinoma of the vulva. Am J Obstet Gynecol 75:834, 1958

73. Ambrosini A, Becagli S, Resta P, et al: Current surgical therapy in vulvar carcinoma and surgical techniques. Eur J Gynaecol Oncol 1:188, 1980

74. Green TH, Ulfelder H, Meigs JV: Epidermoid carcinoma of the vulva. An analysis of 238 cases: Etiology and diagnosis. Am J Obstet Gynecol 75:834, 1958

75. Collins CG, Collins JH, Barclay DL, et al: Cancer involving the vulva. Am J Obstet Gynecol 87:762, 1963

76. Morley GW: Infiltrative carcinoma of the vulva. Results of surgical treatment. Am J Obstet Gynecol 124:874, 1976

77. Cavanagh D, Ruffolo EH, Marsden DE: Gynecologic Cancer. A Clinicopathologic Approach. Appleton-Century-Crofts, E Norwalk, CT, 1985

78. Shepherd JH, Monaghan JM: Clinical Gynecological Oncology. Blackwell Scientific Publications, Oxford, 1985

79. Way S: Carcinoma of the vulva. Am J Obstet Gynecol 79:692, 1960

80. Franklin EW, Rutledge FD: Prognostic facts in epidermoid carcinoma of the vulva. Obstet Gynecol 37:892, 1971

81. Krupp PJ, Lee FY, Batson HWK, et al: Carcinoma of the vulva. Gynecol Oncol 1:345, 1973

82. Homesley H, Bundy B, Sedlis A: Randomized study of radiation therapy versus pelvic node dissection for patients with invasive squamous cell carcinoma of the vulva having positive groin nodes. Presented at the Sixteenth Annual Meeting Society of Gynecologic Oncologists, Miami, February, 1985

83. Annual Report on the Results of Treatment in Gynecological Cancer. Vol. 19. FIGO. Radiumhemmet, Stockholm, Sweden, 1985

84. Phillips B, Buchsbaum HJ, Lifshitz S: Pelvic exenteration for vulvovaginal carcinoma. Am J Obstet Gynecol 141:1038, 1981

85. Frischbier HJ: Die Strahlentherapie des Vulvakarzinoms (Hamburger Methode) p. 151. In Zander J, Baltzer J (eds): Erkrankungen der Vulva. Urban & Schwarzenberg, Baltimore, 1986

86. Boronow RC: Combined therapy as an alternative to exenteration for locally advanced vulvovaginal cancer. Cancer 49:1085, 1982

87. Schmeisser G, Krafft W, Schirmer A, et al: The effectiveness of adjunct bleomycin therapy in vulvar carcinoma. Zentralbl Gynakol 101:350, 1979

88. Kalra JR, Grossmann AM, Krumholz B, et al: Preop-

erative chemoradiotherapy for carcinoma of the vulva. Gynecol Oncol 12:256, 1981

89. Deppe G, Cohen CJ, Bruckner HW: Chemotherapy of squamous cell carcinoma of the vulva: A review. Gynecol Oncol 7:345, 1979

90. Yordan EL, Bonomi PD, Wilbanks GD: Chemotherapy of vulvar and vaginal neoplasms. p. 85. In Deppe G (ed): Chemotherapy of Gynecologic Cancer. Alan R Liss, New York, 1984

91. Pfleiderer A: Zytostatische Therapie des Vulvakarzinoms. p. 194. In Zander J, Baltzer J (eds): Erkrankungen der Vulva. Urban & Schwarzenberg, Baltimore, 1986

92. Andreasson B, Bock JE, Stern KV, et al: Verrucous carcinoma of the vulvar region. Acta Obstet Gynecol Scand 62:183, 1983

93. Japaze H, Van Dinh T, Woodruff JD: Verrucous carcinoma of the vulva: A study of 24 cases. Obstet Gynecol 60:462, 1982

94. Lucas WE, Benirschke K, Lebhertz TB: Verrucous carcinoma of the female genital tract. Am J Obstet Gynecol 119:435, 1974

95. Partridge EE, Murad T, Shingleton HM: Verrucous lesions of the female genitalia. Am J Obstet Gynecol 137:419, 1980

96. Powell JL, Franklin EW, Nickerson JF, et al: Verrucous carcinoma of the female genital tract. Gynecol Oncol 6:565, 1978

97. Rando RF, Sedlacek TV, Hunt J, et al: Verrucous carcinoma of the vulva associated with an unusual type G human papillomavirus. Obstet Gynecol 67:70(S), 1986

98. Stehman FB, Castaldo TW, Charles EH, et al: Verrucous carcinoma of the vulva. Int J Gynaecol Obstet 17:523, 1980

99. Morrow CP, DiSaia PJ: Malignant melanoma of the female genitalia: A clinical analysis. Obstet Gynecol Surv 31:233, 1976

100. Chung AF, Woodruff JM, Lewis JL: Malignant melanoma of the vulva. Obstet Gynecol 45:638, 1975

101. Clark WH Jr, From L, Bernardino EH, et al: Histogenesis and biologic behavior of primary human malignant melanoma of the skin. Cancer Res 29:705, 1969

102. Breslow A: Prognostic factors in the treatment of cutaneous melanoma. J Cutan Pathol 6:208, 1979

103. Bagley RH, Cady B, Lee A, et al: Changes in clinical presentation and management of malignant melanoma. Cancer 47:2126, 1981

104. Baltzer J, Zander J: Das Melanom im Bereich des ausseren genitales aus gynakologischer Sicht. p. 104. In Zander J, Baltzer J (eds): Erkrankungen der Vulva. Urban & Schwarzenberg, Baltimore, 1986

105. Jaramillo BA, Ganjei P, Averette HE, et al: Malignant melanoma of the vulva. Obstet Gynecol 66:398, 1985

106. Leuchter RS, Hacker NF, Voet RL, et al: Primary carcinoma of the Bartholin gland: A report of 14 cases and review of the literature. Obstet Gynecol 60:361, 1982

107. Copeland LJ, Sneige N, Gershenson DM, et al: Adenoid cystic carcinoma of Bartholin Gland. Obstet Gynecol 67:115, 1986

108. Breen JL, Neubecker RD, Greenwald E, et al: Basal cell carcinoma of the vulva. Obstet Gynecol 46:122, 1975

11

Cancer of the Vagina Including DES-Related Lesions

Gunter Deppe
W. Dwayne Lawrence

DYSPLASIA AND CARCINOMA IN SITU OF THE VAGINA (VAGINAL INTRAEPITHELIAL NEOPLASIA)

Vaginal squamous cell dysplasia and carcinoma in situ may occur alone or as a component of multifocal disease involving other lower female genital tract organs, such as the cervix and vulva.[1] In contrast to cervical intraepithelial neoplasia, vaginal dysplasia-carcinoma in situ (vaginal intraepithelial neoplasia) is encountered much less frequently. One relatively recent review of the literature reported fewer than 300 cases of vaginal carcinoma in situ.[2] Epidemiologic studies of vaginal intraepithelial neoplasia are few. Historically, older women have been affected more frequently, with peak incidence in the sixth and seventh decades[3]; however, in the report by Lenehan et al.,[4] one-fourth of patients with vaginal intraepithelial neoplasia were under 50 years of age.

The etiology of vaginal intraepithelial neoplasia is unclear, but the apparent recent increase in its incidence in younger patients may be related to an antecedent or concomitant human papillomavirus (HPV) infection. In the study by Lenehan et al.,[4] 29 percent of patients had histopathologic evidence suggesting HPV effect. Other apparent risk factors for vaginal intraepithelial neoplasia appear to be radiation therapy, chemotherapy, and various immunosuppressive treatments, all of which may also predispose to viral infection.

The natural history of vaginal intraepithelial neoplasia appears to be similar to that of cervical intraepithelial neoplasia in that the epithelium goes through a continuum of changes, beginning with vaginal intraepithelial neoplasia grade I and progressing through grades II to III; the aforementioned degrees of atypia correspond to mild, moderate, and severe dysplasia-carcinoma in situ, respectively. This concept is upheld by the findings of Rutledge,[5] whose study showed the degree of vaginal intraepithelial atypia to progress in severity over time, eventuating in invasive squamous cancer. The transit time for progression from lesser degrees of vaginal intraepithelial neoplasia to invasive squamous cancer is poorly studied but appears to be slow. The effect of HPV on such transit times remains to be elucidated, but some workers have suggested that the papillomavirus may alter the natural history of cervical intraepithelial neoplasia by shortening the transit time through its various grades.[6]

253

In most cases, vaginal intraepithelial neoplasia is asymptomatic, although some patients complain of dyspareunia, vaginal spotting, or leukorrhea. It is usually suspected on the basis of an abnormal Papanicolaou (Pap) smear and confirmed by colposcopically directed biopsies.[3] Vaginal intraepithelial neoplasia has a colposcopic pattern similar to that of cervical intraepithelial neoplasia. Staining the vaginal mucosa with Lugol's solution helps identify the nonstaining abnormal areas. The lesions may be single, occurring most frequently in the upper vagina, or multifocal; typical colposcopic manifestations are acetowhite epithelium with punctation and mosaicism. All such lesions should be biopsied to establish the diagnosis and exclude invasive cancer.

The histologic characteristics of vaginal squamous intraepithelial atypias are similar to those involving other sites in the lower female genital tract. Although some prefer the inclusive term of vaginal intraepithelial neoplasia to characterize such lesions, the older terminology of dysplasia and carcinoma in situ is still in widespread use. In the former case, as in the cervix and vulva, the varying degrees of intraepithelial atypia are graded on a scale of I to III; grades I and II correspond to mild and moderate dysplasia, and grade III groups severe dysplasia and carcinoma in situ under one heading. On microscopic examination, the lesions are graded according to both architectural and cytologic features. The former are judged by the level of the epithelium that is replaced by atypical, or dysplastic, squamous cells.[7] In some cases, the degree of architectural atypia is determined easily, since approximately one-third, one-half, or two-thirds to full thickness of the epithelium are replaced by atypical squamous cells. Evaluation of architectural atypia alone, however, is insufficient and must be accompanied by determination of cytologic atypia; the latter is characterized by increased nucleocytoplasmic ratio, nuclear enlargement and pleomorphism, irregular clumping of chromatin, and the presence of typical and atypical mitotic figures. Mitotic activity is found in increasingly higher levels of the epithelium as the degree of severity increases. The importance of both architectural and cytologic evaluation is underscored by the finding of lesions in which two-thirds to full thickness of the epithelium is replaced by squamous cells showing only mild cytologic atypia.

The normal vaginal mucosa is a moist stratified squamous epithelium that is nonkeratinizing. Accordingly, keratinizing types comprise only 5 to 10 percent of vaginal dysplasias. The hyperkeratosis associated with such lesions, particularly when thick, may signify a benign histopathologic diagnosis if only superficial biopsies are taken.[2]

Koilocytotic, or HPV-related, lesions of the vaginal squamous epithelium are similar to those in other sites of the lower female genital tract (Figs. 11-1 and 11-2). Lesions that contain koilocytes, or halo cells, involving only the intermediate and superficial layers of the squamous epithelium, probably represent papillomavirus infection only. The associated nuclear atypia, present as wrinkled convoluted nuclei, is most likely due to a nucleopathic effect of the virus and does not represent the manifestation of a true dysplasia, or intraepithelial neoplasia (Fig. 11-2). Such le-

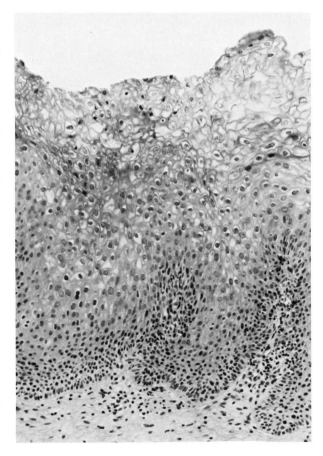

Fig. 11-1 Vagina. Mild koilocytotic dysplasia. The epithelium appears thickened, and the lower third shows cells with a mild degree of nuclear pleomorphism and hyperchromatism. Koilocytes are most prominent in the intermediate and superficial layers. (H & E, ×85.)

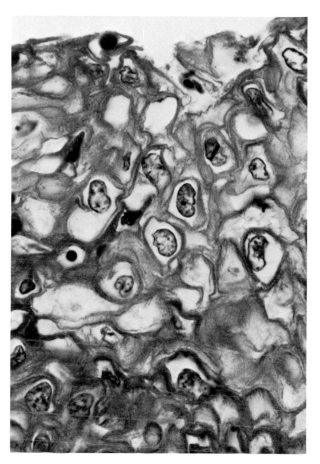

Fig. 11-2 Higher magnification of Figure 11-1, showing superficial layers of epithelium. Koilocytes are characterized by enlarged, convoluted nuclei and paranuclear cytoplasmic halos. Some nuclei are pale and vesicular, whereas others are more hyperchromatic. (H & E, ×450.)

sions may be diagnosed simply as koilocytosis. If, however, koilocytosis is accompanied by significant nuclear pleomorphism, chromatin clumping, or hyperchromatism, the lesion should be evaluated by conventional histologic criteria. Furthermore, the diagnosis should be worded in conventional pathologic terminology, whether in the framework of dysplasia-carcinoma in situ or vaginal intraepithelial neoplasia, and the koilocytotic aspect of the lesions mentioned secondarily, e.g., as severe koilocytotic dysplasia or severe dysplasia with koilocytosis (Fig. 11-1).

Another form of vaginal intraepithelial atypia is that associated with and following radiation therapy for either vaginal, or usually cervical, squamous carcinoma. Such lesions may develop rather rapidly, occurring in less than 6 months postirradiation. Conversely, they may persist for long periods, since cytologic examination as long as 15 years after treatment has revealed their presence.[8] Although atypia secondary to irradiation may persist in the vaginal mucosa, the squamous cells do not have the features of malignancy. Cytologic changes attributed to radiation atypia include nuclear enlargement without a concomitant decrease in the amount of cytoplasm, smudging of chromatin, vacuolization of the cytoplasm, and occasional binucleation.

By contrast, cells of postirradiation dysplasia exhibit large, often hyperchromatic, nuclei but with associated loss of cytoplasm (increased nucleocytoplasmic ratio) and a marked degree of nuclear pleomorphism.[9] Retention of cytoplasmic vacuolization may create confusion with koilocytosis; indeed, one study has indicated that irradiation may reactivate dormant papillomavirus.[10] Microscopic examination of the vaginal stroma often confirms the suspicion of irradiation-related dysplasia, since such features as hyalinization, atypical multinucleated giant cells, and thick-walled hyalinized blood vessels are found.

Treatment

A variety of treatment modalities have evolved for vaginal intraepithelial neoplasia. For many years, the traditional treatment consisted of either local surgical excision or partial or complete vaginectomy. The size and location of the lesion determined the extent of the procedure. Currently, many believe that consideration should be given to the age of the patient as well as to multifocality of lesions when planning therapy.

TREATMENTS USED FOR VAGINAL INTRAEPITHELIAL NEOPLASIA

Local excision
Partial or complete vaginectomy
Cryosurgery
Electrocautery
Intravaginal 5-fluorouracil cream
CO_2 laser

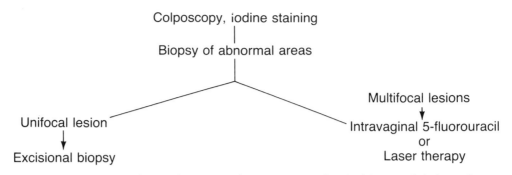

Colposcopy, iodine staining

Biopsy of abnormal areas

Unifocal lesion

Excisional biopsy

Multifocal lesions

Intravaginal 5-fluorouracil
or
Laser therapy

Fig. 11-3 Procedures for the diagnosis and management of vaginal intraepithelial neoplasia.

Colposcopy and staining the vagina with iodine solution help delineate the extent of the abnormalities prior to treatment (Fig. 11-3). Unifocal areas of vaginal intraepithelial neoplasia can be surgically excised, whereas multifocal lesions may require an alternate method of therapy, such as topical 5 percent 5-fluorouracil (5-FU) cream in a white petrolatum base (Efudex). The cream is applied intravaginally with a diaphragm, tampon, or vaginal applicator. The vulva is protected with Vaseline, since an acute chemical inflammation occurs if the vulvar skin is contaminated. By interacting with tumor cell RNA, 5-FU prevents tumor cell replication and causes cell death. The vaginal epithelium undergoes necrosis followed by reepithelialization. Some of the treatment regimens that have been used successfully[11-16] are listed in Table 11-1.

We prefer the treatment regimen as described by Petrilli et al.[15] A 15-g test dose of 5 percent 5-FU is inserted into the vagina; 4 days later, the lesion is inspected. If ulceration is noted, the patient is then instructed to insert 5 g 5-FU cream for five consecutive nights. The patient is followed up to 12 weeks with colposcopic and cytologic evaluation. In the event of persistent disease, an additional course of 5-FU, identical to the first, is prescribed.

If no changes in the vaginal mucosa are present initially, a modified does consisting of 5 g 5 percent 5-FU is prescribed for vaginal insertion each night for 5 days. The patient is re-examined at 12 weeks to assess results.

Severe vaginal ulceration, inflammation, and irritation are common side effects of this treatment. In postmenopausal women especially, treatment courses should last only 4 days because of enhanced mucosal sensitivity in this age group.

The CO_2 laser has been used with increasing frequency to manage vaginal intraepithelial neoplasia; many workers have reported encouraging results.[15,17-20] Power density in the range of 400 to 500 W/cm with a spot size of 1.5 to 2.0 mm is recommended. The lesion and a surrounding 3-mm area of normal-appearing tissue should be vaporized to a depth of only 2 mm, as deeper treatment may injure the bladder.

Intraepithelial neoplasia arising in the vaginal cuff following hysterectomy is notoriously difficult to eradicate. Such lesions may be best treated by everting them with wire sutures or an iris hook. Follow-up examinations are performed at 6, 12, and 24 weeks following treatment. Cytologic and colposcopic examinations should be performed at 12 and 24 weeks; if normal, the patient should be reevaluated every 6 months with cytologic examinations.

Table 11-1 Intravaginal 5-Fluorouracil Treatment for Vaginal Intraepithelial Neoplasia

No. of Patients	Remission (%)	Reference
9	88	Woodruff et al. (1975)[12]
12	100	Ballon et al. (1979)[13]
17	100	Daly and Ellis (1980)[14]
15	80	Petrilli et al. (1980)[15]
27	100	Caglar et al. (1981)[16]

(Modified from Jordan EL, Bonomi PD, Wilbanks GD: Chemotherapy of vulvar and vaginal neoplasms. p. 85. In Deppe G (ed): Chemotherapy of Gynecologic Cancer. Alan R Liss, New York, 1984.)

Cryosurgery and electrocautery are less effective than the CO_2 laser in the management of vaginal intraepithelial neoplasia. Radiotherapy administered with an intravaginal applicator at a dose of 6,000 to 7,000 rad to the mucosa is highly effective but may be accompanied by the complications of subsequent vaginal fibrosis and stenosis. We recommend the use of radiation therapy or extensive surgery only for patients with recurrent multifocal vaginal intraepithelial neoplasia that is unresponsive to other treatment modalities.

The incidence of vaginal intraepithelial neoplasia following hysterectomy for cervical intraepithelial neoplasia is 0.7 to 6.8 percent.[1,21-22] Although vaginal intraepithelial neoplasia following hysterectomy for benign disease occurs infrequently, it does occur spontaneously; in one series, 28 percent of patients with vaginal intraepithelial neoplasia had previously undergone hysterectomy for benign disease.[4] Therefore, we believe that cytologic examination of the vagina should be performed periodically in all patients with a previous hysterectomy, a philosophy not maintained by all gynecologic oncologists.

In high-risk patients, such as those previously treated for cervical intraepithelial neoplasia or cervical squamous cancer, vaginal smears should be obtained at 6- to 12-month intervals. This group includes patients in whom a neovagina has been constructed, especially after vaginectomy for treatment of intraepithelial squamous neoplasia. Recurrent vaginal intraepithelial neoplasia in such patients has been reported.[23] Vaginal intraepithelial neoplasia has the potential for progression to invasive squamous cancer, necessitating close follow-up of patients with such lesions.

SQUAMOUS CELL CARCINOMA

Primary vaginal carcinomas are uncommon, comprising approximately 2 percent of all gynecologic malignancies. Most occur during the sixth and seventh decades of life, and more than two-thirds are encountered in women past the age of 50. The most common histologic type is squamous cell carcinoma, which represents close to 95 percent of such tumors.[24] Other less common malignancies include adenocarcinoma, verrucous carcinoma, small cell carcinoma, diethylstilbestrol (DES)-associated clear cell adeno-

carcinoma, melanoma, sarcoma, and the rare childhood neoplasms, rhabdomyosarcoma and endodermal sinus tumor. Table 11-2 shows the distribution of histologic types in 93 primary cancers of the vagina diagnosed at the University of Pennsylvania during 1958 to 1980.[25]

Before the diagnosis of primary carcinoma of the vagina is made, the possibility of metastasis from another genital malignancy must be excluded. The most common offenders are tumors from the cervix and endometrium, although ovarian cancers uncommonly may spread to involve the vagina as the first manifestation of malignancy.

Although the cause of vaginal squamous cell carcinoma is unknown, proposed etiologies have included chronic irritation associated with procidentia, wearing of pessaries,[26,27] and genital viruses.[28] Previous radiotherapy to the vagina has been disclaimed as an important etiologic factor.[29]

The most common presenting symptom in squamous carcinoma of the vagina is vaginal bleeding, although patients may also complain of vaginal discharge and pelvic pain.[30-35] The nature of the pain depends on the location and size of the tumor. Consequently, carcinomas arising from the anterior vaginal wall may cause urinary symptoms, whereas those in the posterior vagina may be associated with bowel symptoms. The mean delay in the diagnosis ranges from 1 to 11 months.[33,34,36] In 13 to 21 percent of patients with vaginal carcinoma, however, there are no symptoms, and the diagnosis is made incidentally.[31,32,34,35] Consequently, cytologic screening of the vagina every 1 to 2 years should be performed in all post-hysterectomy patients. Pelvic examination as

Table 11-2 Histologic Distribution of Primary Vaginal Cancers: 1958–1980

Histology	%[a]
Squamous carcinoma	81
Adenocarcinoma	10
Sarcoma	6
Melanoma	3

[a] The study consisted of 93 patients.
(Modified from Rubin SC, Young J, Mikuta JJ: Squamous carcinoma of the vagina: Treatment, complications, and long-term follow-up. Gynecol Oncol 20:346, 1985.)

well as colposcopy, iodine staining of the vagina, and biopsy of all suspicious areas are essential. The vaginal speculum should be rotated in order to detect small lesions.

The location of the tumor will determine the pattern of spread. Cancer of the vagina spreads primarily by direct invasion and by lymphatic dissemination. In general, the lymphatics from the anterior wall of the upper and middle portions of the vagina drain into the internal and external iliac lymph nodes, whereas the posterior vaginal lymphatics empty into the obturator, pararectal, and aortic nodes. The lymphatic drainage of the distal vagina is similar to that of the vulva and anus, primarily to the inguinal nodes. Lymphatic communications between upper and lower as well as right and left sides of the vagina can explain the variations of lymphatic involvement in individual patients.

Primary vaginal squamous cell carcinoma most commonly arises from the posterior wall in the upper third of the vagina (Fig. 11-4). In one study, more than one-half occurred in the upper third and approximately two-thirds involved the posterior wall.[24] The anterior wall of the lower third of the vagina is the next most common site of origin. Although this tumor may have any of several appearances on gross examination, the usual one is nodular and ulcerated. Less common forms include a papillary exophytic variety and an insidiously infiltrative flat type that invades the submucosa extensively before becoming evident.

Definitive diagnosis of vaginal squamous carcinoma is established by biopsy of the lesion. Histologically, squamous cell carcinomas of the vagina are similar to those arising in other sites of the lower female genital tract. They may be of either keratinizing or nonkeratinizing types and may be well, moderately, or poorly differentiated. Well-differentiated squamous cell carcinomas frequently show keratinization, although some only exhibit extensive glycogenation. Moderately differentiated squamous cell carcinomas are less likely to be keratinized and may show only focal keratinization, often centrally within nests of tumor. In keeping with their poorly differentiated nature, high-grade squamous cell carcinomas only rarely exhibit keratinization.[37] Some poorly differentiated squamous cell carcinomas are composed of spindle cells virtually indistinguishable from sarcoma, a situation analogous to that seen in other organs, such as the larynx; although these cases usually have foci of moderately differentiated tumor, facilitating the diagnosis, biopsy sampling error may hamper tumor identification in those composed predominantly of sarcomatoid or pseudosarcomatous elements.[38] Immunohistochemical studies are frequently helpful in establishing the correct diagnosis, since the spindle cell elements often stain positively for epithelial markers such as cytokeratin.

Verrucous carcinoma, a unique subtype of squamous cell carcinoma, is a rare finding in the vagina. It has clinical and pathologic features similar to those encountered in the vulva (Chapter 10).

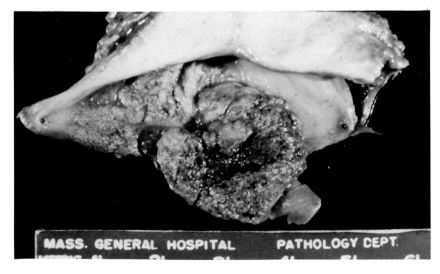

Fig. 11-4 Primary vaginal squamous cell carcinoma. A fungating and necrotic tumor is present in the upper third of the vagina on the posterior wall.

Careful examination of all areas of the vagina and adjacent pelvic organs, including palpation of both inguinal areas, is necessary to rule out continuous spread or metastases from tumors of the cervix, endometrium, vulva, bladder, and rectum. The pretreatment workup and staging procedure should include chest radiography, cystoscopy, sigmoidoscopy, intravenous pyelogram, and barium enema. Computed tomography (CT) of the pelvis and abdomen may detect metastases to pelvic and aortic lymph nodes. Any case demonstrating simultaneous involvement of the vulva, urethra, rectum, or cervix should be classified as originating from those organs.

The staging system of vaginal carcinoma sanctioned by the International Federation of Gynecology and Obstetrics (FIGO) is shown in Table 11-3. The FIGO system is based on clinical examination only, and subsequent surgical findings do not change the stage. The diagnosis of carcinoma of the vagina should be made only if the primary site of the tumor is in the vagina and secondary involvement from either genital or extragenital sites has been excluded. The association between vaginal squamous cell carcinoma and other female genital tract cancers, especially cervical squamous carcinoma, is well documented[39,40]; however, the median interval of 20 years between the diagnosis of invasive cervical carcinoma and subsequent invasive vaginal carcinoma provides strong support for the concept of separate primaries.[40]

Table 11-3 Staging System for Primary Vaginal Cancer

FIGO[a] Stage	Degree of Involvement
0	Carcinoma in situ, intraepithelial carcinoma
I	Carcinoma limited to the vaginal wall
II	Carcinoma involving the subvaginal tissue but not extending onto the pelvic wall
III	Carcinoma extending onto the pelvic wall
IV	Carcinoma extending beyond the true pelvis or involving the mucosa of the bladder or rectum (bullous edema, as such, does not permit a case to be allotted to stage IV)
IVA	Spread of the growth to adjacent organs and/or direct extension beyond the true pelvis
IVB	Spread to distant organs

[a] FIGO, International Federation of Gynecology and Obstetrics.

Treatment

Therapy for invasive carcinoma of the vagina requires individualization, depending on the stage and the location of the tumor. The age of the patient, the results of medical studies, and the desire for preservation of a functional vagina should be considered in planning therapy. The close proximity of bladder, ureters, and rectum may make adequate radiotherapeutic or surgical therapy difficult because of the risk of damage to these organs.

The preferred treatment for most carcinomas of the vagina is radiotherapy.[25,29,32,34,41,42] Patients with small superficial stage I tumors can be treated adequately with intracavitary or interstitial radiation (6,000 to 7,000 rad). In stages I (lesions greater than 2 cm) and II, external beam irradiation is administered to the whole pelvis in the form of 4,000 to 5,000 rad over 4 to 5 weeks followed by an interstitial or intracavitary implant.

Treatment of patients with stage III and IV tumors should consist of 4,000 rad to the whole pelvis and a total of 5,500 rad to the parametrium, combined with interstitial and intracavitary insertions.[29] If the carcinoma involves the lower third of the vagina, 5,000 rad should be added to both groins. Patients with stage I carcinoma involving the upper third of the vagina can be managed with a radical hysterectomy, vaginectomy, and pelvic lymphadenectomy. In selected patients, split-thickness skin grafting is performed in order to maintain vaginal function (Table 11-4). Exenterative surgery is indicated in patients with central recurrence of tumor who have failed primary radiation therapy.

The reported effectiveness of systemic chemotherapy in the treatment of disseminated squamous cell carcinoma of the vagina has been disappointing. Adriamycin, methyl-CCNU, 5-FU, CCNU, and cisplatin have been tried as single agents. Combination chemotherapy with cyclophosphamide, Adriamycin, and 5-FU[43] or cisplatin with 5-FU[11] has been administered in a few cases; complete responses were infrequent and of short duration. A recent phase II trial of cisplatin at 50 mg/m IV every 3 weeks in 26 patients with advanced or recurrent carcinoma of the vagina showed disappointing results.[44] Apparent complete disappearance of an advanced primary vaginal squamous carcinoma with involved inguinal lymph nodes was achieved with three courses of bleomycin, meth-

Table 11-4 Treatment of Invasive Vaginal Cancer

FIGO Stage[a]	Treatment Modality
Stage I <2-cm lesion, upper third of vagina	Vaginal interstitial or intracavitary irradiation or Radical hysterectomy and vaginectomy with pelvic lymphadenectomy and possible split-thickness skin grafting
Stage I >2-cm lesion II III IV	External pelvic beam and vaginal intracavitary or interstitial irradiation

[a] FIGO, International Federation of Gynecology and Obstetrics.

otrexate, and cisplatin in a 52-year-old woman. The chemotherapy was administered prior to radiotherapy.[45]

Five-year survival rates for the various stages of vaginal carcinoma treated with radiation are shown in Table 11-5. These rates relate to the period 1976 to 1978 and encompass the work of 66 investigators.[46] Perez et al.[37] report higher survival, particularly in stage I (90 percent), whereas the results in stage II (32 percent), stage III (40 percent), and stage IV (0 percent) are similar.[19]

Table 11-6 shows the survival rates for different treatment modalities in patients with stage I invasive vaginal cancer.[46] No meaningful conclusion can be drawn from the data because standard criteria were not applied when selecting patients for surgery or radiation. The reported 5-year survival rates, includ-

Table 11-6 Carcinoma of Vagina: Stage I 5-Year Survival and Treatment

Treatment	5-Year Survival (%)
Surgery	83.9
Surgery and radiation	73.9
Radiation	55.6

(Modified from Annual Report on the Results of Treatment in Gynecological Cancer. Vol. 19. FIGO. Radiumhemmet, Stockholm, Sweden, 1985.)

ing all treatment methods, range from 64 to 90 percent (stage I), 29 to 66 percent (stage II), and 0 to 40 percent (stages III and IV).[30] Table 11-7 shows the survival rates for all treatment modalities (FIGO).[46] The incidence of complications following surgery

Table 11-5 Carcinoma of the Vagina: 5-Year Survival with Radiation

Stage	No. of Patients Treated	5-Year Survival (%)
I	124	55.6
II	153	32.7
III	154	38.0
IV	68	4.4

(Modified from Annual Report on the Results of Treatment in Gynecological Cancer. Vol. 19. FIGO, Radiumhemmet, Stockholm, Sweden, 1985.)

Table 11-7 Carcinoma of the Vagina: 5-Year Survival with All Treatment Modalities

Stage	No. of Patients Treated	5-Year Survival (%)
I	179	61.5
II	184	33.7
III	165	25.5
IV	79	8.9

(Modified from Annual Report of the Results of Treatment in Gynecological Cancer. Vol. 19. FIGO. Radiumhemmet, Stockholm, Sweden, 1985.)

and radiotherapy is low in patients with early-stage disease, consisting primarily of vaginal fibrosis and shortening. Major complications such as rectovesicovaginal fistulas are related to stage and radiation dose, generally occurring in patients with more advanced disease.

DES-ASSOCIATED VAGINAL EPITHELIAL CHANGES AND CLEAR CELL CARCINOMA

From 1946 to 1971, physicians prescribed diethylstilbestrol (DES), a nonsteroidal estrogen, to an estimated 2 to 3 million pregnant women. The aim was improved pregnancy outcome in those patients with threatened or habitual spontaneous abortion.[47,48] In 1971, the association between maternal DES therapy during pregnancy and subsequent development of vaginal and cervical clear cell adenocarcinoma in female offspring was substantiated.[49]

DES IN HISTORICAL PERSPECTIVE

1946   First reported suggestion that DES administration prevents repeated abortion.

1953   DES is demonstrated to be of no benefit in pregnancy.

1971   An association between maternal DES use and clear cell adenocarcinoma in their adolescent offspring is shown.

1978   The risk of clear cell adenocarcinoma from maternal DES exposure is estimated to be 1.4 : 1,000 to 1.4 : 10,000.

To study the clinical, epidemiologic, and pathologic aspects of vaginal and cervical clear cell adenocarcinoma, the Registry for Research on Hormonal Transplacental Carcinogenesis was established in 1971. Currently, more than 500 cases have been entered,[50] and the registry now accessions all cases in which cancer of the female genital tract occurs subsequent to prenatal exogenous hormone exposure. Women born after 1940 who have vaginal-cervical clear cell adenocarcinomas and no history of maternal ingestion of hormones are registered as well. Approximately two-thirds of cases have had a history of intrauterine exposure to DES. The risk of the development of clear cell carcinoma in the exposed female offspring is small, approximately 1 : 1,000 to 1 : 10,000. The youngest DES-exposed daughter to develop vaginal clear cell adenocarcinoma was 7 years old at the time of diagnosis and the oldest was 33. The rise in the age incidence curve occurs after age 14 with a peak at age 19.[51] A study of 156 DES-exposed women with clear cell adenocarcinoma and 1,848 DES-exposed control subjects without cancer shows that the relative risk is higher among those daughters whose mothers were given DES before the twelfth week of pregnancy and who had at least one prior spontaneous abortion.[50]

Diethylstilbestrol exposure can lead to various anatomic anomalies, most of which are benign and related to perturbations in normal genital tract development.[52]

EFFECTS ON FEMALE PROGENY FROM IN UTERO EXPOSURE TO DES

Clear cell adenocarcinoma

Adenosis

Cervicovaginal structural changes and their effects
    Transverse ridges
    Cockscombs and septa
    Cervical hoods and collars
    Cervical mucus effects
    Cervical incompetence
    Cervical stenosis (after therapy)

Uterine and tubal structural changes

(Modified from Stillman RJ: In utero exposure to diethylstilbestrol: Adverse effects on the reproductive performance in male and female offspring. Am J Obstet Gynecol 142:905, 1982.)

In the physiologic development of the vagina, the mullerian-derived columnar epithelium is replaced by squamous epithelium from the urogenital sinus. DES administered before the eighteenth week of gestation may inhibit the normal upward progression of the squamous epithelium. Consequently, there is absence of squamous epithelium in the vagina and cervix up to the endocervical canal, with areas of ectopic glandular epithelium (adenosis) persisting in the vagina. An excessive eversion or ectropion may exist on the cervix. The degree of adverse effects is increased if DES is given earlier in pregnancy and at a higher dose; consequently, those exposed prior to the eighteenth week of gestation may have more extensive areas of vaginal epithelial changes.

Vaginal Epithelial Changes

The histologic changes associated with DES exposure have been categorized as vaginal epithelial changes. These include vaginal adenosis and squamous metaplasia, the latter arising by replacement of the former.[53]

Adenosis rarely may involve the surface of the vagina, without underlying stromal involvement, or it may be found exclusively in the stroma; most commonly, however, the condition exists as a combination of the two. The extent of the lesion varies from patient to patient and is probably related to the timing and dosage of DES. In some, the change is manifested by a few scattered glands confined to the stroma; in others, large areas of the vagina are involved by both surface and stromal adenosis. The glandular epithelium of adenosis may resemble that of either the endocervix, fallopian tube, or endometrium. The latter two cell types commonly occur together (tuboendometrial), frequently contain cilia, and are only rarely seen in surface mucosal adenosis. By contrast, endocervical, or mucinous, adenosis is the most frequent type to involve the surface mucosa, although it may be seen in the stroma as well (Fig. 11-5). Tuboendometrial adenosis has been shown to occur with greater frequency in the anterior lower vagina.[54] Nabothian cystlike structures may arise in the vagina secondary to cystic dilation of mucinous glands; these structures are virtually identical to those that occur in the cervix and arise by a common mechanism, obstruction of mucin outflow by surface squamous metaplasia (Fig. 11-6).

The finding of vaginal adenosis, however, is not restricted to DES-exposed females born after 1940, since several studies have documented its presence in women never exposed to the drug. Some of these patients have been postmenopausal[55,56] (Fig. 11-6).

Adenosis can be detected in more than 90 percent of DES-exposed females with vaginal clear cell adeno-

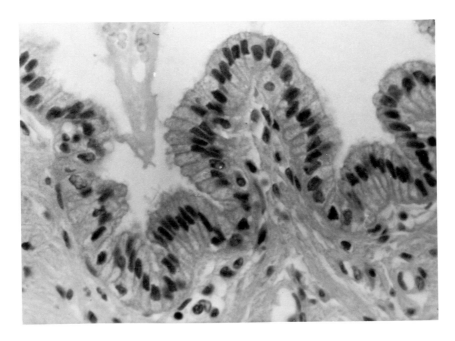

Fig. 11-5 Mucinous adenosis. Tall columnar cells with pale cytoplasm and often basally located nuclei resemble endocervical type epithelium. (H & E, ×450.)

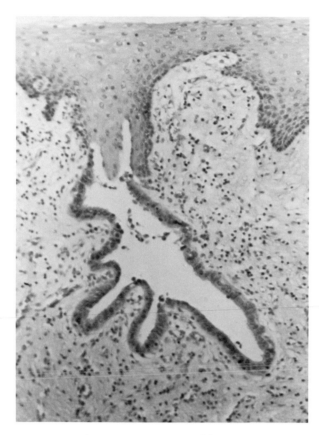

Fig. 11-6 Adenosis in a 56-year-old non-DES-exposed woman. The surface component has been replaced by squamous metaplasia, which is beginning to extend into the underlying tuboendometrial glands. Such blockage of the glandular outlet can lead to the accumulation of secretion and formation of Nabothian-type cysts. (H & E, ×150.)

carcinoma. The extremely low incidence of clear cell adenocarcinoma suggests that, in most cases, adenosis per se is not a premalignant condition. Relatively recent evidence, however, indicates that atypical adenosis may be a precursor to clear cell adenocarcinoma.[57] Such lesions have been identified by serial section studies of vaginal clear cell adenocarcinoma and the surrounding tissues. The glands of atypical adenosis are virtually always of the tuboendometrial type, and their presence in the immediate proximity of the tumor has given rise to speculation that they engender clear cell adenocarcinoma. Glandular atypia is manifested by varying degress of nuclear pleomorphism and hyperchromasia as well as by cellular stratification (Fig. 11-7). Glands of atypical adenosis have been

shown by microspectrophotometric studies frequently to be aneuploid, a pattern commonly associated with malignancy in nonendocrine types of tumors.

The other type of vaginal epithelial change associated with DES-exposure is squamous metaplasia. Coincident with the onset of puberty, the vaginal milieu becomes more acidic, an environment less suitable for the alkaline glandular epithelium of vaginal adenosis; this process is similar to the eversion of alkaline columnar epithelium of the endocervical canal into the acidic vagina and its subsequent replacement by squamous metaplasia. Squamous metaplasia is present in variable amounts within the areas of vaginal adenosis, depending to a great extent on the age of the patient (Fig. 11-8). In younger patients, scattered glands may be partially replaced by an immature squamous epithelium, whereas in older patients especially, most or all of the adenosis has been converted to a squamous epithelium that is heavily glycogenated and virtually indistinguishable from the native vaginal mucosa. Extension of the metaplastic process into glands within the vaginal stroma results in small subepithelial islands and nests of immature squamous epithelium; misinterpretation of microscopic sections in which such foci appear separate from the overlying mucosa has occasionally led to the erroneous diagnosis of invasive carcinoma.

No definitive evidence exists that the large areas of squamous metaplasia arising from replacement of vaginal adenosis and cervical ectropion (transformation zone) result in a greater risk of squamous cell cancer for DES-exposed women. An increased incidence of cervical and vaginal dysplasia, however, was found in 3,980 DES-exposed young women as compared with unexposed control patients. In addition, cervical and vaginal dysplasia were more frequent when squamous metaplasia extended to the outer half of the cervix or onto the vagina.[58]

Clear Cell Carcinoma

Approximately one-fourth of patients with clear cell adenocarcinoma are asymptomatic. Indeed, in a recent study of pregnant patients with clear cell carcinoma, more than one-third had no symptoms prior to diagnosis.[59]

Clear cell adenocarcinoma may arise at any site in the female genital tract, including the ovary, endo-

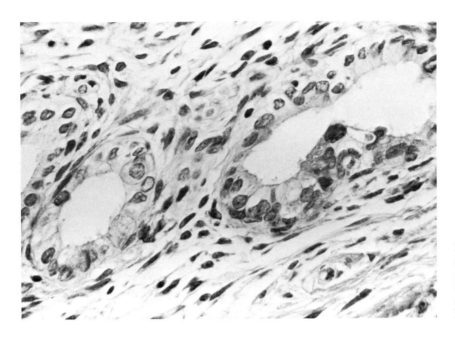

Fig. 11-7 Atypical adenosis in a DES-exposed woman. The glandular cells show focal stratification, nuclear pleomorphism, and prominent nucleoli. (H & E, ×450.)

metrium, cervix, and vagina. In DES-exposed females, clear cell adenocarcinoma has arisen with almost equal frequency in the cervix and vagina, with some investigators reporting a predominance in the vagina (68 percent).[60] In keeping with the most frequent location of vaginal adenosis, clear cell carci-

nomas of the vagina are encountered most often on the anterior upper one-third of the wall. Certainly, however, other sites in the vagina may be involved, and multicentric tumors have been reported.[57] Some clear cell adenocarcinomas have involved only the cervix, particularly the exocervix, and others appar-

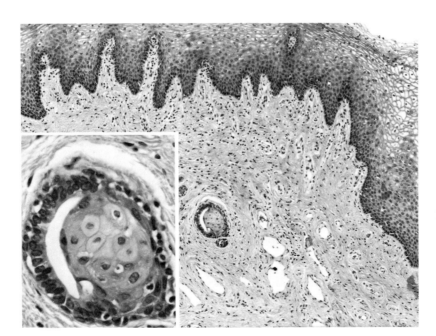

Fig. 11-8 Tuboendometrial adenosis in a DES-exposed woman. The stroma contains bland-appearing tuboendometrial-type glands. (H & E, ×45.) (Inset) Some glands have undergone partial replacement by immature squamous metaplasia. (H & E, ×175.)

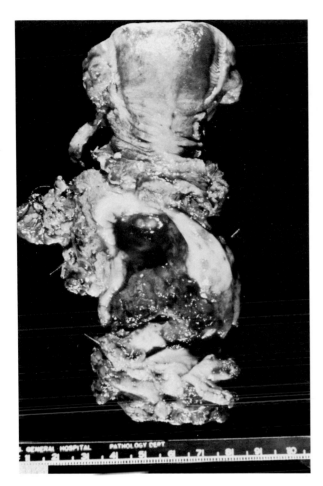

Fig. 11-9 Clear cell adenocarcinoma in a DES-exposed woman. The ulcerated tumor is present at the junction of the upper and middle thirds of the vagina.

ently have arisen from both the cervix and vagina. In a careful and meticulous study of the topographic relationship of vaginal and cervical adenosis to clear cell adenocarcinoma, Robboy et al.[61] emphasized the frequent location of clear cell carcinomas adjacent to the most distal point of glandular extension; these areas warrant especially careful clinical examination.[61]

On gross examination, clear cell adenocarcinoma may vary considerably in size and configuration; some are so small that they may easily be missed on cursory examination and only become evident on subsequent microscopic study. Commonly, small tumors exist as flat, often indurated, lesions. On the other hand, tumors as large as 10 cm in surface area have been reported.[53] Most larger tumors have an exophytic,

nodular, or polypoid configuration, with concomitant friability and necrosis, yet some larger clear cell adenocarcinomas are flattened and indurated, sometimes with ulceration (Fig. 11-9).

On microscopic examination, the clear cell adenocarcinoma may exist as a focal lesion within areas of atypical adenosis, analogous to an adenocarcinoma in situ, or as an overtly invasive tumor. In the latter situation, clear cell adenocarcinoma may be only superficially invasive and relatively restricted to the lamina propria, or it may exhibit transmural invasion of the cervix or vagina (Fig. 11-10). Microscopic study may show a more insidious involvement than suspected on clinical examination or gross inspection at the pathology cutting bench.

Clear cell adenocarcinomas have displayed several different histologic patterns; one pattern may be found exclusively, may form the predominant element, or may be mixed with other histologic types. The histologic appearances are identical with other mullerian tract-derived clear cell carcinomas, such as those from the ovary and endometrium. The most frequently encountered pattern is the tubulocystic type, which, as the name implies, is composed of small tubules and cystic structures. So-called hobnail cells, or cells with bulbous protruding nuclei, often line the lumens but sometimes are joined by low columnar to cuboidal cells (Fig. 11-11). Furthermore, neoplastic cysts may be lined by rather innocuous-appearing flattened cells, an appearance that can engender confusion in the diagnosis, especially on the basis of biopsy alone. Mitotic activity is characteristically, but not invariably, low.

Another pattern of clear cell adenocarcinoma is that of solid sheets of polygonal cells with clear cytoplasm, the latter resulting from loss of glycogen during routine hematoxylin and eosin staining. Periodic acid-Schiff (PAS) stain demonstrates the intracytoplasmic glycogen well; stains for intracytoplasmic mucin are consistently negative, although some staining can occasionally be observed within gland lumens. Other histologic appearances include endometrioid, papillary, and cordlike patterns.

Non-DES-associated adenocarcinoma of the vagina is exceedingly rare. Most probably arise from vaginal adenosis, since studies have shown adenosis to occur in women, some postmenopausal, born prior to the DES era.[55,56] One report described a non-clear cell adenocarcinoma that had developed in a 38-year-old

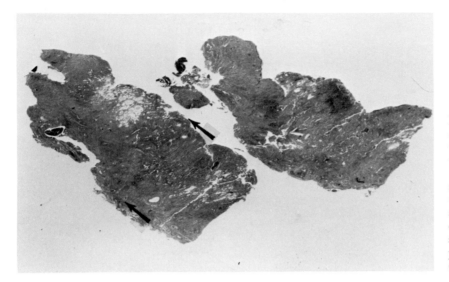

Fig. 11-10 Clear cell adenocarcinoma. Two sagittal sections of vaginal wall from the tumor illustrated in Figure 11-9. The carcinoma shows insidious transmural infiltration (breadth of tumor between arrows; note lower arrow near deep resection margin). Foci of superficial cystic adenosis are present to the left of top arrow. (H & E ×10.)

woman with vaginal adenosis; although there was no history of intrauterine DES exposure, she apparently had taken conjugated estrogen for 10 years despite retention of her ovaries.[62]

TREATMENT

Diethylstilbestrol-exposed women should be followed every 6 months subsequent to the initial screening examination at the time of menarche. Colposcopy is not necessary at every repeat examination. Digital palpation of the vagina and cervix should rule out discrete nodules or indurations, possible early manifestations of clear cell carcinoma. All indurated or unusually firm or cystic areas in the vagina and on the cervix must be biopsied if they are not identified on colposcopy as adenosis or Nabothian cysts. Other cervicovaginal structural abnormalities (e.g., septa, cervical hood) can be detected with the digital examination (see under the Effects on Female Progeny from In Utero Exposure to DES). A Pap smear should be taken from the cervix and vagina. All epithelial changes on the cervix and in the vagina should be sampled. Most often, the atypical colposcopic findings reflect ongoing squamous metaplasia and do not show dysplastic tissue on biopsy.

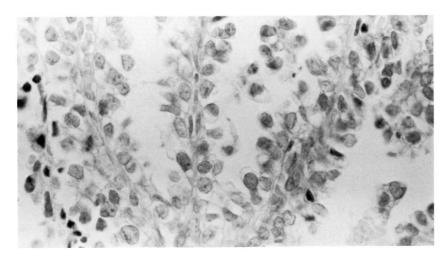

Fig. 11-11 Clear cell adenocarcinoma. The tubulocystic pattern shows prominent hobnail cells and clear cytoplasm. (H & E, ×450.)

RECOMMENDED CLINICAL EXAMINATION AND SCREENING PROCEDURES FOR DES-EXPOSED WOMEN

Inspection of vagina and cervix

Palpation of vagina and cervix

Cytology of vagina and cervix

Iodine staining of vagina and cervix

Colposcopy and vaginal/cervical biopsies, if indicated

Bimanual examination

Colposcopy may assist in the identification of epithelial changes associated with DES exposure and of suspicious areas for biopsy in those with an abnormal Pap smear. In addition, colposcopy can be used to document the extent of cervical and vaginal epithelial changes and to chart their subsequent course. In the absence of a colposcope, areas of intraepithelial neoplasia often can be localized by staining with Lugol's solution and taking a Pap smear. The diagnosis of clear cell adenocarcinoma most often can be accomplished with a digital examination and a Pap smear. Lugol's solution may help outline the limits of the tumor.

The staging is done according to the criteria established by the International Federation of Gynecology and Obstetrics (Table 11-3). More than 50 percent of all patients with vaginal clear cell adenocarcinoma are stage I at the time of diagnosis. The metastatic workup is similar to that for squamous cell carcinoma but should include evaluation of aortic lymph nodes, preferably by CT scan, because of the high recurrence rate at distant sites. Approximately one-third of patients with clear cell adenocarcinoma have presented with recurrent disease in the lungs and supraclavicular lymph nodes.[60] The incidence of positive lymph nodes is related to tumor size and depth of invasion.

The treatment of vaginal clear cell adenocarcinoma should be individualized. Tumor size and location, extent of disease, and patient age must be considered. Treatment for most young patients with stage I and early stage II lesions has consisted of radical hysterectomy, pelvic lymphadenectomy, and partial or complete vaginectomy with reconstruction of the vagina. The ovaries may be preserved, as ovarian metastasis is infrequent.

Primary radiation therapy can accomplish similar results to surgery but has been used more frequently for advanced lesions. Various other therapeutic modalities, including primary exenteration, local resection, and local radiation therapy for preservation of fertility, have been attempted in several patients with varying success.[63]

The 5-year survival for all stages in patients with clear cell adenocarcinoma is 78 percent, as compared with 35 percent for patients with squamous carcinoma of the vagina.[64] This rate may be related to the earlier detection of cancers in DES-exposed patients. An improved 5-year survival rate in patients older than 19 years has been attributed to a higher frequency of the tubulocystic pattern of the tumor in that age group.[65] Five-year survival figures for clear cell adenocarcinoma vary from 87 percent for stage I, 76 percent for stage II, and 37 percent for stage III, with 6-month survival for stage IV disease.[66] Very few recurrences have occurred 3 years or more after primary treatment. Lung and supraclavicular lymph node metastases appear to be more frequent in clear cell adenocarcinoma than in patients with squamous carcinoma of the vagina. Recurrent disease has been treated with radical surgery, irradiation, chemotherapy, or various combinations of these modalities, depending on the site of the tumor.

Exenterative therapy has been used for central recurrent disease in the absence of prior irradiation. Chemotherapy for recurrent systemic disease with various single agent or combination programs has not been effective.

MALIGNANT MELANOMA

The rarity of primary malignant melanoma of the vagina is exemplified by the finding of slightly more than 100 collected cases in the literature.[67] The reported age distribution of malignant melanoma of the vagina has ranged from 22 to 78 years, with most cases occurring past the age of 50.[68,69] Most patients are symptomatic, with the most frequent presenting symptoms being vaginal bleeding and discharge. In spite of these symptoms, however, late diagnosis is common.

Although malignant melanoma of the vagina may arise at any site in the vagina, some studies indicate that most cases occur in the lower one-third of the vagina, with perhaps a slight predisposition for the anterior wall. Vaginal malignant melanoma may be small, measuring less than 1 cm in diameter, or large; in one reported case, the tumor virtually replaced the anterior vaginal wall.[69] The size of the lesion is probably related to the duration of growth before detection and whether ulceration has occurred, the latter giving rise to bleeding, discharge, or pain, either singly or in combination. In postmenopausal women who are not sexually active, malignant melanoma of the vagina may reach considerable dimensions before clinical symptoms appear.

Often malignant melanoma of the vagina has an exophytic growth pattern, occurring as a black, blue-black, or variegated red to yellow polypoid tumor; however, it may also exist as a similarly pigmented flat lesion, with no appreciable mucosal elevation (Fig. 11-12).

On microscopic examination, vaginal malignant melanoma has the same characteristics as those in other body sites, such as the vulva (see Chapter 10). Thus, malignant melanoma of the vagina may exhibit a variety of histologic appearances, including epithelioid, spindled, and alveolar patterns. In addition, there may be regional histologic variation within the tumor; for example, some areas may show a predominance of the alveolar pattern, whereas others may exhibit a sarcomatoid appearance closely resembling a leiomyosarcoma. Malignant melanoma of the vagina may contain varying amounts of melanin, present as yellow-brown pigment. In some cases, the cytoplasm of most tumor cells is filled with melanin, obscuring the nucleus; in others, melanin is only focally present and in small amounts. In so-called amelanotic melanomas, no melanin pigment is evident by light microscopy, and only electron microscopy confirms the diagnosis by revealing the presence of intracytoplasmic premelanosomes, precursors to melanosomes. Amelanotic melanoma, at least according to one study,[70] is the exception rather than the rule in the vagina.

If the overlying squamous mucosa is not ulcerated, one may observe junctional activity as well as the so-called pagetoid spread of melanoma cells into the squamous epithelium. If such changes are not observed, one should entertain the possibility of a vaginal metastasis from another body site. Given the propensity of malignant melanoma to disseminate widely throughout the body, metastasis should be excluded by a careful clinical workup. The rarity of primary malignant melanoma of the vagina mandates caution before considering treatment for this condition.

If such measures suggest the lesion is indeed pri-

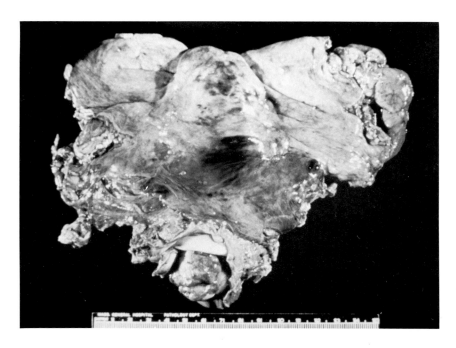

Fig. 11-12 Malignant melanoma. The tumor is present as a flat heavily pigmented lesion of the vaginal mucosa.

mary, the tumor should be measured microscopically in order to determine prognostic parameters. The series reported by Chung et al.[69] suggests that, as in cutaneous melanoma, the depth of invasion dictates the survival of the patient. Using Breslow's methods, originally developed for cutaneous melanoma, Chung and co-workers found that many of their patients had deeply invasive tumors at the time of diagnosis; in fact, 80 percent had level IV lesions. The latter includes lesions invading deeper than 2 mm; level I tumors were confined to the surface epithelium, whereas level II tumors invaded to less than 1 mm and level III between 1 and 2 mm. A staging system as described for vulvar melanomas[71] is best used for vaginal lesions.[69]

Treatment

The primary treatment for vaginal melanomas located in the upper two-thirds of the vagina is radical wide local excision and pelvic lymphadenectomy; lesions in the lower one-third of the vagina may also require a vulvectomy to ensure free resection margins as well as a groin dissection. Exenterative surgery should be performed only to accomplish adequate local radical resection. The role of radiotherapy, chemotherapy, and immunotherapy is unproved, although some workers have espoused radiation therapy for those patients with medical problems that obviate surgery.[72]

Probably as a result of greater public awareness and consequent earlier detection, cutaneous malignant melanoma has lately experienced a respectable increase in the 5-year survival rate; unfortunately, no such case exists for malignant melanoma of the vagina, which still carries a dismal prognosis. The figures for 5-year survival of patients with malignant melanoma of the vagina are generally well below 10 percent.[73]

VAGINAL SARCOMAS (ADULT TYPE)

Primary vaginal sarcoma in adults is extremely rare. In 1985, Peters et al.[74] reported on 51 cases collected from the world literature, in addition to 17 of their own. The most common type is leiomyosarcoma; other less common entities include fibrosarcoma, rhabdomyosarcoma, alveolar soft part sarcoma, neur-

ofibrosarcoma, angiosarcoma, and mixed mesodermal tumor. Each of these tumors exhibits histologic features similar to their counterparts in other organs. In the study by Peters and co-workers, the median age was 57 years. Presenting vaginal symptoms included bloody discharge, pain, and a mass.

Treatment

The treatment of choice in all vaginal sarcomas is surgical resection. Depending on the circumstances, pelvic exenteration may be necessary to ensure wide local excision. Indeed, in the series conducted by Peters and associates, the only patients who were long-term survivors had undergone a pelvic exenteration. Regional lymph node involvement apparently is unusual in patients with vaginal leiomyosarcomas.[75] Radiation therapy appears to have some benefit in achieving local control. The role of chemotherapy needs further investigation.

EMBRYONAL RHABDOMYOSARCOMA (SARCOMA BOTRYOIDES)

In the age group from newborn to 10 years, embryonal rhabdomyosarcoma is the most common malignant tumor arising in the vagina; 85 to 90 percent occur in girls under 5 years of age. Most are encountered between the ages of 1 and 2. The usual presenting symptom in embryonal rhabdomyosarcoma is abnormal vaginal bleeding. In fact, any vaginal bleeding in an infant past the neonatal period is highly suggestive of a malignancy and mandates a complete examination. The commonly used term of sarcoma botryoides refers to the grapelike configuration of the tumor that may be noted on gross examination. As the name implies, such tumors often are polypoid and bulky; when large, they may fill the vaginal cavity and protrude from the introitus (Fig. 11-13). Most embryonal rhabdomyosarcomas are soft and friable, varying in color from pink-red to purple or gray; on section, they frequently present a myxomatous jelly-like surface with hemorrhage.

Embryonal rhabdomyosarcoma probably arises from the undifferentiated mesenchyme of the lamina propria.[76] On microscopic examination, the tumor is composed of primitive-appearing mesenchymal tissue; the ground substance is loose and myxoid, and the

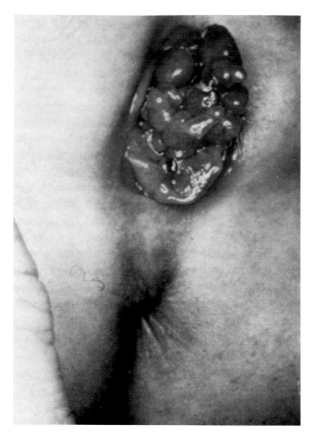

Fig. 11-13 Embryonal rhabdomyosarcoma (sarcoma botryoides). A large polypoid tumor growing in a grapelike configuration protrudes from the vaginal introitus.

cellular component is composed largely of stellate to spindled cells with sparse cytoplasm (Fig. 11-14). A peculiar condensation of such cells immediately beneath the epithelium, designated the cambium layer, is highly characteristic of embryonal rhabdomyosarcoma. Mitotic activity is usually brisk. Primitive skeletal muscle cells, or strap cells, are frequently present, and immunohistochemical stains for myoglobin may show intracytoplasmic positivity within them (Fig. 11-14). The tumor infiltrates the vaginal wall and contiguous pelvic structures. Spread to the regional lymph nodes, as well as the lungs and liver, is common. Embryonal rhabdomyosarcoma is characterized by rapid growth. Left untreated, it will kill the patient within 9 to 18 months after onset of symptoms.

Treatment

Traditionally, treatment has consisted of pelvic exenteration, vaginectomy, and regional lymphadenectomy. In 1975, Hilgers[77] reported that 75 percent of patients with embryonal rhabdomyosarcoma confined to the vagina and 38 percent of patients with extravaginal, but intrapelvic, tumor lived for 2 or more years after pelvic exenteration. More recently, Dewhurst and Ferreira[78] showed that combined treatment with vincristine, actinomycin D, cyclophosphamide, radiation, and extended hysterectomy may be equal to or better than exenterative therapy; three patients treated with this combination were without evidence of disease $1\frac{1}{2}$ to 3 years after therapy.

ENDODERMAL SINUS TUMOR

Endodermal sinus tumor, also known as yolk sac tumor and Teilum tumor, of the vagina is rare. Young and Scully[79] reviewed the literature in 1984 and added 9 patients of their own to the previously reported 48 cases. Most cases occur before the age of 2 years[79]; presenting symptoms include vaginal discharge, usually bloody, and a polypoid tumor (Fig. 11-15). The lesion should be differentiated from embryonal rhabdomyosarcoma, the most common vaginal tumor in infancy. In fact, in the series reported by Copeland et al.,[80] four of their six cases were referred for consultation with a diagnosis of sarcoma botryoides; in that report, two of the cases were restricted to the vagina proper, whereas three involved both vagina and cervix.

On microscopic examination, endodermal sinus tumor of the vagina exhibits the same histologic appearance observed in the ovary as well as other genital and extragenital sites. Festoon, reticular, and solid patterns may predominate or exist as mixed forms. Typical pathognomonic Schiller-Duvall bodies may be identified (Fig. 11-16) and, in all patterns, intracellular and extracellular hyaline bodies and intracytoplasmic glycogen frequently occur. On immunohistochemical staining, α-fetoprotein (AFP) is almost invariably present within cells and provides a reliable marker for endodermal sinus tumor.

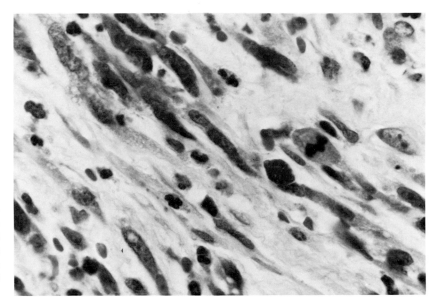

Fig. 11-14 Embryonal rhabdo-myosarcoma (sarcoma bo-tryoides). Elongated, primitive straplike cells are present in a loose myxoid ground substance. A mitotic figure is present at the right. (H & E, ×450.)

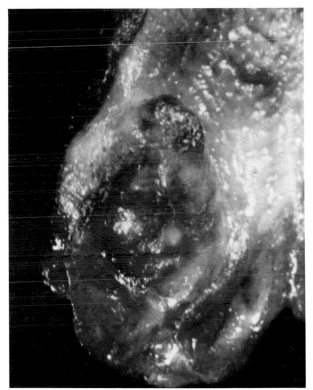

Fig. 11-15 Endodermal sinus tumor is present as a large, irregularly nodular mass arising in the vagina of an infant. Note the normal rugal pattern of the vagina to the upper right.

Treatment

The pretreatment workup of any suspected vaginal malignancy in a young child should include a serum AFP determination. Should the tumor prove to be an endodermal sinus tumor, such a baseline value can be used to plan and monitor therapy.

Until recently, vaginectomy and pelvic exenteration or radiation were the cornerstones of therapy. The current treatment of choice appears to be combination chemotherapy with vincristine, actinomycin, and cyclophosphamide coupled with local excision of the tumor.[80,81] Such an approach is attractive in that it permits preservation of sexual and reproductive function in young patients. Support for this regimen is provided by the report by Copeland et al.[80] in 1985, in which four of six patients with either vaginal or cervical endodermal sinus tumor or both were disease free from 2 to 23 years after vincristine–actinomycin–cyclophosphamide treatment. In addition, Anderson et al.[81] described an infant with vaginal endodermal sinus tumor with no evidence of disease 30 months after completion of vincristine–actinomycin–cyclophosphamide therapy and local excision of the tumor.

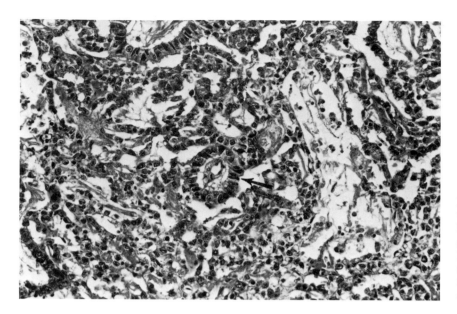

Fig. 11-16 Endodermal sinus tumor with a reticular and trabecular pattern. The arrow denotes a characteristic Schiller-Duvall body containing a central vessel rimmed by primitive-appearing malignant germ cells. (H & E, ×85.)

REFERENCES

1. Gallup DG, Morley GW: Carcinoma in situ of the vagina. A study and review. Obstet Gynecol 46:334, 1975

2. Woodruff JD: Carcinoma in situ of the vagina. Clin Obstet Gynecol 2:485, 1981

3. Benedet JL, Sanders JH: Carcinoma in situ of the vagina. Am J Obstet Gynecol 148:695, 1984

4. Lenehan PM, Meffe F, Lickrish GM: Vaginal intraepithelial neoplasia: Biologic aspects and management. Obstet Gynecol 68:333, 1986

5. Rutledge P: Cancer of the vagina. Am J Obstet Gynecol 97:635, 1967

6. Crum CP, Egawa K, Barrow B, et al: Human papilloma virus infection (condyloma) of the cervix and cervical intraepithelial neoplasia: A histopathologic and statistical analysis. Gynecol Oncol 15:88, 1983

7. Blaustein A, Sedlis A: Diseases of the vagina. p. 59. In Blaustein A (ed): Pathology of the Female Genital Tract. 2nd Ed. Springer-Verlag, New York, 1982

8. Patten SF, Reagan JW, Obenauf M, et al: Postirradiation dysplasia of uterine cervix and vagina: An analytical study of the cells. Cancer 16:173, 1963

9. Hillborne LH, Fu YS: Intraepithelial, invasive and metastatic neoplasms of the vagina. p. 181. In Wilkinson EJ (ed): Pathology of the Vulva and Vagina. Contemporary Issues in Surgical Pathology. Churchill Livingstone, New York, 1987

10. Lowell DM, LiVolsi VA, Ludwig ME: Genital condyloma virus infection following pelvic radiation therapy: Report of seven cases. Int J Gynecol Pathol 2:294, 1983

11. Jordan EL, Bonomi PD, Wilbanks GD: Chemotherapy of vulvar and vaginal neoplasms. p. 85. In Deppe G (ed): Chemotherapy of Gynecologic Cancer. Alan R Liss, New York, 1984

12. Woodruff JD, Parmley TH, Julian CG: Topical 5-fluorouracil in the treatment of vaginal carcinoma in situ. Gynecol Oncol 3:124, 1975

13. Ballon SC, Roberts JA, Lagasse LD: Topical 5-fluorouracil in the treatment of intraepithelial neoplasia of the vagina. Obstet Gynecol 54:163, 1979

14. Daley JW, Ellis GF: Treatment of vaginal dysplasia and carcinoma in situ with topical 5-fluorouracil. Obstet Gynecol 55:350, 1980

15. Petrilli ES, Townsend DE, Morrow CP, et al: Vaginal intraepithelial neoplasia. Biologic aspects and treatment with topical 5-fluorouracil and the carbon dioxide laser. Am J Obstet Gynecol 138:321, 1980

16. Caglar H, Hertzog RW, Hreshchyshyn MM: Topical 5-fluorouracil treatment of vaginal intraepithelial neoplasia. Obstet Gynecol 58:580, 1981

17. Stafl A, Wilkinson EJ, Mattingly RF: Laser treatment of cervical and vaginal neoplasia. Am J Obstet Gynecol 128:128, 1977

18. Capen CV, Masterson BJ, Magrina JF, et al: Laser therapy of vaginal intraepithelial neoplasia. Am J Obstet Gynecol 142:973, 1982

19. Townsend DE, Levine RV, Crum CP: Treatment of

vaginal carcinoma in situ with the carbon dioxide laser. Am J Obstet Gynecol 143:565, 1982

20. Jobson VW, Homesley HD: Treatment of vaginal intraepithelial neoplasia with a carbon dioxide laser. Obstet Gynecol 62:90, 1983

21. Woodruff JD: Treatment of recurrent carcinoma in situ in the lower genital canal. Clin Obstet Gynecol 8:757, 1965

22. Stuart GCE, Allen HH, Anderson RJ: Squamous cell carcinoma of the vagina following hysterectomy. Am J Obstet Gynecol 139:311, 1981

23. Lathrop JC, Ree HJ, McDuff HC Jr: Intraepithelial neoplasia of the neovagina. Obstet Gynecol 65:915, 1985

24. Plentl AA, Friedman EA: Lymphatic System of the Female Genitalia: The Morphologic Basis of Oncologic Diagnosis and Therapy. WB Saunders, Philadelphia, 1971

25. Rubin SC, Young J, Mikuta JJ: Squamous carcinoma of the vagina: Treatment, complications, and long term follow-up. Gynecol Oncol 20:346, 1985

26. Rutledge F: Cancer of the vagina. Am J Obstet Gynecol 97:635, 1967

27. Herbst AL, Green TH, Ulfelder H: Primary carcinoma of the vagina. An analysis of 68 cases. Am J Obstet Gynecol 106:210, 1970

28. Weed JC, Lozier C, Daniel SJ: Human papilloma virus in multifocal, invasive female genital tract malignancy. Obstet Gynecol 62:832, 1983

29. Perez CA, Camel HM: Long term follow-up in radiation therapy of carcinoma of the vagina. Cancer 49:1308, 1982

30. Monaghan JM: The management of carcinoma of the vagina. p. 154. In Shepherd JH, Monaghan JM (eds): Clinical Gynaecological Oncology. Blackwell Scientific Publications, Oxford, 1985

31. Underwood PB, Smith RT: Carcinoma of the vagina. JAMA 217:41, 1971

32. Pride GL, Schultz GE, Chuprevich TW, et al: Primary invasive squamous carcinoma of the vagina. Obstet Gynecol 53:218, 1979

33. Al-Kurdi M, Monaghan JM: Thirty-two years experience in management of primary tumors of the vagina. Br J obstet Gynecol 88:1145, 1981

34. Johnston GA, Klotz J, Boutselis JG: Primary invasive carcinoma of the vagina. Surg Gynecol Obstet 156:34, 1983

35. Benedet JL, Murphy KJ, Fairey RN, et al: Primary invasive carcinoma of the vagina. Obstet Gynecol 62:715, 1983

36. Ball HG, Berman ML: Management of primary vaginal carcinoma. Gynecol Oncol 14:154, 1982

37. Perez CA, Arneson AN, Dehner LP, et al: Radiation therapy in carcinoma of the vagina. Obstet Gynecol 44:862, 1974

38. Steeper TA, Pisciol F, Rosai J: Squamous cell carcinoma with sarcoma-like stroma of the female genital tract. Cancer 52:890, 1983

39. Pride GL, Buchler DA: Carcinoma of the vagina 10 or more years following pelvic irradiation therapy. Am J Obstet Gynecol 127:513, 1977

40. Peters WA, Kumar NB, Morley GW: Carcinoma of the vagina: Factors influencing treatment outcome. Cancer 55:892, 1985

41. Wharton JT, Fletcher GH, Delcos L: Invasive tumors of the vagina: Clinical features and management. p. 345. In Coppleson M (ed): Gynecologic Oncology — Principles and Clinical Practice. Churchill Livingstone, New York, 1981

42. Kucera H, Langer M, Smekal G, et al: Radiotherapy of primary carcinoma of the vagina: Management and results of different therapy schemes. Gynecol Oncol 21:87, 1985

43. Piver MS, Barlow JJ, Dunbar J: Doxorubicin, cyclophosphamide, and 5-fluorouracil in patients with carcinoma of cervix or vagina. Cancer Treatm Rep 64:549, 1980

44. Thigpen JT, Blessing JA, Homesley HD, et al: Phase II trial of Cisplatin in advanced or recurrent cancer of the vagina: A gynecologic oncology group study. Gynecol Oncol 23:101, 1986

45. Katib S, Kuten A, Steiner M, et al: The effectiveness of multidrug treatment by bleomycin, methotrexate and cisplatinum in advanced vaginal carcinoma. Gynecol Oncol 21:101, 1985

46. Annual Report on the Results of Treatment in Gynecological Cancer. Vol. 19. FIGO, Radiumhemmet, Stockholm, Sweden, 1985

47. Smith OW, Smith GV, Hurwitz D: Increased excretion of pregnanediol in pregnancy from diethylstilbestrol with special reference to the problem of late pregnancy accidents. Am J Obstet Gynecol 51:411, 1946

48. Dieckmann WJ, Davis ME, Rynkiewicz IM, et al: Does the administration of diethylstilbestrol during pregnancy have therapeutic value? Am J Obstet Gynecol 66:1062, 1953

49. Herbst AL, Ulfelder H, Poskanzer DC, et al: Adenocarcinoma of the vagina: association of maternal stilbestrol therapy with tumor appearance in young women. N Engl J Med 284:878, 1971

50. Herbst AL, Anderson S, Hubby MM, et al: Risk factors for the development of diethylstilbestrol-associated clear cell adenocarcinoma: A case control study. Am J Obstet Gynecol 154:814, 1986

51. Herbst AL: Diethylstilbestrol exposure — 1984. N Engl J Med 311:1433, 1984

52. Stillman RJ: In utero exposure to diethylstilbestrol: Adverse effects on the reproductive tract and reproductive performance in male and female offspring. Am J Obstet Gynecol 142:905, 1982

53. Robboy SJ, Young RH, Herbst AL: Female genital tract changes related to prenatal diethylstilbestrol exposure. p. 99. In Blaustein A (ed): Pathology of the Female Genital Tract. Springer-Verlag, New York, 1982

54. Robboy SJ, Kaufman RH, Prat J, et al: Pathologic findings in young women enrolled in the National Cooperative Diethylstilbestrol Adenosis (DESAD) Project. Obstet Gynecol 53:309, 1974

55. Kurman RJ, Scully RE: The incidence and histogenesis of vaginal adenosis. Hum Pathol 5:265, 1974

56. Robboy SJ, Hill EC, Sandberg EC, et al: Vaginal adenosis in women born prior to the diethylstilbestrol era. Hum Pathol 17:488, 1986

57. Robboy SJ, Young RH, Welch WR, et al: Atypical vaginal adenosis and cervical ectropion: Association with clear cell adenocarcinoma in diethylstilbestrol-exposed offspring. Cancer 54:869, 1984

58. Robboy SJ, Noller KL, O'Brien P, et al: Increased incidence of cervical and vaginal dysplasia in 3,980 diethylstilbestrol-exposed young women. Experience of the National Collaborative Diethylstilbestrol Adenosis Project. JAMA 252:2979, 1984

59. Senekjian EK, Hubby M, Bell DA, et al: Clear cell adenocarcinoma of the vagina and cervix in association with pregnancy. Gynecol Oncol 24:207, 1986

60. Robboy SJ, Herbst AL, Scully RE: Clear-cell adenocarcinoma of the genital tract in young females. Analysis of 37 tumors that persisted or recurred after primary therapy. Cancer 34:606, 1974

61. Robboy SJ, Welch WR, Young RH: Topographic relation of cervical ectropion and vaginal adenosis to clear cell adenocarcinoma. Obstet Gynecol 60:546, 1982

62. Ray J, Ireland K: Non-clear cell adenocarcinoma arising in vaginal adenosis. Arch Pathol Lab Med 109:781, 1985

63. Wharton JT, Rutledge FN, Gallager HS, et al: Treatment of clear cell adenocarcinoma in young females. Obstet Gynecol 45:365, 1975

64. Herbst AL, Norusis MJ, Rosenow PJ, et al: An analysis of 346 cases of clear cell adenocarcinoma of the vagina and cervix with emphasis on recurrence and survival. Gynecol Oncol 7:111, 1979

65. Herbst AL, Cole P, Norusis MJ, et al: Epidemiologic aspects and factors related to survival in 384 registry cases of clear cell adenocarcinoma of the vagina and cervix. Am J Obstet Gynecol 135:876, 1979

66. Podczaski E, Herbst AL: Cancer of the vagina and fallopian tube. p. 399. In Knapp RC, Berkowitz RS (eds): Gynecologic Oncology. Macmillan, New York, 1986

67. Lee RB, Buttoni L, Dhru R, et al: Malignant melanoma of the vagina: A case report of progression from pre-existing melanosis. Gynecol Oncol 19:238, 1984

68. Deutsch M, Fried AB, Parsons JA, et al: Primary malignant melanoma of the vagina. Oncology 30:509, 1974

69. Chung AF, Casey MJ, Flannery JT, et al: Malignant melanoma of the vagina. Report of 19 cases. Obstet Gynecol 55:720, 1980

70. Morrow CP, DiSaia PJ: Malignant melanoma of the female genitalia: A clinical analysis. Obstet Gynecol Surv 31:233, 1976

71. Chung AF, Woodruff JM, Lewis JL: Malignant melanoma of the vulva. Obstet Gynecol 45:638, 1975

72. Doss LL, Memula N: The radioresponsiveness of melanoma. Int J Radiat Oncol Biol Phys 8:1131, 1982

73. Smith WG: Invasive cancer of the vagina. Clin Obstet Gynecol 24:503, 1981

74. Peters WA, Kumar NB, Anderson WA, et al: Primary sarcoma of the adult vagina. A clinicopathologic study. Obstet Gynecol 65:699, 1985

75. Rastogi BL, Bergman B, Angawall L: Primary leiomyosarcoma of the vagina: a study of five cases. Gynecol Oncol 18:77, 1984

76. Davos I, Abell MR: Sarcomas of the vagina. Obstet Gynecol 47:342, 1976

77. Hilgers RD: Pelvic exenteration for vaginal embryonal rhabdomyosarcoma. A review. Obstet Gynecol 45:175, 1975

78. Dewhurst J, Ferreira HP: An endodermal sinus tumor of the vagina in an infant with seven year survival. Br J Obstet Gynecol 88:859, 1981

79. Young RH, Scully RE: Endodermal sinus tumor of the vagina: A report of nine cases and review of the literature. Gynecol Oncol 18:380, 1984

80. Copeland LJ, Sneige N, Ordonez NG, et al: Endodermal sinus tumor of the vagina and cervix. Cancer 55:2558, 1985

81. Anderson WA, Sabio H, Durso N, et al: Endodermal sinus tumor of the vagina. The role of primary chemotherapy. Cancer 56:1025, 1985

12

Diagnosis and Principles of Treatment of Cancer of the Cervix

S. B. Gusberg
Hugh M. Shingleton

While the mortality from cancer of the cervix has shown a striking decline in the United States during the Papanicolaou (Pap) era, those areas of the world in which screening is less prevalent have not shared this opportunity for secondary prevention. In developing countries, this tumor is still a leading killer of relatively young women. Furthermore, aside from skin cancer, cancer of the cervix is one of the most easily cured malignant tumors in its early clinical stages. If patient, diagnostician, and therapist were all to act in logical accord with current knowledge, cervical cancer would disappear as a world menace (Fig. 12-1).

The accessibility of the uterus to cell and tissue sampling and even to direct physical examination has offered us the opportunity to study incipient uterine cancer, for it has enabled us to learn a great deal about the histogenesis of both cervical and endometrial cancer. It has taught us that most of these tumors have a gradual rather than an explosive onset and that precursors may exist in a reversible form, followed by a stage of surface or in situ development for some years. These phases are most often preclinical or asymptomatic yet are detectable by methods now available[1] (Figs. 12-2 and 12-3). This developmental concept

has persuaded many gynecologists that control of these diseases may be expected in the foreseeable future if global education, economics, and political sophistication attain the level we can now command in diagnostic and therapeutic technology (Fig. 12-4).

Whereas epidemiologic studies convinced us long ago that a sexually transmissible factor is etiologically related to this tumor, the emergence of human papillomaviruses types 16 and 18 as the probable agents has stirred speculation about another avenue of attack, such as vaccination or other antiviral strategies. As the abnormal cellular growth begins, the precursor stages blend into one another without sharp divisions; for this reason, these early phases have been termed cervical intraepithelial neoplasia[2] (Fig. 12-5). The process is slow at first, with the preclinical, preinvasive phases lasting as long as 8 to 10 years. In this phase, the malignant cells are not only small in quantity but different: they lack the quality that ultimately enables them to penetrate the underlying tissues or to metastasize.

The transit of cervical intraepithelial neoplasia to microinvasion and invasive cancer confers a different quality to the emerging tumor, for it now grows more

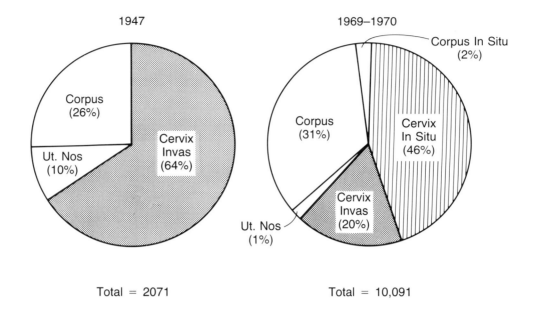

1947

1969–1970

Corpus
(26%)

Ut. Nos
(10%)

Cervix
Invas
(64%)

Corpus In Situ
(2%)

Corpus
(31%)

Cervix
In Situ
(46%)

Cervix
Invas
(20%)

Ut. Nos
(1%)

Total = 2071

Total = 10,091

Fig. 12-1 Distribution of cancers within the total uterus for the national surveys, white females.

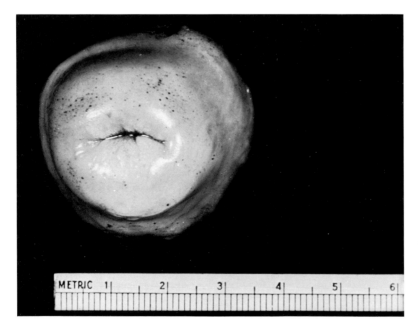

METRIC

Fig. 12-2 Carcinoma in situ in a healthy appearing cervix. Congestion is operative distortion. (Gusberg SB: In Danforth DN (ed): Textbook of Obstetrics and Gynecology. 2nd Ed. Harper & Row, New York, 1971.)

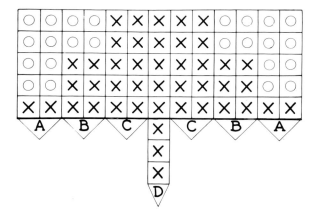

Fig. 12-3 Diagram of histogenesis of cervix cancer. X, active cell with cytologic characteristics of cancer. A, normal epithelium; B, dysplasia; C, cancer in situ; D, early invasion.

rapidly and can cause death within 2 to 3 years by invasion and metastasis, left untreated.

EPIDEMIOLOGY

Although it is clear that one can define a high-risk group for cancer of the cervix, it must be a loose designation without the specificity that would ex-clude persons who do not require screening. This means that our efforts at prevention and early detection must be directed toward all adult women and must even include adolescents who are sexually active.

Family History and Menstrual History

Family history and menstrual history are not significant as they are in the case of endometrial cancer. There are no cancer families with this disease nor is there known endocrine dysfunction.

Marital History

Marital history may be significant, for there is a correlation between early marriage and the incidence of cancer of the cervix. A study by Lombard and Potter[3] found that 44.6 percent of women with cancer of the cervix had married before the age of 20, while only 23.7 percent of matched controls had done so. A correlation also exists with divorce, with 20.7 percent of the cancer group separated and only 5.7 percent of the matched controls having failed marriages. These observations may relate to early onset of sexual activity and the probability of multiple partners. There does not appear to be a correlation between parity and

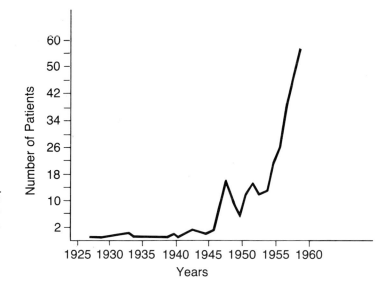

Fig. 12-4 Increase in case findings of cancer in situ with development of cytology laboratory (1946) and its extension (1954).

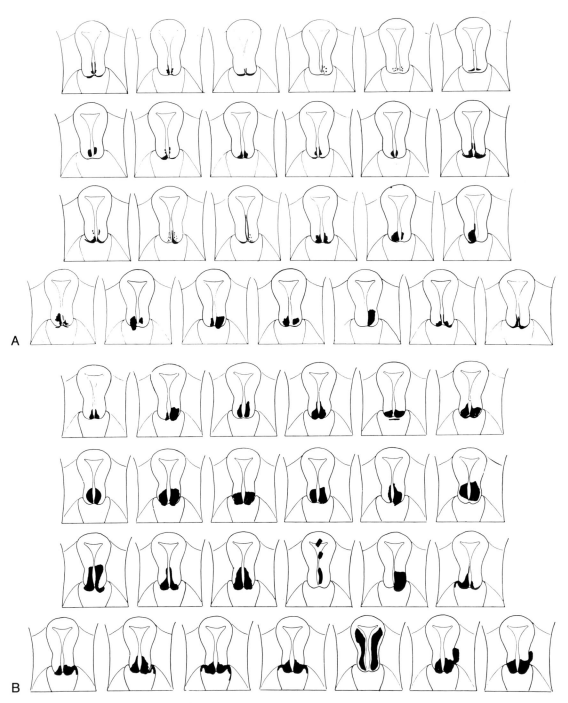

Fig. 12-5 (A) Locations of carcinomas of the cervix showing spread of growth. These are made according to the findings in multiple blocks of specimens removed by radical hysterectomy. **(B)** Locations of tumors of moderate extent. *(Figure continues).*

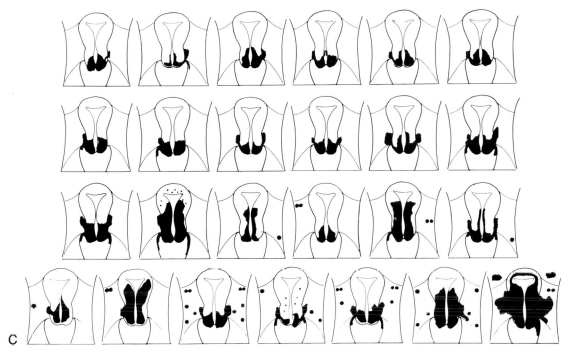

Fig. 12-5 *(Continued).* **(C)** Locations of tumors of greater extent. (Gusberg SB, et al: Obstet Gynecol 2:557, 1953.)

cancer of the cervix, but reported careful statistical analysis sometimes fails to confirm this as a risk factor.

Sexual activity does appear to show a clear correlation to cervical cancer; many reports have demonstrated that early onset of sexual activity after puberty as well as relations with multiple partners place such persons at high risk. Many reports have shown prostitutes to have at least a fourfold relative risk. In a study of 13,000 nuns, Gagnon[4] found no cases of cervical cancer, whereas he found 14 cases of endometrial cancer.

Jewish women seem to be at relatively low risk for squamous carcinoma of the cervix, although satisfactory scientific explanations have not been forthcoming. Many reasons have been offered, including heredity, hygiene, and circumcision. Certainly in the case of circumcision, careful studies have failed to demonstrate a clear correlation in Jewish and Moslem populations, and any difference in U.S. studies might relate to the more common practice of circumcision in the upper than in lower socioeconomic groups.

While there is no clear evidence that diet is a factor, many studies suggest an increased prevalence in the lower socioeconomic groups. In recent years, there have been suggestions of either vitamin C or folic acid deficiency, or both, in those afflicted with this disease, but further studies are needed. In developing countries in which endometrial cancer tends to be rare and confined to the small affluent sector of the population, cancer of the cervix tends to be prevalent.

The etiologic picture that emerges from epidemiologic data is one of a generally sexually transmissible disease, with human papillomavirus types 16 and 18 now considered the most promising etiologic agents. While other papillomaviruses are responsible for genital condylomata, laryngeal papillomas, and other warts, these specific types have been found to relate to cervical cancer. In fact, virologists have found the viral DNA incorporated into the genome of malignant cells in cancer of the cervix. Whether a herpes virus is a cocarcinogenic agent is uncertain. Clearly, other venereal diseases will occur in the same high-risk group. Chronic cervicitis has been indicated in the past, but injury to the cervix by childbirth, diaphragms, pessaries, chemical douches, or even smegma of the male has not found support in hard etiologic evidence.

Although the cervical and vaginal epithelium is under the influence of estrogen, there is no evidence of hormonal correlation in humans. We do not hesitate to offer estrogen therapy to those women we have treated for cervical cancer, should they have symptoms of estrogen deficiency.

Age

Invasive cancer of the cervix, like most cancer, is a disease of advancing age. The peak incidence is at age 45 to 55, at an average age of about 48[1] (Fig. 12-6). This peak is approximately 10 years later than that for carcinoma in situ and a decade earlier than that of cancer of the endometrium. In fact, during the past two decades, the median age for both carcinoma in situ and invasive cancer appears to be getting younger, and dysplasia is now commonly found in young women. The incidence of invasive cancer appears to increase rapidly to age 45, then slow, becoming more or less a flat curve at the age of 60.

Screening

It would seem appropriate, then, for our screening activities to start at the age of initiation of sexual activity and continue throughout that woman's life-time. The necessary frequency of Pap-smear monitoring has traditionally been advised to be an annual event, but this advice, promoted by the American Cancer Society (ACS), has no basis in scientific data. The ACS studied this problem during 1979 to 1980, and issued a general guideline suggesting two annual Pap smears at the age of 20 or earlier if sexually active, followed by cytologic smears at least every 3 years, in accordance with the slow evolution of cervical cancer. This recommendation provoked a great stir in the gynecologic world, having disturbed the annual tradition concerning the quality of commercial laboratories and the allegedly faster transit time of high-risk women.

Such frequency problems are still under study, but no firm evidence has accrued to support the view that high-risk women, who do have a greater prevalence, will have a faster transit time from dysplasia to invasive cancer, an interval that has been shown to vary from 8 to 20 years. The quality control of commercial laboratories may still be a problem, and certification of these laboratories would appear to be a logical answer. Pending this, it would seem appropriate to advise young women to have three or four annual screens before going on the once-every-2-or-3-year interval. In any case, the ACS guidelines published in 1980 emphasized the need for women to be guided by their own physician concerning their interval need. Clearly, women at highest risk may be the most diffi-

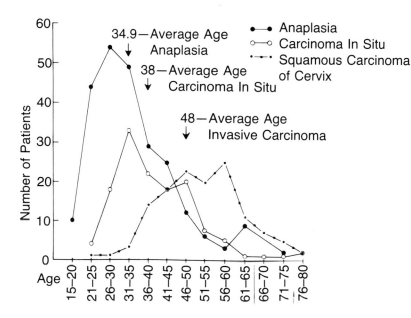

Fig. 12-6 Age incidence of anaplasia (dysplasia), cancer in situ, and invasive carcinoma. (Gusberg SB, McKay DG: Malignant lesions of the cervix and corpus uteri. In Danforth DN (ed): Textbook of Obstetrics and Gynecology. 2nd Ed. Harper & Row, New York, 1971.)

cult to reach for any screening, and a greater effort is required of us in this effort.

DIAGNOSIS

Symptoms

There is no specific symptom that can be called characteristic of cancer of the cervix (Fig 12-7). While bleeding is the only significant symptom, it

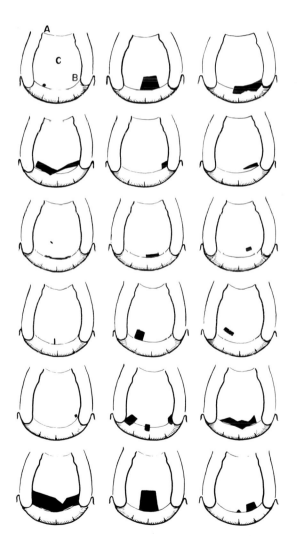

Fig. 12-7 Location of intraepithelial carcinoma of the cervix.

signifies ulceration, a breakthrough on the epithelial surface, whether it be in the canal or on the portio. Unfortunately, some tumors may invade deeply, even spread beyond the cervix without ulcerating the surface, thus without any bleeding[5] (Fig 12-8).

In the case of carcinoma in situ, spontaneous bleeding is rare; a small percentage of patients in this group may have contact staining after coitus, after douching or placing a diaphragm. In general, however, these patients are asymptomatic, and their lesion is discovered only by screening cytology.

Vaginal bleeding with invasive cancer is more reliable, but not necessarily early. One report indicated that in a series of 250 patients with advanced cancer, in whom the tumor had spread to the pelvic wall, 30 percent of patients had experienced bleeding for less than 2 months. Nonetheless, we must teach women the importance of abnormal vaginal bleeding so that they will recognize the need for prompt examination. During the childbearing years, any staining that persists beyond the next expected menstrual flow, and in postmenopausal women any bleeding whatsoever, should be reported.

During the reproductive years, the bleeding symptom may have a gradual onset. It may begin with hypermenorrhea or menorrhagia, but ultimately intermenstrual staining or bleeding will occur. One might say that such metrorrhagia is most characteristic of cervical cancer, because it is lawless—without predictable frequency or duration—unlike that related to dysfunctional bleeding. After the menopause, the onset is usually gradual, starting with staining or even a serosanguineous discharge. It is important to note that abnormal bleeding is the only symptom that can bring a diagnosis of early curable cancer of the cervix.

Malodorous discharge occurs late when saprophytic organisms invade the interstices of cauliflower masses. Pain occurs only when the tumor has reached the pelvic side wall with invasion of nerve trunks and the sacral plexus. In such cases, persistent aching pain may be felt in the lower quadrants or low back, with ultimate sciatic distribution. Hydronephrosis with renal pain or uremia indicates extensive tumor infiltrating the parametrium and obstructing the ureters.

Fistula formation to bowel or bladder is another indication of advanced disease, as is cachexia, for nutrition does not suffer except in widespread tumor. Swelling of the legs usually indicates lymphatic ob-

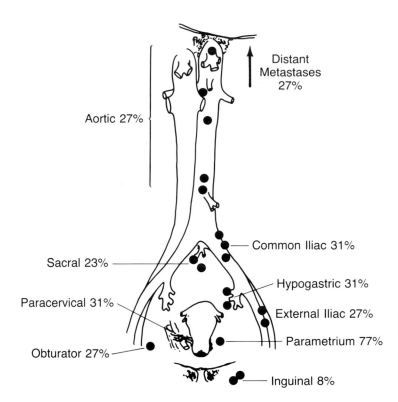

Aortic 27%

Distant
Metastases
27%

Common Iliac 31%

Sacral 23%

Hypogastric 31%

Paracervical 31%

External Iliac 27%

Parametrium 77%

Obturator 27%

Inguinal 8%

Fig. 12-8 Lymph node metastases in untreated cancer of the cervix. (Hendrikson E: The lymphatic spread of carcinoma of the cervix and of the body of the uterus: A study of 420 necropsies. Am J Obstet Gynecol 58:924, 1949.)

struction in main pelvic chains or nodes; it is a symptom of advanced or recurrent disease and an ominous prognostic sign, sometimes acceompanied by ureteral obstruction, evident on pyelograms.

Signs on Physical Examination

The source of a stain may be obscure. The patient may be unable to relate its origin from the bowel, urethra, or vagina. In such a case, a tampon placed against the cervix may be revealing, before one goes on to cystoscopy, sigmoidoscopy, or biopsy of cervix and endometrium.

On examination, one may be confronted by any of the following findings:

Apparently normal cervix: Unless the lesion is entirely endocervical, a normal-appearing cervix, often under suspicion because of an abnormal Pap smear, will usually harbor a carcinoma in situ or microinvasive cancer. Colposcopy with directed biopsy plus endocervical curcttage will frequently make the diagnosis, but conization for biopsy may occasionally be required.

Erosion or ectropion: An ectropion is the red transformation zone without distinction between malignancy and a benign eversion of columnar epithelium.

Ulcer: Ulceration occurs when an invasive tumor destroys the stroma. It will have a granular base and frequently a hard nodular edge (Fig. 12-9). The endophytic type can infiltrate widely with epithelial elements separated by wide bands of fibromuscular tissue (Fig. 12-10). These tumors tend to ulcerate late, but their hardness to palpation may be modified by friability to instrumentation.

Mass: Most cervical cancers will present as a mass, frequently in a so-called cauliflower shape with surface ulceration and necrosis, and general friability except at its edge (Fig. 12-11).

Determination of the extent of these lesions also depends on palpation, especially by rectovaginal examination. This examination enables the examiner to touch the mass vaginally and by rectovaginal palpation to ascertain induration of tumor extension in the parametria and uterosacrals. Clinical examination is to be completed by intravenous pyelogram, cystos-

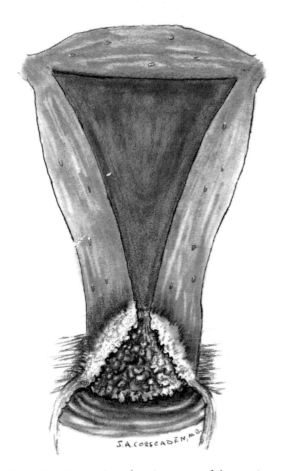

Fig. 12-9 Excavating ulcer in cancer of the cervix.

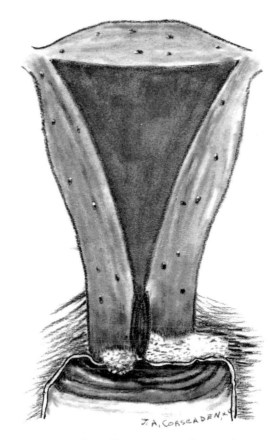

Fig. 12-10 Flat infiltrating type of cervical cancer.

copy, and sigmoidoscopy. The final diagnosis will be made by biopsy. This may be accomplished by any number of sharp cutting double-cup forceps, of which there are a great variety. The Gaylor punch has been a popular and efficient forceps (Fig. 12-12). The friability of the tumor and its paucity of nerve endings make this biopsy relatively painless — a simple ambulatory procedure.

CLINICAL CLASSIFICATION AND STAGING

Such a definition of the extent of the tumor is no mere academic exercise. It affords the oncologist important information regarding:

Quality control: comparison of result with that of other therapists

Individualization: a protocol of treatment

Prognosis: to inform patient and/or relatives of probable outcome

For many years, the tradition of clinical staging has depended on the size (in recent years, volume) of the tumor and is never altered by the surgical or pathologic findings in the excised specimen. This clinical staging has prevailed because many patients harboring this disease were treated by radiotherapy without operation. A recent trend for pretreatment surgical staging by exploratory laparotomy, if its risk-benefit ratio shows it to be significant, could alter the concept of traditional clinical staging. Concurrent with such clinical staging is the knowledge, based on surgical experience, that stage I disease will demonstrate microscopically positive lymph nodes in approximately 15 percent and stage II in about 25 percent of cases.

In 1951, recognizing the need for an international

classification, representatives of the American Medical Association, the American Gynecological Society, the American Association of Obstetricians and Gynecologists, and the editors of The Stockholm Report met to formulate such an international classification. This was adopted by the International Federation of Gynecology and Obstetrics (FIGO) at their congress in Vienna in 1961. At the same time, carcinoma in situ was designated stage 0, for it was considered misleading to include it with invasive cancer.

In communications concerning this tumor, we must remember that stage refers to clinical extent, class to the cytologic interpretation, and grade to the histologic differentiation of the tumor. The most current (1976) FIGO staging is shown in Table 12-1 (see also refs. 1 and 6 and Figs. 12-13 and 12-14.)

Some qualifying explanations are appropriate here. Stage Ia represents those cases in which histologic evidence of stromal invasion is unambiguous. These preclinical lesions are ordinarily diagnosed by conization. Such lesions invading to 3 or 5 mm (depending on which definition one uses) are rarely associated with lymph node metastases. They are consequently ordinarily curable by conservative hysterectomy or, in some cases, by therapeutic conization. The remaining stage I cases should be designated as stage Ib. This

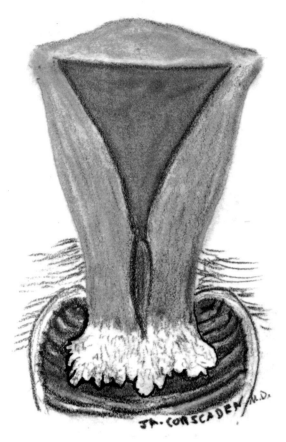

Fig. 12-11 Cauliflower-type cancer of the cervix.

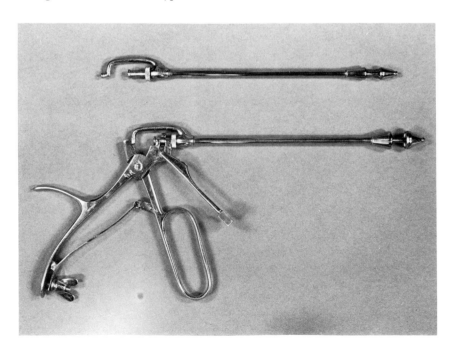

Fig. 12-12 Gusberg endocervical punch.

Table 12-1 International Staging of Cancer of the Cervix

Stage	Description/Features
0	Carcinoma in situ, intraepithelial carcinoma (Cases of stage 0 should not be included in any therapeutic statistics for invasive carcinoma.)
I	Carcinoma strictly confined to the cervix (Figs. 12-13 and 12-14) a. Microcarcinoma—early stromal invasion b. All other stage I (Occult cancer should be marked occ)
II	Carcinoma extending beyond the cervix but has not extended onto the pelvic wall; involves the vagina but not the lower one-third a. No obvious parametrial involvement b. Obvious parametrial involvement
III	Carcinoma extending onto the pelvic wall (On rectal examination, there is no cancer-free space between the tumor and the pelvic wall. The tumor involves the lower one-third of the vagina. All cases with a hydronephrosis or nonfunctioning kidney.) a. No extension onto the pelvic wall b. Extension onto the pelvic wall and/or hydronephrosis or nonfunctioning kidney
IV	Carcinoma extending beyond the true pelvis or clinically involving the mucosa of bladder or rectum. (A bullous edema, as such does not permit a case to be allotted to stage IV.) a. Spread to adjacent organs b. Spread to distant organs

classification includes lesions of all sizes, from small to very large. For years, at the Sloane Hospital for Women (New York City), and more recently at the M.D. Anderson Hospital (Houston, Texas), stage I tumors over 2.5 cm in diameter were classified as stage Ic to distinguish them from smaller lesions with a better prognosis. Such a refinement of the classification of stage I has not gained acceptance by FIGO, however. Current staging suggests that the occult cancer group within stage Ib be considered separately, as these lesions are more likely to be associated with nodal metastases than the stage Ia group and may warrant more aggressive therapy.

Since it is clinically difficult to estimate whether a cancer of the cervix has extended to the corpus (without removing the uterus), extension to the corpus is disregarded in staging. Some treatment centers consider this a bad prognostic sign if it is found, however.

Stage IIa indicates minimal extracervical extension and is still considered an operable stage, whereas stage IIb with parametrial extension is usually transferred for radiotherapy at most institutions.

Stage III indicates wide extension and is generally considered inoperable in the United States. Fixation of the tumor to the side wall will usually defeat surgical removal, although misinterpreted inflammatory induration can make a difference on rare occasions.

Stage IV is widespread disease; metastases that are extrapelvic cannot be controlled by local treatment. At our clinic, we make the distinction between biologic spread, indicating the capacity for embolic extension and geographic spread, which signifies only direct advancement of disease. The designation of stage IVa, spread to contiguous organs such as bowel or bladder, is an example of the latter. Therefore it falls into the category of disease wherein greater excision, or pelvic exenteration, may be curative. Unfortunately, few cervical cancers will involve bladder and bowel by pure anterior or posterior extension without taking the usual route of extension through the parametrium to the pelvic side wall.

With renewed interest in radical surgery for cervical cancer during the 1940s, Meigs and Brunschwig[7] proposed a postoperative classification of disease extent, based on surgical and pathologic findings. They presented the classification of carcinoma of the cervix shown in Table 12-2.

The surgical pathologic classification reflected decreasing likelihood of cure as one moved from class 0 to class F. The classification also suggested prefixes for prior treatment, including PR for preoperative radium planned as part of treatment, R for radium that had been used but failed, S when prior surgery had failed to cure, and RS when both methods had been used unsuccessfully. Clearly, the cumbersome nature of the classification and the fact that treatment of most cancers of the cervix was by radiotherapy made the International Classification the predominating one. When surgery is used, one may use this system or the TNM system (which stands for primary *tumor,* regional lymph *nodes,* and distant *metastasis*) in a supplementary manner, if desired.

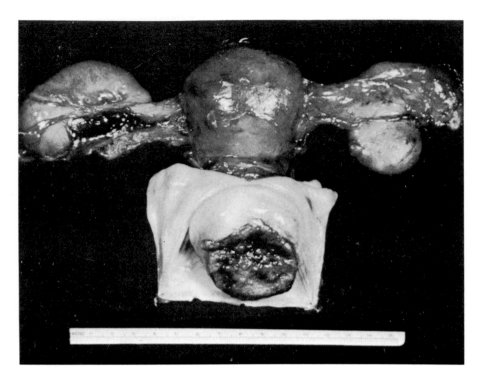

Fig. 12-13 Stage I cancer of the cervix. Note the red raised lesion on the cervix. Such a tumor is readily accessible for punch biopsy. (Gusberg SB, McKay DG: Malignant lesions of the cervix and corpus uteri. In Danforth DN (ed): Textbook of Obstetrics and Gynecology. 2nd Ed. Harper & Row, 1971.)

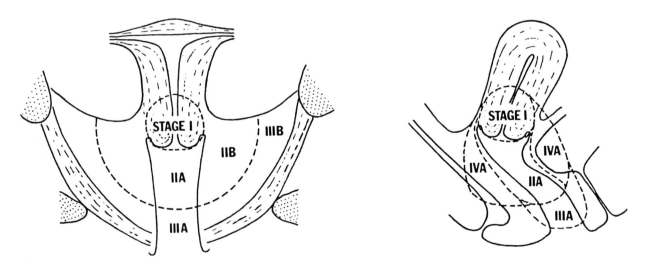

Fig. 12-14 Clinical staging in cancer of the cervix. (Shingleton HM, Orr JW Jr: Cancer of the Cervix: Diagnosis and Treatment. Churchill Livingstone, Edinburgh, 1987.)

PRINCIPLES OF TREATMENT

There is no correlation between the duration of bleeding and the rate of cure, nor is there such a correlation between duration of symptoms and the extent of disease. Virulence factors demonstrable for squamous carcinoma of the cervix include depth of stromal invasion, grade, involvement of vascular spaces, and local migration of lymphocytes to form a round cell collar around the tumor. These parameters can be factored into a treatment protocol. To some extent, they have been overlooked because of the primary importance of the extent of disease (Tables 12-3 and 12-4). Thus, one can anticipate about 100 percent cure in stages 0 and Ia, 90 percent in stage Ib (small), 70 percent in stage Ic (large), 50 to 60 percent in stage

Table 12-2 Surgical and Pathologic Classification of Carcinoma of the Cervix

Class	Description/Features
0	Cancer in situ
A	Carcinoma strictly confined to the cervix
A-o	After positive biopsy of invasive carcinoma, no tumor found in the surgical specimen of the cervix
B	Carcinoma extending from the cervix to involve vagina, except lower one-third; carcinoma extending into the corpus uteri; carcinoma involving upper vagina and corpus; vaginal and/or uterine extension metastatic or by direct spread
C	Carcinoma involving paracervical and/or paravaginal tissues by direct extension or lymphatic channels or in nodes within such tisues; vaginal metastases and/or direct extension into the lower one-third of the vagina
D	Lymph vessel and node involvement beyond paracervical and paravaginal regions, including all lymphatics and/or nodes in the true pelvis, except as described for stage C; metastasis to the tube or ovary
E	Carcinoma penetrating to the serosa, musculature, or mucosa of the bladder and/or colon or rectum
F	Carcinoma involving the pelvic wall (fascia, muscle, bone, and/or sacral plexus)

(Meigs JV, Brunschwig A: A proposed classification for cases of cancer of the cervix treated by surgery. Am J Obstet Gynecol 64:413, 1952.)

Table 12-3 Virulence Factor, Lymphatic Invasion, and Cure Rate with Good RST

Lymphatics	Stage I N	%	Stage II N	%	Total N	%
Negative	28	87.5	53	85.1	81	86.0[a]
Positive	14	53.9	20	30.0	34	39.4[a]

[a] Significant at 0.01 level.
RST, radiosensitivity test.

II, 30 to 40 percent in stage III and possibly 5 percent in stage IV.

PROFILE OF VIRULENCE INDICES IN CANCER OF THE CERVIX

1. Clinical stage
2. Radiosensitivity test (RST)
3. Indices of virulence in biopsy
   a. Lymphatic penetration
   b. Stromal response
   c. Histologic grade

The choice of treatment lies between two excellent modalities, radical surgery or irradiation (Figs. 12-15 through 12-17), while the use of adjuvant chemotherapy is tentative and experimental. The development of the two major forms of treatment is interesting, and it is important to place the individual choice within the context of this background. These methods have developed over a period spanning almost a century as they partook of advancing knowledge of biologic principles and new technology. In fact, the renaissance of radical surgery during the 1940s and 1950s was made practical by the advent of scientific anesthesiology, antibiotics, and blood banks, together with knowledge of surgical physiology bolstering pre- and postoperative care.

Treatment of cancer of the cervix was attempted about a century ago with local applications including chemical cauterization and later cauterization by heat. During the 1860s and 1870s, J. Marion Sims and others removed the cancerous cervix surgically, often

Table 12-4 Biopsy Lymphatics and Lymph Nodes in Cancer of the Cervix

Cervical Lymphatics	Positive Lymph Nodes N	%
Positive (N = 36)	16	44
Negative (N = 67)	3	4

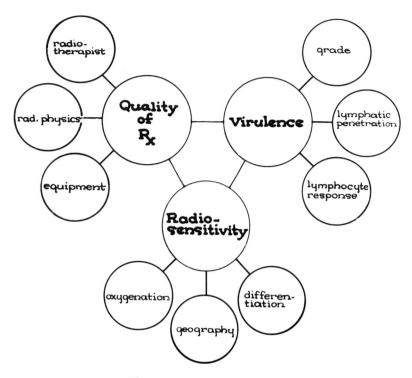

Fig. 12-15 Radiation factors.

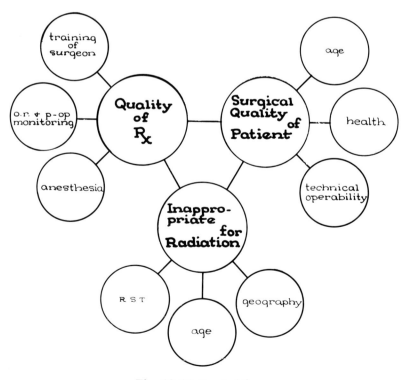

Fig. 12-16 Surgical factors.

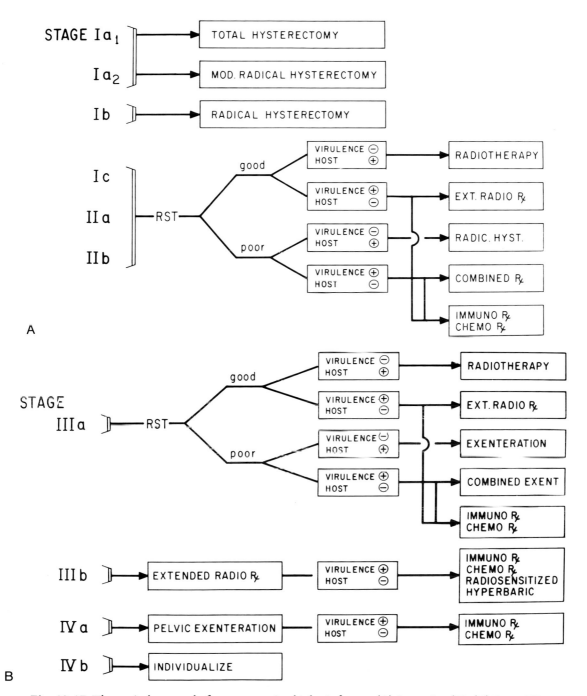

Fig. 12-17 Theoretical protocol of treatment using biologic factors. **(A)** Stages I and II. **(B)** Stages III and IV.

combining this treatment with local application of caustics, such as zinc chloride, sulfuric acid, or bromine. With the discovery of antisepsis, surgeons were tempted further afield, and in 1878 Freund removed the entire uterus by the abdominal route. It soon became clear that this procedure held promise for corpus cancer but was too restricted to cure cancer of the cervix.

In 1895, J. G. Clark and E. Ries,[8] and in 1898 E. Wertheim[9,10] designed and carried out a radical procedure of block dissection that excised the uterus, the surrounding tissue, and ligaments including the regional lymph nodes, taking special care to preserve the uterers. Wertheim's name became attached to the operation that has persisted as the radical Wertheim hysterectomy.

Also in 1895, a seminal year, W. Roentgen discovered the rays that bear his name. The effect on tissues was quickly appreciated, and by 1901 roentgen rays were used clinically, directed at cancer of the cervix by vaginal cone. Injuries and desultory results were apparent because of the imprecision of delivery; it remained for the development of the Coolidge tube in 1913 to open the era of irradiation therapy, delivered with accuracy and some precision.

In 1898 Pierre and Marie Curie discovered radium and its tissue effects soon became apparent (Figs. 12-18 and 12-19), for by 1903, Margaret Cleaves applied it to the treatment of cancer of the cervix. By 1915, principles and techniques of treatment were established by Bailey, C. Regaud, G. Forssell, and Heyman, opening an era of cooperation between surgeons and radiotherapists for the treatment of this tumor. However, surgery gradually gave way to the predominance of radiotherapy for the latter seemed to offer a better result with less injury and less mortality. This was evident by 1930; it was epitomized in 1937 by the words of Fletcher Shaw, one of Britain's most distinguished surgeons, who wrote, "after careful observation of the cases for over 7 years, Professor Dou-

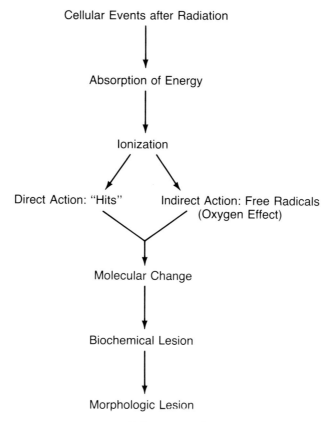

Fig. 12-18 Cellular events after radiation.

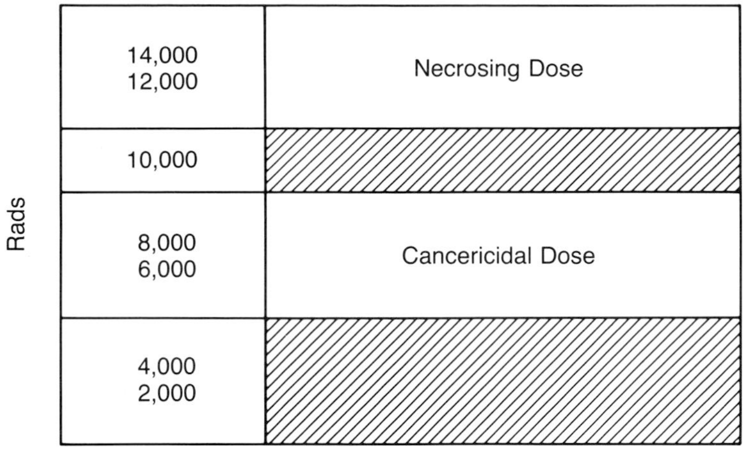

Fig. 12-19 Radiation effect.

gal and I have come to the definite conclusion that radium offers the best chance of cure as well as being the more humane method of treatment. Therefore, strong advocates though we were of operation, we have now abandoned it."

Interstitial radium, radioactive cobalt and gold, and especially cesium have found a place in the radiotherapists's armamentarium, the latter especially with afterloading and the miniaturization of intracavitary sources. Transvaginal x-ray exposure has had its day, while surgeons proposed lymphadenectomy transperitoneally[11] or retroperitoneally[12] after radium therapy.

Vaginal radical hysterectomy, devised by Schauta,[13] in 1904, came to some later prominence because of the high mortality of the abdominal approach and it flourished for some time in the Viennese school. Adler,[14] in 1947, Mitra,[15] in 1959, with extraperitoneal lymphadenectomy, and Navratil,[16] in 1951, continued to advocate this approach, but the near elimination of mortality with the abdominal operation has rendered the vaginal procedure almost obsolete. On the other hand, pelvic exenteration with radical hysterectomy accompanied by removal of bowel and bladder, first introduced by Brunschwig,[17] in 1946, has found a small but well-defined therapeutic place for tumors involving contiguous organs without fixation to the sidewall.

Renewed interest in radical hysterectomy was started in the United States by Meigs of Harvard University in 1944; soon it was enthusiastically adopted by many clinics that realized that surgical adjuvants, including blood banks, antibiotics, and modern anes-

thesiology, permitted greater safety for extended surgery. Sometimes the limitations of radiotherapy were exaggerated, such as the claim that lymph nodes with microscopic disease could not be sterilized. But radiation injuries were evident, and it was clear that some tumors were relatively insensitive to irradiation. It soon became apparent that in skilled hands radical hysterectomy was a relatively safe operation. This trend removed the competition between surgery and irradiation as the primary treatment for cervix cancer. While it was demonstrable that an excellent rate of cure by surgery could be attained by skilled surgeons in good hospitals if one chose subjects who were young, lean, and otherwise fit, one could not compare this result with that of other less favorable patients consigned to radiotherapy. If one chose these treatments impartially, it soon became evident that the cure rate was about the same for either modality as was the rate of complication.

In this atmosphere, several attempts arose to resolve this problem biologically. Glucksmann and Way,[18] in 1948, used serial biopsies to make a radiosensitivity assay and in 1960 the Grahams, then in Boston, evaluated sensitivity of the tumor cytologically. The Sloane Hospital (New York) group, asking the same question, developed a method using cytochemical reactions under a small test dose of irradiation (radiosensitivity testing). Several cellular reactions were found to indicate sensitivity: (1) death and dissolution of cells; (2) maturation of cells or differentiation; and (3) radiocytologic reactions indicating irreversible cell damage, such as increased size of nucleus, increased size of nucleolus, and initial chromatin increase followed by relative decline. Molecular genetics now has the possibility of rendering these observations more precise and more quantitative.

RST RESPONSE

1. Death and degeneration of cells
2. Differentiation
3. Radiocytologic
   a. Enlarged cell and cell nucleus
   b. Enlarged nucleoli (RNA)
   c. Altered chromatin (DNA) — ↑then↓

RST, radiosensitivity test.

In any case, the qualitative nature of radiosensitivity testing, although offering a reasonably accurate and useful appraisal, has failed to be generally accepted, and surgical procedures have increased their scope. The application of radical hysterectomy to young women with this disease offers greater resilience in preserving pelvic tissues for the relatively long life expectancy, if cured; the necessity for intense irradiation for relatively insensitive tumors, increasing the morbidity rate, also suggests the use of surgery for this special group. Therefore most stage Ib and IIa tumors in the United States are treated by surgery unless the patients' general health contraindicates it (Table 12-5). Complex judgments are required when we balance the virulence of the tumor, the technical expertise available, and the sensitivity of the tumor in our effort to offer our patients the maximum opportunity for cure with the minimum complication and dislocation of their lives (Figs. 12-20 through 12-22).[19]

Individualization of treatment, then, should account for all factors biologic and technical, rather than making it dependent entirely on therapeutic fac-

Table 12-5 Radiotherapy and RST in Cancer of the Cervix[a]

RST	Stage I (%) N	Stage I (%) Cure	Stage II (%) N	Stage II (%) Cure	Total (%) N	Total (%) Cure
Good	45	77.5	78	68.8	123	72.1[b]
Poor	14	46.1	33	25.9	47	32.5[b]

[a] Cure = relative cure rate at 3 years plus follow-up.
[b] Significant at 0.01 level.
RST, radiosensitivity test.

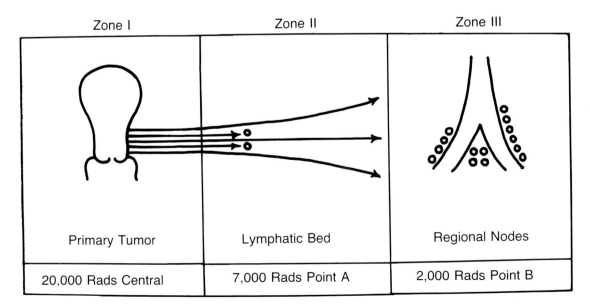

Zone I	Zone II	Zone III
Primary Tumor	Lymphatic Bed	Regional Nodes
20,000 Rads Central	7,000 Rads Point A	2,000 Rads Point B

Fig. 12-20 Zones of treatment for cancer of the cervix with brachytherapy.

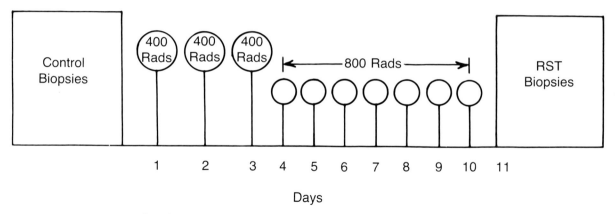

Fig. 12-21 Test dose for radiosensitivity testing of cancer of the cervix. 400 rads × 3 then daily Rx to 2000 rads 10 × 14 cm. Anterior and posterior fields — Betatron (Gusberg SB, Herman GG: Radiosensitivity and virulence factors in cervical cancer. Am J Obstet Gynecol 100:627, 1968.)

tors, such as training, temperament, ancestor worship, departmental policy, or other variables related, sometimes casually, to the physician in charge. In examining factors that could affect individualized treatment, dedifferentiation and invasion of vascular spaces were noted to be significantly virulent; the clinically evident host response attempting to guard against invasion, a collar of lymphocytes that have migrated to the tumor, seemed to form a kind of immunologic barrier (Tables 12-6 and 12-7).

In summary, these principles of treatment may include the use of the following:

1. Applicable biologic data
2. Expert personnel for diagnosis and treatment
3. A planned multidisciplinary approach when indicated
4. Aggressive treatment for especially virulent tumors
5. Individualized treatment to each patient

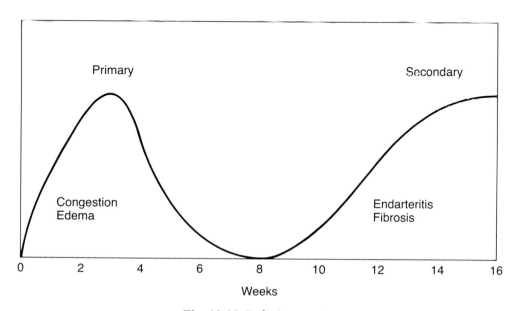

Fig. 12-22 Radiation reaction.

Table 12-6 Good RST and Biopsy Lymphatics: Stages I and II in Cancer of the Cervix

Lymphatics	L + W	
	N	%
Negative (N = 104)	90	86.5
Positive (N = 104)	42	40.4

L, living; W, well

Table 12-7 Stromal Response and Lymph Nodes in Cancer of the Cervix

Lymphocyte Response	Positive Lymph Nodes	
	N	%
Good (N = 36)	5	13.8
Poor (N = 18)	12	66.6

The basic oncologic sciences will constantly nourish the care of patients if we, as clinicians, are prepared to translate new scientific information. We may come to understand better such adjuvant factors as immunotherapy, chemotherapy, and extended irradiation. Surely we have wasted much time in comparing statistically the cure rate after surgery or irradiation, when in fact these excellent modalities should be regarded as complementary, rather than competitive. We must remind ourselves that both surgery and irradiation, no matter how radical, constitute local treatment. We have probably attained the greatest efficiency possible in eradicating local disease with the modalities and search further for advancement.

ADENOCARCINOMA OF THE CERVIX

In general, the principles of diagnosis and treatment applicable to the more common squamous cancers are equally significant for this variation. Most reports indicate equal radiosensitivity of these tumors. While earlier reports favored preoperative radium followed by radical surgery, in current practice the perception of radioresistance by adenocarcinoma, would suggest the same treatment as for squamous cell cancer, stage for stage.

REFERENCES

1. Gusberg SB, McKay DG: Malignant lesions of the cervix and corpus uteri. In Danforth DN (ed): Textbook of Obstetrics and Gynecology, 2nd Ed. Harper & Row, New York, 1971
2. Gusberg SB, Fish SA, Wang Y-Y: The growth pattern of cervical cancer. Obstet Gynecol 2:557, 1953
3. Lombard HL, Potter EA: Epidemiological aspects of cancer of the cervix. II. Hereditary and environmental factors. Cancer 3:960, 1950
4. Gagnon F: The lack of occurrence of cervical cancer in nuns. Proc Natl Cancer Conf 1:625, 1952
5. Henriksen E: The lymphatic spread of carcinoma of the cervix and of the body of the uterus: A study of 420 necropsies. Am J Obstet Gynecol 58:924, 1949
6. Shingleton HM, Orr JW Jr: Cancer of the Cervix: Diagnosis and Treatment. Churchill Livingstone, Edinburgh, 1987
7. Meigs JV, Brunschwig A: A proposed classification for cases of cancer of the cervix treated by surgery. Am J Obstet Gynecol 64:413, 1952
8. Clark JG: A more radical method of performing hysterectomy for cancer of the uterus. Bull Johns Hopkins Hosp 6:120,1895
9. Wertheim E: Zur Frage der Radikaloperation beim Uteruskrebs. Arch Gynakol 61:627, 1900
10. Wertheim E: Ein neurer Beitrag zur Frage der Radikaloperation beim Uteruskrebs. Arch Gynakol 65:1, 1901
11. Taussig FJ: Iliac lymphadenectomy for grade II cancer of the cervix: Technique and 5-year results in 175 cases. Am J Obstet Gynecol 45:733, 1943
12. Nathanson IT: Extraperitoneal iliac lymphadenectomy in treatment of cancer of the cervix. p. 388. In Meigs JV, Sturgis SH (eds): Progress in Gynecology. Grune & Stratton, New York, 1946
13. Schauta F: Die Berechtigung des vaginalen Totalexstirpation bei Gebarmutterkrebs. Monatsscht Geburtshilfe Gynekol (Berlin) 19:475, 1904
14. Adler L: Treatment of cervical cancer. Acta Radiol 28:474, 1947
15. Mitra S: Extraperitoneal lymphadenectomy and radical vaginal hysterectomy for cancer of the cervix (Mitra technique). Am J Obstet Gynecol 78:191, 1959
16. Navratil E: Radical vaginal panhysterectomy and extraperitoneal pelvic lymphadenectomy. Am J Obstet Gynecol 61A(suppl):340, 1951
17. Brunschwig A, Pierce VK: Necropsy findings in patients with carcinoma of the cervix: Implications for treatment. Am J Obstet Gynecol 56:1134, 1948
18. Glucksmann A, Way S, Cherry CP: The 10-year results of individualized treatment of cancer of the cervix

based on the analysis of serial biopsies. J Obstet Gynecol Br Commonw 71:198, 1964

19. Gusberg SB, Herman GG: Radiosensitivity and virulence factors in cervical cancer. Am J Obstet Gynecol 100:627, 1968

SELECTED READINGS

Averette HE, Dudan RC, Ford JH Jr: Exploratory celiotomy for surgical staging of cervical cancer. Am J Obstet Gynecol 113:1090, 1972

Barber HRK: Relative prognostic significance of preoperative and operative findings in pelvic exenteration. Surg Clin North Am 49:431, 1969

Barber HRK, Sommers SC, Rotterdam H, Kwon T: Vascular invasion as a prognostic factor in stage I_b cancer of the cervix. Obstet Gynecol 52:343, 1978

Barron BA, Richart RM: A statistical model of the natural history of cervical carcinoma based on a prospective study of 557 cases. J Natl Cancer Inst 41:1343, 1968

Berek JS, Hacker NF, Fu Y-S et al: Adenocarcinoma of the uterine cervix: Histologic variables associated with lymph node metastasis and survival. Obstet Gynecol 65:46, 1985

Berek JS, Castaldo TW, Hacker NF, et al: Adenocarcinoma of the uterine cervix. Cancer 48:2734, 1981

Boyce JG, Fruchter RG, Nicastri AD, et al: Vascular invasion in Stage I carcinoma of the cervix. Cancer 53:1175, 1984

Brunschwig A, Barber HRK: Extended pelvic exenteration for advanced cancer of the cervix. Long survival following added resection of involved bowel. Cancer 17:1267, 1964

Buchsbaum HJ: Para-aortic lymph node involvement in cervical carcinoma. Am J Obstet Gynecol 113:942, 1972

Cherry CP, Glucksman A: The influence of systemic factors on the reaction to radium treatment of the normal and malignant epithelium of the uterine cervix. Cancer 7:504, 1954

Christopherson WM, Parker JE, Mendez WM, Lundin FE: Cervix cancer, death rates and mass cytologic screening. Cancer 26:808, 1970

Clark JG: A more radical method of performing hysterectomy for cancer of the uterus. Bull Johns Hopkins Hosp 6:120, 1895

Corscaden JA: The treatment of early carcinoma of the cervix. Am J Obstet Gynecol 59:272, 1950

Dubrauszky V: Assessment of radiosensitivity of cancer of the cervix. J Obstet Gynaecol Br Commonw 73:41, 1966

FIGO: Annual report on the results of treatment in gynecological cancer. p. 28. In Pettersson F (ed): International Federation of Gynecology and Obstetrics, Stockholm, 1958

Fletcher GH: Cancer of the uterine cervix. Janeway lecture. 1970. AJR 114:16, 1972

Friedell GH, Parsons L: The spread of cancer of the uterine cervix as seen in giant histological sections. Cancer 14:42, 1961

Gauthier P, Gore I, Shingleton HM, et al: Identification of histopathologic risk groups in Stage I_b squamous cell carcinoma of the cervix. Obstet Gynecol 66:569, 1985

Glucksmann A, Way S, Cherry CP: The 10-year results of individualized treatment of cancer of the cervix based on the analysis of serial biopsies. J Obstet Gynaecol Br Commonw 71:198, 1964

Graham RM: Cytologic prognosis in cancer of the cervix. Am J Obstet Gynecol 79:700, 1960

Gray MJ, Gusberg SB, Guttmann R: Pelvic lymph node dissection following radiotherapy. Am J Obstet Gynecol 76:629, 1958

Gusberg SB: A consideration of the problems of radiosensitivity in cancer of the cervix. Am J Obstet Gynecol 72:804, 1956

Gusberg SB, More DB: Clinical pattern of intraepithelial cancer of the cervix and its pathological background. Obstet Gynecol 2:1, 1953

Gusberg SB, Fish AA, Wang Y-Y: The growth pattern of cervical cancer. Obstet Gynecol 68:1464, 1954

Gusberg SB, Yannopoulis K, Cohen CJ: Virulence indices and lymph nodes in cancer of the cervix. AJR 111:273, 1971

Gusberg SB: The diagnosis of gynecologic cancer. Cancer 51:12, 1983

Johnson LD, Nickerson RJ, Easterday CL, et al: Epidemiologic evidence for the spectrum of change from dysplasia through carcinoma in situ to invasive cancer. Cancer 22:901, 1968

Kaplan IIS: Biochemical basis of reproductive death in irradiated cells. AJR 90:907, 1963

Kaufmann LA, Cuyler WK, Ross RA: Intraepithelial carcinoma of the cervix. Surg Gynecol Obstet 91:179, 1950

Korhonen MO: Adenocarcinoma of the uterine cervix. Prognosis and prognostic significance of histology. Cancer 53:1760, 1984

Kottmeier HL: Current treatment of carcinoma of the cervix. Am J Obstet Gynecol 76:243, 1958

Krieger JS, McCormack LJ: The indications for conservative therapy for intra-epithelial carcinoma of the uterine cervix. Am J Obstet Gynecol 76:312, 1958

McKay DG, Hertig AT, Younge PA: Cervical carcinoma in situ: Statement of the problem. J Int Coll Surg 21:212, 1954

Meigs JV: Results of surgical treatment of cancer of the cervix uteri. AJR 65:698, 1951

Milson I, Chb MB, Friberg LG: Primary adenocarcinoma of the uterine cervix: A clinical study. Cancer 52:942, 1983

Moberg PJ, Einhorn N, Silfversward C, Soderberg G: Adenocarcinoma of the uterine cervix. Cancer 57:407, 1986

Nahas WA, Sharkey FE, Whitney CW, et al: The prognostic significance of vascular channel involvement and deep stromal penetration in early cervical carcinoma. Am J Clin Onc 6:259, 1983

Ostergard DR, Morton DG: Multifocal carcinoma of the female genitals. Am J Obstet Gynecol 99:1006, 1968

Parker RT, Cuyler WK, Kaufmann LA, et al: Intraepithelial (Stage 0) cancer of the cervix. Am J Obstet Gynecol 80:693, 1960

Parsons L, Friedel GH: Radical surgical treatment of cancer of the cervix. Proc Fifth Nat Cancer Conf 5:241, 1964

Petersen O: Spontaneous course of cervical precancerous conditions. Am J Obstet Gynecol 72:1063, 1956

Regan JW: Genesis of carcinoma of the uterine cervix. Clin Obstet Gynecol 10:883, 1967

Ries E: Eine neue operationsmethode des Uterus carcinoma. Z Geburtshilfe Gynaekol 32:266, 1895

Rotkin ID: Sexual characteristics of cervical cancer population. Am J Public Health 57:815, 1967

Rubin IC: Pathological diagnosis of incipient carcinoma of the uterus. Am J Obstet 62:668, 1910

Rutledge FN, Fletcher GH: Transperitoneal pelvic lymphadenectomy following supervoltage irradiation for squamous cell carcinoma of the cervix. Am J Obstet Gynecol 76:321, 1958

Saigo PE, Cain JM, Kim WS, et al: Prognostic factors in adenocarcinoma of the uterine cervix. Cancer 57:1584, 1986

Schauenstein G: Histologiche Untersunchungen uber atypisches Plattenepithel an der Portio und an der Innenflaeche der Cervix uteri. Arch Gynakol 85:576, 1908

Schmitz H: The classification of uterine carcinoma for the study and efficacy of radium therapy. AJR 7:383, 1920

Shaw WF: Radium versus Wertheim's hysterectomy in the treatment of carcinoma of the cervix. Surg Gynecol 64:332, 1937

Taki I, Herman GG, Gusberg SB: A quantitative study of tumor-host response in cervical cancer. Am J Obstet Gynecol 84:1487, 1962

TeLinde RW, Galvin G: The minimal histologic changes in biopsies to justify a diagnosis of cervical cancer. Am J Obstet Gynecol 48:774, 1944

Thornton WN Jr, Fox CH, Smith DE: The relationship of the squamocolumnar junction and the endocervical glands to the site of origin of carcinoma of the cervix. Am J Obstet Gynecol 78:1060, 1959

Twombly GH, Taylor HC Jr: The treatment of cancer of the cervix uteri; A comparison of the radiation therapy and radical surgery. AJR 71:501, 1954

Ulfelder H, Meigs JV: The surgery of advanced pelvic cancer in women. N Engl J Med 246:243, 1952

Warren W, Meigs JV, Severance AO, Jaffe HL: The significance of the radiation reactions in carcinoma of the cervix uteri. Surg Gynecol Obstet 69:645, 1939

Wentz WB, Reagan JW: Survival in cervical cancer with respect to cell type. Cancer 12:289, 1898

Wertheim E: Zur Frage der Radikoloperation beim Uteruskrebs. Arch Gynakol 61:627, 1900

Younge PA: Cancer of the uterine cervix: A preventable disease. Obstet Gynecol 10:469, 1957

13

Treatment of Cancer of the Cervix

Hugh M. Shingleton
Robert Y. Kim

HISTORICAL ASPECTS

Before the twentieth century, cancer of the cervix was a uniformly fatal disease, no curative therapy was available. During the nineteenth century, cervical amputation, application of hot cautery or vaginal packs of caustic chemicals such as bromine or zinc chloride were the only treatments offered the patient. Toward the latter part of the nineteenth century, it became apparent that conservative hysterectomy or cervicectomy was not only dangerous, but ineffective. The introduction of radical surgical procedures by John G. Clark and Ernst Wertheim and the development of radiotherapy during the 1890s offered the first possibility for cure. However, presentation of patients in advanced clinical stages and the dangers of surgery prevented much progress in achieving cures by surgical means.

Radiation Therapy

A number of treatment techniques evolved following the discovery of x-rays (Roentgen, 1895) and radium (Pierre and Marie Curie, 1898). In 1899, two Swedish physicians, Dr. J. T. Stenbeck and Dr. T. A. V. Sjøgreen, claimed the first radiation cure of cancer, a skin tumor on the tip of a patient's nose. The initial use of intracavitary radium (radium bromide in a sealed glass water jacket of a roentgen tube) to treat cancer of the cervix was by Margaret Cleaves in New York in 1903.[1] This afforded the opportunity

to develop radium techniques and to prove the efficacy of radiation therapy in the treatment of cancer of the cervix. By 1913, Coolidge had developed an x-ray tube with a heated tungsten filament, a tungsten target, an effective vacuum, and a peak energy of 140 keV, thus providing the foundation for external x-ray teletherapy. Cobalt-60, delivering 1.2 MeV energy, was introduced during the early 1950s, followed by even higher-energy x-rays (4- to 30-MeV range from linear accelerators and betatrons) in the late 1950s.

Various methods for delivery of radiotherapy for cervical cancer have been advanced over the course of the twentieth century. Major techniques were developed by Forssell at the Radiumhemmet, Stockholm,[2] in 1917, and by Regaud at the Institut du Radium, Paris[3] in 1926. The major difference between these two techniques is the time-dose relationship. The Stockholm technique is characterized by high-intensity radium sources (150 mg radium) with two split-radium insertions. With this technique, vaginal sources are close to the cervix. The Paris technique is characterized by a low-intensity radium source (60 mg) with protraction of a single insertion; the vaginal sources are located further from the cervix through use of larger colpostats or spacers for better depth dose.

In 1938, the Manchester technique was developed by a group at the Holt Radium Institute in Manchester, England. It is a modification of the Paris technique with delivery of a predetermined maximum permissible dose measured in the paracervical tissue (referred to as point A) and at the lateral pelvic wall (referred to as point B). This method, perhaps the most widely used today, consists of two intracavitary applications 2 to 3 weeks apart.

Surgical Therapy

The high mortality and morbidity of the earlier surgical attempts in the late nineteenth and early twentieth centuries led to an era dominated by radiotherapy, beginning in 1903. A rediscovery of surgery occurred during the mid-1940s, promoted primarily by Dr. Joseph Meigs of Boston and Dr. Victor Bonney in England, who proved that surgery could be performed with minimal mortality and with less morbidity and better cure rates than was possible with irradiation. Others advocated intracavitary radium followed (in a few weeks) by abdominal hysterectomy for early-stage disease. Further development of radiotherapy and surgical techniques currently permits the modern oncologist to select treatment suited to the individual patient, using either modality or a combination of the two.

As a consequence of improved therapeutic modalities and treatment of precursor lesions detected by cytologic screening, the mortality of invasive cervical cancer has fallen dramatically in recent years.[3a] Today, the ability to cure more than one-half of patients with cervical cancer worldwide is a dramatic improvement over the earlier part of the twentieth century and past centuries. While one might speculate that uniform application of cytologic screening would permit elimination of cervical cancer as a disease, this seems unrealistic; indeed, subsets of patients with fulminant disease present problems even under ideal screening circumstances.

Precursor Lesions

Although carcinoma in situ was not then recognized, drawings of microscopic sections appearing in the German literature about 1885 suggest that such lesions were observed. Schottlaender and Kermauner[4] described a lesion that translated as "icing on the cake"; they probably were observing some variant of cervical intraepithelial neoplasia. Rubin[5] is credited with suggesting the term carcinoma in situ.

By the 1940s, gynecologists were accepting this entity and advocating treatment for it, but its relationship to invasive carcinoma was unclear. In various papers as well as a debate, Dr. Arthur Hertig and Dr. John McKelvey discussed the relationship which was not accepted until the 1950s. Those lesions that preceded carcinoma in situ were investigated during the late 1950s. Scandinavian physicians had better follow-up of patients than did American and British workers and contributed significantly to these investigations. Initially the preceding lesions were termed anaplasia (a lesion that lacked differentiation), but that term was slowly replaced by dysplasia and its three subdivisions. In 1967, Richart suggested the term cervical intraepithelial neoplasia and defined subdivisions 1, 2, and 3 to replace the terms dysplasia and carcinoma in situ, in 1973.[6,7] Serious efforts have since been made to standardize diagnoses, but this continues to be a problem largely because histologic dividing lines are not absolutely clearcut.

Genital Cytology

It should be noted that clinicians, especially gynecologists, were instrumental in developing cytology as a clinical adjunct. Although Papanicolaou, an anatomist, established and developed the interpretation of the vaginal smear (and subsequently cervical scraping and endocervical aspiration), it was the clinician who refined its applications and most often started the cytology laboratories, frequently under heavy criticism by the pathologists.

In the United States, the early cytology technicians (as they were then called) were an interesting group. Many were doctors' daughters who had been presented to society, did not need to work for their support (fortunately, for what they were paid would not have supported even the most frugal), and whose fathers considered that they ought to be doing something. One Massachusetts pathologist in Fitchburg, who discovered that his wife's cleaning lady was very intelligent, taught her to screen.

Although gynecologists established most cytology laboratories in the late 1940s and in the 1950s, thereafter such laboratories became the province of pathologists. In the early days, physicians trained their own personnel. The American Cancer Society (ACS) became interested; about 1952, the ACS paid a stipend for 3 months to trainees accepted to study and work in a cytology laboratory. Gradually, training programs developed, usually requiring that the applicant have a high school education. On and off over the years, various organizations have subsidized this training. Cytotechnologists have their own organizations, various forms of certification, and laboratories are accredited by national societies. The modern trend is to make cytotechnology training part of a college baccalaureate degree.

ETIOLOGY AND HISTOGENESIS OF CERVICAL CANCER

The literature on this subject is voluminous; Fenoglio and Ferenczy,[8] Baird,[9] and Reid[10] published excellent summaries on this subject. It seems likely that cervical cancer is a sexually transmitted disease based on extensive epidemiologic data. Herpes simplex virus type 2 (HSV-2) has been linked to this type of cancer, based primarily on serologic and immunohistochemical evidence, mostly indirect. More recently, investigators have concentrated on the human papillomavirus in serologic, cytologic, and histologic studies. The association of genital condyloma and cervical intraepithelial neoplasia is strong. Kurman et al.[11] pointed out the similar histology, epidemiology, and relationship to precursor lesions of cancers of the vulva, vagina, and cervix, speculating that all may be caused by human papillomaviruses. Okagaki, et al.[12] using DNA hybridization techniques, demonstrated human papillomavirus in many benign and malignant tumors of all three sites. Other investigators have studied the relationship of *Chlamydia trachomatis* infections and development of cervical intraepithelial neoplasia, as well as the role of protamines (sperm basic proteins) in malignant transformation of cervical and vaginal cells.

Whether some or all of these agents serve as carcinogens or whether they are merely opportunistic infections remains to be established. The epidemiology and etiology of cervical adenocarcinoma are less understood. The possible association of long exposure to oral contraceptive pills, and a reported increase in incidence of adenocarcinoma of the cervix in recent years has been of interest. The relationship of microglandular hyperplasia associated with contraceptive pill use to adenocarcinoma is unknown but may bear further investigation.

GROSS PATHOLOGY

Cancer of the cervix may be derived from any of the tissues normally found in the cervix. Epithelial cancers are usually squamous cell carcinoma, whether derived from squamous epithelium or mature metaplastic epithelium. Adenocarcinoma is derived from the endocervical surface and cleft epithelium and may have a squamous component of varying degrees of atypia. Stromal tumors, including fibrosarcoma and leiomyosarcoma, are rare. The homologous mixed mullerian tumor or carcinosarcoma has both epithelial and stromal components. Rare tumors such as malignant melanoma and lymphoma in addition to carcinoma metastatic to the cervix must be considered.

The gross appearance of invasive cancer of the cervix varies considerably, dependent to some degree on the duration of the disease. Bulky exophytic fungating lesions (Fig. 13-1A) are less commonly seen in developed countries than they were 50 years ago. Left untreated, such lesions may ultimately distend the vagina and fill the pelvis or may ulcerate and slough, producing a copious malodorous vaginal discharge. Infiltrating lesions may ulcerate (Fig. 13-1B); may produce an enlarged cervix not otherwise noticeably abnormal, an irregular nodular cervix; or (when deeply infiltrating from a lesion located in the anatomic endocervical canal) may produce the so-called barrel-shaped cervix. Such expansion of the lower segment and endocervix may result in shortened parametria, complicating assessment of clinical stage. Focal growth may produce a polypoid lesion (Fig. 13-1C).

HISTOPATHOLOGY

Preinvasive and Microscopically Invasive Lesions

It is important to establish a histologic diagnosis prior to institution of therapy. Preinvasive lesions must be distinguished from invasive cancer. These lesions, which have been variously termed mild, moderate, and severe dysplasia and carcinoma in situ and, more recently, cervical intraepithelial neoplasia 1, 2, and 3, vary in their degree of cellular atypia, extent of such atypia and mitotic activity (Fig. 13-2).

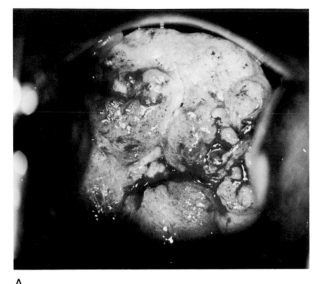

A

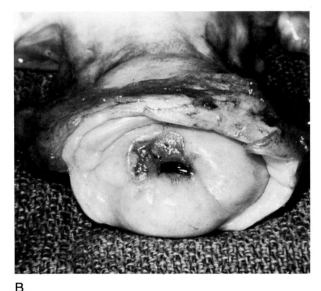

B

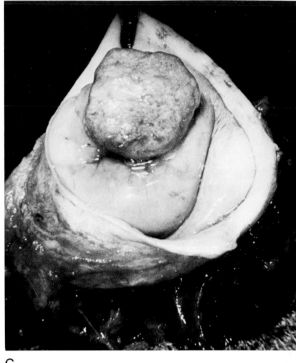

C

Fig. 13-1 (A) Exophytic squamous cell carcinoma involving all quadrants of the cervix. **(B)** One-quadrant superficial ulcerative carcinoma. Maximum depth of invasion in this tumor was 8 mm. **(C)** Radical hysterectomy specimen in which a large polypoid adenosquamous carcinoma extends from the endocervical canal.

Microinvasive Carcinoma

We have recently encountered many patterns of invasion[13] (Figs. 13-3 and 13-4) in a detailed histologic study of 125 women with superficially invading squamous cell carcinoma of the cervix. We were impressed that most microinvasive lesions are multifocal. We concluded that tumor pattern, lesion width, and presence or absence of confluence could be ig-

nored in planning treatment of lesions invading 5 mm or less; we believe that the most important prognostic factor to consider is depth of stromal invasion. Nodal metastases increase in direct proportion to the depth of invasion[13] (Table 13-1). As lesions enlarge (and penetrate more deeply into the stroma), it becomes more important to treat the regional lymph nodes if patients are to have a chance to survive.

Two types of adenocarcinoma in situ have been

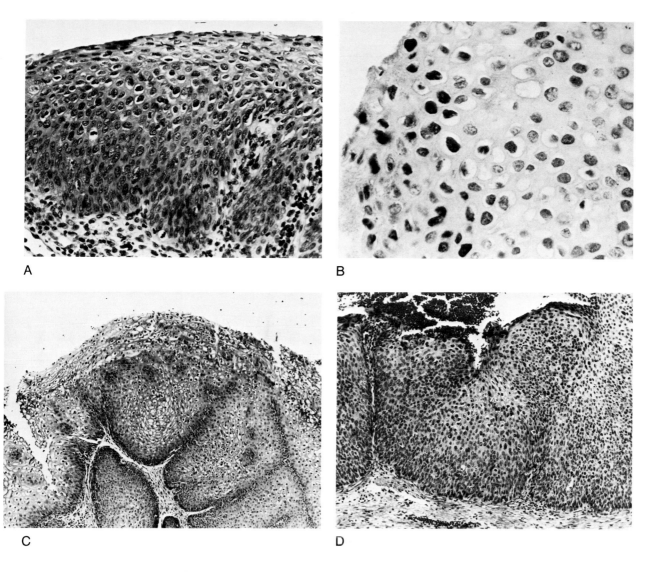

A

B

C

D

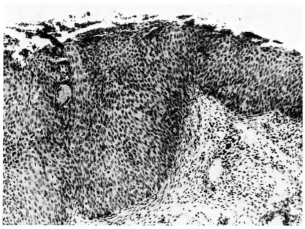

E

Fig. 13-2 **(A)** Moderate dysplasia with mitotic activity extending through about two-thirds of the epithelium. Cytoplasmic alteration in the mature surface cells is consistent with koilocytosis. (H&E ×210.) **(B)** Immunohistochemical stain for human papillomavirus capsid protein on a cervical biopsy section. Dark-stained nuclei represent the site of the viruses. (×340.) **(C)** Koilocytic atypia in which there is cytoplasmic alteration in most of the squamous epithelium. Nuclei vary in size and shape and some cells are binucleate. (H&E ×55.) **(D)** Moderate to severe dysplasia with koilocytic change in some superficial cells. (Note the clear cytoplasm in contrast to the uniform cytoplasm in the carcinoma in situ in E.) (H&E ×85.) **(E)** Carcinoma in situ involving the surface and a cleft in the cervix. Nuclei are relatively uniform but are all atypical and hyperchromatic, and there is absence of the normal squamous cell maturation. (H&E ×85.)

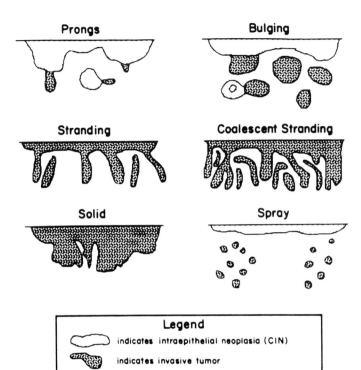

Prongs

Bulging

Stranding

Coalescent Stranding

Solid

Spray

Legend

indicates intraepithelial neoplasia (CIN)

indicates invasive tumor

Fig. 13-3 Patterns of microinvasion. (Simon NL, Gore H, Shingleton HM, et al: A study of superficially invasive carcinoma of the cervix. Obstet Gynecol 68:19, 1986. Reprinted with permission from the American College of Obstetricians and Gynecologists.)

Table 13-1 Stage I Cancer of the Cervix, Nodal Metastases, and Depth of Invasion

Depth of Invasion (mm)	No. of Patients	No. of Patients with Positive Nodes	Positive Nodes (%)
0.0–3.0	43	0	0.0
3.1–5.0	26	1	3.9
5.1–10.0	17	1	5.9
10.1–15.0	19	4	21.0
>15.0	41	18	43.9
Total	146	24	16.4

(Modified from Simon NL, Gore H, Shingleton HM, et al: A study of superficially invasive carcinoma of the cervix. Obstet Gynecol 68:19, 1986. Reprinted with permission from the American College of Obstetricians and Gynecologists.)

described: one consisting of glands lined by hyperchromatic and pseudostratified nuclei and a less common type characterized by large pleomorphic, sometimes clear nuclei containing enlarged nucleoli.[14] Adenocarcinoma in situ can be distinguished from microinvasive adenocarcinoma by limitation of the abnormality to the glandular field, by the constant admixture of normal and abnormal glands, and by lack of stromal response surrounding the abnormal glands.[15] Once glandular or solid cancer budding into the stroma is identified, the lesion qualifies as stage IA, or microinvasive carcinoma. Should a diagnosis of adenocarcinoma in situ be made or suspected on a biopsy, conization of the cervix is recommended in order to rule out invasive adenocarcinoma in a nearby field.

Invasive Squamous Cell Carcinoma

Squamous cell carcinoma has been categorized into subgroups ranging from well differentiated to poorly differentiated. The Reagan-Wentz system classifies squamous cell lesions into large cell keratinizing (with distinct epithelial pearls), large cell nonkeratinizing (sometimes with cytoplasmic kertin but only with very rare pearls, if any), and small cell (possibly neuroendocrine tumors) (Fig. 13-5). The proportion of types varies in several series.

We do not find the Reagan-Wentz classification helpful in therapy planning, nor is tumor grading of

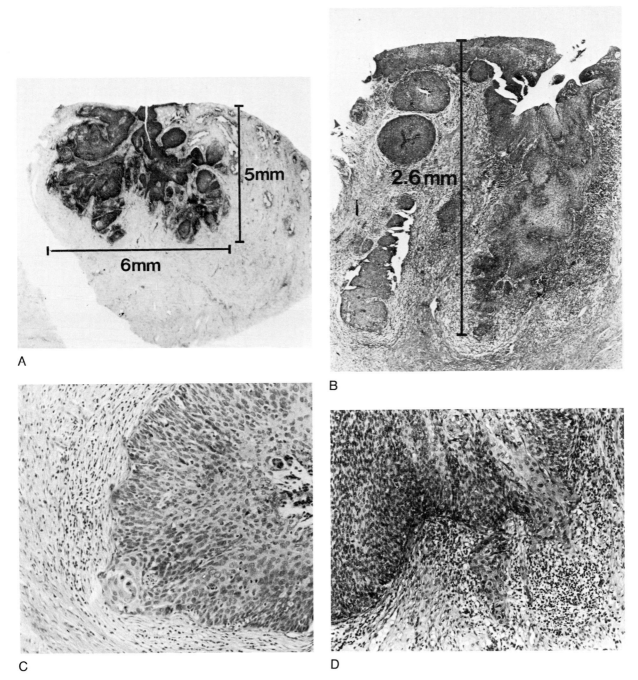

Fig. 13-4 (A) Microinvasive lesion of the solid, often called confluent type. (H&E, ×7.5.) **(B)** This microinvasive carcinoma invades to a depth of 2.6 mm from the surface. Stromal response and inflammatory response to the invading tumor are well illustrated. (H&E, ×31.4.) **(C)** At the margin of a cleft involved by severe dysplasia to carcinoma in situ (CIN 3) are several small pointed foci. That toward the bottom left is differentiating as often happens at the point of invasion. In each of the two foci superior to this, there appears to be a single detached cell. Stromal response is minimal, and there is slight inflammatory response. (H&E, ×125.) **(D)** Inflammatory response is more prominent around the several invasive prongs extending from the solid tumor focus. Whether the main focus is largely within a cleft or an area of invasive carcinoma cannot be determined from this photomicrograph. (H&E, ×125.)

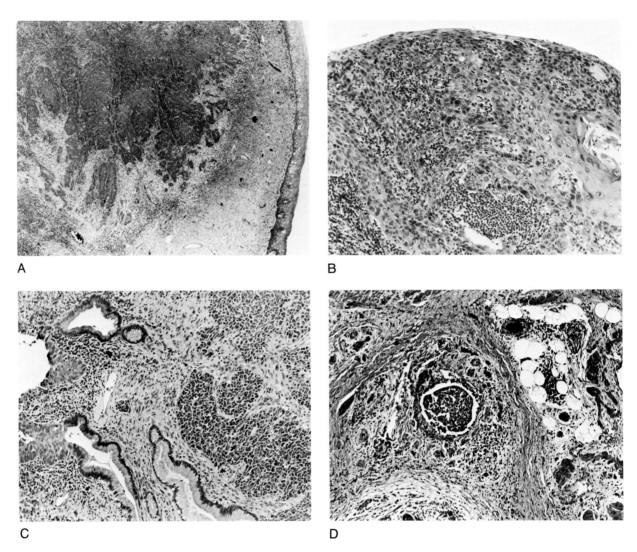

Fig. 13-5 **(A)** Squamous cell carcinoma with altered stroma at its invading borders, extending beneath unremarkable portio epithelium. (Such a tumor may be largely within the endocervix, and such extension beneath the portio epithelium may distort the visible area of cervix only minimally). (H&E, ×35.) **(B)** Prongs of invasion are extending directly from malignant surface squamous epithelium. There is prominent inflammatory response in the subjacent stroma. (H&E, ×140.) **(C)** Groups of poorly differentiated malignant cells invading endocervical tissue. By electromicroscopic studies features characteristic of neuroectodermal differentiation were identified, indicating that this is a small cell undifferentiated carcinoma. It is of interest that there is dysplasia in metaplastic epithelium on the surface and involving cleft mouths. (H&E, ×140.) **(D)** Squamous cell carcinoma extends into a small parametrial blood vessel and is invading its muscular wall. (H&E, ×35.)

prognostic significance in invasive squamous cell carcinoma of the cervix, compared with its value in tumors at other sites. There is no general consensus concerning the predictive value of cellular patterns. Ng[16] and Johansson et al.[17] claim that cure rates with

radiotherapy are better for large cell nonkeratinizing tumors than with large cell keratinizing and small cell tumors. Beecham et al.[18] found no difference in survival for any of these types when they are treated surgically. We have not observed any difference in survival with either of the large cell types, regardless of mode of therapy.

Many attempts have been made to develop a method of determining the degree of malignancy of squamous cell tumors, using a variety of histologic criteria. Such studies have focused on nuclear size, DNA content, tumor morphology, cell types, histologic and nuclear grades, nuclear pleomorphism, mitotic counts, vascular invasion, and stromal response. No system has emerged that offers the simplicity of use to enable adequate evaluation. Pagnini et al.[19] in Padua, and Gauthier et al.[20] in our laboratory, used systems focusing on depth of stromal invasion, lesion diameter, and mode of spread, from which groups at high and low risk of recurrence could be identified. Whereas some investigators[21-23] have predicted a favorable influence with dense lymphocytic infiltrate in the stroma around tumors, Barber et al.[24] and Gauthier et al.[20] found no such association. Histologic scoring systems introduced by Noguchi et al.[25] and Crissman et al.[26] add such time-consuming, costly, multifactorial analyses that they are not practical in the ordinary pathology laboratory; indeed, since they require the entire cervix for study, these analyses are not applicable to the majority of patients with cancer of the cervix.

Invasive Adenocarcinoma

Adenocarcinoma accounts for about 10 percent of cervical cancers. Several cell types, such as endocervical, mucinous, papillary, hobnail/clear cell, and adenoid cystic (Shingleton[27]), may be identified but do not appear to have prognostic significance. Included in this group are adenocarcinomas with a squamous component (histologically benign squamous elements to adenosquamous carcinoma) and the rare collision tumor. It is of interest that dysplasia or squamous cell carcinoma in situ may occur with adenocarcinoma (Fig. 13-6A).

Traditionally, adenocarcinoma has been considered to have a worse prognosis than squamous cell carcinoma, and the idea persists. In our series, cure rates are not significantly different for patients with adenocarcinoma and squamous cell carcinoma treated by either radiation or operation. In addition, we have observed no difference in the rate of metastases to lymph nodes for the two types. In our series of stage IB cervical cancer, 72 patients with large cell keratinizing squamous cell carcinomas, 89 with large cell nonkeratinizing tumors, and 58 with adenocarcinomas, undergoing pelvic lymphadenectomy, had 20.8 percent, 20.2 percent, and 20.7 percent incidence of pelvic node metastases, respectively. The volume of tumor is more important than tissue type in determining prognosis.

Occult Carcinoma

Some tumors arise and grow within the anatomic endocervical canal and thus may be unsuspected until such time as symptoms occur. Squamous cell carcinoma, adenocarcinoma, or mixed tumors may present in this manner. Abnormal bleeding or atypical Papanicolaou (Pap) smears lead to the diagnosis, frequently by curettage. In the amended International Federation of Gynecology and Obstetrics (FIGO) staging system introduced in 1976, these occult lesions were separated from microscopically invasive portio lesions since the occult lesions have lymph node metastasis rates similar to those for stage IB lesions, while the latter group are less likely to be associated with nodal metastases.

Cervical Sarcoma

Histologically, cervical sarcomas including fibrosarcoma, leiomyosarcoma, and carcinosarcoma, are similar to sarcoma in other sites. The rare sarcoma botryoides, generally occurring in children, is beyond the scope of this discussion.

Routes of Spread

Cancer of the cervix appears to spread by direct extension, yet some believe that the parametrial extension commonly thought to represent geographic extension is in fact a combination of coalescent tumor nests, inflammation, and fibrosis. Lymphatic spread by embolization of tumor cells to pelvic and aortic nodes is common as the volume of tumor increases. Direct invasion of blood vessels by tumor (Baltzer et al.[23]) may be a worse prognostic sign than the more common involvement of small lymphatic vessels. Combinations of these routes of metastasis and direct interstitial extension along tissue planes and through body fluids may also occur. The primary nodes drain-

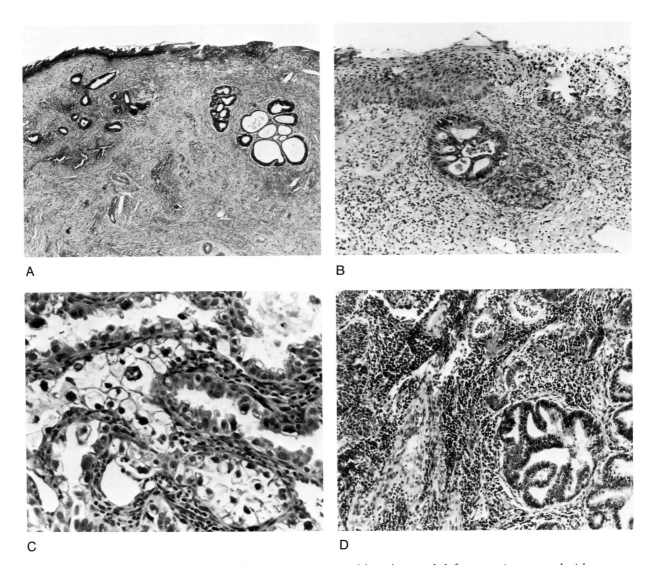

Fig. 13-6 **(A)** This is probably adenocarcinoma in situ although normal clefts are not interspersed with malignant clefts (or glands) in the field of the photomicrograph. There is minimal stromal response to the group on the right (hence questionably invasive). (H&E, ×35.) **(B)** Small focus of adenocarcinoma, a malignant cluster with small gland lumina lying within the main gland, and an adjacent similar focus (tangentially sectioned) lie immediately beneath dysplastic surface squamous epithelium (mild to questionably moderately dysplastic). This combination of atypical findings in cervical squamous and cleft epithelium is not unusual. This glandular focus constitutes adenocarcinoma in situ when appearing alone but could well be part of a larger lesion. (H&E, ×140.) **(C)** Adenocarcinoma of the clear cell pattern. Such tumors were previously classified as mesometanephric carcinoma, until such a pattern was identified in endometrial carcinoma and in transitions from more classic endocervical adenocarcinoma. From this its paramesonephric (mullerian) origin was established. (H&E, ×88.) **(D)** Adenocarcinoma (right) and squamous cell carcinoma (left) with associated prominent inflammation. Whether this is a collision tumor or an adenosquamous carcinoma differentiating into two separate patterns cannot be determined without further evaluation. Making such a differentiation is not important in patient management (H&E, ×140.)

ing the cervix and upper vagina are those located in the parametrial and paravaginal tissues draining to the external iliac, the internal iliac, obturator, and presacral nodes[28] (Fig. 13-7). Further drainage cephalad occurs through the common iliac nodes to the para-aortic nodes. Retrograde spread to the inguinal nodes is less common in cervical cancer than in adenocarcinoma of the corpus. The incidence of pelvic node metastases in stage IB carcinoma varies from 9 to 27 percent and is usually quoted as 15 percent. Given the difficulty in performing a complete pelvic node dissection, the inconsistent study of node specimens by many pathologists, and the chance of false-negative reading in the case of micrometastases, it is likely that the true incidence of pelvic node metastasis for stage IB carcinoma is closer to 25 percent.[29] In stage IIB, incidence of pelvic node metastasis ranges from 16 percent to 50 percent, in stage III 36 percent to 50 percent, and in stage IVA in excess of 50 percent.[28]

Involvement of the secondary nodes along the common iliac vessels and the aorta occurs with increasing frequency as the clinical stage increases[30] (Table 13-2).

Precise knowledge of distribution of nodal metastases in relationship to stage of disease and volume of tumor is a result of an interest in surgical staging during the past two decades. In summarizing six reports between 1971 and 1981 involving 971 patients,[28] differences in clinical and surgical staging were found for 24.1 percent of patients with stage I lesions, 42.9 percent with stage II lesions, 58.9 percent with stage III lesions, and 37.5 percent with stage IV lesions. Although the inaccuracy of clinical staging is apparent, routine surgical staging prior to radiation has not gained a place in the treatment of cervical cancer, since it has not been demonstrated that there is any increased patient survival with the additional knowledge of extent of disease. This may be related to

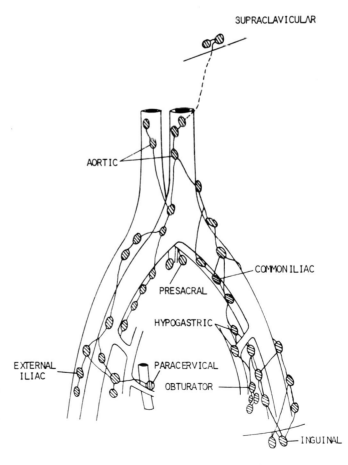

Fig. 13-7 Node groups potentially involved in patients with cervical carcinoma. (Shingleton HM, Orr JW Jr: Cancer of the Cervix: Diagnosis and Treatment. Churchill Livingstone, Edinburgh, 1987.)

Table 13-2 Incidence of Paraaortic Node Involvement in the Various Stages of Cervical Carcinoma

Investigators	Clinical Stage of Tumor				Overall
	I	II	III	IV	
Averette et al. (1972)	3/40	4/18	2/20	1/2	10/80 (12%)
Buchsbaum (1972)	0/23	1/12	7/20	1/2	9/57 (16%)
Nelson et al. (1977)	—	9/63	15/39	0/2	24/104 (23%)
Sudasanam et al. (1978)	11/53	7/43	5/19	0/3	23/218 (11%)
Lagasse et al. (1980)	8/143	23/80	19/64	1/4	51/291 (18%)
Total	22/259 (8%)	44/216 (20%)	48/162 (30%)	3/13 (23%)	117/750 (16%)

(Cavanagh D, Ruffolo EH, Marsden DE (eds): Gynecologic Cancer: A Clinicopathologic Approach. Appleton-Century-Crofts, Norwalk, 1985.)

the ineffectiveness of extended field irradiation and to combinations of surgery, radiation, and chemotherapy in metastatic squamous cell carcinoma. In addition, may women with cervical cancer are elderly or obese, or have medical problems and, indeed, cannot tolerate surgery. Modalities such as computed tomography (CT) scans with directed fine-needle aspiration of enlarged nodes along the aorta have to some degree replaced surgical staging because of their safety and ease of application. Nevertheless, CT scans of the abdomen and pelvis are rather subjective studies and lack sensitivity and specificity[31] in predicting intraabdominal tumor. The same may be said for lymphangiography, which has a high false-negative rate, yet which may be useful in some instances.

TREATMENT OF PRECURSOR LESIONS AND MICROINVASIVE DISEASE

Certain criteria must be met before proceeding with outpatient conservative therapy of cervical dysplasias. In general, the colposcopic examination should permit visualization of the entire transformation zone. There should be minimal or no extension of the lesion into the canal, perferably confirmed by a negative endocervical curettage. The neoplastic lesion should not involve more than two quadrants of the portio. Histologic and cytologic diagnoses should agree and should not suggest invasion. Those patients with histologically proven deep cleft involvement by

the cervical intraepithelial neoplasia lesion are not good candidates for cryosurgical or laser therapy. Furthermore, the patient should agree to adequate follow-up visits; if this seems unlikely, therapeutic conization or hysterectomy might be considered.

Treatment of Cervical Intraepithelial Neoplasia

SURGICAL TREATMENT

A variety of techniques is available for treatment of cervical intraepithelial neoplasia (CIN). Excision may be accomplished by biopsy, conization, or hysterectomy. Excisional biopsy is not uniformly the most reliable treatment, since many patients have large transformation zones and lesions may involve several quadrants. Such treatment can be offered, however, to women with well-demarcated lesions involving one or two quadrants. This treatment should not be considered for the patient who is unlikely to return for frequent colposcopic and cytologic follow-up visits. Therapeutic conization is an acceptable form of treatment for precursor lesions, especially carcinoma in situ, and is widely used, especially outside the United States. Those who defame the use of therapeutic conization point to reports of large percentages of residual CIN in hysterectomy specimens following conization. In most instances, however, such reports fail to analyze the margins of the cone specimens; thus, it is not surprising that residual disease is found in the uterus. It would appear that conization with adequate margins around the lesion is as effective as hysterectomy in treatment of these lesions. On the basis of collected series, about 3.5 percent of CIN patients are expected to have recurrences (as CIN) following conization, yet this incidence is not markedly different from 0.5 to 2 percent recurrence rates following hysterectomy.[32] The rates of invasive carcinoma following conization or hysterectomy for CIN are almost identical (0.5 percent and 0.3 percent, respectively) based on a collected series of 15,071 patients.[28] Hysterectomy has been a popular treatment for CIN in the United States primarily because many of the patients take advantage of hysterectomy for sterilization as well as for treatment of their precursor lesions. Therapeutic conization in this country has been reserved primarily for younger women who desire more children.

CRYOSURGERY AND ELECTROCAUTERY

We favor cryosurgery as treatment over electrocautery because of greater patient acceptance. Cryosurgery can be performed with minimal discomfort, little morbidity, and inexpensive equipment and without anesthesia. Electrocautery is associated with more patient discomfort but is still effective in eradicating CIN as reported by Chanene and Rome[33] and by Schuurmans et al.[34] In Chanen and Rome's report, 1864 patients treated for CIN had only a 2.7 percent failure rate. Schuurmans and co-workers listed a 14 percent initial failure rate in 426 patients and an overall success rate (with some treated two or more times) of 96.6 percent. The results with electrocautery are ostensibly comparable to those obtained with cryosurgery and laser in every way.

Recurrence of CIN after cryosurgery depends somewhat on the degree of severity of the original lesion and the number of quadrants involved. CIN 3 lesions tend to be larger and to have a slightly higher recurrence rate than do CIN 1 lesions (16 percent vs. 7 percent).[35] Treatment other than cryosurgery for lesions involving all four quadrants of the cervix has been suggested, since such lesions recur frequently after cryosurgery.[35] Involvement of the endocervical canal by disease is another factor in failure of cryosurgery. Townsend[35] reported only a 6 percent failure rate in patients with negative endocervical curettages before treatment, whereas 21 percent failed if they

had positive pretreatment endocervical curettage. Thus, the number of cervical quadrants involved, the severity of the dysplasia, and the degree of extension into the endocervical canal are all important in predicting the outcome of treatment by cryosurgery.

We have used cryosurgery extensively at our institution, especially for patients with CIN 1 and 2 lesions; almost three-fourths of such patients are treated by this modality.[36] With CIN 1 and 2 lesions, about 3.5 percent of patients will subsequently require conization or hysterectomy for cryosurgery failure, and we have seen no subsequent invasive tumors. In CIN 3 patients, we have used cryosurgery as treatment in about 30 percent, the remainder being treated by either therapeutic conization or hysterectomy. Using cryosurgery as treatment of CIN 3, we have subsequently performed conization or hysterectomy on 8.9 percent because of recurrent atypical cytologic findings. Overall failure rate, that is, the requirement for additional cryosurgical treatment or other form of treatment to control the disease, is 11 percent in our series of several thousand women treated with cryosurgery, which is similar to that of other reports. Overall success rates (one or several cryosurgical treatments) range from 96 to 98 percent at various centers.[28]

Cryosurgery has definite limitations for a variety of reasons. Equipment may malfunction and the freeze may not be as extensive as is necessary. It is difficult at times to gauge the extent of the freeze and in particular to determine whether the deepest parts of the cervical clefts have been adequately treated. Some patients with a large transformation zone are not suitable for such treatment, since the probe may not fit over the entire lesion. Lesions involving the endocervical canal likewise are often not adequately treated using cryosurgery, since control and extension of the freeze for complete eradication of a premalignant lesion in the anatomic canal may not be possible. The observed failure rates and pitfalls of cryosurgery are such that the treating physician should be cautious in using this technique in populations of women likely to neglect follow-up evaluation. Most large series reported in the United States using cryosurgery have follow-up rates not above 60 to 70 percent, leaving large segments of the treatment group unobserved. For these reasons, we have favored surgical treatment for those with more advanced CIN.

LASER VAPORIZATION

Laser vaporization has certain advantages over cryosurgery, including the more focal and controllable destruction of lesions, less tissue reaction, less transformation zone inversion, and less overall morbidity. Cure rates are equal to that of cryosurgery. The disadvantage of laser therapy for CIN is the greater expense of the equipment and cost to the patient.

Precancerous lesions can be destroyed with greater precision with the laser[37] (Fig. 13-8). The adjacent tissue is left relatively undamaged as compared with the adjacent thermal injury associated with cryosurgery[37] (Fig. 13-9). This accounts for the shorter healing time of the laser-treated areas as compared with areas treated by cryosurgery or electrocautery. Selection criteria of patients for laser vaporization are similar to those used for cryosurgery. One is limited in treating lesions that involve the endocervical canal by laser vaporization. Four quadrant lesions might be

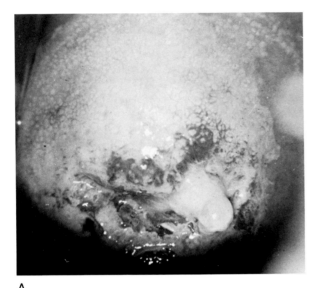

A

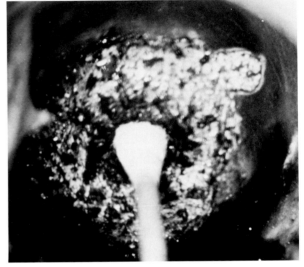

B

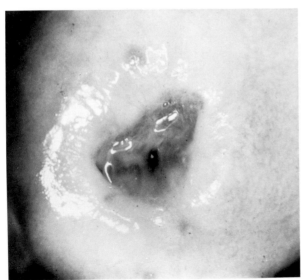

C

Fig. 13-8 Use of laser vaporization for cervical intraepithelial neoplasia. **(A)** Large dyplastic atypical transformation zone. **(B)** During laser vaporization. **(C)** Normal-appearing cervix 2 months later. (Shingleton HM, Hatch KD, Orr JW Jr, et al: Diagnosis and treatment of preinvasive and microscopically invasive squamous cell carcinoma of the cervix: Including comments on surveillance of DES-exposed patients with cytologic atypias. Cancer Bull 35:172, 1983, with permission.)

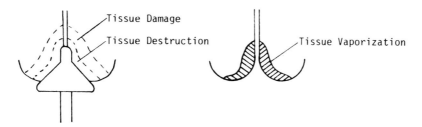

Fig. 13-9 Tissue vaporization by laser causes minimal damage to immediately adjacent tissue, whereas graded damage occurs adjacent to cryoprobe. This accounts for the infection and discharge present after treatment by cryosurgery, compared with a more rapidly healing cleaner cervix associated with laser vaporization. (Shingleton HM, Hatch KD, Orr JW Jr, et al: Diagnosis and treatment of preinvasive and microscopically invasive squamous cell carcinoma of the cervix: Including comments on surveillance of DES-exposed patients with cytologic atypias. Cancer Bull 35:172, 1983, with permission)

more appropriately treated by surgical means, although the laser is superior in this regard as compared with cryosurgery. Laser vaporization is especially helpful in lesions of the vaginal cuff or lateral vagina, which cannot be treated effectively with existing cryoprobes and which otherwise would require surgical excision. Overall, laser vaporization is the superior treatment modality when all the factors enumerated above are considered.

Treatment of Microinvasive Cancer

Stromal invasion to more than 1 mm as isolated projections arising at the base of carcinoma in situ or dysplasia, referred to in the European literature as early stromal invasion, is treated like carcinoma in situ, that is, by therapeutic conization or total hysterectomy (abdominal or vaginal)[28] (Table 13-3). Stromal invasion to 3 mm below the basement membrane, commonly referred to in the American literature as microinvasive, may be treated by conventional hysterectomy. We prefer the abdominal route in order to assess pelvic nodes, but with this degree of invasion one need not dissect pelvic nodes or even sample them unless they are clinically suspicious. In this category, if lymphvascular spaces are involved in the conization specimen, we would include the medial portion of the cardinal ligaments in the operation (modified radical hysterectomy) in order to ensure good margins; this more radical operation is based on the increased chance of recurrence in patients with involvement of

Table 13-3 Choice of Operative Procedure for Cervical Neoplasms Diagnosed by Conization

Histologic Findings	Terminology	Recommended Procedure
Stromal invasion: ≤1 mm as isolated projections arising at base of carcinoma in situ or dysplasia	Focal microinvasion (early stromal invasion)	Total hysterectomy (abdominal or vaginal) or Therapeutic conization
Stromal invasion: ≤3 mm	Microinvasion	Abdominal hysterectomy[a] Pelvic node dissection
Stromal invasion: >5 mm	Invasive carcinoma	Radical hysterectomy Aortic node assessment Pelvic node dissection

[a] If lymphovascular spaces are involved, extended (modified radical) hysterectomy is recommended.
(Shingleton HM, Orr JW Jr: Cancer of the Cervix: Diagnosis and Treatment. Churchill Livingstone, Edinburgh, 1987.)

Table 13-4 Significance of Lymphvascular Space Involvement in Microcarcinoma <5 mm Depth

Investigators	No. of Patients	Recurrence	Deaths
Foushee (1969)	7	1	1
Mussey (1969)	19	2	1
Boyes (1970)	12	1	1
Leman (1976)	12	0	0
Burghardt (1979)	53	2	1
Coppleson (1979)	39	0	0
Iversen (1979)	8	5	NS
Boyce (1981)	10	3	1
Simon (1986)	7	0	0

(Shingleton HM, Orr JW Jr: Cancer of the Cervix: Diagnosis and Treatment. Churchill Livingstone, Edinburgh, 1987.)

the lymphvascular space[37] (Table 13-4). For stromal invasion of 3 to 5 mm below the basement membrane, we also use the modified radical hysterectomy (see Fig. 22-1, Ch. 22). When stromal invasion exceeds 5 mm below the basement membrane, we treat the patient by means of a radical hysterectomy and pelvic node dissection with aortic node assessment.

STAGING AND EVALUATION OF INVASIVE CANCER

The staging classification most widely used is that of FIGO, last modified in 1976 (Table 13-5). Stage IA includes microinvasive carcinoma; the present wording for this lesion may be modified in the future to include both depth and width measurements as part of the definition. All other tumors confined to the cervix but invading beyond the superficial layers are included in stage IB. Stage IIA, that is, involvement of the upper vagina without involvement of the parametrium, is an unusual stage; management often follows that for stage IB. Stage IIB is associated with extension of tumor into the parametrium but without involvement of the pelvic wall; patients with stage IIB and with stage III (AB) tumors are managed in the United States almost exclusively by radiation therapy. Stage IIIB also includes patients with hydronephrosis or nonfunctioning kidney, since such a finding portends a poorer prognosis. In stage IVA, there is invasion of adjacent organs such as the bladder or rectum,

Table 13-5 Staging Classification for Carcinoma of the Cervix[a]

Stage	Description/Features
	Preinvasive Carcinoma
0	Carcinoma in situ, intraepithelial carcinoma (Cases of stage 0 should not be included in any therapeutic statistics for invasive carcinoma.)
	Invasive Carcinoma
I	Carcinoma strictly confined to the cervix (Extension to the corpus should be disregarded.)
Ia	Microinvasive carcinoma (early stromal invasion)
Ib	All other cases of stage I. (Occult cancer should be marked 'occ.')
II	Carcinoma extending beyond the cervix but not onto the pelvic wall. Carcinoma involving the vagina but not the lower one-third
IIa	No obvious parametrial involvement
IIb	Obvious parametrial involvement
III	Carcinoma extending onto the pelvic wall (On rectal examination, there is no cancer-free space between the tumor and the pelvic wall. The tumor involves the lower third of the vagina. All cases with a hydronephrosis or nonfunctioning kidney should be included, unless they are known to be due to another cause.)
IIIa	No extension onto the pelvic wall
IIIb	Extension onto the pelvic wall and/or hydronephrosis or nonfunctioning kidney
IV	Carcinoma extending beyond the true pelvis or showing clinical involvement of the mucosa of the bladder or rectum (A bullous edema as such does not permit a case to be allotted to stage IV.)
IVa	Spread of the growth to adjacent organs
IVb	Spread to distant organs

[a] As adopted by the International Federation of Gynaecology and Obstetrics (1976)

while stage IVB is applied to patients who have distant metastases. The distribution of neoplastic lesions of the cervix can be related to age of the patient (Fig. 13-10).

Patients with invasive cancer, regardless of the tissue type, must undergo a comprehensive evaluation prior to treatment. Chest radiographs and intravenous pyelography (IVP) are routine, while barium enema studies are restricted to patients with advanced stage

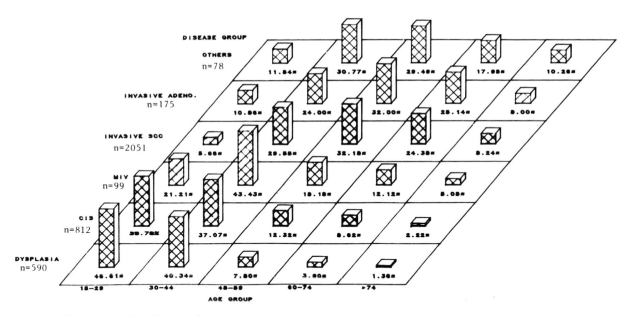

Fig. 13-10 Distribution of neoplastic cervical lesions of the cervix by age in 3,805 women treated at the University of Alabama at Birmingham. (Courtesy of Dr. Seng-Jaw Soong, Biostatistician, Comprehensive Cancer Center.)

Table 13-6 Evaluation of Cervical Cancer Patients

Type of Assessment	Routine Evaluation	Optional Evaluation
Physical assessment	Nodal assessment (supraclavic-ular, inguinal) Abdominal palpation Pelvic assessment (bimanual, rectovaginal)	Delayed sensitivity skin testing Urodynamic testing Pulmonary function studies Electrocardiography Examination under anesthesia
Radiographic imaging	Chest radiography Intravenous pyelography Barium enema[a]	Computed tomography (chest, abdomen, pelvis) Ultrasonography (abdomen, pelvis) Lymphangiography (abdomen, pelvis) Radioisotope scans (renal, liver, bone)
Endoscopic	Cytoscopy Proctosigmoidoscopy	Flexible colonoscopy Retrograde pyelography Bronchoscopy
Hematologic	Packed cell volume White cell count and differential	Coagulation studies Nutritional screen (serum albumin, transferrin)
Blood chemistry	Blood urea nitrogen, creatinine Liver enzymes Electrolytes	Tissue markers

[a] Optional in women under age 50 without history of gastrointestinal disease.

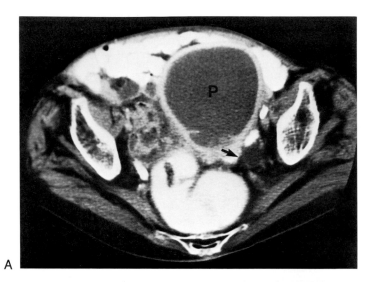

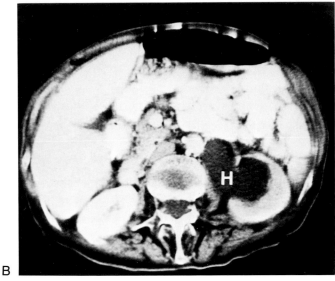

Fig. 13-11 Computed tomography (CT) scans demonstrating tumor. **(A,B)** Pyometra (P) is present in a patient with advanced squamous cell carcinoma. The left ureter (arrow) is obstructed in the pelvis. **(B)** Resultant hydronephrosis (H) is evident. *(Figure continues.)*

disease or postmenopausal women. The value of chest radiographs is obvious, in that therapy would be markedly altered should metastatic disease to the chest be discovered. Intravenous pyelography in itself is essential in that hydronephrosis or a nonfunctioning kidney places the patient in clinical stage III. Proctosigmoidoscopy should be performed if direct extension of tumor to the rectosigmoid is suspected. Cystoscopy is not mandatory in stage I disease but is recommended in lesions involving anterior vaginal wall. Many optional studies are available (Table 13-6). Of these CT scans of the abdomen and pelvis

(Fig. 13-11) and examination under anesthesia may be the most informative. Election of other studies relates to the patient's age, medical condition, nutritional status, and past medical history.

TREATMENT OF INVASIVE CANCER BY RADIATION

Radiation therapy of cancer of the cervix includes two distinct components, each having a different purpose. One is brachytherapy (intracavitary and inter-

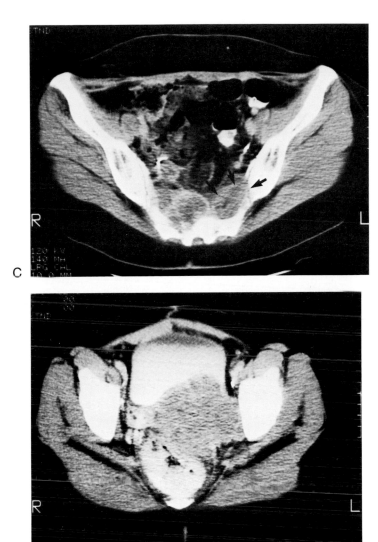

Figure 13-11 *(Continued).* **(C)** Recurrent squamous cell carcinoma invading the sacrum (arrows) of a patient who had been treated surgically for stage IB squamous cell carcinoma. **(D)** A large pelvic tumor mass indenting the base of the bladder of a woman with Stage III squamous cell carcinoma.

stitial radiation therapy), and the other is external radiation therapy.

Intracavitary Radiation Therapy

The primary tumor site and immediate paracervical and vaginal extensions of cervical cancer are treated by brachytherapy. The anatomy of the female pelvis is uniquely favorable for its use. The thick walls of the uterine corpus and endocervix and the pliability of the vaginal vault permit adequate separation between the radiation sources, the rectum, and the bladder. An applicator usually consists of a tandem, which holds the sources within the uterine cavity, and colpostats or ovoids, which hold sources in the vaginal fornices. Currently, afterloading applicators of the Fletcher-Suit type are most commonly used (Fig. 13-12). Afterloading devices facilitate application, since the therapist need not be concerned with radiation exposure and can achieve more optimal dose distribution by selecting the appropriate strength of the isotope sources. Radiographs of the application can be obtained using dummy sources; the active sources will only be inserted after the films have been reviewed

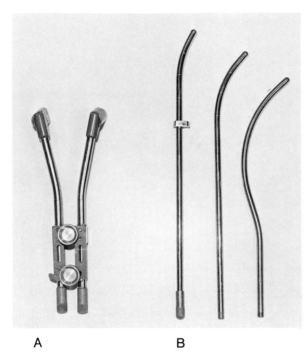

A   B

Fig. 13-12 Fletcher-suit applicator for intracavitary radiation treatment. The vaginal colpostats **(A)** and three different curves of tandem **(B)** are shown.

and the position of the applicator is considered satisfactory. Several isotopes are available, such as radium-226 and cobalt-60, although cesium-137 is most commonly used. The efficacy of the intracavitary treatment is based on the inverse square law, which states that the dropoff in radiation dose is proportional to the inverse of the square of the distance from the radiation source. This rapid dropoff permits the radiotherapist to deliver a high tumor dose to the cervix and still limit the dose to the adjacent organs by minimizing complications.

The Manchester system and the Fletcher system of dose specifications for intracavitary radiation therapy have emerged as the two major approaches in the treatment of cancer of the cervix. The Manchester system is exemplified by the use of point A and point B. Point A was originally defined as 2 cm superior to the lateral vaginal fornix and 2 cm lateral to the cervical canal. Anatomically, it represents the medial parametrium, approximately at the point where the ureter and uterine artery cross. Point B was defined as 3 cm lateral to point A, approximating the region of the

obturator nodes. In clinical practice, dose calculations are often made from radiographs, and point A is taken 2 cm up from the flange of the intrauterine source and 2 cm lateral from the central canal. Because of variation in pelvic anatomy, particularly in women with tumor, these points may not strictly correspond to the anatomic structures indicated, yet they are convenient reference points (Fig. 13-13). The Fletcher system is highlighted by milligram-hours as the key element in the treatment prescription. By setting the fixed-size vaginal colpostats and using defined patterns of radium distribution in the applicators, the dosages to points A and B can be precalculated. Today, however, modern computer techniques permit calculation of dosages to the pelvic nodes as well as to the cervix, bladder, and rectum, using precise isodose distributions (Fig. 13-14).

Interstitial Radiation Therapy

In advanced cancer of the cervix, the associated obliteration of the vaginal fornices or other distortions of the vaginal anatomy may interfere with accurate placement of conventional intracavitary applicators, even after delivery of 5,000 to 6,000 rad to the whole pelvis by external therapy. Syed and Feder, in 1977, developed a technique to solve this problem by placement of transvaginal and transperineal implants. This technique employs a template to guide the insertion of a group of 18-gauge hollow steel needles into the parametrium transperineally, theoretically representing modified interstitial colpostats (Fig. 13-15). This approach holds promise, but long-term studies are needed to demonstrate improved survival rates, particularly in view of increased morbidity, such as higher fistula rates reported by some workers.[39]

External Radiation Therapy

External radiation therapy is directed toward extension of tumor into the extrauterine pelvic soft tissue and lymph nodes, where the influence of intracavitary radiation is minimal. For most patients with small volume cancer, simple anterior and posterior beams 16 cm wide and 16 cm in vertical dimension encompass all necessary tissues. The superior margin of the treatment volume is usually placed at the upper end of the fifth lumbar vertebra (L5). The beam should encompass all vaginal extension of tumor and

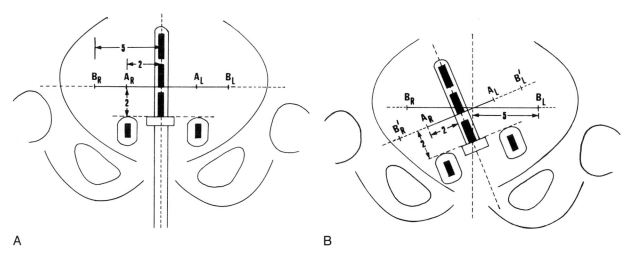

Fig. 13-13 Points A and B with variation in uterine position. **(A)** Uterus in the midline position. The numbers refer to distance in centimeters between various points. **(B)** Uterus in an eccentric position. Points B′ in this instance do not correspond to the region of the obturator nodes.

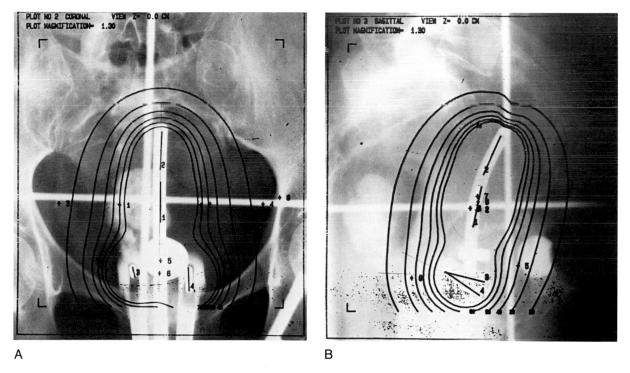

Fig. 13-14 Isodose curves with intracavitary radiation. The isodose curves are shown superimposed over the intrauterine tandem and vaginal colpostats. **(A)** Anterior-posterior view of pelvis. **(B)** Lateral view of pelvis.

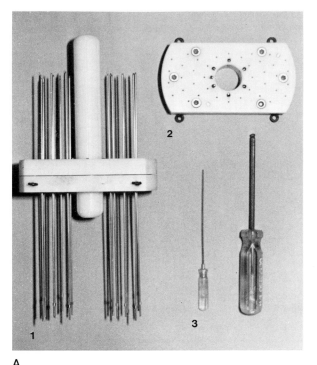
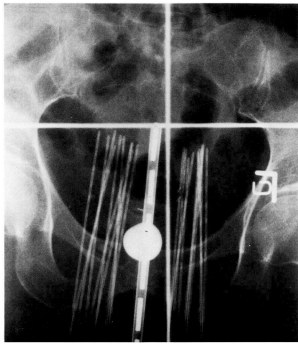

A   B

Fig. 13-15 Syed-Neblett applicator for interstitial-intracavitary implants. **(A)** Applicator with needles (1), perineal template (2), and screwdrivers for tightening needles in the template (3). **(B)** Anterior-posterior view of the pelvis showing interstitial parametrial needles and intrauterine tandem in place.

the entire obturator fossa. The lateral margin is 2.0 cm beyond the lateral margin of the bony pelvic wall at the widest plane of the pelvis. A 3 to 4 cm wide lead shield placed over the area of the intense intracavitary uterine radiation is used to block the rectum and bladder from the external beam employed to boost parametrial radiation dosage (Fig. 13-16). Depending on the clinical situation, the pelvic field can be extended to include the paraaortic nodes. The late subcutaneous fibrosis seen especially in patients with large physical dimensions can be reduced by using a higher-energy beam when possible and also by using a four-port box technique for sparing of the posterior rectal wall and the anterior bladder wall.

Combined Brachytherapy and External Therapy

Optimal treatment should deliver a high central dose to the cervix, paracervical tissue, and parametria as well as a moderate homogeneous dose to the pelvic lymph nodes without exceeding the tolerance doses to the bladder and rectum. The sequence of intracavitary and external radiation is determined by the extent and distribution of the tumor. When the tumor is of limited extent and low in volume (such as in clinical stage I), and the pelvic anatomy is not altered markedly, brachytherapy should be employed initially. However, if the tumor has distorted the pelvic anatomy so as to interfere with good intracavitary placement, external therapy is used initially, in order to shrink the tumor and make the situation more favorable for subsequent brachytherapy.

In women with advanced stages of cancer, external irradiation is the mainstay of treatment; intracavitary irradiation is used only as supplemental treatment, when possible. Suggested radiation therapy for carcinoma of the cervix at our cancer center is shown in Table 13-7. When intracavitary application cannot be used, external irradiation is used alone; 5,000 rad is delivered to the whole pelvis and an additional 2,000 rad through a reduced central pelvic field. The limit-

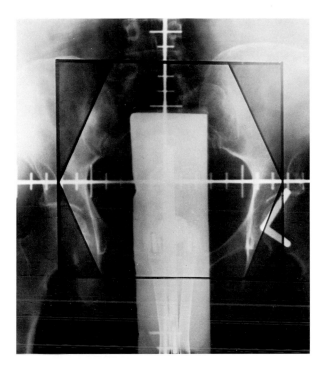

Fig. 13-16 Anterior-posterior pelvic port showing a midline lead block superimposed over the intracavitary applicator.

Table 13-8 Factors to be Considered in Treatment Planning

Technical	Clinical
Total radiation dose	Tumor volume
Daily dose	Cell type and grade
Total number of fractions	Anatomical factors
Field size	Previous surgery
Sequence of therapy	Age
Energy source	Nutritional status
	Systemic disease

ing factors in the treatment of carcinoma of the cervix are the rectum (where the maximum dose should be less than 6,500 rad), the bladder (where the maximum dose should be less than 7,000 rad), and the paracervical tissues (where the maximum dose should not exceed 8,000 rad). Treatment should be adjusted to each individual clinical situation, with consideration of growth patterns, tumor extent, the patient's age, medical and nutritional condition, and the coexistence of systemic disease. Many of these factors affect the tolerance of the patient to therapy (Table 13-8).

Table 13-7 Radiation Therapy for Cancer of the Cervix (University of Alabama at Birmingham)

Stage	Radiotherapy[a] Whole Pelvis (rad)	Intracavitary (Point A)[b] (rad)	Pelvic Sidewall Boost (Midline Shielding) (rad)	Total Dose Point A[b] (rad)	Point B[b] (rad)
IA	None	6,500 (2 imp)	None	6,500	1,625
B (occult)	None	6,500 (2 imp)	3,875	6,500	5,500
B (small)	None[c]	7,000 (2 imp)	3,750	7,000	5,500
	2,000[c]	5,000 (2 imp)	2,250	7,000	5,500
B (bulky) (>4.0 cm)	4,000	4,000 (2 imp)	500	8,000	5,500
IIA	2,000[c]	5,000 (2 imp)	2,250	7,000	5,500
B	4,000[c]	4,000 (2 imp)	500	8,000	5,500
IIIA					
B	5,000[c]	3,000 (2 imp)	250	8,000	6,000
IVA	6,000[c]	2,000 (1 imp)	None	8,000	6,000

[a] Five-day/week fractions of 180 to 200 rad.
[b] Points A and B, defined in text and in Figure 13-13.
[c] Options allowing for differing geometry of tumor in individual patients.
imp, implants (2 weeks apart).

SPECIAL TREATMENT CATEGORIES

Barrel-Shaped Cervical Cancer

Bulky endocervical lesions, which account for approximately 10 percent of stage I and II cancer, are more apt to result in treatment failure. Presumably, local failure relates to the relative radioresistance of bulky tumors to intracavitary applications due to physical principles derived from the inverse square law. In patients with large endocervical lesions (barrel-shaped) of cervical cancer, Durrance and associates[40] recommended an extrafascial conservative hysterectomy 6 weeks following completion of high-dose preoperative radiation. To minimize complications, they recommended no more than 4,000 rad of whole-pelvis radiation therapy in 4 weeks and a single 72-hour intracavitary application of a tandem and ovoids, rather than giving two 48-hour applications. Those patients who underwent adjuvant hysterectomy had fewer central failures compared with a similar group of patients treated by radiation alone. However, this was not a randomized study, and there was no significant increase in survival. We have not favored this combined treatment scheme at our institution, yet many centers in the United States still employ it for patients with barrel-shaped lesions. Complications of combined therapy are not negligible. While Edinger et al.[41] and Gallion et al.[42] reported very few complications in their series, O'Quinn et al.,[43] Blake et al.,[44] and Perkins et al.[45] reported serious complications, such as bowel obstruction or fistula, urologic fistula, or combined (multiple) fistulas in 12.3 to 50 percent of their patients.

Cancer of the Cervical Stump

Cancer of the cervical stump is less commonly encountered than in the early years of the twentieth century, when a supracervical hysterectomy was an acceptable operation. The patient with carcinoma of the cervical stump must be evaluated like the patient who has an intact uterus. The absence of the uterine corpus makes application of the intracavitary radium less effective because the zones of effective radiation do not reach the end of the stump. Therefore, there is a greater emphasis on external whole-pelvis radiation in treatment planning.[46] Whole-pelvis radiation in a dose of 4,000 rad is followed by a standard intracavitary application if the endocervical canal is at least 2 cm in length, allowing a radioactive source in the tandem. Treatment planning should vary with the stage and volume of disease. The 5-year survival rate is about the same as that for cancer of the intact uterus, stage for stage. However, the possibility of complications exists due to expected small bowel adhesions in the deep pelvis following the surgery.

By contrast, if the subtotal hysterectomy was performed less than 2 years before the onset of symptoms of cancer, the control rate is greatly decreased. This most likely reflects the presence of cervical cancer unrecognized at the time of the hysterectomy with delay in treatment.

Inappropriate Simple Hysterectomy

The surprise finding of invasive cancer of the cervix in a surgical specimen after a simple vaginal or abdominal hysterectomy usually follows incomplete evaluation of a young woman who underwent surgery for such conditions as abnormal bleeding, infection, or sterilization or for premalignant conditions such as carcinoma in situ or dysplasia. The term *cut through* is widely used for this situation but should pertain only to those cases in which tumor was at the surgical margins. With the exception of the patient who has microinvasive disease and who may require no further treatment, immediate postoperative radiation therapy offers the best chance of cure[28,45,47] (Table 13-9). The combination of vaginal ovoids and external pelvic radiation therapy permits a high dose to the upper vagina and an adequate dose to the pelvic lymph nodes and parametrial lymphatic vessels. The prognosis correlates well with the extent of disease. It is clear that survival is best if tumor is confined to the surgical specimen, that is, the size of the tumor is small. Alternatively, a surgical approach, that is, radical excision of the upper vagina combined with pelvic lymphadenectomy, might be considered and is described in the discussion on surgical therapy.

Extended Field Irradiation Therapy

Tumor involvement of the lymph nodes, particularly in the paraaortic regions, is of concern. A Gynecologic Oncology Group study confirmed that clinical staging is often inaccurate in determining the

Table 13-9 Survival of Patients with Invasive Cervical Cancer in a Total Hysterectomy Specimen

	Radiation-Completed Treatment					
	Immediate Radiation (no residual)[a]		Immediate Radiation (Residual)[b]		Radiation for Recurrence[c]	
Investigators	No. of Patients	% Survival	No. of Patients	% Survival	No. of Patients	% Survival
Cosbie (1963)	56	71	30	20	23	26
Green (1968)	—	—	—	—	27	26
Andras et al.[47] (1973)	65	89[d]	53	58	—	—
Davy (1977)	48	77	16	38	—	—
Papavasilou (1980)	25	92	7	71	—	—
Perkins et al.[45] (1984)	21	81	15	80	—	—

[a] Negative margins and no clinical evidence of disease at the time of radiotherapy.

[b] Surgical margins involved or no residual cancer clinically apparent.

[c] Clinically recurrent cervix cancer.

[d] Includes 27 patients with microscopic disease.

(Shingleton HM, Orr JW, Jr: Cancer of the Cervix: Diagnosis and Treatment. Churchill Livingstone, Edinburgh, 1987.)

extent of disease in patients with cancer of the cervix: 29 percent of patients with stage II, III, and IV tumors were found to have metastases outside the usual field of pelvic irradiation. Wharton et al.[48] gave 5,500 rad to the paraaortic area in patients with positive paraaortic nodes and noticed severe intestinal complications in 32 of 120 operated patients (27 percent). Because of this problem the radiation dose to the paraaortic area was reduced to 4,500 rad by many therapists. If there is any radiographic evidence of paraaortic adenopathy, a computed tomogram (CT scan) or ultrasound-directed percutaneous needle aspiration may be diagnostic and is not associated with the risk of small bowel adhesions that may result from transperitoneal biopsy of nodes. Alternatively, retroperitoneal staging techniques are available for direct biopsy. The benefits of aortic node irradiation in terms of survival have not been determined conclusively, although most reports suggest a trend toward increased survival with extended field treatment [28,48-50] (Table 13-10).

Postoperative Pelvic Radiation Therapy

About 15 percent of all patients with stage IB cancer of the cervix will be found to have pelvic node involvement by tumor at the time of surgery. The woman found to have metastatic disease in pelvic lymph nodes after a radical hysterectomy presents a unique problem. While postoperative radiation treatment has long been advocated and widely used, its benefits have not been adequately demonstrated.[51,52] Of major concern in those women is the prospect of distal recurrences in addition to local (pelvic) recurrence. Whole-pelvis radiation in a dose of 5,000 rad is given in an effort to achieve local (pelvic) tumor control; the dose per treatment fraction is reduced to 150 to 160 rad in an attempt to lessen the complications of combined irradiation and surgery. Such complications occur in 7 to 28 percent.[53-55] Of these, small bowel damage, bladder dysfunction, and lower leg edema are the most frequently encountered.

COMPLICATIONS OF RADIOTHERAPY

The morbidity resulting from properly conducted radiation therapy in patients with cancer of the cervix is minimal. Although the location of the cervix makes it ideal for intracavitary treatment, the level of tumor dose to the cervix and parametrial area by necessity entails exposure of the adjacent organs to significant (and at times damaging) dosages of radiation. Higher dosages of external pelvic radiation are necessary in

Table 13-10 Extended Field Radiation for Paraaortic Node Metastases

Investigators	No. of Patients	Radiation Dose (rad)	Complications (%)	Survival Time	%	Type of Exp.[a]
Guthrie (1974)	10	5,400	—	2 yr	44	T
Schelhas[49] (1975)	9	6,000	0	—		E
Berman (1977)	4	4,000–5,200	25	—		T
	7	4,000–5,200	0	—		E
Nelson (1977)	48	6,000	48	2 yr	45	T
Wharton et al.[48] (1977)	24	5,500	42	13–38 mo	13	T
Sudarsanam (1978)	21	4,000–4,320	—	19–63 mo	20	T
Averette (1979)	29	4,400–5,000	14	—		T
Bonanno (1980)	18	6,000	26	5 yr	22	T
Hughes (1980)	22	4,500–5,100	9	5 yr	29	T
Ballon (1981)	19	4,320–5,120	0	5 yr[c]	23	E
Buchsbaum (1981)	23	4,650–5,540	—	33–103 mo	22	T
Piver et al.[50] (1983)	21	6,000	62			
	10	4,400–5,000	10	5 yr	10	T
Welander (1981)	31	4,400	20	25–106 mo	26	T
Shah (1982)	4	4,500	—	5 yr	50	T
Tewfik (1982)	23	5,000–5,500	28[b]	45–115 mo	33	T
Komaki (1983)	15	5,000	—	5 yr	40	—
Berman (1984)	98	4,000	—	2 yr	27	T + E
Brookland (1984)	15	4,000–5,000	7	3 yr	40	T
Potish (1984)	21	4,500–5,000	7	3 yr	45	E

[a] T, transperitoneal; E, extraperitoneal.
[b] Intestinal complication.
[c] Projected 5-year survival.
(Shingleton HM, Orr JW Jr: Cancer of the Cervix: Diagnosis and Treatment. Churchill Livingstone, Edinburgh, 1987.)

advanced stages of cancer of the cervix, which in turn may adversely affect both large and small bowel in the pelvis. For example, Strockbine et al.[56] reported 83 complications (8 percent) among 1,030 patients with stage I and II cervical cancer treated at M.D. Anderson Hospital. In this group, there were only 22 patients (2 percent) with serious complications, such as bladder or rectal fistula, vaginal vault necrosis, or obstruction. Among 831 patients with more advanced disease treated with 4,000 rad or more to the whole pelvis, there were 46 severe bowel complications alone (5.5 percent).

Acute Complications

A number of side effects from irradiation are commonly seen during the course of treatment, but these are usually transient and may not lead to permanent injury. Serious skin reaction, important during the orthovoltage era, is seldom a limiting factor in radiation therapy with high-energy machines, unless the beam is striking the skin tangentially. Acute radiation cystitis and proctosigmoiditis, manifested as dysuria, urinary frequency and urgency, and diarrhea, is primarily due to the close proximity of intracavitary sources to the base of the bladder and anterior wall of rectosigmoid. Enteritis or acute injury to small bowel may be a problem, particularly when radiating the paraaortic area. Symptoms of radiation enteritis, including nausea, cramping, and diarrhea, are controlled by antispasmodics and antiemetics, and the patient is placed on a low-residue diet. These symptoms will usually resolve within several weeks of completion of the treatment. The effect of pelvic radiation on bone marrow function is generally not clinically important, although bone marrow suppression is more serious when radiation is given to both the pelvis and paraaortic area.

Delayed Complications

Delayed injuries from pelvic and abdominal irradiation are generally not manifested until 6 to 24 months after completion of the therapy. The varying degree of vaginal and cervical fibrosis is common, due to intensity of the radiation dose, and can cause vaginal stricturing and sexual dysfunction over a period of time, particularly if the patient is sexually inactive following treatment.[57] Postirradiation vaginal stenosis and dyspareunia can be minimized by the use of dilators and estrogen creams. The close relationship of the rectum to the upper vagina and cervix makes it especially vulnerable to injury with intracavitary therapy or with combined internal-external therapy. Proctitis may be mild with superficial ulceration, which persists for years, or it may be severe and require surgical therapy, usually in the form of colostomy. Topical steroids may also be useful in providing symptomatic relief and promoting healing. Radiation sigmoiditis increases in severity and frequency as the dose of external whole-pelvis radiation therapy is raised. It is an infrequent problem when the external therapy is limited to 4,000 rad in 4 weeks. However, the sigmoid is still subject to injury from intracavitary sources because of its relatively fixed position in the hollow of the sacrum and its close association with the uterine corpus.

Rectovaginal fistula is perhaps the most common complication of pelvic radiation requiring surgical intervention. A proximal diverting colostomy is invariably necessary. Surgical closure of the fistula may be difficult, although techniques that bring in new blood supply (omental patches, vulvar flaps) are promising in this situation.

The small bowel is not as commonly injured by standard radiation techniques as is the large bowel, although its dose tolerance is usually less than that of the sigmoid colon. Because of its mobility, however, the small bowel is able to move in and out of the field of irradiation; thus it is thought to receive less than the full dose. The terminal ileum is the most common site of small bowel injury because it is fixed proximal to the ileocecal valve, has a relatively poor blood supply at that point, and is the narrowest portion of the small bowel. Furthermore, the ileocecum is the portion of the small bowel most likely to be adherent in the pelvis as a result of previous surgery or inflammatory disease. The symptoms of the small bowel injuries are usually those of an incomplete bowel obstruction with delayed postprandial cramping, nausea, and vomiting. The management of radiation-induced small bowel injuries is complex and requires fine surgical judgment.[58]

Standard radiation therapy technique should not result in significant fibrosis of the wall of the ureter. Therefore, the appearance of lower ureteral obstruction following judicious radiation treatment suggests progression of tumor or recurrent disease, even in the absence of a palpable mass on pelvic examination. Diagnosis of tumor in this event may be made by needle aspiration or transvaginal biopsy, although laparotomy may be required for such a biopsy.

TREATMENT RESULTS AND FUTURE DIRECTIONS OF RADIOTHERAPY

Cure rates for patients with stage IB and IIA cancers are similar whether treated by radiation or by radical hysterectomy. Five-year survival rates range between 86 to 92 percent for stage IB and 70 to 75 percent for stage IIA. In stage IIB radiation-treated patients, the expected 5-year survival is 60 to 65 percent; in stage IIIB, the 5-year survival rate ranges from 25 to 40 percent.

The anatomic sites of failure in cancer of the cervix after irradiation are closely correlated with tumor stage. Perez et al.[59] analyzed the pattern of radiation failures in 849 patients (Table 13-12) and emphasized better pelvic control with higher radiation dosages in stage IIB and III disease. However, it is evident that in disease beyond stage IIA, the ability to control the tumor in the pelvis is still of significant concern. As the radiation doses increase, there is a diminution in the incidence of pelvic failure but, along with this, an increase in complications. Jampolis et al.[60] analyzed postirradiation recurrences in 916 patients with cancer of the uterine cervix and pointed out that central recurrence was rare in stages IB and IIA (2 percent). Most instances of pelvic recurrence could be attributed to improper placement of the vaginal colpostats, resulting in low doses of radiation to the primary cervical tumor. Parametrial recurrence was correlated in 75 percent of cases with lateral deviation of the tandem without compensation from the external radiation. The overall cause of pelvic failure in patients with stage IIIB disease was bulky parametrial infiltration.

Research efforts are under way using interstitial implants, high linear energy transfer (LET) radiation, hypoxic cell sensitizers, combined hyperthermia-radiation, and intraoperative radiation. Because of the high incidence of distal metastases in patients with stage III and IV cancer of the cervix, it is imperative to develop systemic adjuvant therapy in order to improve the prognosis of such patients. The potential for combined chemotherapy and radiation therapy is hampered by the absence of effective chemotherapeutic agents. However, the combined use of hydroxyurea with radiation therapy holds promise.[61,50] The development of a combined integrated program of surgery, radiation therapy, and adjuvant systemic chemotherapy in those patients at high risk of metastatic disease may have the potential for long-term control of disease for this group of unfortunate women.

SURGICAL TREATMENT

Stage IB Cancer

Radiation therapy and surgery have unique advantages and disadvantages, and treatment must be tailored to the individual patient. Radiation can apply to all patients, and the survival rates for stage I disease are equal to those of surgery. Radiation, however, is associated with serious bowel or bladder damage in 2 to 6 percent of patients and is commonly associated with posttreatment sexual dysfunction due to vaginal stenosis and fibrosis.[57] Complications of radiation may be delayed and difficult to correct. By contrast, surgical treatment permits ovarian conservation, establishes the precise extent of tumor by the surgical staging procedure, and leaves a more functional and less damaged vagina. Surgical complications occur early and are usually more easily correctable. The urologic complications experienced during the 1940s and 1950s have been markedly reduced, wtih urologic fistulas or strictures occurring in fewer than 2 percent of series reported by experienced pelvic surgeons. Since most patients are young and healthy, other operative complications are uncommon. Surgery thus offers a psychologic advantage to the patient with early disease (i.e., complete removal of the cancer) and

is associated with excellent cure rates. In 13 series, including our own, reported between 1973 and 1985 and involving a total of 4,860 nonirradiated patients treated by radical hysterectomy as primary treatment,[28] the mean ureteral fistula rate was 2.3 percent (0 to 5.6 percent), the mean bladder fistula rate was 0.58 percent (0 to 1.4 percent) and the mean operative death rate was 0.45 percent (0 to 1.4 percent). Our own figures in a series exceeding 600 patients are 1.4 percent, 0.23 percent, and 0.23 percent, respectively. We advocate radical surgical excision of stage IB lesion in premenopausal women, especially those with tumors less than 3 or 4 cm in diameter. The operative technique we use is described in Chapter 22.

Special Surgery

Carcinoma of the cervical stump is infrequently seen, since supracervical hysterectomy has become an operation of the past. From a technical viewpoint, surgery in the form of a radical trachelectomy may be used as primary therapy for those with stage I disease. In the earlier years of our surgical series, we performed a number of such operations. Since women with cervical stump carcinoma may be elderly or obese, have medical contraindications to surgery, or have disease extending beyond the cervix, primary operative therapy is rarely selected.

The treatment of patients who are found to have invasive cervical cancer following a conventional total hysterectomy for other indications is discussed under Treatment of Invasive Cancer by Radiation. We have recently reported a series of such patients managed surgically.[62] From a technical viewpoint, there is no difficulty in reoperating and converting the total hysterectomy to (the equivalent of) a radical hysterectomy. In doing so, one grasps the vaginal vault, separates the vagina from the bladder and rectum, isolates the cardinal ligaments, and proceeds with the operation as one would with an intact uterus. We did not encounter any differences in length of surgery, increased intraoperative blood loss, or increased morbidity when comparing these patients with the conventional radical hysterectomy group. We believe that in the case of a young woman, such an operative approach might be considered after the diagnosis of cancer, in order to spare her the long-lasting effects of pelvic irradiation and permit conservation of ovarian function.

TREATMENT OF ADENOCARCINOMA OF THE CERVIX

To some degree, uncertainty regarding the clinical behavior and management of women with primary adenocarcinoma of the cervix persists. We recently reviewed our series of 162 patients evaluated with emphasis on histopathology, clinical features, treatment, and survival.[63] Seventy-seven of these patients underwent radical hysterectomy alone, whereas 65 patients were treated by radiation therapy alone. The remainder were treated with combined radiation and surgery. We have been unable to demonstrate any significant difference in survival when comparing adenocarcinoma patients with squamous cell carcinoma patients matched for stage. Tumor volume as reflected by clinical stage and lesion size is in our opinion the most important prognostic factor.

Adenosquamous carcinomas of the cervix have been reported by a number of authorities to represent more virulent tumors.[64,23] We compared adenocarcinomas of varied histologic patterns with adenosquamous lesions and could find no statistical difference in survival. Women with poorly differentiated adenocarcinoma of the cervix may have a poorer prognosis than do those with poorly differentiated squamous cell lesions of the cervix. We conclude that there is no reason to treat adenocarcinoma of the cervix any differently from squamous cell carcinoma, stage for stage, and our selection of therapy is not altered by the tissue type. We can find no justification for the notion that combined radiation and surgery is the treatment of choice for cervical adenocarcinomas, nor do we necessarily use such combined treatment.

CANCER OF THE CERVIX IN PREGNANCY

Cancer of the cervix complicates pregnancy in 0.02 to 0.4 percent of pregnancies, whereas 0.1 to 7.6 percent of patients with cervical cancer are pregnant at the time of initial diagnosis. In addition, some tumors are diagnosed during the postpartum period. It could thus be stated that between one in 150 and one in 5,000 pregnancies is complicated by invasive cervical cancer.[65] It is particularly important for obstetricians to biopsy cervical lesions encountered in pregnant women. One should not assume that vaginal bleeding during pregnancy is due to benign causes without visualizing the cervix. Cervical cytology and colposcopy are also helpful in finding early invasive tumors or premalignant lesions during pregnancy.

Pregnant women found to have microinvasive lesions should be allowed to deliver before therapy. In this instance, vaginal delivery is not contraindicated. The postpartum cervix after involution will be easier to evaluate than the cervix in advanced pregnancy. For carcinomas of any stage found in the first trimester, therapy should be instituted, ignoring the pregnancy. In those with stage IB lesions in the second trimester, one might consider immediate therapy, depending on the circumstances (patient's parity, religion, size of the lesion). If the lesion is small and the patient is willing to accept a slight additional risk, one might delay therapy until fetal viability. In those with cancer discovered in the third trimester, therapy should begin after delivery, implemented after fetal viability.

Some authorities believe that delays over 4 weeks in patients with clinical lesions are contraindicated. Prem et al.[66] however, allowed five women with early invasive stage I lesions discovered between 20 and 34 weeks to delay therapy and concluded that a planned delay of up to 17 weeks did not adversely affect pregnancy outcome or cancer therapy, as all of his patients survived. Lee et al.[67] reported eight women, seven with advanced cancer, who completed their pregnancies after a planned delay of 1 to 11 weeks (mean 5 weeks). All pregnancies resulted in live births, and none of the patients experienced an advance in clinical stage. The weight of evidence suggests that a planned short therapeutic delay to obtain fetal viability can be undertaken, particularly in patients with early invasive disease. Nevertheless, individualization of therapy is important. It has been established that vaginal delivery is not detrimental to survival of the patients. Since control of bleeding may be a problem is the lesion is advanced, abdominal delivery may be elected in these patients.

Patients with stage IB disease may be treated with radiation therapy as well as by radical surgery (Table 13-11). In more advanced stages, radiotherapy is the treatment of choice. In late pregnancy, once the fetus is delivered (vaginal or abdominally), radiation therapy can begin. There seems to be little benefit of induced abortion prior to initiation of radiation ther-

Table 13-11 Management of Patients with Stage I Cervical Cancer in Pregnancy, According to Time of Detection (University of Alabama at Birmingham)

Histologic Diagnosis[a]	Time of Detection (weeks)	Recommended Treatment
Focal microinvasion	0–40	Delay therapy until viability
Microinvasion		Re-evaluate and treat postpartum
Microcarcinoma	0–12	Institute therapy
	0–26	Consider therapy
		Delay until fetal viability
	27–40	Delay until fetal viability
Carcinoma		Deliver and institute therapy

[a] Refer to Table 13-3 for definitions of each of the histologic diagnoses.

apy in patients in early pregnancy, since patients will abort 3 to 6 weeks after radiation is begun.

The clinical stage is the most important prognostic factor in patients with invasive cancer of the cervix during pregnancy. Five-year survival is not different in patients with stage I disease treated in the first, second, or third trimester or postpartum. The same is true of stage II disease. It would appear from the literature, however, that patients discovered to have cervical cancer in the postpartum period are likely to have more advanced disease than those diagnosed ear-

lier in the pregnancy, presumably due to delay in recognition of the malignant disease during the pregnancy.

RECURRENT CANCER

The disease-free interval of patients whose tumors ultimately recur depends on the original stage and tumor volume, the adequacy of the initial treatment, radiosensitivity of the tumor, the host response, and

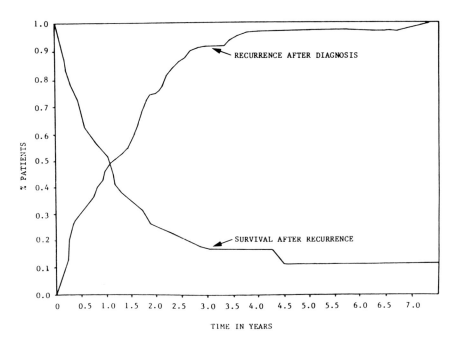

Fig. 13-17 Stage IB cancer of the cervix. Cumulative recurrence rate after diagnosis and survival rate after recurrence. N = 371 patients. (Shingleton HM, Gore H, Soong S-J, et al: Tumor recurrence and survival in Stage IB cancer of the cervix. Am J Clin Oncol 6(3):265, 1983.)

other factors. Eighty percent of recurrences are discovered within 3 years of initial therapy[68,32] (Fig. 13-17).

The terms *recurrent* and *persistent* in reference to the posttreatment behavior of cancer are confusing. In general, active tumor discovered within the first 4 to 6 months post-therapy may be termed persistent cancer, while that found after a disease-free interval of several months is called recurrence. There is no strong evidence that earlier diagnosis of recurrence increases the rate of curability, perhaps related to the tendency for recurrent tumor to be found at distant sites, in the retroperitoneal spaces, or in the central pelvis.[32] (Fig. 13-18, Table 13-12). In our study of 371 patients with stage IB cancer, central pelvic recurrences were encountered in 3 percent of 200 patients treated by an initial surgical approach, while 5 percent of 171 patients treated by radiotherapy recurred centrally. Since this small group of patients includes the only ones potentially curable by pelvic exenteration, it is apparent that the majority of patients who recur will receive experimental chemotherapy unlikely to offer cure or will be treated palliatively. It is thus not surprising that even in those who originally had stage I disease, the cumulative survival rate after recurrence is almost a precise inverse curve from that of cumulative recurrence (Fig. 13-17), the great majority of deaths occurring in the first 3 years after recurrence.

Pelvic Exenteration

When central pelvic recurrence is established following radiation therapy or is found in a patient treated surgically for whom adjunctive radiation therapy has proved unsuccessful, an exenterative procedure might be considered. These massive operations may include removal of all the pelvic viscera (uterus, bladder, rectum, vagina). Such operations should be reserved for women under the age of 70 years in good general health, with small tumor volumes in the central pelvis, and with disease confined to the upper two-thirds of the vagina. Absolute contraindications to exenterative surgery are extrapelvic metastases; the triad of unilateral leg edema, sciatica, and ureteral obstruction; pelvic sidewall fixation by tumor; severe life-limiting medical illness; and the perception that for psychologic or other reasons the patient could not care for herself following surgery (Table 13-13). The procedure should be performed by physicians in hospitals prepared for the major intraoperative and post-

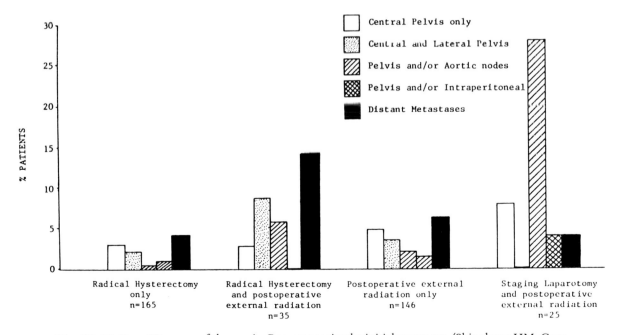

Fig. 13-18 Stage IB cancer of the cervix. Recurrence sites by initial treatment. (Shingleton HM, Gore H, Soong S-J, et al: Tumor recurrence and survival in Stage IB cancer of the cervix. Am J Clin Oncol 6(3):265, 1983.)

Table 13-12 Carcinoma of the Uterine Cervix: Incidence and Patterns of Radiation Therapy Failure

Stage	No. of Cases	5-Year Actuarial Survival NED (%)	Pelvic	Pelvic and DM	Total Pelvic Failures	DM Only
IB	281	87	2 (0.7%)	16 (5.7%)	18 (6.4%)	22 (7.8%)
IIA	88	73	1 (1.1%)	10 (11.4%)	11 (12.5%)	14 (15.9%)
IIB	252	68	22 (8.7%)	22 (8.7%)	44 (17.4%)	38 (15.1%)
III	212	44	31 (14.6%)	45 (21.2%)	76 (35.8%)	39 (18.4%)
IVA	16	—	3 (18.7%)	9 (56.2%)	12 (75%)	3 (18.7%)

NED, no evidence of disease; DM, distant metastases.
(Perez CA, Breaux S, Mados-Jones H, et al: Radiation therapy alone in the treatment of cancer of the uterine cervix: Analysis of tumor recurrence. Cancer 51:1393, 1983.)

Table 13-13 Preoperative Contraindications to Exenteration in Patients with Recurrent Cervical Cancer

Absolute
  Extrapelvic disease
  Triad of unilateral leg edema, sciatica, and ureteral obstruction
  Tumor-related pelvic sidewall fixation
  Bilateral ureteral obstruction (if secondary to recurrence)
  Severe life-limiting medical illness
  Psychosis or the inability of the patient to care for herself
  Religious or other beliefs that prohibit the patient from accepting transfusion
  Inability of physician or consultants to manage any or all intraoperative and postoperative complications
  Inadequate hospital facilities

Relative
  Age over 70 years
  Large tumor volume
  Unilateral ureteral obstruction
  Metastasis to the distal vagina

(Shingleton HM, Orr JW Jr: Cancer of the Cervix: Diagnosis and Treatment. Churchill Livingstone, Edinburgh, 1987.)

operative problems that may be encountered. Further intraoperative contraindications are extrapelvic disease, malignant ascites, metastatic disease in nodes, tumor invasion of major vessels, or documented bowel serosal involvement.

Most patients undergoing exenterative surgery die of cancer thereafter, even though they appeared to have localized disease and were able to survive the "last-chance" operation. It is realistic to note that the more advanced her original clinical stage, the less likely it is that the patient can be cured by an exenterative procedure, although some with original clinical stage III disease have survived. In spite of this, patients who seem to have central pelvic recurrence, who are in generally good condition, and in whom no definite evidence of extrapelvic disease can be demonstrated deserve an exploratory laparotomy to give some chance for long-term survival.

The literature in the past 20 to 30 years has centered on the issue of whether all exenterations should be total (i.e., removal of bladder and rectum with the vagina, uterus, and cervix) (Fig. 13-19) or whether selected patients can be treated by anterior exenteration (the rectum preserved) (Fig. 13-20). We have been successful in using anterior exenteration when small central lesions are confined to the cervix or

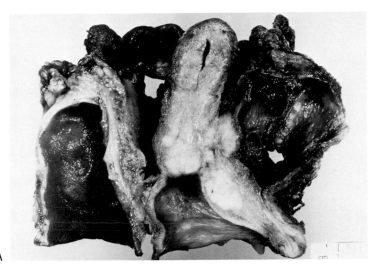

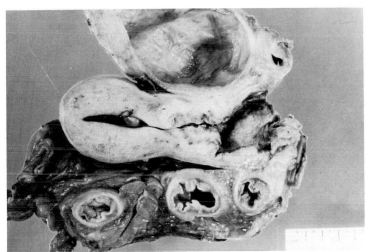

Fig. 13-19 Total exenteration specimens **(A,B)** showing the extent of the operation. Extension of tumor from the cervix is apparent. (Courtesy of Dr. P. T. Taylor, University of Virginia.)

A

B

upper anterior vagina, not involving the rectovaginal septum. We have achieved a 60 percent 5-year survival in 48 such women during the past decade. Our 5-year survival for an additional 53 patients treated by total exenteration has been 29 percent. The 5-year survival reported by others for total exenteration ranges from 20 to 41 percent. The operative mortality varies with the extent of the procedure; we have had a 5.3 percent mortality with anterior exenteration and 12.7 percent for total exenteration. Operative mortality is strictly age related; we have had no operative deaths in women under age 40, whereas we have had 12.2 percent operative mortality in women over age 60. Our overall operative mortality in 164 patients

undergoing pelvic exenteration is 7.3 percent (Table 13-14).

Exenterative surgery is fraught with major acute complications. Infections complicate 30 to 70 percent of cases. Bowel fistulas range from 3 to 26 percent, small bowel obstruction from 4 to 18 percent, and urinary leaks from 1 to 14 percent. Additional late complications of the intestinal and urinary tracts occur as well. It is for this reason that surgical mortality in series reported the last 20 years in America range from 7.7 to 37 percent. Better methods of pelvic closure, antibiotic coverage, and decrease in operative time afforded by the use of stapled anastomoses have improved outcome in recent years. By switching to

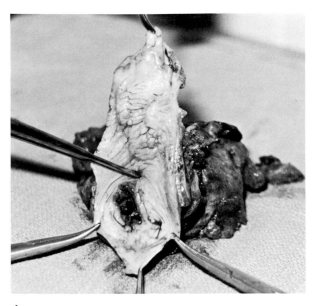

A

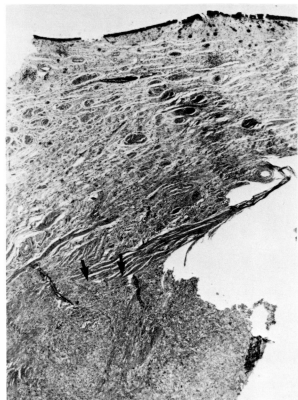

Fig. 13-20 Anterior pelvic exenteration for recurrent cancer. **(A)** The entire anteriolateral vaginal wall, the upper posterior vagina and bladder were removed with this dissection. **(B)** Squamous cell carcinoma (below) persisting in vaginal vault after treatment and invading the muscular wall of the bladder but not extending to submucosa. Arrows indicate advancing margin to tumor. (H&E, ×35.)

B

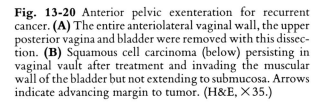

Table 13-14 Operative Mortality Rates and 5-Year Survival Rates for Patients Treated for Advanced or Recurrent Cervical Cancer by Pelvic Exenteration

Investigators	Patients (N)	Operative Mortality (%)	5-Year Survivors (%)
Douglas and Sweeney (1957)	23	4	22
Parsons and Friedell (1964)	112	21	21
Brunschwig (1965)	535	16	20
Kiselow et al. (1967)	153	10	35
Krieger and Embree (1969)	35	11	37
Ketcham et al. (1970)	162	7	38
Symmonds et al. (1975)	198	8	32
Morley and Lindenauer (1976)	34	3	62
Rutledge et al. (1977)	296	14	33
Shingleton et al. (1986)	164	7	44

(Modified from Cavanagh D, Ruffolo EH, Marsden DE (eds): Gynecologic Cancer: A Clinicopathologic Approach. Appleton-Century-Crofts, E. Norwalk, 1985.)

Table 13-15 Single-Agent Cisplatin Trials

Investigators	Treatment (mg/m² q3wk)	Eval. Pts.	% Response	MDR (months)
Bonomi (1982)	50	122	23	3.8
	100	138	27	4.4
	20[a]	121	24	3.7
Lira-Puerto (1979)	100	19	47	3–6+
Hall (1984)	60	22	9	–
Cohen (1982)	3	3	100	–
Thigpen (GOG) (1981)	50	22	50	6
		12	17	6
Rossof (SWOG) (1984)	75	7	0	–
Hayat (1984)	100	11	27	–
Cohen (1982)	120	11	42	4+
Stehman (1984)	50	3	33	–

[a] Exception: 20 mg/m²/day × 5 q3wk.

MDR, mean duration of response; GOG, Gynecologic Oncology Group; SWOG, Southwest Oncology Group.

(Shingleton HM, Orr JW Jr: Cancer of the Cervix: Diagnosis and Treatment. Churchill Livingstone, Edinburgh, 1987.)

Table 13-16 Results of Combination Chemotherapy in Patients with Advanced or Recurrent Cervical Cancer

Regimen	Investigators	No. of Patients	% Response
ADR and BLEO	Bond et al. (1976)	20	35
	de Palo et al. (1976)	15	20
	Greenberg et al. (1977)	11	0
	Piver et al. (1978)	16	6
ADR and CTX	Alberts and Ignoffo (1978)	10	10
	Hanjani and Bonneli (1980)	20	30
ADR, CTX: 5-FU	Sorbe and Frankendal (1982)	27	8
ADR, CTX and 5-FU	Piver et al. (1978)	7	57
	Piver et al. (1980)	34	17
ADR, CTX, and 5-FU, and VCR	Chan et al. (1982)	31	58
ADR, CTX, and PLAT	Lele et al. (1983)	20	20
ADR and MECCNU	Day et al. (1978)	31	45
ADR and MTX	Haid et al. (1977)	16	12
	Guthrie and Way (1978)	39	66
	Papavasiliou et al. (1978)	24	29
	Trope et al. (1980)	24	21
	Von Maillot and Ranger (1982)	22	18
ADR, MTX, and PLAT	Fine et al. (1983)	48	18
ADR, MTX, and VCR	Bone et al. (1976)	21	48
ADR and VCR	Wallace et al. (1978)	57	17
BLEO and MITC	Majima (1977)	10	70
	Miyamoto et al. (1978)	15	93
	Deka et al. (1979)	20	40
	Krebs et al. (1980)	20	40
	Leichman et al. (1980)	19	16

Continued

Table 13-16 Results of Combination Chemotherapy in Patients with Advanced or Recurrent Cervical Cancer *Continued*

Regimen	Investigators	No. of Patients	% Response
	Petrilli et al. (1980)	9	22
	Boice et al. (1982)	23	26
	Greenberg et al. (1982)	18	22
	Trope et al. (1983)	33	36
BLEO, MITC, and VCR	Baker et al. (1978)	50	60
	Baker et al. (1978)	115	41
BLEO, MITC, VCR, and PLAT	Vogl et al. (1980)	13	78
	Alberts et al. (1981)	14	43
	Vermorben et al. (1981)	22	50
	Surwit et al. (1983)	17	47
	Belinson et al. (1985)	21	24
BLEO and MTX	Conroy et al. (1976)	20	60
BLEO, MTX, and CTX	Lira-Puerto et al. (1979)	70	31
BLEO, MTX, and PLAT	Vogl et al. (1979)	9	89
BLEO, MTX, PLAT, and VCR	Rosenthal et al. (1979)	7	57
	Rosenthal et al. (1983)	15	66
BLEO and PLAT	Daghestani et al. (1983)	24	54
	Bloch et al. (1984)	17	53
BLEO, PLAT, and VBL	Friedlander et al. (1983)	33	66
CTX and PLAT	Jobson et al. (1984)	16	42
CTX and VCR	de Palo et al. (1976)	19	11
CTX, ACT D, 5-FU, VCR ARA-C, MTX, and BLEO	Forney et al. (1975)	18	50
MTX and VCR	Hakes et al. (1979)	29	17

ACT D, actinomycin D; ADR, Adriamycin; ARA-C, cytosine arabinoside; BLEO, bleomycin; CTX, cyclophosphamide; 5-FU, 5-fluorouracil; MECCNU, methyl-CCNU; MITC, mitomycin C; MTX, methotrexate; PLAT, diamminedichloroplatinum; VCR, vincristine.
(Shingleton HM, Orr JW Jr: Cancer of the Cervix: Diagnosis and Treatment. Churchill Livingstone, Edinburgh, 1987.)

transverse colon urinary conduits and away from ileal conduits, we have virtually eliminated urinary leaks postoperatively and have reduced acute gastrointestinal (GI) complications, especially small bowel fistula, from 9.7 to 1.9 percent.[69] Small bowel obstruction has also been eliminated for the most part by avoiding the small bowel anastomoses in radiated bowel inherent in the use of ileal conduits.

In spite of its severe morbidity, pelvic exenteration offers a last chance for survival for some patients. Quality of life can be good in spite of the diversions and has been enhanced by techniques developed in recent years for vaginal reconstruction. Fortunately, improvements in radiation therapy during the past 30 years have made pelvic exenteration almost an operation of the past in many major medical centers.

Chemotherapy

Extensive trials using combination chemotherapy have followed earlier trials focussing on many single agents and particularly cisplatin (Table 13-15). Response rates for squamous cell carcinoma using single-agent cisplatin have ranged from 0 to 100 percent, the ordinary response rate quoted being 20 to 40 percent. The mean duration of response varies between 3 and 6 months. Results of combination chemotherapy for advanced or recurrent cervical cancer were summarized (Table 13-16) in our monograph.[28] Platinum combined with Adriamycin, methotrexate with Adriamycin methyl-CCNU, or Adriamycin and Cytoxan seem to offer no superior response to platinum alone. Combinations of bleomycin with methotrexate and/or cytoxan and platinum received some attention during the 1970s, however have not gained popularity, presumably because the earlier encouraging results with small numbers of patients, have not been borne out in larger studies. At this writing, it would appear that there is no effective agent or combination of agents that offers cures to patients with recurrent squamous cell carcinoma or adenocarcinoma of the cervix. Additional trials continue, seeking such an agent or agents.

REFERENCES

1. Cleaves MA: Radium therapy. Chic Med Record 64:601, 1903
2. Forssel G: Ubersicht Uber die Resultate der Kresbehaudlung an Radiumhein in Stockholm, 1910–1915, Fortschr Geb Rontgenstr Nuclearmed Erganzungsband 25:142, 1917
3. Regaud C: Traitement des cancers du col de l'uterus par les radiation: Idée soumaire des methodes et des résultats, indications thérapeutiques. rapport au VII congrès Int chir 1:35, 1926
3a. Ellinger F: Lethal dose studies with x-rays. Med Times 71(5):157, 1943
4. Schottlaender J, Kermauner F: Zur Kenntis des Uteruskarzinomas. S Karger, Berlin, 1912
5. Rubin IC: The pathological diagnosis of incipient carcinoma of the uterus. J Obstet 62:668, 1910
6. Richart RM: Natural history of dysplasia and carcinoma in situ of the cervix. Clin Obstet Gynecol 10:748, 1967
7. Richart RM: Cervical intraepithelial neoplasia. In sommers SC (ed): Pathology Annual. Appleton-Century-Crofts, New York, 1973
8. Fenoglio CM, Ferenczy A: Etiologic factors in cervical neoplasia. Semin Oncol 9:349, 1982
9. Baird PJ: Serological evidence for the association of papillomavirus and cervical neoplasia. Lancet 2:17, 1983
10. Reid R: Genital warts and cervical cancer. II. Is human papillomavirus infection the trigger to cervical carcinogenesis? Gynecol Oncol 15:239, 1983
11. Kurman RJ, Jenson AB, Lancaster WD: Papillomavirus infection of the cervix. II. Relationship to intraepithelial neoplasia based on the presence of specific viral structural proteins. Am J Surg Pathol 7:39, 1983
12. Okagaki T, Twiggs LB, Zachow KR, et al: Identification of human papillomavirus DNA in cervical and vaginal intraepithelial neoplasia with molecularly cloned virus-specific DNA probes. Int J Gynecol Pathol 2:153, 1983
13. Simon NL, Gore H, Shingleton HM, et al: A study of superficially invasive carcinoma of the cervix. Obstet Gynecol 68:19, 1986
14. Gloor E, Ruzicka J: Morphology of adenocarcinoma in situ of the uterine cervix. Cancer 49:294, 1982
15. Ostor AG, Pagano R, Davoren RA, et al: Adenocarcinoma in situ of the cervix. Int J Gynecol Pathol 3:179, 1984
16. Ng ABP: Pathological factors significant in management and prognosis of cervical carcinoma. University of Miami Department of Pathology
17. Johansson O, Johnsson JE, Lindberg LG, Sydsjo A: Prognosis, recurrences and metastases correlated to histologic cell type in carcinoma of the uterine cervix. Acta Obstet Gynecol Scand 55:255, 1976
18. Beecham JB, Halvorsen T, Kolbenstvedt A: Histologic classification, lymph node metastases, and patient survival in Stage IB cervical carcinoma. Gynecol Oncol 6:95, 1978
19. Pagnini CA, Palma PD, DeLaurentiis G: Malignancy grading in squamous carcinoma of uterine cervix treated by surgery. Br J Cancer 41:415, 1980
20. Gauthier P, Gore I, Shingleton HM, Soong S-J: Identification of histopathologic risk groups in early stage cervical cancer. Obstet Gynecol 66:569, 1985
21. Sidhu GS, Koss LG, Barber HRK: Relation of histologic factors to the response of stage I epidermoid carcinoma of the cervix to surgical treatment. Obstet Gynecol 35:329, 1970
22. Gusberg SB, Yannopoulos K, Cohen CJ: Virulence indices and lymph nodes in cancer of the cervix. AJR 3:273, 1971
23. Baltzer J, Lohe KJ, Kopcke W, Zander J: Histological criteria for the prognosis in patients with operated squamous cell carcinoma of the cervix. Gynecol Oncol 13:184, 1982
24. Barber HRK, Sommers SC, Rotterdam, H, Kwon T: Vascular invasion as a prognostic factor in Stage IB cancer of the cervix. Obstet Gynecol 52:343, 1978
25. Noguchi H, Shiozawa K, Tsukamoto T, et al: The postoperative classification for uterine cancer and its clinical evaluation. Gynecol Oncol 16:219, 1983
26. Crissman JD, Makuch R, Budhraja M: Histopathologic grading of squamous cell carcinoma of the uterine cervix: An evaluation of 70 Stage IB patients. Cancer 55:1590, 1985
27. Shingleton HM, Gore H, Soong S-J, Bradley DH: Adenocarcinoma of the cervix. 1. Clinical evaluation and pathologic features. Am J Obstet Gynecol 138:799, 1981
28. Shingleton HM, Orr JW Jr: Cancer of the Cervix:

Diagnosis and Treatment. Churchill Livingstone, Edinburgh, 1987

29. To ACW, Gore H, Shingleton HM, et al: Lymph node metastasis in cancer of the cervix: A preliminary report. Am J Obstet Gynecol 155:388, 1986

30. Cavanagh D, Ruffolo EH, Marsden DE (eds): Gynecologic Cancer: A Clinicopathologic Approach. Appleton-Century-Crofts, E. Norwalk, CT, 1985

31. Kerr-Wilson RHJ, Shingleton HM, Orr JW Jr, Hatch KD: The use of ultrasound and CT scanning in the management of gyn malignancy. Gynecol Oncol 18:54, 1984

32. Shingleton HM, Gore H, Soong S-J, et al: Tumor recurrence and survival in Stage IB cancer of the cervix. Am J Clin Oncol 6:265, 1983

33. Chanen W, Rome RM: Electrocoagulation diathermy for cervical dysplasia and carcinoma in situ: A 15-year survey. Obstet Gynecol 61:673, 1983

34. Schuurmans SN, Ohlke ID, Carmichael JA: Treatment of cervical intraepithelial neoplasia with electrocautery: Report of 426 cases. Am J Obstet Gynecol 148:544, 1984

35. Townsend DE: Cryosurgery for CIN. Obstet Gynecol Surv 34:828, 1979

36. Hatch KD, Shingleton HM, Austin JM Jr: Cryosurgery of cervical intraepithelial neoplasia — Report of 968 patients. Obstet Gynecol 57:692, 1981

37. Shingleton HM, Hatch KD, Orr JW Jr. et al: Diagnosis and treatment of preinvasive and microscopically invasive squamous cell carcinoma of the cervix: Including comments on surveillance of DES-exposed patients with cytologic atypias. Cancer Bull 35:172, 1983

38. Syed AMN, Feder BH: Technique of after-loading interstitial implants. Radiol Clin 46:458, 1977

39. Ampuero F, Doss LL, Khan M, et al: The Syed-Neblett interstitial template in locally advanced gynecological malignancies. Int J Radiat Oncol Biol Phys 9:1897, 1983

40. Durrance FY, Fletcher GH, Rutledge FN: Analysis of central recurrence disease in Stage I and II squamous cell carcinoma of the cervix on intract uterus. AJR 106:831, 1969

41. Edinger DD Jr, Watring WG, Anderson B, Mitchell GW Jr: Residual tumor following radiotherapy for locally advanced carcinoma of the uterine cervix: Prognostic significance. Eur J Gynaecol Oncol 5:90, 1984

42. Gallion HH, van Nagell JR Jr, Donalson ES, et al: Combined radiation therapy and extrafascial hysterectomy in the treatment of stage IB barrel-shaped cervical cancer. Cancer 56:262, 1985

43. O'Quinn AG, Fletcher GH, Wharton JT: Guidelines for conservative hysterectomy after irradiation. Gynecol Oncol 9:68, 1980

44. Blake PR, Lambert HE, MacGregor WG, et al: Surgery following chemotherapy and radiotherapy for advanced carcinoma of the cervix. Gynecol Oncol 19:198, 1984

45. Perkins PL, Chu AM, Jose B, Achino E, Tobin DA: Posthysterectomy megavoltage irradiation in the treatment of cervical carcinoma. Gynecol Oncol 17:340, 1984

46. Nass JM, Brady LW, Glossburn JR, Porasasvinichai S: The radiotherapeutic management of carcinoma of the cervical stump. Int J Radiol Oncol Biol Phys 4:279, 1978

47. Andras EJ, Fletcher GH, Rutledge FN: Radiotherapy of cancer of the cervix following simple hysterectomy. Am J Obstet Gynecol 115:647, 1973

48. Wharton JT, Jones HW III, Day TG, et al: Preirradiation celiotomy and extended field irradiation for invasive cancer of the cervix. Obstet Gynecol 49:333, 1977

49. Schellhas HF: Extraperitoneal para-aortic node dissection through an upper abdominal incision. Obstet Gynecol 46:444, 1975

50. Piver MS, Barlow JJ, Vongtama V, Blumenson L: Hydroxyurea: A radiation potentiator in carcinoma of the uterine cervix. Am J Obstet Gynecol 147:803, 1983

51. Morrow CP, Shingleton HM, Austin JM, et al: Is pelvic radiation beneficial in the postoperative management of Stage Ib squamous cell carcinoma of the cervix with pelvic node metastasis treated by radical hysterectomy and pelvic lymphadenectomy? Gynecol Oncol 10:105, 1980

52. Baltzer J, Kopcke W, Lohe KJ, et al: Surgical treatment of cervix cancer. Treatment results and data on the postoperative course over a minimum of 5 years following surgery and standardized histological examination of the histological material of 1092 patients at 4 university gynecology clinics. Geburtshilfe Fraunheilkd 44:279, 1984

53. Bilek K, Eveling K, Leitsmann H, Seidel G: Radical pelvic surgery versus radical surgery plus radiotherapy for stage Ib carcinoma of the cervix uteri. Preliminary results of a prospective randomized clinical study. Arch Geschwulstforsch 52:223, 1982

54. Kucera H, Skodler W, Weghaupt K: Postoperative radiotherapy of cervical cancer: Complications and implications for the surgical indications. Wien Klin Wochenschr 96:451, 1984

55. Barter JF, Soong S-J, Shingleton HM, et al: Complications of combined radical hysterectomy-postoperative radiation therapy in women with early stage cervical cancer. Obstet Gynecol. In press

56. Strockbine MF, Hancock JG, Fletcher GH: Complications in 831 patients with squamous cell carcinoma of the intact cervix treated with 3000 rads or more whole pelvic irradiation. AJR 108:293, 1970

57. Abitbol MM, Davenport JH: Sexual dysfunction after

therapy for cervical carcinoma. Am J Obstet Gynecol 119:181, 1974

58. Swan RW, Fowler WC Jr, Boronow RC: Surgical management of radiation injury to the small intestine. Surg Gynecol Obstet 142:325, 1976
59. Perez CA, Breaux S, Mados-Jones H, et al: Radiation therapy alone in the treatment of cancer of the uterine cervix: Analysis of tumor recurrence. Cancer 51:1393, 1983
60. Jampolis S, Andras J, Fletcher GH: Analysis of sites and causes of failure of irradiation in invasive squamous cell carcinoma of the intact uterine cervix. Radiology 115:681, 1975
61. Hershchyshyn MM, Aron BS, Boronow RC, et al: Hydroxyurea or placebo combined with radiation to treat Stage IIIB and IV cervical cancer confined to the pelvis. Int J Radiat Oncol Biol Phys 5:317, 1979
62. Orr JW Jr, Ball GC, Soong S-J, et al: Surgical treatment of women found to have invasive cervical cancer at the time of total hysterectomy. Obstet Gynecol 68:353, 1986

63. Kilgore LE, Soong S-J, Gore H, et al: Analysis of prognostic features in adenocarcinoma of the cervix. In Press
64. Adcock LL, Julian TM, Okagaki T, et al: Carcinoma of the uterine cervix FIGO Stage I-B. Gynecol Oncol 14:199, 1982
65. Orr JW Jr, Shingleton HM: Cancer in Pregnancy. Current Problems in Cancer. Vol. VIII. Year Book Medical Publishers, 1983
66. Prem KA, Makowski EL, McKelvey JL: Carcinoma of the cervix associated with pregnancy. Am J Obstet Gynecol 95:99, 1966
67. Lee RB, Neglia W, Park RC: Cervical carcinoma in pregnancy. Obstet Gynecol 58:584, 1981
68. van Nagell JR Jr, Rayburn W, Donaldson ES, et al: Therapeutic implications of patterns of recurrence in cancer of the uterine cervix. Cancer 44:2354, 1979
69. Orr JW Jr, Hatch KD, Shingleton HM, et al: Gastrointestinal complications associated with pelvic exenteration. Am J Obstet Gynecol 145:325, 1983

14

Diagnosis and Principles of Treatment of Cancer of the Endometrium

S. B. Gusberg

Several tumors of the uterine body require our attention, but the predominant lesion continues to be adenocarcinoma of the endometrium. This tumor has come into greater prominence during the past two decades because of its increased frequency and its endocrine relationships. In the United States it has been the most common female genital cancer, with 40,000 new cases anticipated in 1986, while only 16,000 patients with cervix cancer will be newly diagnosed.

The question of optimum treatment for carcinoma of the endometrium continues to be discussed. While individualization of treatment has become commonplace, the role of combined treatment with surgery and irradiation, the possible place of radical hysterectomy, and the roles of adjuvant hormonal or chemotherapeutic medication and lymphadenectomy are still debated, although increasing data will soon force conclusions.

The histogenesis of this lesion, like that of carcinoma of the cervix, is most important for early detection, for it offers the possibility of prevention, especially for those considered hormone dependent or hormone related. In this respect, adenomatous hyperplasia in its various grades of intensity assumes a major role. Just as dysplasia and carcinoma in situ of the

cervix have played a major role in the decrease in mortality from carcinoma of the cervix in Western industrialized countries, where Papanicolaou (Pap) screening is commonplace, recognition of the endo-

---

FACTORS INDICATING HORMONE SENSITIVITY OF ENDOMETRIAL CANCER

1. Obesity
2. Infertility
3. Coincidence of functionary ovarian tumors
4. Coincidence of cystic ovarian syndrome
5. Dysfunctional bleeding
6. Diabetic diathesis
7. Progesterone effect on metastases
8. Ovarian agenesis and replacement estrogen
9. Induction of precursors with estrogen
10. Induction of carcinoma with estrogen
11. Estrogen an immunosuppressant

---

metrial cancer precursor can lead to greater control of invasive endometrial malignancy.

Cancer of the body of the uterus will include tumors arising in the endometrium or in the myometrium. While some have a specific origin, such as adenocarcinoma of the endometrium or leiomyosarcoma of the myometrium, others of mixed origin are grouped for purposes of description. One may group them in the following categories, although most are considered elsewhere in the text:

Adenocarcinoma of the endometrium

Sarcoma of the endometrium (including endolymphatic stromal myosis

Mixed mesodermal tumors

Carcinosarcoma

Rhabdomyosarcoma

Leiomyosarcoma

Hemangioendothelioma

Adenosquamous carcinoma

This does not exhaust the list of possible tumors of the body of the uterus, but it does include most that come under usual consideration. The variety of these tumors has invited classification by the International Federation of Gynecology and Obstetrics (FIGO) and the World Health Organization (WHO) committees of pathologists.

ADENOCARCINOMA OF THE ENDOMETRIUM

Adenocarcinoma of the endometrium is the predominant malignant neoplasm of the uterus, the principal lesion that concerns us for diagnosis and treatment. It may extend to the cervix or invade the myometrium, but its origin is clearly in the endometrial epithelium. It may arise in the fundal or isthmic region, but there is no evidence to indicate a qualitative difference distinguishing tumors from these areas. These tumors may offer differing characteristics from the diagnostic point of view, as small fundal or cornual tumors may be difficult to biopsy by diagnostic curettage, but they should not differ in virulence. In fact, a fractional curettage is a most accurate diagnostic method in general.

INCIDENCE

During the first half of the twentieth century, all tests indicated a predominance of cancer of the cervix over cancer of the endometrium by a ratio of 3:1 or even 6:1. This began to change during the 1950s; by 1953 in New York State outside New York City, where cancer is a reportable disease, the ratio of endometrial cancer to cervix cancer reached 2.13. This changing ratio was reflected in the Third National Cancer Survey (1969), and the reversal of this ratio continued to grow thereafter. The American Cancer Society estimates for 1986 indicate an expectancy of 40,000 new patients with endometrial cancer as opposed to only 16,000 new cases of cervix cancer.

This reversal of the traditional dominance of cancer of the cervix in the United States may be due to an aging population; better nourishment of this population, including a high-calorie, high animal-fat diet; active screening for cervical cancer precursors; and the enthusiasm for long-term administration of estrogen without progestational modification that was popular during the 1960s and early 1970s.

The incidence of carcinoma in situ of the cervix continues to rise, but the mortality rate of invasive cancer of the cervix has dropped dramatically in the United States, presumably because of screening. While the less frequent cervical cancer will cause approximately 7,000 deaths in the United States this year, the more prevalent endometrial tumor will result in about 4,000 deaths. To place these genital tumors in context, we must note that ovarian cancer, without any useful screening technology, will be responsible for approximately 11,500 deaths, breast cancer 37,000 deaths, and lung cancer in females 38,000 deaths in 1986 in the United States. It is interesting, if tragic, to note that with cigarette smoking in women still current, deaths from lung cancer exceeded that from breast cancer in the United States for the first time in 1985.

Environmental effects on cancer incidence are now widely recognized, frequently diminishing the alleged importance of ethnicity. The classic migrant study of Japanese females by Haenszel and Kurihara in 1968, illustrates this well, for these immigrants to the United States tended to assume the tumor characteristics of the host population. The high incidence of stomach cancer in Japan seemed to trend downward toward U.S. levels, while colon, breast, and endometrial cancer rose toward U.S. levels. In the past, endometrial and breast cancer have been rare in Japan, but increasing affluence and assumption of a Western diet, higher in animal fat, have been reported to be coincident with a rising incidence of these tumors by Masabuchi (Fig. 14-1).

Age Incidence

It is well known that endometrial cancer is predominantly a disease of aging postmenopausal women. The peak incidence occurs in the 58- to 60-year age group, approximately 10 years later than the median age for invasive cancer of the cervix and approximately 10 years later than the peak incidence of the endometrial cancer precursor, adenomatous hyperplasia. This incidence is an indication of the relatively slow developmental onset of this and probably other tumors and the opportunity for prevention thereby afforded, especially in high-risk groups.

While 75 percent of endometrial cancer occurs after the age of 50, only 4 percent occurs before age 40. Endometrial cancer is infrequent in young women; when it does occur, it is commonly a well-differentiated hormonal-dependent type. By contrast, cancer of the cervix occurs earlier in reproductive life; its precursors, dysplasia and carcinoma in situ, occur frequently in young women. These observations bear on the problems of screening: while screening for cervical cancer precursors must be directed toward young women especially, detection efforts for endometrial precursors should be aimed principally at the perimenopausal and postmenopausal age group.

Epidemiology of High Risk

In seeking a conceptual basis for the onset of malignancy in the endometrium, one must accept the probable duality of carcinoma types in this area (Fig. 14-2). One type appears to be related to an endocrine dysfunction endogenous or exogenously produced, perhaps constituting 50 to 60 percent of the whole, with

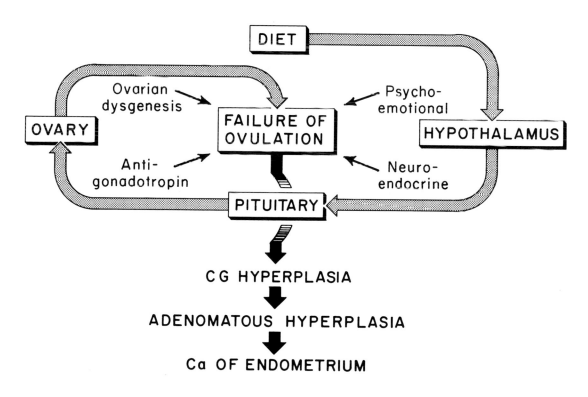

Fig. 14-1 A speculative hypothesis for cancer of the endometrium.

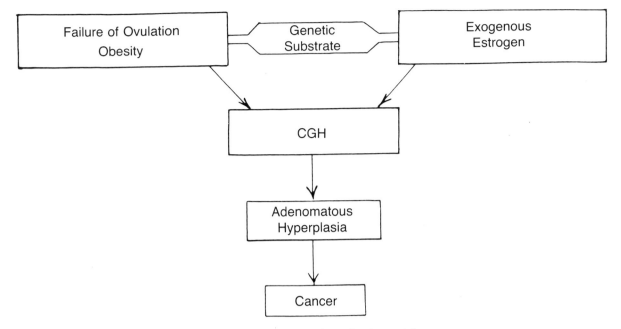

Fig. 14-2 Estrogen relationship of endometrial cancer.

failure of ovulation or lack of progestational modification of constant estrogenic stimulation of the endometrium. This may result in simple hyperplasia, cystic glandular hyperplasia, and finally adenomatous hyperplasia before becoming a true malignancy. This hypothesis suggests a gradual, fairly slow development of this hormone-dependent cancer; it tends to be well differentiated and frequently low in virulence.

The other cancer type may be called autonomous, for it does not relate to an endocrinopathy or any other known factor. Whether the initiator and promotor be viral, chemical, or mutational remains to be discovered. These adenocarcinomas tend to be higher in virulence; some investigators have characterized them as a different cancer, although other properties of this neoplasm do not differ from the rest.

Geographic Distribution

There appears to be an inverse relationship geographically in the frequency of endometrial cancer and cervical cancer. In the highly industrialized countries of the West, a higher frequency of endometrial cancer tends to occur, while developing countries for the most part have a higher incidence of cancer of the cervix with a lower incidence of the endometrial tumor. Japan has been an anomaly in this respect. The traditional concept of these international or even intranational differences as racial or genetically predisposed has given way to greater consideration of environmental differences, with special reference to diet. Indeed, one can relate high frequency of endometrial and even breast cancer to high intake of dietary fat; the change in cancer incidence in emigrants from Eastern to Western countries can be interpreted similarly. Whether dietary calories or dietary fat are specifically responsible is not settled, but the hormonal implications are interesting.

Heredity

Endometrial cancer is one of the lesions that can occur in families. The history of such a tumor in a first-degree relative of the individual under consideration certainly increases her risk; a family history of cancer has been found in 12 to 28 percent of cases. It also correlates with breast cancer in this respect and it has occurred in identical twins at about the same age. No specific genetic marker has been found, but the tendency does seem to bear a genetic substrate.

Economic Status

Traditionally, endometrial cancer has been considered a disease of upper socioeconomic groups, more commonly seen in our hospitals in the private pavilion sector rather than the clinic clientele. This is still true in some parts of the world, as demonstrated in our East-West Study, wherein Asian women with this disease were drawn mainly from the upper socioeconomic classes. Surely developing countries still have a preponderance of cancer of the cervix. In the United States, these frequency tendencies have been disappearing with economic, social, and sexual change tending to obliterate so-called class differences, also bringing more balance to tumor frequency.

Somatotype

That women with endometrial cancer tend to be obese and frequently large in body type has been known for many years. In a study from the Sloane Hospital for Women of The Columbia-Presbyterian Medical Center in New York, subjects with this tumor were on the average 18 lbs (8.1 kg) heavier than those with cancer of the cervix. This was 8.91 times the probable error and therefore significant. This factor has been noted by others, as confirmed in an epidemiologic study by Wynder (1966). It was noted that women who were 30 to 50 lbs (13.5 to 22.5 kg) overweight had a threefold risk of developing endometrial cancer, while those 50 lb (22.5 kg) or more over normal weight had a ninefold risk (see under Hormonal Relationships).

Fertility

In the past, unmarried women were considered more susceptible to this disease, but the data concerning this factor have been conflicting. More appropriate has been the study of infertility, for it seems clear that this deficit, especially related to failure of ovulatin, is significant in placing a woman at high risk for endometrial carcinoma. Many studies during the past four decades have offered clear evidence of infertility as a risk factor. As in the case of other reproductive abnormalities, one must consider the endometrium as a target organ for the proliferative effect of estrogen, with the absence of ovulation and therefore absence of progestin creating an imbalance characterized by a lack of the morphologic antagonist.

CANCER OF THE ENDOMETRIUM: THE HIGH-RISK WOMAN

1. Obese
2. Failure of ovulation
   a. Infertility
   b. Dysfunctional bleeding
   c. Amenorrhea
3. Chronic estrogen intake

Menstrual Disturbance

Menstrual aberration has been commonplace in the history of women with endometrial cancer, both in younger women and in those whose cancer appeared after menopause. In younger women, the cystic ovary syndrome (Stein-Leventhal) resulting in oligoamenorrhea or frank amenorrhea and infertility has been shown to produce higher risk for adenomatous hyperplasia and endometrial carcinoma. These women, sometimes also obese and hirsute, are frequently anovulatory, even when they bleed irregularly. This is also true of the young woman in her 20s with irregular menses since her menarche, also anovulatory and also at higher risk than normal for endometrial carcinoma. Turner's syndrome subjects on long-term estrogen also are at increased risk by a similar mechanism. In our own experience in patients whose cancer appeared before the menopause, one-half give a prior history of disturbed menstruation, chronologically unrelated to the cancer episode.

In those women who cancer appeared after the menopause, menstrual disturbance was also more common than anticipated. Frequent reports of a late menopause in these women have appeared in the past, but other reports have discounted this factor and related it to early symptoms of the developing cancer.

Dysfunctional Bleeding

Dysfunctional bleeding during the menopause does appear to be a significant factor. Again, this appears to be anovulatory bleeding. Irregular, excessive, or prolonged bleeding has been significant in the history of those in whom endometrial cancer later developed. Corscaden and Gusberg (1947) found 39 percent of those with later cancer to have had such dysfunctional bleeding in their perimenopause era. This is three times the expected number. In a prospective study, Randall noted 3.5 times as many neoplasms in dysfunctional bleeders as found in controls.

Similarly, our follow-up study many years ago of women who had had a radiotherapeutic menopause demonstrated almost the same excess. While some attributed this to the irradiation, the common factor appeared to be the dysfunctional bleeding; in fact, in this study all women in whom endometrial cancer developed after the radiotherapeutic menopause had been treated for excessive bleeding, while no patient for whom the menopause was induced for other reasons than bleeding did so (Fig. 14-3). Those patients who were treated with radiation for conditions other than perimenopausal bleeding included patients with fibroids, endometriosis, dysmenorrhea, or some nongenital disorders. It was especially noteworthy in this study that many of the patients in whom cancer developed in later life were found to have had adenomatous hyperplasia during their perimenopausal episodes of bleeding. The bleeding symptom at this time of life frequently indicates overstimulation of the endometrium by irregular estrogen secretion without modification by progesterone. In a study of patients with

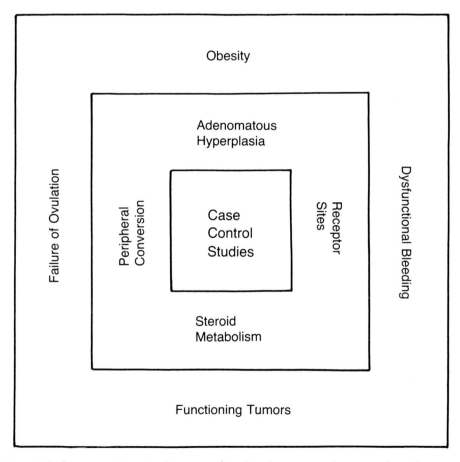

Fig. 14-3 Risk factors and the development of studies that support hormone dependence in some endometrial carcinomas.

dysfunctional bleeding unrelated to subsequent cancer, only 11 percent were found to have evidence of ovulation.

Diabetes and Hypertension

These coincident disorders have been reported through the years in patients with endometrial carcinoma, although most studies seem to indicate a casual rather than a causal relationship. In fact, all three disorders appear to share symptoms of obesity and the maturity of age (Fig. 14-4). While Benjamin and others have reported carbohydrate intolerance in subjects with this tumor, frank diabetes has varied from one series to another, some supporting, others denying this correlation. After controlling for age, weight, and socioeconomic status, Kaplan and Cole found a relative risk of 2.8 associated with a history of diabetes. Hypertension is found in about 50 percent of endometrial cancer patients, a figure that correlates with age, obesity and would appear unrelated to the cancer.

HORMONAL RELATIONSHIPS

The hormonal dependence of some endometrial cancers has been recognized and discussed for almost four decades (Figs. 14-5 and 14-6). This observation has rested on evidence of a developmental relationship between constant estrogenic stimulation and a deficit or progestational modification necessary to modify and protect the endometrium. This can result in the cancer precursor, adenomatous hyperplasia, and ultimately invasive endometrial adenocarcinoma. It may be important to re-emphasize that not all such endometrial tumors are so conditioned for almost 40 percent appear to be autonomous and free of hormonal connotation.

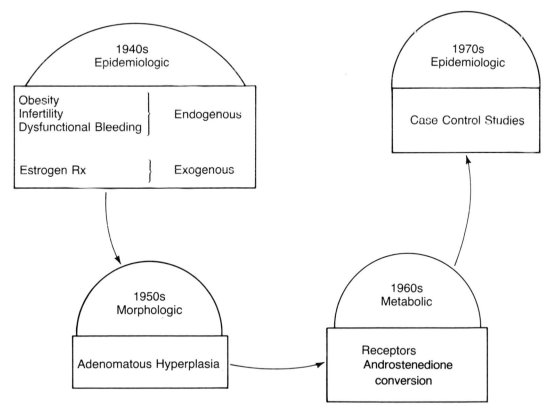

Fig. 14-4 Unmodified estrogen and endometrial carcinoma. The chart shows progressive acceptance of hormone dependence with advanced technology.

PROGESTIN-ESTROGEN ANTAGONISM

Oral contraception = ↓ Adenomatous hyperplasia and endometrial cancer

Postmenopausal E and P = ↓ Adenomatous hyperplasia and endometrial cancer

Progestin in obesity = ↓ Adenomatous hyperplasia and endometrial cancer

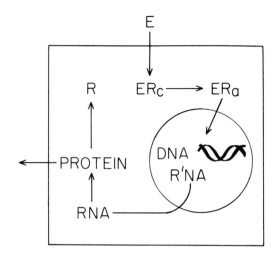

Fig. 14-6 E_2 receptor.

Epidemiology and Morphology

Our observation of a high-risk group, characterized by obesity, infertility due to failure of ovulation, dysfunctional uterine bleeding, or prolonged estrogen administration provided us with a basis for a definition of adenomatous hyperplasia as a cancer precursor (Table 14-1 and Fig. 14-7), and the relationship of this cancer to estrogen many years ago, in fact in 1947 (Table 14-2). When we found similar tissue change in postmenopausal subjects who harbored estradiol-producing theca-granulosa cell tumors (Fig.14-8) or younger women in whom ovulation had failed due to the cystic ovary syndrome (Stein-Leventhal type), we were persuaded that constant estrogenic stimulation at whatever level without progestational maturation and differentiation, in some individuals could bring the physiologic proliferative, mitogenic effect of es-

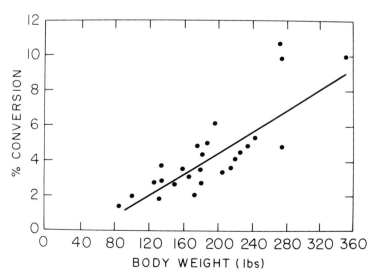

Fig. 14-5 Correlation of conversion with body weight, androstenedione to estrone in postmenopausal women. (Siiteri PK, MacDonald PC: Handbook of Physiology. Williams & Wilkins, Baltimore.)

Table 14-1 Adenomatous Hyperplasia: Prospective Studies

Investigators	Cases	Follow-up Years	Progression to Cancer (%)
Novak and Rutledge (1948)	8	15	12.5
Hertig et al. (1949)	64	1–11	9.4
Marrubini (1949)	60	3.5–14	8.3
Te Linde et al. (1953)	14	10 (mo)–23	100.
Arfwedson and Winblad (1953)	7	1–2.5	28.6
Copenhaver (1959)	23	1–5	34.8
Campbell and Barter (1961)	128	1 (wk)–9	22.7
Gusberg and Kaplan (1963)	68	1–10	11.8
Buehl et al.	7	1–8	28.6
Wentz (1966)	86	3–8	17.4
Chamlian and Taylor (1970)	97	1–30	14.
Total	562		18.5

(Modified from Gusberg SB, Chen SY, Cohen CJ: Endometrial cancer: Factors influencing choice of treatment. Gynecol Oncol 2:308, 1974.)

tradiol to this pathologic state (Fig. 14-9). Recognition of adenomatous hyperplasia as a precancerous lesion (Tables 14-3 and 14-4) offered gynecologists an opportunity for early detection and prevention in the 1950s which was accepted, but the hormonal implication did not curb enthusiasm for estrogen as a youth promoter during the 1950s and 1960s in the United States.

Metabolism

These morphologic observations were further supported by advances in steroid metabolic technology in the 1960s and 1970s:

1. Steroid-receptor studies in target cells gave us insight into the estrogenic proliferative capacity of

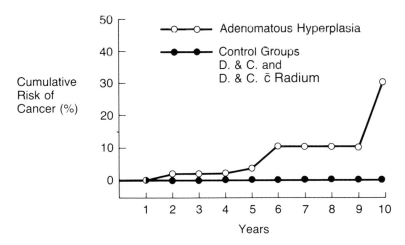

Fig. 14-7 Probability of cancer of the endometrium after adenomatous hyperplasia. At the end of the seventh year, the percentage of cancer in the hyperplasia group is statistically different from the percentage of cancer in the control groups at the 0.01 level of significance.

Table 14-2 Milestones in Estrogen and Endometrial Cancer Research

Investigators	Finding
Isvesco (1912)	An estrogenic extract
Allen-Doisy (1923)	Isolation of estrogen
Zondek (1926)	Therapeutic use
Cook, Dodds, and Hewitt (1937)	Synthesis of DES
Shorr, Robinson, and Papanicolaou (1939)	Therapeutic use of DES
Gusberg (1947)	Adenomatous hyperplasia precursor and estrogen related
Wilson (1963)	Menopause as a deficiency disease
Brush, Taylor, King, and Kalinga (1968)	Receptor site
MacDonald, Gordin, and Siiteri (1969)	Androstenedione conversion
MacDonald and Siiteri (1973); Hausknecht-Gusberg 1974)	Estrone and endometrial cancer
Smith-Prentice, Thompson, and Hermann (1975)	Epidemiology

the postmenopausal endometrium even into old age and the means to arrest it by progestational agents.

2. Steroid metabolism in target cells and serum became increasingly appreciated. The induction of progesterone receptors by estradiol, the repression of estradiol receptors by progestins, and the initiation of 17-β-estradiol dehydrogenase activity by progesterone that also encourages lesser estrogenic activity in the target cell by conversion of estradiol to the weaker estrogen estrone and its transport out of the cell, all clarified the steroid ebb and flow in the target epithelium. In addition, studies of serum estradiol-binding capacity in health and disease helped clarify these steroid-target cell relationships.

3. The role of obesity as a high-risk factor for adenomatous hyperplasia and endometrial cancer was clarified by the observation of the peripheral aromitization of the adrenal prehormone androstenedione to estrone in postmenopausal women. That one could correlate the level of conversion to estrone to the degree of obesity also indicated that the production rate of estrogen in grossly obese postmenopausal women was of a significant magnitude. Clearly, the absence of progesterone in these women is a key factor in endometrial proliferation.

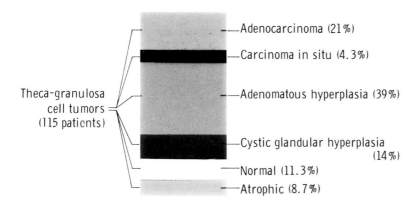

Theca-granulosa cell tumors (115 patients)

— Adenocarcinoma (21%)
— Carcinoma in situ (4.3%)
— Adenomatous hyperplasia (39%)
— Cystic glandular hyperplasia (14%)
— Normal (11.3%)
— Atrophic (8.7%)

Fig. 14-8 Most intense stage of proliferation reached in endometrium stimulated by functioning ovarian tumors.

POST MENOPAUSAL ESTROGENS

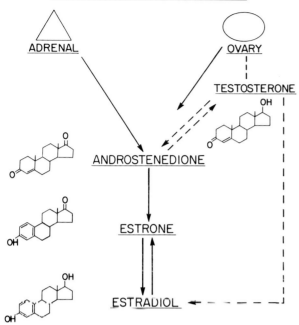

Fig. 14-9 Sex steroid metabolism in postmenopausal women.

Table 14-4 Progression of Precursors

Disorder	%
Cystic glandular hyperplasia	~1–3
Adenomatous hyperplasia	~20
Severe (atypical) adenomatous hyperplasia	~25

found readily, were quite revealing. They showed a 4- to 14-fold relative risk of developing endometrial cancer in those taking estrogen for more than 2 years, over their age-matched controls.

Although there have been dissenters from the conclusions of these observations, epidemiologists have generally accepted this estrogenic risk as valid because (1) the relative risk in those studies tended to be in the same general range, (2) the controls were chosen well, (3) the risk was time related; and (4) the risk was dose related. Thus, the circle of evidence appeared to return to epidemiology for its closure.

Gardner et al. (1957) noted that tumors appearing in hormone-dependent tissues (breast, endometrium, prostate), although disproportionally prevalent, occur at a time of life when these organs were involuting or atrophic. One must then speculate whether (1) some of these tumors are hormone dependent, (2) the endocrinopathy occurred earlier with fixation of tissue in a cancer-ready state for those genetically predisposed; (3) the stimulus continues, as we have shown; or (4) some inhibiting mechanism has been removed (e.g., estrogen, like other steroids, is an immunosuppressant). There is some experimental support for each of these factors.

Epidemiology

Finally, during the 1970s more sophisticated epidemiology came to bear upon this question with case-control studies of this tumor. These studies, frequently in retirement communities where postmenopausal subjects on long-term estrogen were

Table 14-3 Studies Leading to Concept of Adenomatous Hyperplasia as a Cancer Percursor

Investigators	Finding
Cullen (1900)	Atypical change indicates cancer nearby
Meyer (1923)	Case reports: conversion to cancer
Taylor Jr (1932)	Significance of postmenopausal hyperplasia
Novak and Yui (1936)	Emphasis postmenopausal hyperplasia
Gusberg (1947)	Names and defines adenomatous hyperplasia era of the developmental concept of cancer
Novak and Rutledge (1948)	Affirm distinction from cystic glandular hyperplasia and cancer
Hertig and Sommers (1949)	Confirm and separate carcinoma in situ

Animal Models

In a conference on hormone-tumor relationships, held in 1956, one well-known investigator stated that "the experimental evidence for classifying estrogenic hormone as a carcinogen is as good as that for methylchlocanthrene." Certainly there have been many reports of estrogen dependence in animal tumors.

Greene (1941) reported the development of endometrial tumors in infertile rabbits, and others have induced adenomatous hyperplasia endometrial cancer in those animals and other species with estrogen administration. Taki and co-workers (1966) in Japan showed estrogen dependence and progesterone protection.

Cancer of the endometrium has not been produced, to my knowledge, in subhuman primates. However, most studies have suffered from species variation with apparent lack of the appropriate genetic substrate in these animals and the relatively short duration of most experiments of this type in these relatively long-lived animals.

Human Therapeutic Response

The evidence supplied by reports of therapeutic benefits with progestins in advanced endometrial cancer must be considered. Although Kelley and Baker (1960) and others have since used pharmacologic rather than physiologic doses to arrest metastatic disease, its hormonal implications must be invoked. Furthermore, the evidence of reversability of adenomatous hyperplasia by progestins or wedge resection of the ovary or induction of ovulation by gonadotropin in young women is significant. Even its prevention by progestin in high-risk persons must be included.

Adenomatous Hyperplasia and the Developmental Concept

Cystic glandular hyperplasia is a benign reaction of the endometrium to estrogenic stimulation without progestational modification. It may accompany dysfunctional bleeding at menarche or menopause and also at other times during reproductive life. Any unmodified estrogenic stimulus, endogenous or exogenous, can produce this hyperplastic change, and it will usually regress following the termination of the endocrine imbalance.

There is some evidence that it is the earliest change in the development of endometrial cancer; for susceptible individuals with a continuing stimulus, it may be converted to adenomatous hyperplasia and thereafter, to true cancer. The percentage of those with cystic glandular hyperplasia in whom endometrial cancer develops is small, but the percentage of those with endometrial cancer who have harbored cystic glandular hyperplasia in their past is significant.

Adenomatous Hyperplasia

We described this lesion and its estrogenic connotation in 1947, but there were suggestions before and refinements since that have augmented our knowledge of this endometrial cancer precursor. In his book on cancer of the endometrium published in 1900, Cullen describes an unusual endometrial change coexisting with carcinoma that suggested malignancy nearby, and Backer (1904) reported a patient subjected to repeated curettage for irregular bleeding in whom carcinoma finally developed. Robert Meyer (1923) reported several cases of early carcinoma arising in hyperplastic epithelium as did Schroeder (1929); Hintz did not in a short follow-up series. Thereafter, Taylor (1932) and Novak and Yui (1936) emphasized the importance of postmenopausal hyperplasia.

Armed with the then (1947) fairly recent knowledge of the developmental stages of carcinoma of the cervix and the recognition that most cancers probably develop slowly rather than explosively, with long preclinical preinvasive phases, we were enabled to recognize and define adenomatous hyperplasia as an endometrial cancer precursor. In the following years, Novak and Rutledge emphasized the difficulty in discriminating between this hyperplastic lesion and well-differentiated adenocarcinoma, while Hertig and associates fractionated the group into mild ones they were willing to call adenomatous and the intense form, which they called carcinoma in situ.

Surely biologic concepts are more important than semantic discussions of taxonomy, but classification remains important. We have preferred the designations adenomatous hyperplasia grades I, II, and III as a unifying principle for we have seen cancer follow each grade without intervening stages (Fig. 14-10). We have also preferred the term adenomatous hyperplasia grade III, rather than atypical hyperplasia, because of

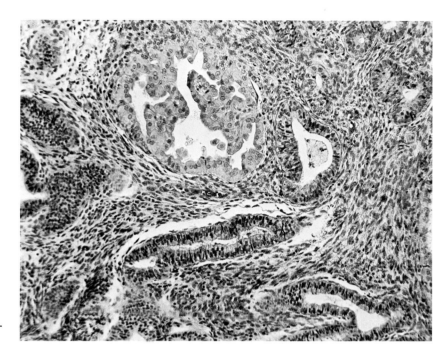

Fig. 14-10 Early focus of adenomatous hyperplasia.

the imprecision of the latter except by indirection; we have avoided the term carcinoma in situ for intense hyperplasia of this variety because of the imprecise criteria for invasion in the endometrium, and because the lesion is reversible in some, by the administration of a progestin or restoration of ovulation.

Mild (grade 1) adenomatous hyperplasia: This entity may be a general or focal lesion; there is moderate glandular crowding and pseudostratification of epithelium. Beginning intraluminal infolding and budding are also seen (Fig. 14-11).

Moderate (grade II): Increased crowding of glands re-

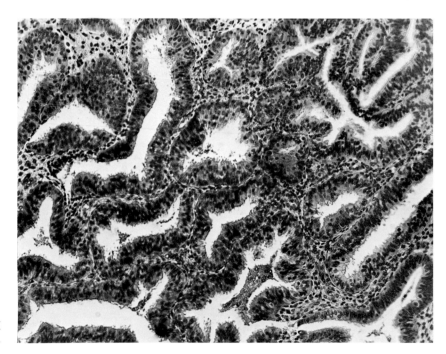

Fig. 14-11 Example of grade I adenomatous hyperplasia: mild.

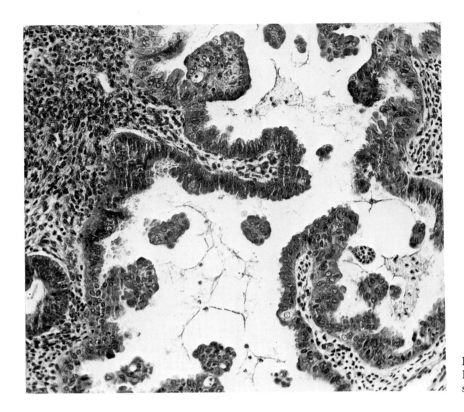

Fig. 14-12 Example of grade III adenomatous hyperplasia: severe.

duces intervening stroma, giving a sort of micro-follicular pattern in some instances; pseudostratification and intraluminal budding are more marked.

Marked (grade III): Adenomatous hyperplasia exhibits intense intralumimal budding and pseudostratifica-tion and the epithelium assumes an eosinophilic pallor with syncytium-like masses frequent on the surface. Some pathologists have emphasized ana-plastic cytologic changes recently, but surely the histologic configuration is clearly diagnostic. We

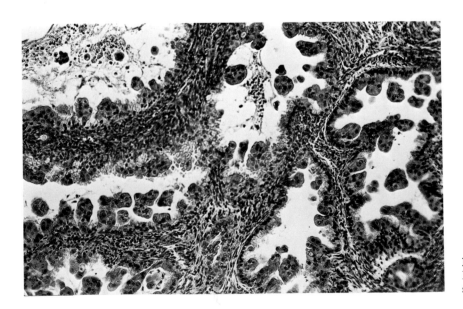

Fig. 14-13 Example of grade III adenomatous hyperplasia; severe.

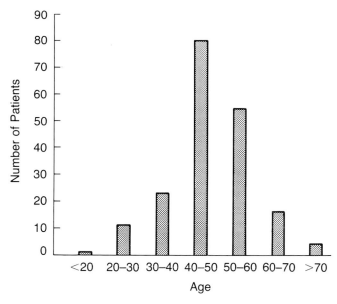

Fig. 14-14 Age incidence in adenomatous hyperplasia.

may call this stage 0 carcinoma of the endometrium (Figs. 14-12 and 14-13).

Many contributions have been made to this subject since its definition in the 1940s and evidence has accrued that approximately 20 percent of these lesions can progress to invasive cancer if untreated. The recognition of a cancer precursor and its frequent dysfunctional etiology offers the opportunity for both primary and secondary prevention. With peak years for adenomatous hyperplasia in the perimenopausal age group of the late 40s (Fig. 14-14) and the median age for invasive endometrial cancer in the late 50s, one must believe that endometrial cancer also has a long preclinical phase in many cases, similar to that of cancer of the cervix. Since the histogenesis of these uterine tumors is known as well or better than other human cancers, one can assume from such evidence and that of investigational tumors in laboratory animals that this is a general phenomenon.

DETECTION AND DIAGNOSIS

Bleeding is a symptom of ulceration; endometrial tissues are soft and they erode easily. While 10 percent of patients with endometrial carcinoma will note a serous discharge or a blood-streaked watery discharge before actual bleeding, frank bleeding is, in fact, the first and principal symptom of this disease. Since most of these patients are postmenopausal, there will usually be a clear onset, sometimes scant or moderate in amount. It is difficult to ignore such a symptom for most health educated women, but our era of the estrogenized menopause and its frequent induction of some escape bleeding may cause confusion for patient and physician alike. The course of the bleeding is unpredictable for frequency, duration, and amount, but heavy bleeding is unusual. The interval after the menopause when bleeding must be called postmenopausal is arbitrary, but an interval of a year, a flow of unusual amount or duration, or the absence of habitual molimina for that woman may be indices that indicate significance. The causes of postmenopausal bleeding in our experience are found to be malignant in one-third, benign in about another one-third, and of unknown origin in the last third.

Premenopausal or perimenopausal bleeding accompanies endometrial cancer in a small minority of patients. Lawless bleeding that is intermenstrual is easier to define than hypermenorrhea or menorrhagia, but it is unwise in any case to administer treatment without an endometrial biopsy, whether it be ambulatory or a formal curettage in the hospital. One aberration may be observed, but a repetition suggests a pattern that must be documented by a tissue sample.

Pain is an unimportant symptom of uterine cancer for early diagnosis, usually indicating widespread disease or involvement of nerve trunks laterally. Thus, this symptom is infrequently seen and cannot be considered important in our search for early disease.

Pelvic examination is also considered of minor value in this disease for the uterus is frequently normal in size and symmetrical in configuration. As the tumor grows, the shape of the uterus may become more globular and larger in size, but in such a circumstance the examiner may find it difficult on examination alone to distinguish this enlargement from that of a fibroid. The fibroid will make the uterus hard or nodular rather than boggy, but postmenopausal regression of fibroids reduces the significance of this sign as well.

The High-Risk Woman

Most precursors of endometrial cancer are seen in the perimenopausal period; they are frequently encountered during the course of a curettage necessary for the exclusion of organic disease during the investigation of dysfunctional bleeding. If a woman does develop a proliferative lesion of her endometrium, the menopause may be a point at which fixation will take place for the rest of her life. Therefore, we should pay special attention and offer some surveillance to those at the highest risk for later endometrial malignancy. The characteristics of such subjects include

1. Obesity
2. Diabetic tendency
3. Infertility
4. Dysfunctional bleeding
5. Adenomatous hyperplasia
6. Prolonged estrogen administration

Few attempts have been made to screen perimenopausal women for endometrial disease, but some examinations have revealed silent asymptomatic lesions. It would seem appropriate to initiate such screening activity for a tumor in which a high-risk grouping is clearly defined.

REQUIREMENTS FOR SCREENING ENDOMETRIAL CARCINOMA

1. Accuracy for carcinoma and adenomatous hyperplasia
2. Satisfactory specimen for cancer and hyperplasia
3. Acceptable to patients
4. Free of complications
5. Inexpensive
6. Technically efficient

Technology of Sampling

Various sampling techniques has been studied and made available in greater breadth and depth in recent years (Table 14-5).

*Pap smear cytologic sample:*So accurate for cancer of the cervix, it has but a 50 percent rate of accuracy in the detection of endometrial cancer in most laboratories. Some cytopathologists ascribe greater accuracy to the endocervical sample or the vaginal pool sample, but most will find it unsatisfactory.

Table 14-5 Endometrial Carcinoma: Diagnostic Accuracy of Detection Techniques

Technique	Morphology	Patients	Accuracy
Endometrial aspiration	Cytologic	12,480	88.5
Endometrial lavage	Cytologic	2,805	81.6
Jet wash			
Direct smear	Cytologic	2,258	86.7
Millipore	Cytohistologic	1,234	75.0
Cell Block	Cytohistologic	4,701	87.5
Endometrial biopsy	Histologic	1,679	87.4
Aspiration curettage (Vabra)	Histologic	1,135	97.5

(Modified from Vuopola S: Diagnostic accuracy in endometrial carcinoma. Acta Obstet Gynecol Scand 56(suppl 70):1, 1977.)

Cytologic sample taken through a cannula from the endometrial cavity: This sample offers a considerable degree of accuracy in the diagnosis of cancer, whether taken by aspirating syringe or by the so-called jet wash, that is, irrigation. While it can disclose frank cancer in some hands, its ability to detect precursor lesions, especially adenomatous hyperplasia, has not been significant in most laboratories.

Cytologic sample obtained by abrasion: As in the case of cannula samples; these techniques while primarily cytologic, do frequently obtain histologic fragments that are diagnostically useful.

Aspiration curettage: This technique has been found most successful by us, and this method is widely used in the United States for detection and even diagnosis following symptoms. This method, originating in Europe and adopted in the United States can be performed with a minimum of discomfort on an outpatient, ambulatory basis. We can obtain, by the use of a 3-mm probe and a small attached suction pump, a histologic sample that is virtually the equivalent of that obtained by formal diagnostic curettage. It avoids hospitalization and anesthesia, although some apply a local anesthetic, and it is not only accurate for the detection of cancer but is highly efficient in the disclosure of adenomatous hyperplasia. Since in the case of endometrial screening, as is true for cervical screening, the objective is the detection of the precancerous lesion, we have preferred this histologic method over cytologic techniques. In most women, this probe can be passed into the uterine cavity with minimal or no discomfort; those who have some annoyance usually find it acceptable, although a local anesthetic can be used if necessary.

Fractional curettage under anesthesia: This is the standard by which we judge all other diagnostic techniques, for it is accurate, complete, and virtually free of complications and sequelae. It makes the final judgment of the volume of tumor, size of the cavity, and spread to the cervix and offers a complete biopsy for analysis. The experienced surgeon can frequently make a gross judgment on the state of the endometrium by inspection of the tissue obtained; hyperplastic tissue, although thicker than normal, will come away in strips, while cancer appears in chunks or pieces, coarsely granular and friable. This type of tissue is susceptible to frozen section if necessary.

USE OF ASPIRATION CURETTAGE IN ENDOMETRIAL SCREENING
1. Ease of interpretation
2. Successful in obtaining sample (90%)
3. Acceptable to patient (90% accept again)
4. Detects precursors (91.7% accuracy)
5. Detects carcinoma (97.5% accuracy)
6. Side effects insignificant (7 perforations in 4,500 patients)

Hysterography

The use of radiopaque dye for diagnostic radiography has increased in popularity recently for disclosure of tumor volume and depth and spread to the cervix. In the hands of those experienced with this method, it offers some added parameters, but others have considered it more favorable for cancer dissemination and to be no more accurate than the data obtained by careful fractional curettage. We have used hysterography for those patients who have resumed bleeding after a negative curettage, on the chance that an endometrial polyp or small submucous fibroid has been missed.

Hysteroscopy

Advancing optical technology has offered an endoscopic instrument that can be passed through the cervix to the endometrial cavity to visualize the extent and location of the tumor and again its possible spread. It is also alleged to be useful for direction a biopsy instrument to the most favorable locus for biopsy. Hysteroscopy is another addition to the diagnostic array that can be brought to bear upon treatment planning and decision making.

PATHOLOGY

Gross Pathology

The adenocarcinoma may be a diffuse process spreading superficially about the endometrial cavity, or it may be a focal polypoid mass arising at any point in this cavity. Before spreading to deeper invasion, it tends to spread about the cavity and to expand it before deep invasion, although the uterus rarely increases in size to more than that of a 3-month pregnancy before the patient comes to treatment. The tumor mass is usually soft and friable and comes away piecemeal on curettage for it has lost normal tissue cohesion.

Histology

The lesion is usually confined to the glandular elements of the epithelium and it differs from the proliferation of hyperplasia in that it has invaded basement membranes and occupied the stromal areas. The tumor is now invasive, although it is not necessary for it to invade myometrium for such invasive properties. Ultimately it may do so, but it is important to stress that the majority (approximately 70 percent) are tumors of low virulence and stay local for long periods of time.

Most of these tumors are adenocarcinoma, but some may have benign squamous metaplasia and are called adenoacanthoma. These do not differ in virulence from the usual adenocarcinomas. However, several varieties do connote great virulence, including adenosquamous tumors in which both elements are malignant, clear cell tumors, and papillary carcinoma.

The grading of the adenocarcinoma of the endometrium, relating to its dedifferentiation or lack of it, is crucial, for it relates closely to the prognosis and therfore the need for increasing aggression of the treatment plan. From grade I, the highly differentiated form with glandular structures that do not vary greatly from the norm in spite of their abnormal proliferative tendencies, through grades II and III, wherein increasing differentiation is seen, one can encounter some masses of tumor cells without gland formations, without normal architecture, and increasingly with cellular anaplasia (Fig. 14-15 through 14-18). In grade III, there is complete loss of architecture, no gland formation, and frequent invasion of myometrium or beyond. It may be difficult to distinguish those cells microscopically from malignant squamous elements and from sarcoma, except with special staining. Thus, the virulent forms of endometrial cancer include

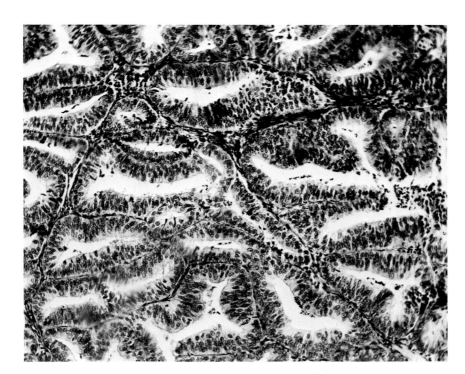

Fig. 14-15 Well-differentiated cancer of the endometrium.

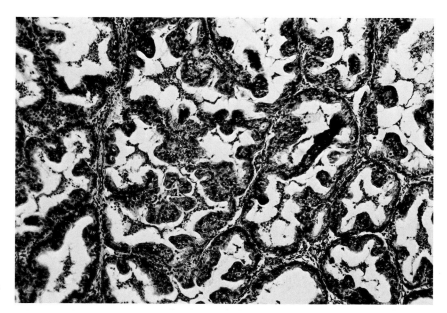

Fig. 14-16 Estrogen effect in cancer of the endometrium.

Grade III adenocarcinoma
Adenosquamous carcinoma
Papillary carcinoma
Clear cell carcinoma

Fortunately, in most series, the diffentiated adenocarcinomas predominate for these aggressive forms are relatively infrequent.

SPREAD OF ADENOCARCINOMA

Direction

Adenocarcinoma may spread in any of several ways (Fig. 14-19):

1. *Along the surface of the uterine cavity:* In this case, it may ultimately reach the endocervix or fallopian tubes.

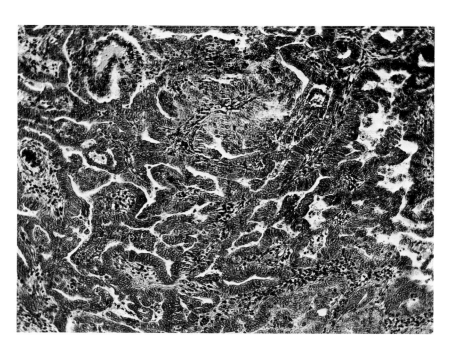

Fig. 14-17 Moderately differentiated cancer of the endometrium.

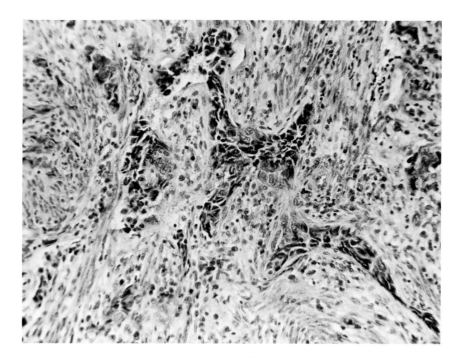

Fig. 14-18 Anaplastic cancer of the endometrium.

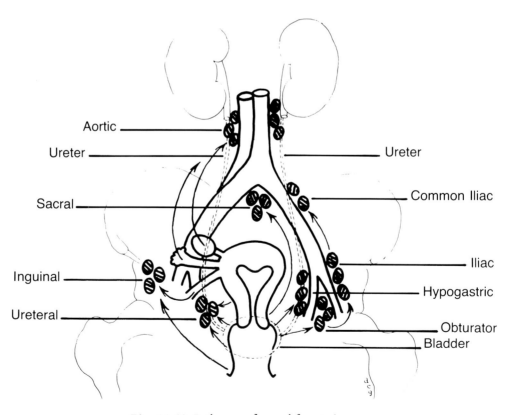

Aortic

Ureter

Sacral

Inguinal

Ureteral

Ureter

Common Iliac

Iliac

Hypogastric

Obturator

Bladder

Fig. 14-19 Pathways of spread for uterine cancer.

2. *Directly into the myometrium:* If this invasion is deep, it may extend to the peritoneum or pick up lymphatics to invade the upper broad ligament and beyond (Table 14-6).
3. *Free transplant to ovary or peritoneal cavity:* This occurs via cells escaping from the fallopian tube.
4. *Blood vessels (veins):* These have been shown to contain emboli offering an explanation for distant metastasis to lung, bone, or other sites.
5. *Lymphatic system:* This is an important vehicle for spread:
   a. It is seen from the fundus and upper uterus through the broad ligament to the ovary or directly to the paraaortic nodes and occasionally along the round ligaments to the inguinal nodes.
   b. It can spread from the isthmus and cervix to the deep pelvic nodes, including the iliac, obturator, and hypogastric nodes, and occasionally the sacral nodes.
   c. Because of the rich anastomosis of subserosal lymphatics, one may encounter a variation in lymph node metastasis, especially in retrograde fashion, as may be the case with vaginal metastasis. It cannot be assumed that paracervical lymphatics are free of tumor cells, because the endometrium is the primary site of the tumor. Therefore, treatment if radiotherapeutic, should cover this area, and, if surgical, should be radical.
   d. Extension of the cancer to the cervix creates a special problem that must be resolved therapeutically because of the possible parametrial direction of spread to pelvic lymph nodes or vagina. By spread to cevix, we mean to cervical substance, rather than tumor hanging into the cervical canal, which is frequently mistaken for true cervical spread.

Rate of Spread

The rate of metastasis varies greatly, but one must note again that the prognosis for most cancers of the endometrium is very good and the cure rate very high because these tumors tend to be well differentiated and tend to stay local. Some virulent tumors do spread quickly and lethally, but these probably do not constitute more than 15 percent of the whole (Table 14-7).

ENDOMETRIAL CANCER: DELAY IN CONTROL DUE TO HISTORIC FALLACIES

Fallacies:

1. That cancer of the corpus is always a benign cancer and that women will report postmenopausal bleeding promptly
2. That postmenopausal bleeding accompanying the popular cosmetic estrogen is always physiologic
3. That all corpus cancer could be treated best by one modality
4. That the Papanicolaou smear covers all uterine cancer surveillance
5. Slow acceptance of adenomatous hyperplasia as a significant cancer precursor
6. Reluctance to accept a staging that includes appropriate virulence factors.

Table 14-6 Cancer of the Corpus: Myometrial Invasion

Grade	No. of Patients	Local Disease (%)	Deep Invasion (%)
I	160	56.8	20.6
II	79	49.3	34.1
III	58	25.8	53.4

Table 14-7 Clinical Appraisal of Tumor Virulence

Stage	Description
I	Localized dependent tumor
II	Geographic spread
III	Biologic spread
IV	Widespread autonomous tumor

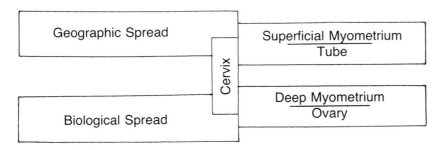

Fig. 14-20 Extension of tumor and virulence.

Metastasis to Tube and Ovary

In one of our studies of 251 patients, 25 patients had microscopic adnexal disease, and 11 had metastatic lesions that were clinically manifest.

It is important to distinguish extension to the tube or ovary, which may be geographic, that is, accidental surface spread and highly curable, from embolic, lymphatic, biologic spread, which may indicate high virulence (Fig. 14-20). In a series from the Sloane Hospital, microscopic adnexal involvement still allowed a 76 percent rate of cure, whereas in those with gross involvement, a 45 percent rate of only 5-year survival was found.

Lymph Node Metastasis

Traditionally, the lymph nodes were ignored in cancer of the endometrium in the belief that if regional nodes were involved, there would be distant metastases as well and treatment would be futile. In that past era, the study conducted by Finn, and the autopsy study by Henriksen (1949) seemed to support the view that this tumor stayed local for an extended period and that when it did leave the primary site, it spread widely.

Once again, gynecologic oncologists need the reminder that irradiation or surgery no matter how radical tend to be local or regional treatment while cancer is frequently a general disease. The advent of effective chemotherapy urged us to look at the node problem more closely.

Schwartz and Brunschwig (1957) found involved pelvic lymph nodes in 13 of 96 patients treated by radical hysterectomy. Liu and Meigs (1965) found regional node involvement in 4 of 33 cases in which the tumor was limited to the endometrial cavity, but 7 of 14 cases had nodal involvement in which the endo-

metrial lesion had extended to the cervix. Kottmeier's series (1959) confirmed those findings, while a literature review by Morrow et al. (1973) showed an incidence of pelvic node involvement to be 10.6 percent in FIGO stage I and 36.5 percent in FIGO stage II. In a personal Oxford series Stallworthy (1971) reported an incidence of 41 percent pelvic node involvement in those patients with cervix extension.

Further analysis of these problems came with the current trend for pretreatment surgical staging: node sampling or lymphadenectomy was studied by Creasman and collaborators (1976) in the Gynecologic Oncology Group, demonstrating, as might be anticipated, an increased incidence of positive pelvic and aortic nodes with enlargement of the cavity, dedifferentiation, and deep myometrium invasion.

Thus, the virulence factors for endometrial cancer that we defined in 1964 appear to be significant:

1. Undifferentiated tumor
2. Enlarged cavity
3. Extension to cervix
4. Deep myometrial invasion

We must use these parameters for treatment planning and prognosis.

SUGGESTED READINGS

Antunes CMD, Stolley PD, Rosenshein NG, et al: Endometrial cancer and estrogen use. N Engl J Med 300:9, 1979

Atkinson WB, Gusberg SB: Histochemical studies on abnormal growth of human endometrium. I. Alkaline phosphatase in hyperplasia and adenocarcinoma. Cancer 1:248, 1948

Backer J, Zentralbl Gynakol 22:735, 1904

Benjamin F, Casper DJ: Alternations in carbohydrate metabolism induced by progesterone in cases of endometrial carcinoma and hyperplasia. Am J Obstet Gynecol 94:991, 1966

Christopher WM, Mendez WM, Lundin FEJ, Parker JE: A ten-year study of endometrial carcinoma in Louisville, Kentucky. Cancer 18:554, 1965

Cohen CJ, Gusberg SB, Koffler D: Histologic screening for endometrial cancer. Gynecol Oncol 2:279, 1974

Corscaden JA, Gusberg SB: The background of cancer of the corpus. Am J Obstet Gynecol 53:419, 1947

Corscaden JA, Fertig JW, Gusberg SB: Carcinoma subsequent to the radiotherapeutic menopause. Am J Obstet Gynecol 51:1, 1946

Creasman WT, Boronow RC, Morrow CP, et al: Adenocarcinoma of the endometrium: Its metastatic lymph node potential. Gynecol Oncol 4:239, 1976

Cullen TS: Cancer of the uterus: Its pathology, symptomatology, diagnosis and treatment; also The Pathology of Diseases of the endometrium. WB Saunders, Philadelphia, 1900

Dunn JE Jr: Geographic considerations of endometrial cancer. Gynecol Oncol 2:114, 1974

Finn WF: Time, site and treatment of recurrences of endometrial carcinoma. Am J Obstet Gynecol 60:773, 1950

Gardner, Hertz et al: Role of hormones in origin and control of abnormal neoplastic growth. Proc Am Cancer Soc Conf. Cancer Res 17:481, 1957

Greene HSN: Uterine adenomata in the rabbit. III. Susceptibility as a function of constitutional factors. J Exp Med 73:273, 1941

Gusberg SB: Precursors of corpus carcinoma: Estrogens and adenomatous hyperplasia. Am J Obstet Gynecol 54:905, 1947

Gusberg SB, Hall RE: Precursors of corpus cancer. III. The appearance of cancer of the endometrium in estrogenically conditioned patients. Obstet Gynecol 17:397, 1961

Gusberg SB, Kaplan AL: Precursors of corpus cancer. IV. Adenomatous hyperplasia as Stage O carcinoma of the endometrium. Am J Obstet Gynecol 87:662, 1963

Gusberg SB, Kardon P: The response of the endometrium to theca-granulosa cell tumors. Am J Obstet Gynecol 3:633, 1971

Gusberg SB: Precursors of corpus carcinoma: Estrogens and adenomatous hyperplasia. Am J Obstet & Gynecol 54:905, 1947

Gusberg SB, Milano C: Detection of endometrial cancer and its precursors. Cancer 47:1173, 1981

Gusberg SB: The changing nature of endometrial cancer. N Engl J Med 302:729, 1980

Gurpide E, Hausknecht R, Vandewiele RL, Lieberman S: Estimation of the rates of secretion and peripheral inter-

conversion of estrogens. p. 32. In Proceedings of the Forty-fifth Meeting of Endocrine Society, 1963

Haenzel W, Kurihara M: Studies of Japanese migrants. J Natl Cancer Inst 40:43, 1968

Hausknecht RU, Gusberg SB: Estrogen metabolism in patients at high risk for endometrial cancer. II. Am J Obstet Gynecol 116:98, 1973

Henriksen E: The lymphatic spread of carcinoma of the cervix and the body of the uterus, a study of 420 necropsies. Am J Obstet Gynecol 58:924, 1949

Hertig AT, Sommers SC, Bengloff H: Genesis of endometrial carcinoma; carcinoma-in-situ. Cancer 2:964, 1949

Hintze O: Klinische Nachuntersuchung an 24 Fällen schwerer Hyperplasie der Korpusschleimhaut. Zentralbl Gynäkol 53:2396, 1929

Huggins C: Proceedings of conference on hormone-related tumors. Cancer Res 25:1053, 1965

Jensen EV: Proceedings of the International Congress of Biochemists, Vienna, 1958. Pergamon Press, London, 1960

Kaplan SD, Cole P: Epidemiology of cancer of the endometrium. Quoted by MacMahon (1974).

Kelley RM, Baker WH: Progestational agents in the treatment of carcinoma of endometrium. Proc Am Assoc Cancer Res 3:125, 1960

Kistner RW: Histological effects of progestins on hyperplasia or cancer in situ of the endometrium. Cancer 12:1106, 1959

Koss LG, Schreiber K, Oberlander SG et al: Detection of endometrial carcinoma and hyperplasia in asymptomatic women. Obstet Gynecol 64:1, 1984

Kottmeier HL: Carcinoma of the Female Genitalia. Williams & Wilkins, Baltimore, 1953

Kottmeir HL: Carcinoma of the corpus uteri: Diagnosis and therapy. Am J Obstet Gynecol 78:1127, 1959

Liu W, Meigs JV: Radical hysterectomy and pelvic lymphadenectomy. Am J Obstet Gynecol 69:1, 1965

Longcope C: Metabolic clearance and production rates of estrogens in post-menopausal women. Am J Obstet Gynecol 111:778, 1971

MacDonald PC, Siiteri, PK: Relation between extraglandular production of estrone and endometrial neoplasia. Gynecol Oncol 2:259, 1974

MacDonald PC, Gordon JM, Siiteri PK: Proceedings of the International Congress. Endocrinology 184:770, 1969

MacMahon B: Risk factors for endometrial cancer. Gynecol Oncol 2:122, 1974

Masubuchi K (1974): Proceedings of the U.I.C.C. International Cancer Congress, Florence.

Meyer R: Ueber seltenere gutartige and zweifelhafte. Epithelveranderung der Uterusschleimhaut im vVergleich mit der inhen ahnlichen Karzinomforemen; Endometritis; Schleimhauthyperplasie. Z Geburtshilfe Gynakol 85:440, 1923

Morrow CP, DiSaia PJ, Townsend DE: Current management of endometrial cancer. Obstet Gynecol 42:399, 1973

Novak E, Rutledge R: Atypical endometrial hyperplasia simulating adenocarcinoma. Am J Obstet Gynecol 55:46, 1948

Novak E, Yui E: Relation of endometrial hyperplasia to adenocarcinoma of uterus. Am J Obstet Gynecol 32:674, 1936

Randall CL: Adenocarcinoma of the uterus. In Kimbrough RA (ed): Gynecology. JB Lippincott, Philadelphia, 1965

Rubin BL, Gusberg SB, Butterfly J, et al: Screening test for estrogen dependence of endometrial carcinoma. Am J Obstet Gynecol 114:660, 1972

Schroeder R: Zentralbl Gynakol 46:2396, 1929

Schwartz AE, Brunschwig A: Radical pan-hysterectomy and pelvic node excision for carcinoma of the corpus uteri. Surg Gynecol Obstet 105:675, 1957

Sherman AI, Arneson AN: Cancer of the endometrium. Am J Med Sci 228:701, 1954

Southam AL, Richart RM: Prognosis for adolescents with menstrual abnormalities. Am J Obstet Gynecol 94:637, 1966

Speert H: The premalignant phase of endometrial carcinoma. Cancer 5:927, 1952

Stallworthy JA: Surgery of endometrial cancer in the Bonney tradition. Ann R Coll Surg Engl 48:293, 1971

Taki I, Iijima I, Doi T, et al: Histochemistry of hydrolytic and oxidative enzymes in the human and experimentally induced adenocarcinoma of the endometrium. Am J Obstet Gynecol 94:86, 1966

Taylor HC Jr: Endometrial hyperplasia and carcinoma of the body of the uterus. Am J Obstet Gynecol 23:309, 1932

TeLinde RW, Jones HW, Galvin GA: What are the earliest endometrial changes to justify a diagnosis of endometrial cancer? Am J Obstet Gynecol 66:973, 1967

Thiery M, Willighagen RG: Enzyme histochemistry of adenocarcinoma of the endometrium including hormone-induced changes. Am J Obstet Gynecol 99:173, 1967

Tseng L, Gusberg SB, Gurpide E: Estradiol receptor and 17 beta dehydrogenase in normal and abnormal human endometrium. Ann NY Acad Sci 286:190, 1977

Twombly GH, Scheiner S, Levitz M: Endometrial cancer, obesity and estrogenic excretion in women. Am J Obstet Gynecol 82:424, 1961

Whitehead MI, Townsend PT, Pryse-Davies J, et al: Effects of estrogens and progestins on the biochemistry and morphology of the post-menopausal endometrium. N Engl J Med 305:1599, 1981

Wynder EL, Escher G, Mantel N: An epidemiological investigation of cancer of the endometrium. Cancer 19:489, 1966

15

Treatment of Cancer of the Endometrium

S. B. Gusberg

Advancement in knowledge of cancer of the endometrium has been impeded by several persistent concepts:

That endometrial cancer is always a relatively benign malignancy, easily cured

That women will report postmenopausal bleeding promptly, especially that accompanying long-term estrogen administration, which may indeed be physiologic

That all tumors of this type should be treated by one modality

Slow acceptance of adenomatous hyperplasia as a significant cancer precursor

Reluctance to accept virulence factors in the international staging in the past

Studies of this neoplasm in the more recent past have modified or corrected these erroneous ideas and have led to more logical treatment, especially more individualization and an international convention of classification concepts that allows comparison of data and increasing quality control.

PREVENTION

Preventive measures may be applied differentially in an effort to establish surveillance of high-risk persons and reduce or modify promoting factors that are

known. To do this we must:

1. Recognize the high-risk factors
2. Restrict the promiscuous use of estrogen without control
3. Treat adenomatous hyperplasia appropriately
4. Screen all women at the menopause

High-Risk Women and Periodic Examination

We have discussed the factors that place persons at increased risk of endometrial cancer, including obesity, infertility, dysfunctional bleeding with failure of ovulation, perhaps with accompanying mild diabetes, or subjection to prolonged estrogen administration (Figs. 15-1 and 15-2).

Surveillance of such women must include a careful history to elicit a possible abnormal bleeding episode that they have ignored as well as periodic sampling of the endometrium by aspiration curettage at the menopause and every year or two thereafter. No treatment should be offered a perimenopausal woman without an endometrial biopsy of this type.

The obese woman may require special attention in view of the fact that she may have a significant production rate of estrogen endogenously. One can reduce endometrial stimulation by the periodic admin-

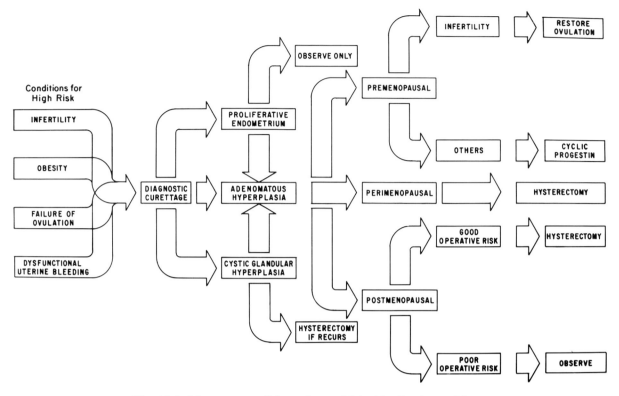

Fig. 15-1 Management of the patient at high risk of endometrial cancer.

istration of a progestin; 10 mg medroxyprogesterone for 10 to 14 days every 3 months will usually suffice, but monitoring the endometrium with tissue biopsy may reveal individual variation and the special requirement of some more sensitive subjects.

Estrogen

While the capricious use of estrogen for cosmetic purposes has decreased, the introduction of the concept that osteoporosis can be prevented or reduced by

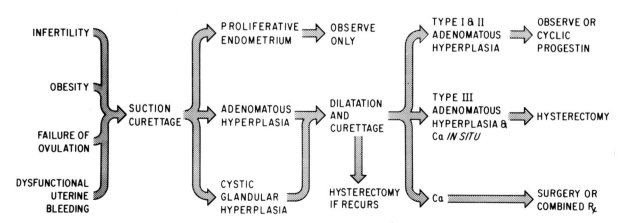

Fig. 15-2 Management of the high-risk menopausal patient. Detection of precursors and their treatment.

the prophylactic use of steroids has given such hormonal treatment renewed support. Since the osteoporosis-prone woman cannot be defined as yet, this so-called hormonal support is offered to all postmenopausal women by many physicians.

It is demonstrable that progestins are antagonists of estrogen at the morphologic level. The metabolic basis for this lies in the progesterone inhibition of E_2 receptors and its stimulation of estradiol beta dehydrogenase that converts E_2 to E_1 and clearance of estrogen from the target cell thereafter. Evidence of the efficacious use of progestin in the clinical context comes from reports that the use of the combined oral contraceptive pill during active reproductive life will diminish the later incidence of endometrial carcinoma; in a similar manner 10 mg medroxyprogesterone acetate for 10 to 14 days each month or every second or third month has been demonstrated to reduce the incidence of adenomatous hyperplasia and endometrial carcinoma in those women on long-term estrogen replacement.

One difficulty with such a regimen of estrogen modified by progestin is the frequent induction of bleeding. This is considered undesirable by most women and sometimes confusing by their physicians, who are then faced with the need to discriminate between the probably hormonally induced phenomenon or some pathologic aberration, if the bleeding becomes irregular. An alternative strategy for estrogen replacement in these women is the continued use of estrogen without progestin but accompanied by monitoring with aspiration curettage every year or two, depending on the sensitivity or stimulation of the endometrium incurred. This regimen will usually avoid regular bleeding and permit control of any tendency toward induction of hyperplasia.

Treatment of Adenomatous Hyperplasia

Treatment of adenomatous hyperplasia or stage 0 carcinoma of the endometrium depends on the age and reproductive needs of the patient. In young women, frequently the subject of failure of ovulation with the cystic ovary syndrome, cycling with 10 to 20 mg medroxyprogesterone acetate (Provera) for 14 days each month will usually cause reversion of the endometrium to normal within four or five cycles. In these young subjects, if infertility is also a problem,

the induction of ovulation with a gonadotrophin will be more appropriate, for it can accomplish both missions.

In the perimenopausal woman, in which age group most of these lesions occur, the milder grades (I and II) of adenomatous hyperplasia may be treated effectively in some by medroxyprogesterone acetate in 10 to 20 mg/day dosage for 3 to 4 months with regression, but this should be monitored by repeat curettage at the end of treatment. The more intense forms (grade II and especially III) of this cancer precursor at this time of life are better treated by hysterectomy, unless there is a medical contraindication to surgery. In such a situation when the untreated recurrent precursor carries a prospect of a 20 to 25 percent risk of future cancer, removal of the uterus not only cures the usually recurrent bleeding but confers the benefit of prophylaxis.

In the postmenopausal woman, in whom the induction of adenomatous hyperplasia is the result of estrogen administration, merely discontinuing the estrogen will usually result in regression of the overstimulated endometrium. If this fails to occur in 4 months, on repeat biopsy or curettage, one can administer a progestin for 4 additional months before advising surgery, or continue hormonal treatment longer or more intensively, if surgery is contraindicated.

Clearly, primary or secondary prevention is most applicable to hormone-dependent tumors. Early detection by screening is the only strategy applicable to the autonomous tumors.

CURATIVE TREATMENT

In the past, carcinoma of the endometrium has been cured by irradiation, hysterectomy (conservative or radical, vaginal or abdominal), and combinations of irradiation and surgery. Some (Corscaden and Tovell (1953)) have even noted cure with subtotal hysterectomy, but this excellent cure rate relates not to the casual treatment, which one must condemn, but to the tiny lesions cited, so small as to be overlooked in some cases, mostly treated long ago, and found accidentally in the removed specimen.

Historically, after the technique for removal of the uterus was established in the nineteenth century, it was noted that a considerable number of patients with endometrial cancer were cured by this procedure, whereas those with cancer of the cervix usually failed. Thereafter, the surgical approach to this disease gained increasing favor.

Radium application was used as early as 1914 for the treatment of endometrial cancer as well as cancer of the cervix; it became clear that irradiation was very effective in the treatment of the cervix, and it gradually replaced the radical Wertheim procedure in most clinics. However, it was not accepted as an important treatment for endometrial disease, for which surgery continued to gain favor. Regaud's (1922) studies of the radioresistance of the adenomatous structures of bull's testes convinced him that all adenomatous tissues, benign or malignant, are resistant to irradiation. Furthermore, the results of the treatment by hysterectomy appeared quite satisfactory, and by 1930 it was stated commonly that "radium was for the cervix and hysterectomy for the corpus." But Forsell and later Heymann and co-workers in Stockholm persisted with irradiation for endometrial cancer and achieved excellent results.

In the United States, gynecologists watched the success of treatment with both irradiation and surgery and reasoned that combining both might improve the cure rate further. Stimulated by early clinical trials by Healy and Brown (1939), Corscaden and Tovell, reported later in 1954, and Arneson (1948), American gynecologists adopted this method of combined treatment which became the standard treatment for endometrial adenocarcinoma in the United States and in other parts of the world. It did appear, during that era, to give a better result than either modality alone.

When radical hysterectomy could be performed with relative safety, it became briefly prominent in some clinics to satisfy the philosophy that malignant lesions, if treated surgically, should undergo radical treatment. This surgical fashion was short-lived, however, doomed to failure by the age, habitus, and infirmity of many of the subjects and the modest results of treatment, no greater than that with conservative surgery.

STAGING AND CLASSIFICATION

When we decide on treatment for any malignant tumor, we usually depend on clinical staging to aid this decision. Not only does staging help with protocols of treatment, but it enhances quality control by enabling comparison of cure rates between institutions. For some years, these advantages of staging were inhibited by an international convention that lumped all tumors "confined to the corpus" into stage I, thus incorporating almost all operable tumors into that category, ignoring factors of virulence that could separate them and encouraging one treatment for all.

At one point, a classification used at the Radiumhemmet in Stockholm based on operability seemed useful:

The operable patient: one with an apparently local removable tumor who was in otherwise good health and therefore a good surgical subject

The technically operable patient: one whose disease appeared eradicable but who was not a fit surgical subject either because of poor general health or because of obesity of a degree that complicated operability to the point of hazard

The inoperable patient: one whose disease appeared to be beyond removal, by virtue of invasion of contiguous organs, fixation, or distant metastases

With the years, as surgery and its adjuvants increased operability, clinics varied considerably in their approach to judgments concerning the safety of operation in particular cases, and these designations lost any possible universality they might have attained in the past.

FIGO

The Cancer Committee of the International Federation of Obstetrics and Gynecology (FIGO) recommended the following staging in 1961:

Stage I: carcinoma confined to the corpus

Stage II: carcinoma involving the corpus and cervix

Stage III: carcinoma extending outside the uterus but not outside the true pelvis

Stage IV: carcinoma extending outside the true pelvis or obviously involving the mucosa of bladder or rectum

This classification designed for statistical reporting to the international Annual Report in Stockholm never achieved the widest acceptance, for it contained important deficiencies:

1. Almost all treatable tumors were to be included in stage I, equating the tiny localized disease with a tumor that filled and enlarged the uterine cavity.

2. There was not a straight-line decrement of cure rate for frequently stage II tumors would have a poorer outlook than some stage III disease where tumor was outside the uterus but not outside the pelvis. The concept of virulence, expressed by separating geographic extension from biologic extension (metastasis), was not used, as may be seen in the comparison of the FIGO curve with our virulence-based classification.

3. Tumor differentiation, a significant factor in virulence, was not included; thus, an important parameter for planning treatment and comparing result was omitted in their effort to reach as many reporting clinics as possible in this international effort.

Virulence Classification

The virulence-based classification enables one to define an order or progression in making a logical clinical classification. A local, so-called dependent tumor is one of low virulence that can share the biologic, endocrinologic, and enzymatic properties of the host tissue. Geographic spread implies local invasion; it may be a mere morphologic accident without biologic significance, it may have spread by chance, and it may retain low virulence, permitting surgical encompassment by increased surgical radicality with a high degree of success. By contrast, biologic spread indicates an order of invasiveness that permits lymphatic permeation, lymph node metastasis, and a decline in curability. In such a lesion, even radical surgery or irradiation may fail, for the tumor has become autonomous, does not share host tissue biochemical properties, and curability is beyond the scope of regional treatment.

An illustration of such differences may be seen in geographic spread to the fallopian tube, where we attained a 76.7 percent cure rate, whereas biologic spread (metastasis) to the adjacent ovary carried only a 29.8 survival rate.

Our studies (1964, 1966) of endometrial cancer virulence (Fig. 15-3) enabled us to use three preoperative parameters to define a sliding-scale clinical classification on the basis of three factors:

Size of uterine cavity
Involvement of cervix
Histologic differentiation

These factors are easily obtained by sounding the uterine cavity, indicating most frequently the size of the tumor, fractional curettage to ascertain cervix involvement, and analysis of curettings, frequently on a frozen-section basis. More formal review of curettings permits definition of the adenosquamous, clear cell or papillary tumors with increased virulence; postoperative analysis may demonstrate deep myometrial penetration indicating an increasing order of virulence and decreasing prognosis.

Our virulence classification allowed better comparison of results for clinical studies than the prior FIGO staging and formed the basis for increasing consideration of individualization of treatment over the former lock-step approach.

In fact, in 1971, the FIGO Committee incorporated these proposed virulence factors that had proved significant, publishing the new International Classification for Endometrial Cancer. This staging has now come into wide acceptance, for it supports logical prognosis and comparative studies; in addition, it has encouraged the individualization of treatment that we strongly sought, now increasingly recognized and used, as evident from recent reports.

Stage I	Uterus normal size	
Stage II	Uterus mildly enlarged up to 2 1/2 months or 10 cm. depth	Downstage for anaplastic tumor or cervix involvement
Stage III	Uterus markedly enlarged over 3 months or 10 cm. depth	
Stage IV	Contiguous organs involved or distant metastases	

Fig. 15-3 Virulence classification of endometrial cancer showing a sliding scale using three preoperative parameters.

FIGO CLASSIFICATION OF VIRULENCE
FACTORS IN ENDOMETRIAL CANCER

Stage I: Tumor confined to corpus
    Not enlarged: <8 cm in depth of canal
        G_1 Well differentiated
        G_2 Moderately differentiated
        G_3 Poorly differentiated
    Enlarged: ≥8 cm in depth
        G_1
        G_2
        G_3
Stage II: Involvement of corpus and cervix
Stage III: Extension outside uterus but not
    outside the true pelvis
Stage IV: Involvement of bladder or rectum or
    distant metastasis

TREATMENT MODALITIES

Hysterectomy

Alone or combined with irradiation has been recognized as the primary treatment for endometrial cancer; it is now universally accepted as such in the United States and in most other parts of the world. The operation generally utilized is a total abdominal hysterectomy by the extrafascial technique and bilateral salpingo-oophorectomy. While surgery for benign tumors may use an intrafascial approach, leaving the fascial investment to which the uterosacral, vesicouterine, and cardinal ligaments are attached, hysterectomy for endometrial cancer should remove the cuff of lymphatics about the isthmus and cervix. The excision is still close to the uterus, and dissecting the ureters is not required for the uterine vessels are ligated medial to them.

The removal of a vaginal cuff is often advocated on the thesis that this is an area of recurrence, but logic dictates the improbability of its importance; local lesions will not require it, and for more aggressive tumors it will be inadequate. The individualization of treatment required in such instances is described below.

Preliminary ligation of the fallopian tubes may be advantageous in preventing spill of cancer cells, for it is difficult to prevent manipulation of the specimen, even in the hands of the most seasoned surgeons. By the same token, we have avoided doing supplementary operations such as prophylactic appendectomy at the time of a cancer operation for spread of tumor cells by instruments is not unknown.

Ligature closure of the cervix before hysterectomy has been practiced, but not by our group. Theoretically, it is also meant to prevent spill into the vagina or cuff, but the diagnostic curettage has already spilled many cells into the vagina, and statistically significant results do not indicate a correlation.

In most cases, cancer operations should be done through a vertical suprapubic or paramedian incision. The Pfannenstiehl cosmetic approach should not be used. In very obese subjects, a transverse incision including separation of the tendinous insertions of the rectus muscle will provide adequate exposure.

Radical Hysterectomy (with Lymphadenectomy)

It was inevitable in this surgical era that radical surgery would be applied to this tumor. With increasing surgical lattitude due to antibiotic, anesthesiologic, and chemical advances, blood bank support, and cancer of other sites treated with radical surgery, it was necessary to defend the use of conservative hysterectomy for this disease. The lymph nodes and parametrial lymphatic channels seemed vulnerable, and some groups attempted routine radical hysterectomy and lymphadenectomy. Meigs and Brunschwig in the United States and Stallworthy and the Oxford group, especially in the United Kingdom, carried out such a program but this experiment was doomed to failure and this practice has not been followed except in special circumstances. The obesity, advanced age, and frequent circulatory deficiency of these subjects add to the hazard of such a procedure; the parametrium should not be a conventional pathway of spread, except in those with deep myometrial involvement or spread of tumor to the isthmus or cervix. Furthermore, these clinical trials failed to show an increased rate of cure over more conventional treatment.

Vaginal Hysterectomy

Vaginal hysterectomy is mentioned only to be dismissed. It has not been popular due to the inability to explore the abdomen and sometimes an inadequate approach to removal of the adnexal structures. Although it has been offered as useful for obese subjects, we have found the obesity to be as great an impediment from below as above. In general, good cancer surgery requires gentleness and care in surgical manipulation; this means adequacy of exposure, which is difficult to obtain by the vaginal route.

Exenteration

Ultraradical operations have been performed for endometrial cancer, but insufficient cases have accrued to form the basis of a judgment concerning its applicability. The embolic nature of advanced adenocarcinoma suggests that such a strategy will rarely be successful unlike the case of squamous cancer of the cervix wherein direct extension plays a greater role.

RADIATION

A radiotherapeutic technique was developed in Stockholm during the 1930s designed for patients found unsuitable for primary surgery, therefore referred for treatment to the Radiumhemmet, regarded as the prime radiotherapeutic hospital there. This method of uterine radium packing was finally reported by Heyman and colleagues (1941) and elaborated by Kottmeier (1959). In those years, it was used as a definitive treatment and an absolute cure rate of 63.3 percent was attained with 68.2 percent survival in the operable group. The Stockholm method also made provision for postoperative vaginal application for those operated before coming to the Radiumhemmet with an 80.4 percent survival in those undoubtedly earlier and healthier patients and a 40 percent 5-year survival in patients treated with irradiation for vaginal recurrence.

There seemed little remaining doubt that radiation was capable of destroying this tumor tissue effectively, but its use as primary treatment never overcame the primacy of surgery for this disease. To this day, it has remained a secondary treatment for the currently infrequent inoperable patient, except in its usefulness as an adjuvant treatment.

Preoperative Radiation

With knowledge of the radiosensitivity of endometrial cancer, some clinics (principally American) began to combine preoperative irradiation, followed

in 4 to 6 weeks by total abdominal hysterectomy and bilateral salpingo-oophorectomy. This trend actually started as early as the 1930s, but a substantial series was first reported by Corscaden and Tovell in 1954. Significant improvement of combined over straight surgical treatment was noted in a series by Arneson (1953), our own study (1966), the earlier report of Corscaden, and other series. Some disagreed, but during that era, comparative figures were difficult of analysis because the virulence factors of differentiation, size, cervical involvement, and deep myometrial penetration were not considered or stated. In addition, in most clinics all cases of endometrial cancer were treated by the same method of their choice.

Advocates of preoperative radiation (the combined method) proposed several advantages:

1. Diminution in the size of the corpus to improve operative clearance
2. Fibrosis of the uterus to prevent operative dissemination
3. Destruction of vitality of surface tumor in the cavity to reduce implantation metastases and operative dissemination
4. Sealing lymphatics and vascular channels to prevent operative spread
5. Devitalization of the vaginal vault as a tumor receptor site
6. Radiation of fresh, well-oxygenated tumor tissue
7. Apparent improvement in the cure rate

In our own series, during the preindividualization era, we did note a diminution in vaginal recurrence and an improvement in cure rate in patients subjected to the combined mode over those treated by hysterectomy alone, in spite of the fact that some subtly early cases did have surgery only.

Discussion concerning the value of combined treatment continues to this day, but much of the evidence lacks adequate material and proper staging. In the earlier reports, there appeared to be clear evidence that the combined method had an advantage in the more aggressive tumors with enlarged uteri, invasion of myometrium, and dedifferentiation.

Technique of Preoperative Radiation

This method may employ radium (or equivalent isotopes, frequently cesium in modern usage) or external x-irradiation. We may use the Stockholm method as a prototype for it has been used very effectively there and imitated widely with minor variations; one can illustrate this method with the use of radium, although radium equivalents are used mostly in modern miniaturization with isotopes.

The Stockholm Packing Method

The Stockholm Packing method is traditional treatment, usually given in divided doses, with two applications usually 3 weeks apart, approximately 10 radium tubes (8 mg each) packed into the cavity tightly, for approximately 1,500 mg hr, in each sitting for the average patient with the smallest of the three filters (9- to 15-mm filter diameters). Larger or smaller applications are chosen to suit the size of the cavity. A total dose of 3,000 gamma rads is given at 1.5 cm from the nearest applicator in the cavity. A vaginal cylinder is also applied to attain a dose of approximately 1,800 gamma rads at a point 1 cm beneath the surface of the vaginal mucosa.

In patients with advanced disease, in an era when the Radiumhemmet used a radiotherapeutic plan for definitive treatment, external radiation was used to supplement the radium application, but 1,600 rads only were given to each of four pelvic portals.

Our own method has developed by the use of standard-size tubes for endometrial cavity packing (Campbell applicators, 10-mg radium tubes or cesium equivalent) with vaginal ovoids placed in the upper third of the vagina (Fig. 15-4). Our application is a single one with 7 to 10 tubes packed into corpus and cervix for 5,000 to 7,000 mg/hr. This will give a dose of approximately 3,300 gamma rads at the radiotherapeutic point 1.5 cm from the cavity and the 2 × 15 mg ovoids in the fornices give 2,400 gamma rads to the vaginal radiotherapeutic point 1 cm lateral to the vaginal surface. We have occasionally supplemented this with a half-pelvic cycle by the Betatron to add 2,750 rads bringing the dosage to a theoretical cancercidal level.

We have restricted radiation in this way to the upper third of the vagina on the principle that coverage of possible remote metastases in the lower vagina should be reserved for the occasional palliative plan, rather than expose the usual patient to the hazard of undue radiation trauma for equivocal therapeutic advantage. In the case of patients with a cavity more

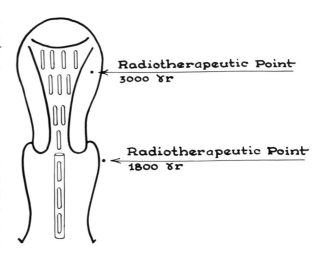

Fig. 15-4 Packing technique in the Stockholm method of radium application or its equivalent.

than $2\frac{1}{2}$ months gestation in size, we have always preferred any preoperative radiation to be given by external x-ray beam. Though some have practiced immediate operation after preoperative radium, we have preferred a 4-week interval before surgery. This would seem to confer excellent radiation benefit, the time is chosen after the primary radiation blush (hyperemia and edema) has begun to subside and before the secondary fibrosis (6 to 8 weeks) begins. This does not mean that any technical difficulty of earlier operation cannot be overcome in the modern surgical era.

In the United States filtration of radium tubes has been accomplished with 0.5 mm of platinum, which is said to filter out all the β-rays. At the Curie Institute in Paris 1.0 mm of platinum was said to cause less injury, while in Stockholm 3 mm of lead is used equivalent to 1.5 mm of platinum.

The distribution of sources concerns the question of use of a tandem in the cavity vs the packing method. We have preferred the latter because of the differential dosage with tandems in the midline as opposed to lateral lying positions due to cavity distortion (Fig. 15-5). In the past, several studies have testified to the efficiency of the Packing method. Nolan, Arneson, and others have shown greater efficiency for multiple sources over tandem applications with less residual cancer in the operative specimen. We believe that this eradication will confer a greater benefit in cure.

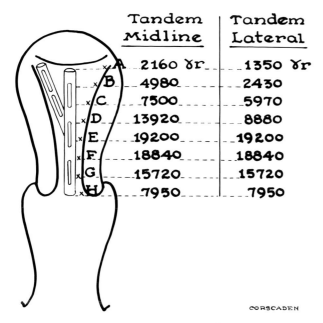

	Tandem Midline	Tandem Lateral
A	2160 δr	1350 δr
B	4980	2430
C	7500	5970
D	13920	8880
E	19200	19200
F	18840	18840
G	15720	15720
H	7950	7950

CORSCADEN

Fig. 15-5 Radium tandem in cancer of the endometrium showing variation of dosage by geography of placement.

External Radiotherapy

External radiotherapy has come to increasing prominence in both preoperative and postoperative usage in recent years, for its general pelvic distribution, while lacking the intracavitary intensity of local radium or its isotope equivalent, can bathe the entire

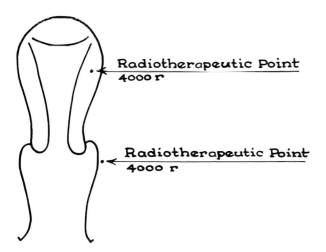

Radiotherapeutic Point
4000 r

Radiotherapeutic Point
4000 r

Fig. 15-6 External radiation of carcinoma of the endometrium.

pelvic area at risk in a homogeneous way, 4,000 to 4,500 rads TD have been used generally without sequellae of note and without hindrance to the usual surgery (Fig. 15-6). In addition to the benefit to the uterine and vault bloc preoperatively, one can confer coverage to the pelvic lymph nodes and even cover the paraaortic nodes postoperatively by cephalad field extension. Indication for its use postoperatively is discussed below.

Postoperative Radium to the Vaginal Vault

This method has been used in Stockholm for many years as treatment for those patients operated before referral to the Radiumhemmet, with an excellent rate of cure, apparently better than the usual result but also apparently earlier disease, for they were subjected first to primary surgery in an atmosphere where combined treatment had become important. In other parts of the world, discussions concerning preoperative versus postoperative radiation have continued without sufficient evidence for resolution of the problem. In an effort to settle this problem Graham (1963) reported an apparently randomized series in which he concluded that the cure rates were equivalent. Advocates of postoperative vault radium have offered the following as advantages:

No delay in operation

Fresh tissue for study of invasion

Same reduction in vault recurrence

One hospitalization

In recent years, this postoperative method has yielded to the use of postoperative external irradiation.

COMPLICATIONS OF RADIATION

Injuries from standard methods of radiation for endometrial cancer are rare. In the past, the use of intracavitary radium has suffered from undertreatment rather than overtreatment, and radiation complications have been uncommon. The threat of uterine perforation with a radium or cesium tube must be remembered, and the possibility that a past laparotomy could bring a loop of bowel adherent to the uterus or to another vital focus like the aorta into the intense radiation field should be held ever-present. However, with care in planning, precise probing of the uterine cavity and even afterloading, so that ajustment of applications can be made immediately, there should be little risk of significant radiation injury. This contrasts with the radiation treatment of cancer of the cervix, where complications are not rare. We like to remember the aphorism that the worst complication of cancer treatment is persistence or recurrence of cancer.

Table 15-1 Corpus Cancer, Stage I: Lymph Nodes[a]

Stage and Grade	Pelvic Nodes Positive (%)	Aortic Nodes Positive (%)
IA		
G_1	2.6	2.6
G_2	6.9	3.5
G_3	16.7	8.3
IB		
G_1	3.9	0.0
G_2	14.3	4.8
G_3	54.0	46.0

[a] Total 140 patients, stage I. Pelvic nodes positive: 11.4%; aortic nodes positive: 5.7%.
(Creasman W, Boronow R, Morrow CP, et al. Gynecol Oncol 4:239, 1976.)

SELECTION OF TREATMENT: INDIVIDUALIZATION

Knowledge of the virulence factors and their relation to tumor aggression and prognosis led to our current mode of individualized treatment based upon preoperative and operative findings (Tables 15-1 and 15-2; Figs. 15-7 and 15-8).

Preoperatively

The size of the uterine cavity is an index, if imperfect, of the volume of tumor growth for this tumor tends to grow locally for long periods of time, without extension or metastasis. This parameter is easily estimated by sounding the depth of the cavity.

Tumor involvement of the cervix or isthmus is important, for it can indicate possible need for treatment of parametrial lymphatic channels and deep pelvic nodes (Table 15-3; Fig. 15-9). This extension may be diagnosed by fractional curettage, though some utilize hysteroscopy.

Dedifferentiation of Tumor

This is another index of possible deep myometrial penetration or possible node involvement that serves notices that such a more aggressive tumor requires

Table 15-2 Individualized Treatment for Endometrial Cancer[a]

Stage	
IAG_1	TAH + BSO
IBG_1	TAG + BSO + vault radium
IAG_2 and IAG_3 IBG_2 and IBG_3	TAH + BSO + Iliac-aortic selective lymphadenectomy + XRT
II and III	Preoperative radium + XRT + TAH + BSO + selective lymphadenectomy OR Preoperative radium + radical hysterectomy + selective lymphadenectomy
IV	Individualized treatment

[a] Chemotherapy is applicable for positive aortic nodes, and XRT is given for positive pelvic nodes.
TAH, total abdominal hysterectomy; BSO, bilateral salpingo-oophorectomy; XRT, external radiation therapy.
(Modified from Gusberg SB: Treatment of corpus cancer. Cancer 38:603, 1976)

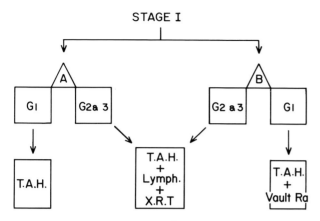

Fig. 15-7 Treatment protocol for stage I carcinoma of the endometrium. **(A)** With cavity < 8 cm in depth; **(B)** With cavity ≥ 8 cm in depth; G_1, well differentiated; G_2, moderately differentiated; G_3, anaplastic; TAH, total abdominal hysterectomy; Lymph, lymphadenectomy; XRT, external radiotherapy; vault Ra, internal vault radiotherapy.

Table 15-3 Corpus Cancer: Incidence of Pelvic Node Metastases — Combined Statistics

Stage[a]	No. of Patients[b]	% Positive
I	369	10.6
II	85	36.5

[a] Based on FIGO staging.
[b] Corrected survival = 31.2% in stage I.
(Morrow CP, DiSaia PH, Townsend DE: Current management of endometrial cancer. Obstet Gynecol 42:399, 1973.)

more aggressive treatment. One can frequently use frozen-section analysis for this appraisal, although some protocols of treatment allow time for permanent sections in the pathology laboratory.

Operative and Postoperative Data

Such data permit observation of myometrial invasion and node involvement. Clearly these data will be obtained in the more aggressive tumors where node sampling in the pelvic (especially common iliac) and paraaortic areas has become part of an extended surgical procedure.

CLASS I: TUMORS OF LOW AGGRESSION

Differentiated adenocarcinomas in a cavity less than 8 cm in depth will require in general only surgical treatment by extrafascial hysterectomy and bilateral salpingo-oophorectomy. This group will comprise approximately 70 percent of the whole and in general one can attain a cure rate of approximately 90 percent (Table 15-4).

CLASS II: TUMORS OF HIGHER AGGRESSION

By virtue of dedifferentiation, large size, deep myometrial penetration, or special histology (adenosquamous, clear cell or papillary) are best treated by hysterectomy and bilateral salpingo-oophorectomy together with pelvic and aortic lymph node sampling, peritoneal washing, and diaphragmatic scraping for later analysis. Adjuvant external pelvic irradiation is

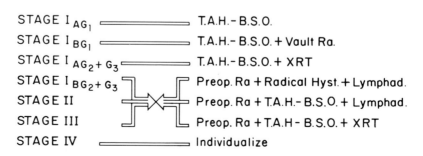

Fig. 15-8 Treatment protocol for corpus cancer. XRT, external radiotherapy; TAH, total abdominal hysterectomy; BSO, bilateral salpingo-oophorectomy; Preop Ra, preoperative radium or equivalent; Lymphad, lymphadenectomy.

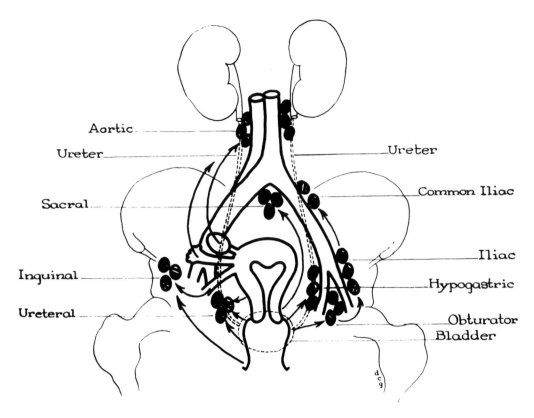

Aortic

Ureter

Sacral

Inguinal

Ureteral

Ureter

Common Iliac

Iliac

Hypogastric

Obturator
Bladder

Fig. 15-9 Lymph node groups draining uterus: corpus and cervix.

Table 15-4 Corpus Cancer, Stage I: Treatment and Methods

Treatment	No. of Patients	5-yr Survival (%)	Adjusted 5-yr Survival[a] (%)
Primary surgery	150	90.7	95.9
Preoperative radium	130	89.2	93.5

[a] Adjusted for mortality in general population.
(After Bean HA, et al: Carcinoma of the endometrium in Saskatchewan. Gynecol Oncol 6:503, 1978.)

Table 15-5 Corpus Cancer: Radical Hysterectomy and Lymphadenectomy

Investigators	No. of Patients	5-yr Survival (%)
Winterton (1959)	99	76
Hawksworth (1964)	167	69
Lees (1969)	76	63
Stallworthy (1971)	131	71

significant and chemotherapy added for those with positive aortic nodes or peritoneal involvement. Phosphorus-32 has been used by some for positive cytology of washings and aortic radiation for positive aortic nodes.

CLASS III: TUMORS INVOLVING THE CERVIX

These tumors deserve special consideration, as deep pelvic lymphatic channel must be considered. The choice of treatment here allows several courses of action

Preoperative radium followed by radical hysterectomy and lymphadenectomy — will be applicable to few patients because of health, age, or habitus (Table 15-5)

Preoperative irradiation by full cervix and corpus patterns followed by conservative hysterectomy.

Such protocols of individualization offer the patient with a tumor of low virulence, the majority, a high rate of cure with a treatment that confers this benefit with a very low exposure to complication, while assigning the individual with an aggressive tumor the opportunity for cure with an aggressive approach to therapy.

Thus, the trend toward individualization and surgery first, begun in the early 1960s by our reports has been confirmed and re-emphasized by reports by Wade et al. (1967), Nelson and Koller (1969), Stallworthy (1971), and Rutledge (1974), while Boronow (1969), Morrow et al. (1973), and Underwood et al. (1974) used similar factors with minor variation. A Canadian group reporting from two clinics with apparently identical material showed an equivalent high cure rate in those treated primarily by surgery (70 percent of the group), using postoperative radiation for the remainder 30 percent, who required it by virtue of factors of tumor aggression. Once again, this report emphasized the efficacy of surgery alone for the majority, while supporting the value of adjuvant irradiation for the minority with more virulent tumors.

PROGNOSIS

If one uses a virulence type of clinical classification, a steady decrement in cure rate can be shown, from 84.3 percent in stage I in our series to 12.5 percent in stage IV, a stage-for-stage equivalent to that seen in cancer of the cervix or indeed for most solid tumors elsewhere in the body. By FIGO staging analysis, one can expect a cure rate above 98 percent for stage IA and reduction thereafter, although some will report a better rate of survival in stage III than in stage II (Table 15-6 and 15-7).

Although it is still difficult to analyze many survival figures from around the world because the new I FIGO classification has come slowly into acceptance, and results clearly vary according to the composition of the material in any one clinic, we get the best broad-based view from the Stockholm annual report. These data offer a survival rate varying from 52.5 to 88.6 percent in those clinics with significantly large patient accrual (Table 15-8). We find once again that differentiation is a most important virulence factor for

Table 15-6 Carcinoma of the Endometrium: Results by Stage and Year

Stage	Patient Treatment Period/(% 5-Year Survival)			
	1962–1968 (Vol. 16) (%)	1969–1972 (Vol. 17) (%)	1973–1975 (Vol. 18) (%)	1976–1978 (Vol. 19) (%)
I	71.9	73.6	74.2	75.1
II	49.7	55.7	57.4	57.8
III	30.7	31.3	29.2	30.0
IV	9.3	9.2	9.6	10.6
Total	63.0	65.4	66.6	67.7

(FIGO: Annual Report, Stockholm, Vol. 19.)

Table 15-7 Carcinoma of the Endometrium: Stage, Grade, and Result

Histologic Grade	Stage I No. Treated	Stage I 5 yr Survival N	Stage I 5 yr Survival (%)	Stage II No. Treated	Stage II 5 yr Survival (%)	Stage III No. Treated	Stage III 5 yr Survival (%)	Stage IV No. Treated	Stage IV 5 yr Survival (%)
I	3,665	2,918	79.6						
II	2,287	1,678	73.4						
III	886	508	58.7						
Not Graded	1,017	738	72.6						
Total	7,835	5,842	74.6	1,352	57.2	614	32.4	296	10.5

(FIGO: Annual Report, Stockholm, Vol. 19.)

Table 15-8 Carcinoma of the Endometrium

Institution (City)	No. Treated	% Survived After 5 yr
Melbourne	279	64.1
Vienna	312	52.5
Saskatchewan	262	84.8
Toronto	560	78.6
Vancouver	445	83.7
Winnipeg	370	81.7
Brno, Czech	235	78.6
Helsinki	253	74.7
Leipzig	204	63.5
Kiel	229	72.6
Munich, Ist Clinic	226	57.1
Munich, Grosshadern	264	66.0
Debrecen, Hungary	215	70.3
Oslo	678	84.1
Lodz	200	83.2
Gothenburg	508	77.8
Stockholm	541	80.2
New Haven	211	76.5
Leningrad	201	88.6
Ljubljana	310	73.7
Zagreb	236	80.5

(FIGO: Annual Report, Stockholm, Vol. 19.)

in stage I disease the 5-year survival drops from 79.6 percent in grade I tumors to 58.7 percent in grade 3 tumors.

It is also important to remember that the world view offered by this Stockholm report indicates a slow advance in control, for total cure rate has reached only 67.7 percent in the 1983 analysis from the earlier report of the 1962 to 1968 analysis, which showed a 63.0 percent 5-year survival. We must not be complacent about the cure of this disease, although some individual institutions have reported relatively high cure rates, reaching 90 percent for stage I disease.

HORMONAL TREATMENT

Recurrence

Kelly and Baker (1960) reported that pharmacologic doses of progestin could induce regression of metastatic endometrial cancer. This was especially true for lung metastasis, somewhat less effective in bone disease, and rather poorly active in regional soft tissue recurrence. Medroxyprogesterone caproate (Delalutin) at a dose of 500 mg twice a week has been most widely used, although in recent years Provera 200 mg/day or Megace 160 mg/day have been used with equal effect. At least 12 weeks of such a loading dose is required, after which maintenance therapy may be modified for an indefinite period.

Much experience with this treatment has been reported since that time with a regression rate of 31 to 34 percent overall. Pulmonary nodules may regress completely, and the regression may persist for long periods, as much as 2 to 5 years. Several factors concerning response have come from this earlier experience:

1. Pulmonary metastases are most favorable for such treatment.
2. Bone metastases are less favorable, and soft tissue recurrence is still less responsive.
3. Those subjects with a prolonged interval from primary disease to recurrence are favorable for such treatment.
4. Differentiated lesions respond better than undifferentiated ones.
5. Recurrent disease is more responsive than primary metastatic disease.
6. In contrast to chemotherapy these hormonal regimens have low toxicity and the medication is well tolerated over long periods; therefore, few patients will abandon treatment.

Advances in knowledge of steroid metabolism have made assay of estrogen and progesterone receptors important in the primary tumor and, if possible, in the recurrence. It can be demonstrated in this tumor, as in breast cancer, that those with high levels of progesterone receptor will usually respond to progestin therapy, while those with low levels or absence of receptors will usually fail (Fig. 5-10). Unfortunately, experience has shown that poorly differentiated tumors contain receptors only infrequently. Since these are the most virulent tumors, the prognosis for these patients is poor, while the differentiated tumors with high levels of receptors are readily cured by surgery without resort to hormonal treatment.

Studies are under way in an attempt to increase the cytosol and nuclear estradiol receptor and progesterone receptor levels or to prevent their decrease in some cases by priming with estrogen before treatment

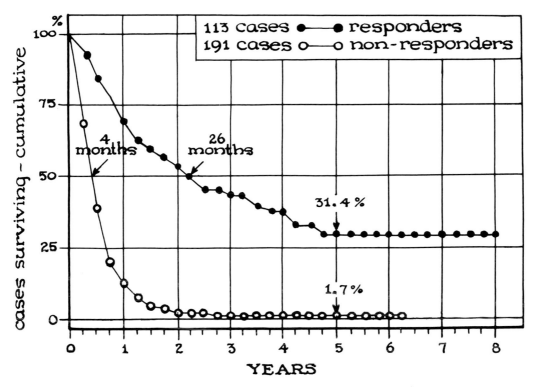

Fig. 15-10 Metastatic endometrial cancer survival after progestin treatment. (Refenstein EC: Treatment of advanced endometrial cancer with hydroxyprogesterone correate. Gynecol Oncol 2:377, 1974.)

with progestin, or by administration of tamoxifen, a nonsteroidal synthetic antiestrogen that can increase the progesterone receptor.

Antiestrogens such as tamoxifen can also block the proliferative stimulus of estrogen by blocking its interaction with receptor though a small percentage of tumors will have estrogen receptors without progesterone receptors. Endometrial carcinoma unresponsive to progestin or to cytotoxic chemotherapy may respond to tamoxifen.

The hormonal milieu can be deterred further by aminoglutethimide. This reduces all adrenal steroid production by blocking the primary conversion of cholesterol to pregnenolone and it selectively inhibits androstenedione aromitization to estrone. Replacement therapy with corticosteroid is necessary. Reports are now appearing of its use alone or in combination with tamoxifen in advanced endometrial disease, but most efforts are still investigational and require appropriate clinical trials to establish therapeutic value.

Our group has shown that the induction of 17 β-dehydrogenase by a test dose of Provera, 60 mg/day for 3 days, will also offer an index of tumor responsiveness to progestin. One can say that the disappointment over the poor prognosis of less differentiated tumors that may fail hormonal therapy, must by tempered by the precision of therapeutic choice allowed, offering the opportunity to switch to another cytotoxic nonhormonal chemotherapy.

The role of androgens in the etiology and treatment of endometrial cancer is speculative. In vitro studies show an inhibitory effect of androsterone on growth of these tumor cells in tissue culture, and a specific cytosol receptor for dehydrotestosterone has been demonstrated. Such studies have not provided a substantial basis for renewed clinical trials where earlier ones have failed.

Primary endometrial cancer has also been the recent target of hormonal treatment although reports have been sporadic or generally poorly controlled. Occasionally, this disease appears in young women.

These tumors often appear to be hormone dependent for they occur in subjects with failure of ovulation and they tend to be well differentiated and local. Because of the low virulence of such tumors, some have been tempted to offer hormone treatment alone by large and continuous doses of progestin in an effort to spare these young women hysterectomy with loss of fertility and even castration. Theoretically, such an effort would appear worthwhile, but reports of success have been fragmentary, and some of the lesions successfully treated, on review have proven to be adenomatous hyperplasia. A careful clinical trial is needed, but case finding is small, some tumors are more virulent, and few gynecologists have been willing to take the risk of delayed treatment and persistent disease.

There are some young patients who will plead to take this risk. If such a trial is to be made in a patient with failure of ovulation and typical hormonal intolerance, she should be counseled carefully about the risk/benefit ratio. Fractional curettage under anesthesia is necessary for complete tissue sampling to seek possible heterogeneity of the tumor because of the importance of tumor differentiation, and of course, receptor assay is now mandatory. A program of treatment may be planned with daily progestin in the order of 50 to 100 mg medroxyprogesterone acetate, or 40 mg megestrol acetate, with repeat endometrial biopsy in 3 months and formal curettage in 6 months for monitoring. If no disease is found in 6 months, treatment may be continued at half-dose and another curettage performed at 1 year.

Two negative curettage samples would persuade us to offer maintenance therapy of 10 mg Provera daily for another 6 months and then to allow escape for possible return to normal ovulation and fertility. Clearly, one would abandon the trial if curetted tissue were positive at 6 months or 1 year and advise surgical treatment. Hormonal treatment alone in these young women must be regarded as investigational, to be undertaken, if at all, in a controlled clinical trial by experts.

Adjuvant hormonal treatment has been used in primary disease, after standard surgical treatment and several favorable, if tentative, reports have been published. That progestin can help all such patients is unproven as yet, but the knowledge that high levels of progesterone receptor (≥ 50 fmoles/mg protein) in recurrent or metastatic disease usually indicate responsiveness to progestin has induced the hope that a subgroup can be found in primary disease that can be helped by adjuvant hormonal treatment after standard therapy. This might possibly benefit all such individuals, but it would be most important in those with high virulence factors or advanced disease at the onset.

CHEMOTHERAPY

Cytotoxic chemotherapy may be useful for disseminated disease that is not hormone dependent and for patients with positive paraaortic lymph nodes in combination with a progestin. Since the action of such chemotherapy is mediated by means other than steroid receptors, this modality of treatment can be used in both receptor-positive and receptor-negative tumors. Some recent studies have attempted to correlate response to chemotherapy with differentiation of the tumor, steroid receptor status, and location of the tumor. Most studies show chemotherapy to be most effective in poorly differentiated tumors (G_2 and G_3 lesions). One recent study showed that tumors with low steroid receptor levels responded better to cytotoxic chemotherapy, independent of histologic differentiation. If these studies are confirmed, treatment decisions can be made on a more rational basis, offering chemotherapy or hormonal therapy or combinations based on these parameters.

Adriamycin has been the drug most frequently studied in the management of advanced or recurrent endometrial carcinoma. As a single agent, it has induced response rates in the range of 19 to 37 percent. It has been used in combination with Cytoxan, Cytoxan and cisplatin, and Cytoxan and 5-fluorouracil (5-FU) with a similar range of response in controlled trials from 16 to 37 percent.

5-FU has also been studied extensively as a single agent and in combination. As a single agent, the response rate is about 20 percent. In combination with Adriamycin and cyclophosphamide and combined with melphalan, the response rates have been similar, about 35 percent.

Cisplatin has also been shown to have some activity in this disease, but the optimum dose and use as a single agent or in combination have not yet been adequately reported for analysis.

The superiority of combination therapy over single-agent Adriamycin has not been established. It is possible that chemotherapeutic agents in combination with hormonal medication, the formulation based on receptor data, tumor cell differentiation, and other parameters will permit future improvement in the response rate.

SELECTED READINGS

Anderson DG: Management of advanced endometrial adenocarcinoma with medroxyprogesterone acetate. Am J Obstet Gynecol 92:87, 1965

Arneson AN: An evaluation of the use of radiation in the treatment of endometrial cancer. Bull NY Acad Med 29:395, 1953

Arneson AN, et al: The use of multiple sources of radium within the uterus in the treatment of endometrial cancer. Am J Obstet Gynecol 55:64, 1948

Boronow R: Cancer of the corpus—Treatment at M.D. Anderson Hospital. p. 35. In Cancer of the Uterus and Ovary. Year Book Medical Publishers, Chicago, 1969

Brunschwig A, Murphy AI: The rationale for radical panhysterectomy and pelvic node excision in carcinoma of the corpus uteri. Am J Obstet Gynecol 68:1482, 1954

Corscaden JA: Gynecol Cancer. 2nd Ed. Williams & Wilkins, Baltimore, 1956

Corscaden JA, Tovell HMM: The management of carcinoma of the corpus. Am J Obstet Gynecol 68:737, 1954

DiSaia P, Creasman W: Clinical Gynecologic Oncology. CV Mosby, St. Louis, 1981

Graham JB: Discussed in Boutelis et al. Am J Obstet Gynecol 85:994, 1963

Gusberg SB: The problem of staging endometrial cancer. Obstet Gynecol 28:305, 1966

Gusberg SB, Yannopoulos D: Therapeutic decisions in corpus cancer. Am J Obstet Gynecol 88:157, 1964

Hawksworth W: The treatment of ca of the body of the uterus. Proc R Soc Med 57:467, 1964

Healy WR, Brown RL: Experience with surgical and radiation therapy in carcinoma of the corpus uteri. Am J Obstet Gynecol 38:11, 1939

Heyman J, Benner S: Further experiences with radiotherapy in cancer of the corpus of the uterus. Acta Radiol (Stockh) 27:328, 1946

Heyman J, Reuterwall O, Benner S: The radiumhemmet experience with radiotherapy of the corpus of the uterus: Classification, method treatment, and results. Acta Radiol (Stockh) 22:14, 1941

Kelley RM, Baker WH: Role of progesterone in human endometrial cancer. Cancer Res 25:10, 1965

Kennedy BJ: Progestogens in the treatment of carcinoma of the endometrium. Surg Gynecol Obstet 127:103, 1968

Kistner RW, Griffiths CT, Craig JM: Use of progestational agents in the management of endometrial cancer. Cancer 18:1563, 1965

Kottmeier HL: Carcinoma of the corpus uteri: Diagnosis and therapy. Am J Obstet Gynecol 78:1127, 1959

Liu W, Meigs JV: Radical hysterectomy and pelvic lymphadenectomy. Am J Obstet Gynecol 69:1, 1965

Morrow CP, DiSaia PH, Townsend DE: Current management of endometrial cancer. Obstet Gynecol 42:399, 1973

Nolan JF, Dorough ME, Anson JH: The value of preoperative radiation therapy in Stage I carcinoma of the uterine corpus. Am J Obstet Gynecol 96:663, 1967

Parsons L, Cesare F: Wertheim hysterectomy in the treatment of endometrial carcinoma. Surg Gynecol Obstet 108:583, 1959

Pratt JH, Symmonds RE, Welch JS: Vaginal hysterectomy for carcinoma of the fundus. Am J Obstet Gynecol 88:1063, 1964

Regaud C: Influence de la durée d'irradiation sur les effets determinés dans le testicule par le radium. Compt Rend Soc Biol 86:787, 1922

Reifenstein EF: Treatment of advanced endometrial cancer with hydroxyprogesterone correate. Gynecol Oncol 2:377, 1974

Rutledge F: Role of radical hysterectomy in adenocarcinoma of the endometrium. Gynecol Oncol 2:331, 1974

Simon N: Afterloading and radium substitutes. Gynecol Oncol 2:324, 1974

Stallworthy JA: Surgery of endometrial cancer in the Bonney tradition. Ann R Coll Surg Engl 48:293, 1971

Underwood PB Jr, Fenn JO, Wallace K, Travis E: Adenocarcinoma of endometrium. Role of pre-operative radiation in Stage I disease. Gynecol Oncol 2:71, 1974

Wade JE, Kohorn EI, Morris JMcL: Adenocarcinoma of endometrium. Am J Obstet Gynecol 99:869, 1967

Wentz WB: Effect of a progestational agent on endometrium hyperplasia and endometrial cancer. Obstet Gynecol 24:370, 1964

Whitehead MK, Townsend PT, Pryce-Davies J, et al: Effect of estrogens and progestins on biochemistry and morphology of post-menopausal endometrium. N Engl J Med 305:1599, 1981

16
Cancer of the Ovary

Gunter Deppe
W. Dwayne Lawrence

Ovarian cancer is the sixth most common cancer in women, accounting for about 4 percent of all female cancers. It is the leading cause of gynecologic cancer death in the United States and results in 5 percent of all deaths due to cancer. In fact, estimates are that 19,000 new ovarian cancer cases will be diagnosed in 1987 and that, of that number, 11,700 women will die of their disease; the latter figure exceeds the deaths due to endometrial and cervical cancer combined. The incidence rate for ovarian cancer rises with age and the greatest number of cases are found in the age group 55 to 60 years. The relative 5-year survival rate for both black and white women with ovarian cancer is 38 percent; this figure represents diagnoses through 1983, with follow-up on all patients through 1984.[1]

EPIDEMIOLOGY

Several recent studies have attempted to identify the high-risk patient for ovarian carcinoma. Epithelial ovarian cancer is principally a disease of industrialized Western civilization. In the United States, it occurs predominantly in older Caucasian women of northern European descent. The increasing incidence of this disease in better developed countries may be related to dietary and environmental factors, since immigrants moving from developing countries to more industrialized areas reportedly develop a higher incidence of ovarian cancer.[2,3] Environmental factors appear to be more important than ethnic factors in the genesis of ovarian cancer. Beral et al.[4] reported an inverse correlation between the national ovarian cancer mortality and the average completed family size; high death rates and small families have been observed in Sweden and Denmark, whereas low ovarian cancer death rates and large families have been seen in Bulgaria, Spain, and Japan.

RISK FACTORS FOR EPITHELIAL OVARIAN CANCER

High Risk
   Member of ovarian cancer-prone family
   More than 40 ovulation years
   Mother or sister with ovarian cancer

Significant Risk
   Age above 45 with nulliparity, or first pregnancy after age 30
   Late menopause
   Regular perineal exposure to talc

(Modified from Smith LH, Ol RH: Detection of malignant ovarian neoplasms: A review of the literature. 1. Detection of the patient at risk; clinical, radiological and cytological detection. Obstet Gynecol Surv 39:313, 1984.)

The concept of incessant ovulation, that is, the more frequently a female ovulates, the greater her risk of developing ovarian cancer, was first introduced by Fathalla.[5] Factors that decrease the rate of ovulation or prevent it, such as pregnancy before age 25, early menopause, and the use of oral contraceptives, appear to be protective against the development of ovarian cancer.[6] A diet rich in vitamin A and fiber may lessen the risk of ovarian cancer. Indeed, Byers et al.[7] reported a diminished intake of fiber and vitamin A by ovarian cancer patients aged 30 to 49 years. The protective effect of mumps was first suggested by West[8]; conversely, Cramer et al.[9] suggested that mumps may increase the risk of ovarian cancer.

Other possible risk factors include a history of ionizing irradiation to the pelvis, exposure to asbestos, and dusting the genital area with talc.[2,3] A positive family history of ovarian cancer is known to increase the likelihood of contracting this disease; in fact, the risk is increased by 20-fold in women with a sister or mother who had ovarian cancer.[10] Prophylactic oophorectomy might be considered for women with such a family history, once childbearing is completed. Such treatment, however, does not guarantee against the development of pelvic carcinoma. Indeed, Tobacman et al.[11] reported the occurrence of disseminated intraabdominal malignancy indistinguishable from ovarian cancer in 3 of 28 females, 1, 5, and 11 years following oophorectomy. These cases probably represent the development of pelvic serous carcinoma, arising from coelomic metaplasia, or endosalpingosis, of the peritoneum.

Ovarian cancer has been linked with carcinoma of the breast, endometrium, and colon. Either a short interval between the diagnosis of ovarian cancer and the subsequent development of breast, colon, or endometrial cancer, or their simultaneous occurrence, suggest a common etiology.[12,13]

SYMPTOMS

The woman with early ovarian cancer may have no, or only mild, symptoms unless a pathologic accident occurs such as torsion, intracystic hemorrhage, rupture, or possibly infection of the tumor. Insidious signs of early ovarian cancer as described by Barber[14] are shown below.

1. Vague abdominal discomfort
2. Dyspepsia
3. Flatulence
4. Bloating
5. Digestive disturbances

These gastrointestinal (GI) manifestations are nonspecific and may precede the diagnosis for several months. Any physician is obligated to rule out ovarian cancer in a woman who presents with continuous GI complaints that cannot be diagnosed. The usual manifestations associated with advanced disease are as follows:

Abdominal distention
Abdominal pain
Pelvic mass
Vaginal bleeding

Barber[14] draws attention to the following triad as an aid in the diagnosis of ovarian cancer:

1. Age 35 years or older
2. Persistent unexplained GI symptoms
3. Long history of ovarian imbalance and malfunction

In approximately two-thirds of cases, ovarian carcinoma has spread to involve contiguous pelvic and abdominal organs by the time of diagnosis. Such patients frequently present to the physician with the complaint of increasing abdominal girth secondary to either ascites or tumor mass, or both, and abdominal pain. Some patients experience vaginal bleeding.

SPREAD

Ovarian carcinoma spreads most commonly by intraperitoneal implantation and contiguous growth of tumor cells; lymphatic and hematogenous dissemination, however, may also occur.

The major pathway of dissemination is along the right paracolic gutter to the undersurface of the right hemidiaphragm. Obstruction of the diaphragmatic lymphatic system by tumor cells contributes to the development of ascites by impairing lymphatic drainage of the peritoneum. Transdiaphragmatic spread to lymph nodes on the thoracic surface of the diaphragm may lead to pleural effusion. Indeed, a right-sided malignant pleural effusion is frequently the first extraperitoneal manifestation of ovarian cancer. Often there is contiguous growth of tumor with extension to adjacent bowel, pelvic peritoneum, bladder, rectosigmoid, cecum, ileum, and omentum. Ovarian carcinoma usually invades superficially, with growth confined to the surface of the involved organs; mucosal involvement of the bladder and bowel is rare.

Small bowel obstruction in ovarian cancer patients is frequently caused by extrinsic compression of the bowel by large tumor masses and involvement of the myenteric plexus, leading to impaired motility. Increasing intraperitoneal tumor volume and progressive starvation contribute to death from ovarian carcinoma.

Retroperitoneal spread of primary ovarian cancer may occur through lymphatic pathways along the ovarian blood vessels to the paraaortic lymph nodes, through the lymphatic trunks within the broad ligament to the external iliac and hypogastric lymph nodes, or infrequently along the round ligaments to the external iliac and the inguinal lymph nodes. Wu et al.[15] found an overall incidence of positive retroperitoneal lymph nodes in 42 of 74 patients (57 percent) with various types of ovarian malignancies.

The hematogenous spread of ovarian cancer to the liver, bones, and central nervous (CNS) appears to be a late phenomenon. A recent review by Larson et al.[16] identified CNS metastases in only 13 of 4,456 patients with ovarian carcinoma.

PREOPERATIVE WORKUP

In the assessment of the patient with suspected ovarian cancer, several diagnostic studies are helpful before the patient undergoes surgical staging. Good clinical judgment, however, is necessary to select the most useful tests to avoid delay of the surgical exploration.

A complete history and physical examination, including a Papanicolaou (Pap) smear and rectovaginal examination, is recommended. Routine laboratory evaluation, with a complete blood count (CBC) and

---

PREOPERATIVE EVALUATION IN PATIENTS WITH OVARIAN CARCINOMA

History and physical examination
Papanicolaou smear of cervix
Complete blood count
Renal function tests
Liver function tests
β-hCG, alphafetoprotein, CA 125
Chest radiography
Intravenous pyelogram
Proctosigmoidoscopy
Barium enema
Upper GI series and small bowel series

---

hepatic and renal function tests, should be ordered. Serum markers, such as alphafetoprotein (AFP) and human chorionic gonadotropin (hCG), should be ordered as well, if the surgeon suspects a germ cell tumor. CA 125 may be useful in monitoring the subsequent course of the patient if the tumor is a carcinoma.[17]

The preoperative evaluation must include a chest radiograph. An intravenous pyelogram (IVP) is helpful to define the pelvic mass and to rule out ureteral obstruction or a pelvic kidney. A barium enema, an upper GI series, and an endoscopic bowel examination may identify a primary bowel carcinoma or impending obstruction secondary to an ovarian tumor. Ultrasound, computed tomography (CT), and lymphangiogram are unable to characterize tissue or detect masses less than 1 cm in diameter; therefore, they are seldom of significant help in the preoperative assessment and should not replace exploratory laparotomy as the definitive staging investigation.

STAGING

Staging of primary ovarian carcinoma is based on findings at clinical examination and/or surgical exploration. The Cancer Committee of the International Federation of Gynecology and Obstetrics (FIGO) recommends that both histologic and cytologic examinations be used in the staging when effusions are present; furthermore, biopsies should be taken from suspicious areas outside the pelvis. The most recently approved FIGO staging system (1985) for primary carcinoma of the ovary is outlined in Table 16-1.[18]

Primary Surgical Staging

Metabolic or hematologic abnormalities should be corrected prior to surgery. A mechanical and antibiotic bowel prep should be ordered for all patients with known or suspected ovarian tumor, since bowel resection may be necessary to accomplish adequate debulking.

The abdomen should be opened with a vertical midline incision and curved around the umbilicus. Consequently, extension of the incision cephalad for adequate assessment of the upper abdomen may be easily accomplished.

On entering the peritoneal cavity, any ascites encountered should be aspirated and sent for cytologic evaluation. If no free fluid is present, differential washings for cytologic examination are obtained from the cul-de-sac, from both lateral and paracolic gutters and the subdiaphragmatic areas. About 100 ml of normal saline is instilled for selective irrigation of each space. A soft rubber catheter connected to a bulb syringe is used for irrigation of the subphrenic spaces.

Next, the pelvic organs are inspected. Unless the primary tumor is unequivocally malignant or metastatic implants are present, the ovarian tumor is re-

Table 16-1 FIGO Staging System for Primary Carcinoma of the Ovary

Stage	Description/Features
I	Growth limited to the ovaries
IA	Growth limited to one ovary; no ascites; no tumor on the external surface; capsule intact
IB	Growth limited to both ovaries; no ascites; no tumor on the external surfaces; capsules intact
IC[a]	Tumor either stage IA or IB but with tumor on the surface of one or both ovaries; or with capsule ruptured; or with ascites present containing malignant cells or with positive peritoneal washings
II	Growth involving one or both ovaries with pelvic extension
IIA	Extension and/or metastases to the uterus and/or tubes
IIB	Extension to other pelvic tissues
IIC[a]	Tumor either stage IIA or IIB, but with tumor on surface of one or both ovaries; or with capsule(s) ruptured; or with ascites present containing malignant cells or with positive peritoneal washings
III	Tumor involving one or both ovaries with peritoneal implants outside the pelvis and/or positive retroperitoneal or inguinal nodes; superficial liver metastasis equals stage III; tumor limited to the true pelvis but with histologically proven malignant extension to small bowel or omentum
IIIA	Tumor grossly limited to the true pelvis with negative nodes but with histologically confirmed microscopic seeding of abdominal peritoneal surfaces
IIIB	Tumor of one or both ovaries with histologically confirmed implants of abdominal peritoneal surfaces none exceeding 2 cm in diameter; nodes negative
IIIC	Abdominal implants greater than 2 cm in diameter and/or positive retroperitoneal or inguinal nodes
IV	Growth involving one or both ovaries with distant metastases; if pleural effusion present, there must be positive cytology to allot a case to stage IV; parenchymal liver metastasis equals stage IV

[a] To evaluate the impact on prognosis of the different criteria for allotting cases to stage IC or IIC, it would be of value to know whether (1) rupture of the capsule was (a) spontaneous or (b) caused by the surgeon, or (2) the sources of malignant cells detected was (a) peritoneal washings or (b) ascites.

sected and sent for frozen-section examination. If the tumor proves to be malignant, careful systematic examination of all visceral and parietal peritoneal surfaces is carried out. This should include the paracolic gutters, the entire small bowel serosa from the ligament of Treitz to the ileocecal valve and its mesentery, the entire serosa of the large bowel and its mesentery, the omentum, the diaphragm, the anterior surfaces of the kidneys, and other visceral organs, including the pancreas, spleen, stomach, and liver. Lysis of adhesions from previous operations may be necessary to gain adequate access to these organs. A laparoscope may aid in inspection of the liver surface and diaphragm. Biopsy of visible lesions and scrapings for cytology should be obtained. If the omentum is not grossly involved, an infracolic omentectomy or large omental biopsy should be performed. We have found the LDS mechanical stapling device useful for this procedure. A total omentectomy is indicated if the omentum is replaced by tumor.

Selective paraaortic and pelvic lymphadenectomy should only be performed for proper staging or debulking. In the presence of abdominal implants greater than 2 cm in diameter or distant metastases, routine aortic and pelvic lymphadenectomy is not justified. A total abdominal hysterectomy and bilateral salpingo-oophorectomy is the preferred operation unless the patient desires to maintain her childbearing capacity and the ovarian carcinoma is stage IA and histologically well differentiated. An appendectomy frequently is included because adenocarcinoma of the appendix at times cannot be clinically differentiated from ovarian carcinoma.[19]

The goal of surgery in the treatment of ovarian cancer is to remove all the tumor, if possible, or to reduce tumor masses to 2 cm or less in diameter; to accomplish these objectives, bowel resection with anastomosis or diversion, or partial bladder resection with reimplantation of ureters may be necessary.

A retroperitoneal approach often permits adequate debulking. Mainly, the experience and judgment of the gynecologic oncologist will determine the extent of surgical debulking. The biologic aggressiveness and manner of spread of some cancers, however, make significant debulking impossible.

Improved survival rates may be related to successful cytoreductive surgery[20-25] (Table 16-2). Prospective randomized studies will be necessary, however, to assess the significance of surgical debulking.[26,27] After

Table 16-2 Correlation of Residual Tumor Size and Survival (Survival – Months)

Tumor Size (<2 CM)	Tumor Size (>2 CM)	No. of Patients
28	11	102
27	15	104
22	6	47
39	22	56

(Data from refs. 20–23.)

the surgical procedure, the volume, location, measurement, and number of residual tumor masses should be accurately recorded.

PATHOLOGY OF COMMON EPITHELIAL TUMORS

The common epithelial tumors are indeed the most common types of ovarian tumors, comprising two-thirds of all ovarian neoplasms and more than three-fourths of all malignant ovarian tumors. The epithelial component of the term reflects their supposed origin from the surface epithelium of the ovary. Although it appears deceptively innocuous on microscopic examination of the normal ovary, the latter has extraordinary metaplastic capabilities and its derived tumors can accurately mimic virtually any other tissue in the female genital tract. Thus, the relatively complex classification of common epithelial tumors that has evolved as new information about them has come to light. Since recognizing that the underlying ovarian stroma may also represent a neoplastic component, workers have added even more subtypes. Besides the contribution of the stroma, other criteria used to classify common epithelial tumors include (1) the cell type (i.e., serous, mucinous, endometrioid, clear cell, or transitional—Brenner); (2) the degree of malignancy (i.e., benign, borderline, or malignant); and (3) the architectural growth characteristics (i.e., exophytic and growing on the surface of the ovary and/or endophytic and growing into a cyst). Table 16-3 shows the World Health Organization (WHO) classification of common epithelial tumors of the ovary, derived from using these various criteria. A given tumor may show varying combinations of many of these characteristics; for example, an ovarian carcinoma may show areas of borderline neoplasia to

Table 16-3 WHO Histologic Classification of Epithelial
Tumors of the Ovary

A. Serous tumors
   1. Benign
      a. Cystadenoma and papillary cystadenoma
      b. Surface papilloma
      c. Adenofibroma and cystadenofibroma
   2. Borderline
      a. Cystadenoma and papillary cystadenoma
      b. Surface papilloma
      c. Adenofibroma and cystadenofibroma
   3. Malignant
      a. Adenocarcinoma, papillary adenocarcinoma, and papillary
         cystadenocarcinoma
      b. Surface papillary carcinoma
      c. Malignant adenofibroma and cystadenofibroma

B. Mucinous tumors
   1. Benign
      a. Cystadenoma and papillary cystadenoma
      b. Surface papilloma
      c. Adenofibroma and cystadenofibroma
   2. Borderline
      a. Cystadenoma and papillary cystadenoma
      b. Surface papilloma
      c. Adenofibroma and cystadenofibroma
   3. Malignant
      a. Adenocarcinoma and cystadenocarcinoma
      b. Malignant adenofibroma and cystadenofibroma

C. Endometrioid tumors
   1. Benign
      a. Adenoma and cystadenoma
      b. Adenofibroma and cystadenofibroma
   2. Borderline
      a. Adenoma and cystadenoma
      b. Adenofibroma and cystadenofibroma
   3. Malignant
      a. Carcinoma
         i. Adenocarcinoma
         ii. Adenoacanthoma
         iii. Malignant adenofibroma and cystadenofibroma
      b. Endometrioid stromal sarcomas
      c. Mixed mesodermal tumors

D. Clear cell tumors
   1. Benign
      a. Adenofibroma
   2. Borderline
   3. Malignant
      a. Carcinoma and adenocarcinoma

Continued

Table 16-3 WHO Histologic Classification of Epithelial
Tumors of the Ovary *Continued*

E. Brenner tumors
   1. Benign
   2. Borderline
   3. Malignant

F. Mixed epithelial tumors
   1. Benign
   2. Borderline
   3. Malignant

G. Undifferentiated carcinoma

H. Unclassified epithelial tumors

WHO, World Health Organization, 1973.

coexist with overtly invasive tumor; in addition, although the carcinoma is predominantly of serous type, foci of endometrioid carcinoma may be present.

Serous cystadenomas are variable in size but can reach large proportions. The external surface of the ovary is often smooth, pink-tan, and glistening, with a delicate vascular pattern. Many serous cystadenomas are unilocular, but occasional multiloculated forms are encountered. On section, the cyst is filled with a clear to straw-colored fluid, sometimes having a mucoid consistency. Examination of the inner cyst lining shows it to be smooth and glistening, although small papillary excrescences, generally few in number, may be present. Noncystic benign serous tumors, termed serous surface papillomas, may be encountered, arising from the surface of the ovary in the form of similar small papillary excrescences; although such lesions are usually focal, they may at times be widespread over the ovarian surface.

Microscopically, the serous cystadenomas are characterized by a cyst wall composed of either fibrous tissue or ovarian cortical stroma. The lining of the cyst wall is composed of epithelial cells closely resembling those of the fallopian tube; the epithelium varies in height from flattened to cuboidal to columnar, probably depending in large part on the intracystic fluid tension. Cilia are easily identified; psammoma bodies, small rounded calcific bodies with a laminated concentric internal structure, may be seen. Nuclear atypia is minimal. Serous papillomas arising from the cortical surface of the ovary have a similar histologic appearance.

Serous cystadenofibromas share many gross features with serous cystadenomas and may represent a subtype of the latter. As the name implies, the tumor is cystic and usually unilocular and frequently contains a clear serous-type fluid. Serous cystadenofibromas

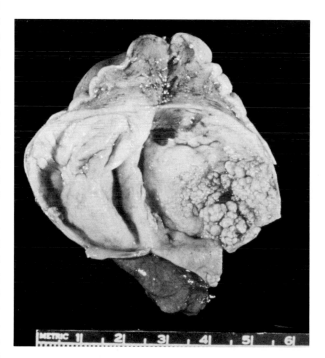

Fig. 16-1 Serous cystadenofibroma. The ovary has been bisected, exposing a cyst wall that is largely smooth and glistening; however, numerous broad blunt papillae project into the cyst cavity and did not appear grossly to involve the underlying cyst wall on section.

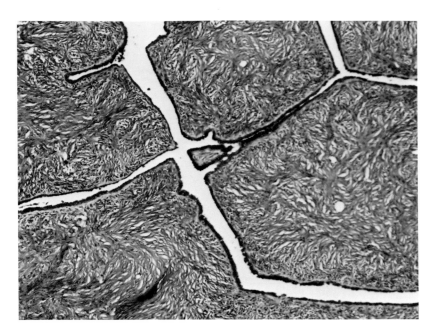

Fig. 16-2 Serous cystadenofibroma showing knobby blunt papillae composed predominantly of fibrous tissue, lined by an innocuous epithelium. On higher magnification, the latter was composed of pseudostratified columnar cells with cilia, reminiscent of tubal epithelium. (H&E, ×30.)

vary in size but have a mean diameter of approximately 10 cm. On section, the cyst wall contains variable numbers of rounded, firm, stubby projections extending into the cystic spaces (Fig. 16-1); the papillae usually cover less surface area than do those identified in serous cystadenoma and serous borderline tumors. On microscopic examination, serous cystadenofibromas are composed of broad, blunt papillae with a densely fibrous core covered by an innocuous lining of serous-type epithelium (Fig. 16-2). The papillae project into the lumen from the fibrous cyst wall and sometimes show extensive edema of the stromal cores.

The serous cystadenoma of borderline malignancy likewise may exist primarily as a cystic neoplasm or as a papillary exophytic growth projecting from the cor-

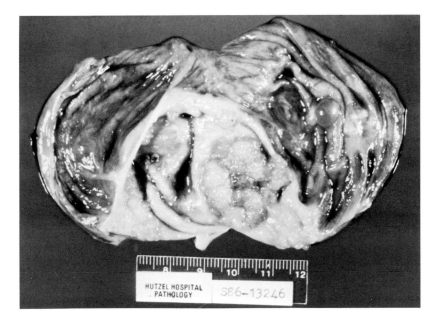

Fig. 16-3 Serous cystadenoma of borderline malignancy in which much of the inner cyst lining is smooth and glistening. However, irregularly shaped papillary excrescences that were soft and yellow project centrally into the cystic space.

tical surface of the ovary. The external surface of the ovary involved by the pure cystic form may appear similar to the serous cystadenoma; in addition, a similar clear serous to slightly yellow fluid may be present; however, serous borderline tumors more often contain a fluid having a thick mucoid consistency, at times raising the question of a mucinous tumor on gross examination. The cyst lining of the serous cystadenoma of borderline malignancy has more of its surface area occupied by exophytic delicate papillary excrescences than the serous cystadenoma; indeed, much of the lining may be occupied by the soft pink-tan tumor (Fig. 16-3). The histologic appearance of this tumor is characteristic; an exuberant markedly complex papillary tumor arises from the cyst wall and shows no evidence of underlying stromal invasion. The papillae are composed of fibrovascular cores lined by a serous type of epithelium showing cellular stratification, tufting, varying degrees of nuclear atypia, and generally low mitotic activity. The degree of papillarity is so striking that the plane of sectioning results in small, apparently detached, pinched-off buds of serous epithelium, a characteristic finding in these tumors (Fig. 16-4). Another trait, also arising from the extreme degree of infolding and papillarity, is the presence of areas of pseudoinvasion. Such areas, characterized by apparently isolated islands of glandular epithelium within the ovarian stroma, may be shown by serial section study actually to be connected to the ovarian cyst lining. A desmoplastic stromal reaction in such foci is virtually never seen in the serous cystadenoma of borderline malignancy; its presence is a more ominous sign of true invasion.

Serous papillary cystadenocarcinomas are complex neoplasms, frequently showing an admixture of both cystic and solid components; the former are commonly multiloculated and the inner surfaces entirely filled by exuberant papillary excrescences (Fig. 16-5). Necrosis and hemorrhage are often seen. The tumor may extend through the surface and form friable and necrotic papillary excrescences. Indeed, the tumor may replace one or both ovaries entirely and show spread to the adnexae and uterus. Serous papillary carcinomas often are large, more than one-half of which measure greater than 15 cm at the time of diagnosis.

On microscopic examination, serous carcinomas, as opposed to serous borderline tumors, show frank invasion of the ovarian stroma. Such foci of invasion

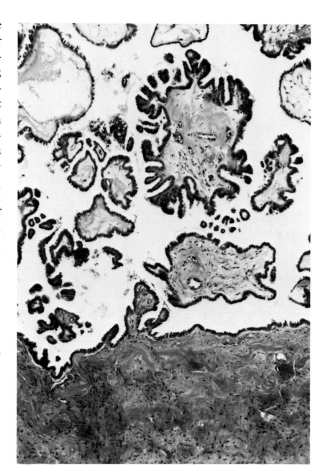

Fig. 16-4 Serous cystadenoma of borderline malignancy showing papillary fibrovascular stalks arising from the underlying cyst wall with no evidence of stromal invasion; the proliferating serous epithelium focally forms apparently detached pinched-off buds of tumor. (H&E, ×30.)

frequently are accompanied by a desmoplastic stromal response. Some workers grade ovarian serous carcinomas on a scale of 1 to 3, roughly corresponding to well, moderately, or poorly differentiated. Well-differentiated serous carcinomas have a predominant or exclusively papillary pattern; poorly differentiated serous tumors grow as solid sheets of anaplastic cells with minimal to virtually no papillarity; the moderately differentiated tumors are intermediate between the two and exhibit loss of fine papillarity with coarsening and fusion of papillae (Fig. 16-6). Psammoma bodies are present in approximately one-third of serous carcinomas.

As a group, mucinous neoplasms of the ovary tend

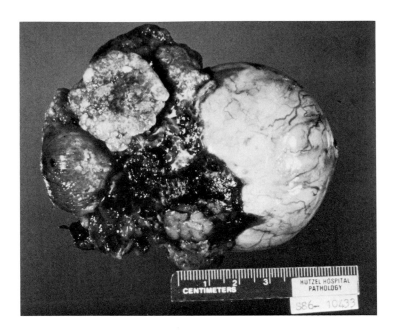

Fig. 16-5 Serous papillary cystadenocarcinoma showing a large fungating irregular tumor, with necrosis and hemorrhage, projecting from the ovarian surface. Section showed the tumor to have a cystic component.

to form the largest of the common epithelial tumors. Benign mucinous tumors are infrequently bilateral (fewer than 5 percent) and are multilobulated. Section shows them often to be multiloculated, in contrast to the characteristic uniloculation seen in benign serous tumors. The thin cyst walls usually have a smooth surface, and the locules contain fluid ranging from watery and mucoid to thick, viscid, and almost gel-like. On microscopic examination, the variably-sized cysts of the mucinous cystadenoma are lined by a single row of tall columnar epithelial cells with basally located nuclei. Little to no pseudostratification and crowding of cells are seen. The cells contain abundant intracytoplasmic mucin and are usually of endocervi-

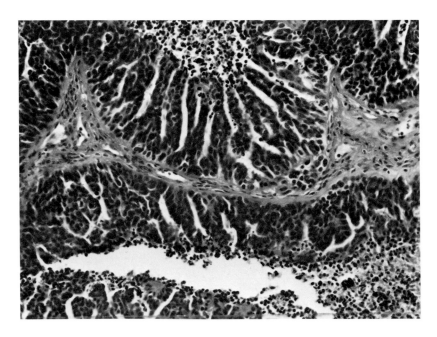

Fig. 16-6 Serous papillary carcinoma in which the tumor forms papillary projections and elongate cleftlike spaces. Central necrosis is prominent. (H&E, ×60.)

cal type, although GI-type mucinous epithelium, complete with goblet cells and Paneth cells, may be encountered.

On gross examination, mucinous borderline tumors (mucinous cystadenomas of borderline malignancy) are generally large and have a smooth external surface; as opposed to serous borderline neoplasms, mucinous borderline tumors rarely, if ever, display surface involvement. On section, mucinous borderline tumors are commonly multiloculated, displaying a more complex array of cysts than mucinous cystadenoma (Fig. 16-7). The contents of the variably sized cysts vary from clear and stringy mucoid fluid to viscid inspissated mucus. Some degree of papillarity may be present; necrosis is uncommon.

On microscopic examination, the mucinous borderline tumor may vary considerably from one area of the tumor to another; some foci may represent benign mucinous cystadenoma, lined by a single row of mucinous columnar cells, whereas others are more characteristic of the mucinous borderline tumor. The latter contain more complex cysts, many of which display papillary infolding, lined by stratified mucinous epithelium (Fig. 16-8). The epithelium is generally stratified two to three cell layers in thickness and nuclear atypia, manifested by hyperchromatism and pleomorphism, is usually present. The papillary formations may be delicate and fingerlike or tufted. As in the serous borderline tumors, there is no stromal invasion, but rather intracystic proliferation. Determination of stromal invasion, however, is more difficult in mucinous borderline tumors, since the cysts themselves are surrounded by stroma; a desmoplastic stromal reaction around irregular aggregates of mucinous glands is a helpful feature in identifying true stromal invasion.

Mucinous cystadenocarcinomas tend to be large heavy tumors, often measuring up to 40 to 50 cm in diameter. Section displays a markedly complex and varied surface; different areas resemble both the benign mucinous cystadenoma and the mucinous borderline tumor, and numerous variably sized cysts are present. Solid and necrotic areas as well as papillarity are more common and often represent the invasive component of the tumor.

Microscopically, mucinous cystadenocarcinomas may be well, moderately, or poorly differentiated. Differentiation between a mucinous borderline tumor and a well-differentiated adenocarcinoma may

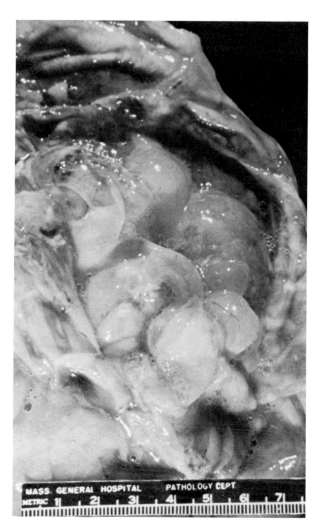

Fig. 16-7 Mucinous cystadenoma of borderline malignancy in which the cystic ovary has been opened and variably sized locules are present. A stringy mucoid fluid imparts a glistening appearance to the inner surface of the tumor.

be difficult. In the opinion of Hart and Norris,[28] intracystic stratification of cells greater than three layers within a mucinous borderline tumor warrants the diagnosis of carcinoma; this finding has clinical significance, since metastasis in that series occurred in such tumors without demonstrable invasion.[28] The finding of overt stromal invasion, present as irregular nests and cords of cells or as solid collections of back-to-back glands, mandates a diagnosis of adenocarcinoma. Well-differentiated mucinous adenocarcinomas are composed almost exclusively of

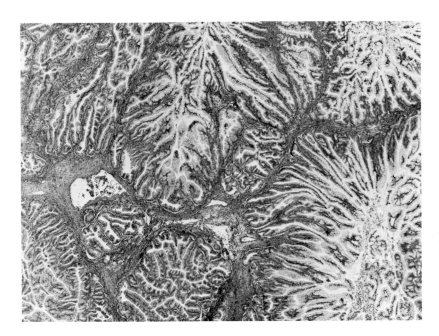

Fig. 16-8 Mucinous cystadenoma of borderline malignancy in which the locules are lined by a markedly complex papillary mucinous epithelium. No destructive invasion of the stroma was present. (H&E, ×12.)

well-developed glands lined by tall, columnar, crowded cells, often containing abundant intracytoplasmic mucin. Moderately and poorly differentiated adenocarcinomas show progressive loss of the ability to form glands, and in the latter much of the tumor grows in sheets with few to no readily identifiable glands.

According to several investigators, rupture of a benign or borderline mucinous tumor of the ovary virtually never results in pseudomyxoma peritonei; spillage of a mucinous carcinoma, however, can result in compromised survival of the patient. Most cases of pseudomyxoma peritonei are present at the initial surgical procedure, and the ovarian mucinous tumor is frequently accompanied by a mucocele of the appendix. The histology of the ovarian mucinous tumor as well as the tumor throughout the pelvic and abdominal cavities is often that of a mucinous borderline tumor. The appendiceal mucocele may contain mucinous epithelium varying in appearance from hyperplastic to a mucinous borderline tumor. The appendix may or may not show rupture or transmural extension of the tumor.

Endometrioid carcinomas possess no distinctive gross features to permit their delineation from other common epithelial tumors of the ovary. Many have cystic as well as solid components, frequently accompanied by hemorrhage and necrosis. Papillarity may

occur and is sometimes extensive. The presence of mucinous fluid within cysts may suggest the possibility of a mucinous tumor. Some endometrioid carcinomas are accompanied by, and apparently arise from, ovarian endometriosis; presence of the latter, however, is not a requisite for the diagnosis of endometrioid carcinoma. In fact, concomitant endometriosis is not identified in most endometrioid carcinomas. At times, however, endometrioid carcinomas may be seen arising from the wall of an endometriotic cyst, usually containing so-called "chocolate" fluid.

Microscopically, endometrioid carcinomas closely resemble their uterine counterparts, being composed of tubular-type glands (Fig. 16-9). In fact, to retain the purity of the designation endometrioid, ovarian carcinomas should not be designated as such unless endometrial type tubular glands are identified, if only focally, within the tumor. In addition, the presence of either benign or malignant squamous elements within the neoplastic glands virtually ensures the diagnosis of endometrioid carcinoma.

Concomitant endometrial adenocarcinoma and ovarian endometrioid carcinoma is a well-recognized phenomenon. Such an occurrence has been reported in approximately one-fifth to one-half of cases and most are probably best classified as separate primaries. Support for the latter theory is provided by the sometimes small noninvasive and well-differentiated

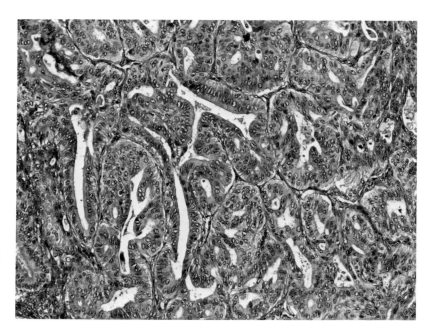

Fig. 16-9 Endometrioid carcinoma consisting of closely packed tubular glands identical to those of an endometrial adenocarcinoma. Cribriform areas, or glands-within-glands, are present. (H&E, ×60.)

tumors of the endometrium and the relatively good outcome in these patients, a finding that would be unexpected if one of the tumors represented a metastasis from the other.

Clear cell adenocarcinoma has no characteristic gross features, except that it is the common epithelial tumor of the ovary most frequently associated with, and arising from, ovarian endometriosis. Therefore,

an ovarian malignancy arising within a "chocolate" cyst has a higher likelihood of being a clear cell carcinoma, rather than an endometrioid carcinoma (Fig. 16-10). On microscopic examination, clear cell carcinomas have the same histologic patterns as those of other sites in the female tract; the tumor may grow in sheets of cells with clear cytoplasm, the clearing of the cytoplasm due to leaching out of intracytoplasmic

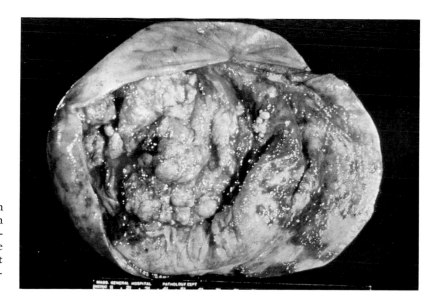

Fig. 16-10 Clear cell carcinoma in which the cystic ovary has been opened to reveal an irregular polypoid soft tumor arising from the lining. Darker areas within the cyst wall proved to be old blood associated with an endometriotic cyst.

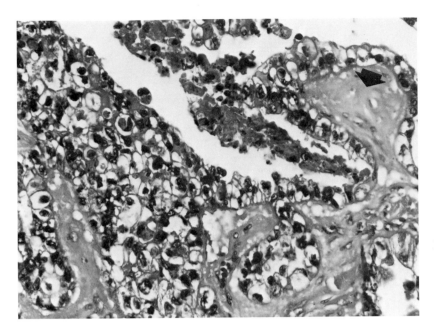

Fig. 16-11 Clear cell carcinoma showing solid sheets and nests of cells with clear cytoplasm and enlarged hyperchromatic nuclei. A papilla shows stromal hyalinization (arrow). (H&E, ×120.)

glycogen during processing or as peg or hobnail cells with prominent bulbous cellular apices (Fig. 16-11).

The Brenner tumor varies in size from a microscopic lesion, often discovered incidentally, to a large mass totally replacing the ovary. Although cystic forms of Brenner tumor are rarely encountered, most resemble fibromas and are firm, somewhat nodular, and yellow-gray on cut section.

On microscopic examination, the Brenner tumor is composed of varying proportions of fibrous elements and islands or nests of epithelial cells. The latter resemble transitional cells of the urinary tract (urothelium) and have oval "coffee-bean" nuclei with central grooves, resembling those of the granulosa cell tumor. Small cystic spaces lined by cuboidal mucinous-type cells may be found centrally within the urothelial nests.

A relatively common occurrence is the coexistence of a Brenner tumor with another cystic ovarian tumor; of the latter, the two most common such neoplasms appear to be cystic teratomas and mucinous cystadenomas.[29]

Both borderline and malignant forms of Brenner tumor have been described. The former has a histologic appearance similar to a grade I papillary transitional cell carcinoma, and the latter shows features of either a high-grade transitional cell or squamous cell carcinoma. The association of benign Brenner tumor with the carcinoma substantiates the origin of the latter from the former.

CHEMOTHERAPY

Traditional chemotherapy for ovarian carcinoma has consisted of single alkylating agents[30-34] (Table 16-4). Melphalan has been used most frequently be-

Table 16-4 Single-Agent Chemotherapy in Ovarian Cancer

Drug	No. of Patients	Response (%)
Alkylating Agents[30-33]		
Melphalan	494	47
Chlorambucil	280	50
Thiotepa	144	64
Nitrogen mustard	81	31
Cyclophosphamide	126	49
Antimetabolites[34]		
5-Fluorouracil	126	29
Methotrexate	34	18
Miscellaneous[34]		
Hexamethylmelamine	215	24
Doxorubicin	102	33
Cisplatin	190	32

Table 16-5 Combination Chemotherapy Versus Alkylating Agents in Advanced Epithelial Ovarian Cancer

Regimen	Response Rate (%)	Investigators
Hexamethylmelamine Cyclophosphamide Methotrexate 5-Fluorouracil	75	Young et al.[35]
OR		
Melphalan	54	
Cyclophosphamide Hexamethylmelamine 5-Fluorouracil	83	Delgado et al.[36]
OR		
Melphalan	58	
Doxorubicin Melphalan	67	Trope[37]
OR		
Melphalan	40	
Doxorubicin Cyclophosphamide	47	Omura et al.[38]
OR		
Melphalan	38	

cause of its ease of administration and reliable activity. No single alkylating agent has proved superior to another. Smith and Rutledge[30] reported a 47 percent response rate and 16 percent of responding patients alive at 5 years.

Several nonalkylating agents that have demonstrated activity against ovarian carcinoma include doxorubicin, hexamethylmelamine, cisplatin, 5-fluorouracil (5-FU), and methotrexate. Two newer platinum analogues, carboplatin and iproplatin, contain significantly less nephrotoxicity and neurotoxicity and are less commonly associated with vomiting. They may exhibit activity similar to cisplatin in the treatment of advanced or recurrent ovarian carcinoma.

The knowledge that various chemotherapeutic drugs act by different mechanisms led to studies on the effects of combination chemotherapy on ovarian cancer. Although most of these studies have shown combination chemotherapy to elicit a higher overall response rate[35-38] (Table 16-5) than single-agent therapy, no definitive survival advantage has been identified.

Numerous combinations containing cisplatin have been used in the treatment of epithelial ovarian cancer[39-42] (Tables 16-6 and 16-7). The important contribution of cisplatin in combination chemother-

Table 16-6 Combination Chemotherapy Including Cisplatin in Stage III/IV Ovarian Cancer

Regimen	Pathologic Complete Remissions N	Pathologic Complete Remissions %	Partial and Complete Response (%)	Investigators
Cyclophosphamide Doxorubicin Cisplatin	13	20	76	Omura et al.[39]
Cyclophosphamide Hexamethylmelamine 5-Fluorouracil Cisplatin	10	20	75	Louie et al.[40]
Cisplatin Adriamycin	13	43	76	Cohen et al.[41]
Cyclophosphamide Hexamethylmelamine Adriamycin Cisplatin	14	30	98	Greer et al.[42]

Table 16-7 Typical Dose and Schedule Used in Chemotherapy for Epithelial Ovarian Carcinoma

Regimen	Dose and Schedule (mg/M² IV q3wk)
Cyclophosphamide	500
Cisplatin	50
Doxorubicin	50
Cyclophosphamide	600
Cisplatin	100
Cisplatin	50–100

apy has been proved in three recent studies. In a randomized trial of cyclophosphamide versus cyclophosphamide plus cisplatin at the Mayo Clinic, the 2-year survival rate for cyclophosphamide alone was 19 percent compared with 62 percent for the combination.[43] A randomized trial from the Netherlands Cancer Institute (cyclophosphamide, hexamethylmelamine, Adriamycin, and cisplatin versus hexamethylmelamine, cyclophosphamide, methotrexate, and 5-FU) showed a statistically significant higher response rate, disease-free survival, and overall survival for the regimen containing cisplatin.[44]

Furthermore, the superiority of cisplatin combination chemotherapy has been statistically demonstrated in a randomized trial conducted by the Gynecologic Oncology Group.[39] One hundred twenty patients received cyclophosphamide and doxorubicin, while one hundred seven were treated with cyclophosphamide, doxorubicin, and cisplatin. The three-drug regimen achieved a statistically significant improved survival time (19.7 versus 15.7 months), and a complete response rate (51 percent versus 26 percent). In patients with stage III and IV ovarian cancer, a combination chemotherapy regimen can achieve an overall average response rate of 60 to 80 percent. Approximately 25 percent of these patients will have complete pathologic remission.

Patients receiving cisplatin combination chemotherapy benefit from a prolonged median survival time and progression-free interval compared with those treated without cisplatin; however, an increased cure rate of cisplatin-based combination chemotherapy has not been shown.

Drug regimens that add hexamethylmelamine to the combination of cyclophosphamide, doxorubicin, and cisplatin show no improvement in results.[42,44]

The toxicities of less active agents may prohibit the optimal use of cisplatin. Whether doxorubicin functions as a beneficial component of combination chemotherapy for ovarian cancer has not been elucidated.

Cyclophosphamide and cisplatin alone produced excellent results.[43] A randomized trial comparing cisplatin and chlorambucil with cisplatin, chlorambucil, and doxorubicin found no advantage from the addition of doxorubicin.[45] Conversely, doxorubicin and cisplatin were reported to be the most active agents in a study comparing doxorubicin and cisplatin with the three-drug regimen.[46] In a randomized trial, using cyclophosphamide and cisplatin with or without doxorubicin, the clinical complete response rate for cyclophosphamide and cisplatin was 20 percent, compared with 40.6 percent for cyclophosphamide, doxorubicin, and cisplatin. In 79 patients who underwent a second-look operation, 39.5 percent of the patients receiving cyclophosphamide plus cisplatin had a complete response in comparison with 62.2 percent of patients treated with the three-drug regimen. The better surgical complete response rate of the latter was statistically significant, but it did not improve survival or progression-free interval.[47]

The optimal point at which to perform second-look surgery is unknown, although the stage of the original tumor, the amount of residual tumor left at the primary operation, and the number of chemotherapy courses have been suggested to correlate with negative second-look procedures. Some workers have suggested that a second-look exploratory laparotomy be performed[48] after 12 courses of chemotherapy, usually about 1 year after the initial surgery; recently, however, others have proposed that the interval should be shortened to six to eight courses, or 6 months.[39,49,47,50] Patients with negative second-look operations have a recurrence rate of approximately 30 percent over the following 5 years.[51] Consolidation therapy using intraperitoneal chemotherapy or abdominopelvic radiation needs to be further investigated in this group of patients.

SINGLE-AGENT SECOND-LINE CHEMOTHERAPY

Many different single chemotherapeutic agents have been evaluated in the treatment of patients with advanced refractory ovarian carcinoma,[52,53] yet only a

Table 16-8 Active Single Agents in Advanced Refractory Ovarian Cancer

Drug	Evaluable Patients	Response (%)
Cisplatin[54,55]	21	42
	19	31
Carboplatinum[56]	28	25
Iproplatinum[57]	16	25
Hexamethylmelamine[58-60]	16	25
	49	16
	18	0
Bleomycin[61]	24	17
Etoposide[62]	22	31
Dianhydrogalactitol[63]	39	15

few drugs have demonstrated significant activity[54-63] (Table 16-8). Several investigators have reported favorable responses with high-dose cisplatin in patients who had failed on lower dosage of the drug. Cisplatin, at a dose of 120 mg/m², produced responses in 4 of 20 patients.[64] Similarly, 2 of 9 patients responded to cisplatin at a dose of 110 mg/m².[65]

Ozols and Young[66] administered high-dose cisplatin (40 mg/m²/day for 5 days in 250 ml 3 percent saline and 6 L/day saline hydration) to 19 previously treated patients with refractory ovarian cancer. Six of 19 patients (31 percent) responded to therapy (two clinically complete responses and four partial responses). The median duration of response was 5 months. The median survival for patients who responded to such therapy was 16 months, in contrast to 4 months for patients who failed treatment.

The dose of cisplatin appears to be a critical factor in the successful treatment of patients with advanced ovarian cancer; however, the use of high-dose cisplatin therapy is impaired by the dose-limiting toxic effect of peripheral neuropathy. The cisplatin analogue carboplatin was administered in a high dose (800 mg/m²) every 35 days in 30 patients with refractory ovarian cancer.[67] Objective responses were observed in 8 patients (27 percent), but no response occurred in patients who had progressive disease on cisplatin-containing regimens. The primary toxicity was myelosuppression, and there was no clinically apparent nephrotoxic or neurotoxic cross-resistance between cisplatin and carboplatin. Thus, carboplatin may be an alternative to cisplatin in the treatment of some patients with ovarian cancer who have preexisting renal dysfunction or have a potential to develop neurotoxicity.

SECOND-LINE COMBINATION CHEMOTHERAPY FOR ADVANCED OVARIAN CARCINOMA

Currently, no combination of drugs provides a significant survival advantage or better response rate than does a single agent in previously treated patients with advanced ovarian cancer. Active combination chemotherapeutic regimens[68-71] are listed in Table 16-9. Most of these patients had failed therapy with alkylating agents. Although some patients apparently respond to second-line chemotherapy, long-term survival is unlikely to result from this treatment.

Table 16-9 Active Second-Line Combination Chemotherapy in Advanced Ovarian Cancer

Regimen	No. of Patients	Response (%)	Investigators
Cyclophosphamide Hexamethylmelamine Doxorubicin Cisplatin	35	45	Kane et al.[68]
Hexamethylmelamine Doxorubicin Cisplatin	27	63	Vogl et al.[69]
Cisplatin Doxorubicin	24	42	Briscoe et al.[70]
Doxorubicin 5-Fluorouracil Hexamethylmelamine Cisplatin	29	48	Alberts et al.[71]
5-Fluorouracil Hexamethylmelamine Cisplatin	74	31	Alberts et al.[71]

INTRAPERITONEAL CHEMOTHERAPY

Intraperitoneal administration of chemotherapeutic agents has a potential role in the treatment of patients with ovarian cancer who have either microscopic or minimal residual intraabdominal tumor masses (<2 cm). This technique permits direct application of high concentrations of drugs to the tumor, obviating unacceptable host toxicity. Listed below are the properties of ideal drugs for intraperitoneal chemotherapy.

PROPERTIES OF IDEAL DRUGS FOR INTRAPERITONEAL CHEMOTHERAPY

1. Absence of local peritoneal toxicity
2. Steep dose-response relationship
3. Low peritoneal permeability
4. Capability of direct tumor kill
5. Rapid clearance from the plasma

Clinical trials with a small number of patients have been performed using 5-FU, methotrexate, doxorubicin, ara-C, melphalan, mitomycin C, and cisplatin.[72] With the exception of doxorubicin, which causes peritonitis at modest intraperitoneal doses, all other tested agents can be administered with acceptable associated toxicity. Cisplatin appears to be the drug of choice for intraperitoneal administration because of its lack of significant peritoneal toxicity and its activity in ovarian cancer. Twenty-three patients with small-volume residual tumor were treated intraperitoneally with 50 mg/m² cisplatin in 2 L fluid after cisplatin containing chemotherapy; six patients had a pathologically confirmed complete remission.[73]

Intravenous thiosulfate is an agent protective against cisplatin nephrotoxicity. Used with the intraperitoneal instillation of cisplatin, it permits administration of higher doses of intraperitoneal cisplatin, ranging from 150 mg to 270 mg/m².[74] A complete remission in 30 percent of 21 patients with minimal residual ovarian cancer following IV cisplatin combination chemotherapy has been achieved.[75]

Whether the potential benefit of thiosulfate, exposing the tumor to a higher concentration of cisplatin, outweighs the possible risk of diminished tumoricidal activity needs to be investigated. Prospective randomized studies will be necessary to compare intraperitoneal chemotherapy with or without intravenous chemotherapy to standard chemotherapy in patients who have primary or refractory ovarian cancer and minimal residual disease.

BIOLOGIC RESPONSE MODIFIERS

Biologic response modifiers are agents that may favorably alter the course of cancer, primarily through modification of the host response to tumor.[76] The biologic response modifiers include interferons; thymic hormones; immunomodulating agents, such as bacillus Calmet-Guerin (BCG), *Corynebacterium parvum*, and levamisole; tumor vaccines; monoclonal antibodies; cytotoxins; and tumor necrosis factor. Several preliminary adjuvant studies in the treatment of ovarian cancer have used a variety of systemic biologic response modifiers (BCG, *C. parvum*) and combination chemotherapy; the results have been inconclusive with regard to the contribution of biologic response modifiers to activity.[77-79]

Human lymphoblastoid interferons were given to 36 patients with recurrent ovarian carcinoma. Adverse reactions were acceptable and two patients had a complete response. Three patients had a partial response, while 14 patients had stable disease.[80] Intraperitoneal administration of β-interferon (IF_β) in eight patients with advanced ovarian cancer completely inhibited the formation of ascites in four of seven patients with effusions.[81] Although these early results are promising, further trials are necessary to establish a clinical role for biologic response modifiers in ovarian cancer.

HORMONAL THERAPY

Fifty to 75 percent of common epithelial ovarian carcinomas have either estrogen or progesterone receptors, or both.[82] Progestins are occasionally used to treat patients with advanced refractory ovarian carcinoma. Sikic et al.[83] administered megestrol acetate (800 mg/day PO for 4 weeks followed by 400 mg/day until tumor regression) to 47 patients with ovarian carcinoma; all had failed initial chemotherapy and 37 had received cisplatin-containing combination regimens. One complete and three partial responses were observed. The overall response rate was 8 percent, lasting 4 to 18 months. Using high-dose megestrol acetate in a similar fashion, Geisler[84,85] observed a response in 10 of 22 patients (45 percent), the duration lasting 4 to 65 months. Most of his patients had received only a single alkylating agent prior to hormonal therapy.

The Eastern Cooperative Oncology Group evaluated the response to administration of weekly medroxyprogesterone acetate (1,000 mg IM) in 19 patients with refractory ovarian carcinoma. None of the patients responded.[86] The major side effects in most trials of high-dose progestins are increased appetite and weight gain. Megestrol acetate can be used for palliation in patients with advanced ovarian carcinoma who have failed cytotoxic chemotherapy; the optimal dose and its potential use with primary combination chemotherapy or irradiation needs to be investigated further.

Meyers et al.[87] evaluated the antiestrogen tamoxifen in the treatment of ovarian carcinoma; these workers obtained a complete remission of 18 months and two partial responses in three patients who had failed prior cytotoxic chemotherapy. Of 813 patients treated with tamoxifen after chemotherapy failure, Schwartz et al.[88] noted a partial response for 8 weeks in one patient and prolonged stabilization for up to 100 weeks in four patients. No objective tumor regression was found in 23 tamoxifen-treated patients with ovarian carcinoma who had undergone prior chemotherapy. These patients were given 20 to 40 mg tamoxifen PO daily for a minimum of 8 weeks[89]; in 19 patients, the tumor remained stable for a period of 8 to 47 weeks, with a median duration of 17 weeks. The only toxicities noted were weight gain and edema. The duration of disease stabilization apparently was not related to the presence of estrogen or progesterone receptors. The small number of patients does not permit any conclusions; however, tamoxifen may stabilize the tumor for several weeks without significant toxicity in some patients with refractory ovarian carcinoma.

ROLE OF RADIOACTIVE ISOTOPES

Radioisotopes are instilled into the peritoneal cavity along with 1 L normal saline. The procedure is performed under fluoroscopy to ensure adequate distribution of contrast material; in the absence of adhesions, the radioisotopes should follow the dissemination routes of ovarian cancer and spread over all serosal surfaces.

Currently, radioactive phosphorus, a pure β-ray emitter with a half-life of 14 days, is administered at a dose of 15 to 20 MIC on the seventh to fourteenth postoperative day. Penetration and concentration occurs in the superficial 2 mm of tissue surfaces, and there is negligible systemic absorption. Intestinal obstruction and fistula formation are the major complications. In one series reported in the literature, radioactive gold, which has a half-life of 2.7 days and emits γ- as well as β-rays, was administered and 5-year survival rates ranging from 90 to 95 percent were achieved for patients with stage I ovarian cancer.[90,91]

The better utilization of chemotherapy largely has replaced the use of radioisotopes in the treatment of ovarian cancer; however, patients with ovarian cancer who are macroscopically free of disease and who have no adhesions to cause loculations may be treated by this method. In this selected group of patients, isotope therapy may accomplish results comparable to other treatment modalities.

RADIATION THERAPY

Several investigators have explored the use of external radiation therapy as a treatment modality for ovarian cancer[92-94] (Table 16-10). Since ovarian cancer spreads over all peritoneal surfaces, including the diaphragm, liver, and kidney, large radiation fields are required, and the tumoricidal dose usually exceeds the normal tissue tolerance. The moving strip and the open-field technique have been used for irradiation of the whole abdomen. With the abdominal strip technique, the abdomen is divided into a series of 2.5-cm contiguous segments, and the field is moved from one end to the other. At any one time, only a 10-cm segment of the abdominal cavity receives irradiation. The kidneys are shielded from the back as is the right side of the liver. The total dose to each strip

Table 16-10 Randomized Trials of Radiotherapy in Ovarian Cancer

Stage	Regimen	Radiotherapy Dose (Rad)	Five-Year Survival (%)	Investigators
I–III	Moving strip vs. Melphalan	2,800 abdomen +2,000 pelvis	71	Smith et al.[92]
IB–III	Pelvis vs.	4,500	47	Dembo et al[93]
	Pelvis + chlorambucil vs.	4,500	45	
	Moving strip	2,250 abdomen +2,250 pelvis	78	
IB–III	Moving strip vs. Open field	2,250 abdomen +2,250 pelvis 2,250 abdomen 2,250 pelvis	No difference	Dembo[94]

is limited to 2,600 to 2,800 rad delivered in eight fractions.

In the open-field technique, the whole abdomen is treated in one treatment portal, without liver shielding but with posterior kidney shielding, after 1,500 cGy. With both techniques, a pelvic boost (−2,250 cGy in 10 fractions) is given.

Both methods were compared in a randomized study at the Princess Margaret Hospital.[94] The investigators concluded that the moving strip and open-

Table 16-11 Postoperative Treatment in Patients with Epithelial Ovarian Cancer

Stage	Grade	
IA	1	No therapy
IA	2	Cisplatin
IB,C	1,2 (and residual disease <2 cm)	Cyclophosphamide
IIA,B,C		±Doxorubicin
		OR
		Abdominopelvic Radiation
		OR
		Intraperitoneal ^{32}P
IA,B,C	3 (and residual disease <2 cm)	Cisplatin
IIA,B,C		Cyclophosphamide
IIIA,B		±Doxorubicin
		OR
		Abdominopelvic Radiation
IA,B,C	3 (and/or residual disease >2 cm)	Cisplatin
IIA,B,C		Cyclophosphamide
IIIC		±Doxorubicin
IV		

field technique are equally effective; however, there were more late complications with the moving strip technique. The open-field technique is simpler and has a shorter duration of treatment. They also suggested that external radiation, a technique that encompasses the entire peritoneal contents, is the method of choice. Furthermore, patients with large residual tumor masses or spread outside the abdomen or involvement of the liver parenchyma should not primarily receive irradiation. Finally, they stressed that the dose of irradiation should be within limits of tolerance for the liver and bowel.

Whole abdominal irradiation has been attempted to salvage patients who have been treated previously with combination chemotherapy and are found to have persistent ovarian carcinoma at the second-look operation. In a series of 51 patients, including his own, who were discovered to have microscopic residual disease at second-look operation, Peters et al.[95] found 12 (24 percent) with disease-free survival; many of these patients, however, have been followed for less than 5 years.

Both chemotherapy and radiotherapy appear to be active and can be used in the postoperative treatment of ovarian cancer (Table 16-11). Irradiation techniques that include the entire peritoneal cavity can benefit, and sometimes cure, patients with minimal residual tumor volume. Prospective trials are necessary to determine whether (1) initial postoperative irradiation is preferable to chemotherapy for patients with minimal residual tumor, and (2) irradiation should be used simultaneously with chemotherapy or as consolidation therapy in patients with negative second-look operation but a high risk of relapse. The latter is more commonly associated with a poorly differentiated tumor, an advanced stage of tumor, or a large tumor mass prior to onset of chemotherapy.

IN VITRO DRUG-SENSITIVE TESTING

The use of a human tumor stem cell assay to identify active chemotherapeutic agents for individual patients with ovarian cancer offers potential advantages; however, the selection of chemotherapy on the basis of the assay has often been of limited value because of inadequate specimen growth. Since it has not been shown that assay-guided therapy is superior to empiri-

cal drug choice by the treating physician,[96] such an assay currently must be considered an investigational procedure.[96,97]

BORDERLINE OVARIAN TUMORS

The serous cystadenoma of borderline malignancy, also known as carcinoma of low malignant potential, is a tumor that is intermediate, in both its histologic appearance and biologic behavior, between the overtly benign and malignant serous neoplasms.[98] Whichever term is applied, there is justification for its existence, since patients with such tumors generally have a much better prognosis than do those with overtly malignant serous neoplasms. In fact, early studies claimed 10-year survivals of 79 to 91 percent for these tumors as opposed to approximately 25 percent for invasive serous carcinoma.[99] Even in the face of postoperative residual disease within the pelvis, patients with serous borderline tumor still had a 10-year survival of 75 percent, compared with 5 percent for overt serous cancer.

In a more recent study by Bostwick et al,[100] 109 patients with ovarian serous borderline tumors diagnosed from 1958 to 1982 were reviewed. The histologic types were 73 serous, 30 mucinous, and 6 mixed seromucinous. To date, only four patients had died of tumor. Patients with initial stage III serous borderline tumors recurred more frequently (64 percent) than did patients with lower-stage tumors (12 percent). Recurrences generally occurred within 5 years after the initial diagnosis, but recurrent tumor was diagnosed up to 19 years later. In a study of 76 patients with low malignant-potential tumors of the ovary, survival was similarly related to stage. Patients with stages II and III had a significantly lower survival than did those with stage I lesions. Mucinous tumors were less frequently bilateral (12.8 percent) than were serous tumors (48.3 percent).[101]

Of 61 patients (37 serous, 19 mucinous, and 5 mixed seromucinous) with stage IA borderline ovarian tumors, 41 were treated with total abdominal hysterectomy and bilateral salpingo-oophorectomy. Twenty-one were treated with cystectomy and unilateral salpingo-oophorectomy. After a mean follow-up of 89 months (range 36 to 244 months) subsequent recurrences developed in three patients treated conservatively and in two patients who had undergone an abdominal hysterectomy and bilateral salpingo-oophorectomy. At the time of the report, all 61 patients were alive and free of disease.[102]

Mucinous borderline ovarian tumors are frequently stage I. Staging includes inspection of all peritoneal surfaces, cytologic washings of the abdomen and pelvis, scraping or biopsy of the diaphragm, and a sampling of the pelvic and aortic lymph nodes.

Women with stage IA tumors who desire preservation of fertility may be treated by unilateral salpingo-oophorectomy if surgical staging, including evaluation of the contralateral ovary, shows no tumor. Hysterectomy and bilateral salpingo-oophorectomy with tumor debulking is recommended for patients with stages IB to IV.

For stage IA tumors, no adjuvant therapy is indicated because of their excellent prognosis.[102] The appropriate postoperative treatment for patients with high-stage borderline tumors remains controversial. The Gynecologic Oncology Group is currently conducting a study of the natural history of patients with ovarian tumors of low malignant potential. Melphalan is given to patients in the presence of clinically evident tumor or gross residual disease following surgery or if the patient is found to have progressive disease at the time of second-look laparotomy. Cisplatin chemotherapy is administered in patients who fail on melphalan therapy. Randomized prospective multiinstitutional studies are necessary to compare the results of debulking surgery alone with chemotherapy and irradiation therapy. Such studies, as well as investigation of the role of second-look procedures in the management of ovarian borderline neoplasia, are mandatory to define the best treatment.

GERM CELL TUMORS OF THE OVARY

According to the U.S. Third National Survey of ovarian cancer, germ cell tumors represent fewer than 5 percent of ovarian malignancies when considering all age groups.[103] Germ cell tumors, however, account for approximately two-thirds of malignant ovarian tumors in females under the age of 20. Furthermore, approximately 80 percent of germ cell tumors in patients younger than 10 years are malignant.[104] Much of the early work on the histogenesis of germ cell tumors was done by Teilum,[105] who proposed that such neoplasms originate from primordial germ cells and could give rise, in the female, to either dysger-

minoma or tumors of totipotential cells; the latter could then differentiate into embryonal carcinoma, which in turn could form neoplasms of extraembryonic structures (endodermal sinus tumor and choriocarcinoma), or embryonic structures (teratoma) (Fig. 16-12). Various combinations of germ cell tumors may ensue.

The World Health Organization established the currently accepted classification of germ cell tumors of the ovary in 1973.[106]

Significant characteristics of malignant ovarian germ cell tumors include rapid growth, frequent production of tumor markers (hCG, AFP, LDH), predilection for lymphatic and hematogenous spread, frequent mixtures of germ cell types and, with the

---

WORLD HEALTH ORGANIZATION HISTOLOGIC CLASSIFICATION OF MALIGNANT GERM CELL TUMORS OF THE OVARY

I. Germ cell tumors
 A. Dysgerminoma
 B. Endodermal sinus tumor
 C. Teratomas
  1. Immature malignant teratoma
  2. Mature cystic teratoma with malignant transformation
  3. Monodermal or highly specialized
   a. Struma ovarii
   b. Carcinoid
   c. Strumal carcinoid
   d. Others
 D. Embryonal carcinoma
 E. Choriocarcinoma
 F. Combination germ cell tumor
II. Mixed germ cell and sex cord stromal tumors
 A. Gonadoblastoma
 B. Others
III. Germ cell tumors arising in dysgenetic gonads
 A. Pure gonadal dysgenesis
 B. Mixed gonadal dysgenesis
 C. Turner's syndrome
 D. Testicular feminization

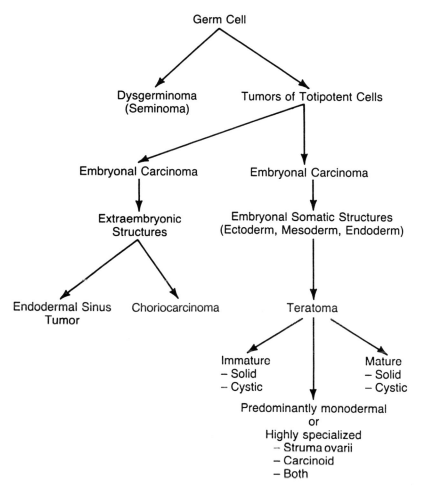

Fig. 16-12 Germ cell tumors of the ovary. (Modified from Teilum G: Classification of endodermal sinus tumor (mesoblastoma vitellinum and so-called embryonal carcinoma of the ovary). Acta Pathol Microbiol Scand 64:407, 1965.)

exception of dysgerminomas, predominantly unilateral development.

DIAGNOSIS AND WORKUP

The child, adolescent, or young woman with a malignant germ cell tumor typically presents with acute or chronic abdominal pain and a pelvic mass. Prior to puberty, an enlarged ovary may appear as an abdominal mass rather than a pelvic mass. After ruling out pregnancy, the workup should include the studies listed below. Often, time is critical and may not permit a thorough preoperative workup, since patients may present with an acute abdomen due to torsion or rupture of a rapidly growing, friable, malignant tumor.

METASTATIC WORKUP FOR OVARIAN GERM CELL MALIGNANCIES

Routine blood studies

Serologic tumor markers
  Human chorionic gonadotropin
  Alphafetoprotein
  Lactic dehydrogenase

Chest radiograph

Intravenous pyelogram

Optional studies (depending on clinical situation):
  Barium enema
  Sonogram
  Lymphangiogram
  CT scan

DYSGERMINOMA

Dysgerminoma is the most common malignant ovarian germ cell tumor, comprising more than 50 percent of such neoplasms. In a review of 158 dysgerminomas from the Johns Hopkins Hospital and Emil Novak Ovarian Tumor Registry, the patients ranged in age from 4 to 45 years; however, approximately 90 percent of patients were under age 30.[107] About one-third of all ovarian cancers discovered during pregnancy are dysgerminomas.[108,109] Approximately 14 percent of dysgerminomas have other malignant germ cell elements, usually immature teratoma, endodermal sinus tumor, and choriocarcinoma;[110] the latter two may produce AFP or hCG, respectively. Some patients with ovarian dysgerminomas have been reported to have elevated serum lactate dehydrogenase.[111,112]

Compared with other malignant germ cell tumors, dysgerminoma displays several characteristic features[113]:

1. Propensity for lymphatic metastasis
2. Unique radiosensitivity
3. Occult bilateral disease in 20 percent of stage I tumors

Dysgerminomas are predominantly unilateral and are more commonly encountered in the right ovary; however, at least 15 to 20 percent of dysgerminomas are bilateral. Dysgerminoma usually occurs in normally developed young women but occasionally may be associated with gonadoblastoma in dysgenetic gonads, Turner's syndrome, testicular feminization, ambiguous genitalia, and hermaphroditism.[110,114-116] At least one-half of gonadoblastomas have a coincident dysgerminoma, and there is purportedly a greater incidence of bilaterality in such tumors. The contralateral dysgerminoma may be microscopic in size and either not appreciated grossly at the time of surgery or missed by random biopsy. This supposition is supported by the subsequent occurrence of a dysgerminoma in up to 10 percent of contralateral ovaries in patients treated with unilateral oophorectomy for dysgerminoma.

On gross examination dysgerminomas form rounded to ovoid, often bosselated, masses around which a gray to white capsule may be appreciated. The capsule is usually intact; however, rupture occasionally may occur, especially in larger tumors. Dysgerminomas may vary in size from microscopic up to 15 cm in diameter. Section of the tumor shows it to be solid, firm, and rubbery, with a lobulated appearance; the color may vary among tumors, but most appear gray to pink-yellow to tan (Fig. 16-13). Cyst formation may occur rarely. The presence of hemorrhage and a more variegated appearance raises the question of other germ cell elements and mandates liberal sampling of different areas.

On microscopic examination, the typical dysgerminoma is composed of sheets and nests of large round to oval monotonous cells with pale eosino-

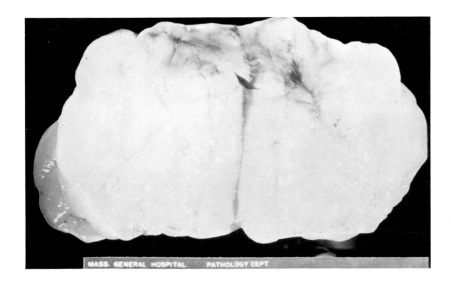

Fig. 16-13 Dysgerminoma. The ovary has been replaced by a lobulated tumor that on section was firm, gray-tan, and homogeneous.

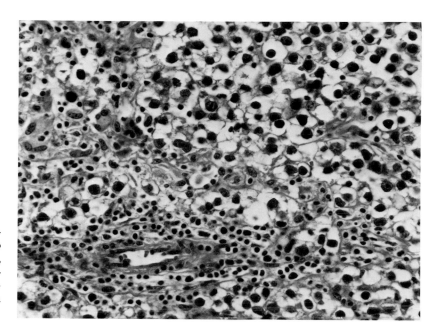

Fig. 16-14 Dysgerminoma showing sheets of monotonous round to oval cells with clear cytoplasm, centrally placed nuclei, and prominent nucleoli. A characteristic lymphocytic infiltrate is present within the fibrous septae. (H&E, ×120.)

philic to clear cytoplasm; the clearing of the cytoplasm is due to the presence of abundant intracytoplasmic glycogen (Fig. 16-14). Dysgerminoma is histologically identical to its testicular homologue, the seminoma. Varying numbers of lymphocytes frequently are observed in the stroma and in some cases they are so abundant as to form lymphoid follicles. Even sarcoid-type noncaseating granulomas may occur. Another cell type that may be seen in dysgerminoma is the syncytiotrophoblast-type giant cell; such cells may even elaborate significant quantities of hCG and be confused with choriocarcinoma. Diagnosis of the latter, however, also requires the presence of cytotrophoblast and significantly worsens the prognosis, whereas the mere presence of syncytiotrophoblast-type cells appears to have no influence on clinical outcome. Dysgerminoma may be confused with other entities, such as clear cell carcinoma, undifferentiated carcinoma, and histiocytic large cell lymphoma.

Selected patients with stage IA disease may be treated with unilateral salpingo-oophorectomy. All patients who do not fulfill the criteria listed below are treated most effectively with a total abdominal hysterectomy and bilateral salpingo-oophorectomy followed by irradiation.[117] A lymphangiogram or CT scan is required when patients have not undergone careful surgical and pathologic examination of pelvic and paraaortic lymph nodes. Postoperative radiation therapy consists of 2,500 to 3,000 rad to the whole abdomen and a boost of 1,500 rad to the pelvis and

---

DYSGERMINOMA: CRITERIA FOR CONSERVATIVE TREATMENT

1. Unilateral, nonadherent, encapsulated, unruptured tumor
2. Tumor size < 10 cm in diameter
3. Pure dysgerminoma
4. No ascites or positive cytologic washings
5. No evidence of extraovarian disease
6. Negative lymph nodes, negative contralateral ovary, and negative staging biopsies
7. Desire to retain fertility
8. No evidence of dysgenetic gonads or a 46, XY karyotype
9. Patient agreement for close follow-up

(Modified from Gershenson DM, Wharton JT, Kline RC, et al: Chemotherapeutic complete remission in patients with metastatic ovarian dysgerminoma. Cancer, 58:2594, 1986.)

paraaortic region. If the paraaortic lymph nodes are involved, the mediastinal and supraclavicular lymph nodes should receive 2,500 rad.

Survival in patients with dysgerminoma ranges from 75 to 90 percent.[107,117]Most recurrences occur within 2 years following initial treatment and abdominal, pelvic, paraaortic, and supraclavicular lymph nodes are the most frequent sites.[118] If possible, patients with recurrent tumor should be surgically debulked and receive subsequent irradiation or chemotherapy.

Cytotoxic chemotherapy has not been used frequently to treat dysgerminoma because of the exquisite radiosensitivity of the tumor. Several drug combinations have been used in the treatment of recurrent or metastatic ovarian dysgerminoma; the active combinations[119-123] are summarized in Table 16-12. Many of these reports are single case descriptions, yet

Table 16-12 Combination Chemotherapy Active in Ovarian Dysgerminoma

Agents	Investigators
Dactinomycin 5-Fluorouracil Cyclophosphamide	Krepart et al.[119]
Vincristine Bleomycin	Cohen and Goldsmith[120]
Vincristine Dactinomycin Cyclophosphamide	Weinblatt and Ortega[121]
Vinblastine Bleomycin Cisplatin	Jacobs et al.[122]
Vincristine Methotrexate Bleomycin Cisplatin Etoposide Dactinomycin Cyclophosphamide Vinblastine Hydroxyurea Chlorambucil	Newlands et al.[123]
Etoposide Bleomycin Cisplatin	Gershenson et al.[117]

it is probably reasonable to conclude that chemotherapy is helpful in the treatment of metastatic dysgerminoma; it can preserve fertility and may be successful as adjuvant therapy. The role of chemotherapy and its comparative effectiveness with radiation therapy will require prospective randomized multiinstitutional trials.

ENDODERMAL SINUS TUMOR OF THE OVARY

First described by Schiller[124] in 1933 as mesonephroma ovarii, this histologically unique tumor has been labeled with a variety of names, including angioreticuloma, mesoblastoma, embryonal cell carcinoma, extraembryonal teratoma, and malignant endothelioma.

Teilum[105,125] confirmed its extraembryonic nature and named the tumor endodermal sinus tumor since the glomerulus-like structure resembles papillae of the endodermal sinus in the rat placenta. It is the second most common malignant germ cell tumor and is encountered most frequently in young females, particularly from the first to third decades of life. Endodermal sinus tumor may be located at any point along the migratory path of the germ cell, accounting for some of the reports of extragonadal tumors. The tumor is capable of producing AFP in amounts that appear correlative with tumor volume.

Endodermal sinus tumor is most commonly unilateral and, like the dysgerminoma, favors the right ovary. Metastatic involvement of the contralateral gonad is not unusual, however, and careful inspection of the other ovary, with biopsy of any suspicious lesion, is mandatory before consideration of conservative therapy. Most endodermal sinus tumors are relatively large and bulky tumors, measuring more than 10 cm in diameter and frequently weighing more than 500 g.[116] Although they may be predominantly solid, cystic degeneration is a frequent phenomenon. Larger tumors, especially, tend to exhibit considerable hemorrhage and necrosis. Many endodermal sinus tumors have already spread beyond the ovary by the time of surgery; all too commonly, exploratory laparotomy shows the pelvis to be filled with soft, friable, and gelatinous tumor.

On microscopic examination, endodermal sinus tumors may exhibit a variety of histologic patterns;

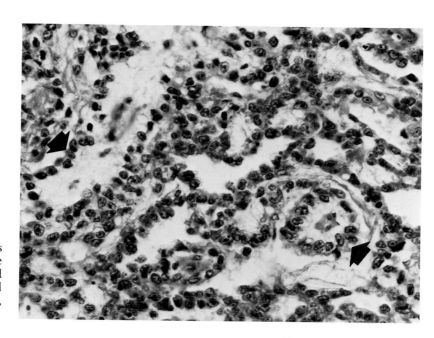

Fig. 16-15 Endodermal sinus tumor. The tumor forms a delicate reticular and trabecular pattern and pathognomonic Schiller-Duvall bodies (arrows) are present. (H&E, ×120.)

one pattern may predominate, or there may be a mixture of the different types. A loose myxomatous reticular pattern is seen in many endodermal sinus tumors, as are the characteristic Schiller-Duvall bodies; the latter mimic the endodermal sinus of the rat placenta and are composed of an elongate loose fibrovascular stromal core with a central blood vessel and a rim of primitive germ cells (Fig. 16-15). The cells may show clear cytoplasm due to the loss of glycogen and/or lipid during tissue processing. Extracellular and intracellular hyaline droplets are a frequent occurrence within endodermal sinus tumors. The droplets often stain positively with immunohistochemical stains for AFP and α_1-antitrypsin. In keeping with its highly malignant nature, the cells composing an endodermal sinus tumor are primitive and anaplastic with hyperchromatic and pleomorphic nuclei. Mitotic activity is usually brisk.

EMBRYONAL CARCINOMA

In the relatively recent past, the term embryonal carcinoma was used interchangeably with endodermal sinus tumor. In 1976, however, Kurman and Norris[126] described embryonal carcinoma as a distinct pathologic entity in the ovary. Embryonal carcinoma is characterized by production of both tumor markers,

AFP and hCG. Accordingly, symptoms of hormonal stimulation, such as precocious pseudopuberty, abnormal uterine bleeding, and amenorrhea, occur frequently.

Pure embryonal carcinoma is distinctly uncommon in the ovary, in contrast to its homologue in the testis, and more often represents a component within an ovarian mixed germ cell tumor. Embryonal carcinoma is encountered more commonly in young females; cases have been seen in prepubertal children under 5 years of age as well as in women in their mid-twenties. The average age of patients with embryonal carcinoma is 15 years as compared with 19 years for endodermal sinus tumor. As with most other germ cell tumors, it is usually unilateral.

On gross inspection, pure embryonal carcinoma is solid and gray-white; however, larger tumors especially may exhibit significant necrosis and hemorrhage. Embryonal carcinoma may coexist with other germ cell elements; accordingly, areas of hemorrhage may represent foci of choriocarcinoma. All the variegated areas of a germ cell tumor should be sampled liberally to ensure that the most prognostically significant malignant elements are recognized.

Microscopically, embryonal carcinoma has a similar appearance to its testicular counterpart. It represents the most poorly differentiated form of germ cell tumor; consequently, many embryonal carcinomas are composed of solid sheets of large anaplastic cells with abundant pale to clear cytoplasm and large, often hyperchromatic, nuclei. Numerous mitotic figures are usually present. This particular pattern, especially when the embryonal carcinoma is pure, may be confused with dysgerminoma. The former has less well-defined cell borders than dysgerminoma and lacks the characteristic lymphocytic infiltrate; distinction between the two is vital, however, due to their markedly different clinical courses. Glandlike and tubular patterns also may be seen in embryonal carcinoma, as well as papillary areas. Certain foci within embryonal carcinoma may differentiate toward endodermal sinus tumor, as well as choriocarcinoma, and indeed, such areas may stain positively for AFP and hCG, respectively. Hyalin droplets are a frequent occurrence in many embryonal carcinomas.

IMMATURE TERATOMA

Immature teratomas are rare as opposed to their mature benign counterparts, the mature cystic teratomas (Fig. 16-16); the latter, in fact, are the most commonly encountered ovarian tumor, yet immature teratoma comprises fewer than 1 percent of all ovarian teratomas. Like other germ cell tumors, immature teratoma may exist in a pure form or coexist in variable proportions with other germ cell elements in a

given tumor. Although immature teratoma may arise in the third decade, most appear in the first two decades of life. The almost invariable unilaterality of the immature teratoma is important in this regard, since the contralateral gonad may be conserved. A mature cystic teratoma rarely is present in the opposite ovary at the time of surgery or develops subsequently.

Gross examination often reveals the immature teratoma to be large at the time of discovery, ranging from 10 to 30 cm in diameter, and lobulated (Fig. 16-17). Although the tumor is essentially solid, careful inspection of the sectioned surface may show numerous small cystic structures scattered throughout the gray-tan to brown tissue. Grossly recognizable mesenchymal elements, such as bone and cartilage, may be present. In larger tumors, necrosis and hemorrhage may be prominent. Neural elements form a prominent component of many immature teratoma and are represented grossly by soft grayish tissue. The tumor may have extended through the surface of the ovary and invaded contiguous structures so that capsular adhesions may be present.

On microscopic examination, immature teratoma is characterized by the presence of tissue arising from all three germ layers: ectoderm, mesoderm, and endoderm. A common finding is the presence of mature elements within an immature teratoma; indeed, some of the latter are composed almost exclusively of mature teratoma and the immature elements comprise a

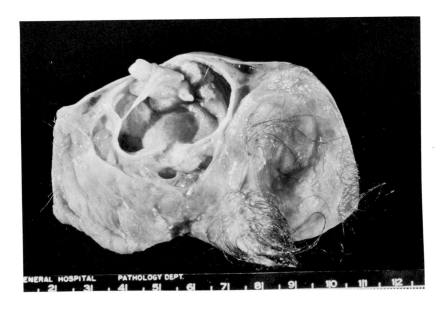

Fig. 16-16 Mature cystic teratoma (dermoid cyst). The ovarian cyst has been opened to reveal hair and well-formed teeth.

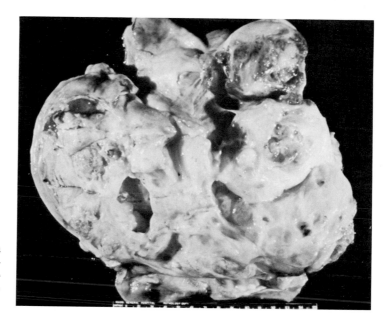

Fig. 16-17 Immature teratoma showing an ovary that has been replaced by a large irregular and focally cystic mass that has a variegated appearance after sectioning. Foci of necrosis are present.

minor component. Whatever the proportion of immature elements, they are represented by embryonic ectoderm, mesoderm, and endoderm; the first is commonly in the form of immature neural tissue, the degree of atypia of which frequently dictates the overall grade of the tumor (Fig. 16-18). Such tissue may be in the form of neuroblastic tissue, neuroepithelium, and atypical glia. Embryonic-appearing bone and cartilage, primitive mesenchyme, and immature GI and bronchial epithelium may constitute the mesodermal and endodermal derivatives.

Histologic grading of immature teratoma probably has prognostic value; currently, immature teratomas are graded according to the amount of immature tumor present as well as by its degree of atypia. The former is important clinically, since a given teratoma

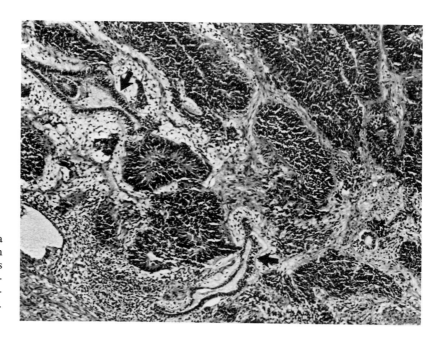

Fig. 16-18 Immature teratoma showing immature epithelium in the form of irregular neurotubules and rosettelike structures. Endodermal glandular elements are interspersed among them (arrows). (H&E, ×30.)

Table 16-13 Grading Systems for Immature Teratoma

Grade	Description
0	All tissues mature; no mitotic activity
1	Abundant mature tissue, but some immaturity mainly glial with loose primitive mesenchyma; mitoses present, but neuroepithelium absent or restricted to one low-power field (×40) per slide
2	Greater immaturity, with neuroepithelium not exceeding three low-power fields per slide
3	Severe immaturity, with neuroepithelium found in four or more low-power fields per slide and frequently merging with sarcomatous stroma

(Norris HJ, Zirkin HJ, Benson WL: Immature malignant teratoma of the ovary. Cancer 37:2359, 1976.)

may be largely composed of mature elements. This fact again underscores the necessity of liberal sampling of ovarian tumors, especially in the age group of patients susceptible to the development of germ cell tumors. Histologic assessment of the degree of differentiation within the immature elements is important in determining the grade of immature teratoma; brisk mitotic activity and immature neural elements usually are seen in more poorly differentiated tumors. A grading system of 0 to 3 is based on the aforementioned histologic evaluation[127] (Table 16-13).

Other germ cell elements including endodermal sinus tumor, embryonal carcinoma, and choriocarcinoma, may coexist with immature teratoma, representing another reason for proper sampling.

Immature teratoma should not be confused with malignant mixed mullerian tumor, which may arise rarely as a primary ovarian tumor or, more commonly, by metastasis. Malignant mixed mullerian tumors occur almost exclusively in postmenopausal women and would be exceedingly unusual in the age group likely to develop immature teratoma. In addition, coexistent mature elements are not present in malignant mixed mullerian tumor, and the latter often is composed of high-grade typical adenocarcinoma and sarcomas identical to rhabdomyosarcoma, chondrosarcoma, and osteogenic sarcoma rather than immature embryonic tissue.

POLYEMBRYOMA OF THE OVARY

Polyembryoma is an exceedingly rare germ cell neoplasm first described by Peyron[128] in a testicular teratoma. It may exist in either a pure form or, more commonly, as a component of a mixed germ cell tumor. The great majority of the few reported cases have existed in the latter category. As with other germ cell tumors, polyembryoma occurs primarily in young children and adolescents and less commonly in women in early reproductive life. Unilaterality is the rule. Since polyembryoma may have an associated trophoblastic component, serum levels of hCG and hPL may be elevated and result in endocrinologic symptoms. Takeda et al.[129] reported a case of polyembryoma of the ovary in a 9-year-old girl who presented with vaginal bleeding and pseudopuberty. Both the serum hCG and AFP were elevated.

On gross examination, polyembryomas are commonly solid tumors, varying in color from pink to gray; hemorrhage and necrosis are frequently present.

The microscopic picture of polyembryoma is quite distinctive; in the pure form, large numbers of so-called embryoid bodies, in varying stages of development, are found throughout the tumor. These structures are so designated because they recapitulate the early embryo, containing in the better-developed forms an embryonic disc, an amniotic cavity, and a yolk sac with associated extraembryonic mesenchyme. Less well-developed and atypical embryoid bodies may be present. In the type of polyembryoma mixed with other germ cell elements, the embryoid bodies are scattered among the various germ cell elements and teratomatous tissues.

NONGESTATIONAL OVARIAN CHORIOCARCINOMA

Primary choriocarcinoma of the ovary may arise on a gestational or nongestational basis. In the former case, the tumor may represent the rare sequela of a primary (ectopic) ovarian pregnancy or, more commonly, a metastasis from a primary uterine choriocarcinoma. Nongestational choriocarcinoma is seen more frequently than gestational engendered ones, however, and more likely represents one component of a mixed germ cell tumor. Bilateral choriocarcinomas are highly unusual. At least one-half of ovarian choriocarcinomas occur in young children, adolescents, and young adults. Those arising in prepubertal girls are almost certainly of germ cell origin, even when not accompanied by other germ cell elements.

Abdominal pain and distention, nausea, vomiting, and menstrual irregularities are frequently the presenting symptoms. A concurrent abdominopelvic mass and positive pregnancy test lead to an initial presumptive diagnosis of intra- or extrauterine pregnancy; the latter can usually be ruled out by ultrasonography. The general principles of preoperative workup and surgical therapy are similar for all nondysgerminomatous ovarian germ cell malignancies (Fig. 16-19). Serum hCG is always elevated in ovarian choriocarcinoma and should be used as a tumor marker to evaluate response to treatment. If other germ cell elements are present, determination of serum AFP and/or LDH levels may be helpful in monitoring the patient's course.

On gross examination, choriocarcinomas, whether pure or mixed, are characterized by hemorrhage and are usually solid but friable and necrotic. In a mixed germ cell tumor, the gross appearance of the remainder of the tumor depends on its components.

On microscopic examination, ovarian choriocarcinoma appears no different from those arising in other body sites. The presence of recognizable cytotrophoblast, as well as syncytiotrophoblast, is a requisite for the diagnosis, since syncytiotrophoblastic elements may be seen in a variety of other germ cell tumors. Cytotrophoblast, usually centrally arranged, is composed of round to polygonal cells with clear cytoplasm; syncytiotrophoblast rims the cytotrophoblast and is composed of large eosinophilic cells containing multiple nuclei. In the better differentiated forms of choriocarcinoma, a plexiform arrangement of the

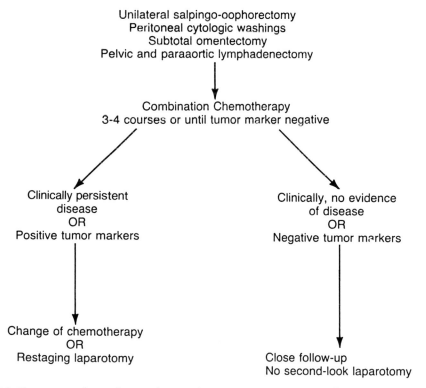

Fig. 16-19 Treatment schema for nondysgerminomatous ovarian germ cell malignancies (stage IA).

syncytiotrophoblast and cytotrophoblast may be seen; however, in poorly differentiated tumors there is less distinction between the two. Because of its hemorrhagic tendency, the presence of choriocarcinoma may be masked; consequently, particular attention should be paid to areas within, and especially at, the borders of markedly hemorrhagic areas within germ cell tumors.

STRUMA OVARII

Struma ovarii is defined as a monodermal mature teratoma composed predominantly of thyroid tissue; the latter may exist in the form of unremarkable thyroid tissue or in a hyperplastic or adenomatous form. Thyrotoxicosis is an uncommon complication. Malignant struma ovarii, present as a papillary or follicular carcinoma, is exceedingly rare and metastasis seldom occurs.[130]

CARCINOID

Primary ovarian carcinoids are unusual, are frequently associated with other teratomatous elements, and occur in fewer than 1 percent of ovarian teratomas.[131] Generally, these are unilateral tumors, although occasionally the opposite ovary may contain a benign teratoma or mucinous cystadenoma. The insular and trabecular forms are the most common histologic patterns. Approximately 30 percent of primary ovarian carcinoids with the insular pattern have been accompanied by the carcinoid syndrome of flushing, cyanosis, diarrhea, and hypertension. Since the venous return from the ovaries empties directly into the vena cava, bypassing the liver, patients with primary ovarian carcinoids may demonstrate manifestations of the carcinoid syndrome in the absence of metastatic disease. Primary ovarian carcinoids have a low malignant potential but must be differentiated from metastatic carcinoids that are almost always bilateral and associated with metastases to the peritoneum and liver.

On gross examination, primary ovarian carcinoids, whether of the insular or trabecular type, are often large and may measure up to 25 cm in diameter. They are almost invariably unilateral, although the contralateral ovary may contain a mature cystic teratoma.

When a carcinoid arises in a mature cystic teratoma, it appears as a well-defined solid yellow to gray-tan firm mass with a homogeneous cut section, surrounded by the other gross elements typical of mature teratoma.

On microscopic examination, the insular and trabecular carcinoids have different growth patterns; the former exhibits discrete islands and nests of uniform cells with ample cytoplasm and round to oval bland-appearing nuclei. Small glandlike structures, or acini, appear as punched-out spaces within islands of tumor. The cytoplasm may contain neurosecretory granules that stain positively by silver stains and have a characteristic ultrastructural appearance. Such midgut-type carcinoids may be confused with granulosa cell tumors (since the acini resemble Call-Exner bodies), metastatic GI tumors of the Krukenberg type (especially the relatively recently described tubular Krukenberg tumor), and metastatic carcinoid tumors. The latter group, however, are practically always bilateral and result in numerous scattered metastatic nodules within the ovary. Careful workup of such patients usually reveals the primary, which is commonly in the GI tract.

The trabecular pattern of carcinoid tumor is histologically distinct from the insular pattern and is characterized by elongated ribbons and cords of cells one to two layers in thickness. Cells within the cords have ample cytoplasm and round to oval bland-appearing central nuclei. The supporting stroma of the tumor often is densely fibrotic. The cytoplasm frequently contains refractile red-orange to brown granules that may be accentuated by silver stains or confirmed as neurosecretory granules by electron microscopic study. Trabecular carcinoid of the ovary may be confused with several entities, including primary endometrioid carcinoma, Sertoli-Leydig cell tumor and tubular Krukenberg tumor.

STRUMAL CARCINOID

An even rarer tumor than the primary ovarian carcinoid, strumal carcinoid represents an intimate admixture of thyroid tissue and carcinoid.[132] Occasionally, another ovarian tumor, most frequently a mature teratoma, is found in the opposite ovary.

Grossly, strumal carcinoid often is discovered as a variably sized yellow-tan mass in the wall of a mature cystic teratoma, or less commonly, a mature solid teratoma. On microscopic examination, strumal carcinoid is composed of a mixture of thyroid and carcinoid elements; the former may exist in the form of histologically normal appearing thyroid or as one of the variants of a follicular adenoma. In most cases, the carcinoid component of the tumor exhibits only a trabecular pattern; combinations of trabecular and insular carcinoid occur in the next order of frequency, and only rarely do pure insular forms arise.

There is considerable variability in the proportions of struma and carcinoid from case to case; some are composed virtually entirely of either component, whereas almost equal mixtures of the two constitute others. In most strumal carcinoids, the tumor types merge almost imperceptibly, and carcinoid elements are seen closely intermingling with thyroid tissues; less commonly, the two are in close juxtaposition without an admixture of elements.

MIXED GERM CELL TUMORS OF THE OVARY

Mixed germ cell tumors of the ovary are defined as neoplasms that contain at least two or more malignant germ cell elements. In Kurman and Norris's series,[133] dysgerminoma was the most common component (80 percent), followed in frequency by endodermal sinus tumor (70 percent), immature teratoma (50 percent), choriocarcinoma (20 percent), and embryonal carcinoma (15 percent). The most common combination was dysgerminoma and endodermal sinus tumor. Patients ranged in age from 5 to 33 years, with a median age of 16 years.

MALIGNANT TRANSFORMATION OF MATURE TERATOMAS

Mature cystic teratomas are benign tumors containing tissues of ectodermal, mesodermal, and endodermal origin. Malignant transformation may be suspected at the time of surgery by the presence of adhesions, thickened areas or solid nodules in the cyst wall, necrosis, or rupture. Malignant transformation occurs in 1 to 2 percent of benign teratomas, usually in postmenopausal women in the sixth or seventh decade. Any component of a teratoma may undergo ma-

lignant transformation; however, most are squamous cell carcinomas. Other malignancies that occur with any regularity are struma ovarii and carcinoid tumors.

Grossly, mature cystic teratomas harboring a malignant tumor are generally larger than the usual benign form. Such neoplasms are usually unilateral, and a benign mature cystic teratoma may be present in the contralateral ovary. A mature cystic teratoma containing a squamous cell carcinoma may show a large fungating exophytic tumor filling the cyst and extending through the wall to form tumor masses; the latter may grow into contiguous pelvic organs and form adhesions, an ominous sign of malignancy. Necrosis and hemorrhage may be present as well.

On microscopic examination, the most frequent tumor arising in mature cystic teratoma is squamous cell carcinoma, a not unexpected finding, considering the relatively large amount of squamous epithelium within most dermoid cysts. Occasionally, squamous cell carcinoma in situ, either alone or adjacent to invasive squamous cell carcinoma, is seen. Tumors that have been reported in mature cystic teratoma include, among others, sarcomas, adenocarcinomas, melanomas, basal cell carcinomas, and carcinoids.

TREATMENT OF NONDYSGERMINOMATOUS OVARIAN GERM CELL MALIGNANCIES

Approximately 75 percent of germ cell tumors are unilateral. Therefore, unilateral salpingo-oophorectomy after proper surgical staging (Fig. 16-17) is justified in young women who have stage IA tumors and are desirous of preservation of fertility. Patients with more advanced disease should undergo hysterectomy and bilateral salpingo-oophorectomy with debulking of the tumor (Fig. 16-20). In highly selected patients with advanced stages of disease, a normal contralateral ovary and uterus occasionally may be preserved.

Various combinations of postoperative chemotherapy have been used. The Gynecologic Oncology Group treated 76 patients with malignant germ cell tumors, using vincristine, actinomycin, and cyclophosphamide. Twenty-nine patients had endodermal sinus tumor, 2 had embryonal carcinoma, 17 had malignant mixed germ cell tumor, and 28 had immature teratoma. Fifty-four patients, treated with this three-

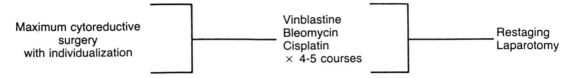

Fig. 16-20 Treatment schema for advanced nondysgerminomatous ovarian germ cell malignancies.

drug regimen after removal of all gross tumor were disease free at the time of that report. Conversely, another report describes 15 of 22 (68 percent) patients with incompletely resected germ cell tumors who failed treatment. Vincristine–actinomycin–cyclophosphamide chemotherapy appears to be considerably less effective in patients with bulky residual disease.[134]

Using vinblastine, bleomycin, and cisplatin as first-line treatment in 13 patients with pure or mixed malignant ovarian germ cell tumors, Taylor et al[135] reported 13 patients to be alive and free of disease from 20 months to 8 years after the initial diagnosis. One patient died of bleomycin-induced pulmonary toxicity.

Several investigators reported on the efficacy of the more toxic combination of vinblastine, bleomycin, and cisplatin using differing drug doses.[136-138] Initial short-term responses have been obtained with combinations of etoposide, actinomycin, and cyclophosphamide[136] (Table 16-14) or vincristine, methotrexate, bleomycin, and cisplatin in patients who failed with vincristine–actinomycin–cyclophosphamide and Platinol-vinblastine-bleomycin[136] (Table 16-14).

Table 16-14 Chemotherapy for Germ Cell Tumors

Regimen	Dosage	Investigators
Etoposide	100 mg.M² IV, days 1–5	Newlands et al.[136]
Actinomycin	0.5 mg IV, days 3, 4, and 5	
Cyclophosphamide	500 mg/M² IV, day 5	
Vincristine	Day 1: Oncovin (vincristine) 1 mg/M² IV Methotrexate 100 mg/M² IV, followed by Methotrexate 200 mg/M² as a 12-hour infusion	Newlands et al.[136]
Bleomycin	Day 2: Bleomycin 15 mg as 24-hour infusion, folinic acid rescue, 24 hours after the start of methotrexate in a dose of 15 mg every 12 hours for 4 doses	
	Day 3: Bleomycin infusion 15 mg by 24-hour infusion	
Cisplatin	Day 4: Mannitol, 3 gr magnesium sulfate IV, and hydration at 1 l/hr for 3 hours, then Cisplatin 120 mg/M² IV by infusion, followed by diuresis with Mannitol at 1 l/hr for 3 hours; hydration until patient stops vomiting	
Methotrexate	0.3 mg/kg, IV daily for 5 days, every 3 weeks (all three drugs)	
Actinomycin	8–12 μg/kg	
Cyclophosphamide	3 mg/kg	
Vincristine	1.5 mg/M², IV every 2 weeks	Slayton et al.[134]
Actinomycin	350 μg/M², IV daily ×5, every 4 weeks	
Cyclophosphamide	150 mg/M², IV daily ×5, every 4 weeks	
Vinblastine	6 mg/M², IV every 3 weeks	
Bleomycin	20 U/M² (max. 30 units) IV weekly	
Cisplatin	20 mg/M², IV daily ×5 every 3 weeks	

Prospective randomized multiinstitutional trials will be necessary to define which of the various drug combinations is superior.

Combination chemotherapy with methotrexate, actinomycin D, cyclophosphamide, or chlorambucil is being used routinely to treat early-stage choriocarcinoma of the ovary[139] (Table 16-14). Postoperative chemotherapy is advocated for patients with immature teratoma of grade II or III and for patients with malignant ascites or ruptured immature teratomas of any grade.[127] The Gynecologic Oncology Group postoperatively treated 37 patients with completely resected immature teratoma with vincristine–actinomycin–cyclophosphamide, and only two patients have failed treatment.[134] This three-drug regimen of chemotherapy is recommended only for patients with totally resected stage IA immature teratomas of grade II and III.

In patients with stage IA disease, a second-look laparotomy is seldom necessary (see Fig. 16-19). Conservative surgery and intensive short-term chemotherapy can achieve nearly 100 percent survival rates in patients with stage IA tumors, often preserving fertility. In those patients with initially elevated tumor markers that subsequently normalize during treatment, second-look laparotomy may be omitted, provided those markers are obtained monthly. The vincristine–actinomycin–cyclophosphamide regimen (Table 16-14) can be used in patients who are optimally debulked with no gross residual disease. If no tumor markers are present, 6 to 12 courses are administered. If tumor markers are available, at least one course of consolidation chemotherapy after tumor markers have become negative is indicated. The vinblastine–bleomycin–cisplatin regimen (Table 16-14) appears to be effective therapy for patients with more advanced immature teratomas and nondysgerminomatous ovarian germ cell malignancies, suboptimally debulked with gross residual disease. In those patients having tumors with serum markers, such as hCG and AFP, treatment should continue until all tumor markers have returned to normal; at least one, or if possible several, consolidation courses should be administered. In the absence of tumor markers, the optimal duration of treatment is unknown. Six courses of chemotherapy are suggested. Cumulative toxicity from cisplatin, manifested by nephrotoxicity and neurotoxicity, and bleomycin-induced pulmonary toxicity and myelosuppression will limit the duration of treatment with the vinblastine–bleomycin–cisplatin regimen. Since only 50 percent of patients with advanced disease are cured with combined surgery and chemotherapy, a second-look laparotomy should be performed in those patients at the completion of therapy. Thus, the status of the tumor may be adequately assessed and a decision made regarding the need for further therapy. Patients with negative second-look laparotomies should be seen and have tumor markers measured at least every 3 months for 2 years, then every 6 months for 5 years.

SEX CORD-STROMAL TUMORS

Ovarian sex cord-stromal tumors are derived from the gonadal stroma and account for approximately 3 percent of all ovarian tumors. They may consist of stromal cells, theca cells, granulosa cells, Sertoli cells, and Leydig cells either singly or in various combina-

---

CLASSIFICATION OF SEX CORD-STROMAL TUMORS

Granulosa-stromal cell tumors
    Granulosa cell tumor
    Tumors in the thecoma-fibroma group
    Thecoma
    Fibroma - fibrosarcoma
        Fibroma
        Cellular fibroma
        Fibrosarcoma
        Sclerosing stromal tumor
        Unclassified
Sertoli-Leydig cell tumors (androblastomas)
    Well differentiated
    Intermediate differentiation
    Poorly differentiated with heterologous elements
    Gynandroblastoma
    Sex cord tumor with annular tubules
    Unclassified

(Young RH, Scully RE: Ovarian sex cord-stromal tumors: Recent progress. Int J Gynecol Pathol 1:101, 1982.)

tions.[140] Many of these tumors are hormonally active and produce androgens, estrogens, progestogens, and other corticosteroids.

The WHO has proposed the term sex cord-stromal tumors to include those neoplasms formerly categorized as gonadal stromal tumors, sex cord mesenchyme tumors, and mesenchymomas. The nomenclature for this group of neoplasms has been controversial mainly due to dispute over the embryologic origin of granulosa, Sertoli, theca, and Leydig cells. Sex cord-stromal tumors are composed of these four cell types either in pure form or mixed in different combinations and degrees of differentiation; fibroblast-like cells derived from the specialized ovarian stroma also engender neoplasms that compose the stromal category of such tumors.

The sex cords are thought to give rise to the granulosa cell tumor and the Sertoli cell tumor, both of which have largely epithelial growth patterns, whereas the ovarian stroma, which contains not only supporting fibroblastic tissue but also specialized stromal cells, produces fibromas, thecomas and Leydig cell tumors.

Sex cord-stromal tumors are relatively uncommon as compared with the prevalence of the common epithelial tumors. The former comprise only 3 to 5 percent of all ovarian tumors yet they account for a substantial majority of the hormonally active neoplasms.

Granulosa Cell Tumors

Granulosa cell tumors are uncommon low-grade malignant neoplasms composed of granulosa cells, either alone or mixed with theca cells and fibroblasts. Granulosa cells in significant numbers are an essential feature for the diagnosis, yet the latter two cell types may comprise a substantial portion of the tumor. Granulosa cell tumors are hormonally active, most commonly estrogenic, neoplasms that may occur over a wide age range; however, the adult form is seen frequently in postmenopausal women, who may present with abnormal uterine bleeding. The endometrium in such patients may show hyperplasia or well-differentiated adenocarcinoma. The woman of reproductive age complains of menstrual perturbations such as menometrorrhagia or oliogomenorrhea; amenorrhea, especially when accompanied by breast enlargement and swelling, may raise the question of pregnancy in these patients. Conversely, the prepubertal patient presents with signs of isosexual precoc-

ity, including vaginal bleeding, accelerated growth, and breast development. Many of these patients (70 percent) have a clinically and histologically distinctive type of granulosa cell tumor designated the juvenile granulosa cell tumor; such tumors have a relatively benign clinical course, despite their aggressive histologic appearance, and must be recognized to preclude overly aggressive therapy.

Most granulosa cell tumors are unilateral, and 90 percent are stage I at the time of diagnosis. Although several different pathologic criteria have been investigated in order to predict biologic behavior, only tumor size appears significant. Although tumors less than 5 cm in diameter have been reported to have a uniformly good prognosis (10-year survival of 73 to 100 percent), there is a significant worsening of the prognosis in granulosa cell tumors measuring 6 to 15 cm in diameter (10-year survival of 57 to 63 percent). In one series, the 10 year survival dropped to 34 percent when the tumor was larger than 15 cm in diameter. Survival rate was not corrected for stage in these studies, however. Conversely, in a study from the Radiumhemmet, there was no statistically significant difference in 10-year survival between stage I granulosa cell tumors measuring 5 cm or less and those of larger size.[140-142] Studies to correlate nuclear atypia, mitotic activity, histologic pattern, and degree of differentiation with prognosis have yielded conflicting results.[141] Rupture of the tumor, however, has been associated with a significant worsening of the prognosis; in fact, Bjorkholm and Silfversward found the 25-year survival rate to drop from 86 to 60 percent in patients with unruptured versus ruptured stage I granulosa cell tumors, respectively. In the more acute situation, rupture may lead to hemoperitoneum that may be life-threatening.

The prognosis for patients with stage I disease is better than for those with metastatic disease; in one study, the relative 10-year survival rate for stage I granulosa cell tumor was 96 percent, as compared with 20 percent for patients with advanced stages of disease.[143]

On gross examination, granulosa cell tumors may have a variable appearance; probably the most commonly encountered one is that of a large multicystic mass, the cysts of which are variably sized containing serosanguineous fluid or frank blood (Fig. 16-21). A solid component may be present within the tumor and may be various shades of gray to yellow, the intensity of the latter dependent on the relative amount of lipid

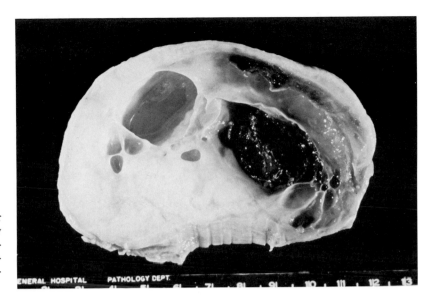

Fig. 16-21 Granulosa cell tumor showing an ovary replaced by tumor that is focally firm and homogeneous but in other areas contains variably sized cysts, some containing blood.

present. Indeed, large amounts of lipid, in addition to imparting a bright yellow color, may also result in a soft consistency. Conversely, those granulosa cell tumors containing less lipid and more fibromatous tissue are usually gray-tan and have a firm consistency. Less common forms include a large unilocular cyst and a multiloculated thin-walled cyst containing a serous-type fluid; the latter may be mistaken for a serous cystadenoma on gross inspection.[98] This tendency to cyst formation probably accounts for the common phenomenon of rupture, either spontaneously or during attempts at surgical removal.

On microscopic examination, granulosa cell tumors display several different patterns, some of which may be confused with other tumors. The most common is the microfollicular pattern, characterized by islands of granulosa cells containing angular irregularly disposed nuclei; many exhibit the distinctive nuclear grooves that impart to them the well-known "coffee-bean" appearance (Fig. 16-22). Within the islands and nests of granulosa cell tumors are small punched-out acinus-like structures known as Call-Exner bodies; these are rounded spaces, containing wispy eosinophilic material formed by the haphazard arrangement of nuclei to form a glandlike space.[98] The Call-Exner bodies must be differentiated from the true gland formation of adenocarcinoma, the acini of insular carcinoid tumors, and the spaces within adenoid cystic carcinomas.

As the name implies, the macrofollicular pattern is composed of large cysts containing watery eosinophilic fluid, the thin trabeculae of the cyst walls being lined by an attenuated layer of granulosa cells rimmed by theca cells. Both the architectural and the cytologic characteristics of this form of granulosa cell tumor are reminiscent of a follicular cyst.

The watered silk growth pattern is composed of elongate and anastamosing thin strands and cords of cells somewhat resembling the early sex cords of the developing male gonad. Less well-differentiated forms of granulosa cell tumors include a diffuse type in which granulosa cells grow in solid sheets without well-defined epithelial configurations; the nuclei, however, retain their angularity as well as their characteristic grooves.

The aforementioned juvenile granulosa cell tumor, a relatively recently described subtype, deserves special mention since its recognition may have clinical importance. As the name implies, the juvenile form occurs primarily in children and young adults; indeed, in the series by Young et al.[144] 85 percent occurred within the first two decades. The apparent immaturity of the granulosa cells in the juvenile form, manifested by often hyperchromatic nuclei and brisk mitotic activity, may result in the erroneous diagnosis of a more poorly differentiated tumor; another reason for overdiagnosis is the extensive luteinization of the granulosa cells, resulting in large eosinophilic cells with copious cytoplasm. In this age group, the most likely error would be the misdiagnosis of a malignant

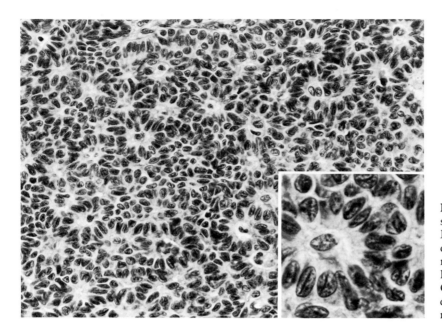

Fig. 16-22 Granulosa cell tumor showing numerous glandlike Call-Exner bodies, formed by granulosa cells loosely arranged around a connective tissue space. (H&E, ×120.) Inset: Higher magnification of Call-Exner body with granulosa cells containing coffee bean-shaped nuclei. (H&E, ×300.)

germ cell tumor with consequent aggressive surgery and chemotherapy.

Thecomas

Thecomas more often occur in women in or after the fifth decade; they are almost invariably unilateral. Estrogenic manifestations are frequently present and are the same as those of the granulosa cell tumor.

Grossly, the typical thecoma is a unilateral firm to rubbery solid tumor that varies in color from shades of yellow to orange, the intensity of which depends on the amount of contained lipid. Section shows it to be relatively homogeneous, often lobulated, and fairly well delineated from the surrounding ovarian tissue.

Thecomas are derived from the ovarian stromal cell and they, like other sex-cord stromal tumors, often contain minor granulosa cell elements. As their name implies, thecomas resemble the ovarian theca cell. Thecomas may exist in typical and luteinized forms. The former are characterized by the intimate admixture of two cell types; the more prominent is composed of plump oval cells with ample pale vacuolated cytoplasm containing abundant lipid. Intermixed are fibroblastic-type spindle cells, forming scattered hyalinized plaques of collagen.

The luteinized thecoma is distinguished from the typical thecoma only by the presence of nests of large, polygonal cells with pale eosinophilic cytoplasm (lutein cells); the remainder of the tumor resembles the typical thecoma. Many of the reported cases of malignant thecoma may actually represent other tumors, including diffuse granulosa cell tumors and the rare ovarian fibrosarcomas; caution should be exercised before making the diagnosis of malignant thecoma.

Fibroma

Ovarian fibromas usually occur in patients after the age of 40, are unilateral, and do not produce hormones. Fibromas may occur in young women with the basal cell nevus syndrome; the latter is characterized by bilateral, calcified, and multinodular ovarian fibromas, together with odontogenic keratocysts and basal cell carcinomas, which initially occur at a very early age and continue to occur throughout life.[140,145] Meig's syndrome (ascites and pleural effusion) accompanies approximately 1 percent of ovarian fibromas[140]; the pleural effusion and ascites disappear on removal of the fibroma.

Fibromas are usually unilateral, varying in size from focal microscopic tumors to large neoplasms that totally replace the ovary. The fibroma is frequently difficult to section and, in those cases with extensive calcification, may be impossible to cut until after decalcification (Fig. 16-23). The cut surface is

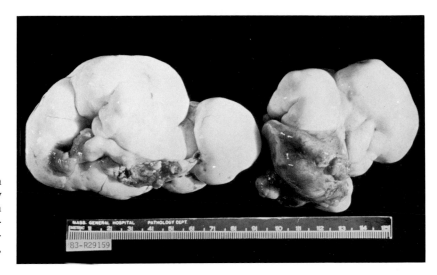

Fig. 16-23 Fibroma showing both ovaries replaced by an irregularly knobby and convoluted tumor with a glistening porcelain-white external and cut surface. Section revealed both ovaries to be firm, whorled, and homogeneous.

relatively homogeneous and whorled and may show foci of edema. Although calcification is fairly unusual, its presence, especially when extensive, should alert the clinician to investigate the patient for the basal cell nevus syndrome.

On microscopic examination, the typical fibroma shows interlacing bundles of spindle-shaped fibroblast-type cells; in contrast to the thecoma, the cells of which are plump, the cells of the fibroma have sparse cytoplasm, are relatively fewer in number than the thecoma, and are set in a background of dense collagen.

Mitotic activity within fibromas is generally low to absent; however, Prat and Scully[146] have reported recurrence in fibromas with increased cellularity and mitotic counts ranging from 1 to 3 per 10 high-power fields (HPF); furthermore, these workers concluded that cellular fibromatous tumors with more than four mitotic figures per 10 HPF should be classified as fibrosarcomas, since they tend to pursue a more aggressive clinical course. Such tumors were generally larger and more often adherent to contiguous organs.[146]

Treatment of Granulosa Cell Tumors

The standard treatment for the ovarian granulosa cell tumor is abdominal hysterectomy and bilateral salpingo-oophorectomy. Children and young women with stage IA tumors, however, should be treated by unilateral salpingo-oophorectomy if the opposite ovary appears normal and results of other staging biopsies (e.g., omentum, peritoneal washings, paraaortic lymph nodes) are negative. In one study, patients with ruptured tumors received postoperative irradiation to the pelvis and abdomen, and 80 percent were alive at 10 years.[147] The benefit of adjuvant radiation of chemotherapy in stage I tumors has not been proved. Patients with metastatic or recurrent tumors should be surgically debulked; if residual tumor masses are less than 2 cm, either postoperative radiation therapy or chemotherapy should be administered. The superiority of either method has not been established. Those patients with bulky residual tumor

Table 16-15 Combination Chemotherapeutic Regimens Active in Granulosa Cell Tumors

Regimen	Investigators
Doxorubicin Bleomycin	Barlow et al.[148]
Cisplatinum Doxorubicin	Jacobs et al.[149]
Dactinomycin 5-Fluorouracil Cyclophosphamide	Schwartz and Smith[147]; Slayton et al.[150]
Cisplatin Vinblastine Bleomycin	Colombo et al.[151]

masses or who have failed radiation therapy should receive chemotherapy. Combinations[147-151] that have shown positive results in a few patients are listed in Table 16-15.

Sertoli-Leydig Cell Tumors

Sertoli-Leydig cell tumors are rare neoplasms that occur most commonly between 20 and 40 years of age, although about 10 percent are encountered in perimenopausal or postmenopausal women[141]; the great majority of tumors diagnosed as Sertoli-Leydig cell tumors in this age group, however, are actually other types of primary or metastatic neoplasms. In one series of 36 cases,[152] the average age was 23 years, with a range of 4 to 67 years.

Sertoli-Leydig cell tumors frequently produce androstenedione and testosterone, leading to secondary amenorrhea, decreased breast size, hirsutism, acne, temporal balding, and clitoral hypertrophy. Estrogenic effects are rare. Novak and Long[153] described hormonal manifestations in 98 of 111 patients with Sertoli-Leydig cell tumors, and virilization was reported in 18 of 36 such patients by Young.[152] Manifestations of virilization usually regress or disappear after treatment. All the patients in the latter series had unilateral tumors with an average diameter of 14 cm.

Sertoli-Leydig cell tumors have no characteristics that permit their gross distinction from other types of sex cord-stromal tumors. Like most of the latter, Sertoli-Leydig cell tumors are virtually always unilateral. They may exhibit great variability in size, ranging from microscopic to more than 20 cm in diameter,[154] but most measure less than 10 cm in diameter at the time of discovery. Sertoli-Leydig cell tumors frequently appear to have a capsule and on section have a lobulated configuration. The cut section reveals either a predominantly solid or cystic neoplasm; solid areas vary in color from gray-tan to yellow, the latter being seen more frequently in tumors with large quantities of lipid.

Some tumors, especially the more aggressive ones, contain a more prominent cystic component; others are composed virtually entirely of either a unilocular cyst or multilocular cysts; larger tumors may have a higher frequency of cystic change. As in granulosa cell tumors, the cysts often contain serosanguineous fluid or clotted blood.

Microscopic examination shows Sertoli-Leydig cell tumors to display a wide variety of histologic patterns; the well-differentiated forms recapitulate the seminiferous tubules, forming either hollow structures or solid cords and tubules reminiscent of these seen in the embryonic male gonad. A less common but nonetheless distinctive form of tumor is the Sertoli cell tumor with lipid storage, in which the

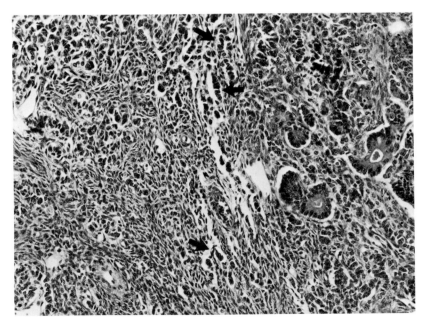

Fig. 16-24 Sertoli-Leydig cell tumor showing intermediate differentiation with heterologous elements. Much of the tumor is composed of sheets of spindled cells with foci of solid sex cords resembling the embryonic testis (arrows). Heterologous elements in the form of mucinous gastrointestinal-type glands are seen in the right portion of the photomicrograph. (H&E, ×60.)

tubular lining cells are pale and vacuolated; this appearance is attributable to the large amount of intracytoplasmic lipid that is lost during processing of the tissue.

Leydig cells are interspersed in variable numbers among and intimately associated with the Sertoli cell tubules. In some tumors, only scattered groups of Leydig cells are seen, whereas in others they represent a prominent contribution, equal to or greater than that of the tubular component.

The moderately differentiated forms of Sertoli-Leydig cell tumors currently have been designated as of intermediate differentiation. Although better differentiated hollow tubules may be seen in such tumors, the epithelial element more commonly is found in the form of thin cords and solid tubules similar to those of the embryonic testis; the latter may merge imperceptibly with the stromal elements, consisting of an intimate admixture of spindle and round cells (Fig. 16-24). In addition, easily identifiable Leydig cells may be scattered throughout the tumor.

Quite a variety of histologic patterns may result from the various combinations of different epithelial and stromal elements in the intermediate Sertoli-Leydig cell tumor; therefore, no one, or even several, histologic patterns typify them.

In the poorly differentiated form the stromal component predominates, and so much resembles a spindle cell sarcoma that in the earlier literature, it was described as sarcomatoid. Given the even greater rarity of pure ovarian sarcomas however, such a histologic appearance should raise the question of poorly differentiated Sertoli-Leydig cell tumors. Focal epithelial elements, as well as Leydig cells, usually may be identified after careful searching within the spindle cell stroma. Rarely, the epithelial element appears sufficiently anaplastic to warrant the diagnosis of Sertoli cell carcinoma.

Confusion in the diagnosis of intermediate and poorly differentiated forms is further abetted by the presence of heterologous elements, which may occur in either. Such elements occur in about 20 percent of Sertoli-Leydig cell tumors and include mucinous glands, skeletal muscle, and cartilage; these may be present in benign or atypical forms as well as malignant ones, such as embryonal rhabdomyosarcoma.[152] Sertoli-Leydig cell tumors with immature skeletal muscle and/or cartilage appear to have a poor prognosis. In a study by Prat et al.[155] 8 of 10 patients with such elements died.

The presence of heterologous elements, especially in young females, may cause confusion with teratoma, particularly immature teratoma. Other pathologic entities that may be confused with Sertoli-Leydig cell tumors include primary and metastatic carcinoid tumors, endometrioid carcinomas of the ovary, and the Krukenberg tumor, often metastatic from the stomach (Fig. 16-25 through 16-27). In the

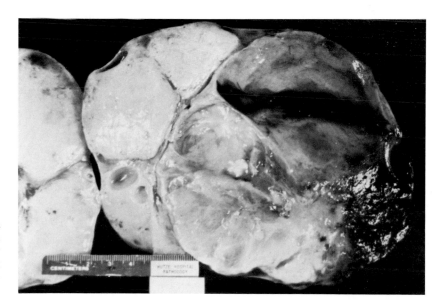

Fig. 16-25 Krukenberg tumor in a 30-year-old woman showing an ovary replaced by a lobulated tumor that was firm and yellow-tan. Cyst formation and hemorrhage (right) are present.

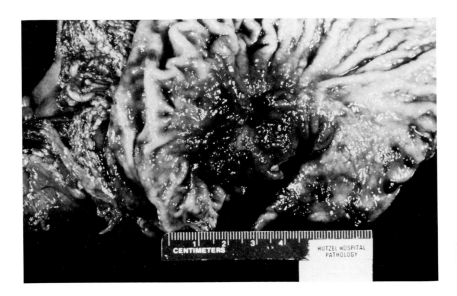

Fig. 16-26 Stomach showing a large ulcerated carcinoma in the gastric antrum.

latter instance, the metastatic adenocarcinoma may be present typically as signet ring-type cells, but also as tubular type glands (especially in the so-called tubular Krukenberg tumor)[156] that simulate Sertoli tubules. The prominent stromal luteinization elicited by both types of Krukenberg tumors mimics Leydig cells.

Treatment of Sertoli-Leydig Cell Tumors

The treatment for Sertoli-Leydig cell tumors is primarily surgical. In young women with stage IA disease, unilateral salpingo-oophorectomy may be

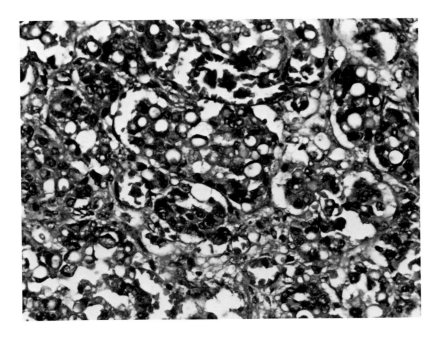

Fig. 16-27 Krukenberg tumor showing metastatic poorly differentiated adenocarcinoma invading the ovarian parenchyma in nests of signet-ring cells with clear cytoplasm and eccentric nuclei. (H&E, ×120.)

performed after a careful exploration of the entire pelvis and abdomen and with negative findings in the contralateral ovary and negative staging biopsies. A total abdominal hysterectomy and bilateral salpingo-oophorectomy is the surgical procedure of choice for (1) patients who have stage IA tumors and who do not wish to retain fertility, and (2) women with all other stages.

The benefit of adjuvant chemotherapy or radiation therapy is unproved, although the combination of vincristine, actinomycin D, and cyclophosphamide has been helpful in a few patients with metastatic disease.[147] More aggressive chemotherapy with bleomycin, vinblastine, and cisplatin (see Table 16-14) or radiation therapy after surgical debulking is recommended for widespread primary or recurrent Sertoli-Leydig cell tumors.

REFERENCES

1. Silverberg E, Lubera J: Cancer Statistics 1987. Cancer 37:2, 1987
2. Smith LH, Ol RH: Detection of malignant ovarian neoplasms: A review of the literature. 1. Detection of the patient at risk; clinical, radiological and cytological detection. Obstet Gynecol Surv 39:313, 1984
3. Greene MH, Clark JW, Blayney DW: The epidemiology of ovarian cancer. Semin Oncol 11:209, 1984
4. Beral V, Fraser P, Chilvers C: Dose pregnancy protect against ovarian cancer: Lancet 1:1083, 1978
5. Fathalla MF: Incessant ovulation: A factor in ovarian neoplasia. Lancet 2:163, 1971
6. Dicker RC, Webster LA, Layde PM, et al: Oral contraceptive use and the risk of ovarian cancer. JAMA 249:1596, 1983
7. Byers T, Marshall J, Graham S, et al: A case control study of dietary and non-dietary factors in ovarian cancer. J Natl Cancer Inst 71:681, 1983
8. West RO Epidemiologic study of malignancies of the ovaries. Cancer 19:1001, 1966
9. Cramer DW, Welch WR, Cassalls S, et al: Mumps, menarche, menopause and ovarian cancer. Am J Obstet Gynecol 147:1, 1983
10. Franceschi S LaVecchia C, Mangioni C: Familial ovarian cancer: Eight more families. Gynecol Oncol, 13:31, 1982
11. Tobacman JK, Tucker MA, Kase R, et al: Intraabdominal carcinomatosis after prophylactic oophorectomy in ovarian cancer prone families. Lancet 2:795, 1982
12. Reimer RR, Hoover R, Fraumeni JF Jr, et al: Second primary neoplasms following ovarian cancer. J Natl Cancer Inst 61:1195, 1978
13. Eifel P, Henriskson M, Ross J, et al: Simultaneous presentation of carcinoma involving the ovary and uterine corpus. Cancer 50:163, 1982
14. Barber HRK: Ovarian cancer: Diagnosis and management. Am J Obstet Gynecol 150:910, 1984
15. Wu PC, Qu JY, Lang JH, et al: Lymph node metastasis of ovarian cancer: A preliminary survey of 74 cases of lymphadenectomy. Am J Obstet Gynecol 155:1103, 1986
16. Larson DM, Copeland LJ, Moser RP, et al: Central nervous system metastases in epithelial ovarian carcinoma. Obstet Gynecol 68:746, 1986
17. Bast RC Jr, Klug TL, St. John E, et al: A radioimmunoassay using a monoclonal antibody to monitor the course of epithelial ovarian cancer. N Engl J Med 309:883, 1983
18. Staging Announcement: FIGO Cancer Committee, West Berlin, September 1985. Gynecol Oncol 25:383, 1986
19. Buchsbaum HJ, Lifshitz S: Staging and surgical evaluation of ovarian cancer. Semin Oncol 11:227, 1984
20. Griffiths CT, Parker LM, Fuller AF: Surgical resection of tumor bulk in the primary treatment of ovarian carcinoma. Natl Cancer Inst Monog 42:101, 1975
21. Wharton JT, Herson J: Surgery for common epithelial tumors of the ovary. Cancer 48:582, 1981
22. Hacker NF, Berek JS, Lagasse LD, et al: Primary cytoreductive surgery for epithelial ovarian cancer. Obstet Gynecol 61:413, 1983
23. Stehman FB, Ehrlich LH, Einhorn LH, et al: Long term follow-up and survival in Stage III-IV epithelial ovarian cancer treated with Cis-dichlorodiammine platinum, adriamycin and cyclophosphamide (PAC). Proc Am Soc Clin Oncol C-593, 1983
24. Griffiths CT, Parker LM, Fuller AF: Role of cytoreductive surgical treatment in the management of advanced ovarian cancer. Cancer Treatm Rep 63:235, 1979
25. Day TG, Smith JP: Diagnosis and staging of ovarian carcinoma. Semin Oncol 2:217, 1975
26. Wharton JT, Edwards CL, Stringer CA: Techniques for surgical staging and cytoreductive surgery. Clin Obstet Gynecol 28:800, 1985
27. Richardson GS, Scully RE, Nikrui N, et al: Common epithelial cancer of the ovary. N Engl Med J 312:415, 1985
28. Hart WR, Norris HJ: Borderline and malignant mucinous tumors of the ovary. Histologic criteria and clinical behavior. Cancer 31:1031, 1973

29. Czernobilsky B: Common epithelial tumors of the ovary. p. 11. In Roth L, Czernobilsky B (eds): Tumors and Tumor-like Conditions of the Ovary. Contemporary Issues in Surgical Pathology. Vol. 6. Churchill Livingstone, New York, 1985

30. Smith JP, Rutledge F: Chemotherapy in the treatment of cancer of the ovary. Am J Obstet Gynecol 107:691, 1970

31. Parker RT, Parker CH, Wilbanks GD: Cancer of the ovary: Survival studies based upon operative therapy, chemotherapy and radiotherapy. Am J Obstet Gynecol 108:878, 1970

32. Young RC: Chemotherapy of ovarian cancer: Past and present. Semin Oncol 2:267, 1975

33. Decker DG, Mussey E, Malkasian GD Jr, et al: Cyclophosphamide in the treatment of ovarian cancer. Clin Obstet Gynecol, 11:382, 1968

34. Thigpen T: Single agent chemotherapy in the management of ovarian carcinoma. p. 115. In Alberts DS, Surwit EA (eds): Ovarian Carcinoma. Martinus Nijhoff, Boston, 1985

35. Young RC, Chabner BA, Hubbard SP: Prospective trial of melphalan (L-PAM) versus combination chemotherapy (hexa-CAF) in ovarian adenocarcinoma. N Engl J Med 299:1261, 1978

36. Delgado G, Schien P, MacDonald J, et al: L-PAM vs cyclophosphamide, hexamethylmelamine, and 5-fluorouracil (CHF) for advanced ovarian cancer. Proc Am Assoc Cancer Res 20:434, 1979

37. Trope C: A prospective and randomized trial comparison of melphalan vs. adriamycin-melphalan in advanced ovarian carcinoma. Proc Am Soc Clin Oncol 22:469, 1981

38. Omura GA, Morrow CP, Blessing JA, et al: A randomized comparison of melphalan versus melphalan plus hexamethylmelamine versus adriamycin plus cyclophosphamide in ovarian carcinoma. Cancer 51:783, 1983

39. Omura GA, Blessing JA, Ehrlich CE, et al: A randomized trial of cyclophosphamide and doxorubicin with or without cisplatin in advanced ovarian carcinoma. A Gynecologic Oncology Group Study. Cancer 57:1725, 1986

40. Louie KG, Ozols RF, Myers CE, et al: Long-term results of a cisplatin-containing combination chemotherapy regimen for the treatment of advanced ovarian carcinoma. J Clin Oncol 4:1579, 1986

41. Cohen CJ, Bruckner HW, Goldberg JD, et al: Improved therapy with cisplatin regimens for patients with ovarian carcinoma (FIGO III and IV) as measured by surgical end-staging (second-look surgery). The Mount Sinai experience. Clin Obstet Gynecol 10:307, 1983

42. Greco FA, Julian CG, Richardson RL, et al: Advanced ovarian cancer: Brief intensive combination chemotherapy. Obstet Gynecol 58:199, 1981

43. Decker DG, Fleming JR, Malkasian GD, et al: Cyclophosphamide plus cisplatin in combination: Treatment program for Stage III or IV ovarian carcinoma. Obstet Gynecol, 60:481, 1982

44. Neijt JP, Van der Burg MEL, Vriesendorp R, et al: Randomized trial comparing two combination chemotherapy regimens (Hexa-CAF vs CHAP-5) in advanced ovarian carcinoma. Lancet 2:594, 1984

45. Barker GH, Wiltshaw E: Randomized trial comparing low-dose cisplatin and chlorambucil with low-dose cisplatin, chlorambucil and adriamycin in advanced ovarian carcinoma. Lancet 2:747, 1981

46. Bruckner HW, Cohen CJ, Goldberg J, et al: Ovarian cancer: Comparison of adriamycin and cisplatin + cyclophosphamide. Proc Am Soc Clin Oncol C-594:152, 1983

47. Conte PF, Bruzzone M, Chiara S, et al: A randomized trial comparing cisplatin plus cyclophosphamide versus cisplatin, doxorubicin and cyclophosphamide in advanced ovarian cancer. J Clin Oncol 4:965, 1986

48. Schwartz PE, Smith JP: Second-look operations in ovarian cancer. Am J Obstet Gynecol 138:1124, 1980

49. Wils J, Blijham A, Naus C, et al: Primary or delayed debulking surgery and chemotherapy consisting of cisplatin, doxorubicin, and cyclophosphamide in Stage III-IV epithelial ovarian carcinoma. J Clin Oncol 4:1068, 1986

50. Copeland LJ, Gershenson DM, Wharton JT, et al: Microscopic disease at second-look laparotomy in advanced ovarian cancer. Cancer 55:472, 1985

51. Gershenson DM, Copeland LJ, Wharton JT, et al: Prognosis of surgically determined complete responses in advanced ovarian cancer. Cancer 55:1129, 1985

52. Stanhope RC, Smith JP, Rutledge F: Second trial drugs in ovarian cancer. Gynecol Oncol 5:52, 1977

53. Weiss GR: Second-line chemotherapy for ovarian cancer. Clin Obstet Gynecol 29:665, 1986

54. Piver MS, Barlow JJ, Lele SB, et al: Cis-diamminedichloroplatinum (11): Second line induction chemotherapy in advanced ovarian carcinoma. J Surg Oncol 24:329, 1983

55. Bruckner HW, Cohen CJ, Wallach RC, et al: Treatment of advanced ovarian cancer with cis-dichlorodiammine platinum (11): Poor risk patients with intensive prior therapy. Cancer Treatm Rep 62:555, 1978

56. Evans BD, Raju KS, Calvert AH, et al: Phase II study of JM 8, a new platinum analog, in advanced ovarian carcinoma. Cancer Treatm Rep 67:997, 1983

57. Bramwell VHC, Crowther D, O'Malley S, et al: Ac-

tivity of JM9 in advanced ovarian cancer: A phase I-II trial. Cancer Treatm Rep 65:409, 1985

58. Bonomi PD, Mladineo J, Morrin B, et al: Phase II trial of hexamethylmelamine in ovarian carcinoma resistant to alkylating agents. Cancer Treatm Rep 63:137, 1979

59. Omura GA, Greco FA, Birch R: Hexamethylmelamine in mustard-resistant ovarian adenocarcinoma. Cancer Treatm Rep 65:530, 1981

60. Stehman FB, Ehrlich CE, Callangan MF: Failure of hexamethylmelamine as salvage therapy in ovarian epithelial adenocarcinoma resistant to combination chemotherapy. Gynecol Oncol 17:189, 1984

61. Blackledge G, Lawton F, Buckley H, et al: Phase II evaluation of bleomycin in patients with advanced epithelial ovarian cancer. Cancer Treatm Rep 68:543, 1984

62. Kuhnle H, Achterrath W, Frischkorn R: Krankheitsorientierte Phase II studie mit Etoposid (NSC 141540) bei cisplatin-refraktaren Ovarialkarzinomen. Tumor Diagn Ther 5:152, 1984

63. Stehman FB, Bolm J, Blessing JA, et al: Phase II trial of galactitol 1,2:5,6-dianhydro (NSC 132313) in the treatment of advanced gynecologic malignancies: A Gynecologic Oncology Group Study. Gynecol Oncol 15:381, 1983

64. Bruckner HW, Wallach R, Cohen CJ, et al: High-dose cisplatin for refractory ovarian cancer. Gynecol Oncol 12:64, 1984

65. Barker GH, Wiltshaw E: Use of high dose cis-dichlorodiammineplatinum (11) following failure on previous chemotherapy for advanced carcinoma of the ovary. Br J Obstet Gynaecol 88:1192, 1981

66. Ozols RF, Young RC: High-dose cisplatin therapy in ovarian cancer. Semin Oncol 12:21, 1985

67. Ozols RF, Ostchega Y, Curt G, et al: High-dose carboplatin in refractory ovarian cancer patients. J Clin Oncol 5:197, 1987

68. Kane R, Harvey H, Andrews T et al: Phase II trial of cyclophosphamide, hexamethylmelamine, adriamycin and cis-dichlorodiammine platinum (11) combination chemotherapy in advanced ovarian carcinoma. Cancer Treatm Rep 63:307, 1979

69. Vogl SE, Berenzweig M, Kaplan BH, et al: The CHAD and HAD regimens in advanced ovarian cancer: Combination chemotherapy including cyclophosphamide, hexamethylmelamine, adriamycin and cis-dichlorodiammineplatinum (11). Cancer Treatm Rep 63:311, 1979

70. Briscoe KE, Pasmantier MW, Ohnuma T, et al: Cis-dichlorodiammineplatinum (11) and adriamycin treatment of advanced ovarian cancer. Cancer Treatm Rep 62:2027, 1978

71. Alberts DS, Hilgers RD, Moon TE, et al: Combination chemotherapy for alkylator-resistant ovarian carcinoma: A preliminary report of a Southwest Oncology Group trial. Cancer Treatm Rep 63:301, 1979

72. Brenner DE: Intraperitoneal chemotherapy: A review. J Clin Oncol 4:1135, 1986

73. Cohen CJ: Surgical considerations in ovarian cancer. Semin Oncol 12:53, 1985

74. Howell SB, Pfeifle C, Wung W, et al: Intraperitoneal cisplatin with systemic thiosulfate protection. Ann Intern Med 97:845, 1982

75. McVie JG, ten Bokkel Huinink WW, Aartsen E, et al: Intraperitoneal chemotherapy in minimal residual ovarian cancer with cisplatin and IV sodium thiosulfate protection. Proc AM Soc Clin Oncol 4:125, 1985

76. Mihich E: Future perspectives for biological response modifiers: A viewpoint. Semin Oncol 13:234, 1986

77. Alberts DS, Moon TE, Stephens RA, et al: Randomized study of chemoimmunotherapy for advanced ovarian carcinoma: A preliminary report of a Southwest Oncology Group Study Cancer Treatm Rep 63:325, 1979

78. Creasman WT, Gall SA, Blessing JA, et al: Chemoimmunotherapy in the management of primary Stage III ovarian cancer: A Gynecologic Oncology Group Study. Cancer Treatm Rep 63:319, 1979

79. Rao B, Wanebo HJ, Ochoa M, et al: Intravenous corynebacterium parvum: an adjunct to chemotherapy for resistant advanced ovarian cancer. Cancer 39:514, 1977

80. Abdulhay G, DiSaia PJ, Blessing JA, et al: Human lymphoblastoid interferon in the treatment of advanced epithelial ovarian malignancies: A Gynecologic Oncology Group Study. Am J Obstet Gynecol 152:418, 1985

81. Rambaldi A, Introna M, Colotta F, et al: Intraperitoneal administration of interferon B in ovarian cancer patients. Cancer 56:294, 1985

82. Schwartz PA, Merino MJ, Livolsi VA, et al: Histopathologic correlations of estrogen and progestin receptor protein in epithelial ovarian carcinomas. Obstet Gynecol 66:428, 1985

83. Sikic BI, Scudder SA, Ballon SC, et al: High-dose megesterol acetate therapy of ovarian carcinoma: A phase II study by the Northern California Oncology Group. Semin Oncol 13:26, 1986

84. Geisler EH: The use of high-dose megestrol acetate in the treatment of ovarian adenocarcinoma. Semin Oncol 12(suppl 1):20, 1985

85. Geisler EH: Megestrol acetate for palliation of advanced ovarian carcinoma. Obstet Gynecol 61:95, 1983

86. Slayton RE, Pagano M, Creech RH: Progestin therapy for advanced ovarian cancer: A phase II Eastern

Cooperative Oncology Group Trial. Cancer Treatm Rep 65:895, 1981

87. Meyers AM, Moore GE, Major F: Advanced ovarian carcinoma: Response to antiestrogen therapy. Cancer 48:2368, 1981

88. Schwartz PE, Keating G, MacLusky N, et al: Tamoxifen therapy for advanced ovarian cancer. Obstet Gynecol 59:583, 1982

89. Shirey DR, Kavanagh JJ Jr, Gershenson DM, et al: Tamoxifen therapy of epithelial ovarian cancer. Obstet Gynecol 66:575, 1985

90. Piver MS: Radioactive colloids in the treatment of Stage IA ovarian cancer. Obstet Gynecol 40:42, 1972

91. Buchsbaum HJ, Keetel WC, Latourette HB: The use of radioisotopes as adjunct therapy of localized ovarian cancer. Semin Oncol 2:247, 1975

92. Smith JP, Rutledge FN, Deldos L: Postoperative treatment of early cancer of the ovary: A random trial between postoperative irradiation and chemotherapy. Natl Cancer Inst Monog 42:149, 1975

93. Dembo AJ, Bush RS, Beale FA, et al: Ovarian carcinoma: Improved survival following abdominopelvic irradiation in patients with a completed pelvic operation. Am J Obstet Gynecol 134:793, 1979

94. Dembo AJ: Radiotherapeutic management of ovarian cancer. Semin Oncol 11:238, 1984

95. Peters WA III, Blasko JC, Bagley CM Jr, et al: Salvage therapy with whole-abdominal irradiation in patients with advanced carcinoma of the ovary previously treated by combination chemotherapy. Cancer 58:880, 1986

96. Hanauske AR, VonHoff DD: The value of the human tumor cloning assay in ovarian cancer. Clin Obstet Gynecol 29:638, 1986

97. Ozols RF, Young RC: Chemotherapy of ovarian cancer. Semin Oncol 11:251, 1984

98. Scully RE: Tumors of the ovary and maldeveloped gonads. In Atlas of Tumor Pathology. Second series. Fascicle 16. Armed Forces Institute of Pathology, Washington, DC, 1979

99. Santesson L, Kottmeier HL: General classification of ovarian tumours. p. 1. Gentil F, Junqueira AC (eds): UICC Monograph Series. Vol. 11: Ovarian Cancer. Springer-Verlag, New York, 1968

100. Bostwick DG, Tazelaar HD, Ballon SC, et al: Ovarian epithelial tumors of borderline malignancy. A clinical and pathologic study of 109 cases. Cancer 58:2052, 1986

101. Kliman L, Rome RM, Fortune DW: Low malignant potential tumors of the ovary: A study of 76 cases. Obstet Gynecol 68:338, 1986

102. Tazelaar HD, Bostwick DG, Ballon SC, et al: Con-servative treatment of borderline ovarian tumors. Obstet Gynecol 66:417, 1985

103. Weiss NS, Homonchuk, Young JL: Incidence of the histologic type of ovarian cancer: The US Third National Cancer Survey, 1969–1971. Gynecol Oncol 5:161, 1977

104. Norris HJ, Jensen RD: Relative frequency of ovarian neoplasms in children and adolescents. Cancer 30:713, 1972

105. Teilum G: Classifications of endodermal sinus tumor (mesoblastoma vitellinum and so-called "embryonal carcinoma" of the ovary. Acta Pathol Microbiol Scand 64:407, 1965

106. Serov SF, scully RE, Sobin LH: International histologic classification of tumors. No. 9: Histological Typing of Ovarian Tumors. World Health Organization, Geneva, 1973

107. Gordon A, Lipton D, Woodruff JD: Dysgerminoma: A review of 158 cases from the Emil Novak ovarian tumor registry. Obstet Gynecol 58:497, 1981

108. Novak ER, Lambrou CD, Woodruff JD: Ovarian tumors in pregnancy. Obstet Gynecol 46:401, 1975

109. Karlen JR, Akbari A, Cook WA: Dysgerminoma associated with pregnancy. Obstet Gynecol 53:330, 1979

110. Norris HJ, Adam AE: Malignant germ cell tumors of ovary. p. 680. In Coppleson M (ed): Gynecologic Oncology. Churchill Livingstone, Edinburgh, 1981

111. Liu TL, Lian LJ, Deppe G: Serum lactic dehydrogenase (SLDH) in germ cell malignancies of the ovary. Gynecol Oncol 19:355, 1984

112. Awais GM: Dysgerminoma and serum lactic dehydrogenase levels. Obstet Gynecol 62:99, 1983

113. Kurman RJ, Norris HJ: Malignant germ cell tumors of the ovary. Hum Pathol 8:551, 1977

114. Schwartz IS, Cohen CJ, Deligdisch L: Dysgerminoma of the ovary associated with true hermaphroditism. Obstet Gynecol 56:102, 1980

115. Talerman A: Gonadoblastoma and dysgerminoma in two siblings with dysgenetic gonads. Obstet Gynecol 38:416, 1971

116. Talerman A: Germ cell tumors of the ovary p. 581. In Blaustein A (ed): Pathology of the Female Genital Tract. Springer-Verlag, New York, 1982

117. Gershenson, DM, Wharton JT, Kline RC, et al: Chemotherapeutic complete remission in patients with metastatic ovarian dysgerminoma. Cancer 58:2594, 1986

118. Gershenson DM: Malignant germ-cell tumors of the ovary. Clin Obstet Gynecol 28:824, 1985

119. Krepart G, Smith JP, Rutledge F, et al: The treatment of dysgerminoma of the ovary. Cancer 41:986, 1978

120. Cohen SM, Goldsmith MA: Prolonged chemotherapeutic remission of metastatic ovarian dysgerminoma. Report of a case. Gynecol Oncol 5:299, 1977

121. Weinblatt ME, Ortega JA: Treatment of children with dysgerminoma of the ovary. Cancer 49:2608, 1982

122. Jacobs AJ, Harris M, Deppe G, et al: Treatment of recurrent and persistent germ cell tumors with Cisplatin, Vinblastine and Bleomycin. Obstet Gynecol 59:129, 1982

123. Newlands, ES, Begent RHJ, Rustin GJS, et al: Potential for cure in metastatic ovarian teratomas and dysgerminomas. Br J Obstet Gynaecol 89:551, 1982

124. Schiller W: Mesonephroma ovarii. Am J Cancer 35:1, 1939

125. Teilum G: Endodermal sinus tumors of the ovary and testis. Comparative morphogenesis of the so-called mesonephroma ovarii (Schiller) and extraembryonic (yolk sac-allantoic) structures of the rat's placenta. Cancer 12:1092, 1959

126. Kurman RJ, Norris HJ: Embryonal carcinoma of the ovary: A clinicopathologic entity distinct from endodermal sinus tumor resembling embryonal carcinoma of the adult testis. Cancer 38:2420, 1976

127. Norris HJ, Zirkin HJ, Benson WL: Immature malignant teratoma of the ovary. Cancer 37:2359, 1976

128. Peyron A: Faits nouveaux relatifs à l'origine et à l'histogénèse des embryomes. Bull Cancer (Paris) 28:658, 1939

129. Takeda A, Ishizuka T, Goto T, et al: Polyembryoma of the ovary producing alpha fetoprotein and hCG. Immunoperoxidase and electron microscopic study. Cancer 49:1878, 1982

130. Yannopoulos D, Yannopoulos K, Ossowski R: Malignant struma ovarii. Pathol Annu 11:403, 1976

131. Robboy SJ, Norris HJ, Scully RE: Insular carcinoid primary in the ovary. A clinicopathologic analysis of 48 cases. Cancer 36:404, 1975

132. Arhelger RB, Kelly B: Strumal carcinoid. Report of a case with electronmicroscopical observations. Arch Pathol Lab Med 97:323, 1974

133. Kurman RJ, Norris HJ: Malignant mixed germ cell tumors of the ovary. A clinical and pathologic analysis of 30 cases. Obstet Gynecol 48:579, 1976

134. Slayton RE Part RC, Silverberg SG, et al: Vincristine, dactinomycin and cyclophosphamide in the treatment of malignant germ cell tumors of the ovary. A Gynecologic Oncology Group Study. (A final report.) Cancer 56:243, 1985

135. Taylor MH, DePetrillo AD, Turner AR: Vinblastine, bleomycin and cisplatin in malignant germ cell tumors of the ovary. Cancer 56:1341, 1985

136. Newlands ES, Begent RHJ, Rustin GJS, et al: Chemotherapy for malignant ovarian germ cell tumors. p 133. In Bleehen NM (ed): Ovarian Cancer. Springer-Verlag, Berlin, 1985

137. Williams S, Slayton R, Silverberg S, et al: Response of malignant ovarian germ cell tumors to Cis-platinum, Vinblastine and Bleomycin (PVB). Proc Am Soc Clin Oncol C-509, 1981

138. Gershenson DM, Kavanagh JJ, Copeland LJ, et al: Treatment of malignant nondysgerminomatous germ cell tumors of the ovary with Vinblastine, Bleomycin and Cisplatin. Cancer 57:1731, 1986

139. Creasman WT, Soper JT: Assessment of the contemporary management of germ cell malignancies of the ovary. Am J Obstet Gynecol 153:828, 1985

140. Young RH, Scully RE: Ovarian sex cord-stromal tumors: Recent progress. Int J Gynecol Pathol 1:101, 1982

141. Young RH, Scully RE: Ovarian sex cord-stromal and steroid cell tumors. p. 43. In Roth L, Czernobilsky B (eds): Contemporary Issues in Surgical Pathology. Vol. 6: Tumor and Tumorlike Conditions of the Ovary. Churchill Livingstone, New York, 1985

142. Scully RE: Sex cord-stromal tumors. p. 581. In Blaustein A (ed): Pathology of the Female Genital Tract. Springer-Verlag, New York, 1982

143. Bjorkholm E, Silfversward C: Prognostic factors in granulosa cell tumors. Gynecol Oncol 11:261, 1981

144. Young RH, Dickersin GR, Scully RE: Juvenile granulosa cell tumor. A clinicopathologic analysis of 125 cases. Am J Surg Pathol 8:575, 1984

145. Gorlin RJ, Vickers RA, Kelln E, et al: The multiple basal cell nevi syndrome. Cancer 18:89, 1965

146. Prat J, Scully RE: Cellular fibromas and fibrosarcomas of the ovary. A comparative clinicopathologic analysis of seventeen cases. Cancer 47:2663, 1981

147. Schwartz PE, Smith JP: Treatment of ovarian stromal tumors. AM J Obstet Gynecol 125:402, 1976

148. Barlow JJ, Piver MS, Chuang JT, et al: Adriamycin and Bleomycin alone and in combination in gynecological cancer. Cancer 32:735, 1973

149. Jacobs AJ, Deppe G, Cohen CJ: Combination chemotherapy of ovarian granulosa cell tumor with Cisplatinum and Doxorubicin. Gynecol Oncol 14:294, 1982

150. Slayton R, Johnson G, Brady L, et al: Radiotherapy and chemotherapy in malignant tumors of the ovarian stroma. Proc Am Soc Clin Oncol 21:430, 1980

151. Colombo N, Sessa C, Landoni F, et al: Cisplatin, vinblastine and bleomycin combination chemotherapy in metastatic granulosa cell tumor of the ovary. Obstet Gynecol 67:265, 1986

152. Young RH, Prat J, Scully RE: Ovarian Sertoli-Leydig cell tumors with heterologous elements. Gastrointes-

tinal epithelium and carcinoid. A clinicopathologic analysis of thirty-six cases. Cancer 50:2448, 1982

153. Novak ER, Long JH: Arrhenoblastoma of the ovary. A review of the ovarian tumor registry. Am J Obstet Gynecol 92:1082, 1965

154. Fox H, Langley FA: Tumors of the Ovary. Yearbook Medical Publishers, Chicago, 1976

155. Prat J, Young RH, Scully RE: Ovarian Sertoli-Leydig cell tumors with heterologous elements. II. Cartilage and skeletal muscle. A clinicopathologic analysis of twelve cases. Cancer 50:2465, 1982

156. Bullow A Jr, Arseneau J, Prat J, et al: Tubular Krukenberg tumors: A problem in histopathological diagnosis. Am J Surg Pathol 5(3):225, 1981

17

Cancer of the Fallopian Tube

Gunter Deppe
John M. Malone, Jr.
W. Dwayne Lawrence

Primary carcinoma of the fallopian tube is rare, accounting for only 0.31 percent[1] to 1.8 percent[2] of all gynecologic malignancies. To date, approximately 1,200 cases of fallopian tube carcinoma have been reported,[3] but the experience of any one institution is limited.

The diagnosis of primary fallopian tube carcinoma is complicated by the close anatomic proximity of the tube to the ovary and uterus and its characteristic histology, which may be similar to papillary adenocarcinoma of either the endometrium or the ovary. Differentiation between a primary tubal or primary ovarian malignancy may be extremely difficult; the diagnostic criteria suggested by Finn and Javert[4] may be helpful, however, in determining a tubal origin:

1. The tubal carcinoma should arise from the endosalpinx.
2. The histologic pattern should resemble the epithelium of the tubal mucosa.
3. Transition from benign to malignant epithelium should be present.
4. The endometrium and ovaries should be normal or should contain a malignant neoplasm that by its histologic appearance, small size, and distribution appears to be metastatic from a tubal primary.

Although tubal carcinoma has been reported to occur in both premenopausal and postmenopausal women ranging from 17 to 82 years of age, it most frequently occurs in the fifth decade, with a mean age of 52 years.

The most commonly reported symptom in patients with fallopian tube carcinoma is vaginal bleeding or abnormal vaginal discharge. Most patients present with one or more of the symptoms comprising the classic triad of abdominopelvic pain or pressure, abnormal vaginal discharge, and a pelvic mass or abdominal distention. Hydrops tubae profluens, profuse watery discharge following colicky pelvic pain, has been described as pathognomonic of tubal carcinoma.[6] The pelvic pain is thought to be secondary to tubal distention by carcinoma.

An abnormal Papanicolaou (Pap) smear from the cervix with normal findings on colposcopy, cone biopsy, or endometrial curettage is suggestive of fallopian tube carcinoma. Most patients, however, have a normal Pap smear. Preoperative diagnosis of fallopian tube carcinoma is rarely made, and more often the diagnosis is established at the time of an exploratory laparotomy performed for an adnexal or pelvic mass that was indistinguishable from the uterus. Henderson et al.[7] reported ovarian carcinoma and uterine

427

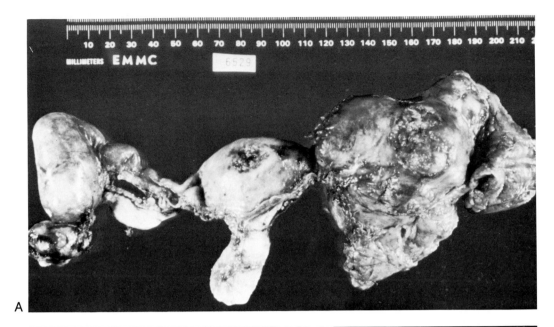

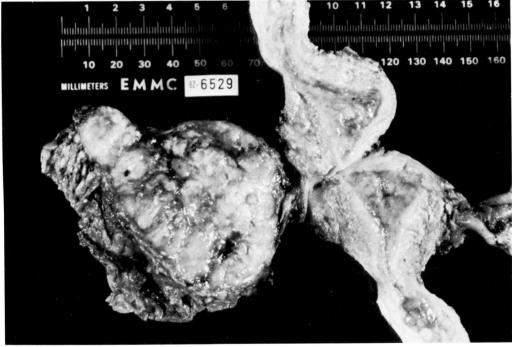

Fig. 17-1 Primary fallopian tube carcinoma. **(A)** Bilateral view. Both tubes are markedly enlarged; the left tube is virtually totally replaced by tumor and the right shows distal involvement. **(B)** Left fallopian tube, posterior view. Cut section of primary fallopian tube carcinoma shows replacement of the tube by necrotic yellow tumor that was soft and friable. (Courtesy of John S. Kaiser, M.D., Dahl-Chase Pathology Associates, Eastern Maine Medical Center, Bangor.)

18

Gestational Trophoblastic Disease and Gestational Choriocarcinoma

John T. Soper
Charles B. Hammond

Gestational trophoblastic disease (GTD) is a term that encompasses a spectrum of clinical and histologic entities, referring to a group of neoplastic disorders arising from the human placenta. This broad term includes the histologic entities of partial and complete hydatidiform mole, placental site tumor, invasive mole (chorioadenoma destruens), and gestational choriocarcinoma. Clinical presentations of GTD range from uncomplicated evacuation of molar gestation with spontaneous human chorionic gonadotropin (hCG) titer regression, proliferative sequelae after molar evacuation with local involvement of the uterus, or widely disseminated metastatic choriocarcinoma following term pregnancy and requiring multiagent chemotherapy.

These neoplasms are unique in their genetic composition, since they are derived from the paternal genome with occasional maternal contribution. hCG is secreted by these neoplasms and serves as a sensitive marker that correlates well with the clinical course. Malignant forms of GTD are among the most sensitive human solid malignancies, responding to a wide variety of chemotherapeutic regimens. This chapter discusses current concepts important in the management of GTD.

BENIGN GTD: MOLAR GESTATION

Two distinct types of molar gestations have recently been described, partial and complete hydatidiform moles, which have distinct cytogenetic origin, pathologic features, and clinical behavior. It is unclear from the literature whether partial mole represents a neoplastic placental disorder or whether this represents an extreme form of hydropic degeneration of the placenta in abnormal pregnancies. Until larger series of patients with partial molar pregnancies are studied, it is prudent to consider this as a variant of hydatidiform mole, carrying the possible risk of becoming malignant. Most patients with molar gestations do not require chemotherapy; following evacuation, patients can be safely monitored with serial hCG-titer surveillance until spontaneous titer regression occurs or until the patient develops criteria for instituting chemotherapy.

Partial Hydatidiform Mole

Approximately 1 percent of all human gestations have triploidy and result in spontaneous abortion. Recently, it has been recognized that a portion of these

Table 18-1 Partial Versus Complete Hydatidiform Mole

Analyses	Partial Hydatidiform Mole	Complete Hydatidiform Mole
Cytogenetic	Triploidy Paternal + maternal origin	Diploidy 46XX most common paternal origin
Pathology		
Hydropic villi	++	++++
Trophoblastic proliferation	Focal – slight	Slight – marked
Fetus, amnion or fetal vessels	+	—
Clinical		
"Mole" clinical diagnosis	Rare	Common
Uterus large for dates	Rare	30–50%
Malignant sequelae	Rare	10–25%

abnormal gestations exhibit histologic features in common with hydatidiform mole; these have been described as partial hydatidiform moles. A comparison of cytogenetic, pathologic, and clinical features of partial and complete moles is given in Table 18-1. Partial moles are often associated with a fetus or amniotic membranes. Gross examination shows a mixture of normal and edematous or swollen villi. Microscopic features include intermingled normal and hydropic chorionic villi with focal mild hyperplasia of trophoblastic elements.[1-3] Scalloping of hydropic villi is common with occasional trophoblastic inclusions in the stroma. Fetal vessels are usually observed with nucleated fetal erythrocytes within the vessels.[3,4] Normal amniotic membranes are often identified microscopically, even when a fetus has not been identified.

The cytogenetic origin of most partial moles appears to be complete triploidy with both maternal and paternal chromosomal markers.[4,5] Partial moles are almost always associated with one haploid maternal and two haploid paternal sets of chromosomes. Presumably, this results from dispermic fertilization of a haploid ovum or fertilization of a haploid ovum with a diploid sperm.[4,5]

Clinically, patients with partial hydatidiform mole present with uterine size that is small or appropriate for gestational age (SGA or AGA).[4,6,7] Frequently, the clinical diagnosis is spontaneous abortion or missed abortion. Often ultrasound is unable to identify the hydropic villi characteristic of hydatidiform mole, and the diagnosis is not suspected until after evacuation of the pregnancy. Initial hCG titers are often lower than those seen in patients with complete hy-

datidiform mole, and a prompt postevacuation regression of hCG titer usually occurs.[6-8] In contradistinction to complete moles, which have a 10 to 30 percent incidence of malignant sequelae, malignant complications following partial hydatidiform mole have rarely been reported. In one series of 47 patients with partial hydatidiform mole, Szulman and associates[6] treated only one patient, while Berkowitz et al.[7] treated 8 (9.9 percent) of 81 patients with chemotherapy for malignancy after evacuation of partial mole.

Although patients with partial hydatidiform mole appear to have a low incidence of malignant sequelae and prompt hCG titer regression,[8] it is recommended that all undergo hCG-titer surveillance following evacuation, similar to that recommended for patients with complete hydatidiform mole. Frequently, pathologists are not familiar with the diagnosis of partial hydatidiform mole. In addition, patients with coexistent normal gestation and a twin complete hydatidiform mole have been recorded. Therefore, the identification of a fetus in conjunction with molar changes of the placenta does not necessarily guarantee that the patient has a partial hydatidiform mole.

Complete Hydatidiform Mole

Complete hydatidiform mole is identified macroscopically by edema and swelling of all chorionic villi with the lack of a fetus or amniotic membranes, except in the rare case of coexistent normal gestation and hydatidiform mole. Microscopically, essentially all the chorionic villi are hydropic with marked interstitial edema. No fetal vessels are identified in the stroma of the chorionic villi. Proliferation of both cytotrophoblasts and syncytotrophoblasts is identified histologically. Although Hertig and Sheldon classified complete hydatidiform moles on the basis of trophoblastic proliferation and suggested that the amount of trophoblastic proliferation is predictive of malignant sequelae,[9] the histologic features of a complete hydatidiform mole do not dictate the subsequent clinical course for individual patients.[10] All complete hydatidiform moles secrete hCG, and this marker is used to monitor regression following evacuation.

Complete moles are almost uniformly diploid with paternal chromosomal markers.[11,12] The majority are 46,XX although a small portion have 46,XY karyotype.[13,14] This finding implies that the most common origin of complete hydatidiform moles is fertilization of an empty egg by a haploid sperm with reduplication of the chromosomal complement.[4,11,12] A few complete hydatidiform moles result from dispermic fertilization of an empty egg.[13,14] It has been suggested that complete hydatidiform moles with a 46,XY karyotype may have a malignant predisposition, compared with 46,XX moles[15,16]; however, these data require confirmation with larger series of patients.

In contrast to partial hydatidiform moles (Table 18-1), approximately one-third to one-half patients with complete hydatidiform mole have uterine enlargement more than expected for gestational dates.[4,6,17,18] Patients often present with vaginal hemorrhage and spontaneous abortion of the typical hydropic vesicles. The clinical diagnosis is most often molar gestation.[4,6] Theca lutein cysts are detected clinically in approximately 20 percent of patients with complete hydatidiform mole.[17,18] Hyperemesis, pregnancy-induced hypertension, and hyperthyroidism are occasionally observed.[6,17] The clinical diagnosis of molar gestation is supported by ultrasound. Ultrasound of the uterus provides documentation of diffuse hydropic villi, giving a characteristic appearance on ultrasound.

Epidemiology of Hydatidiform Mole

There is considerable geographic variation in the incidence of hydatidiform mole. In general, a much lower incidence is recorded in industrialized nations than in underdeveloped nations, ranging from an incidence of 1 to 2,000 pregnancies in the United States to 1 to 120 in Asia.[19] Some, but not all, of this variation may be accounted for by the methodology of studies reporting the incidence of molar gestation, since many studies were reported from the experience at referral centers and may overestimate the true incidence of molar pregnancy in their general population. Racial differences may account for some of the observed geographic variation in the incidence of hydatidiform mole, as suggested by McCorristen's observation that Japanese migrants to Hawaii have an incidence of molar gestation intermediate between that of native Hawaiians and native Japanese.[20]

Maternal age appears to influence the risk of hydatidiform mole. Several studies have suggested that the risk of having a molar gestation increases with increasing maternal age,[21,22] while other studies have suggested an increased risk for younger women or adolescents.[21,23] The impact of paternal age on the incidence of hydatidiform mole is difficult to separate from the effect of maternal age.[22]

Nutritional factors may be important in the etiology of hydatidiform mole. Protein deficiency[24] has been implicated as a possible cause. Nutritional causes may explain, in part, the observed geographic differences in the incidence of hydatidiform mole and changing incidence among migrant populations.[20] Recently, a case-controlled study by Berkowitz and associates[25] has implicated dietary deficiency of animal fat and fat-soluble carotene as a possible risk factor for hydatidiform mole.[25] Other nutritional factors may be identified in the future as important in the etiology of molar gestation.

Finally, genetic causes have been considered possible causative factors for the development of hydatidiform mole. Many studies have documented a markedly increased risk for recurrent molar gestation in pregnancies following evacuation of hydatidiform mole.[17,22] However, no major differences in ABO blood types or HLA antigens were found between patients with hydatidiform mole or malignant GTD and normal controls.[17,26] The interactions of environmental and possible genetic risk factors required to produce a molar gestation remain speculative.

Management of Molar Gestation

The basic tenets for managing a patient with hydatidiform mole include (1) establishing the diagnosis, (2) evacuating the molar gestation, and (3) providing adequate hCG-titer monitoring after evacuation to aid in the early detection of malignant GTD. Although patients with an unevacuated hydatidiform mole frequently have marked elevation of hCG titer, a single titer is not to be relied on to establish the diagnosis of hydatidiform mole, since comparable elevations are occasionally seen in patients with multifetal gestations. Although amniography, arteriography, and other radiographic techniques were used in the past to establish the diagnosis of hydatidiform mole, ultrasound is currently the diagnostic method of choice for evaluation of patients with suspected hydatidiform mole. Ultrasound of the patient with hydatidiform mole gives a characteristic image of multiple echogenic regions within the uterus corresponding to hydropic villi and focal hemorrhage.

Evaluation of the patient prior to evacuation of hydatidiform mole is aimed at preparing the patient for the evacuation procedure, obtaining baseline hCG-titer information, screening for occult metastatic disease, and screening for associated hyperthyroidism. We recommend the following studies as initial evaluation for patients with hydatidiform mole:

1. Complete physical examination and pelvic examination
2. Complete blood count (CBC)
3. Blood chemistries, including renal, hepatic, and thyroid function tests
4. Baseline serum hCG titer
5. Chest radiography
6. Pelvic ultrasound

The currently recommended technique for evacuation of molar pregnancy is suction curettage, or dilatation and curettage (D&C).[21] Occasional patients who do not desire preservation of reproductive function may benefit from primary hysterectomy as the method of choice for evacuation of hydatidiform mole. Hysterotomy or induction of labor are no longer considered desirable methods of evacuation in these patients. Tow[27] reported that abdominal hysterotomy resulted in greater blood loss than D&C when used for evacuation of hydatidiform mole. Others have cited increased postoperative morbidity and the need for repeat cesarean section following hysterotomy as additional reasons for avoiding this form of uterine evacuation.[17] Several studies have suggested that hysterotomy is associated with a higher incidence

of persistent disease requiring therapy after evacuation of molar pregnancy than D&C.[17,21,27] For these reasons, we recommend that hysterotomy not be used as the primary method for evacuation of hydatidiform mole.

Suction D&C offers a safe, rapid, effective method for evacuation of hydatidiform mole in almost all patients. Oxytoxic agents are given after cervical dilatation and partial evacuation to aid in postoperative hemostasis. Suction D&C has a low complication rate in patients with uterine size at less than 16 weeks. Twiggs et al.[28] noted a 27 percent incidence of acute pulmonary complications after D&C in patients with uterine size of 16 weeks or larger. They identified multiple factors associated with the development of pulmonary complications including trophoblastic deportation, preeclampsia, fluid overload, anemia, and hyperthyroidism. A small series of patients studied hemodynamically were found to have a transient impairment of left ventricular function associated with the D&C, which may have contributed to these pulmonary complications when combined with vigorous iatrogenic fluid replacement.[29] Patients with uterine enlargement also had a higher incidence of post-evacuation hemorrhage. We recommend that baseline arterial blood gases (ABGs) be obtained and that a laparotomy set and facilities for hemodynamic monitoring be available during evacuation of patients with hydatidiform mole complicated by uterine enlargement of more than 16 weeks' size.

Primary hysterectomy is a reasonable alternative for termination of molar gestation in patients who have completed childbearing. Hysterectomy reduces the incidence of malignant sequelae after evacuation of mole from approximately 20 percent following suction curettage to 3.5 percent after hysterectomy.[17] Hysterectomy does not, however, in any way eliminate the need for careful follow-up or complete hCG-titer surveillance after evacuation of hydatidiform mole, since malignant GTD may develop in some patients even after hysterectomy.

Induction of labor with oxytoxic agents or prostaglandins is not recommended as a method for molar evacuation.[21] Complete uterine evacuation may not occur following induction of labor. In addition, induction of uterine contractions prior to evacuation may lead to embolization of trophoblastic elements. Stone and Bagshawe[21] reported a higher incidence of malignant GTD following induction of labor for molar evacuation than in patients treated with suction D&C.

Theca lutein cysts are clinically detected in approximately 20 percent of patients with molar gestations.[17,18] These cysts are thin walled and highly vascular. They usually regress spontaneously after molar evacuation, usually over an interval of several weeks. It is preferable to avoid operation or ovarian manipulation in patients with uncomplicated theca lutein cysts. Occasionally, the cyst may become unduly large and undergo torsion, infarction, or rupture. Under such circumstances, oophorectomy may be life-saving.

Prophylactic methotrexate or actinomycin D chemotherapy has been used in some studies at the time of molar evacuation and decreases the incidence of malignant sequelae.[17,30-32] Although prophylactic chemotherapy may decrease the incidence of malignant GTD following molar evacuation in pregnancies with high-risk molar gestations, it does not eliminate the chance of subsequent malignancy and does not eliminate the need for hCG-titer surveillance. In addition, significant morbidity[17,30] and mortality following prophylactic chemotherapy have been observed[33] (C B Hammond, personal communication). Therefore, we do not recommend prophylactic chemotherapy at the time of molar evacuation in patients with uncomplicated hydatidiform mole when reliable hCG-titer surveillance is available.

Surveillance After Molar Evacuation

With the advent of sensitive hCG assays, histologic evaluation of hydatidiform mole has assumed less importance in predicting potential malignant postmolar sequelae. Currently, several sensitive hCG assays are available, measuring the β-subunit of hCG by radioimmunoassay (RIA)[34,35] or by immunoradiometric assay.[36] These assays are able to detect elevated hCG levels above baseline variations of pituitary gonadotropins. These sensitive hCG assays should be used to monitor patients with GTD following evacuation of hydatidiform mole and during therapy of patients with malignant GTD. The practice of following patients after evacuation of hydatidiform mole with urinary or serum pregnancy screening tests is to be condemned, since these assays do not have sufficient

sensitivity to permit detection of normal hCG levels (negative or absent).

Recommendations for surveillance following evacuation of hydatidiform mole include the following:

1. Baseline physical examination, pelvic examination, and chest radiography
2. Serum β-hCG titer every 1 to 2 weeks following evacuation until hCG titer is normal
3. hCG titer 2 to 4 weeks following first normal titer to confirm spontaneous titer regression
4. hCG surveillance after titer regression every 1 to 2 months for 6 to 12 months following first negative hCG titer

Most patients undergo hCG-titer regression to normal limits and require no further therapy. We recommend strict contraception during hCG-titer surveillance to avoid intercurrent pregnancy, which would interfere with hCG-titer surveillance.

Stone and associates[37] initially observed that patients using oral contraceptives after molar evacuation appear to have a higher incidence of malignant sequelae than do patients using barrier methods of contraception. Subsequent investigators have reported no significant difference in malignant sequelae among patients who use oral contraceptives or barrier methods following evacuation of hydatidiform mole.[38-40] Morrow and colleagues[40] observed an apparent decreased risk in women using oral contraceptives after molar evacuation. By contrast, Yuen et al.[39] noted a trend toward increased postmolar GTD among women using oral contraceptives containing more than 50 μg estrogen.[39] Since oral contraceptives are the most reliable form of contraception, we have not avoided oral contraceptives for patients after evacuation of hydatidiform mole.

After completion of hCG-titer surveillance, patients are allowed to achieve pregnancy if desired. Patients are at modestly increased risk of recurrent molar gestation in subsequent pregnancies.[17,22] We recommend that these patients undergo early screening of future pregnancies with ultrasound to exclude the possibility of recurrent molar gestation. In subsequent pregnancies, the placenta should be histologically evaluated, and an hCG titer should be obtained 6 to 8 weeks postevacuation to exclude the possibility of choriocarcinoma.

Malignant GTD Following Molar Evacuation

Malignant sequelae following evacuation of hydatidiform mole consists of intrauterine molar proliferation (retained mole), invasive mole (chorioadenoma destruens), and metastatic GTD. The purpose of hCG-titer surveillance is to detect trophoblastic proliferation before the development of complications related to local proliferation, uterine invasion, or distant metastasis.

Before effective chemotherapy against GTD was developed, Delfs[41] noted that in 11 (9 percent) of 119 patients with molar pregnancies, malignant sequelae eventually developed, requiring hysterectomy. Many series of patients reported since the development of chemotherapy have been reported[17,18,41-48] (Table 18-2), with a wide range of frequency of patients requiring therapy after molar evacuation. The observed differences in the reported frequency of therapy may reflect inclusion of partial moles in some studies, a different incidence of metastatic disease in these patient populations, or different hCG-titer regression criteria used to define proliferative disease and assign therapy in various studies.

Before the development of sensitive hCG assays, clinical and pathologic risk factors were often used to follow patients after evacuation of molar pregnancy. Histologic assessment of trophoblastic proliferation yields high- and low-risk groups of molar gestations[9] but is of little value in determining the need for therapy in individual patients.[10,17] Uterine enlargement,

theca lutein cysts, respiratory distress syndrome following molar evacuation, and postevacuation uterine bleeding are associated with a higher frequency of postmolar malignant GTD.[17,18] Prompt uterine involution and regression of theca lutein cysts are favorable prognostic signs, but the definitive method for predicting the development of postmolar malignant GTD is observation of the hCG-titer regression pattern.

Most authorities recommend that patients be followed after evacuation of hydatidiform mole with serial hCG titers and that therapy be instituted for either a rise or plateau in hCG titer appearance of metastases, or histologic evidence of malignant GTD (chorioadenoma destruens or choriocarcinoma). Some investigators have used more conservative criteria, relying on longer-term trends of hCG-titer regression. By contrast, occasional investigators have recommended instituting therapy based solely on persistence of measurable hCG at an arbitrary interval following evacuation of hydatidiform mole.

Bagshawe and associates[44] used extremely conservative criteria to institute chemotherapy and treated only 16 (6 percent) of 280 patients. Patients in this series with vaginal or lung metastases were treated only if hCG titers rose or if complications from metastases developed. Patients with an hCG-titer plateau were apparently observed over several weeks and were also not treated unless the hCG titer rose. This is in contrast to the frequent recommendation that patients be treated if a titer plateau persists over three consecutive weekly hCG titers.[17,18,42,48]

Kohorn[49] also recently suggested that plateauing hCG titers may be safely followed beyond a 2-week interval if reliable hCG-titer follow-up is available. Six (5 percent) of 131 patients followed after evacuation of hydatidiform mole in his series had an hCG-titer plateau for more than 2 weeks during hCG-titer surveillance. Subsequently, spontaneous hCG-titer regression developed in all these patients. In addition, five (14 percent) of 37 patients treated with chemotherapy had an immediate prechemotherapy hCG-titer fall of greater than 25 percent from a prior plateau.[49] These data would suggest that some patients with a plateauing hCG titer after evacuation of a hydatidiform mole can be safely monitored with serial hCG titers over several weeks and that a significant number of these patients enter spontaneous hCG-titer remission.

Table 18-2 Incidence of Malignant Gestational Trophoblastic Disease After Evacuation of Hydatidiform Mole

Series	Number of Patients	Patients Treated (%)	Metastatic Tumor (%)
Delfs[41]	119	9	—
Brewer et al.[42]	51	22	9
Goldstein[43]	116	20	22
Bagshawe et al.[44]	280	6	
Curry et al.[17]	347	20	17
Morrow et al.[18]	121	26	12
Hatch et al.[45]	212	32	18
Schlaerth et al.[46]	77	36	25
Kohorn[47]	127	27	6
Lurain et al.[48]	738	19	15

Some investigators have initiated therapy after hydatidiform mole if hCG titers remained elevated beyond an arbitrary length of time. Morrow and associates[18] instituted therapy if hCG titers persisted at 8 weeks after molar evacuation. Hatch and colleagues[45] treated most patients with detectable hCG at 12 weeks postevacuation. Although these reports may cover a different patient population, as reflected by the incidence of metastatic GTD, the incidence of patients treated in their series is somewhat higher than reported in other series in which therapy was instituted on the basis of hCG titer alone and not on the basis of persistent titer at an arbitrary time after molar evacuation (Table 18-2).

Delfs[41] noted that 22 percent of her patients had a positive hCG titer 60 days after molar evacuation, 42 percent of whom required hysterectomy. Curry and associates[17] reported that 40 percent of patients with persistent titer of 60 days eventually required therapy.[17] Likewise, Lurain and associates[48] noted that 322 (47 percent) of 738 patients followed after evacuation of hydatidiform mole had elevated hCG titer 60 days postevacuation. Only 36 percent of these patients subsequently required chemotherapy. These data suggest that, although patients with persistent hCG titer beyond 60 days after molar evacuation are at an increased risk of proliferative sequelae, most can still be safely followed with serial hCG testing.

We recommend that for patients with hydatidiform mole, pre- and postevacuation hCG titers be obtained as a baseline and that these patients be screened for metastases with chest radiography and physical examination. The patient should be followed with hCG titers at 1- to 2-week intervals with physical examination and chest radiography every 2 to 4 weeks, as long as hCG titers are elevated. Patients are treated with chemotherapy according to the following criteria:

1. hCG titer rise
2. hCG titer plateau for three consecutive weekly titers (x, x + 7 days, x + 14 days)
3. Appearance of metastasis
4. Histologic evidence of chorioadenoma destruens or choriocarcinoma

On the basis of these criteria, our incidence for therapy of postmolar malignant GTD has remained approximately 20 percent[17] (C B Hammond, personal communication).

MALIGNANT GTD

Malignant GTD consists of a spectrum of clinical and histologic entities. Since the development of effective chemotherapy, precise histologic definition has seemed less important in assigning therapy. Patients are often diagnosed and treated on the basis of hCG titer without a specific histologic diagnosis. The spectrum of clinical entities included in malignant GTD ranges from proliferative sequelae following hydatidiform mole (retained mole), invasive mole (chorioadenoma destruens), metastatic GTD following molar pregnancy or normal pregnancy, and trophoblastic choriocarcinoma.

Histologically, retained mole and invasive mole consist of hydropic villi with trophoblastic proliferation. Endometrium is present between the trophoblastic elements and myometrium in retained mole, while trophoblastic elements are in direct contact with the myometrium in invasive mole. Choriocarcinoma consists of undifferentiated sheets of intermingled cytotrophoblastic and syncytotrophoblastic elements. Both invasive mole and choriocarcinoma may metastasize and be identified in histologic sections of distant metastases. Frequently, a patient will have only invasive mole involving the uterus but distant metastases showing the histologic appearance of choriocarcinoma.

A rare histologic variant of GTD termed placental site tumor has been described.[49] These tumors consist of invasive neoplasms derived predominantly from cytotrophoblastic elements that are locally invasive and that rarely have the tendency to metastasize. Uterine perforation is common, however. These neoplasms secrete hCG at a very low level in contrast to other forms of GTD and tend to be resistant to chemotherapy.[50]

Diagnosis and Staging Studies

The diagnosis of malignant GTD is made when a patient has a rising or plateauing hCG titer following evacuation of hydatidiform mole or shows the appearance of metastases following evacuation of hydatidiform mole.[17,18,42-48] Likewise, the histologic diagnoses of chorioadenoma destruens or choriocarcinoma are criteria for malignant GTD. In certain situations, the key to the diagnosis of GTD lies in considering the possibility of the diagnosis. Approximately

50 percent of malignant GTD follows molar pregnancy. This population is generally identified promptly through the use of serum hCG monitoring. The remaining 50 percent follows nonmolar gestations and is divided roughly equally into GTD occurring after abortion or ectopic pregnancy, and GTD that occurs after term gestation. Often, these patients present with atypical symptoms referable to distant metastases[51,52]: Gastrointestinal (GI) or urologic bleeding, hemoptysis, or cerebral hemorrhage may be initial symptoms. In these circumstances, the diagnosis of GTD is facilitated by a high index of suspicion coupled with serum hCG testing. The possibility of metastatic GTD should be considered in any woman in the reproductive age group presenting with metastases to lungs, brain, or liver from an unknown primary site of malignancy.

The recommended clinical, laboratory, and radiographic evaluation of a patient with malignant GTD consists of the following routine:

1. Physical and pelvic examinations
2. Baseline hCG titer
3. Complete blood count and baseline chemistries
4. Chest radiography
5. Brain scan, i.e., computed tomography (CT) or radionuclide
6. Liver scan, i.e., CT or radionuclide
7. Pelvic ultrasound
8. Optional radiographic tests, as indicated
9. Diagnostic surgical procedures, as indicated

A general physical and pelvic examination may yield useful information about metastatic disease. A baseline neurologic evaluation is necessary to permit close monitoring of changes in neurologic function during therapy of GTD metastatic to the brain; however, the clinical neurologic examination is relatively insensitive in detecting occult central nervous system (CNS) metastases or in assigning the extent of CNS involvement. Likewise, the examination of lungs and abdomen may not detect pulmonary or hepatic metastases. Vaginal metastases are initially detected by pelvic examination, but other pelvic findings must be evaluated separately to distinguish pelvic metastases from theca lutein cysts of the ovaries. Pretherapy hCG titer is important in assigning the patient to a prognostic category and for reference during therapy. The hematologic, renal, and hepatic functions are necessary as baseline tests; only rarely will hepatic metastases be diagnosed on the basis of liver function tests. Thyroid function is also determined to diagnose the rare patient with secondary hyperthyroidism significant enough to require therapy until control of GTD results in euthyroidism.

Approximately 50 percent of patients with malignant GTD have pulmonary metastases detected by routine chest radiographs.[53] The clinical significance of small pulmonary metastases detected only by whole-lung tomography or CT scans of the lungs is unknown. These latter studies are not recommended as routine procedures but may be used to delineate questionable lesions detected on chest radiographs. Since CNS and hepatic metastases have occasionally been encountered without clinical or radiographic evidence of pulmonary or vaginal metastases,[54-56] the remainder of the radiologic studies are strongly recommended regardless of whether abnormalities are detected by chest radiography or physical examination. Rapid-sequence CT scans of the brain are more sensitive in detecting small metastases than are radionuclide scans. Brain CT scans are able to distinguish metastatic GTD from other abnormalities.[54,55] Abdominal CT and ultrasound of the pelvis can provide a combined survey of the pelvis and abdomen for possible involvement of other viscera. Pelvic ultrasound should be used prior to an aggressive radiographic evaluation or chemotherapy in the patient with suspected GTD to exclude pregnancy as the cause of an elevated hCG titer. Since metastases of GTD are highly vascular, the abdominal CT with contrast provides a reliable screen for hepatic metastases.[56] The role of magnetic resonance imaging (MRI) studies is not yet fully defined.

Arteriography is not used routinely for initial staging, since false-negative and false-positive findings have been reported.[57] Also, the arteriographic abnormalities of GTD may persist long after therapy has produced remission.[57] Selective arteriography is therefore reserved as an optional diagnostic tool to delineate lesions of unclear etiology detected by other imaging techniques.

A potentially useful study for detecting CNS metastasis is lumbar puncture with simultaneous serum and cerebrospinal fluid (CSF) hCG determinations.

Bagshawe and Harland[58] reported that the plasma-CSF ratio is normally greater than 60 : 1 in the absence of CNS metastasis from GTD, while the ratio was less than 60 : 1 in 29 of 33 patients with CNS metastasis.[58] These workers noted that in some patients a fall in plasma/CSF hCG ratio developed before radiographic documentation of CNS metastasis. Other investigators have reported falsely lowered plasma-CSF hCG ratios among patients undergoing first-trimester abortion without GTD and in patients with nonmetastatic GTD.[59] We have used CSF hCG determinations most frequently to evaluate patients in whom resistance to chemotherapy developed with residual disease documented by elevated serum hCG titer but in whom the site of disease has remained obscure.

Operative procedures may sometimes be useful in the therapy of patients with malignant GTD but are rarely indicated for staging or diagnosis alone. Dilatation and curettage might theoretically debulk intrauterine disease and limit the amount of chemotherapy necessary to induce remission in patients with nonmetastatic disease. We have not advocated pretherapy D&C, since patients with uterine malignancy are at risk of uterine perforation and intraperitoneal hemorrhage. We have used curettage on an individual basis only for patients with significant vaginal bleeding. Routine pretherapy D&C was evaluated by Berkowitz and colleagues[60] in 37 patients in whom nonmetastatic GTD developed after evacuation of hydatidiform mole. Twenty (54 percent) patients had no tissue detected by D&C, 19 of whom achieved sustained remission with limited chemotherapy. Patients having intrauterine disease with a worsened histology by Hertig and Sheldon's criteria were at risk of failure of initial chemotherapy.[60] None of the patients in this series suffered uterine perforation, and no other complications of pretherapy D&C were reported.

Laparoscopy has been advocated by some investigators for delineation of the extent of pelvic and intra-abdominal disease,[61] but we have not found this approach justified as a routine procedure for staging purposes. Craniotomy or thoracotomy are rarely justifiable in order to establish the primary diagnosis of malignant GTD, since this diagnosis can be made, after the exclusion of pregnancy, on the basis of an elevated hCG titer with radiographic evidence of metastasis.

Finally, it should be re-emphasized that all cases of malignant GTD must be evaluated thoroughly; selection of initial therapy and subsequent survival are largely dependent on identification of poor prognostic factors in patients with metastatic disease.

Clinical Staging of GTD

The clinical staging system is currently used at our center.[62-65] Once the staging studies are complete, the patient is considered to have nonmetastatic GTD if there is no evidence of extrauterine metastasis. This category is not divided into good-prognosis and poor-prognosis categories, since these patients have achieved essentially 100 percent remission rates according to current chemotherapeutic regimens. It is also noted that the histologic diagnosis of choriocarcinoma, although mandating treatment, does not change the initial choice of therapy. If there is any clinical or radiographic evidence of extrauterine metastasis, the patient is staged as having metastatic GTD. This diagnosis is further divided into good-prognosis and poor-prognosis categories on the basis of prognostic factors that would predict failure of primary single-agent chemotherapy with methotrexate or actinomycin D. The rationale for each category is discussed below.

PRETREATMENT hCG TITER

Initially, Hertz and associates[66] found no relationship between initial level of hCG and remission rates in patients with metastatic GTD treated with single-agent methotrexate or vinblastine. However, Ross and colleagues[67] observed that patients with low hCG titer had a 91 percent remission rate compared with 41 percent if the initial titer was elevated. Bagshawe[68] reported that patients with an initial hCG titer of less than 10,000 IU/24-hr urine had a 97.5 percent remission rate, progressively falling to 39 percent when the initial hCG titer was greater than 1,000,000 IU/24-hr urine. In considering all patients with metastatic GTD, Lurain et al.[69] observed an 88 percent remission rate in patients with a pretreatment titer of less than 100,000 IU/24-hr urine, falling to 75 percent in patients with an hCG titer of greater than 100,000 IU/24-hr urine.[69] These studies suggest that an initial hCG titer is a reflection of tumor volume and that increasing titer correlates with a poorer prognosis.

PROGNOSIS FOR NONMETASTATIC AND METASTATIC GESTATIONAL TROPHOBLASTIC DISEASE

1. Nonmetastatic GTD
   a. Not defined in terms of good versus poor prognosis — see text
2. Metastatic GTD
   a. Good prognosis
      1. Immediate pretreatment hCG-titer level less than 40,000 mIU/ml serum β-hCG
      2. Less than 4-month duration of symptoms of malignant disease
      3. No evidence of brain or liver metastasis
      4. No significant prior chemotherapy
      5. No antecedent term pregnancy
   b. Poor prognosis
      1. Immediate pretreatment hCG titer greater than 40,000 mIU/ml serum β-hCG
      2. Greater than 4-month duration of symptoms of malignant disease
      3. Brain and/or liver metastasis
      4. Failed prior chemotherapy
      5. Antecedent term pregnancy

DURATION OF DISEASE

Hertz and colleagues[66] noted that 72 percent of patients treated within 4 months of an antecedent pregnancy achieved remission, compared with 32 percent of patients treated with a longer duration of disease. Ross et al.[67] reported 85 percent remission rate when there was short duration and 61 percent remission rate in women with greater than 4-month duration of disease. Bagshawe[68] noted that survival decreased linearly over a range of less than 4 months to greater than 24 months. In considering patients with metastatic disease, Lurain and associates[69] found that 89 percent versus 70 percent of patients achieved remission, again using 4 months as the criterion for prolonged duration of disease. The studies by Ross et al.[67] and Lurain et al.[69] found that duration of disease

and hCG titer combined to identify low-risk (short-duration, low-titer) and high-risk (long-duration, high-titer) populations of patients, while patients with one favorable and one unfavorable factor were at intermediate risk.

BRAIN AND LIVER METASTASES

The presence of liver or brain metastases from GTD is associated with poor outcome.[67,68] Bagshawe,[68] in 1976, reported that only 11 of 23 patients who presented with brain metastases survived, while none of 20 in whom brain metastases developed while receiving chemotherapy survived. In 1983, the same investigators reported improved survival rates for both groups (80 percent for patients with early and 25 percent for patients with late brain metastases); however, this was still lower than their overall survival.[70] Patients with brain metastases are at risk of early mortality due to hemorrhage and late deaths due to the development of resistance to other forms of therapy. Therefore, most investigators have used a combination of both chemotherapy and specific therapy directed against brain metastases in the form of either whole-brain irradiation or intrathecal chemotherapy. Using these approaches, improved survival rates have been realized for patients presenting with brain metastases; however, brain metastases developing during therapy are an extremely poor prognostic feature.

Liver metastases are also indicative of poor prognosis, even with aggressive therapy.[71,72] These also have a tendency to rupture and may result in massive intraabdominal hemorrhage.

FAILURE OF PREVIOUS CHEMOTHERAPY

Failure of prior therapy is an extremely poor prognostic feature. A combination of resistance to chemotherapy and fibrosis around sites of residual tumor may contribute to poor survival results in these patients.[71] Hammond et al.[63] and Lurain et al.[69] noted that patients with metastatic GTD and poor prognostic factors who were initially treated with single-agent chemotherapy had poor survival, even when multiagent chemotherapy was used for salvage, in contrast to an enhanced survival of patients with poor-prognosis disease treated initially with multiagent chemotherapy. The single most important aspect of the clinical staging system is the identification of patients at risk of failure of single-agent chemotherapy. This permits individualization of therapy, with intense multiagent chemotherapy used initially in patients with poor-prognosis features.

ANTECEDENT TERM OR NONMOLAR PREGNANCY

Before the development of effective chemotherapy for GTD, several investigators noted an association between decreased survival and antecedent term pregnancy. Using single-agent chemotherapy, Hertz et al.[66] and Ross et al.[67] found identical survival for patients with antecedent mole and term gestations; however, survival rates were lower than those reported in more recent series; this observation may reflect a lack of effective combination chemotherapy for their high-risk patients. Bagshawe[68] reported no significant difference in survival among patients with antecedent mole, abortion, or term gestation and reported remission rates of 77 percent, 86 percent, and 80 percent respectively. He did, however, incorporate the type of antecedent pregnancy into his prognostic scoring system. Miller and associates[73] noted that 15 of 20 patients with GTD after term pregnancy were in the poor-prognosis metastatic GTD category on presentation and that these patients had a significantly worse outcome than all other poor-prognosis patients (47 percent versus 75 percent survival). They concluded that term pregnancy was an additional, not a confounding, poor-prognosis factor. Recently, Olive

and colleagues[74] reported that the risk of term pregnancy appeared to be related to other high-risk factors, such as prolonged duration of disease or high hCG titer, which were frequently associated with antecedent term pregnancy. After correcting for other high-risk factors, these workers concluded that the type of antecedent pregnancy is not important in determining prognosis. Patients with an antecedent nonmolar gestation must be critically evaluated for other risk factors, since these patients often have a long interval between delivery and recognition of malignant GTD. Most frequently, these patients will have metastatic disease with other associated high-risk factors and should be treated accordingly.

Prognostic Scoring Index

The prognostic scoring index uses both the FIGO anatomic staging system[75] for GTD and a weighted scale for arriving at a low-risk or high-risk index. The FIGO anatomic staging system is as follows[76]:

Stage I: Confined to the uterine corpus
Stage II: Vaginal or pelvic metastases
Stage III: Pulmonary metastases
Stage IV: Other extrapelvic metastases

The scoring index (Table 18-3) is based on Bagshawe's analysis of prognostic factors among his patient population.[68] In addition to using a weighted scale for the risk factors already discussed, such as duration of disease, pretherapy titer, and metastatic

Table 18-3 Prognostic Scoring of Gestational Trophoblastic Disease

Factor	0	1	2	3
Antecedent pregnancy	Hydatidiform mole	Nonmole abortion; ectopic	Term pregnancy	
Interval (months) between end of antecedent pregnancy and initial therapy	<3	3–6	7–12	>12
hCG value at initial therapy	$<10^3$	10^3-10^4	10^4-10^5	$>10^5$
ABO blood group (patient)			B or AB	
Largest tumor (cm)	<2		2–5	>5
Site of metastasis		Lung	GI tract kidney, spleen	Brain–liver
Number of metastasis identified		1–4	4–8	>8
Previous chemotherapy			Failed prophylactic	Failed therapeutic

Low risk: Prognostic score ≤7
High risk: Prognostic score >7

site, the system identifies a graded range of additional risk factors. Ectopic pregnancy and abortions are considered intermediate risks between molar and term pregnancy. Blood types B or AB are considered additional risk factors. The size of the largest tumor and number of metastatic sites and considered as well. Following computation of risk factors, a patient is considered to be at low risk if the score is less than or equal to 7 or at high risk if the score is greater than 7. The greatest value for this staging system may be in identifying patients who are at an extremely poor risk even when treated with aggressive multiagent chemotherapy[76]; it may prove useful in the future in identifying patients requiring more intensive chemotherapy than currently used methotrexate-based regimens.

THERAPY FOR MALIGNANT GTD

Nonmetastatic GTD

Before the development of effective chemotherapy, surgical therapy for even nonmetastatic GTD was unsatisfactory. Brewer and associates[77] noted poor survival following hysterectomy as therapy for nonmetastatic persistent mole or choriocarcinoma. Since the introduction of methotrexate as effective therapy for GTD,[78] most centers have reported essentially 100 percent cure rates for patients with nonmetastatic GTD. Methotrexate and actinomycin D have been the principal agents used in the therapy of this disease; however, oral VP-16 has recently been used with great success. Currently, many centers are investigating options for chemotherapy that would retain a high remission rate for this disease and limit toxicity or expense.

METHOTREXATE

Since the 1950s, methotrexate has been used in the therapy of GTD and has resulted in an almost 100 percent cure for patients with nonmetastatic disease. Methotrexate, 0.4 mg/kg IM × 5 days recycled every 12 to 14 days, was originally used as primary therapy in 58 patients with nonmetastatic GTD at the National Cancer Institute (NCI).[79] Only four (7 percent) patients developed resistance to first-line therapy; three of four patients were salvaged with second-line

actinomycin D. Toxicity to this regimen included significant incidence of alopecia, mucositis, neutropenia, thrombocytopenia, cutaneous and GI toxicity, and mesothelitis. However, there were no therapy-related deaths. With additional reports of excellent cure rates of nonmetastatic GTD using single-agent methotrexate,[43,64,65,69,80] alternative regimens have been explored to limit toxicity.

ACTINOMYCIN D

Goldstein et al.[81] used actinomycin D, 9 to 13 μg/kg/day IV × 5 days recycled at 12- to 14-day intervals, as primary therapy for 12 patients with nonmetastatic GTD. In two patients with nonmetastatic GTD therapy was changed to methotrexate, and all 12 achieved sustained remission. A later report from the same institution noted 94 percent remission with actinomycin D as primary therapy of 31 patients with nonmetastatic GTD.[82] The most common side effects were nausea and vomiting reported in two-thirds of patients, as well as alopecia and transient marrow depression. No therapy-related deaths were reported. Most reports have used actinomycin D as salvage therapy for nonmetastatic GTD resistant to initial methotrexate regimens.

METHOTREXATE PLUS FOLINIC ACID

Bagshawe and Wilde[83] first proposed methotrexate plus folinic acid as therapy for GTD. The rationale for folinic acid administration is rescue of the dihydrofolate reductase block induced by methotrexate, permitting administration of a higher dose of methotrexate, with subsequent rescue of normal tissues by folinic acid. Recently, Rotmensch et al.[84] evaluated serial methotrexate levels during rescue therapy with methotrexate plus folinic acid. It was concluded that dosing with alternating methotrexate and folinic acid resulted in subtherapeutic and subtoxic trough methotrexate levels with higher peak methotrexate levels than could be achieved with daily methotrexate administration.[84] This finding showed therapeutic effect and limited toxicity rather than rescue of normal tissues with folinic acid. Various dose schedules using methotrexate plus folinic acid have been used.

Goldstein and associates[85] used methotrexate, 1 mg/kg IM, on days 1, 3, 5, and 7, alternating with folinic acid, 0.1 mg/kg IM, on days 2, 4, 6, and 8. A single cycle of chemotherapy was administered for nonmetastatic GTD, and the pattern of hCG-titer regression was followed. For patients who showed a progressive decrease in hCG titer and who went into remission, no further therapy was given. For those whose hCG titer plateaued for more than 3 weeks or was re-elevated, treatment was reinstituted. Alternative therapy with actinomycin D was used for salvage therapy. Berkowitz and colleagues[86] treated 106 patients with nonmetastatic GTD or low-risk metastatic GTD using this regimen. Seventy-two (80.9 percent) of 94 patients with nonmetastatic GTD achieved remission with one cycle of chemotherapy, while 12 (13.5 percent) required a second course to achieve remission. Alternative therapy was required for five (5.7 percent) patients.[86] Patients with nonmetastatic GTD were more likely to respond to this regimen than were those with low-risk metastatic disease. Only three of seven patients with an hCG titer greater than 50,000 mIU/m responded versus 79.9 percent with lower hCG titers. Toxicity was extremely limited, with mild marrow suppression observed in fewer than 10 percent of patients. Previously, Berkowitz and Goldstein[87] attempted to improve the response rate by increasing the methotrexate dose to 1.5 mg/kg, alternating with folinic acid, 0.15 mg/kg. There was no significant improvement in response rate, but the higher dose rate yielded 30 percent significant hepatic or hematologic toxicity and was subsequently abandoned. These investigators did not give chemotherapy following induction of remission and have not reported recurrence data in their studies.

Methotrexate plus folinic acid has also been administered as repetitive cyclic chemotherapy until remission is achieved. At this center, Smith et al.[88] and Mutch et al.[89] used methotrexate, 1.0 mg/kg, on days 1, 3, 5, and 7 and folinic acid, 0.1 mg/kg/24 hr, following each dose of methotrexate. Wong and associates[90] used the same schedule but administered folinic acid rescue 30 hours after each dose of methotrexate. In these reports, cycles of chemotherapy were repeated at 14- to 15-day intervals until remission was achieved as determined by hCG-titer surveillance or until evidence of resistance was noted. Smith and associates[89] reported a higher failure rate with methotrexate plus folinic acid than with conventional single-agent methotrexate, 27.5 percent versus 7.7 percent, respectively. Myelosuppression and hepatic

toxicity were more frequently encountered among patients with single-agent methotrexate than among those treated with methotrexate plus folinic acid rescue. Four (10.3 percent) of 39 patients treated with single-agent methotrexate had therapy changed to actinomycin D because of significant toxicity.[88] All patients in this series who failed with initial methotrexate plus folinic acid or with methotrexate alone were salvaged using single-agent chemotherapy. Reporting from the same institution, Mutch and associates[89] confirmed a persistent 26 percent failure rate for methotrexate plus folinic acid as primary chemotherapy for nonmetastatic GTD. Eight (80 percent) of 10 patients who failed with initial methotrexate plus folinic acid chemotherapy had pulmonary micrometastases documented on pulmonary CT scanning; this feature was considered a poor-prognosis factor for success of this regimen, since 8 (50 percent) of 16 patients with pulmonary micrometastases detected by CT scanning failed initial chemotherapy.[89]

Wong and associates[90] also compared single-agent methotrexate with methotrexate plus folinic acid rescue as therapy for patients with nonmetastatic and low-risk metastatic GTD. These workers observed a lower failure rate for methotrexate plus folinic acid than for conventional single-agent methotrexate but noted significantly increased hepatic toxicity in the methotrexate plus folinic acid-treated rescue group. Their protocol differed somewhat from that used by Smith et al.[88] in that folinic acid was administered 30 hours following methotrexate.[90] In addition, a high

Table 18-4 Therapy for Nonmetastatic Gestational Trophoblastic Disease[a,b]

Agent	Dose	Day
Initial therapy		
Methotrexate	1.0 mg/kg IM	1, 3, 5, 7
Folinic acid	0.1 mg/kg IM	2, 4, 6, 8 (24 hr after methotrexate)
OR		
Methotrexate	0.4 mg/kg IM	1–5
Salvage therapy		
Actinomycin D	9–13 μg/kg IV	1–5

[a] Chemotherapy is recycled after a minimum 7 days off of therapy until normal hCG titer.
[b] One cycle of maintainence chemotherapy given after first negative hCG titer.

endemic rate of hepatitis was found among their patient population. No randomized study has prospectively evaluated toxicity or efficacy of methotrexate plus folinic acid versus single-agent methotrexate in the therapy for nonmetastatic GTD.

We recommend the cyclic repetitive methotrexate plus folinic acid regimen as initial therapy for patients with nonmetastatic GTD (Table 18-4), since an acceptable cure rate is achieved with this regimen with minimal associated toxicity. Alternatively, conventional methotrexate can be used as initial therapy. We have reserved actinomycin D as salvage therapy for patients who have failed with initial methotrexate regimens in therapy for nonmetastatic GTD (Table 18-4).

ACTINOMYCIN D BOLUS

Petrilli and Morrow[91] first proposed using a single intravenous bolus of actinomycin D (40 μg/kg = 1.25 mg/M^2) administered every 2 weeks. The rationale for the bolus regimen was that actinomycin D has a long half-life and that the total dose administered was equivalent to the more traditional 5-day course of actinomycin D. This regimen has subsequently been evaluated by Twiggs[92] and Petrilli et al.[93] Petrilli and Morrow[91] compared actinomycin D, 500 μg IV × 5 days, recycled every 2 weeks versus the bolus regimen. Three of 15 patients failed 5-day actinomycin D versus one of five patients treated with the actinomycin D bolus. Toxicity was similar in both therapy arms. Twiggs[92] subsequently treated 12 patients with the bolus regimen and reported that all patients entered remission after an average 4.8 cycles of chemotherapy. There was one episode of significant thrombocytopenia in his patient population, which Twiggs considered cost-effective chemotherapy with an acceptable remission rate and acceptable toxicity. Petrilli and associates[93] reported that 29 (94 percent) of 31 patients achieved remission after an average 4.4 cycles of bolus actinomycin D chemotherapy. There was no grade 3 or 4 hematologic or hepatic toxicity and only a 10 percent incidence of grade 3 GI toxicity. Further investigations using bolus actinomycin D or methotrexate are being conducted by the Gynecologic Oncology Group to determine whether this is cost-effective chemotherapy for the treatment of nonmetastatic GTD.

VP-16

Wong and colleagues[94] used oral VP-16 (etoposide), 200 mg/M^2 × 5 days, recycled at 12- to 14-day intervals, and treated 48 patients with nonmetastatic and 12 patients with low-risk metastatic GTD. Fifty-nine (98 percent) of 60 patients achieved remission using this regimen. One patient was changed to the methotrexate plus folinic acid regimen due to intolerable GI toxicity. All patients developed alopecia. Other toxicity consisted of mild to moderate neutropenia, stomatitis and nausea, but toxicity was generally limited.[94] Oral VP-16 is not currently available in the United States, and further experience will be required to determine its efficacy in the chemotherapy of nonmetastatic GTD.

SUMMARY

Nonmetastatic GTD has an excellent prognosis with essentially 100 percent cure rates using currently available chemotherapeutic regimens. Future investigations are needed to compare regimens in a prospective manner to identify cost-effective regimens of modest toxicity that will retain a high cure rate for these patients.

Good-Prognosis Metastatic GTD

Single-agent methotrexate or actinomycin D has been used as primary therapy for patients with metastatic GTD since the late 1950s (Table 18-5). Among patients without poor prognostic features, the cure rate for patients with good-prognosis GTD approaches 100 percent using these agents.[43,62–69] Therapy using either agent as initial treatment appears to be equally effective. Approximately 40 to 50 percent of patients will fail primary therapy with either agent, and most can be salvaged with the alternative single-agent regimen. Multiagent chemotherapy is reserved for patients who have failed with both single-agent chemotherapeutic regimens.

Methotrexate alternating with folinic acid rescue as used in the therapy of nonmetastatic GTD has been reported in patients with good-prognosis metastatic GTD. Although the report by Wong et al.[90] indicates that patients can be cured with this regimen, Berkowitz et al.[86] found that patients with nonmetastatic GTD were more likely to respond to methotrexate

Table 18-5 Therapy for Metastatic Good-Prognosis Gestational Trophoblastic Disease[a,b]

Agent	Dose	Day
Initial therapy		
Methotrexate	0.4 mg/kg IM	1–5
OR		
actinomycin D	9–13 μg/kg IV	1–5
Salvage therapy		
Alternative single-agent chemotherapy		
Combination chemotherapy for patients failing methotrexate and Actinomycin D regimens		

[a] Chemotherapy is recycled after a minimum 7 days off of therapy until normal hCG titer.
[b] Two cycles of maintainence chemotherapy given after first negative hCG titer.

plus folinic acid chemotherapy than were patients with good-prognosis metastatic disease. Furthermore, the recent report by Mutch et al.[89] indicating a 50 percent failure of primary methotrexate plus folinic acid among patients with pulmonary metastases detected only by CT scan of the lungs casts doubt on the efficacy of this regimen in treating patients with metastatic disease. Currently, the Gynecologic Oncology Group is studying the relative efficacy of single agent methotrexate versus methotrexate plus folinic acid regimens in patients with good-prognosis metastatic GTD.

Poor-Prognosis Metastatic GTD

Patients with metastatic GTD who have poor prognostic features have enhanced survival and decreased toxicity when treated initially with multiagent chemotherapeutic regimens.[63,69] It should be emphasized that all patients with malignant GTD must be evaluated thoroughly, since the choice of initial therapy and subsequent survival are largely dependent on making or excluding the diagnosis of poor-prognosis metastatic GTD. Methotrexate-based combination chemotherapy consisting of methotrexate, actinomycin D, and chlorambucil (or cyclosphosphamide) and the modified Bagshawe protocol have been used most frequently in the therapy for patients with poor-prognosis metastatic GTD. Recently, reports of either cisplatin or VP-16-containing regi-

mens have indicated that these agents may be useful in first-line therapy for patients with poor-prognosis metastatic GTD; however, comparative studies have not been performed to evaluate toxicity or efficacy of these regimens.

The methotrexate–actinomycin D–chlorambucil (or cyclophosphamide) regimen (Table 18-6) was originally proposed by Li[95] for patients with testicular choriocarcinoma and was later adopted for use as salvage therapy for patients with GTD. Subsequently, Hammond et al.[63] demonstrated that initial multiagent therapy with methotrexate–actinomycin D–chlorambucil was preferable to single-agent therapy in the group of patients with poor-prognosis features. Various institutions have achieved long-term complete remission rates of 60 to 80 percent in these patients using methotrexate–actinomycin D–chlorambucil as standard initial therapy.[64,65,69,71,96,97]

This regimen uses methotrexate, 0.3 mg/kg IM, actinomycin D 8 to 10 μg/kg IV, and chlorambucil, 0.2 mg/kg PO, or cyclophosphamide, 3 to 5 mg/kg IV, each given daily for five consecutive days (Table 18-6). Each treatment cycle is repeated after 9 to 14 days off therapy, as toxicity allows. The toxicity of this regimen is considerable. Often, cumulative toxicity requires a change to single-agent chemotherapy following two or more cycles of methotrexate–actinomycin D–chlorambucil after initial tumor control and stabilization of the patient have been achieved.[63]

Table 18-6 MAC Chemotherapy for Metastatic Poor-Prognosis Gestational Trophoblastic Disease[a–c]

Agent	Dose	Day
Methotrexate	0.3 mg/kg IM	1–5
Actinomycin D	8–10 μg/kg IV	1–5
Chlorambucil	0.2 mg/kg PO	1–5
or		
Cyclophosphamide	3–5 mg/kg IV	1–5

MAC = methotrexate–actinomycin–chlorambucil or cyclophosphamide.
[a] Chemotherapy is recycled after a minimum 9 days off of therapy until normal hCG titer.
[b] Three cycles of maintainence chemotherapy are given after first normal hCG titer.
[c] If hCG titer control achieved, may change to single-agent chemotherapy to limit toxicity after two or more cycles of MAC.

Berkowitz and colleagues[98] modified the triple-agent regimen, substituting methotrexate, 1.0 mg/kg, alternating with folinic acid for four doses. Survival and toxicity similar to that observed with standard methotrexate–actinomycin D–chlorambucil chemotherapy was reported in a single study using a modified version of this chemotherapy as the only treatment arm.[98] No comparative studies have been conducted to evaluate either regimen or to compare the effectiveness of methotrexate–actinomycin D–chlorambucil to methotrexate combined with actinomycin D as initial therapy for these patients.

Bagshawe[99] initially reported a 9- to 10-day chemotherapeutic regimen using hydroxyurea, vincristine, intermediate-dose methotrexate with folinic acid rescue, actinomycin D, cyclophosphamide, melphalan, and Adriamycin. Subsequently, this regimen was modified by both Surwit et al.[100] and Weed et al.[101] to reduce the length of the treatment cycle and to increase the amount of actinomycin D in the regimen (Table 18-5). The modified Bagshawe protocol (Table 18-7) was initially used at this center as salvage therapy for patients with poor-prognosis metastatic GTD who developed resistance to methotrexate–

actinomycin D–chlorambucil. The initial report of a remission rate of 83 percent among six patients with acceptable toxicity led to the recommendation of the modified Bagshawe protocol as primary chemotherapy for patients with poor-prognosis metastatic GTD.[100] Further experience with this protocol yielded a sustained remission rate of 56 percent among 18 patients with considerably higher toxicity levels.[101] Bagshawe[102] reported 75 percent survival among high-risk patients treated initially with the modified Bagshawe protocol.[101] The Gynecologic Oncology Group is currently conducting a randomized trial comparing methotrexate–actinomycin D–chlorambucil versus the modified Bagshawe protocol as primary therapy in patients with poor-prognosis metastatic GTD.

Recently, Bagshawe's group used a complex alternating regimen consisting of VP-16, methotrexate with folinic acid rescue, and actinomycin D alternating with cyclophosphamide and vinblastine (EMA CO). Initially, this combination was used as salvage therapy for patients with drug-resistant GTD with significant response rates.[102,103] This led to the use of EMA CO as initial chemotherapy among high-risk

Table 8-7 Modified Bagshawe Protocol Chemotherapy[a,b]

Day	Agent	Dose	Schedule (hr)
1	Hydroxyurea	500 mg PO	0600, 1200, 1800, 2400
	Actinomycin D	200 μg IV	1900
2	Vincristine	1 mg/M² IV	0700
	Methotrexate	100 mg/M² IV bolus	1900
	Methotrexate	200 mg/M² IV 12-hr infusion	1900
	Actinomycin D	200 μg IV	1900
3	Actinomycin D	200 μg IV	1900
	Cyclophosphamide	500 mg/M² IV	1900
	Folinic acid	14 mg IM	1900
4	Folinic acid	14 mg IM	0100, 0700, 1300, 1900
	Actinomycin D	500 μg IV	1900
6, 7	No treatment		
8	Doxorubicin	30 mg/M² IV	1900
	Melphalan	6 mg/M² PO	1900
	OR		
	Cyclophosphamide	500 mg/M² IV	1900

[a] Chemotherapy is recycled after a minimum 9 days off of therapy.
[b] Day 8 is omitted if significant hematologic toxicity is present.

patients. Bagshawe[102] reported an increased complete remission rate among patients with high-risk GTD using this regimen, as compared with historic controls at his institution, and has been impressed with the lack of significant toxicity. However, comparative studies have not yet systematically evaluated the efficacy or toxicity of this regimen.

Patients with poor-prognosis metastatic GTD require complex integration of various therapeutic modalities including chemotherapy, surgery, and radiation therapy in their treatment. A sensitive hCG-titer assay must be readily available to assist clinicians in the management of these patients. It is strongly recommended that patients with poor-prognosis metastatic GTD be treated at a trophoblastic disease center by physicians experienced in the management of these patients.

Salvage Chemotherapy for GTD

The development of drug resistance during therapy of poor-prognosis GTD presents a multitude of problems to the clinician. These patients generally have depleted nutritional reserves and significant accumulated marrow toxicity and often have anatomically resistant disease. Each case must be constantly reevaluated for metastatic sites amenable to surgical resection or irradiation. Carefully selected adjuvant surgical procedures may result in the ultimate cure of metastatic GTD, which is apparently resistant to chemotherapy. Prior chemotherapy must be carefully evaluated for selection of agents and for regimens to which the malignancy has not been exposed and that can be rapidly recycled. Often, the limiting factor in therapy for these patients is accumulated toxicity from prior therapy. Tumor escape can develop both through drug resistance and when recycling of chemotherapy is delayed due to toxicity.

The largest experience with salvage chemotherapy at this institution has been with the modified Bagshawe protocol. Among 18 patients with poor-prognosis metastatic GTD treated with this protocol through 1979, a prolonged remission rate of 56 percent was reported; 16 of these patients had received significant previous treatment.[101] Many other agents and combination of agents have been tried as salvage therapy at this institution, including actinomycin D, Adriamycin, bleomycin, cisplatin, vinblastine, vincristine, high-dose methotrexate with folinic acid res-

cue, modifications of the Einhorn regimen, VP-16, intraarterial perfusion with chemotherapeutic agents, and bone marrow transplantation following high-dose BCNU.[71] Responses have been seen to many of these agents, but complete remissions have been few in number.

Various combinations of vinblastine, bleomycin, and cisplatin modeled after the Einhorn regimen for testicular carcinoma have been reported as salvage therapy of GTD with anecdotal sustained remissions.[104,105] Despite initial enthusiasm for this regimen,[71] we have not observed a significant sustained remission rate among patients treated with modified Einhorn regimens as salvage therapy, which is the experience of others.[69,96] The EMA CO regimen was initially developed as salvage therapy for patients with poor-prognosis metastatic GTD. Given the high level of activity against GTD exhibited by VP-16 and VP-16-containing regimens,[102,103] it is clearly rational to treat patients with drug-resistant GTD, using VP-16.

Treatment of Brain and Liver Metastasis

In addition to chemotherapy, we recommend the use of adjuvant radiation therapy for the initial treatment of brain and liver metastasis.[54,55,65,71] Whole-brain irradiation of approximately 2,000 to 3,000 total rad over 10 days is begun concomitantly with initial chemotherapy when brain metastases are diagnosed. Brace[106] initially demonstrated that whole-brain irradiation to 2,000 rad resulted in long-term survival in 29 patients with GTD metastatic to the brain, while an additional five patients had eradication of CNS metastasis as determined by subsequent radiographic or autopsy evaluation. Furthermore, CNS radiation permitted stabilization of neurologic signs and symptoms, so that chemotherapy could be continued in most patients. Using this combined approach, a survival rate of 40 to 50 percent for patients with brain metastases from GTD has been achieved.[54,55] The prognosis for patients in whom brain metastases develop during chemotherapy may be worse than for patients initially presenting with brain metastases. However, Weed and Hammond[54] reported three of seven survivors in patients treated for CNS metastases that had developed during therapy.

Intrathecal administration of methotrexate has been advocated by Bagshawe for prophylaxis and therapy for CNS metastases.[68,70] Intrathecal chemotherapy could overcome the problem of delivering methotrexate across the blood-brain barrier. Experimentally, however, metastatic implants in the CNS result in increased permeability of the blood-brain barrier.[107] Intrathecal chemotherapy and whole-brain irradiation have not been prospectively evaluated for efficacy but, given the propensity for early hemorrhage into CNS metastases,[70] it is rational to incorporate one of these forms of therapy to prevent early mortality from CNS metastases.

Craniotomy is not often required for the primary therapy or diagnosis of brain metastases due to GTD and usually proves unsuccessful when used alone. However, neurosurgical consultation should be obtained early in the course of therapy in the event that craniotomy is required for stabilization during therapy.

Patients with liver metastases have also had these lesions treated with whole organ radiation therapy at our institution.[71,72] A total of approximately 2,000 rad is delivered in divided fractions over 10 days to keep within the limits of hepatic radiation tolerance. This is less than a tumorocidal dose but does appear to decrease the potential for hemorrhage from liver metastases during chemotherapy. Some investigators have not used hepatic irradiation unless ongoing hemorrhage is present, to avoid exacerbation of hepatic chemotherapy toxicity.[69] Others have advocated selective occlusion of the hepatic artery through ligation or embolization.[108] Barnard et al.[72] reported that 12 of 13 patients who received chemotherapy and hepatic radiation were able to tolerate full doses of chemotherapy, with significant hepatotoxicity developing in only one patient. Patients with hepatic metastasis have a dismal prognosis and require aggressive chemotherapy and careful monitoring during therapy to maximize chances for survival.

SURGICAL THERAPY FOR MALIGNANT GTD

Before the advent of chemotherapy, patients with malignant GTD were usually treated with either surgery or irradiation, and overall survival was poor.[80] Most women with malignant GTD died of rapidly progressing disease, within 1 year of diagnosis. Although the importance of surgery as the primary mode of therapy for malignant GTD has decreased, surgical intervention is required in some patients to control complications of metastases or resect foci of drug-resistant disease. In addition, hysterectomy may be indicated as part of primary therapy for selected patients. We have performed adjuvant surgical procedures under coverage of chemotherapy to reduce the potential for tumor embolization and metastases caused by surgical manipulation.[64]

Hysterectomy

Both primary and delayed hysterectomy play a role in the management of patients with nonmetastatic and metastatic GTD. Hammond et al.[64] observed that patients with nonmetastatic or good-prognosis metastatic GTD treated initially with hysterectomy combined with chemotherapy achieved remission after a shorter duration of hospital stay and a decrease in the number of courses of chemotherapy required to achieve remission. Delayed hysterectomy was required for approximately 10 percent of patients in these categories, and all patients were eventually cured. Chemotherapy alone, however, was successful in curing approximately 85 percent of patients with nonmetastatic and good-prognosis metastatic GTD. Therefore, patients in these categories who desire preservation of childbearing capacity should be treated initially with chemotherapy alone.[64] Among women with poor-prognosis metastatic GTD, preservation of childbearing capacity must be of secondary importance, but primary or delayed hysterectomy does not appear to be as beneficial as in patients with nonmetastatic or good-prognosis metastatic GTD.[64]

Thoracotomy

Thoracotomy with pulmonary resection has been the most frequently used procedure for extirpation of distant drug-resistant metastases.[64] Although thoracotomy can be performed safely in most patients under the cover of chemotherapy, caution must be exercised. Radiographic evidence of tumor regression may lag behind hCG-titer response.[53] Although patients with persistent pulmonary nodules may be at increased risk of recurrent GTD, there is little justification for extirpation of pulmonary metastases that persist during chemotherapy with a falling hCG titer or that persist into hCG-titer remission.[109]

Many investigators have reported success with pulmonary resection of solitary nodules in highly selected women with drug-resistant disease.[109-113] Before submitting a patient to thoracotomy, it is important to exclude the possibility of disease elsewhere. We recommend CT evaluation of brain, thorax, and abdomen, as well as simultaneous serum and CSF β-hCG titers in search of occult extrapulmonary disease. If the patient has not had hysterectomy, active pelvic GTD should be investigated with arteriography.

Indications for a planned pulmonary resection for therapy of GTD have been reviewed by Tomoda and associates.[113] These workers proposed several criteria: (1) good surgical candidate, (2) primary malignancy controlled (uterus removed or no evidence of pelvic disease by arteriography), (3) no evidence of other metastatic sites, (4) solitary pulmonary lesion, and (5) persistent hCG titer of less than 1,000 mIU/ml. In their series, 14 (93 percent) of 15 patients who satisfied these criteria survived after pulmonary resection, compared with none of four patients who had one or more unfavorable clinical feature.[113] Other investigators have reported that prompt hCG-titer remission following pulmonary resection predicts a favorable outcome.[108-113]

Craniotomy

Brain metastases are clinically detected in 8 to 15 percent of patients with metastatic GTD. Since these metastases are highly vascular and have a tendency for central necrosis and hemorrhage, acute neurologic deterioration may develop. Major goals of therapy are early detection of brain metastases through radiographic studies, stabilization of the patient's neurologic status, and institution of therapy. Craniotomy with resection of brain metastases is usually performed for patients requiring decompression in the presence of CNS hemorrhage. Craniotomy and resection of drug-resistant lesions is justified only in carefully selected patients.

Other Surgical Procedures

Other surgical procedures may be indicated in individual patients to correct bowel obstruction, drain abscesses, and other complications of disease or ther-

apy.[64] When extirpation of a drug-resistant disease focus is planned, resection is performed under coverage of chemotherapy to decrease the risk of potential embolization and establishment of new metastases during surgery. The combination of chemotherapy and surgery has not been observed to increase complications related to surgery.[64]

MONITORING THERAPY OF GTD

During therapy of GTD, hematologic, renal, and hepatic indices should be monitored carefully. Unless a patient is receiving salvage therapy for drug-resistant or recurrent GTD, a new cycle of therapy should be withheld unless the total white blood count (WBC) is greater than 3,000/mm^3 or a neutrophil count is greater than 1,500/mm^3, the platelet count is greater than 100,000/mm^3, and hepatic indices are normal. Radiographic studies of metastatic lesions and pelvic examinations should be repeated frequently to monitor response to therapy.

More important than radiographic surveillance is close follow-up of hCG-titer response during therapy. Sensitive hCG-titer assays should be obtained at least at 1-week intervals during therapy. Chemotherapy should be changed if the hCG titer has not dropped at least 25 percent following a treatment cycle or when toxicity will not permit an adequate dosage or frequency of administration.

hCG Titer Remission and Surveillance

Complete remission is defined as three consecutive weekly hCG titers in the normal range. Long-term surveillance consists of hCG titers every 2 weeks for the first 3 months after completion of therapy, every month for 3 months, and every 2 months for the next 6 months. Although in most patients with recurrences an elevated hCG titer develops within a few months after completion of therapy, late recurrences will develop in a few cases.[114,115] We therefore recommend that hCG titers be repeated at 6-month intervals indefinitely. Patients are counseled to avoid pregnancy through the first year of hCG-titer surveillance; most are treated with oral contraceptives to avoid low-level interference with the hCG assay caused by luteinizing hormone (LH).

PREVENTION OF RECURRENT GTD

Despite the fact that hCG monitoring gives a sensitive index of disease status in patients with GTD, recurrence may develop even after hCG-titer remission is achieved. Surwit and Hammond[115] reported recurrence rates of 3 percent, 0 percent, and 26 percent among patients with nonmetastatic, metastatic good prognosis, and metastatic poor prognosis GTD. The mean length of maintenance chemotherapy in patients with metastatic disease in whom recurrent GTD developed was 1.2 cycles; only one had received three cycles beyond the first negative hCG titer.[115] Bagshawe[99] advocated two to eight cycles of chemotherapy after titer remission, depending on the rate of hCG regression during therapy. He observed a decrease in the recurrence rate at his institution from 9 percent to 3 percent after routinely administering maintenance chemotherapy to patients in titer remission. Likewise, Lurain et al.[69] cited a reduction in recurrence rate from 18.2 percent to 3.1 percent when a policy of routine administration of two cycles of maintenance chemotherapy was instituted. We individualize maintenance chemotherapy according to the clinical stage of disease and difficulty of achieving remission. We recommend administering one cycle of maintenance chemotherapy for patients with nonmetastatic GTD, two cycles for patients with good-prognosis metastatic GTD, and three cycles for patients with poor-prognosis metastatic GTD.[65] Since 1979, the recurrence rate for patients with poor-prognosis metastatic GTD at our institution has decreased from 26 percent to 11.6 percent,[65] suggesting that this approach is beneficial.

REPRODUCTION AFTER THERAPY FOR GTD

Since chemotherapy without hysterectomy is often successful in the therapy of women with nonmetastatic and good-prognosis metastatic GTD, a relatively large proportion of women in these diagnostic categories will require counseling about the potential effects of chemotherapy on subsequent pregnancies. Several reports have documented that there is little if any increased risk of congenital malformation in infants resulting from subsequent pregnancies in these patients.[64,116,117] Hammond et al. reported that 67 (46 percent) of 146 patients treated for nonmetastatic

or good-prognosis metastatic GTD with chemotherapy alone subsequently had 83 pregnancies.[64] Sixty-seven (81 percent) of term pregnancies resulted in 69 living children, with nine (11 percent) spontaneous abortions and two (2.4 percent) recurrent molar gestations.[64] Berkowitz et al.[117] observed an apparent slight increase in the incidence of spontaneous abortion in their population of patients previously treated for nonmetastatic GTD, which they attributed to closer monitoring of possible pregnancies after therapy for GTD. They also reported an increased incidence of repeat molar gestation in their patient population.[117]

Patients who have received intensive therapy for poor-prognosis metastatic GTD often undergo hysterectomy during therapy[65] or may occasionally have ovarian failure resulting from prolonged multiagent chemotherapy. Hammond et al.[64] observed that only 4 (21 percent) of 19 patients with uterine conservation in this category of patients were able to conceive after therapy.

Pregnancies after therapy for GTD may result in increased morbidity. Major obstetric complications were reported in 9 percent of 82 term or premature deliveries reported by Berkowitz et al.[117] while Hammond et al.[64] reported no apparent increase in obstetric complications. Van Thiel and associates[118] observed that the incidence of placenta accreta was markedly increased in women previously treated with GTD compared with reports in normal obstetric populations.

We recommend that women who have been treated successfully for GTD be advised that pregnancy should be deferred for at least one full year of hCG-titer surveillance. They should be reassured regarding the incidence of congenital malformations and recurrent GTD in subsequent pregnancies. Ultrasound should be performed early in pregnancy to exclude the possibility of recurrent molar gestation and that a chest radiograph and serum hCG titer be obtained 6 to 8 weeks postpartum to screen for the rare case of choriocarcinoma developing after a subsequent pregnancy.

SUMMARY

Gestational trophoblastic disease is a term that encompasses a spectrum of clinical and pathologic entities caused by neoplasms of the human trophoblast. Most cases of GTD can be successfully treated, with reproductive capacity preserved following treatment. Future research in molar gestation is needed to delineate etiologic factors and to refine indications for institution of chemotherapy. Clinical research in malignant GTD is needed to refine and expand the currently available chemotherapeutic strategies to permit reduction in toxicity for women with low-risk disease and provide enhanced survival for women in the highest risk categories.

REFERENCES

1. Szulman AE, Surti U: The syndromes of hydatidiform moles. I. Cytogenetics and morphologic correlations. Am J Obstet Gynecol 131:665, 1978

2. Szulman AE, Surti U: The syndromes of hydatidiform moles. II. Morphologic evolution of the complete and partial mole. Am J Obstet Gynecol 132:20, 1978

3. Szulman AE, Philippe E, Bone A, et al: Human triploidy: Association with partial hydatidiform moles and non-molar conceptuses. Hum Pathol 12:1016, 1981

4. Szulman AE: Syndromes of hydatidiform moles: Partial versus complete. J Reprod Med 29:788, 1984

5. Jacobs PA, Szulman AE, Finkhouser J, et al: Human triploidy: Relationship between paternal origin of the additional haploid complement and development of partial hydatidiform mole. Ann Hum Genet 46:223, 1982

6. Szulman AE, Surti U: The clinicopathologic profile of the partial hydatidiform mole. Obstet Gynecol 59:597, 1982

7. Berkowitz RS, Goldstein BP, Bernstein MR: Natural history of partial molar pregnancy. Obstet Gynecol 66:677, 1983

8. Smith EB, Szulman AE, Hinshaw W, et al: hCG levels in complete and partial moles and in non-molar abortuses. Am J Obstet Gynecol 149:129, 1984

9. Hertig AT, Sheldon WM: Hydatidiform mole: A pathologicoclinical correlation of 200 cases. Am J Obstet Gynecol 53:1, 1947

10. Elston CW: The histopathology of trophoblastic tumours. J Clin Pathol 29 (suppl 10):111, 1977

11. Kajii T, Ohama K: Androgenetic origin of hydatidiform mole. Nature (Lond) 268:633, 1977

12. Jacobs PA, Wilson CM, Sprinkle JA, et al: Mechanism of origin of complete hydatidiform moles. Nature (Lond) 286:714, 1980

13. Ohama K, Kajii T, Okamoto E, et al: Dispermic origin of XY hydatidiform moles. Nature (Lond) 292:551, 1981

14. Surti U, Szulman AE, O'Brien S: Complete (classic) hydatidiform mole with 46,XY karyotype of paternal origin. Hum Genet 51:153, 1979

15. Kajii T, Kurashige M, Ohama K, Uchino F: XX and XY complete moles: Clinical and morphologic correlations. Am J Obstet Gynecol 150:57, 1984

16. Wake N, Seki T, Fujita H, et al: Malignant potential of homozygous and heterozygous complete moles. Cancer Res 44:1226, 1984

17. Curry SL, Hammond CB, Tyrey L, et al: Hydatidiform mole: Diagnosis, management and long-term follow-up in 347 patients. Obstet Gynecol 45:1, 1975

18. Morrow CP, Kletzky OA, DiSaia PJ, et al: Clinical and laboratory correlates of molar pregnancy and trophoblastic disease. Am J Obstet Gynecol 128:424, 1977

19. Bagshawe KD, Lawler SD: Choriocarcinoma. p. 909. In Schothenfeld DF, Frauemini JF (eds): Cancer Epidemiology and Prevention. WB Saunders, Philadelphia, 1982

20. McCorristen CC: Racial incidence of hydatidiform mole. Am J Obstet Gynecol 101:377, 1968

21. Stone M, Bagshawe KD: An analysis of the influence of maternal age, gestational age, contraceptive method, and the primary mode of treatment of patients with hydatidiform mole and the incidence of subsequent chemotherapy. Br J Obstet Gynaecol 46:782, 1979

22. Yen S, McMahon B: Epidemiologic features of trophoblastic disease. Am J Obstet Gynecol 101:126, 1968

23. Bandy LC, Clarke-Pearson DL, Hammond CB: Malignant potential of gestational trophoblastic disease at the extreme ages of reproductive life. Obstet Gynecol 64:395, 1984

24. Acousta-Sison M: Observations which may indicate the etiology of hydatidiform mole and explain its high incidence in the Philippines and Asiatic countries. Philos J Surg Specialt 14:280, 1959

25. Berkowitz RS, Cramer D, Bernstein M, et al: Case-control study of molar pregnancy. Gynecol Oncol 17:253, 1984 (abst)

26. Berkowitz RS, Horning-Rohen J, Martin-Alosco S, et al: HLA antigen frequency distribution in patients with gestational choriocarcinoma and their husbands. Placenta 3 (suppl 3):263, 1981

27. Tow WSH: The place of hysterotomy in the treatment of hydatidiform mole. Aust NZ J Obstet Gynecol 7:97, 1967

28. Twiggs CB, Morrow CP, Schlaerth JB: Acute pulmonary complications of molar pregnancy. Am J Obstet Gynecol 135:189, 1979

29. Cotton DB, Bernstein SG, Read JA, et al: Hemodynamic observations in evaluation of molar pregnancy. Am J Obstet Gynecol 138:6, 1980

30. Ratnam SS, Teoh ES, Dawood MY: Methotrexate for

prophylaxis of choriocarcinoma. Am J Obstet Gynecol 111:1021, 1971

31. Goldstein DP: Prevention of gestational trophoblastic disease by use of actinomycin D in molar pregnancies. Obstet Gynecol 43:475, 1974

32. Goldstein DP, Berkowitz RS, Bernstein MR: Management of molar pregnancy. J Reprod Med 26:208, 1981

33. Bagshawe KD, Golding PR, Orr AM: Choriocarcinoma after hydatidiform mole. Studies related to effectiveness of follow-up practice after hydatidiform mole. Br Med J 2:733, 1969

34. Vaitukaitis JL, Braunstein GD, Ross GT: A radioimmunoassay which specifically measures human chorionic gonadotropin in the presence of human luteinizing hormone. Am J Obstet Gynecol 113:751, 1972

35. Clayton LA, Tyrey L, Weed JC Jr, et al: Endocrine aspects of trophoblastic neoplasia. J Reprod Med 26:192, 1981

36. Patillo RA, Hussa RO: The hCG assay in the treatment of trophoblastic disease. J Reprod Med 29:802, 1984

37. Stone M, Dent J, Kardana A, et al: Relationship of oral contraceptives to development of trophoblastic tumour after evacuation of a hydatidiform mole. Br Med J 83:913, 1976

38. Berkowitz RS, Goldstein DP, Marean AR, et al: Oral contraceptive and postmolar trophoblastic disease. Obstet Gynecol 58:474, 1981

39. Yuen BH, Burch P: Relationship of oral contraceptives and the intrauterine devices to the regression of concentrations of the beta subunit of human chorionic gonadotropin and invasive complications after molar pregnancy. Am J Obstet Gynecol 145:214, 1983

40. Morrow P, Nakamura R, Schlaerth J, et al: The influence of oral contraceptives on the postmolar human chorionic gonadotropin regression curve. Am J Obstet Gynecol 151:906, 1985

41. Delfs E: Chorionic gonadotropin determinations with hydatidiform mole and choriocarcinoma. Ann NY Acad Sci 80:125, 1959

42. Brewer JI, Torok EE, Webster A, et al: Hydatidiform mole. A follow-up regimen for the identification of invasive mole and choriocarcinoma and for selection of patients for treatment. Am J Obstet Gynecol 101:557, 1968

43. Goldstein DP: The chemotherapy of gestational trophoblastic disease. Principles of clinical management. JAMA 220:209, 1972

44. Bagshawe KD, Wilson H, Dublou P, et al: Follow-up after hydatidiform mole: Studies using radioimmunoassay for urinary human chorionic gonadotropin (hCG). J Obstet Gynaecol Br Commonw 80:461, 1973

45. Hatch KD, Shingleton HM, Austin JM Jr, et al: Southern Regional Trophoblastic Disease Center, 1972-1977. South Med J 71:1334, 1978

46. Schlaerth JB, Morrow CP, Kletzky OA, et al: Prognostic characteristics of serum human chorionic gonadotropin titer regression following molar pregnancy. Obstet Gynecol 58:478, 1981

47. Kohorn EI: Hydatidiform mole and gestational trophoblastic disease in southern Connecticut. Obstet Gynecol 58:478, 1981

48. Lurain JR, Brewer LI, Torok EE, et al: Natural history of hydatidiform mole after primary evacuation. Am J Obstet Gynecol 145:591, 1983

49. Kohorn EI: Criteria toward the definition of nonmetastatic gestational trophoblastic disease after hydatidiform mole. Am J Obstet Gynecol 142:416, 1982

50. Driscoll SG: Placental-site chorioma. The neoplasm of the implantation-site trophoblast. J Reprod Med 29:821, 1984

51. Hammond CB, Hertz R, Ross GT, et al: Diagnostic problems of choriocarcinoma and related trophoblastic neoplasms. Obstet Gynecol 29:224, 1967

52. Magrath IT, Golding PR, Bagshawe KD: Medical presentations of choriocarcinoma. Br Med J 2:633, 1971

53. Libshitz HI, Baber CE, Hammond CB: The pulmonary metastases of choriocarcinoma. Obstet Gynecol 49:412, 1977

54. Weed JC, Hammond CB: Cerebral metastatic choriocarcinoma: Intensive therapy and prognosis. Obstet Gynecol 55:89, 1980

55. Weed JC, Woodward KT, Hammond CB: Choriocarcinoma metastatic to the brain: Therapy and prognosis. Semin Oncol 9:208, 1982

56. Snow JM Jr, Goldstein HM, Wallace S: Comparison of scintigraphy, sonography and computed axial tomography in hepatic neoplasms. AJR 32:915, 1979

57. Maroulis GB, Hammond CB, Johnsrude IS, et al: Arteriography and infusional chemotherapy in localized trophoblastic disease. Obstet Gynecol 45:397, 1975

58. Bagshawe KD, Harland S: Immunodiagnosis and monitoring of gonadotropin producing metastases in the central nervous system. Cancer 38:112, 1976

59. Goldstein DP, Berkowitz RS: Nonmetastatic and low-risk metastatic gestational trophoblastic neoplasms. Semin Oncol 9:191, 1982

60. Berkowitz RS, Goldstein DP, Driscoll SG, et al: Pretreatment curettage — A predictor of chemotherapy response in gestational trophoblastic neoplasia. Gynecol Oncol 10:39, 1980

61. Berkowitz RS, Goldstein DP, Bernstein MR: Laparoscopy in the management of gestational trophoblastic neoplasms. J Reprod Med 24:261, 1980

62. Hammond CB, Parker RT: Diagnosis and treatment of trophoblastic disease. A report from the Southeastern Regional Trophoblastic Disease Center. Obstet Gynecol 35:132, 1970

63. Hammond CB, Borchert LG, Tyrey L, et al: Treatment of metastatic trophoblastic disease: Good and poor prognosis. Am J Obstet Gynecol 115:4, 1973

64. Hammond CB, Weed JC, Currie JL: The role of operation in the current therapy of gestational trophoblastic disease. Am J Obstet Gynecol 136:844, 1980

65. Hammond CB, Clarke-Pearson DL, Soper JT: Management of patients with gestational trophoblastic neoplasia: Experience of the Southeastern Regional Trophoblastic Disease Center. p. 369. In Patillo RD, Hussa RO (eds): Human Trophoblastic Neoplasms. Plenum Press, New York, 1984

66. Hertz R, Lewis JL Jr, Lipsett MB: Five years' experience with the chemotherapy of metastatic choriocarcinoma and related trophoblastic tumors in women. Am J Obstet Gynecol 82:631, 1961

67. Ross GT, Goldstein DP, Hertz R, et al: Sequential use of methotrexate and actinomycin D in the treatment of metastatic choriocarcinoma and related trophoblastic tumors in women. Am J Obstet Gynecol 93:223, 1965

68. Bagshawe KD: Risk and prognostic factors in trophoblastic neoplasia. Cancer 38:1373, 1976

69. Lurain JR, Brewer JI, Torok EE, et al: Gestational trophoblastic disease: Treatment results at the Brewer Trophoblastic Disease Center. Obstet Gynecol 60:354, 1982

70. Athanassion A, Begent RH, Newlands ES, et al: Central nervous system metastases of choriocarcinoma. 23 years' experience at Charing Cross Hospital. Cancer 52:1728, 1983

71. Surwit EA, Hammond CB: Treatment of metastatic trophoblastic disease with poor prognosis. Obstet Gynecol 55:565, 1980

72. Barnard DE, Woodward KT, Yancy SG, et al: Hepatic metastases of choriocarcinoma: A report of 15 patients. Gynecol Oncol 25:73, 1980

73. Miller JM, Surwit EA, Hammond CB: Choriocarcinoma following term pregnancy. Obstet Gynecol 53:207, 1979

74. Olive DL, Lurain JR, Brewer JI: Choriocarcinoma associated with term gestation. Am J Obstet Gynecol 148:711, 1984

75. Pettersson F (ed): Annual Report on the Results of Treatment in Gynecological Cancer. Vol 19. International Federation of Gynecology and Obstetrics. Stockholm, Sweden, 1985

76. Goldstein DP, Berkowitz RS: Staging system for gestational trophoblastic tumors. J Reprod Med 29:792, 1984

77. Brewer JI, Eckman TR, Dolkart RE, et al: Gestational trophoblastic disease. Am J Obstet Gynecol 109:335, 1971

78. Li MC, Hertz R, Spencer DB: Effects of methotrexate upon choriocarcinoma and chorioadenoma. Proc Soc Exp Biol Med 93:361, 1956

79. Hammond CB, Hertz R, Ross GT, et al: Primary chemotherapy for nonmetastatic gestational trophoblastic neoplasms. Am J Obstet Gynecol 98:71, 1967

80. Brewer JI, Eckman TR, Dolkart RE, et al: Gestational trophoblastic disease: A comparative study of the results of therapy in patients with invasive mole and choriocarcinoma. Am J Obstet Gynecol 109:335, 1971

81. Goldstein DP, Winig P, Shirley RL: Actinomycin D as initial therapy of gestational trophoblastic disease: A re-evaluation. Obstet Gynecol 39:341, 1972

82. Osathanondh R, Goldstein DP, Pastor-Side GB: Actinomycin D as the primary agent for gestational trophoblastic disease. Cancer 36:863, 1975

83. Bagshawe KD, Wilde CE: Infusion therapy for pelvic trophoblastic tumours. J Obstet Gynaecol Br Commonw 71:565, 1964

84. Rotmensch J, Rosenshein N, Danehower R, et al: Plasma methotrexate (MTX) levels in patients with gestational trophoblastic neoplasia (GTN) treated by various methotrexate regimens. Am J Obstet Gynecol 148:730, 1984

85. Goldstein DP, Sarocco P, Osathanondh R, et al: Methotrexate with citrovorum factor rescue for gestational trophoblastic disease. Obstet Gynecol 51:93, 1978

86. Berkowitz RS, Goldstein DP, Bernstein MR: Methotrexate with citrovorum factor rescue as primary therapy for gestational trophoblastic disease. Cancer 50:2024, 1982

87. Berkowitz RS, Goldstein DP: Methotrexate with citrovorum factor rescue for nonmetastatic gestational trophoblastic neoplasms. Obstet Gynecol 54:725, 1979

88. Smith EB, Weed JC Jr, Tyrey L, et al: Treatment of nonmetastatic gestational trophoblastic disease: Results of methotrexate alone versus methotrexate-folinic acid. Am J Obstet Gynecol 144:88, 1982

89. Mutch DG, Soper JT, Baker ME, et al: Role of computed axial tomography of the chest in staging patients with nonmetastatic gestational trophoblastic disease. Obstet Gynecol 68:348, 1986

90. Wong CC, Cho YC, Ma HK: Methotrexate with citrovorum factor rescue in gestational trophoblastic disease. Am J Obstet Gynecol 152:59, 1985

91. Petrilli ES, Morrow CP: Actinomycin D toxicity in the treatment of trophoblastic disease: A comparison

of the five-day course to single-dose administration. Gynecol Oncol 9:18, 1980

92. Twiggs LB: Actinomycin D scheduling in nonmetastatic gestational trophoblastic neoplasia: Cost-effective chemotherapy. Gynecol Oncol 16:190, 1983

93. Petrilli ES, Twiggs LB, Curry SL, et al: Single-dose actinomycin D treatment for nonmetastatic gestational trophoblastic disease. Gynecol Oncol 23:244, 1986 (abst)

94. Wong LC, Chao YC, Ma HK: Primary oral etoposide therapy in gestational trophoblastic disease: An update. Cancer 58:14, 1986

95. Li MG: Management of choriocarcinoma and related tumors of uterus and testis. Med Clin North Am 45:661, 1961

96. Gordon AN, Gershenson DM, Copeland LJ, et al: High-risk metastatic gestational trophoblastic disease. Obstet Gynecol 65:550, 1985

97. Lurain JR, Brewer JI: Treatment of high-risk gestational trophoblastic disease with methotrexate, actinomycin D, and cyclophosphamide chemotherapy. Obstet Gynecol 65:830, 1985

98. Berkowitz RS, Goldstein DP, Bernstein MR: Modified triple chemotherapy in the management of high-risk metastatic gestational trophoblastic tumors. Gynecol Oncol 19:173, 1984

99. Bagshawe KD: Treatment of trophoblastic tumours. Ann Acad Med 5:273, 1976

100. Surwit EA, Suciu TN, Schmidt HJ, et al: Case report. A new combination chemotherapy for resistant trophoblastic disease. Gynecol Oncol 8:110, 1979

101. Weed JC Jr, Barnard DE, Currie JC, et al: Chemotherapy with the modified Bagshawe protocol for poor prognosis metastatic trophoblastic disease. Obstet Gynecol 59:377, 1982

102. Bagshawe KD: Treatment of high-risk choriocarcinoma. J Reprod Med 29:813, 1984

103. Newlands ES, Bagshawe KD: The role of VP16-213 (Etoposide; NSC-141540) in gestational choriocarcinoma. Cancer Chemother Pharmacol 7:211, 1982

104. Schlaerth JB, Morrow CP, DePetrillo AD: Sustained remission of choriocarcinoma with cis-platinum, vinblastine, and bleomycin after failure of conventional combination chemotherapy. Am J Obstet Gynecol 136:983, 1980

105. Hainsworth JD, Burnett LS, Jones HW, et al: Resist-

ant gestational choriocarcinoma: Successful treatment with vinblastine, bleomycin, and cisplatin (VBP). Cancer Treatm Rep 67:393, 1983

106. Brace KC: The role of irradiation in the treatment of metastatic trophoblastic disease. Radiology 91:540, 1968

107. Ausmen JI, Levin VA, Brown WE, et al: Brain tumor chemotherapy. J Neurosurg 46:155, 1977

108. Grumbine FC, Rosenshein NB, Brewerton, MD, et al: Management of liver metastasis from gestational trophoblastic neoplasia. Am J Obstet Gynecol 137:959, 1980

109. Wong LC, MA HK: Persistent chest opacity in trophoblastic disease: Is thoracotomy justified: Aust NZ J Obstet Gynaecol 23:237, 1983

110. Shirley RL, Goldstein DP, Collins JJ Jr: The role of thoracotomy in the management of patients with chest metastases from gestational trophoblastic disease. J Thorac Cardiovasc Surg 63:545, 1971

111. Edwards JJ, Makey AR, Bagshawe KD: The role of thoracotomy in the management of the pulmonary metastases of gestational choriocarcinoma. Clin Oncol 1:329, 1975

112. Sink JD, Hammond CB, Young WG: Pulmonary resection in the management of pulmonary metastases from choriocarcinoma. J Thorac Cardiovasc Surg 81:830, 1981

113. Tomoda Y, Arii Y, Kaseki S, et al: Surgical indications for resection in pulmonary metastasis of choriocarcinoma. Cancer 46:2723, 1980

114. Vaughn TC, Surwit EA, Hammond CB: Late recurrences of gestational trophoblastic neoplasia. Am J Obstet Gynecol 138:73, 1980

115. Surwit EA, Hammond CB: Recurrent gestational trophoblastic disease. Gynecol Oncol 12:177, 1981

116. Van Thiel DH, Ross GT, Lipsett MB: Pregnancies after chemotherapy of trophoblastic neoplasms. Science 169:1326, 1970

117. Berkowitz RS, Goldstein DP, Bernstein MR: Management of nonmetastatic trophoblastic tumors. J Reprod Med 26:219, 1981

118. Van Thiel DH, Grodin JM, Ross GT: Partial placenta accreta in pregnancies following chemotherapy for gestational trophoblastic neoplasia. Am J Obstet Gynecol 112:54, 1972

19

Sarcoma and Lymphoma

Alan N. Gordon
Raymond H. Kaufman

SARCOMA

The prevalence of sarcoma arising in the female genital tract is exceedingly low, accounting for 1 percent or less of malignant neoplasms of the female genital tract. This is low, despite the abundant connective tissue supporting the epithelium of the female genital tract and the mesodermal origin of most tissues of the female genital tract. Any single institution will have limited experience with these rare tumors; therefore, prospective studies have been difficult. Over the past two to three decades, however, some consensus has been reached regarding classification of these tumors. Retrospective studies of large numbers of cases in single centers have also yielded clinical information, and multicentered studies have yielded further prospective information about the clinical behavior of these unusual neoplasms.

In 1959, Ober[1] provided the first widely accepted scheme for classifying uterine sarcomas, which consisted of five major groups (Table 19-1). Group 1 includes leiomyosarcomas; group 2 mesenchymal sarcomas, divided into either pure or mixed lesions and/or homologous or heterologous tissues; group 3 blood vessel sarcomas; group 4 lymphomas; and group 5 unclassified sarcomas. This classification has provided the basis for other classifications, with slight modifications, used by later investigators. Many authorities have applied this basic classification to sarcomas arising in other parts of the female genital tract because of

their similar embryologic origins. Nevertheless, this classification scheme is somewhat complex and difficult for clinical use. The Gynecologic Oncology Group has therefore further simplified the classification for use in clinical studies, a simplified version that has been accepted by many authorities.[2] This classification is divided into five simple groups: leiomyosarcoma; endometrial stromal sarcoma; mixed mesodermal homologous; mixed mesodermal heterologous; and uterine sarcoma, type not specified, In discussing the various sarcomas arising in the female genital tract, we follow the Gynecologic Oncology Group's classification and discuss the types of sarcomas not by their location, but by histology, since the latter is similar regardless of the site of origin throughout the female genital tract.

LEIOMYOSARCOMA

Leiomyosarcomas are malignant tumors arising from smooth muscle. As such, they most often arise within the uterus, although they may develop in the wall of the vagina, the fallopian tube, or on the vulva. Christopherson et al.[3] reported an incidence rate of 0.67 per 100,000 women aged 20 years or older in a review of a population-based registry. Corscaden and Singh[4] reported a prevalence of 0.13 percent in patients undergoing surgery for leiomyomas. However, the frequency of sarcoma in patients operated on for

Table 19-1 Classification of Uterine Sarcoma

I. Leiomyosarcoma
  A. In leiomyoma
  B. Diffuse in uterine wall
II. Mesenchymal sarcoma
  A. Homologous, pure
    1. Endometrial stroma sarcoma
    2. Stromatous endometriosis (endolymphatic stromal myosis)[a]
    3. Sarcoma botryoides (no heterologous elements)
  B. Heterologous, pure
    1. Rhabdomyosarcoma
    2. Chondrosarcoma
    3. Osteosarcoma
    4. Liposarcoma
  C. Homologous, mixed (carcinosarcoma)
    1. Adenocarcinoma plus stromal sarcoma
    2. Adenoacanthoma plus stromal sarcoma
    3. Squamous carcinoma plus stromal sarcoma
    4. Sarcoma botryoides plus neoplastic epithelium, without heterologous elements
  D. Heterologous, mixed
    1. Carcinosarcoma (with one or more heterologous elements)
    2. Mixed mesenchymal sarcoma
      a. Stromal sarcoma with heterologous elements
      b. Heterologous elements without mesenchymal myxomatous stromal sarcoma
    3. Sarcoma botryoides with heterologous elements
III. Blood vessel sarcoma[b]
  A. Hemangiosarcoma (hemangioendothelioma)
  B. Hemangiopericytoma [a]
IV. Lymphomas
  A. Reticulum cell sarcoma
  B. Lymphosarcoma
  C. Leukemic infiltration
V. Unclassified sarcoma

[a] Not uniformly malignant.
[b] Lymphangiosarcoma has also been reported.
(Ober WB: Uterine sarcomas: histogenesis and taxonomy. Ann NY Acad Sci 75:568, 1959.)

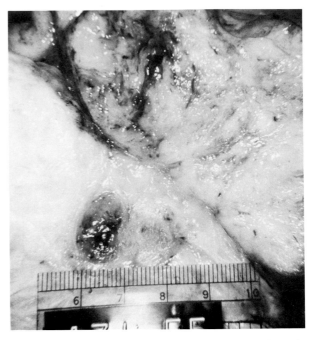

Fig. 19-1 Leiomyosarcoma arising de novo within the myometrium.

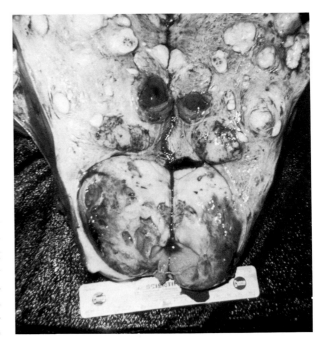

Fig. 19-2 Leiomyosarcoma arising in the uterus with leiomyomata.

leiomyoma varies depending on the diagnostic criteria used for the diagnosis of leiomyosarcoma. Different diagnostic criteria also result in widely varying survival rates in different reported series of leiomyosarcoma. Stearns and Sneeden[5] introduced the term secondary to describe sarcoma arising in a leiomyoma, as opposed to a primary leiomyosarcoma or one arising diffusely within the uterus (Figs. 19-1 and 19-2) These designations may cause confusion. Spiro and Koss[6] noted that patients with sarcomas arising within

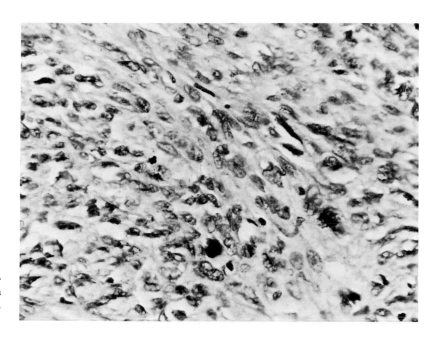

Fig. 19-3 Leiomyosarcoma. Scattered atypical mitoses are noted in this pleomorphic cellular tumor. (H&E, ×400.)

leiomyomas have a more favorable prognosis. The latter tumors are often better differentiated and are therefore more easily recognized as sarcomas arising within leiomyomas.

The diagnostic criteria for leiomyosarcoma centered on the degree of cellular and nuclear pleomor-phism, the presence of giant cells, and the number of mitoses (Figs. 19-3 and 19-4). Spiro and Koss,[6] Bartsich et al.,[7] and Silverberg[8] suggested that the diagnosis be based on grade or degree of cellular atypia. At the same time, Silverberg[8] noted that the number of mitoses is related to survival. As early as 1919, Proper

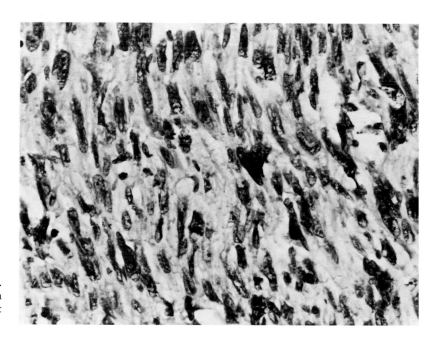

Fig. 19-4 Cellular leiomyoma. Markedly pleomorphic pattern noted. Scattered mitoses are present in this field. (H&E, ×400.)

and Simpson[9] and. 1 year later, Evans,[10] made efforts to predict the behavior of this tumor based on the number of mitoses per volume of tumor. Taylor and Norris[11] found that all tumors with less than 10 mitoses per 10 high-powered field (hpf) behave in a benign manner, regardless of the degree of atypism. In their study, only 3 of 36 patients whose tumors contained greater than 10 mitoses in 10 hpf were alive without evidence of disease, with only two women alive longer than 2 years after initial treatment. Kempson and Bari[12] noted that 9 of 12 patients with more than 10 mitoses per 10 hpf developed metastases and died. All patients with fewer than 5 mitoses per 10 hpf survived, while all patients whose tumors contained 5 to 10 mitoses per 10 hpf developed metastases and died.[12] However, all patients in this latter group had marked cellular atypism. Although these workers concluded that mitoses are most important, the difference between their group with 5 to 10 mitoses, and Taylor's may have been the presence of atypism. Recent studies have suggested a compromise in diagnostic criteria whereby all tumors with greater than 10 mitoses per 10 hpf are considered sarcomas as well as those with 5 to 9 mitoses per 10 hpf with associated atypia.[13]. The use of more strict criteria has excluded, in some instances, as many as 50 percent or more of the original cases classified as sarcoma.[3,14,15]

The mean age at diagnosis in most reported series is 52 to 55, with a range from 26 to 86.[3,8,11,14–23] Several investigators have reported a trend toward better survival in younger patients, either by age or by menopausal status.[8,16,22] However, in one series, younger age was reported to be more often associated with a lower stage, a factor that may be related to the better prognosis seen in these younger women.[16]

A review of presenting symptoms from several recent reports reveals that abnormal uterine bleeding (postmenopausal bleeding or abnormal menstrual history) is by far the most common presenting symptom [8,14,18,19,21–23] (Table 19-2). Other presenting symptoms, in order, are abdominal discomfort or pain, a sensation of increasing abdominal girth, and weight loss. When leiomyosarcoma occurs in the vagina, most patients present with the mass as the major symptom.[24] Since bleeding is a common presenting complaint in the older population, a woman will often undergo dilatation and curettage (D&C) for diagnostic purposes. Nevertheless, most investigators have noted that this procedure detects the neoplasm in

Table 19-2 Presenting Symptoms in Leiomyosarcoma[a]

Symptom	N	%
Abnormal bleeding	82	65.5
Pain	47	37.6
Increasing abdomen	27	21.6
Decreasing weight	5	4.0
Other	8	6.4
Patients	125	100.0

[a] Many patients reported more than one symptom.
(Data from Silverberg,[8] Barter et al.,[21] Vardi and Tovell,[22] and Montague et al.[23])

only 20 to 60 percent of cases.[21,22] Five percent or less of patients with leiomyosarcoma give a history of previous radiation therapy for benign or malignant disease.[3,16,18,19] This is much less often than is seen in patients with mixed mesodermal sarcomas.

Recently, investigators retrospectively staged patients with sarcoma according to the International Federation of Gyneocology and Oncology (FIGO) staging system for carcinoma of the uterine corpus. According to this format, most patients have been found to have clinical stage I disease, that is, disease confined to the uterine fundus.[16–18,20–22] These recent reports have demonstrated that 63 percent of cases present as stage I disease (Table 19-3). A review of the literature suggests that the most important factor related to prognosis appears to be whether the disease is confined to the uterus. In a study of cases of sarcoma arising in leiomyoma, Montague et al.[23] found all patients with extrauterine disease to have died. Aaro et al.[19] similarly noted that the prognosis was worse if disease extended to or beyond the serosa of the uterus; they recommended an anatomic staging system. Silverberg[8] reported all patients with disease beyond the limits of the apparent leiomyoma to have died. Salazar

Table 19-3 Leiomyosarcoma: Stage at Presentation

Stage	N	%
I	99	63
II	9	6
III	23	15
IV	26	16
Total	157	100

(Data from Kahanpaa et al.,[16] Wheelock et al.,[17] Salazar et al.,[18] Marchese et al.,[20] Barter et al.,[21] and Vardi and Tovell.[22])

et al.[18] also reported that the extent of the disease was the best indicator of patient survival. In these reports, in which stage I disease was separated from other clinical stages, patients with limited disease had a better survival. In some reported series, the only survivors were those with localized disease.[12,17,19,20,22] A review of reported survival rates (Table 19-4) reveals a 5-year survival rate of 50 percent for stage I disease, compared with 39.5 percent for all stages combined.

The standard surgical treatment for leiomyosarcoma has consisted of total abdominal hysterectomy with bilateral salpingo-oophorectomy. Bilateral salpingo-oophorectomy has been almost universally performed because most patients present at or after the menopause. However, Aaro et al.[19] reported that 7 of 9 patients in their series who had not had the ovaries removed remained without evidence of disease after 5 years, as compared with an overall 55 percent 5-year survival rate. Moreover, there is no evidence of significant recurrence within the ovary or evidence of spread of disease to the ovary in the pesence of widespread disease.

The diagnosis of leiomyosarcoma may be suggested at the time of exploration by obvious extrauterine disease. Taylor and Norris[11] reported that leiomyosarcomas occur more often as solitary lesions than in association with multiple leiomyomas. According to these investigators, many of the leiomyosarcomas reported in association with multiple leiomyomata are actually cellular leiomyomas. In fact, Silverberg[8] compares the possibility that leiomyosarcomas arise exclusively from leiomyomas because they both occur in the same uterus with the belief that spontaneous generation of mice results from a mixture of cloth and fermeting grain. Kurman and Norris[26] recently described a variation of leiomyosarcoma, which they have termed epithelioid leiomyosarcoma. These lesions are encountered as isolated tumors in 77 percent of cases. Histologically, these lesions contain rounded to polygonal cells, often arranged in a cordlike pattern. There may also be vacuolization of the cytoplasm; in some areas, clear cells may be seen. These tumors, however, appear to behave like other leiomyosarcomas. Subsequent reports from Buscema et al.[27] failed to uncover any notable difference between these and common leiomyosarcomas.

More recent reports of survival rates still demonstrate a wide range of variation in 5-year survival, varying from 20 to 60 percent.[3,8,16,21-23,25] In patients who succumb to disease, a large percentage have distant recurrence or persistence of disease. Kahanpaa et al.[16] reported that 5 of 17 patients who were treatment failures had distant recurrences. More recent series have revealed distant failure rates as high as 67 to 90 percent.[14,28] These high failure rates seem to reflect the propensity of sarcomas for hematogenous dissemination. Although the number of patients in each group was small, Salazar et al.[18] noted that patients treated with surgery plus radiation fared no better than those treated with surgery alone.

Some investigators have noted an increased survival in patients with leiomyosarcoma as compared with patients with mixed mesodermal sarcoma.[18,25] This increased survival may be due to the larger number of patients with tumor confined to the uterus in patients with leiomyosarcoma. By contrast, Kahanpaa et al.[16] and Wheelock et al.[17] found similar survival rates for leiomyosarcomas and mixed mesodermal tumors. Since survival rates for these tumors appear to be similar, the use of adjuvant radiotherapy and chemotherapy for advanced disease are discussed together under Mixed Mesodermal Tumors.

Mixed Mesodermal (Müllerian) Tumors

Multiple terms have been used throughout the years to describe these sarcomas. The most recent classification still uses a differentiation between mixed mullerian tumors based on the presence of heterologous elements and carcinosarcomas containing only homologous elements. Earlier studies from the Armed Forces Institute of Pathology (AFIP) suggested that there may be a somewhat better outcome in patients with homologous elements only.[29,30]

Table 19-4 Leiomyosarcoma: Survival

	Survival					
	2 yr		5 yr		10 yr	
Stage	N	%	N	%	N	%
I	21/27	78	53/106	50	11/23	48
II–IV	8/24	33	92/261	25	1/22	5
All	29/51	57	145/367	40	12/45	27

(Data from Christopherson et al.,[3] Silverberg,[8] Kempson and Bari,[12] Wheelock et al.,[17] Salazar et al.,[18] Aaro et al.,[19] Marchese et al.,[20] Vardi and Tovell,[22] Montague et al.,[23] and Schwartz et al.[25])

However, several reviews from the M. D. Anderson Hospital[31,32] and recent reviews by Peters et al.[33] and Mascadaet et al.[34] have failed to reveal any difference in survival for patients with homologous versus heterologous tumors when corrected for stage and depth of invasion in the myometrium.[17,19] These lesions can occur anywhere along the genital tract. The uterus seems to be the most common site, although mixed mesodermal tumors are seen in ovary,[35,36] fallopian tube,[37] cervix,[38] and vagina.[39] Sarcoma botryoides is a form of mixed mesodermal tumor that occurs in the infantile vagina. However, because these tumors follow a different clinical course, they are discussed under a separate heading (see Rhabdomyosarcoma).

The age of most patients with mixed mesodermal tumors seems to be somewhat later than for patients with leiomyosarcoma, occurring for the most part in the mid- to later 60s.[16,17,20,29-34] Most patients present with vaginal bleeding, as is also observed in patients with other genital tract sarcomas.[12,17,19,20] In some cases, the lesion will be seen as a mass protruding through the cervix, similar to a prolapsed fibroid[12] (Fig. 19-5). In one report, almost 50 percent of patients had cervicovaginal smears that were at least

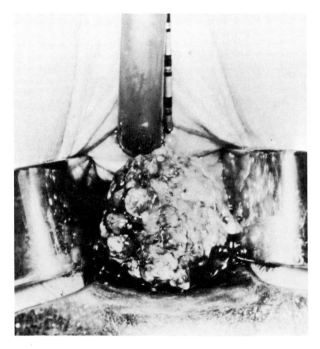

Fig. 19-5 Mixed mesodermal sarcoma prolapsing through the cervix in a postmenopausal woman.

suspicious for cancer.[16] Findings on D&C have shown evidence of cancer in 50 percent[16] to better than 90 percent[17] of cases. Approximately 10 to 30 percent of patients have a history of prior pelvic irradiation, somewhat higher than that seen in association with other sarcomas.[17,19,29,30,33]

Approximately 50 to 60 percent of patients present with what is clinically thought to be stage I disease[20,32-34] (Fig. 19-6). At surgery, however, many patients are found to have more extensive disease and often have abdominal metastases.[32,33] As observed with leiomyosarcoma, virtually all survivors have disease limited to the uterus.[12,19,20,30,32,33] Although some studies have shown improved survival in patients having tumors with only homologous elements[30] (Figs. 19-7 and 19-8) most series show equal survival rates for patients with homologous and heterologous elements.[17,19,31-34] Persons diagnosed as having carcinosarcoma appear to have somewhat better survival than do patients with heterologous tumors, because a higher percentage of the former tumors are limited to the uterus. This seems to be the major predictor of survival.[12,19,32,33] Some reviews have suggested improved survival in patients with heterologous tumors in which chondrosarcoma is the only sarcomatous element.[12] This has been noted in cases with more limited invasion, which may account for the improved survival seen in patients with this type of tumor.[33]

Mixed mesodermal tumors occurring in the ovary or fallopian tube have a clinical presentation similar to that seen with ovarian cancer.[35,36] Stage I disease is an exceedingly rare occurrence. Only 20 percent of patients will survive beyond 1 year.[35,36] Somewhat better survival has been noted in patients with stage I disease, but long-term survival is unusual. No difference in survival has been noted between homologous and heterologous tumors.[36] Responses to chemotherapy have been seen,[40] but long-term survival has been noted only in isolated case reports.[37,41]

The survival rates for mixed mesodermal tumors using both crude and actuarial survival methods vary from 27 percent to 55 percent at 5 years.[16-19,25,30,32] Although the failure rate increases with advancing clinical stage, the surgical stage based on whether the disease is localized to the uterus appears to be the major prognostic factor. The 5-year survival rate with disease confined to the uterus is about 50 percent, whereas it is only 10 percent or less when disease

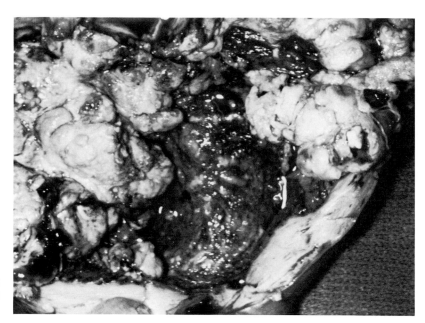

Fig. 19-6 Large polypoid mass filling the endometrial cavity. The tumor was limited to the uterus.

extends beyond the uterus.[32,33] When analyzing survival rates for disease localized to the uterus, the depth of invasion in some studies appears to be significant. Even involvement of the cervix does not appear to be as important as depth of invasion in regard to prognosis.[33] Although the reported 5-year survival rates for mixed mesodermal tumors are slightly lower than those for leiomyosarcomas, the differences are not statistically significant.[16-19] One series reported a lower late survival rate, that is, at 5 and 10 years,[16] and the M. D. Anderson group noted a tendency toward later recurrence, especially distant metastases, in patients with mixed mesodermal tumors.[32]

Regardless of the treatment modality, the possibil-

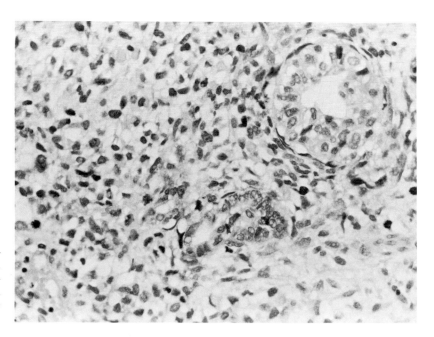

Fig. 19-7 Mixed mesodermal sarcoma arising within the uterus. The tumor was composed of homologous elements. Both stromal and glandular components are noted. (H&E, ×250.)

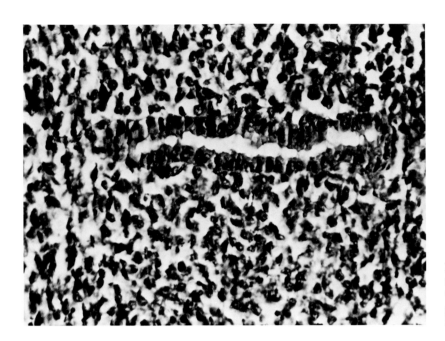

Fig. 19-8 Homologous mixed mesodermal sarcoma arising within the ovary. Both stromal and glandular components are seen. (H&E,×250.)

ity of distant failure seems to be a major problem in treating these tumors. Among patients who have recurrences, 50 to 87 percent involve distant failure,[19,20,25,28,42] These high failure rates, similar to those seen in patients with leiomyosarcoma, make treatment difficult. Even with this tendency toward distant (i.e., hematogenous) dissemination, these tumors can spread via the lymphatics. In a small series, DiSaia et al.[43] demonstrated a 35.7 percent frequency of positive pelvic and paraaortic lymph nodes in apparent stage I cases.[43] Six of the 10 patients with positive lymph nodes had the diagnosis established by microscopic examination. Peters et al.[33] also found a 15 percent frequency of positive lymph nodes in patients with apparent stage I disease.

THERAPY

In patients with ovarian and tubal mixed mesodermal sarcoma, therapy is similar to that used in treating epithelial carcinomas. Tumor-debulking surgery should be followed by adjuvant chemotherapy, even in early-stage disease. Chemotheraphy can be either vincristine–actinomycin–Cytoxan or an Adriamycin-based combination. However, the development of an effective chemotherapeutic regimen is still awaited.[35–37] Patients presenting with vaginal lesions usually require pelvic exenteration, and distant failure

is and will remain a significant problem until such time as an effective chemotherapy regimen is developed.[39]

In patients with uterine disease, the cornerstone of therapy is total abdominal hysterectomy with bilateral salpingo-oophorectomy, just as it is in patients with leiomyosarcoma. When disease appears to be confined to the uterus, a careful search should be made for extrauterine tumor. This should include the nodal areas[43] and peritoneal surfaces.[32,33] DiSaia et al.[31] reported that radiation therapy combined with hysterectomy resulted in higher survival than surgery alone, and Gilbert et al.[44] also reported that there seemed to be an advantage to adjuvant pelvic radiation in patients with mixed mesodermal tumors. This was not true for leiomysarcomas, in which radiation did not appear to improve survival.[44] However, both studies failed to show any statistical improvement in survival with the addition of pelvic radiation. DiSaia et al.[31] noted that distant failure still remains a problem. In a recent review from the M. D. Anderson Hospital, where almost all patients with mixed mesodermal tumors received pelvic radiation, the low pelvic failure rate of only 13 percent was attributed to the use of radiation therapy. Salazar et al.[18,28] also found that the frequency of isolated pelvic failure using adjuvant radiation was only 13 percent. On the other hand, they found no improvement in survival in patients receiving surgery plus radiation compared to patients treated by surgery alone. It is well documented that radiation therapy can cure localized disease.[28] The addition of pelvic radiation in the treatment of mixed mesodermal tumor and in leiomyosarcoma may lower the pelvic failure rate by controlling disease within the radiation field, but with the high frequency of suboccult, distant disease, survival is not affected by the addition of this adjuvant therapy.

Patients who present with disease beyond the uterus or are found to have extrauterine disease at the time of hysterectomy have been treated with chemotherapy following their surgical procedure. Various chemotherapeutic regimens have been used, often borrowing from results reported in the treatment of extragenital sarcomas (Table 19-5). Adriamycin has often been used as a single agent; nevertheless, complete responses have been rare and partial response rates have ranged from 6 to 15 percent.[45-48] Median survival reported in these series has ranged from only 7.2 to 11.6 months,[45-47] in spite of the fact that in many series the patients had received previous radiotherapy or chemotherapy.[46,47] In two randomized reports by the Gynecologic Oncology Group, the addition of either Cytoxan[45] or DTIC[46] to Adriamycin did not result in increased response rates or increased survival times. The addition of these agents only resulted in a somewhat higher frequency of toxicity. Piver et

al.[49] reported an overall response rate of 23 percent using multiagent therapy in previously treated patients but reported no long-term survivors, even among responders. Seltzer et al.[50] recently reported on the combination of adriamycin with cisplatin with a 50 percent response rate in six patients. However, follow-up on these patients is still short. Piver et al.[51] recently reported on the use of cisplatin in combination with DTIC and noted an overall 35-percent response rate in heavily pretreated patients. Hannigan et al.[52] found a 13 percent complete response rate and a 16 percent partial response rate using vincristine–actinomycin–Cytoxan chemotherapy. Complete responders had a median survival of 16 months, a significant improvement compared with the survival of partial responders. Two patients remained free of disease at 3 and 5 years; however, toxicity was significant. One-third of patients required hospitalization at some time during therapy, and 11 percent of patients died due to toxicity.[52] Hannigan et al.,[52] along with Muss et al.,[45] noted that measurable disease was important in predicting survival; that is, longer survival was seen in patients without measurable disease. This is probably a reflection of the tumor burden, rather than a beneficial effect from the chemotherapy. With randomized studies failing to show any improvement with multiagent therapy, future studies will certainly have to stratify for measurable disease. Muss et al.[45]

Table 19-5 Chemotherapy in Metastatic Sarcomas

Therapy	Eval.Pts. (N)	CR (%)	PR (%)	Surv. (months)	PFI (months)
Adria[45]	26	4	15	11.6[a]	5.1[a]
Adria[46]	80	6	10	7.7[a]	10.0
Adria[47]	39	0	10	7.2	—
Adria[48]	17	0	6	—	—
Adria, Cy[45]	26	8	12	10.9[a]	4.9[a]
Adria, DTIC[46]	66	11	14	7.3[a]	8.0
CyVADIC[49]	26	12	12	—	—
Adria, DDP[50]	6	50	33	9.0	9.0
DDP, DTIC[51]	20	20	15	—	—
VAC[52]	45	13	16	—	—

[a] Includes patients without measurable disease.
CR, complete responders; PR, partial responders; Surv median survival; PFI, progression free interval; Adria, Adriamycin; Cy, cytoxan; DTIC, dimethyltriazenoimidazole carboxamide; CyVADIC, cytoxan–vincristine–Adriamycin–dimethyltriazenoimidazole carboxanide; DDP, cisplatin; VAC, vincristine–actinomycin D–cytoxan.

stated that most combination regimens using the drugs currently available probably will not significantly improve survival. Significant improvement in survival will depend on the development of more active single agents.

The poor survival rates seen in patients with advanced and recurrent disease, together with the failure of radiotherapy to improve survival due to distant disease spread, suggest a possible role for prophylactic chemotherapy. Buchsbaum et al.[53] used adjuvant vincristine, actinomycin D, and Cytoxan in 17 patients. Five patients were alive without evidence of disease, compared with one of 14 patients in a group of historic controls. Piver et al.[49] studied Adriamycin in a small series of patients and found no advantage and increased toxicity in the treated patient group. In comparing patients who received either vincristine–actinomycin D–Cytoxan or Adriamycin alone or in combination with vincristine and cyclophosphamide, Hannigan et al.[54] found no advantage over the patients receiving adjuvant therapy. Several patients in Hannigan's study, however, had either positive lymph nodes or disease present in the margins of the surgical specimens. Even if survival rates are corrected for patients with negative margins and nodes, the results indicate no advantage to adjuvant therapy, with a 60.7 percent 5-year survival rate in the treated group, compared with a 54.5 percent 5-year survival rate for patients receiving no adjuvant therapy. Recently, Kohorn et al.[55] reported an 80 percent survival in patients receiving adjuvant therapy, compared with historic controls who had a 28 percent survival; and Van Nagell et al.[56] reported 71 percent of patients alive and well using vincristine–actinomycin–Cytoxan as adjuvant therapy, compared with 18 percent alive and well without adjuvant therapy in historic controls. Both studies, however, were not randomized, used historic controls, and follow-up was short. The administration of this three-drug regimen and Adriamycin has not been without toxicity.[49,52] As noted in previous studies, patients with nonmeasurable disease have demonstrated improved survival over those with measurable disease.[45,52] Because the improved survival suggested by nonrandomized studies may merely show that chemotherapy modifies the disease course,[52] longer-term studies in randomized series are necessary to prove increased survival with adjuvant therapy.

Rhabdomyosarcoma

The rhabdomyoblast can give rise to several different types of neoplasms that have been classified by Horn and Enterline[57] as either embryonal, botryoid, alveolar, or pleomorphic. The polypoid appearance of the botryoid tumor is due to the location of the embryonal-type cells under the mucous membrane, allowing for early detection and the typical grape like appearance. Many reports list these tumors with mixed mesodermal sarcomas because the latter often contain rhabdomyoblasts. However, the different presentation and clinical behavior of the rhabdomyosarcomas justify a separate classification.[58]

Sarcoma botryoides, or embryonal rhabdomyosarcoma, is probably the most common form of rhabdomyosarcoma encountered in gynecology. These lesions can arise almost anywhere in the body. One of the most common locations is the genital canal, with lesions occasionally seen in the head and neck area.[58] Eighty percent of patients present with either vaginal bleeding or a mass protruding from the vagina.[58] (Fig. 19-9). Hilgers et al.[58] reported a mean age of 27.5 months, with 90 percent of patients presenting before the age of 5. Nevertheless, patients are sometimes

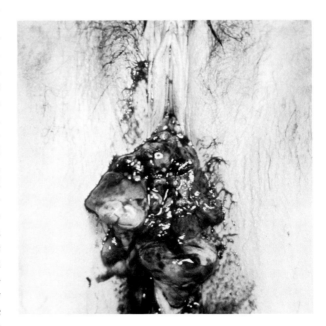

Fig. 19-9 Sarcoma botryoides. The tumor arose in the cervix in an 18-year-old woman. Mass is seen protruding through the introitus.

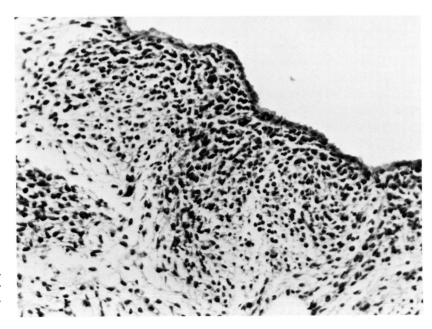

Fig. 19-10 Sarcoma botryoides. Poorly differentiated stromal elements making up a cambian layer. (H&E, ×150.)

seen in late adolescence or older, and patients in this older age group tend to have disease at the upper end of the genital canal — the upper vagina, the cervix, or the uterine corpus.[38,59] Microscopically, the lesions show an intact mucosa with the underlying cambian layer infiltrated by typical elongated strap cells consistent with rhabdomyoblasts (Figs. 19-10 and 19-11). Cross-striations may or may not be easily detectable, even with special stains.

In reviewing the literature and the experience at Memorial Sloan-Kettering Hospital, Daniel et al.[60] considered surgical excision the treatment of choice. Because of subclinical extension of the tumor into the submucosal area beyond the visible primary lesion and

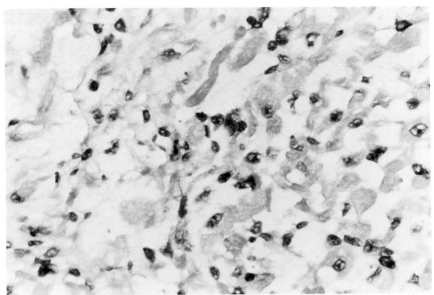

Fig. 19-11 Sarcoma botryoides. The section demonstrates characteristic rhabdomyoblasts. Cross-striations were identified in these cells. (H&E, ×400.)

what these workers believed was often multifocal disease, exenteration was suggested as the treatment of choice. Later, in reviewing the experience at the Mayo Clinic and the literature, Hilgers et al.[58] also concluded that the tumor is best treated by combined pelvic exenteration and pelvic lymphadenectomy because a large percentage of patients had lymph node disease at time of recurrence or lymph node disease at autopsy. These investigators also recommended that chemotherapy and radiation therapy be used only in patients with recurrences.[58] Although Hilgers et al.[58] did find 14 reported patients in the literature who were treated with hysterectomy and vaginectomy, including five 10-year survivors, they also noted that among these patients there was minimal delay between onset of symptoms and treatment. These patients were also found to have superficial involvement of the vagina without local extension.[58]

In 1975, the Intergroup Rhabdomyosarcoma Study group recommended a staging system for classifying patients with rhabdomyosarcoma. Subsequently, many investigators have used this staging system in describing and detailing cases[61] (Table 19-6). Hilgers[62] used this staging scheme in reviewing cases of pelvic exenteration and found a 75 percent survival rate for cases with disease localized to the vagina, compared with a 37 percent survival rate in patients with disease localized to the pelvis but extending beyond the vagina. Most recurrences were regional, occurring at a mean of 9.7 months after surgery, and no significant difference in survival was noted in patients who had lymph node dissections, as compared to those who did not.[62] They concluded that while extenteration is effective for treating localized disease, coordinated therapy with surgery and chemotherapy and/or radiation therapy is better than surgery alone.

Rivard et al.[63] reviewed all cases of childhood rhabdomyosarcoma of the pelvis reported through 1975 and retrospectively staged patients according to the Intergroup staging scheme. They found that prior to 1970 the median survival in 17 patients was 6 months. In a group of nine patients treated wtih chemotherapy and/or x-ray therapy prior to surgery, five were still alive without evidence of disease from 12 to 16 months after onset of treatment, with the median not yet reached.[63] In addition, only three of these patients required surgery and all were treated with local excisions only (either total abdominal hysterectomy or vaginectomy). No exenterations were performed.[63]

Kumar et al.[64] reported on three patients who were treated with total abdominal hysterectomy, bilateral salpingo-oophorectomy, and vaginectomy only, two of whom received preoperative radiation and chemotherapy and one of whom received postoperative radiation therapy and chemotherapy. All three patients were alive without disease 32 to 54 months after treatment.[64]

Ortner et al.[65] reported on a patient with a stage I cervical lesion treated by total abdominal hysterectomy with a wide cervical cuff, followed by chemotherapy with vincristine – actinomycin D – Cytoxan, who remains in remission after 31 months. These recent reports[63-65] have all suggested that combining chemotherapy with radiotherapy is advantageous. They concluded that this approach not only permits a less extensive procedure than exenteration in treating patients with advanced disease, but also allows more conservative surgery in the management of patients with earlier disease. Preliminary studies from the Intergroup Rhabdomyosarcoma Study tends to support this thesis. The study group reported that 92 percent of patients with group 1 disease who were treated for 2 years with vincristine – actinomycin D – Cytoxan) remained without evidence of disease, with a med-

Table 19-6 Intergroup Rhabdomyosarcoma Study Clinical Staging System

Group	Description
1	Localized disease, completely resected
	A. Tumor confined to muscle or organ of origin
	B. Infiltration beyond site of origin, but regional nodes not involved
2	Gross excision
	A. With microscopic residuum (tumor found by pathologist at margin)
	B. Regional disease completely resected that involves nodes or extends into an adjacent organ
	C. Regional disease plus involved nodes grossly resected, but with evidence of microscopic residuum
3	Incomplete resection or biopsy with gross residual disease
4	Distant metastatic disease present at onset

(Maurer HM: The intergroup rhabdomyosarcoma study (NIH): Objectives and clinical staging. J Pediatr Surg 10:977, 1975.)

ian follow-up of 72 weeks.[66] Group 3 and 4 patients were treated with intensive pulse vincristine–actinomycin–Cytoxan or the regimen plus Adriamycin, followed by radiation after 6 weeks; 81 percent of patients responded favorably with either complete regression (noted in more than one-fourth of patients even before the start of radiation) or partial response (noted in approximtely one-half of all patients who received radiation therapy).[66] Copeland et al.[59] recently observed these trends. This study and the results of the Intergroup study[66] all seem to show that multifocal origin is rare and that extensive surgery, if based on the premise of a multifocal origin, is not justified.

The role of radiotherapy remains unclear. The Intergroup Study demonstrated no improvement in survival in patients with localized disease who received radiotherapy versus those who did not.[66] Patients presenting with localized disease could be treated with wide excision following by vincristine–actinomycin–Cytoxan chemotherapy, perhaps even with preservation of fertility.[59,66] Patients with more extensive disease could be pretreated with chemotherapy and/or radiation therapy, if necessary, in an effort to avoid more extensive surgery, that is, exenteration. Although the frequency of lymph node metastasis is reportedly higher in genital rhabdomyosarcomas (in the range of 19 percent) than is found in tumors from other locations (in the range of 2 percent),[66] the frequency of nodal spread as related to stage of disease was not reported in this study. The higher occurrence of lymph node disease may be a reflection of several patients with more advanced stages of disease. In a previous report by Hilgers et al.[58] emphasizing lymph node metastasis, all patients with nodal spread had recurrent disease, or recurrent disease was noted as autopsy, reflecting an advanced stage of disease.

The alveolar variant of rhabdomyosarcoma was originally described by Horn and Enterline.[57] This tumor is characterized by multiple flat cells often protruding into the lumen of epithelialized-like lined spaces. While this entity has not received much notice in gynecologic literature, Copeland et al.[67] recently reported a series of eight patients with this morphologic variety of tumor. These lesions occurred more frequently in adolescents and usually were vulvar and perineal in location. The major differential diagnosis was sarcoma botryoides or endodermal sinus tumor.

Copeland's group noted a tendency for this tumor to metastasize early, with the breast being a commonly reported site. Only two patients were without evidence of disease 7 and 12 years post therapy. Both patients had undergone complete excisions of tumor followed by radiation therapy and the three-drug regimen. Five patients died in less than 9 months' time. Therefore, the question as to whether these lesions respond equally as well to chemotherapy as other varieties of sarcoma botryoides remains unanswered.

Stromal Sarcoma

Stromal sarcomas are most often encountered in the endometrium, although they may also arise from ovarian stroma. They account for only a small percentage of sarcomas of the genital tract.[16-18] As is observed with leiomyosarcomas, differentiating this malignant neoplasm from its more benign counterpart may be difficult. The problem has been further complicated by the use of multiple terms to describe the benign stromal tumors, such as stromal endometriosis,[68] uterine stromatosis,[69] endometrial stromatosis,[70] and uterine endolymphatic stromal myosis.[71] All the latter as well as the malignant stromal tumors are believed to arise from neoplastic proliferation of endometrial stromal cells.[72] Stromal sarcoma is characterized as a highly cellular neoplasm with a monotonous-appearing cell population (Figs. 19-12 and 19-13). These tumors must be differentiated from hemangiopericytoma and reticulum cell sarcoma (large cleaved cell lymphomas).[12,59,72]

Norris and Taylor[72] described two patterns of infiltration of stromal tumors. A pushing pattern is associated with solitary nodules and has a very low recurrence rate. None of the patients with this pattern developed recurrences; they were designated as stromal nodules by Norris and Taylor. Similar results have been reported by other investigators.[70] These tumors are adequately treated by total abdominal hysterectomy.[72] In patients whose tumors are associated with infiltrating borders, the most predictable measure of malignancy appears to be the mitotic figure count. A diagnosis of sarcoma is made for those neoplasms having more than 10 mitoses per 10 hpf, whereas a diagnosis of stromatosis is reported when fewer than 10 mitoses per 10 hpf is observed. In reviewing cases at AFIP, Norris and Taylor[72] found a 100 percent survival rate at the end of 10 years in

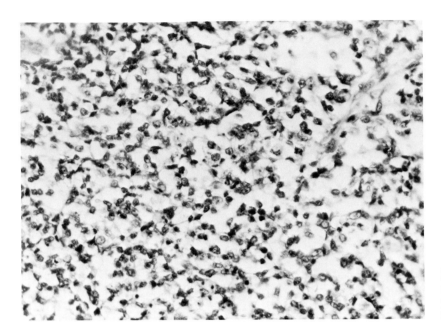

Fig. 19-12 Stroma sarcoma. Note the monotonous-appearing cell population with features of endometrial stroma. (H&E, ×250.)

patients with lesions of fewer than 10 mitoses per 10 hpf versus a 55 percent survival rate at 5 years for patients with lesions with a higher mitotic count. Similar findings were reported by Kempson and Bari,[12] who noted that all lesions with fewer than 5 mitoses per 10 hpf were benign and associated with a pushing rather than an infiltrating margin.

Stromatosis and stromal sarcoma have been reported to occur in all age ranges, varying from the second to the eighth decade. The most common presenting complaint is abnormal vaginal bleeding (either menometrorrhagia or postmenopausal bleeding), which is reported in 75 to 100 percent of patients.[69,70,73] While disease is most often confined to

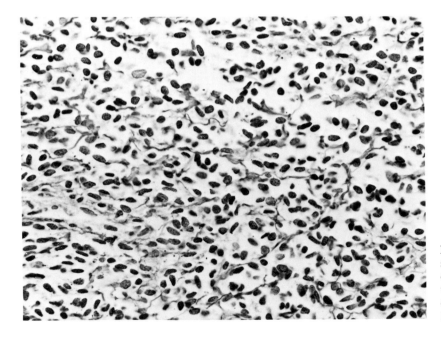

Fig. 19-13 Endometrial stromal sarcoma. Monotonous appearance of cells with a loose reticulum network running around groups of cells and between individual cells. (Recticulum stain, ×400.)

the uterus at the time of presentation in both stromatosis and stromal sarcoma,[16,33,71] extrauterine disease can be found. In patients found to have stromatosis, total abdominal hysterectomy is the cornerstone of therapy and all nodules, including tumor in the adnexal veins, must be removed.[68,70] Fifty-five percent of patients with stromatosis confined to the endometrium, however, will have recurrences, with approximately 80 percent of recurrences found in the pelvis.[71] In patients with metastatic disease, partial responses following oophorectomy have been described,[68,69] although the value of removing the normal-appearing ovary at hysterectomy remains unproved. Descriptions of complete regression of stromatosis with progesterone therapy[69] and a 46 percent response rate with hormonal therapy have been noted in reviewing the literature. Piver et al.[71] recommended postoperative progesterone therapy, even for patients with disease localized to the uterus. Responses to chemotherapy have been less rewarding, and radiation therapy has been shown to control only local (pelvic) disease.[71] Because of the different criteria for diagnosing sarcoma, reported 5-year survival rates have ranged from 9 to 61 percent for all stages.[12,15,17,18,72] Yoonessi and Hart[73] reported on six patients treated by gross excision who had recurrences within 22 months, none of whom responded to either radiation therapy, progesterone therapy, or nitrogen mustard. By contrast, Kahanpaa et al.[16] found only a 33 percent recurrence rate, all of which were local, with three-fourths of these patients surviving. However, the low mitotic count they reported in patients with stage I disease suggests that patients with stromatosis were included in their report.[16] Owing to the high recurrence rate, Yoonessi and Hart[73] recommended surgery followed by radiation therapy for all patients. Peters et al.[33] noted that survival was the same for patients with endometrial stromal sarcoma as for patients with mixed mesodermal tumors.

It appears that radiation therapy may reduce local recurrence rates, as with mixed mesodermal tumors, but endometrial stromal sarcoma remains a systemic disease. With the small numbers of patients involved in any series, there are no data to support the use of one chemotherapy regimen over another, and most of the data are extrapolated from series involving sarcomas in general.[45,46,49,52] Despite their different histology, stromal sarcoma arising in the uterus can probably be treated in a similar manner to a mixed mesodermal tumor or a leiomyosarcoma.

If stromal sarcomas arise in the ovary, clinical differentiation from epithelial ovarian cancer can be difficult. However, the microscopic picture on frozen section is distinctively different. As in endometrial stromal sarcomas, the lesions are represented by monotonous-appearing elongated cells characterized by nuclear pleomorphism along with a high mitotic index. The surgical approach is aimed at debulking the tumor, with emphasis placed on the restoration of GI function and maintaining the integrity of the urinary tract. As with other sarcomas, the clear superiority for cure or long-term remission with any particular chemotherapy regimen has yet to be demonstrated.[49,51]

Other Sarcomas

Because of the vast quantity of connective tissue present, virtually any form of sarcoma can arise at any site along the female genital tract. Almost all types have been reported; however, interpretation of older reports is difficult because of recent changes in terminology[74] as well as improvements in the histopathology techniques in differentiating between the various histologic subtypes.

Hemangiopericytomas have been described within the uterus as well as in other sites along the genital canal. This lesion often presents as a pelvic mass or as an enlarged uterus associated with menometrorrhagia. These are vascular lesions, yet have been described as being easy to enucleate. The differential diagnosis usually consists of stromatosis or hemangioendothelioma. Wilbanks et al.[75] noted that when the lesions are confined to the uterus they behave in a benign manner. However, outside the uterus, they appear to be somewhat more malignant. Only three of seven cases presenting with extrauterine disease were alive after 2 years of follow-up. This may be due to the ease with which uterine tumors can be excised with wide tumor-free margins.

Epithelioid sarcoma has been described in case reports as usually localized to the vulva.[76,77] Clinically, they appear as slowly enlarging nodules with some necrosis and ulceration of the overlying skin.[77] These tumors often appear to be encapsulated. Microscopically, they consist of small cells that are sarcomatous to epithelioid in appearance. Because they appear encapsulated, removal by simple local excision may be carried out, which may result in failure of therapy.[77] Local recurrences are usually noted early, with distant recurrences seen late in the course of disease. These results, reported in earlier series, have led investigators to recommend wide local excision of all lesions.[76]

Alveolar soft part sarcomas were recently described, both in the vulva[78] and in the vagina.[79] These unusual lesions are generally seen on the extremities of young adults. In many cases, they also are thought to be encapsulated or to have a pseudocapsule. Microscopically, they appear as cellular clusters separated by fibrocollagen septae, along which there are loosely aggregated cells with an eosinophilic granular cytoplasm. The cell of origin is uncertain, although either muscle or paraganglion cells have been considered.[78] Wide local excision is the recommended therapy, and radiotherapy may decrease local recurrence. However, no adequate chemotherapy has yet been reported.[78]

Malignant fibrous histiocytoma has been described in the broad ligament[80] and on the vulva.[81,82] Many of the fibrosarcomas reported in the past may have been malignant fibrous histiocytomas that were misdiagnosed.[82] These can present as ulcers with inward-rolling edges or as pelvic masses, depending on their location. Microscopically, they appear as storiform collections of fibrous elements with histiocytic cells mixed in varying degrees.

Despite improvements in classification of the various forms of sarcoma, the treatment involved appears to be the same, regardless of the histologic type. As recommended by DiSaia et al.[74] and Davos et al.,[82] extensive wide local excision or radical excision with sampling of the nodes is the mainstay of therapy. Radiotherapy may play some role in reducing local recurrence. However, because most of these tumors are susceptible to hematogenous dissemination, further

advance in treatment of systemic disease awaits the development of effective chemotherapeutic agents.

LYMPHOMA

Although involvement of internal and external genitalia by lymphomas is often seen at autopsy and in late stages of disease, initial manifestation of lymphoma in the genital canal is an unusual occurrence. In reviewing the files of the AFIP, Chorlton et al.[83] found that the ovary was the site of initial manifestation of lymphoma in approximately 1 in 500 cases, whereas the uterus and vagina were the sites of involvement once in every 730 lymphomas.[84] Most reports have therefore been limited to either single cases or small series of patients. There has often been considerable confusion in the gynecologic literature because of the use of older terminology, especially the terms lymphosarcoma and reticulum cell sarcoma and, until recently, a failure to use newer classification schemes, such as those proposed by Rappaport et al.[85] and recently modified, and the classification for Hodgkin's disease[86] (Table 19-7). The gynecologic literature has also been slow in adopting the Ann Arbor staging for Hodgkin's disease and lymphomas[87] (Table 19-8). Most reports tend to stage by the FIGO staging for the particular organ involved. Crisp et al.[88] reported that with the increasing incidence of lymphomas we may see an increase in pelvic disease; therefore, gynecologists should be aware of the manifestations of lymphomas. They also noted that less extranodal disease is seen with Hodgkin's disease and that most cases seen will be of the non-Hodgkin's variety. The diagnosis may be difficult to establish but should be suspected in cases of enlarging, asympto-

Table 19-7 Classification of Lymphomas

Non-Hodgkin's Lymphoma		Hodgkin's Disease
Follicular (Nodular)	Diffuse	
Lymphocytic, well differentiated	Lymphocytic, well differentiated	Lymphocytic predominance
Lymphocytic, poorly differentiated	Lymphocytic, poorly differentiated	Nodular sclerosis
Mixed, lymphocytic and large cleaved cell	Mixed, lymphocytic and large cleaved cell	Mixed cellularity
Large cleaved cell	Large cleaved cell	Lymphocytic depletion
	Burkitt's lymphoma	
	Undifferentiated	

(Modified from Rappaport et al.[85] and Lukes et al.[86])

Table 19-8 Staging of Lymphoma

Stage	Description
I	Involvement of a single lymph node region or of a single extralymphatic organ or site (I_E)
II	Involvement of two or more lymph node regions on the same side of the diaphragm or localized involvement of a single extralymphatic organ or site and of one or more lymph node groups on the same side of the diaphragm (II_E)
III	Involvement of lymph node groups on both sides of the diaphragm or accompanied by involvement of a single extralymphatic organ or site (III_E) or involvement of the spleen (III_S) or both (III_{SE}).
IV	Diffuse or disseminated involvement of one or more extralymphatic organs or tissues with or without lymph node involvement: liver involvement.

(Carbone PP, Kaplan HS, Musshoff K, et al: Report of the committee on Hodgin's disease staging classification. Cancer Res 31:1860, 1971.)

matic, retroperitoneal masses; in patients with chylous ascites; or in cases in which the Papanicolaou (Pap) smear shows marked inflammatory changes. Although many authorities have doubted the existence of primary lymphoma in genital organs, the initial presentation of disease in the genital organs may bring the patient to the attention of the gynecologist. While laparotomy may often be required for further diagnosis, the surgeon should understand that radical surgery is not curative for a lymphoma. Adequate staging should be done, including biopsies of all nodal groups.[88]

Non-Hodgkin's lymphoma involving the lower genital canal (uterus, cervix, vagina) has been reported under many terms, such as lymphosarcoma or reticulum cell sarcoma.[89-94] Many of these cases have been initially misdiagnosed. However, the authors[89-94] have noted that the lesions tend to present early and are responsive to therapy.[94] Several recent reviews have shown that abnormal bleeding is the most common symptom associated with genital tract lymphoma, occurring in 54 to 70 percent of patients.[84,95,96] The lesions in the lower genital canal tend to present as expansile lesions, enlarging the cervix or uterus or vagina and causing discomfort.[95,96] The major differential diagnoses are sarcoma and undifferentiated carcinoma, either primary or metastatic.[84,95] Careful examination will demonstrate that in lymphoma the cells infiltrate around the normal structures (cervical glands, vessels) without destroying the normal tissue, as sarcomas or carcinomas do[84] (Fig. 19-14). The use of a touch prep will often help differentiate lymphoma from carcinoma or sarcoma.[95] While it may be difficult to distinguish a

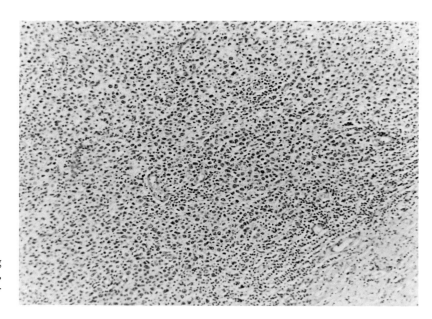

Fig. 19-14 Lymphoma involving the cervix. A diffuse, lymphocytic, well-differentiated malignant lymphoma. (H&E, ×100.)

granulocytic sarcoma from a lymphoma, the use of special stains is helpful.[92,95] This lesion must be distinguished as it represents a form of acute myelogenous leukemia, which always requires systemic chemotherapy or bone marrow transplantation. Although the FIGO staging system does show some correlation wth prognosis, the Ann Arbor staging system is much more accurate in prognosis.[84,95] In fact, almost 75 percent of patients present with stage IE disease in the lower genital canal if the uterus, cervix, and vagina are considered as a single organ.[95] This appears to be a reasonable assumption, since they will all fall within the local radiation field. Harris and Scully[95] recently reported an overall 73 percent 5-year survival rate for all patients and an 89 percent 5-year survival rate for stage IE disease. Twelve stage IE patients treated with local therapy alone were without any evidence of relapse. These results are similar to extranodal non-Hodgkin's lymphoma reported for other organs. Local control for stage I disease, if adequately staged, can be obtained with radiation therapy[95,96] or even with hysterectomy without radiotherapy if disease is truly stage IE.[94] Disease also involving other lymphnode groups, stage II and beyond, requires radiation therapy and/or chemotherapy, depending on the stage of disease, with chemotherapy required in diffuse disease.

Ovarian involvement as an initial manifestation of disease and as the place of origin has been questioned even more than primary involvement of the lower genital canal.[83] Ovarian involvement is certainly seen more commonly at autopsy as a late manifestation of diffuse disease. When it occurs as an initial presentation, most cases seem to occur between the ages of 20 and 50.[97] The median age of occurrence is 38.[83] In contradistinction to the lower genital canal, gynecologic symptoms were unusual, with only 15 percent of patients presenting with abnormal bleeding.[83] An abdominal or pelvic mass is seen in 80 percent of patients,[83] and back pain or increasing abdominal girth is the most common symptom.[97] Approximately 50 percent of cases are unilateral and at least one-half of cases exhibit extraovarian disease at the time of diagnosis.[83] Almost all histologic types of lymphoma may be seen in the ovary (Fig. 19-15); however, if Burkitt's lymphoma is present, it is usually a manifestation of disseminated disease.[83] The differential diagnosis in ovarian lesions includes dysgerminoma, granulosa cell tumor, or metastatic cancer.[97] The use of touch preps may be helpful in establishing the diagnosis. Rotmensch and Woodruff[97] reported only a 7 percent survival at 5 years in a series of 55 patients, although many did not have adjuvant therapy. Using the Ann Arbor staging, Chorlton et al.[83] reported that for stage IE disease, 1-year survival was 45 percent and 5-year survival 22 percent. This is worse than the survival seen with other extranodal lymphomas.[83] However, many patients in this referral series were

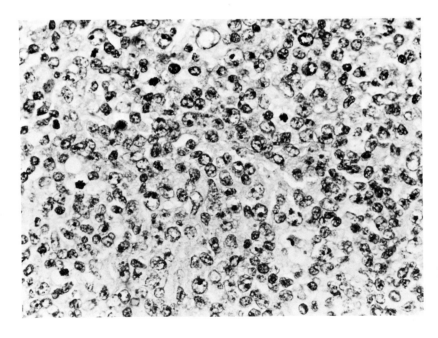

Fig. 19-15 Lymphoma involving the ovary. Note diffuse, mixed lymphocytic and large cleaved cell tumor. (H&E, ×400.)

probably inadequately staged. These data appear to suggest that all lymphomas involving the ovary behave aggressively and should be treated with systemic chemotherapy.

REFERENCES

1. Ober WB: Uterine sarcomas: Histogenesis and taxonomy. Ann NY Acad Sci 75:568, 1959

2. DiSaia PJ, Creasman WT: Sarcoma of the uterus. p. 178. In Clinical Gynecologic Oncology. CV Mosby, St. Louis, 1984

3. Christopherson WM, Williamson EO, Gray LA: Leiomyomosarcoma of the uterus. Cancer 29:512, 1972

4. Corscaden JA, Singh BP: Leiomyosarcoma of the uterus. Am J Obstet Gynecol 75;149, 1958

5. Stearns HC, Sneeden VD: Leiomyosarcomas of the uterus. Am J Obstet Gynecol 95:374, 1966

6. Spiro RH, Koss LG: Myosarcoma of the uterus: A clinicopathological study. Cancer 18:571, 1965

7. Bartsich EG, Bowe ET, Moore JG: Leiomyosarcoma of the uterus: A 50-year review of 42 cases. Obstet Gynecol 32:101, 1968

8. Silverberg SG: Leiomyosarcoma of the uterus: A clinicopathologic study. Obstet Gynecol 38:613, 1971

9. Proper MS, Simpson BT: Malignant leiomyomata. Surg Gynecol Obstet 29:39, 1919

10. Evans N: Malignant myomata and related tumors of the uterus. Surg Gynecol Obstet 30:225, 1920

11. Taylor HB, Norris HJ: Mesenchymal tumors of the uterus. Arch Pathol Lab Med 82:40, 1966

12. Kempson RL, Bari W: Uterine sarcomas: Classification, diagnosis and prognosis. Hum Pathol 1:331, 1970

13. Hendrickson MR, Kempson RL: Surgical pathology of the uterine corpus. p. 468. In Bennington JL (ed): Major Problems in Pathology. WB Saunders, Philadelphia, 1980

14. Hart WR, Billman JK: A reassessment of uterine neoplasms originally diagnosed as leiomyosarcomas. Cancer 41:1902, 1978

15. Burns B, Curry RH, Bell MEA: Morphologic features of prognostic significance in uterine smooth muscle tumors: A review of 84 cases. Am J Obstet Gynecol 135:109, 1979

16. Kahanpaa KV, Wahlstrom T, Grohn P, Heinonen E, Nieminen U, Widholm O. Sarcomas of the uterus: A clinicopathologic study of 119 patients. Obstet Gynecol 67:417, 1986

17. Wheelock JB, Krebs HB, Schneider V, Goplerud DR: Uterine sarcomas: Analysis of prognostic variables in 71 cases. Am J Obstet Gynecol 151:1016, 1985

18. Salazar OM, Bonfiglio TA, Patten SF, et al: Uterine sarcomas: Natural history, treatment and prognosis. Cancer 42:1152, 1978

19. Aaro LA, Symmonds RE, Dockerty MB: Sarcoma of the uterus: A clinical and pathologic study of 177 cases. Am J Obstet Gynecol 94:101, 1966

20. Marchese MJ, Liskow AS, Crum CP, et al: Uterine sarcomas: A clinicopathologic study 1965–1981. Gynecol Oncol 18:299, 1984

21. Barter JF, Smith EB, Szpak CA et al: Leiomyosarcoma of the uterus: Clinicopathologic study of 21 cases. Cynecol Oncol 21:220, 1985

22. Vardi JR, Tovell HMM: Leiomyosarcoma of the uterus: Clinicopathologic study. Obstet Gynecol 56:428, 1980

23. Montague ACW, Swartz DP, Woodruff JD: Sarcoma arising in a leiomyoma of the uterus. Am J Obstet Gynecol 92:421, 1965

24. Rastogi BL, Bergman B, Augervall L: Primary leiomyosarcoma of the vagina: A study of five cases. Gynecol Oncol 18:77, 1984

25. Schwartz Z, Dgani R, Lancet M, Kessler I: Uterine sarcoma in Israel: A study of 104 cases. Gynecol Oncol 20:354, 1985

26. Kurman RJ, Norris HJ: Mesenchymal tumors of the uterus. VI. Epithelioid smooth muscle tumors including leiomyoblastoma and clear-cell leiomyoma: A clinical and pathologic analysis of 26 cases. Cancer 37:1853, 1976

27. Buscema J, Carpenter SE, Rosenshein NB, Woodruff JD: Epithelioid leiomyosarcoma of the uterus. Cancer 57:1192, 1986

28. Salazar OM, Bonfiglio RA, Patten SF, Keller BE, Feldstein ML, Dunne ME, Rudolph JH: Uterine sarcomas: Analysis of failure with special emphasis on the use of adjuvant radiation therapy. Cancer 42:1161, 1978

29. Norris HJ, Roth E, Taylor HB: Mesenchymal tumors of the uterus. II. A clinical and pathologic study of 31 mixed mesodermal tumors. Obstet Gynecol 28:57, 1966

30. Norris HJ, Taylor HB: Mesenchymal tumors of the uterus. III. A clinical and pathologic study of 31 carcinosarcomas. Cancer 19:1459, 1966

31. DiSaia PJ, Castro JR, Rutledge FN: Mixed mesodermal sarcoma of the uterus. AJR 117:632, 1973

32. Spanos WJ, Wharton JT, Gomez L, et al: Malignant mixed mullerian tumors of the uterus. Cancer 53:311, 1984

33. Peters WA III, Kumar NB, Fleming WP, Morley GW: Prognostic features of mixed tumors of the endometrium. Obstet Gynecol 63:550, 1984

34. Mascadaet MA, Waxman M, Fruchter RE, et al: Prognostic factors in malignant mesodermal (mullerian)

mixed tumors of the uterus. Gynecol Oncol 20:32, 1985

35. Hanjani P, Peterson RO, Lipton SE, Nolte SA: Malignant mixed mesodermal tumors and carcinosarcoma of the ovary. Report of eight cases and review of the literature. Obstet Gynecol Surv 38:537, 1983

36. Dictor M: Malignant mixed mesodermal tumor of the ovary. Obstet Gynecol 65:720, 1985

37. Deppe G, Zbelle E, Friberg J, Thomas W: Combination chemotherapy for mixed mesodermal tumor of the fallopian tube. Cancer 54:1517, 1984

38. Rotmensch J, Rosenshein NB, Woodruff JD: Cervical sarcoma: A review. Obstet Gynecol Surv 38:456, 1983

39. Peters WA, Kumar NB, Anderson WA, Morley GW: Primary sarcoma of the adult vagina: A clinicopathologic study. Obstet Gynecol 65:699, 1985

40. Lele SB, Piver S, Barlow JJ: Chemotherapy in the management of mixed mesodermal tumors of the ovary. Gynecol Oncol 10:298, 1980

41. Carlson JA, Day TG: Five year survival following combination radiotherapy and chemotherapy for recurrent mixed mesodermal sarcoma of the ovary. Gynecol Oncol 22:129, 1985

42. Spanos WJ, Peters LJ, Oswald MJ: Patterns of recurrence in malignant mixed mullerian tumor of the uterus. Cancer 57:155, 1986

43. DiSaia PJ, Morrow CP, Boronow R, et al: Endometrial sarcoma: Lymphatic spread pattern. Am J Obstet Gynecol 130:104, 1978

44. Gilbert HA, Kagen AR, Lagasse L, Jacobs MR, Tawa K: The value of radiation therapy in uterine sarcoma. Obstet Gynecol 45:84, 1974

45. Muss HB, Bundy B, DiSaia PJ, et al: Treatment of recurrent or advanced uterine sarcoma: A randomized trial of doxorubicin versus doxorubicin and cyclophosphamide. (A phase III trial of the Gynecologic Oncology Group.) Cancer 55:1648, 1985

46. Omura GA, Major FJ, Blessing JA et al: A randomized trial of adriamycin with and without dimethyl triazenoimidazole carboxamide in advanced uterine sarcomas. Cancer 52:626, 1983

47. Hannigan EV, Freedman RS, Elder KW, Rutledge FN: Treatment of advanced uterine sarcoma with adriamycin. Gynecol Oncol 16:101, 1983

48. Piver MS, Barlow JJ, Lele SB, Yazigi R: Adriamycin in localized and metastatic uterine sarcoma. J Surg Oncol 12:263, 1979

49. Piver MS, DeEulis TG, Lele SB, Barlow JJ: Cyclophosphamide, vincristine, adriamycin and dimethyl-triazenoimidazole carboxamide (CYVADIC) for sarcoma of the female genital tract. Gynecol Oncol 14:319, 1982

50. Seltzer V, Kaplan B, Vogl S, Spitzer M: Doxorubicin and cis-platinum in the treatment of advanced mixed mesodermal uterine sarcoma. Cancer Treatm Rep 68:1389, 1984

51. Piver MS, Lele SB, Patsner B: Cis diamminedichloroplatinum plus dimethyl-triazenoimidazole carboxamide as second and third line chemotherapy for sarcomas of the female pelvis. Gynecol Oncol 23:371, 1986

52. Hannigan EV, Freedman RS, Elder KW, Rutledge FN: Treatment of advanced uterine sarcoma with vincristine, actinomycin D, and cyclophosphamide. Gynecol Oncol 15:224, 1983

53. Buchsbaum HJ, Lifshitz S, Blythe JG: Prophylactic chemotherapy in stages I and II uterine sarcoma. Gynecol Oncol 8:346, 1979

54. Hannigan EV, Freedman RS, Rutledge FN: Adjuvant chemotherapy in early uterine sarcoma. Gynecol Oncol 15:56, 1983

55. Kohorn EI, Schwartz PE, Chamber JT, et al: Adjuvant therapy in mixed mullerian tumors of the uterus. Gynecol Oncol 23:212, 1986

56. Van Nagell JR Jr, Hanson MB, Donaldson ES, Gallion HH: Adjuvant vincristine dactinomycin and cyclophosphamide therapy in stage I uterine sarcomas: A pilot study. Cancer 57:1451, 1986

57. Horn RC Jr, Enterline HT: Rhabdomyosarcoma: A clinicopathological study and classification of 39 cases. Cancer 11:181, 1958

58. Hilgers RD, Malkasian GD, Soule EH: Embryonal rhabdomyosarcoma (botryoid type) of the vagina. A clinicopathologic review. Am J Obstet Gynecol 107:484, 1972

59. Copeland LJ, Gershenson DM, Saul PB, et al: Sarcoma botryoides of the female genital tract. Obstet Gynecol 66:262, 1985

60. Daniel WW, Koss LG, Brunschweig A: Sarcoma botryoides of the vagina. Cancer 12:74, 1959

61. Maurer HM: The intergroup rhabdomyosarcoma study (NIH): Objectives and clinical staging. J Pediatr Surg 10:977, 1975

62. Hilgers RD: Pelvic exenteration for vaginal embryonal rhabdomyosarcoma: A review. Obstet Gynecol 45:175, 1975

63. Rivard G, Ortega J, Hittle R, et al: Intensive chemotherapy as primary treatment for rhabdomyosarcoma of the pelvis. Cancer 36:1593, 1975

64. Kumar APM, Wrenn EL, Fleming ID, et al: Combined therapy to prevent complete pelvic exenteration for rhabdomyosarcoma of the vagina or uterus. Cancer 37:118, 1976

65. Ortner A, Weiser G, Haas H, et al: Embryonal rhabdomyosarcoma (botryoid type) of the cervix. A case report and review. Gynecol Oncol 13:115, 1982

66. Maurer HM, Moon T, Donaldson M, et al: The intergroup rhabdomyosarcoma study: A preliminary report. Cancer 40:2015, 1977

67. Copeland LJ, Sneige N, Stringer CA, et al: Alveolar rhabdomyosarcoma of the female genitalia. Cancer 56:849, 1985

68. Hunter WC, Nohlgren JE, Lancefield SM: Stromal endometriosis or endometrial sarcoma. A re-evaluation of old and new cases, with especial reference to duration, recurrences, and metastases. Am J Obstet Gynecol 72:1072, 1956

69. Baggish MS, Woodruff JD: Uterine stromatosis. Clinicopathologic features and hormone dependency. Obstet Gynecol 40:487, 1972

70. Hart WR, Yoonessi M: Endometrial stromatosis of the uterus. Obstet Gynecol 49:393, 1977

71. Piver MS, Rutledge FN, Copeland L, et al: Uterine endolymphatic stromal myosis: A collaborative study. Obstet Gynecol 64:173, 1984

72. Norris HJ, Taylor HB: Mesenchymal tumors of the uterus: I. A clinical and pathological study of 53 endometrial stromal tumors. Cancer 19:755, 1966

73. Yoonessi M, Hart WR: Endometrial stromal sarcomas. Cancer 40:898, 1977

74. DiSaia PJ, Rutledge F, Smith JP: Sarcoma of the vulva. Report of 12 patients. Obstet Gynecol 38:180, 1971

75. Wilbanks GD, Szymanska Z, Miller AW: Pelvic hemangiopericytoma. Report of 4 patients and review of the literature. Am J Obstet Gynecol 123:555, 1975

76. Piver MS, Tsukada Y, Barlow J: Epithelioid sarcoma of the vulva. Obstet Gynecol 40:839, 1972

77. Hall DJ, Grimes MM, Gopelrud DR: Epithelioid sarcoma of the vulva. Gynecol Oncol 9:237, 1980

78. Shen JT, D'Ablaing G, Morrow CP: Alveolar soft part sarcoma of the vulva. Report of first case and review of the literature. Gynecol Oncol 13:120, 1982

79. Kasai K, Yoshida Y, Okumura M: Alveolar soft part sarcoma in the vagina. Clinical features and morphology. Gynecol Oncol 9:227, 1980

80. Dieste MC, Lynch GR, Gordon A, et al: Malignant fibrous histiocytoma of the broad ligament. A case report and literature review. Gynecol Oncol 28:225, 1987

81. Hensley GT, Friedrich EG: Malignant fibroxanthoma: A sarcoma of the vulva. Am J Obstet Gynecol 116:289, 1973

82. Davos I, Abell MR: Soft tissue sarcomas of vulva. Gynecol Oncol 4:70, 1976

83. Chorlton I, Norris HJ, King FM: Malignant reticuloendothelial disease involving the ovary as a primary manifestation: A series of 19 lymphomas and 1 granulocytic sarcoma. Cancer 34:397, 1974

84. Chorlton I, Karnei RF Jr, King FM, Norris HJ: Primary malignant reticuloendothelial disease involving the vagina, cervix and corpus uteri. Obstet Gynecol 44:735, 1974

85. Rappaport H, Winter WJ, Hicks EB: Follicular lymphoma: A re-evaluation of its position in the scheme of malignant lymphoma based on a survey of 253 cases. Cancer 9:792, 1956

86. Lukes RJ, Carver LF, Hall TC et al: Report of the nomenclature committee. Cancer Res 26:1311, 1966

87. Carbone PP, Kaplan HS, Musshoff K, et al: Report of the committee on Hodgkin's disease staging classification. Cancer Res 31:1860, 1971

88. Crisp WE, Surwitt EA, Grogan TM, Freedman MF: Malignant pelvic lymphoma. Am J Obstet Gynecol 143:69, 1982

89. Buchler DA, Kline JC: Primary lymphoma of the vagina. Obstet Gynecol 40:235, 1972

90. Wright CJE: Solitary malignant lymphoma of the uterus. Am J Obstet Gynecol 117:114, 1973

91. Cihak RW, Hamada J: Primary reticulum cell sarcoma of the uterus: A case report and review of the literature. Cancer 33:1039, 1974

92. Kapadia SB, Krause JR, Kanbour AI, Hartsock RJ: Granulocytic sarcoma of the uterus. Cancer 41:687, 1978

93. Tunca JC, Reddi PR, Shah SH, Slack ST: Malignant non-Hodgkin's type lymphoma of the cervix uteri occurring during pregnancy. Gynecol Oncol 7:385, 1979

94. Steinfeld AD: Histiocytic lymphoma of the cervix. Gynecol Oncol 8:97, 1979

95. Harris NL, Scully RE: Malignant lymphoma and granulocytic sarcoma of the uterus and vagina: A clinicopathologic analysis of 27 cases. Cancer 53:2530, 1984

96. Komaki R, Cox JD, Hansen RM, et al: Malignant lymphoma of the uterine cervix. Cancer 54:1699, 1984

97. Rotmensch J, Woodruff JD: Lymphoma of the ovary: Report of twenty new cases and update of previous series. Am J Obstet Gynecol 143:870, 1982

20

Cancer of the Breast: Diagnosis

George W. Mitchell
Marc J. Homer

Discouraging statements to the effect that the mortality from breast cancer, or from cancer in general, has not significantly decreased in more than 40 years have appeared frequently in the medical literature and in the lay press, suggesting that treatment modalities, however innovative, continue to prove ineffective and that early diagnosis has not improved results. Advocates of a holistic approach to breast care have recommended prevention in the form of macrobiotic diets, vitamins, and progestins and the strict avoidance of alcohol, tranquilizers, and methylxanthines. Although prevention should not be decried, it does not confer immunity, nor is it rational to assume that early disease will necessarily share the same fate as advanced disease or that small lesions are prognostically as dangerous as large ones. If present trends continue, breast cancer will afflict one out of every 11 females born today, and it is unlikely that a means will be found in the near future to reduce the incidence. Figures also show that for a large population of women who have been screened for breast cancer, a significant reduction in mortality from the disease can be achieved by early diagnosis. It is therefore, imperative, to make the effort necessary to educate women and their physicians concerning the symptoms and signs of breast cancer and the need for thorough examinations.

SCREENING AND DIAGNOSIS BY EXAMINATION

Screening by self-examination of the breast should be a frequent routine for all women past the thelarche and should be taught by the most appropriate informed counselor, whether mother, sister, nurse, or physician. The examination is best done on a monthly basis for greater familiarity with tissue patterns, preferably immediately following menses in the reproductive-age group. If the educational process is begun early, objections will be fewer and anxiety decreased; accuracy improves as confidence grows. In the physician's office, videotapes provide the clearest objective description of the examination; these should be reinforced by a positive attitude on the part of medical personnel.

Screening examinations of the breasts by professionals should be a routine part of every general physical examination. How often breast examinations per se should be done is a matter of conjecture, since data are not available to prove the possible advantage of examinations more often than the usually recommended once a year. It seems unlikely, however, that increasing the frequency of examinations would provide benefit other than the allaying of anxiety, since the doubling time of individual tumors is variable and chronologic stage of development in any given instance unpredictable. Well-trained paramedical personnel are able to perform screening examinations with an accuracy comparable to that of physicians.

The breast examination is performed on patients unencumbered by jewelry and clothing above the waist, and in both the seated and supine positions. Inspection of the breasts is done first, with the patient raising her arms above her head or clasping her hands behind her neck, while retracting her shoulders. The following must be noted: nipple and skin retraction, raised skin lesions, excoriations and ulcers, erythema, venous congestion, asymmetry, and edema. The heavy pendulous breast may have to be further elevated manually to ascertain the characteristics of the underside. For cancer detection, the most important considerations are unilateral nipple retraction or deviation that is not congenital, skin dimpling, or a red scaly eruption over the areola, which may be indicative of Paget's disease. Skin lesions have the same connotation on the breast as elsewhere on the body, and many are manifestations of a general systemic process.

To assist accurate palpation the patient should place her hands on her hips and relax her shoulder muscles. Palpation is begun on the neck, followed by the supra- and infraclavicular areas, to rule out enlarged lymph nodes. Each breast in turn is then pressed against the chest wall with the flats of the examiner's fingers, making sure that no part of the breast is omitted; it is best to do this in a ritualized way, either clockwise or counter clockwise, ending beneath the nipple and then compressing the breast between the examiner's hands, while drawing it away from the chest wall, in an attempt to detect lesions close to the muscle.

Examination of the axillae can be done with the patient either seated or supine, depending on individual preference. One method is to take the patient's left hand to draw her arm diagonally forward, while the examiner's right hand palpates along the insertion of the pectoralis major muscle, the medial surface of the latissimus dorsi muscle, and upward to the apex of the space between them. The procedure is done in the reverse on the other side, taking the patient's right hand and palpating with the left.

With the patient reclining, it is helpful to use a towel or pillow to prop up the shoulder on the side to be examined. Each breast is examined with the ipsilat-

eral arm extended above the head, and again with the arm at the side. The examination proceeds as previously described, pressing all parts of the breast against the chest wall until there is reasonable certainty that no suspicious lesions exist. The time required to do an adequate examination depends, to some extent, on the experience of the examiner, the size of the breasts and the demands of the patient, but a minimum of 3 to 5 minutes is essential. Positive findings of any kind, surface or internal, should be charted, preferably on a predrawn diagram, and a description of the results of examination should appear in the record.

The interpretation of palpable findings requires experience, and even experienced hands yield false-positive and false-negative rates. A discrete mass, of whatever size, must be subjected to further investigation. Areas of thickening, usually most prominent in the upper outer quadrants, wax and wane with variations in the menstrual cycle and are often tender. The term fibrocystic disease has been applied to these condensations of breast tissue, and their role in the possible future development of breast cancer has been a matter of prolonged debate. The microcystic form, containing ductal and glandular dilatations less than 2 mm in diameter, is present in most female breasts; the gross changes that can be noted by physical examination are only a quantitative expression of cellular secretion in an individual hormonal milieu. The term fibrocystic change avoids the connotation of a premalignant condition as well as the health insurance problems related to the previous terminology. However, dominant projections from any generally thickened area must be considered suspicious.

The benefits of breast self-examination and periodic professional examination, whether by physicians or by paramedical personnel, have been evaluated statistically during the past 10 years in terms of both early diagnosis of cancer and survival. Even though approximately 80 percent of American women discover their own breast cancers, early opposition to the widely publicized breast self-examination technique included the probable lack of compliance, the anxiety effect produced, the greater likelihood of accidental rather than programmed discovery, and variability in size and shape of the breast preventing accurate diagnosis. More recent criticisms of breast self-examination have come from the Breast Cancer Detection Demonstration Project (BCDDP) and other studies, which demonstrate that cancers are discovered later by this technique and that, because of delay, the prognosis is worse when the patient has been the diagnostician. They also indicate that the size and stage of lesions discovered by breast self-examination are not lower than those diagnosed by other methods.

A breast lesion must be at least 1 cm in diameter to be easily palpable; at that time, it probably represents approximately 8 years of preclinical growth and is therefore being diagnosed too late. When discovered by professionals, the average size of the palpable lesion is 2.5 cm, and the likelihood of distant metastases of lymph node involvement is approximately 50 percent. Professional screening is probably superior to breast self-examination but is not comparable in precision to the sophisticated diagnostic technology now available, which has the capacity to detect the presence of subclinical disease. It will remain the primary screening technique until the logistic and economic problems of applying high-resolution radiologic methods to all women in the age groups at risk have been solved. The deficiences of the method should serve to stimulate more careful attention to it on the part of both patients and doctors.

Other studies of large numbers of patients indicate that, in addition to being cheaper and relatively less threatening, professional and self-examinations provide earlier diagnosis and longer survival than would occur without them.

MAMMOGRAPHY

The fact that a breast lump, when first palpable, may represent a stage of the disease already beyond the likelihood of the survival of its bearer has led to a concentrated effort to develop diagnostic technology that can detect cancer in its preclinical form. The 5-year BCDDP has shown that tumors were detected at earlier biological stages in the development of breast cancer and at stages more amenable to definitive therapy than less rigorous projects have been able to achieve. Diagnostic modalities in use at that time were relatively primitive compared with those now available but showed improved results over those obtained by regular breast examination. In the same broad study, 42 percent of neoplasms were detected only by mammography and were nonpalpable, while 9 percent were detected only by physical examination

and were mammographically negative. The advantages of routine screening for breast cancer were also demonstrated by a study conducted by the Health Insurance Plan of New York during the 1960s. A 25 percent reduction in mortality was demonstrated in women over 50 years of age as compared with a control group. The study involved periodic screening by both physical examination and x-ray mammography, while the control group received only customary medical care. Although further randomized control studies both of early diagnosis and survival are needed, current evidence shows that screening by physical examination and mammography is advantageous and that, of the two, mammography is far more sensitive. Information obtained from these and other studies led to further refinements of radiologic techniques and attempts to extend their usefulness to increasing numbers of women. The American Cancer Society has set guidelines for the mammographic screening of asymptomatic women.

AMERICAN CANCER SOCIETY GUIDELINES FOR SCREENING

1. Baseline mammograms for all women at age 35 to 40 years
2. Mammography at 1- or 2-year intervals from 40 to 49 years
3. Annual mammograms for women 50 years or older

In spite of the educational effort that has been made to implement these guidelines and the fear inspired by the high incidence of breast cancer, only 5 percent of women in the United States over the age of 50 actually undergo screening mammography on a regular basis, and only one-third have ever had a mammogram for any reason. The logistic load that full implementation of the American Cancer Society (ACS) guidelines would impose on departments of radiology would be impossible to bear, and the economic implications are equally staggering. In the only cost analysis that has been made, the cost per cancer found was $9,046; for each curable cancer, $26,961; and for each death averted, $61,100. Although these costs seem high, in an idealistic society they must be matched against the costs of the prolonged management of advanced breast cancer and the societal disruptions associated with it.

Compliance with ACS guidelines has been further obstructed by the specter of the known cancerogenic effect of ionizing irradiation. The scarce data bearing on this issue have come from studies of persons exposed to high doses of irradiation, including patients who have undergone radiation therapy or fluoroscopic studies for benign conditions and survivors of the explosions at Hiroshima and Nagasaki. Extrapolating from these data, the National Research Council (NRC) estimated that an additional six cancers per year per rad per one million women might be expected after a 10-year latency period. Since approximately 120,000 new cases of breast cancer develop each year from all causes, it is apparent that diagnostic radiography has a relatively slight influence on the incidence of the disease, and this must be weighed against the demonstrable beneficial effect of regular screening on early diagnosis, and probably on survival. A linear relationship between breast cancer and the extremely low doses used in state-of-the-art dedicated mammography equipment has not been proved. However, even if this relationship exists, the potential risk of developing breast cancer from these low radiation doses is comparable to the risks of daily living. This theoretical risk has been compared with the risk of death from flying 1,200 miles or driving 180 miles in a car. Nevertheless, it is the responsibility of the radiologist to keep the dose of radiation from the unit to a minimum and to limit multiple exposures to the lowest number compatible with providing accurate diagnosis.

In the presence of symptoms and signs suggestive of malignant breast disease, the need for diagnostic mammography is more clearly defined than for screening. Since only a small fraction of women will have been screened by mammography, most will be radiographed for diagnosis of a suspected or known condition, further emphasizing the necessity for physical examination in screening. Most of the listed indications are obvious, and there is no limiting factor of age in ordering diagnostic mammography, but in the gray zone are decisions to order films based on questionable thermograms or sonograms, patient requests in lower age groups, family history, or even the recommendations of radiologists to repeat examina-

tions at intervals of less than 6 months. Such decisions must be predicated upon the merits of each individual case, with the medicolegal consequences of incorrect diagnosis in mind. Histologic identification of the lesion is imperative, if either the physical examination or the mammogram is positive or suspicious, and, in some instances, even if both are negative, as may be the case with a bloody nipple discharge, when no other objective evidence of disease is present. In the event that physical examination is conclusive for the presence of malignancy, mammography should also be done to determine the extent of the disease, whether it is multifocal, and whether it is present in the contralateral breast.

INDICATIONS FOR DIAGNOSTIC MAMMOGRAPHY

Dominant mass
Discrete thickening
Bloody nipple discharge
Change in previous lesion
Localized skin puckering
Unilateral deviated nipple
Noninfectious erythema
Discrepancy in professional opinions
Prebiopsy evaluation
Patient request
Positive thermography or ultrasonography

During the past 15 years, great improvements have been made in the techniques of x-ray mammography. The use of high-resolution x-ray film has made good-quality images possible with a much lower dose than was previously required, and formerly indistinct soft tissue masses are now well defined. Xeromammography employs an aluminum plate coated with selenium, which, when exposed to the rays and properly treated, can be viewed in ordinary room light. It provides good detail, and it is excellent for visualizing the microcalcifications often associated with breast cancer (Fig. 20-1).

Film-screening mammography is the other major imaging modality in wide use. New technology lead-

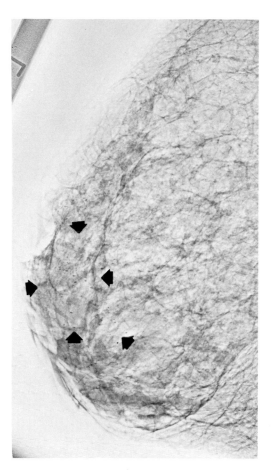

Fig. 20-1 Xeroradiogram showing a cluster of microcalcifications, which were proved to be associated with an invasive carcinoma.

dedicated units. Many variables can have a detrimental effect on the quality of mammographic interpretation, including the training of radiologic technologists, the anatomy and position of the patient, the degree of exposure, and the development of the image receptor. To be sure that all the necessary areas to be viewed are covered, patients must be examined by a trained person before the films are taken. Radiologists trained in mammographic interpretations are necessary to provide accurate diagnosis. A second opinion from a more experienced mammographer may be indicated in the presence of an indeterminate lesion. A diagnostic accuracy of at least 90 percent should be achieved in cases that are clinically suspicious.

The effort to diagnose breast cancer in a preclinical phase, when it is theoretically more curable, has introduced a new terminology to radiologic reports that poses a dilemma both for radiologists and surgeons. Some data have suggested that dense breasts, in which fibrocystic change predominates, are more susceptible to the future development of cancer. They are certainly more difficult to evaluate because of their relative impenetrability. This has led to attempts to predict the probability of developing malignancy on the basis of densities produced by parenchymal patterns in the breast. Categorization of these patterns was attempted by Wolfe, who divided them into four classes. The classification was based on two retrospec-

ing to the development of fast x-ray film combined with rare earth screens allows exquisite resolution at very low radiation dose. The recent introduction of grid technology and magnification provides even greater diagnostic sensitivity. As a general rule, film-screen mammography is superior for resolving mass densities in the breast. Electron beam mammography has the advantage of using a very low dose of irradiation but is not widely available because of the complexity and expense of the equipment and its tendency to dysfunction.

Although film-screen mammography and xeroradiography can be performed using standard x-ray equipment, optimal results can be obtained only with equipment especially designed for mammography. Mammography should be performed only on such

MAMMOGRAPHIC PARENCHYMAL PATTERNS (WOLFE)	
N1	Primarily fat with few areas of increased density
P1	Mostly fat with prominent anterior ducts to one-fourth breast volume
P2	Severe involvement with prominent duct pattern greater than one-fourth breast volume
DY	Severe involvement with dysplasia often obscuring underlying duct pattern

tive studies, each with a large number of patients, with results indicating a significant relative risk in both the P2 and DY categories, but much higher in the latter. Further description of the four classes emphasized the quantitative degree of density as an important risk factor, as well as the prominence of linear and nodular patterns of ducts in the breast. The term, dysplasia, which was used to describe generalized density, has since confused many physicians of all disciplines, who erroneously equate the term with a microscopic histologic entity.

Both the study and the terminology have since evoked widespread controversy. Approximately 18 other studies have produced variable results; the validity of each of these has been further analyzed statistically without resolving the issue. It is possible that some increased risk might be associated with dense mammographic parenchymal patterns, but final proof is lacking; at this time, the presence or absence of these patterns should not be used to determine individual patient management or to serve as markers for more rigorous screening of populations assumed to be at greater risk.

In the detection of actual breast cancers, mammography is the only imaging technique that can accurately determine the pesence of lesions less than 1 cm in diameter. With very small lesions, the differentiation between benign and malignant is often extremely difficult, but a true-positive rate approaching 20 to 30 percent occurs with lesions that are nonpalpable but mammographically suspicious. Biopsy is indicated when the physical examination is positive, even though mammograms may be negative, since the false-negative rate of mammography is 10 percent. When mammograms are positive and physical and histologic findings negative, careful follow-up evaluation with further radiographs and possible rebiopsy, is indicated.

Obvious cancers often have a typical spiculated appearance, even if clinically occult. They may be multifocal in the same breast or present in both breasts (Fig. 20-2). When clusters of microcalcifications (less than 1 mm in diameter) are seen localized in a certain area, they are usually assumed to be associated with early malignancy, although they can also accompany benign processes. These and other findings suspicious of early cancer but clinically undetectable must be marked with a needle inserted under radiologic guidance as close as possible to the suspicious area in order

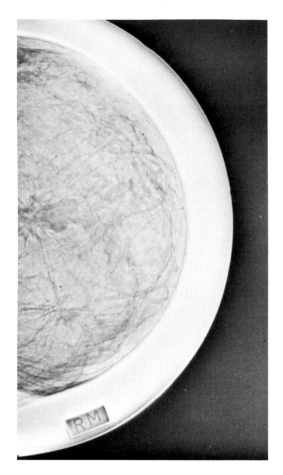

Fig. 20-2 Xeroradiogram showing two spiculated lesions in the same breast, typical of carcinoma.

to facilitate precise excision at the time of biopsy. A wire is passed through the needle, which has been inserted percutaneously, and is then stabilized at the tissue level by a hook at the end and, at the skin level, by a locking device, until the time of surgery. A dye marker can also be injected through the needle. The Homer Mammalok is a convenient all-purpose instrument (Fig. 20-3).

Mammographic reports tend to reflect the fact that there are major areas of disagreement among mammographers. This circumstance is compounded by the scarcity of experts in the field experienced enough to avoid overreading and to present recommendations in a manner compatible with the findings and satisfactory to the surgeon. Rather than use terms such as normal or abnormal, or positive and negative, which have no significance, since each women's breasts are

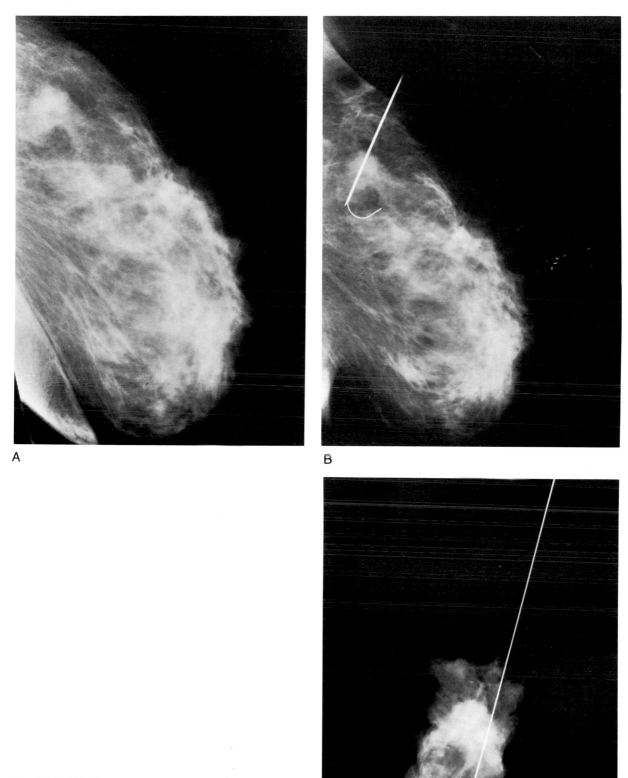

Fig. 20-3 **(A)** Film-screen mammogram showing invasive carcinoma 1.5 cm beneath the skin, presenting as a spiculated lesion without a palpable mass. **(B)** Same as A showing localization of lesion with Mammalok needle. **(C)** Radiograph of specimen with needle after removal.

unlike any others, a concise description of exactly what is seen is more appropriate, followed by a recommendation for follow-up or biopsy. (A mammographer never recommends that a biopsy not be done.) It is of the utmost importance to confer with the mammographer and establish a continuing line of communication in order to prevent misunderstanding either on the basis of semantics or intent. This is all the more urgent in the current medicolegal climate.

STAGING

Standardization of the staging taxonomy for breast cancer has received much attention, and the TNM system is replacing stages I to IV in many institutions. It is important for the diagnostician to be familiar with both and to be able to correlate them (Table 20-1). T0 refers to "unmeasurable" primary disease, T1 to lesions less than 2 cm in diameter, and T2 to lesions between 2 and 5 cm. N designates nodal involvement and M distant metastases. Nodal involvement is usually categorized in levels, I, II, and III. All are beneath the clavicle and the pectoralis major. Level I nodes lie in the outer axillary compartment just medial to the latissimus dorsi. Level II nodes lie just lateral to and beneath the insertion of the pectoralis minor, and level III nodes lie medial to the pectoralis minor close to the sternoclavicular junction. The size of the primary lesion can best be ascertained preoperatively by mammography and the presence of enlarged lymph nodes by computed tomography (CT) scan. Final staging is surgical and pathologic.

BIOPSY

Until 20 years ago, biopsies were done in the hospital, under general anesthesia, and a biopsy positive for the presence of cancer was immediately followed by the mastectomy of the surgeon's choice. Chronologic separation of biopsy from definitive surgery was thought to result in the spread of cancer cells into the breast and throughout the body. As a result of a number of studies indicating that this was not necessarily the case, biopsies were more and more frequently done in an outpatient ambulatory facility or private office, and definitive treatment was delayed for a few days or weeks to allow the patient to consider the various treatment options. The delay was also thought to decrease the emotional stress caused by the patient's not knowing whether she would awake from the anesthesia with or without her breast and to enable the pathologist to read permanent rather than frozen sections with less chance of error. Outpatient biopsy using local anesthesia has now become firmly established, resulting in better patient compliance and reduction of cost. It has also encouraged the performance of biopsies by gynecologists, family practitioners, and others, with the result that the biopsy and the secondary surgery, if the biopsy proves positive, are frequently done by different individuals. So long as mastectomy was to be performed when cancer was present, the use of the two-stage technique entailed no risk to the patient. The current enthusiasm for conservative surgery designed to preserve the breast, when the cancer is in a T1 or early T2 category, has, in certain instances, necessitated an alteration in this practice.

Table 20-1 Staging.

Clinical Stage	Pathologic Stage	TNM Equivalent		
I	I	T1	N0	M0
II	II	T0		
			N1	
		T1		M0
		T2	N0 or N1	
III	III	T3		
			Any N	
		T4		M0
		Any T	W/N2 and N3	
IV	IV	Any T	Any N	W/M1
Bilat.	Bilat.	Any T or N with M2		

In the office, needle aspiration of breast lesions is a simple maneuver that can be done without analgesia, and often without local anesthesia. It is indicated for the evacuation of macrocysts and for differentiating between solid and cystic lesions (Fig. 20-4). Fluid aspirated from cysts is usually acellular, of a yellowish-brown color, and nonviscous. Although it is usually difficult to make an accurate diagnosis on centrifuged specimens of this material, it should be sent to the laboratory because of the remote possibility that an intracystic hyperplastic or malignant lesion may be present. Cells from solid lesions may be obtained by passing a skinny needle through the tumor in several different planes while maintaining constant suction with a syringe. This material is blown on a slide and sent to pathology. Interpretation of such a specimen is often difficult and, unless a strongly positive diagnosis is made by an expert pathologist, the presence of suspicious cells should lead to a more definitive biopsy.

Because of the need to insert a needle of larger caliber, core biopsies should be done with local anesthesia. A variety of instruments is available for this purpose. The needle is inserted percutaneously into the lesion; the cutting mechanism is introduced, and a core of tissue taken for histologic section. If a specimen of 2 mm or greater has been obtained, it should provide a trustworthy diagnosis. To prevent pneumothorax, needles should be inserted tangential to the chest wall, and facilities for the management of accidental pneumothorax should be available. Core biopsies sometimes cause bleeding, with resultant ecchymoses, but this can usually be controlled by the application of a tight binder. When cancer is identified by needle biopsy, open biopsy is unnecessary, and the size of the lesion is the criterion on which the decision to direct the patient toward conservative lumpectomy or a mastectomy is based.

When needle biopsy is negative, open biopsy is indicated. If the probability of benign disease is high, a circumareolar incision is made, even if it is subsequently necessary to tunnel outward for 3 or 4 cm in order to resect the lesion. Especially for disease in the upper breast, circumareolar incisions give better cosmetic results than radial incisions. When clinical and mammographic evidence suggests the presence of malignancy, a semilunar incision, parallel to the areola, is made directly over the lesion, if it is less than 4 cm in diameter and therefore within the arbitrary limit for lumpectomy. The more direct approach ensures adequate exposure for complete resection with margins free of disease. Larger tumors, for which mastectomy would probably be advised should they prove malignant, are approached by an incision placed so as not to obstruct the path of the subsequent mastectomy incision. Wedge biopsies of such large

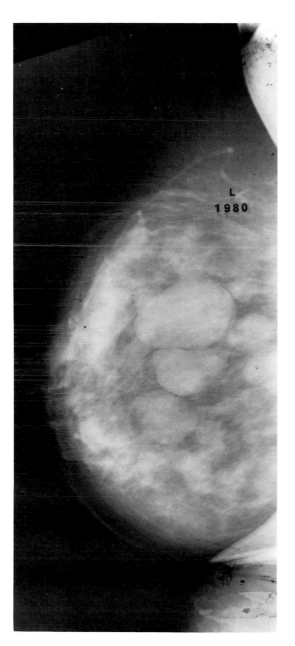

Fig. 20-4 Film-screen mammogram showing presence of multiple macrocysts.

tumors may be advisable rather than an attempt to perform a complete excision, which may result in greater morbidity and the possibility of incomplete resection.

Lumpectomy as a reasonable alternative to mastectomy for small cancers has increased the complexity of open biopsy by making it essential to perform a complete excision and to confirm this by careful pathologic examination of the margins of resection. For this purpose, it is helpful to the pathologist to mark the boundaries of the specimen with sutures or clips in four places or to ink the entire specimen. When histologic extension of disease to the margins of resection is noted, futher removal of more breast tissue in the area must be done, either immediately or in a second operation, the former being preferable. Frozen-section diagnosis may be assumed to be 98 percent correct in the best hands under these circumstances; the advisability of performing the operation in a facility where this expertise is available is obvious.

The data showing the beneficial effect of adjunctive chemotherapy on time of first recurrence and survival in patients with stage II disease have made it necessary to extend diagnostic surgery from the primary lesion to the axilla, currently thought to be the most likely site of early metastasis. Nodes at levels I and II are removed through an incision extending obliquely across the base of the axilla from the edge of the pectoralis major to the edge of the latissimus dorsi. Although sampling of these nodes is simpler and quicker, complete dissection of the nodes at levels I and II is far more satisfactory because of the notorious tendency of the disease to skip certain areas. It is also possible to resect level III nodes by retracting the insertion of the pectoralis major and severing the pectoralis minor just proximal to its insertion, but these nodes are found to be positive in less than two percent of cases when levels one and two are negative.

The necessity to perform axillary dissection in all instances when breast-sparing surgery is contemplated has led to a return to the concept of a one-stage operation under general anesthesia, including total removal of the primary lesion and regional lymphadenectomy, sometimes in continuity. For patients who object to any procedure beyond local excision, the alternative is to perform open biopsy, wait for the permanent sections, and, if the lesion is positive, proceed later with axillary dissection and the removal of any additional breast tissue that may be considered

necessary. In some states, a one-stage two-step procedure is prohibited by law unless all treatment options have been fully explained to the patient. It must be emphasized that the open diagnostic biopsy is also the recommended treatment for all patients who may be candidates for conservative surgery.

PATHOLOGY

The pathologic interpretation of tissues removed from the breast by biopsy, when equivocal or couched in ominous terms, has caused consternation among patients and confusion among surgeons and has contributed to the controversy regarding the implications of the term, fibrocystic disease. Funded by a grant from the ACS, the Cancer Committee of the College of American Pathologists reached a consensus on a taxonomy designed to solve the fibrocystic disease problem (Table 20-1). This consensus quantitates the relative risk in three different categories of benign breast disease. Cellular hyperplasia and the prevalence of atypical cells are the determining factors rather than cystic changes and simple proliferation. When these warning signs exist, closer follow up by physical examination and mammography is indicated. Pathologic reports sent to surgeons should indicate descriptively whether or not these changes are present.

Most breast malignancies are adenocarcinomas, either of the ductal or lobular variety, and an in situ form of each is recognized. On the basis of circumstantial evidence, the potential for in situ lesions to progress to invasion is definite, but data are lacking to show clearly the frequency with which this occurs and the time lag to invasion. The process is thought to be often multicentric and bilateral. When a diagnosis in one of these categories is returned, there is time for due consideration of the management alternatives in each individual case.

In the last decade, the term minimal breast cancer entered the literature and may be encountered in reports from pathology. Included in this category are all noninvasive ductal and lobular carcinomas and invasive carcinomas up to 0.5 cm in diameter. The purpose of this definition is to designate a group of tumors that are not likely to have metastasized and that are therefore curable by local treatment. Approximately 10 percent of all breast cancers are within these boundaries.

In the pathologic description of invasive carcinomas, many terms are used to denote patterns of growth, connective tissue involvement, and leukocyte infiltration. For the most part, these have relatively little impact on survival, whereas anaplasia, lymphatic and vascular invasion, and attachment to muscle are markers of a poorer prognosis.

The pathologist must receive the entire specimen after resection. It is the pathologists's responsibility to have the radiologist take additional films to determine whether calcifications noted before surgery are present in the specimen. The pathologist must also send at least 1 g of tumor tissue to the laboratory for the estrogen and progesterone receptor studies so important to the management of future problems. Unless an organizational protocol to accomplish these purposes is rigidly followed, essential information may be lost.

OTHER DIAGNOSITC AIDS

Although mammography, including both film-screen and xeromammography, is unequivocally the keystone on which the diagnosis of early breast cancer is made, the need for a more accurate, less invasive method has led to the development of some new techniques and the modification and recycling of old techniques. Breast clinics, both institution-based and free-standing, offering a multiplicity of diagnostic choices, have proliferated recently; many contend that if one diagnostic modality is good, two or more offer even greater security. Costs are increased accordingly, and it is difficult to justify additional procedures that only confirm positive findings but do not alter patient management.

ULTRASOUND

Comparison with mammography has generally shown ultrasound to be relatively inadequate in detecting occult malignant disease. In the detection of minimal breast cancer, its inability to visualize microcalcifications is a definite liability. For this reason, ultrasound has no role as a screening technique. It can, however, reliably distinguish between solid and cystic masses and is useful as an adjunct to mammography in reducing the number of surgical biopsies in favor of aspiration or observation (Fig. 20-5).

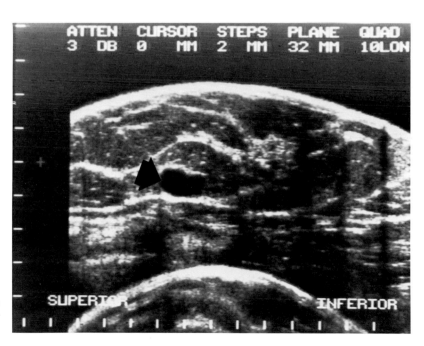

Fig. 20-5 Ultrasonogram showing well-defined mass that is clearly cystic.

THERMOGRAPHY

Thermographic interpretation of breast disease is based on the observation that many breast tumors have a higher temperature than that of surrounding normal tissue, either as a result of direct conduction to the skin, where measurements are taken, or by convection with the venous blood draining the tumor. First measured with handheld sensors that provide a pictorial representation of the infrared (IR) radiation, the variations in temperature are used not only to detect the presence of cancer but also to predict the risk of future development of the disease (Fig. 20-6).

The interpretation of thermograms depends on the amount of contrast between hot and cold or black and white as it appears on the screen. (By electronic inversion, hot or cold may be depicted either black or white.) Isotherm devices are used to give a uniform shade to all areas having the same temperature, and it is then possible to read from a scale variations from the norm that might represent disease.

To increase the contrast between normal and ab-cally depressing the temperature of normal tissue without concomitantly affecting diseased areas, but artifacts due to varying vascularity interfere with interpretation. Known as graphic stress telethermometry, this process has had a considerable vogue.

Another variation of the same principle is liquid crystal thermography. The patient's breasts are placed in direct contact with a cholesteric plate that transmits temperature changes to a camera, which codes these changes in color on a film. Interpretation requires great experience.

The improvement in thermographic technology has been commendable, but rigorously controlled prospective studies of the methods are necessary before its use in breast cancer diagnosis can be accepted. Although some studies extol its efficacy in the detection of cancer, the incidence of false-positive diagnoses is too high, leading to unnecessary surgery, and it fails to locate many cases of early disease. Its use as a screening tool remains controversial and unproved.

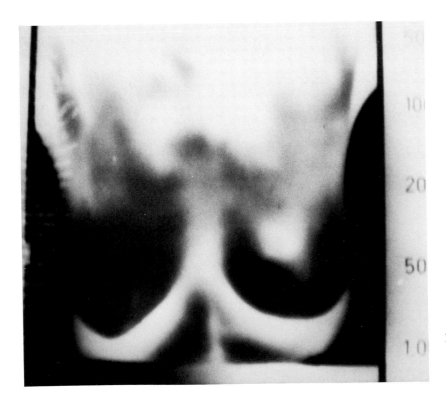

Fig. 20-6 Thermogram showing large white hot spot beneath the left areola that proved to be carcinoma.

DIAPHANOGRAPHY

Transillumination of the breast with fiberoptic light sources is now being used in many clinics as a noninvasive screening tool. Its accuracy in cancer detection is about 60 percent, but this does include some nonpalpable lesions. Light scanning is affected by breast size but not by architecture. The chief difficulty is in the diagnosis of lesions of less than 1 cm; for this reason, it is not adequate as a routine screening method and is unnecessary as an adjunct to mammography. The few preliminary studies that have been done do not demonstrate an advantage of this over exisiting techniques, except in its noninvasiveness.

MAGNETIC RESONANCE IMAGING

Available for only the past 4 years, magnetic resonance imaging (MRI) has been the subject of only a few preliminary studies of its effectiveness in the diagnosis of breast disease. It can differentiate solid from cystic lesions, detect small noncalcified masses in dense breasts, and delineate parenchymal patterns. The chief disadvantage is its inability to define calcifications, either benign or malignant. However, it is an exciting modality still in its infancy, and the major research now in progress will define its role in the near future.

DUCTOGRAPHY

Direct injection of radiopaque material into the duct system of the breast to demonstrate the presence and location of nonpalpable intraductal lesions still has some proponents in Europe but has been discontinued in most institutions in this country. In some instances, the radiography shows a clear pattern, but in others it is misleading, and the process is rather painful to the patient. It is generally assumed here that unilateral nipple discharge containing red blood cells requires open dissection of the ducts and removal of any lesion encountered. At surgery, the localization of such lesions is usually not difficult.

SUGGESTED READINGS

Baker LH: Breast cancer detection demonstration project: Five year summary report. Cancer 32:194, 1982

Baker RR: Out-patient breast biopsies. Ann Surg 185:543, 1976

Barrett AH, Myers PC, Sadowsky NL: Microwave thermography in the detection of breast cancer. AJR 134:365, 1980

Billings KJ: Status of mammography in breast cancer screening. Postgrad Med J 79:89, 1986

Boyd NF, O'Sullivan B, Fishell E, et al: Mammographic patterns and breast cancer risk: Methodologic standards and contradictory results. J Natl Cancer Inst 72:1253, 1984

Caffee HH, Benfield JR: Data favoring biopsy of the breast under local anesthesia. Surg Gynecol Obstet 140:88, 1975

Cancer Committee of the College of American Pathologists. Is "fibrocystic disease" of the breast precancerous? Arch Pathol Lab Med 110:171, 1986

Consensus Conference: Adjuvant chemotherapy for breast cancer. JAMA 254:3461, 1985

Dash N, Lupetin AR, Daffner RH, et al: Magnetic resonance imaging in the diagnosis of breast disease. AJR 146:119, 1986

Deschenes L, Fabia J, Meisels A, et al: Fine needle aspiration biopsy in the management of palpable breast lesions. Can J Surg 21:417, 1978

Dupont WD, Page DL: Risk factors for breast cancer in women with proliferative breast disease. N Engl J Med 312:146, 1985

Feldman JG, Carter AC, Nicastri AD, et al: Breast self-examination, relationship to stage of breast cancer at diagnosis. Cancer 47:2740, 1981

Fisher B: Reappraisal of breast biopsy prompted by the use of lumpectomy JAMA 253:3585, 1985

Fisher B, Bauer M, Margolese R, et al: Five-year results of a randomized clinical trail comparing total mastectomy and segmental mastectomy with or without radiation in the treatment of breast cancer. N Engl J Med 312:665, 1985

Fletcher SW, O'Malley MS, Bunce LA: Physicians' abilities to detect lumps in silicone breast models. JAMA 253:2224, 1985

Foster RS, Costanza MC: Breast self-examination practices and breast cancer survival. Cancer 53:999, 1984

Frank JW, Mai V: Breast self-examination in young women: more harm than good? Lancet 2:654, 1985

Frazier TG, Murphy JT, Furlong A: The selected use of ultrasound mammography to improve diagnostic accuracy in carcinoma of the breast. J Surg Oncol 29:231, 1985

Gautherie M: Thermobiological assessment of benign and malignant breast diseases. Am J Obstet Gynecol 147:861, 1983

Gautherie M, Gros CM: Breast thermography and cancer risk prediction. Cancer 45:51, 1980

Geslien GE, Fisher JR, DeLaney C: Transillumination in breast cancer detection: Screening failures and potential. AJR 144:619, 1985

Goldberg IM, Schick PM, Pilch Y, et al: Contact plate thermography. Arch Surg 116:271, 1981

Greene FL, Hicks C, Eddy V et al: Mammography, sonomammography, and diaphanography (Lightscanning) Am Surg 51:58, 1985

Hall FM: Screening mammography — Potential problems on the horizon. N Engl J Med 314:53, 1986

Harper P, Kelly-Fry E: Ultrasound visualization of the breast in symptomatic patients. Radiology 137:465, 1980

Harris WG: Ductography for nipple discharge (Letter). Lancet 1:110, 1984

Health and Public Policy Committee, American College of Physicians: The use of diagnostic tests for screening and evaluating breast lesions. Ann Intern Med 103:143, 1985

Hindle WH, Navin J: Breast aspiration cytology: A neglected gynecologic procedure. Am J Obstet Gynecol 146:482, 1983

Homer MJ: The mammography report. AJR 142:643, 1984

Homer MJ: Nonpalpable breast abnormalities: A realistic view of the accuracy of mammography in detecting malignancies. Radiology 153:831, 1984

Homer MJ: Nonpalpable breast lesion localization using a curved-end retractable wire. Radiology 157:259, 1985

Homer MJ, Smith TJ, Marchant DJ: Outpatient needle localization and biopsy for nonpalpable breast lesions. JAMA 252:2452, 1984

Horwitz RI, Lamas AM, Peck D: Mammographic parenchymal patterns and risk of breast cancer in postmenopausal women. Am J Med 77:821, 1984

Hutter RVP: Goodbye to "fibrocystic disease." N Engl J Med 312:179, 1985

Kline TS, Neal HS: Needle aspiration biopsy: A critical appraisal. JAMA 239:36, 1978

Kopans DB, Meyer JE, Sadowsky N: Breast imaging. N Engl J Med 310:960, 1984

Love SM, Gelman RS, Silen W: Fibrocystic "disease" of the breast — A nondisease? N Engl J Med 307:1010, 1982

Mitchell GW Jr: Benign and malignant diseases of the breast. p. 183. In TeLinde's Operative Gynecology. 6th Ed. JB Lippincott, Philadelphia, 1985

Mitchell GW Jr, Homer MJ: Outpatient breast biopsies on a gynecologic service. Am J Obstet Gynecol 144:127, 1982

Moore FD: Breast self-examination. N Engl J Med 299:304, 1978

Moskowitz M: Mammographic parenchymal patterns: More controversy. JAMA 247:210, 1982

Moskowitz M, Feig SA, Cole-Beuglet C, et al: Evaluation of new imaging procedures for breast cancer: Proper process. AJR 140:591, 1983

Moskowitz M, Fox SH: Cost analysis of aggressive breast cancer screening. Radiology 130:253, 1979

Moskowitz M, Milbrath J, Gartside P, et al: Lack of efficacy of thermography as a screening tool for minimal and Stage I breast cancer. N Engl J Med 295:249, 1976

Mueller CB: Surgery for breast cancer. N Engl J Med 312:712, 1985

Rosner D, Blaird D: What ultrasonography can tell in breast masses that mammography and physical examination cannot. J Surg Oncol 28:308, 1985

Saba JEY, Duchesneau RH: Magnetic resonance imaging of the human breast. Rad Clin North Am 22 4:859, 1984

Saltzstein SL: Potential limits of physical examination and breast self-examination in detecting small cancers of the breast. Cancer 54:1443, 1984

Schwartz GJ, D'Ugo DM, Rosenberg AL: Extent of axillary dissection preceding irradiation for carcinoma of the breast. Arch Surg 121:1395, 1986

Shapiro S: Evidence on screening for breast cancer from a randomized trial. Cancer 29:2772, 1977 (Healthy Insurance Plan of New York)

Sickles EA: Mammographic features of 300 consecutive nonpalpable breast cancers. AJR 146:661, 1986

Sickles EA: Mammographic features of "early" breast cancer. AJR 143:461, 1984

Snyder RE, Watson RC, Cruz N: Graphic stress telethermometry (GST^{tm}). Am J Diagn Gynecol Obstet 1:197, 1979

Tabar L, Dean PB: Mammographic parenchymal patterns. JAMA 247:185, 1982

Walker GM, Foster RS, McKegney CP, et al: Breast Biopsy — A comparison of outpatient and inpatient experience. Arch Surg 113:942, 1978

Wertheimer MD, Costanza ME, Dodson TF, et al: Increasing the effort toward breast cancer detection. JAMA 255:1311, 1986

Whitehead J, Carlile T, Kopecky KJ, et al: Wolfe mammographic parenchymal patterns. Cancer 56:1280, 1985

Wolfe JN: Breast patterns as an index of risk for developing breast cancer. AJR 126:1130, 1976

Wolfe JN: Risk for breast cancer development determined by mammographic parenchymal pattern. Cancer 37:2486, 1976

Section III
SURGICAL PROCEDURES

21

Introduction to Pelvic Surgery — Pre- and Post-Operative Care

James W. Orr, Jr.

Improved anesthetic techniques, the introduction of broad-spectrum antibiotics, modern blood-banking facilities, nutritional supplementation, and the incorporation of cardiovascular monitoring and support techniques have expanded the indications and application of specific surgical procedures for patients with gynecologic malignancy. With these changes and the evolution of surgical knowledge, operations may now be offered to many patients who might previously have been denied the benefit of a surgical procedure. However, this progress arrives at a time of maximum consciousness concerning health care costs. The physician and patient must formulate and agree on a plan that considers surgical risks, medical benefits, as well as the potential cost-effective benefits of each procedure.

Perioperative preparation and postoperative care of women undergoing gynecologic surgery requires a basic understanding of the physiology of the complex interactions of associated medical and surgical illness. The gynecologic surgeon must understand the alterations associated with anesthesia and surgery and must evaluate specific patient risks or the risk factors involved. The gynecologic surgeon should utilize appropriate preoperative and postoperative diagnostic studies. All available resources must be incorporated, so that appropriate diagnostic or therapeutic interventions are made at an optimal time to minimize each woman's surgical risk.

The hallmark of the competent gynecologic surgeon involves the ability to select or tailor the specific procedure for the individual patient. The gynecologic oncologist has less choice in patient selection and may enter the operating suite in a less than optimal situation. Regardless, the outcome of any surgical procedure is directly related to the adequacy of the surgical plan and the appropriateness of the operative technique. The occurrence of intraoperative or postoperative complications, which may or may not be related to the plan or technique, is the major modifier of surgical outcome.

The surgical plan must be formulated before the patient enters the operating suite. While the time involved varies related to the urgency of the procedure, a diligent preoperative search for coexisting or confounding medical problems must be undertaken. Decisions regarding each patient variable, its possible adverse effect on surgical outcome, and the necessary intervention to modify this effect should be made. Despite the vast array of available diagnostic studies, a thorough history and complete physical examination remain a most sensitive detector of coexisting disease.

In fact, routine screening laboratory studies are rarely (<1 percent) abnormal when not suspected on the basis of history or examination. These abnormal studies are even less likely to effect surgical outcome than those associated with an abnormal examination. It is therefore crucial that each surgeon develop a systematic format to evaluate current or past medical problems. The omission of any information such as drug allergies or current medications (i.e., aspirin) can have potential disastrous effects on surgical outcome. Once potential problems are identified, a specific intervention can be implemented or an appropriate consultation sought. Many potential problems may surface during postoperative surveillance and, in most situations, the medical consultant should continue the evaluation during postoperative convalescence.

Attention to the medical aspects of each woman's illness takes precedence; however, the gynecologic surgeon cannot, and should not, overlook the importance of psychic preparation and preoperative counseling. A cancer diagnosis is associated with anxiety and depression and may evoke a bleak outlook from the patient's standpoint. Specific procedures involving the reproductive tract may be psychologically equated with a loss of femininity. The fears and loss of control associated with anesthesia may contribute to a feeling of helplessness. These situations necessitate preoperative discussion with the patient detailing the anatomic and physiologic changes associated with the operation. Combating misconceptions or misinformation regarding the diagnosis and surgical procedure are best undertaken preoperatively with the patient and her sexual partner in a quiet private situation that minimizes interruption.

Preoperative information and instruction also has medical importance, as it can decrease postoperative pain and anxiety, increase postoperative ambulation, and allow patients increased participation in their postoperative respiratory care. A concerned, frank discussion detailing the necessity of preoperative evaluation and the progression of postoperative care permits the patient to understand the benefits of the procedure and to anticipate the various interventions.

While the physician's thoughts, plans, and actions are important, the final results of each surgical procedure rely on the effort of the total health care team. During the perioperative period, women undergoing abdominal hysterectomy receive an average of 16 drugs. The number is 9 following vaginal hysterectomy. Medication errors are known to occur in as many as 25 percent of physician orders, and a delay or omission in medication administration may render the best surgical plan ineffective. For example, poor or inappropriate timing of the administration of prophylactic antibiotics diminishes their effectiveness. This type of omission in specific situations may counteract the best surgical skill and technique. The psychological impact of the team effort is important. The patient's hospital interactions primarily involve nonphysician members of the health care team who must continue to provide an understanding approach to the patient's disease and surgical procedure. Appropriate explanations and concern avoid patient confusion and facilitate recovery.

The technical aspects of the individual procedure involve less actual time than the surgical plan but are of equal importance. Surgical skill, experience, intraoperative decision making, and judgments correlate with the risks of specific complications, such as infection. In addition some procedures, such as ovarian debulking, are probably best performed by those physicians with specific expertise or experience. Gynecologic oncologists are likely to perform an optimal cytoreductive surgical debulking in 78 percent of patients with advanced-stage ovarian carcinoma. Nononcologists may lack specific skills such as those required for gastrointestional (GI) surgery. In fact, the nongynecologic oncologist may perform optimal resection in 20 percent of these patients. While this may not affect long-term survival, an optimal resection correlates with increased response rates and longer progression-free intervals. Finally, while the actual technique of cutting and tying is important, the gynecologic surgeon must appropriately incorporate new techniques or instrumentation as they evolve. Modifications using stapling devices, alternative suture material, or other innovations that either shorten or improve outcome must be the goal.

Regardless of the plan or surgical technique, intraoperative and postoperative complications as a result of the procedure or associated medical illness continue to occur and result in significant patient morbidity, mortality, and cost. Specific methods of prophylaxis may not be available for rare complications, such as septic pelvic thrombophlebitis. However, prophylaxis is available for postoperative infections, which are more common, increase hospital stay by as much as 10 days, and increase the patient's drug exposure by

Table 21-1 Influence of Infectious Morbidity Following Hysterectomy

	Afebrile	Minor Infection	Major Infection
Drug doses (antipyretics and analgesics)	13.6	30.1	91.1
Hospital days	4.2	5.7	17.6
Costs (dollars)	1,805	2,719	8,347

(Modified from Schwartz, Obstet Gynecol 54:284, 1979.)

as much as sixfold (Table 21-1). Importantly, each drug administered has the potential to cause major or minor adverse effects and increase the risk for poor outcome. In addition, following radical or ultradical surgery, the occurrence of one complication, such as pelvic infection, may increase the risk of other problems such as a urinary leak. Immobilization and catabolic losses of these secondary complications further increase cost and risks to the patient.

On an individual patient basis, the prevention of complications remains a most important goal of each physician. However, in the United States, 673,000 women undergo hysterectomy and 632,000 women undergo dilation and curettage (D&C). These two operations are the second and third most common surgical procedures performed and the decreased risk associated with the incorporation of specific methods of prophylaxis may have a profound impact on national health care costs. Even a 1 percent decrease in the morbidity of a procedure should lead to more effective use of the health care dollar.

THE ROLE OF SURGERY IN CANCER TREATMENT

Radiation and chemotherapy are potential and effective methods of cancer therapy, but surgery maintains an important role in the management of most women with a gynecologic malignancy. A diagnostic, curative, staging, or palliative surgical procedure has a role in the treatment of most of these cases.

Current predictions indicate that the diagnosis of invasive cancer of the cervix, endometrium, and ovary will be established in more than 70,000 women in 1987. Conservative estimates indicate that at least another 200,000 women will require treatment for premalignancy disease of the reproductive tract.

Diagnostic procedures, including D&C and conization (71,000/year), are considered low-risk operative procedures and are often performed on an outpatient basis. Infectious or hemorrhagic complications are rare; however, anesthetics are required and may be associated with serious complications. Quoted mortality rates for these procedures are low, approaching 0.01 in 1,000. Even in these low-risk procedures, the surgeon may adversely influence operative complications by simple maneuvers, such as the injection of vasoconstrictors during vaginal operations. Although intended to decrease operative blood loss, there is little evidence to support this practice, and its routine use potentially alters blood supply during the time of contamination and may actually increase the risk of infectious complications. Also, the injection of vasoconstrictors is associated with significant cardiovascular alterations and a high incidence (50 percent) of ventricular irritability. While specific patients may be susceptible to these cardiovascular complications, the adverse effects of vasoconstrictor use in most situations apparently outweigh its benefits. Avoiding their routine use seems prudent.

Curative surgery is the goal in patients with premalignant or early-stage invasive cervix cancer and in patients with endometrial carcinoma. Preoperative preparation must be geared to accommodate the possibility of additional surgery or a more radical dissection. If total hysterectomy is required following conization, infectious morbidity is decreased if the procedure is performed early (within 48 hours) or delayed until 6 weeks. The use of frozen-section conization may eliminate delay. However, the physician and patient must be prepared to stop the surgical procedure if equivocal results are reported after pathologic evaluation of the conization specimen. If radical hysterectomy is required, this interval is not important, and the radical procedure can be performed at any interval following conization without increasing the risk of infection, blood loss, or hospital stay. In this latter situation, cancer treatment can proceed without delay and decrease the associated psychic stress.

Ovarian cancer operations, although occasionally curative, are usually considered a resection and staging procedure as most of these women require additional therapy. Optimal resections require extended procedures involving the GI or urinary tracts in as many as 30 percent of patients. Intraoperative judgment and alteration of a specific procedure may potentially avoid later morbidity. This may be as simple as incorporating permanent suture material in the fascial closure. An en bloc closure might protect the incision during the administration of postoperative chemotherapy. The interposition of an omental flap or graft may provide new pelvic blood supply and reduce the risk of small bowel injury during postoperative radiation therapy.

The use of frozen-section conization may eliminate delay. However, the physician and patient must be prepared to stop the surgical procedure if equivocal results are reported after pathologic evaluation of the conization specimen.

Finally, surgical procedures may have an important role in the palliative care of women with gynecologic cancer. Urgent procedures may not allow for optimal preoperative preparation; however, the decision to operate is as important as the decision is to resect or bypass the GI tract when treating small bowel obstruction. These judgments in palliative care are as important as those associated with other procedures, as they are intended to relieve pain and to restore quality of life outside of the hospital.

SURGICAL STRESS

Anesthesia and surgery create a significant physiologic stress on virtually every organ system. Proper understanding of a woman's response to this stress requires knowledge of the normal woman's physiologic makeup and permits appropriate intervention.

Water constitutes approximately 50 ± 15 percent of a young women's body weight. With age, this total percentage of body water decreases as the proportion of fatty tissues (with less water per gram than muscular tissues) increases. In fact, water as the percentage of total body weight approximates 57 percent in an 18-year-old but falls to 46 percent in a 60-year-old. Body water can be functionally divided into three compartments. Intracellular water composes 30 to 40 percent of the individual woman's body weight, while extracellular water makes up approximately 20 percent of total body weight. The latter is composed of the plasma or intravascular volume, which represents approximately 5 percent of body weight; lymphatic volume, which approximates 2 percent; and interstitial volume, which represents 13 percent of body weight. An additional fluid compartment, the third space, which consists of intestinal contents and joint and pleural fluid, contributes to these patient volumes as well. Under normal condition, this latter volume is not clinically significant. In general, these third-space fluids are considered immobile and are relatively unresponsive to the normal physiologic mechanisms that allow and govern fluid flux. Postoperatively, particularly in those patients with ascites, pleural effusion, extensive pelvic dissection, or prolonged intestinal ileus, these volumes may increase dramatically, influence hemodynamic status, and require monitoring and appropriate fluid replacement.

The normal chemical composition of intravascular, intracellular, and interstitial fluids differs significantly (Table 21-2). Postassium and magnesium are the primary intracellular cations, while phosphates and proteins are the principal anions. Extracellular fluid contains sodium as its principle cation, with chloride and magnesium as its principal anion. The extracellular fluid compartment volume is determined primarily by the total-body sodium content. In most instances, the interstitial-plasma volumes are considered interchangeable, and the intravascular ad-

Table 21-2 Fluid Composition (mEq/L)

Cations	Anions	Plasma		Interstitial		Intracellular	
Na+	Cl−	142	103	144	114	10	
K	HCO3−	4	27	4	30	150	10
Ca	SO4²−/PO4²−	5	3	3	3		
Mg	HPO4³−/SO4²−	3	—	2		40	150
	Organic acids		5		5		
	Protein		16		1		40
Total		154	154	153	153	200	200

ministration of crystalloids will equilibrate. Clinically, this becomes important, as the intravenous administration of isotonic fluids may acutely contribute to intravascular volume but later distribute to the interstitial (three-parts) and intravascular (one-part) compartments. Thus, 1 L of isotonic fluid may acutely maintain intravascular volume; however, with time and equilibration, 750 ml will move to the interstitial space and contribute to peripheral edema. Since dextrose solutions distribute through total body water, only one-half of the infused free-water fluid remains in the intravenous space. These complicated interactions, and particularly the distribution of the extracellular fluids, are determined by the balance between plasma and the interstitial oncotic and hydrostatic pressures. Osmotic pressures relate to the actual number of particles present in solution in the individual fluid compartment. The total number of osmotically active particles in each compartment varies between 290 and 310 mOsm. Effective oncotic pressures are dependent on those substances that fail to pass through the semipermeable cellular membranes. In general, dissolved proteins are primarily responsible fo effective osmotic pressures. Water flux is associated with any alteration in effective oncotic pressure. Thus, hypernatremia will usually result in a flux of water from the intracellular to extracellular compartment; however, clinically, most losses and gains of body fluids are from the extracellular compartment. As a general rule, hypotonicity is associated with expansion and hypertonicity with contraction of the intracellular fluid compartment. Clinically, hypernatremia always implies a hypertonic state. However, hyponatremia cannot always be equated with hypotonic states.

The boundaries of three fluid compartments are not rigid but are governed by a number of active and passive forces. Interstitial-intracellular ion flow is governed by active transmembrane transport mechanisms and concentration differences, as well as transmembrane potential differences. Volume interchange between the intravascular and interstitial compartments is determined primarily by Starling forces and their modifications. This interplay between hydrostatic and oncotic forces is much more important than ion distribution (Gibbs-Donnan equilibrium) in determining compartmental volumes.

In health, fluid volume in these compartmental boundaries is largely regulated by the pressure and perfusion of the kidney, modulated by antidiuretic hormone (ADH) and aldosterone. The GI tract may have an important passive role in this regulation, as GI losses may markedly alter renal perfusion. Aldosterone, a product of the adrenal gland (zona glomerulosa), influences the renal absorption of sodium and is essential in the maintenance of a circulating volume during times of decreased intravascular volume (dehydration, hemorrhage). Its serum levels are regulated by adrenocorticotropic hormone (ACTH) renin, and possibly input from myocardial stretch receptors. Hyperaldosteronism is common during the postoperative period and is predominantly related to alterations in effective arterial blood volume. ADH, a product of the supraoptic and paraventricular nucleus of the hypothalamus, increases water absorption by increasing the permeability of the renal collecting ducts to water. The primary physiologic stimulus for ADH release is a rise in body fluid tonicity. Fear, pain, hemorrhage, injury, and osmoreceptors are important factors that stimulate its production and release. Large decreases (10 to 15 percent) in blood volume are associated with dramatic increases in ADH release. The increased ADH secretion has a major role in intraoperative and postoperative water retention.

Alterations in acid-base homeostasis may profoundly alter cardiovascular function, cell membrane permeability, cellular metabolism, or cerebral blood flow. Clinical effects occur after the pH falls to less than 7.2. Despite normal daily metabolic production of 20,000 mmoles carbonic acid and 80 mmoles nonvolatile acids, the free hydrogen ion concentration of body fluids is fixed within a relatively narrow range. The normal arterial pH of 7.35 to 7.45 is maintained by the kidneys, the lungs, and seven buffer systems. Proteins and phosphates are the primary intracellular regulatory mechanism, while the Bicarbonate-carbonic acid system is the primary extracellular regulatory system. In the absence of coexisting disease, preoperative acid-base alterations are unusual. Postoperative manipulations, including volume depletion or nasal gastric suction, can result in significant acid-base abnormalities. Associated hyperaldosteronism results in renal hydrogen ion secretion, making metabolic alkalosis the norm. Obtaining an arterial pH and referring to specific nomograms (Fig. 21-1) aids in making a specific diagnosis and calculation of specific defects or excess. The primary therapy for acid-base disturbances should be guided by the primary etiology and, unless alterations are severe, replacement or correction may be undertaken slowly.

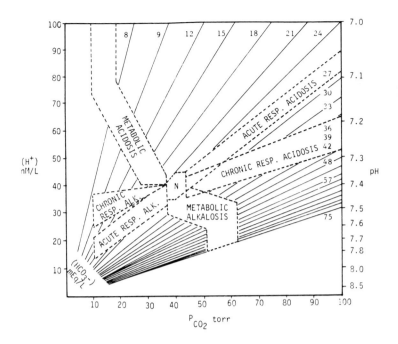

Fig. 21-1 Values for pH, PCO_2, and HCO_3 are plotted. The point at which any two values intersect is then evaluated in relationship to the appropriate areas that represent the confidence limits, as determined by review of the literature, for the predicted response of a group of persons to a given preturbation in PCO_2 (respiratory disturbances) or HCO_3 (metabolic disturbances). If a value falls outside a denoted area, a mixed disturbance is likely. HCO_3 values from the directly measured pH and PCO_2 can be calculated. (Modified from Golberg M: Computer based instruction and diagnosis of acid-based disorders. JAMA 223:269, 1973. Copyright 1973, American Medical Association.)

BUFFER SYSTEMS

Plasma
  Inorganic phosphate
  Bicarbonate
  Plasma protein

Red Cell
  Hemoglobin
  Oxyhemoglobin
  Inorganic phosphate
  Bicarbonate

Replacement Fluids

In the usual postoperative state, fluid losses for a 70-kg woman vary between 2,000 to 2,500 ml/day. At least 800 ml/day urine production is required for solute excretion, maintaining a urine osmolality of <1,400 mOsm. Insensible pulmonary losses approach 800 ml/day; insensible losses from perspiration, which is sodium free, and GI losses average 300 ml/day. An additional 400 to 600 ml is usually required to replace other losses, such as those that occur related to temperature elevation. These later losses increase 10 percent for each 1°F increase in body temperature. In individual circumstances, losses from other sources (Table 21-3) may be excessive and require replacement.

Postoperative replacement of electrolytes and calories is also necessary. Under optimal conditions, the normal kidney can excrete less than 10 mEq sodium per day, while potassium excretion averages 15 to 20 mEq/day. These minimal requirements exist; however, additional electrolyte losses occur, and at least 75 to 100 mEq sodium and 40 to 60 mEq potassium is usually replaced daily. In general, potassium concentrations of greater than 40 mEq/L are avoided in an attempt to minimize patient discomfort. In the postoperative catabolic state, 100 g dextrose is administered daily in an effort to avoid ketosis.

Currently, a number of parenteral replacement or maintenance fluids are available (Table 21-4). However, reliance on any formula or single clinical sign to determine the adequacy of volume and electrolyte replacement is fraught with problems. Any effective postoperative plan for fluid administration must begin early and be altered to detect and correct preoperative deviations from normal fluid or electrolyte

Table 21-3 Potential Fluid Losses

		Cation		Anion	
Type	Volume (ml/24 hr)	Na (mEq/L)	K (mEq/L)	Cl (mEq/L)	HCO₃ (mEq/L)
Saliva	1,500 (500–2,000)	10 (5–10)	26 (10–30)	10 (5–15)	30 (25–30)
Stomach	1,500 (100–4,000)	60 (10–100)	10 (0–30)	130 (8–150)	—
Pancreas	400 (100–800)	140 (113–185)	5 (3–10)	75 (50–90)	115 (95–115)
Bile	300 (50–800)	145 (130–160)	5 (3–12)	100 (90–180)	35 (30–40)
Small intestine	2,000 (1,000–3,000)	140 (80–150)	5 (2–8)	104 (90–110)	30 (30–40)
Colon	—	60	30	40	—
Lymphadenectomy drainage	300 (100–7,000)	135	4.0	107	—

Table 21-4 Composition of Parenteral Fluids (mEq/l)

	Cation					Anion		
Solution	Na	K	Ca	Mq	NH₄	Cl	HCO₃⁻	HPO₄³⁻
Extracellular fluid	142	4	5	3	0.3	103	27	3
Ringer's lactated solution	130	4	2.7			109	28ᵃ	
0.9% sodium chloride (normal saline)	154					154		
0.45% sodium chloride (half-normal saline)	77					77		
M/6 sodium lactate	167						167ᵃ	
M (molar) sodium lactate	1,000						1,000ᵃ	
3% sodium chloride	513					513		
5% sodium chloride	855					855		
0.9% ammonium chloride					168	168		

ᵃ Lactate in solution is converted to bicarbonate.

balance profiles. Existing volume deficits may be isotonic (loss of equal sodium and water), hypertonic (loss of water in excess of electrolytes), or hypotonic (loss of electrolytes in excess of water). Prediction of individiual deficits should be made before replacement and correction should proceed as clinically indicated. In general, one-half the indicated deficit is replaced; the parameters are remeasured and deficits recalculated. Once deficits have been replaced, maintenance fluids plus ongoing losses should be monitored and replaced with the appropriate parenteral fluids. Any drain or suction output should be measured, as replacement may be necessary. Following pelvic lymphadenectomy, closed suction drainage losses may approach 7,000 ml during the first postoperative week. While average losses are less, women with excessive output or with associated medical illness may experience significant hemodynamic alterations.

Neuroendocrine-Metabolic Response

The complex physiologic response to anesthesia and surgical procedures is a result of neuroendocrine and metabolic changes modulated by individual end-organ response. Primary (initiated by the injury) or secondary (initiated by pain in response to the injury) stimuli may affect these responses. Hypovolemia, related to preoperative deficits, blood loss, or extracellular fluid sequestration, is a most important primary stimulus. Atrail stretch receptors sense the volume of venous return, and aortic or carotid stretch receptors sense cardiac output. Nervous projections from the receptors to the brain stem and hypothalamus are vital in the initiation of specific neural and hormonal functions intended to maintain or protect volume status. Pain, another primary stimulus, may have local effects by releasing kinins, histamines, and prostaglandins. Opioid transmitters may mediate central effects. Hypoxia, sensed by chemoreceptors in the carotid, aorta, and medulla and emotional factors regulated by the limbic system are also capable of contributing to the neuroendocrine response. These primary neuroendocrine and metabolic responses can also be moderated by secondary stimuli. Temperature changes (sensed in the preoptic area), serum glucose levels (detected in the hypothalamus), and blood-volume restitution are thought to be important secondary stimuli. Additional factors, including analgesics, volume administration, and sepsis, are capable of altering the final response.

The neuroendocrine response involves an interaction among vasopressin, ACTH, growth hormone, prolactin, thyroid-stimulating hormone (TSH), and gonadotropins. End-organ effects can be correlated to altered levels of cortisol, aldosterone, thyroxine, catecholamines, glucagon, insulin, and renin.

Classically, three distinct phases of recovery have been defined. After injury by accident or surgical design, an initial ebb phase is followed by a flow of vitality and finally by an anabolic phase. The initial homeostatic response during the ebb phase, which usually lasts less than 36 hours, is related to the internal priority of maintaining adequate circulatory volume. Sympathetic stimulation, with its hemodynamic alterations as well as metabolic expression, predominates. Altered tissue perfusion and impaired thermoregulation result in reduced heat production and a reduced respiratory quotient. Hyperglycemia, secondary to cortisol-, epinephrine-, and glucagon-induced glycogenolysis is common. Hepatic glycogen stores are small, and muscle glycogen cannot be converted to glucose because of the lack of the enzyme glucose VI phosphatase in muscle. Renal blood flow, which may be reduced by one-half of nonoperative perfusion levels results in transient hyperaldosteronism and elevated angiotensin II levels. Aldosterone promotes sodium absorption in exchange for potassium and hydrogen ions in the renal distal tubule. This phenomena of acid urine excretion contributes to the normal postoperative metabolic alkalemia and is related in part to the intracellular movement of potassium and hydrogen ion.

The flow phase is characterized by catabolism and heat production and the body's attempt to provide energy. Energy requirements parallel the extent of injury and may be 10 to 50 percent greater than the normal resting metabolic needs. Temperature elevation may increase these needs dramatically. Initial energy needs are met by hepatic glycogen stores, which are depleted within 24 to 48 hours. Gluconeogenesis, predominantly in the liver and kidney, results from protein degradation. Although all endogenous proteins, including liver polypeptides, digestive enzymes, and albumin, are used, skeletal muscle is the chief contributor. Alanine and glutamine serve as the primary substrates. Transamination results in urinary nitrogen losses, which approach 10 g/day. In the nonstressed patient, nitrogen losses are minimized. Metabolic alterations permit later energy needs to be met by fat oxidation, fatty acid release, formation of acetyl coenzyme A, and glycerol. In the postoperative patient, this adaptation does not occur, and hypercatabolism predominates. The administration of carbohydrate alone has only a minor protein-sparing effect.

The anabolic phase is characterized by restoration of depleted protein. At this time, continued bed rest may be detrimental, as it increases nitrogen losses and increases excretion of calcium, which may predispose the patient to the development of osteoporosis.

End-Organ Response

In response to neuroendocrine and metabolic alteration, individual organs undergo profound functional changes related to anesthesia and surgery.

PULMONARY

Postoperative pulmonary dysfunction occurs in as many as 80 percent of patients. Changes occur in lung volume, ventilatory pattern, gas exchange, and lung-defense mechanisms. Impaired oxygenation and elimination of carbon dioxide results from increased dead-space ventilation, loss of compliance, mismatch of ventilation and perfusion, and alteration in chest wall and diaphragm mechanics. Shallow breathing, absent sigh breaths, reduced surfactant and microatelectasis result in a progressive decrease in functional residual capacity to levels below closing volumes (Fig. 21-2). This leads to premature small airway and alveolar closure and gas trapping. Anesthetics and intubation result in desquamation of the respiratory epithelium, a decrease in mucus velocity and a reduced clearance of bacteria from airways. Atelectasis is associated with depressed phagocytic activity of alveolar macro-

phages. Lowered vital capacity, forced expiratory volume, and function residual volume occur frequently and contribute to postoperative hypoxemia. These alterations are maximal during the first 2 postoperative days and gradually improve over the ensuing week but may last longer. These pulmonary changes are greater after an upper abdominal incision are are influenced by postoperative pain, ileus, abdominal distention, and narcotics.

CARDIOVASCULAR

Induction of anesthesia stresses cardiovascular mechanics. Even at low concentration, inhalation anesthetics depress myocardial function. While the majority directly depress contactility, most anesthetics also modify neural control of vascular tone. This vasodilation can result in a drop in systemic blood pressure and myocardial perfusion. Avoiding intraoperative hypotension is important, as episodes of hypoperfusion measured as a 33 percent drop in blood pressure for a 10-minute interval is associated with a fivefold increase in cardiac deaths. Cellular function is also altered, as anesthesia decreases metabolic rate and oxygen consumption.

Anesthesia is arrhythmogenic, and the incidence of

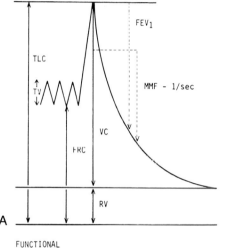

Fig. 21-2 Lung-pressure relationships **(A)** depict total lung capacity (TLC) when the lungs are fully expanded. Residual volume (RV) is the amount of gas in the lungs following maximal expiration. Vital capacity (VC), the volume between total lung capacity and residual volume, is determined by the balance of forces generated by respiratory muscles as well as lung and chest-wall mechanics. Dynamic measurement of airflow resistances may include forced expiratory volume in 1 second (FEV) or maximal mid-expiratory flow (MMF). Normal lung compliance **(B)** suggests that closing capacity (CC) of the airway is usually below the functional residual capacity. However, this relationship may be altered dramatically in either direction leading to premature airway closure and inefficient respiratory mechanics. (Modified from Craig DB: Postoperative recovery of pulmonary function. Anesth Analg 60:46, 1981. Reprinted with permission from IARS.)

MYOCARDIAL KINETICS

Oxygen demand increased
  Tachycardia
  Tachyarrhythmia
  Fever
  Hypothermia
  Volume Overload
  Shivering

Oxygen supply decreased
  Hypoxemia
  Anemia
  Bradycardia
  Hypotension
  Hypovolemia

intraoperative arrhythmias varies from 27 to 84 percent. Only about 5 percent are clinically important, with supraventricular dysrhythmias being most common. Appropriate monitoring, maintaining the appropriate depth of anesthesia and sympathetic blockade, and manipulating myocardial kinetics to maintain a favorable oxygen supply-and-demand ratio should decrease these risks.

Renal

Anesthetics predictively decrease renal blood flow by 30 to 70 percent of preanesthesia values. Smaller alterations occur in the glomerular filtration rate; however, direct or indirect (myocardial depression) may be responsible. Intraoperative urinary osmolality is increased secondary to vasopressin release. This lessened ability to handle free water is associated with less renal autoregulation.

Gastrointestinal

Altered GI function associated with anesthesia and surgery includes ileus, lessened hepatic perfusion, and stress-related bleeding. Specific methods of anesthesia may affect these alterations. Regional anesthesia has been reported to lessen the risk of postoperative ileus and favorably alter blood flow and healing. Regardless of methods, an empty GI tract is a prerequisite to a safe anesthetic, and preparation includes maintenance of a nil per os (NPO) status.

Hematologic

Anesthesia adversely affects the function of white blood cells (WBCs). Cell-mediated immunity as well as T- and B-cell levels are reduced by as much as 50 percent. Lymphocyte responsiveness and chemotactic activity are also decreased. Both phagocytic function and levels of antibody production are defective after major surgical procedures. Fibronectin, an α_2-surface glycoprotein that has an important role in the opsonic activity of the reticuloendothelial system, is also lowered following surgical procedures.

Anesthetics, perioperative drugs, and transfusions may reduce oxyhemoglobin affinity. Fortunately the tissue effect on oxygen supply is not generally clinically significant.

Central Nervous System

Cerebral blood flow is determined by the complex interaction of perivascular hydrogen ion concentration, the effects of local metabolites, serum osmolality, PCO_2, and PO_2 levels, and systemic blood pressure. Cerebral blood flow and cerebral metabolic rate may be altered by specific anesthetics. Typically, the hydrocarbons increase blood flow, decrease metabolic rate, and in effect increase intracranial pressure. While not usually deemed important during gynecologic surgery, these problems with altered cerebral blood flow or increased pressures assume more importance in older women, in those with vascular disease, or in those with proven or suspected cerebral metastatic disease.

Psychologic

The psychic stress of surgery, particularly when it relates to a cancer diagnosis, may be overwhelming and impede physical recovery. The woman undergoing cancer treatment may consider herself a burden and feel that she has lost control of her role in the family. The surgeon must relate the indications as well as the expectations for the operative procedure. Postoperative drains, intravenous lines, and intubations are better tolerated if their use and benefits are explained preoperatively. The physician must be sensitive to the patient's needs and realize that every interaction impacts on the patient-physician relationship. Even attitudes exhibited during morning rounds are important. The physician who sits, listens without interruption, and establishes a sense of privacy during bedside examinations is more likely to be received positively by the patient. Honesty in the discussion concerning the need for additional therapy and realistic projections concerning long-term prognosis and management are essential. Using justifiable optimism, the surgeon must establish and maintain a position as the patient's advocate and partner during perioperative care as well as during long-term management.

COMPLICATIONS

MORTALITY

Mortality, the ultimate surgical complication, is most commonly related to the patient's disease process (78 percent) but may be related to surgical (18 percent) or anesthetic management (3 percent). The overall risk of anesthetic or intraoperative death in any surgical procedure approaches 0.3 percent. Approximately 10 percent of anesthetic-related deaths occur during induction, and 85 percent of anesthetic deaths are due to some error in management. Hypoxia has an important role in approximately 50 percent of anesthetic deaths. Fatal anesthetic events occur intraoperatively in approximately 55 percent of patients and in the postoperative period in 35 percent of patients. In the former, risks are increased twofold during induction and sixfold with emergency procedures. In these latter instances, more than one-half of postoperative deaths occur after the patient leaves the recovery room. This latter fact suggests the need for continuing appropriate patient monitoring and consultation during the postoperative interval.

The major causes of intraoperative or postoperative death include cardiac arrest, pneumonia, sepsis, embolic phenomena, and renal failure. Individual patient risks are directly related to the nature and duration of the surgical illness, the extent of the underlying disease, patient age, the urgency of the surgical procedure, and the experience of the surgical team. Patient-related risks of surgical mortality can be correlated with the American Society of Anesthesiologists (ASA) physical status scale (Table 21-5).

The mortality rate per 1,000 population for simple procedures such as D & C is 0.1. This rate rises to 0.25 per 1,000 for hysterectomy and to 0.3 per 1,000 for ovariectomy. Radical hysterectomy carries a mortality risk of 3 per 1,000, while exenterative procedures have a mortality rate of 70 to 80 per 1,000.

Other potentially nonfatal surgical complications can be divided into those that occur intraoperatively and those that occur postoperatively. The latter may be further divided into early and late complications.

Intraoperative Complications

CARDIAC ARREST

Intraoperative cardiac arrest is a rare problem, with a reported incidence ranging between 1 in 3,444 to 1 in 825 operative procedures. However, 50 to 80 percent of these events are fatal, and cardiac areests account for approximately one-fifth of all anesthetic mortalities. The risk of death following a cardiac arrest correlates with the patient's ASA classification. Contrary to opinion, regional anesthetics are not necessarily associated with a decreased risk of this or other cardiovascular complications. In fact, in specific circumstances, the relative risk for cardiac arrest may be

Table 21-5 Mortality Associated with Physical Status

	ASA[a]				
	I	II	III	IV	V
48-hour mortality (%)					
Elective	0.07	0.24	1.4	7.5	8.1
Emergency	0.16	0.51	3.4	8.3	9.5
N = 68,388					
6-week mortality (%)					
Elective					
Low-Risk	0.03	0.31	1.9	5.6	20.0
Medium-Risk	0.02	1.7	7.2	17.2	31.4
High-Risk	2.2	5.4	14.6	20.5	42.4
N = 856,000					

[a] ASA status:
    I   Healthy
    II   Mild systemic disease
    III   Severe, but not incapacitating disease
    IV   Incapacitating disease
    V   Moribund
(Modified from Feigal DW, Blaisdell FW: The estimation of surgical risk. Med Clin North Am 63:1131, 1979. Reprinted with permission from WB Saunders Co.)

increased by as much as fourfold with regional anesthetics.

The risk of cardiac arrest during maintenance of anesthesia is probably equal to that during induction. Implicated mishaps include anesthetic overdose, airway mismanagement, inadequate volume replacement, or inadequate ventilation. There is no apparent correlation between risk and specific anesthetic agent or premedication. Most of these cardiac arrests occur during the extremes of life, with children and patients in their fifth decade at greatest risk. The latter risk is likely related to the effects of coexisting medical disease. Cardiac arrest during abdominal surgery is less frequently encountered than during thoracic surgery. Women with significant cardiac disease are at greater risk, and efforts to identify and methods to monitor cardiac function should be incorporated into the surgical plan. When identified, methods to enhance cardiac performance or to modify the operative procedure should be considered.

Essential intraoperative monitoring consists of an ECG monitor and frequent blood pressure recording. Noninvasive measurements of tissue oxygen levels, oxygen saturation, or invasive methods, including an arterial line or pulmonary artery catheter, should be considered for those patients with significant cardiac risk factors or in those women undergoing high-risk or lengthy procedures that might be associated with significant blood loss. This intensive monitoring allows for early detection and appropriate intervention in those clinical situations.

ARRHYTHMIA

Almost all anesthetics are arrhythmogenic, and intraoperative cardiac arrhythmias commonly occur. Approximately 30 percent occur during induction. This risk is highest during intubation, however, regional anesthetics do not consistently decrease these risks. The incidence is lowest (16.3 percent) in patients without preoperative arrhythmias and increases in patients with known preoperative arrhythmias (26.6 percent), as well as in patients with known cardiac disease (34.4 percent). Age, when corrected for preexisting heart disease, does not affect this risk. Fortunately, most arrhythmias are transient, and only 5 percent of intraoperative arrhythmias are considered clinically significant. However, if an arrhythmia occurs in a patient with heart disease, the risk of ventricular irritability and hemodynamic alteration may

approach 80 percent. While most require no specific therapy, the occurrence of hemodynamically compromising arrhythmias requires immediate attention and appropriate medical or electrical treatment. Therapy based on an understanding of physiologic mechanisms should be instituted after an accurate ECG diagnosis, with an awareness of the sympathetic dominance present. Any contributing clinical factor, such as hypoxia, hypercapnia, pain, hypovolemia, or electrolyte abnormality, should be identified and corrected. In general, patients requiring antiarrhythmic therapy should continue their medication without interruption. Administration of a morning preoperative dose should be considered.

With the exception of those patients with documented paroxysmal arrhythmias or those with coronary artery disease and complex ectopy, perioperative antiarrhythmic prophylaxis is rarely indicated. Patients with accepted indications for cardiac pacing require appropriate preoperative evaluation and intervention. Asymptomatic patients with bifascicular conduction disease do not require pacing unless the need of a pulmonary artery catheter is contemplated.

HEMORRHAGE

Intraoperative hemorrhage requiring transfusion occurs in as many as 8 percent of patients undergoing vaginal hysterectomy and in approximately 15 percent of patients after abdominal hysterectomy. Blood loss during radical hysterectomy averages 1,500 ml and approaches 3,000 ml following exenterative or ultraradical procedures. The physician must realize that the actual measurement of suction losses is inaccurate, as 15 to 42 percent of intraoperative blood losses are immeasurably lost on gowns and drapes. In addition, 38 percent of women enter radical surgical procedures with significant intravascular volume deficits and are at increased risk to require intraoperative resuscitation. Intraoperative monitoring of vital signs and urine production may be sufficient to ensure the maintenance of adequate intravascular volume and avoid hypotension. In most situations, the measurement of hemoglobin and hematocrit serves little purpose, as changes in these parameters generally require time. Specific values prior to vascular equilibration may be falsely assuring and may not reflect acute blood loss. Other methods of monitoring vascular volumes may be necessary during lengthy operative procedures, those procedures with a risk of sudden massive blood loss, surgery in those with coexisting disease, or in situations such as urinary diversion that do not permit surveillance of the usual clinical parameters. Pulmonary artery catheters or other invasive methods to measure vascular volume, filling pressures, or related cardiac function may be necessary. These methods permit early detection of volume deficits or cardiac dysfunction and guide medical intervention or resuscitation.

Any surgical procedure can be associated with significant clinical blood loss. Technical factors including inadequate exposure or improper isolation and ligation of tissue pedicles make up the majority of problems. Only on occasion is an intraoperative bleeding problem related to a coagulopathy. This problem may be unavoidable, but anatomic awareness and dissection of the retroperitoneal spaces often permit proper exposure, vascular ligation, and control of the hemorrhage even in the most difficult situations. Pelvic oozing may require hypogastric artery ligation. This procedure effectively converts arterial pressures to venous pressures and often controls serious bleeding. Potential injury to the ureter and adjacent vascular structures can be avoided with careful surgical technique. Laceration of major abdominal or pelvic vessels is less common but serious. Vascular repair requires specific training and special instrumentation. Acute control can be accomplished with pressure; however, vessel repair should not be delayed.

Repair of a major arterial injury requires isolation of the involved segment and maintenance of the distal arterial circulation, which may require systemic anticoagulation. Coexisting venous injuries should be repaired first to establish improved outflow. The goal of arterial reconstruction with primary reanastamosis, lateral repair, repair with angioplasty, or graft replacement is to restore flow without narrowing the vessel lumen. Direct suture repair of most venous injuries is generally the method of choice. The fragility of the venous walls makes repair hazardous, and partial occlusion clamps may be necessary.

Clotting abnormalities, drug-induced platelet aggregation defects, or congenital deficits of specific clotting factors are rarely the cause of intraoperative or postoperative bleeding. Fortunately, these conditions are rare, and the vast majority (99 percent) of these abnormalities can be detected by history and physical or preoperative laboratory screening. Drug-induced platelet abnormalities may persist for 7 to 10 days and drug cessation. Elective delay of surgery may

be prudent. Consumptive coagulopathies rarely occur after a single volume transfusion, as clotting elements are only reduced to 75 percent of normal levels. However, clinical bleeding does occur after a two-volume blood transfusion, reducing clotting elements to only 10 percent of original levels.

Unless unusual circumstances exist, blood replacement is rarely necessary until losses exceed 1,000 ml. However, hemodynamic changes can occur earlier with lesser losses, and the decision to transfuse must be individualized. Patients capable of doubling their cardiac output can tolerate removal of 20 percent of their blood volume without demonstrable hemodynamic or tissue effects. Earlier blood replacement may be required if the preoperative hemoglobin is low or if associated medical disease necessitates an increase in oxygen-carrying capacity. In general, hemoglobin levels of 10 g/d provide adequate tissue levels of oxygen for normal metabolic requirements. Ventricular function stabilizes, and coronary blood flow is maximal with hematocrits of 32 percent. Lower levels of hemoglobin may be associated with abnormal distribution of blood flow and subendocardial ischemia.

Blood-component therapy (Table 21-6) permits specific replacement and is considered the appropriate method of transfusion therapy. Stored whole blood rapidly loses specific coagulation factor activity, has altered levels of 2,3-DPG, and is associated with reduced red blood cell (RBC) survival. Crystalloid solutions are added as needed for volume expansion. The use of blood substitutes, such as Fluosol, has not yet been clinically successful. Crystalloid infusion offers immediate intravascular volume resuscitation; however, later equilibration occurs in a 3:1 ratio of extravascular and intravascular distribution. In these situations, peripheral edema may occur in the absence of normal vascular volumes.

In urgent circumstances, colloid or other protein administration may allow for more rapid intravascular resuscitation. Its use is more expensive, impairs cardiopulmonary function, reduces the levels of nonalbumin proteins, and decreases the activity of nonalbumin proteins, including immunoglobulins and coagulants. High-molecular-weight Dextran or solutions such as Heta Starch may be used for rapid vascular resusitation.

In general, most gynecologic procedures do not require that cross-matched blood be available. A blood type and screen that facilitates recognition of the presence of specific or unusual antibodies will usually suf-

Table 21-6 Blood-Component Therapy

Component	Approximate Volume (ml)	Indication	Risk	Comment
Whole blood[a]	500	Acute replacement of massive losses	Hepatitis; allergenic proteins, volume overload	Hematocrit of 39%
Packed red blood cells[b]	250	Hemoglobin elevation	Hepatitis	Hematocrit of 75%; increase patient hematocrit by 3–4%/unit; fewer febrile reactions than whole blood
Platelet concentrate	50	Thrombocytopenia	Hepatitis Rh isoimmunization	Increase platelet count by 7,500/units; may not benefit those with immune thrombocytopenia
Cryoprecipatate	40	Hemophilia A vonWillebrands Hypofibrinogenemia	Hepatitis	Increase fibrinogen level by 10 mg/dl/unit; concentrated source of I, V, VIII, XIII; concentrated fibronectin
Fresh-frozen plasma	200	Volume expansion	Hepatitis	Contains most clotting factors, but not concentrated
Serum albumin	250	Volume expansion		Available in 5% or 25% solution; minimal risk of hepatitis

[a] Stored whole blood has a diminished post-transfusion red blood cell survival, diminished platelet viability and diminished levels of factors V and VIII.

[b] Leukocyte—poor red blood cells may benefit who have repeated nonhemolytic febrile transfusion reactions. Washed red blood cells may be necessary in patients known to develop anaphylactic or severe allergic reactions to plasma components of blood.

fice, as type-specific blood can be crossed rapidly and is readily available. In radical or ultraradical procedures, where average blood loss exceeds 1,000 ml, the prudent surgeon will have blood available.

INJURY

Although rare, intraoperative injury to the GI or urinary tract occurs, and the incidence can be correlated to the indications for the primary procedure. Gastrointestinal injury occurs in approximately 0.40 percent of gynecologic procedures performed for benign indication; however, this incidence may approach 30 percent in surgical efforts designed to resect ovarian cancer. Careful opening of the abdominal incision, adequate exposure, and sharp dissection of intraabdominal adhesions are all methods designed to minimize this risk.

Small intestinal laceration injury is associated with a low level of bacterial contamination (Table 21-7), and a layered primary repair can usually be performed. Sutures placed in an axis perpendicular to the laceration decrease the risk of stenosis. Following radiation therapy, small bowel injury, particularly in the terminal ileum, may require a more extensive procedure, as blood supply is altered and healing adversely affected. In those instances, resection of the injured bowel with

Table 21-7 Bacterial Flora

Site	Number	Comment
Stomach	$0-10^4$	Gram-positive cocci and *Lactobacillus* (anaerobes rare)
Duodenum	$0-10^4$	Gram-positive cocci and *enterococcus* (anaerobes rare)
Jejunum	$0-10^4$	G-positive cocci (anaerobes rare)
Ileum	$1 \times 10^{4-5}$	Aerobes plus anaerobes coliforms, *Bacteroides, Clostridium* (aerobic cocci rare)
Colon	$10^{10}-10^{11}$	90% anaerobes; 10% aerobes and facultative bacteria
Vagina	10^9	90% anaerobes; 10% aerobes and facultative bacteria

an ileoascending colostomy to promote new blood supply may be appropriate. Decreasing intraabdominal contamination with irrigation or administering parenteral antibiotics are two methods used to combat potential infection.

Large intestinal injury results in higher levels of bacterial contamination that potentially interfere with healing. In the absence of preoperative mechanical bowel preparation, diversion of the fecal stream proximal to the repair may be necessary. Broad-spectrum parenteral antibiotic coverage and irrigation should decrease the risk of infection. Antibiotic irrigation may benefit those patients with massive intraabdominal contamination. Previous radiation therapy significantly alters intestinal healing, and primary repair or reanastomosis in heavily irradiated bowel is fraught with the risk of anastomotic breakdown, fistula formation, and poor healing. Anastomotic blood supply can be improved by incorporating nonirradiated bowel into the anastamosis or by a wrap with an omentum flap.

The stapling devices can be incorporated into almost any GI procedure; their use is associated with a significant saving of operative time and decreased operative contamination. Staples have no adverse effect on healing and improve anastomotic blood supply.

Those patients undergoing a GI operation often have a preexisting nutritional deficit or will be exposed to long postoperative intervals of inadequate caloric intake. Some women with a borderline or abnormal nutritional status may benefit from the addition of parenteral or enteral hyperalimentation. These therapies should be strongly considered and instituted

early in those situations in order to decrease operative risks.

The prophylactic use of nasal intubation of the GI tract following routine gynecologic procedures or repair is unnecessary. Only 6 to 8 percent of these patients benefit from GI suction; the remainder are subjected to discomfort with little benefit in terms of intestinal ileus or early return of bowel function.

The true incidence of urinary injury is probably unknown, as many silent injuries may go unnoticed. However, urinary tract injury is reported to occur in as many as 1.4 percent of patients undergoing vaginal hysterectomy. Bladder injury is most common; however, ureteral injury occurs in 0.2 percent of women undergoing operative procedures for benign gynecologic conditions. This figure increases dramatically in procedures performed for malignant disease. Ureteral injury occurs in 1 to 7 percent of patients undergoing radical hysterectomy, and 2 percent of patients undergoing ovarian debulking procedures require urinary resection. Adequate exposure and sharp dissection should reduce the incidence of bladder injury. Ureteral injury is less likely if the retroperitoneal spaces are dissected and the ureters visualized. Attention to the relationship of the ureters to the infundibulopelvic ligament, uterine artery, and the lateral vagina should reduce the risk of injury.

Recognition of urinary tract injury is of particular importance, as repair and appropriate drainage are usually associated with good results. The installation of sterile milk or some other marker will determine the presence and distinguish the site of injury without staining the surrounding tissues. Most of the bladder (80 percent) can be resected and repaired, with resultant normal function. Avoiding the placement of intravesical suture, a watertight repair and postoperative drainage are the standard. Urinary injury and coexistence of a urinary tract infection mandate appropriate antibiotic. Tolerance doses of radiation increase the risk of poor healing. Repair of a bladder injury in this situation might include prophylactic attempts to transport new pelvic blood supply (omental wrap). Longer bladder drainage seems prudent.

Ureteral injuries may result from devascularization, ligation, crushing, or incisional injury. Devascularization injuries may not become clinically evident until 7 to 10 days postoperatively. When ureteral dissection is necessary, an effort should be made to avoid interference with its longitudinal vascular supply. Ligation or crush injuries require recognition and attention. Immediate deligation or unclamping the ureter avoids the necessity to resect the injured segment in 66 percent of patients. If persistent blanching occurs or ureteral peristasis does not cross the injured site, resection, reanastomosis, or reimplantation are necessary. If the ureteral injury occurs in the distal one-third, reimplantation with bladder mobilization via a psoas hitch or Boari flap is usually performed. Transvesical ureteroureterostomy or transureteral ureterostomy is a procedure of choice, if the injury is higher.

Percutaneous nephrostomy drainage or the placement of transvesical ureteral stents permits nonoperative salvage of remaining renal function or potential diversion following the late recognition of a ureteral ligation or injury. Later internalization of these stents can be sucessfully performed, completely avoiding the need for an open surgical procedure.

Intraoperative neurologic injury to the sciatic or femoral nerve can occur as a result of retractor trauma. Using stirrups or other surgical positions (frog's leg) may be associated with sciatic stretch injury or peroneal nerve injury. Although pressure nerve injury may not be apparent until convalescence, attention to the retractor placement can avoid pressure on the psoas muscle and the retroperitoneal nerves. Stirrup placement must be inspected prior to draping so as to minimize pressure, particularly on the lateral tibial area near the peroneal nerve. Fortunately, most stretch- or pressure-related problems resolve with time.

Intraoperative crush or laceration nerve injuries most commonly occur to the genitofemoral (L1, L2) or obturator (L2, L3, L4) nerve. Injury to the genitofemoral nerve results during pelvic lymphadenectomy, as the nerve is situated parallel to the lateral external iliac nodal chain. This injury results in anesthesias and paresthesias over the mons pubis and ipsilateral anterior medial thigh. Careful dissection of the obturator space decreases the risk of nerve injury. Loss of obturator nerve function results in an inability to adduct the ipsilateral lower limb. This loss can usually be compensated for by other adductor muscles.

Postoperative Complications

ARREST

Alterations in pulmonary physiology predispose the lungs to numerous complications. Ventilation-perfusion abnormalities affect pulmonary closing pressures (Fig. 21-2) and increase the risk of postoperative atelectasis. Patients with obstructive pulmonary disease are at greater risk than those with restrictive pulmonary disease for the development of pulmonary complications. Even with these predisposing factors, diligent preoperative preparation and postoperative care can decrease the rate of pulmonary complica-

Table 21-8 Respiratory Insufficiency

Mechanics	Normal	Insufficiency
Respiratory rate (min)	12–20	>35
Tidal volume (cc/kg)	6	<3
Vital capacity (cc/kg)	70	<15
Inspiratory force (cmH$_2$O)	20–40	<20
Ventilation		
PaCO$_2$ (mmHg)	35–45	>55
Physiologic deadspace (V$_D$/V$_T$)	0.4	>0.6
Oxygenation		
PaO$_2$ (mmHg)	60–95	<100 on F$_I$O$_2$ = 100
A-aO$_2$ (mmHg)	5–15	>450 on F$_I$O$_2$ = 100
Pulmonary shunt (%) (QS/QT)	5–6	30
Perfusion		
Cardiac index	3.0 ± 0.5	<2
Mixed venous oxygen (mmHg)	40	<30

(Modified from Hammond GL: Acute respiratory failure. Surg Clin North Am 60:1133, 1980. Reprinted with permission from WB Saunders Co.)

tions. Postoperative respiratory care must emphasize sustained maximum inspiration to increase alveolar inflation and maintain a near-normal functional residual capacity. Intermittent positive-pressure breathing, blow bottles, and endotracheal stimulation are only variably effective and may be harmful. Incentive spirometry is the most effective postoperative maneuver to decrease the risk of atelectasis. Once inflated, alveoli tend to remain open for at least 1 hour; consequently, any effective pulmonary maneuver should be scheduled on an hourly basis during the patient's waking hours.

Postoperative pulmonary infection occurs in approximately 0.4 percent of patients undergoing total hysterectomy for benign indications. This incidence is 2 percent after radical hysterectomy, 3 percent after exenteration, and 3 percent after ovarian debulking procedures. These risks are increased in the immunocompromised patient (malignancy, malnutrition) and in those patients undergoing long (more than 3 hours) operative procedures. Prophylactic antibiotics are not effective in decreasing these risks. However, postoperative ambulation combined with deep inspiration may decrease these risks. If pneumonia occurs, unusual organisms may be responsible, and broad-spectrum antibiotic coverage should be considered in the immunocompromised patient.

In the absence of preexisting disease or coexisting complication, respiratory insufficiency (Table 21-8) is a rare complication following nonradical surgical procedures. However, this is not true of longer procedures requiring high-volume blood replacement or ultraradical procedures whereby postoperative respi-

ratory compromise may complicate recovery in 25 percent of patients. Preoperative risk factors have been defined, and appropriate intervention can successfully alter these risks. Specific preoperative testing (Table 21-9) can determine the likelihood of postoperative pulmonary complications and should be performed in those patients deemed at risk by history and physical examination. Abnormal studies should prompt either appropriate consultation or modification of the surgical plan, or both. Specific methods of intervention may decrease these risks.

METHODS TO DECREASE PULMONARY RISK

Stop smoking (> 2 weeks)

Antibiotic treatment of pulmonary infection or chronic bronchitis

Bronchodilators for those with spasm

Preoperative psychological preparation and teaching of required respiratory maneuvers

Minimize anesthesia time

Maintain nutritional status

Maximize postoperative inspiration, ambulation

Maintain adequate but not excessive analgesia

(Modified from Harmon E, Lillington G: Pulmonary risk factors in surgery. Med. Clin North Am 63:1289, 1979.

Table 21-9 Tests Predicting Increased Risk of Pulmonary Complications

Study	Abnormality
Maximum breathing capacity	<50% of predicted
Preoperative forced expiratory volume (1 second)	<2.0 L
Predicted postoperative forced expiratory volume (1 second)	<0.8 L
$PaCO_2$	>50 mmHg
Electrocardiogram	Abnormal
Pulmonary wedge pressures	>30 mmHg

(Modified from Harmon E, Lillington G: Pulmonary risk factors in surgery. Med Clin North Am 63:1289, 1979. Reprinted with permission from WB Saunders Co.)

Postoperative deep venous thrombosis or pulmonary thromboembolism remains a significant problems following gynecologic surgery. Depending on the methods of detection (Table 21-10), and the risk of the population, it occurs as frequently as 29 to 50 percent (Table 21-11). Clinically, thrombosis above the popliteal is more likely to result in thromboembolus, and fibrinogen scan (nonclinical) detected calf thromboses will extend proximally in approximately 20 percent of patients. Thrombus in the proximal deep venous system is of serious clinical significance, as one-half of these women may develop pulmonary embolic phenomena. Detection is important, as untreated women with pulmonary thromboembolism

Table 21-10 Venous Thrombosis: Methods of Detection

Method	Comment
Clinical	Insensitive and inaccurate unless clinical symptoms are present: Treatment based only on the clinical diagnosis should rarely be undertaken.
Venography	Reference method for diagnosis, but limited visualization of abdominal venous system: Pain, phlebitis, and hypersensitivity reactions can occur.
^{125}I fibrinogen scanning	Sensitive and specific screening test for new clot in distal extremity: Diagnostic delay of 72 hours and insensitivity to proximal vein thrombosis limit its diagnostic value.
Plethysmography	Not sensitive for nonocclusive thrombi: Study is altered by other conditions (i.e., compression) that alter venous flow. It is sensitive in clinically suspicious cases.
Doppler ultrasound	Sensitive and accurate for the diagnosis of proximal vein thrombosis: This potentially versatile test requires subjective expertise.

(Modified from Farquharson DIM, Orr JW Jr: Prophylaxis against thromboembolism in gynecologic patients. J Reprod Med 29:845, 1984.)

Table 21-11 Risk Factors for the Development of Venous Thrombosis

Risk	Example	Thrombosis % Calf	Thrombosis % Proximal	Fatal Embolism
Low	Minor surgery			
	20-year-old	0.8	<1	<0.02
	40-year-old	2.9		
Moderate	Minor surgery			
	60-year-old	9.1		
	Major surgery			
	40-year-old	6.3	2–8	0.1–0.7
	60-year-old	18.3		
	>60-year-old	36.4		
High	Major surgery			
	40-year old with other risk factors[a]	40–80	10–20	1–5

[a] Approximate increased risk for those women with varicose veins (3X), previous DVT (4X), infection (2X), cancer (4X), estrogens (7X), obesity (2X), operative time of greater than 3 hours (2X).

(Modified from Farquharson DIM, Orr JW Jr: Prophylaxis against thromboembolism in gynecologic patients. J Reprod Med 29:845, 1984.

have a 40 percent chance of recurrence and at least a 20 percent mortality. The initial event may not be fata, but 75 percent of patients who die as a result of pulmonary thromboembolism have evidence of a recent prior embolus. Although common during hospitalization, as many as 50 percent of pulmonary emboli occur after initial discharge.

The risk of thrombogenesis is governed by Virchow's triad of altered blood flow, blood coagulation, and intimal damage. The latter commonly occurs during pelvic operations for malignancy. The usual intimal protection against thrombosis may be related to the effects of electrostatic repulsion, secretion of fibronectin, local production of prostacyclin, plasminogen activator, or heparinoids. Damage to endothelium that occurs during retroperitoneal or nodal dissection results in the exposure of collagen microfibrils and basement membranes, increases local coagulability, and predisposes the patient to thrombogenesis.

Vascular or venous stasis occurs with regional or general anesthesia, and 50 percent of postoperative deep venous thrombosis develops within 24 hours of surgery. The major risk of stasis begins at the time of induction and, to be effective, any method designed to prevent thrombosis or emboli should be incorporated prior to that time. Methods of prophylaxis have included minidose heparin, dextran, venoconstrictors, and various physical methods. Although minidose heparin has been proclaimed as the prophylactic method to decrease thrombosis, its efficacy in the prevention of emboli following gynecologic surgery has not been documented. However, its use during radical gynecologic procedures has been associated with an increased risk of bleeding and lymphocyst formation. Pneumatic calf compression appears to be a promising effective method of prophylaxis. Compression stockings are intermittently inflated to 40 to 60 mm Hg, resulting in a twofold increase in venous blood velocity and increase in systemic fibrinolytic activity. Prospective and retrospective reports indicate its benefit and suggest the need to continue use of these stockings for at least 3 postoperative days. Although cumbersome, these stockings are tolerated well, and this physical method is of equal or superior benefit as subcutaneous minidose heparin, without subjecting the patient to potential risks. Until information to the contrary exists, the use of a low-morbidity physical method of prophylaxis should be recommended routinely. Other prophylactic methods such as dextran, dihydroergotamine, and coumadin therapy remain of uncertain benefit in the gynecologic patient.

Most postoperative pulmonary emboli probably go unrecognized; however, clinical suspicion mandates evaluation. The clinical diagnosis of emboli with systemic anticoagulation is unacceptable, as it may be associated with a risk of bleeding as high as 25 percent. In some situations (CNS bleeding), the mortality rate of heparin-associated bleeding approaches 50 percent. In fact, heparin is the leading cause of drug-related deaths in an otherwise healthy population. For this reason, a pulmonary evaluation is recommended prior to anticoagulation. If the ventilation-perfusion scan is normal, no additional evaluation is necessary. However, 14 percent, 63 percent, 86 percent, and 18 percent of patients will have angiographic demonstration of pulmonary with low, moderate, high, or indeterminate probability scans. The scan will alert the angiographer to the most suspicious area, and the study will require the injection of less dye. The importance of documentation becomes most important if symptoms persist after anticoagulation, and a caval filter or interruption is required.

CARDIOVASCULAR

Cardiovascular complications can occur following benign gynecologic procedures; however, cardiovascular disease is a common coexisting medical illness, often complicating cancer surgery. Although patients with heart disease generally tolerate surgery, associated complications can be life-threatening. Recognition of cardiovascular problems and alteration of the medical management or the surgical plan can decrease these risks.

Preexisting cardiac disease poses an eightfold increase in the risk of postoperative myocardial infarction. Temporal relationship is important, as patients undergoing surgical procedures within 3 months of a previous infarction have a 37 percent risk of reinfarction. If surgery is delayed from 3 to 6 months, this risk falls to 16 percent and, if delayed to 6 months, this risk falls to 4.7 percent. Subsequent risk decreases little with further delay. Unless emergent, surgery should be delayed, as mortality rates for a postoperative reinfarction approaches 70 percent. At least three recent reports suggest that patients undergoing recent successful coronary artery bypass grafting are not at increased risk of cardiovascular complications.

The risk of cardiac death is 5 to 20-fold increased in women with any sign or symptoms of heart disease; Goldman and co-workers (1982) determined the major cardiac risk factors associated with postoperative cardiovascular morbidity (Table 21-12). In addition, noncardiac factors, including abdominal surgery and procedures lasting longer than 3 hours, increase the risk of postoperative cardiac morbidity. Using this index (Table 21-13), the risk of life-threatening or cardiac death may be predicted. Although overall cardiovascular risks can be calculated, variables not associated with postoperative cardiac complications include hyperlipidemia, smoking, diabetes, hypertension, atherosclerotic vascular disease, and mitral valve disease. In addition ECG stress testing is not reliably predictive of cardiovascular morbidity.

Development of postoperative pulmonary edema is ominous, with mortality rates approaching 45 percent. These risks are increased in older patients with perioperative ventricular dysfunction, an abnormal ECG, and valvular disease. A history of stable angina

Table 21-12 Cardiovascular Risk Factors

Criteria	Points
History	
Age >70 years	5
Recent MI (≤6 months)	10
Examination	
S3 gallop or jugular venous distention	11
Aortic stenosis	3
Electrocardiogram	
Nonsinus rhythm (excluding PACs)	7
>5 PVCs/min	7
General status	
$PaO_2 <60$; $PaCO_2 >50$	3
Serum $K^+ <3.0$	
Serum $HCO_3 <20$ mEq/l	
BUN >50; Cr >3.0 mEq/dl	
Chronic liver disease	
Patient bedridden	
Operation	
Abdominal, thoracic	3
Emergency	4

MI, myocardial infarction; PAC, premature atrial contractions; PVC, premature ventricular contractions.

(Modified from Goldman L: Cardiac risks and complications of noncardiac surgery. Ann Intern Med 98:504, 1983.)

or β-blocker therapy does not increase these risks. Preoperative ionotropic support with lanoxin should be considered in those patients with a previous history of pulmonary edema, signs or symptoms of ventricular dysfunction, the presence of nocturnal angina, atrial fibrillation with a rapid ventricular response, and frequent episodes of paroxysmal atrial or junctional tachycardia.

Patients with valvular disease or congenital defects are at increased risk of developing endocarditis. Most gynecologic procedures are clean contaminated, and antimicrobial prophylaxis consisting of a penicillin plus an aminoglycoside should be administered perioperatively. Those patients requiring anticoagulation for prosthetic values should have their oral anticoagulants discontinued 24 to 48 hours prior to their surgical procedure. Protection against thromboembolic phenomena can be accomplished with the administration of perioperative heparin. Under no circumstance should anticoagulation be completely reversed, as the risk of cardiac death in these situations is markedly increased.

Patients with hypertension may have other coexisting diseases. In their absence, diastolic pressure below 110 mm Hg is not associated with increased cardiovascular risks. In this group of patients, it is important that preoperative medications be continued to prevent rebound hypertensive effects.

While careful history, physical examination, and routine diagnostic studies may suffice in the usual gynecologic patient, those with abnormal findings and those who are older, obese, or undergoing radical surgical procedures often require additional studies. In fact, only 17 percent of patients undergoing radical gynecologic procedures are without associated medical problems.

The risk of postoperative cardiac death is increased 10-fold in patients over 70 years of age and, if reoperation is needed in the older woman, mortality rates approach 100 percent. These factors are becoming increasingly important, as almost 10 percent of the U.S. population is older than 65 years of age.

In one recent report, using intensive preoperative

Table 21-13 Cardiac Risk Index

Class (# patient)	Point Total	No or Minimal Complications (N = 943) (%)	Life-threatening Complication (N = 39) (%)	Cardiac Death (N = 19) (%)
I (537)	≤5	99	0.7	0.2
II (316)	6–12	93	5	2
III (130)	13–25	86	11	2
IV (18)	>26	22	22	56

(Modified from Goldman L, Caldera DL, Nussbaum SR et al: Multifactorial index of cardiac risk in noncardiac surgical procedures. N Engl J Med 297:845, 1977.)

evaluation, Babu (1980) found that only 33 percent of older (> 68 years) patients had normal left ventricular function. Volume deficits (preload) were present in 27 percent of cases, and vasodilatory agents (afterload reduction) were required in 13 percent of patients. Ionotropic support was required in 17 percent of patients, and the remainder had some form of combination therapy. Importantly, 93 percent of patients showed improved ventricular function and the delay (usually less than 3 days) had no apparent adverse effect on outcome.

Del Curcio and Cohn (1980) evaluated 148 elderly patients who were normal by standard evaluation. Intensive invasive evaluation indicated that only 13.5 percent of patients had a normal hemodynamic cardiovascular status. Twenty-two percent of these patients were severely compromised, and the remainder (63.5 percent) had mild to moderate deficits. Postoperative mortality risks paralleled these deficits. While no patient with a normal profile died, the mortality rate with mild to moderate abnormalities was 8.5 percent. All those patients with severe compromise who underwent the original planned surgical procedures died. These studies indicate the need for continuously monitoring and evaluating the cardiovascular status of older patients, as their associated medical illness predisposes them to numerous postoperative complications.

At least 50 percent of obese patients have associated medical problems and react to anesthesia with a more pronounced ventricular dysfunction. Decreased tidal capacity, lowered tidal volume, increased work of breathing coupled with long operative procedures, and increased blood loss in these cases results in a marked increase in perioperative cardiovascular and pulmonary morbidity and mortality.

In any of these patients, intraoperative attention to hypotension, perfusion, and cardiovascular performance is mandatory. Maintaining optimal myocardial kinetics in certain risk groups may necessitate invasive monitoring, including pulmonary artery catheters or other methods of monitoring oxygen delivery. Successful treatment during the postoperative period may require continued intensive monitoring to define problems accurately and permit continuous assessment and appropriate early intervention before physiologic reserves are exhausted. The intensity and duration of the initial and continued monitoring should be in proportion to the predictability of the patient's

convalescence. Most patients have a short, uneventful postoperative course, postoperative evaluation of cardiovascular status focuses on urine output, blood pressure, and hematocrit. Occasionally, a central venous pressure is measured. Unfortunately, these parameters may not predict the patient's clinical status if there is coexisting cardiovascular disease or serious illness. In fact, heart rate, mean arterial pressure, hematocrit, and central venous pressure are not early predictors of cardiovascular morbidity. These parameters become abnormal late in clinical management, making it less likely that early intervention will prove successful.

PATIENTS WHO MAY BENEFIT FROM INTENSIVE CARDIOVASCULAR MONITORING

Elderly

Obese

Cardiovascular disease

Pulmonary disease

Undergoing extensive or ultraradical surgical procedure

Critically ill patient who has failed initial clinical management

Requires positive-pressure ventilation

While healing is not directly influenced, the hematocrit should be stabilized at about 32 percent to maximize oxygen availability and ventricular function. A urine output of 30 ml/hr should be the minimal accepted volume, as outputs approaching 2 ml/kg/hr are to be expected if postoperative cardiovascular parameters are normalized.

Central venous pressures are less likely to be meaningful in patients with cardiovascular disease; optimal central monitoring in these patients requires insertion of a pulmonary artery catheter. Although routine use is not advocated, those with serious cardiovascular disease or those who fail to respond to initial clinical management are prime candidates. In these situations, the ability to define important cardiovascular parameters clinically is only 50 to 60 percent. Intraoperatively or postoperatively, patients with cardiovascular

Table 21-14 Complications of Pulmonary Artery Catheterization

Complication	Comment
Venous insertion injury	Risk decreased with increased experience; postinsertion chest radiograph to evaluate pneumothorax
Cardiac dysrhythmias	Rhythm monitored during insertion; rare hemodynamic instability
Infection	Careful attention to insertion site; minimize duration of use
Thrombotic endocardial vegetations	Minimize duration of use
Pulmonary parenchymatic damage	Constant monitoring to avoid continued wedge; postinsertion chest radiograph
Trauma to cardiac conduction system	Continuous monitoring to evaluate dysrhythmia
Mechanical knotting	
Balloon rupture	Avoidance of excessive wedging
Ventilator disconnect	Attention to details during measurements

disease may require large-volume crystalloid replacement. The resultant and peripheral edema makes clinical assessment difficult. In these situations, the catheter permits evaluation and appropriate intervention. Prior to insertion, it is important to recognize potential complications and methods to avoid them (Table 21-14).

In addition, patients with significant cardiovascular disease might benefit from serial electrocardiograms (ECG), as the risk for infarct and other cardiovascular problem is greatest during the first 7 postoperative days. During this time, serial ECGs should be obtained in high-risk patients, as 50 percent of postoperative infarctions are silent. Cardiac enzymes may be necessary.

Patients with New York Heart Association classification III or IV disease may benefit from coronary artery bypass surgery, and patients with significant aortic or mitral valvular heart disease may require valve replacement prior to abdominal surgery. The interval between procedures may be quite short without adversely affecting surgical outcome.

RENAL

Postoperatively, the kidneys perform a central role in maintaining body water, regulating electrolytes and acid-base balance, controlling pressure, and excreting metabolic wastes and drugs. These functions imply the importance of certain precautions in those patients with renal insufficiency. Maintenance of normal postoperative function remains important, as many of these women require additional therapy with potentially nephrotoxic drugs, such as antibiotics or antimitotic agents.

In general, the degree of reduction of glomerular filtration rate (GFR) rather than the type of renal disease is the most important factor in estimating surgical risk. Those patients with mild (GFR > 50 ml/min) or moderate (GFR > 25 < 50 ml/min) renal dysfunction require close attention to electrolyte, drug, and fluid therapy. Those with severe renal dysfunction (GFR < 10 ml/min) have often developed extrarenal manifestations, such as anemia, hypertension, and coagulation defects, and are at significant risk at the development of postoperative infection. In fact, patients on dialysis have a surgical mortality rate of 2 to 4 percent.

Preoperative evaluation of the blood urea nitrogen is not the most accurate index of renal function, as this parameter is heavily dependent on other factors, such as increased protein load, hypercatabolism, GI intestinal bleeding, or urinary flow rate. The blood creatinine, a product of creatinine phosphate metabolism, is a better index but is closely related to muscle mass. The complete cessation of renal function leads to increased serum creatinine, roughly 1 to 2 mg/dl/day. Less significant daily rises suggest some remaining function, while greater rises suggest the presence of increased catabolism.

Patients on dialysis should undergo hemodialysis within the 24 hours prior to surgery. Dialysis may be required immediately following surgery, as these patients have an impaired ability to respond to sodium, water loads, or fluid shifts. In addition, potassium balance may be disturbed. The associated metabolic acidosis should be corrected preoperatively.

In some patients, renal insufficiency or oliguria develops during the postoperative period. Adequate function requires the production of at least 400 ml urine per day as an obligatory volume to excrete the daily metabolic osmotic load of 500 mOm. Urine output per se is not a good index of renal function; however, if metabolic products are in constant production, a doubling of blood creatinine levels represent a halving of the GFR.

Postoperative renal failure can be therapeutically and diagnostically classified into renal, prerenal, and postrenal causes. Prerenal failure, results from inadequate perfusion and is the most common cause of oliguria. Renal etiologies include primary or secondary glomerular diseases and tubulointerstitial disease, including acute tubular necrosis. Predisposing factors to the latter include advancing age, volume concentration, and recent myocardial infarction. Drug-induced interstitial nephritis is becoming a more common renal etiology. Postrenal etiologies include bladder outlet, catheter obstruction, or complete ureteral occlusion (unilateral or bilateral). These are rare and should present clinically as anuria. Renal ultrasonography can determine the presence of hydronephrosis.

Postoperative evaluation and early attention to oliguria are important, as the development of renal failure, depending on the clinical setting, is associated with mortality rates as high as 80 percent. Initial physical examination may detect evidence of prerenal causes, such as cardiac dysfunction or vascular volume contraction. Urinalysis with a specific gravity greater than 1,010 suggests a prerenal etiology. Additional diagnostic studies (Table 21-15) may be necessary, and the fractional excretion of sodium may be the most helpful. These diagnostic indices are of little value if obtained within 24 hours of diuretic administration.

The correction of postoperative prerenal volume deficits may require immediate rapid infusion of crystalloid or blood. Third-space losses or other deficits may require large volumes of crystalloid. In the absence of clinical cardiac failure, volume challenge and not diuresis should be the primary therapy. Prognosis is improved in nonoliguric renal insufficiency, and efforts to rehydrate may be guided by vital signs, central venous pressure, or pulmonary capillary wedge pressure. Once hydration is accomplished, renal output may be increased with furosemide or mannitol diuresis.

When unresponsive renal insufficiency develops, early consultation, attention to electrolyte and acid-base status, early dialysis, minimizing catabolic needs, and meeting caloric requirements become important therapeutic goals. All drugs being administered should be reviewed. Dosages should be altered or drugs discontinued in an effort to minimize nephrotoxicity.

GASTROINTESTINAL

Postoperative GI complications rarely occur following nonradical gynecologic surgery. However, GI obstruction occurs in 8 to 10 percent of patients undergoing ultraradical surgical procedures. These risks are related to the operative indications and previous therapy (i.e., radiation).

The degree and duration of postoperative ileus may be related to retroperitoneal dissection, retroperitoneal hematoma, or electrolyte abnormalities. Routine

Table 21-15 Diagnostic Urinary Parameters in Acute Renal Insufficiency

	Prerenal	Renal	Postrenal
Urine osmolality	≥500	≤350 (ATN)	NA
$\frac{\text{Urine}}{\text{Plasma}}$ osmolality	>1.3	<1.1	NA
Urine sodium (mEq/L)	<20	>40	NA
$\frac{\text{Urine}}{\text{Plasma}}$ urea	>8	<3 (ATN) >8 (GN)	<3
$\frac{\text{Urine}}{\text{Plasma}}$ creatinine	>40	<20 (ATN) >40 (GN)	<20
Fractional excretion of sodium	>1%	>2% (ATN)	>2%

ATN; acute tubular necrosis; GN, glomerular nephritis.
(Modified from Goldstein MB: Acute renal failure. Med Clinic North Am 67:1325, 1983. Reprinted with permission from WB Saunders, Co.)

nasogastric tube suction is of no benefit in this problem but creates a potential alteration of electrolytes and volume changes and results in significant patient discomfort. Fewer than 8 percent of patients will require some form of GI suction to control symptoms following major surgical procedures.

In some clinical situations, it becomes difficult to differentiate between the presence of an ileus and small bowel obstruction. In general, small bowel obstruction rarely occurs before the fifth postoperative day. Adhesions are not likely to be firm enough to cause obstruction prior to this time. In these situations, the diagnosis can be established by the use of an upper GI series, as dye should transverse the ileocecal value within 2 hours. Slow transit may be associated with ileus, but long delays are usually related to obstruction. In the absence of previous radiation, postoperative GI obstruction can be successfully managed by intubation, suction, volume resuscitation, and nutritional support in 84 percent of patients. This form of conservative therapy is less likely to be successful following radiation therapy or in patients with disseminated ovarian cancer. The former requires early surgical intervention. If surgical therapy is required, lysis or adhesion or intestinal resection and reanastamosis should be performed in an effort to preserve intestinal vascular supply. If radiation injury is present, an intestinal bypass or resection is usually necessary. While the optimal procedure may vary, related to intraoperative findings, any involved, heavily irradiated bowel should be resected, particularly if necrosis is present. Intestinal bypass procedures in this situation may treat the initial problem successfully, but secondary or repeat operative procedures are more likely to be needed.

Routine GI stress prophylaxis is unnecessary; however, those patients at risk or those undergoing radical procedures should receive antacids in an attempt to maintain gastric pH about 3.5. This regimen can effectively reduce the incidence of upper GI bleeding from 25 to 5 percent.

HEALING

Abnormal healing is a potential complication of any surgical procedure. While problems such as superficial wound separation may be relatively frequent, they are not as serious as a fascial dehiscence or evisceration. Although the latter occurs in fewer than 1 percent of cases, mortality rates approach 20 to 40 percent. Following surgical injury, a lag phase of 5 to 7 days occurs before bodily tissues exhibit any tensile strength. Healing rates of individual tissues differ, with an intrapersonal variation of tissue strengths of 5- to 10-fold. With the characteristics of the multiple tissues involved in gynecologic cancer surgery, it becomes imperative that the surgeon understand the characteristics of available sutures (Table 21-16) and incorporate proper closure techniques to aid postoperative recovery.

The surgeon must consider specific environmental factors, including humidity, temperature, infection, and oxygen tension, all of which influence wound healing. Nutritional deficits adversely affect healing and predispose the wound to infection. Previous therapy including chemotherapy and radiation therapy can adversely affect healing. Closure technique using deadspace closure or tightly tied sutures result in poor healing and increased risks of infection and morbidity.

There is no need for a layered abdominal closure, as en bloc suture closure imparts optimal tissue tensile strength. In those situations in which the patient is at risk of poor healing, the author prefers the use of permanent suture material for fascial closure. The decision to close the abdominal incision with an interrupted or continuous technique should be individualized. The latter saves operative time but may result in a slight increase in the risk of poor healing. In general, the use of small-diameter (2-0) synthetic sutures is potentially beneficial in decreasing tissue reaction, pain, and infection; during the pelvic portion of the operation, larger-diameter sutures are used for fascial closure. While the decision to use a specific incision is related to patient (cosmetic, previous incision) and physician (exposure, indication) needs, appropriate closure results in distribution of stress. While a midline incision closed with a far and near technique offers the strongest closure (Table 21-17) transverse incisions are subjected to fewer physiologic stresses and clinically perform well.

ENDOCRINE

Endocrine problems can present significant risks to postoperative patients. Diabetics frequently have significant associated medical problems, including arteriosclerosis, renal disease, and coronary artery disease.

Table 21-16 Suture Materials

Material	Tensile Strength	Knot Security	Reactivity	Days to 10% of Tensile Strength
Permanent				
Manufactured				
Steel	4	4	1	
Polyamides (Nylon)	3	3	1	
Polyesters (Dacron)	3	3	1	
Polyolefins (Prolene)	3	1	1	
Natural				
Silk	2	3	3	
Cotton	2	2	2	
Linen	2	2	2	
Absorbable				
Catgut	1	2	3	5
Chromic catgut	1	3	3	28
Polyglycolic acid	2	2	1	28
Polydioxonone sulfate	3	2	1	56

Neutrophil dysfunction increases the risk of postoperative infections, and autonomic neuropathy may make them susceptible to respiratory depression.

Normally, the surgically stressed nondiabetic becomes hyperglycemic and develops deficiencies of insulin and C peptide. The hyperglycemic episodes may be exaggerated in the diabetic. In general, the operative procedure should be scheduled in the early morning, and management should be aimed at avoiding ketosis, hyperglycemia, or hypoglycemia. The subcutaneous administration of one-third to one-half of the patient's usual dose is intermediate-acting insulin and the initiation and continuous administration of intravenous dextrose is probably the method of standard management. Plasma glucose levels should be monitored regularly with a reflectance photometer or re-

Table 21-17 Fascial Incision Strength

Type Incision	Total Closure Strength (Indexed)
Midline (wide en bloc closure)	3.2
Transverse Incision	2.1
Midline (ordinary closure)	1.5
Paramedian	1.0

(Modified from Tera H, Aberg C: Acta Chir Scand 142:349, 1976.)

agent strips during the procedure to avoid hypoglycemia or hyperglycemia.

Glucose-insulin infusions can be administered. When manipulating the patient's normal caloric intake and insulin requirements, units of insulin per calorie can be calculated. With a known caloric intake, insulin dosage can be administered continuously. Insulin may bind to the intravenous glass or tubing, but doses may be increased as needed. Monitoring of blood serum levels remains important, as healing appears to be improved with sugar levels maintained at less than 200 mg percent. Lower levels also decrease the risk of initiating an osmotic diuresis.

Patients who are controlled with diet or oral hypoglycemic agents may require perioperative insulin. Those patients on long-acting oral hypoglycemics, such as chlorpropamide ($t_{\frac{1}{2}}$ = 60 hours), should have those agents discontinued 3 to 4 days preoperatively to avoid hypoglycemia. In additon to glucose control, other medical problems must be addressed. Because cardiovascular disease is common, obtaining serial postoperative ECGs may detect specific problems, as myocardial infarction in these patients is frequently silent.

The normal response to surgery includes an increase in the production of cortisol. Serum levels commonly increase 5- to 10-fold and may reach 100 mg/dl. Primary Addison's disease is uncommon; however, patients may have iatrogenic adrenocortical insufficiency related to previous or current steroid administration. Patients with any significant medical illness should be carefully questioned regarding the prior use of steroids. While different regimens such as qod administration may decrease the risk of adrenal suppression, current recommendations indicate that perioperative steroid administration should be part of routine care for those patients currently on steroids, for those with treatment (at least 1 month) during the last 6 months, or for those who have received at least 1 g cortisol during the last 6 months. Importantly, adrenal suppression may continue for 1 year and may not be predicted by initial steroid dose or interval. If questions exist, perioperative stress steroid coverage should be instituted, as adrenal insufficiency may be subtle or have a clinical presentation suggesting cardiovascular disease. Cortisone acetate is not the drug of choice, as it has a short half-life. Replacement administration of intravenous hydrocortisone hemisuccinate, 100 mg started the night before surgery and given at 6-hour intervals during the 24 to 48 hours of perioperative stress achieves serum levels compatible with those of control subjects.

Surgical procedures in untreated patients with hyperthyroidism or in those thought to have mild disease may precipitate thyroid storm. Awareness of the symptoms associated with thyroid disease and liberal preoperative thyroid function studies are important in decreasing these risks. Euthyroidism should be the goal and achieved preoperatively. In elective procedures, several months of therapy with propylthiouracil or methimazole may be required. In more emergent situations, iodines and β-blockers should be stated preoperatively, and antithyroid medication is instituted early during the postoperative period.

Surgical procedures in the hypothyroid woman may be associated with cardiovascular complications and myxedema coma. If symptoms are elicited and thyroid function studies document deficiencies, treatment should be started with 25 to 50 mg L-thyroxine.

Patients with diabetes insipidus can compensate for their defects, if they have access to water. This diagnosis should be suspected in patients with elevated urinary output and may be established by measuring urinary osmolality during water deprivation. Intramuscular administration of aqueous vasopressin (6 to 10 units) at 2 to 6 hours is adequate replacement therapy. Longer-acting synthetic analogues such as DDAVP can be administered via nasal spray if postoperative urine outputs exceed 250 ml/hr for 2 hours.

INFECTION

The risk of postoperative pelvic or wound infection is complex and associated with many potential factors. Following benign gynecologic procedures, this risk is 8 to 10 percent. After radical operation, this risk approximates 10 percent, and after ultraradical surgery this risk approaches 40 to 60 percent. Importantly, the development of a postoperative infection is associated with a marked increase in patient drug exposure, cost of hospitalization, and psychologic morbidity.

FACTORS INFLUENCING THE RISK OF POSTOPERATIVE INFECTION

Age
Associated medical illness
Urgency of procedure
Surgical experience
Preoperative hospitalization
Method of hair removal
Method of incision
Duration of surgery
Antibiotics
Suture material (type, amount)
Suture placement
Use of cautery
Use of drains
Deadspace closure
Use of perioperative oxygen
Nutritional deficits
Use of vasoconstrictors

The risk of developing infection is related to the number and character of pathogenic organisms and specific host factors. Every incision offers an appropriate culture medium with ischemic tissue, blood and serum. Laboratory models require contamination with 10^5 organisms/g of tissue to produce infection consistently; these levels are readily approached in many gynecologic procedures. Even the prepared vagina may harbor as many as 10 potential pathogens per patient.

There is little question that prophylactic antibiotics benefit many patients undergoing gynecologic cancer procedures (Table 21-18). While single-dose therapy is appropriate in total procedures, additional antibiotic doses, bowel preparation, or intraabdominal irrigation may be helpful in radical procedures that result in higher levels of bacterial contamination.

Attempts to minimize preoperative hospitalization and shaving should result in decreased risk of wound infection. If necessary, hair removal should be performed as close to the time of procedure as possible. Clipping is preferable to shaving. A single bold incision results in less potential deadspace than do multiple sawtoothed incisions. The former is associated with decreased risk of infection. Maintaining hemostasis is important, but excessive use of cautery probably increases the risk of infection. The risk of infection correlates directly with the type, size, and length of suture material. Evidence suggests that polyglyco-

Table 21-18 Prophylactic Antibiotics in Radical Surgical Procedures

Site/Disease	Suggestion
Cervical Cancer	
Conization	Rarely indicated
Total hysterectomy	First- or second-generation cephalosporin (<3 doses)[a]
Radical hysterectomy	First- or second-generation cephalosporin (<3 days)
Pelvic exenteration	Bowel preparation[b]
	Intraoperative irrigation
	Second-generation cephalosporin (<5 days)
	Septra DS with stent removal (<3 days)
Endometrial Cancer	
Hysterectomy plus lymphadenectomy	First- or second-generation cephalosporin (<3 doses)
Ovarian Cancer	
Primary resection	Bowel preparation[b]
	Intraoperative irrigation
	First- or second-generation cephalosporin (<3 doses)
Second-look	Rarely indicated
Palliative (or secondary) resection	Second-generation cephalosporin
	Intraoperative irrigation
Vulvar Cancer	
Vulvectomy (± node dissection)	Cephalosporin (<3 doses)[c]
Trophoblastic Disease	
Suction evacuation	Doxycycline (1 week)

[a] Flagyl may be used in the penicillin-allergic patient.
[b] Mechanical plus antibiotic.
[c] Good gram-positive coverage.

lic acid sutures decrease the risk of infection. Smaller sutures, 2-0 in diameter are suitable for almost all gynecologic procedures.

While pelvic drainage has been associated with lowered risk of pelvic infection after vaginal hysterectomy, this is not true of radical hysterectomy or extended pelvic procedures. In addition, in the absence of gross contamination, subcutaneous skin drains are of little or no benefit in decreasing the risk of infection in the usual clean contaminated hysterectomy incision.

Longer-duration surgery, older age, and immunocompromise are factors associated with increased risk of infection. While the procedure should not be hurried, each part of the surgical technique should be designed to make progress toward completion of the operation.

There is no question that the presence of malnutri-tion increases the risk of infectious complications after bowel surgery. Recent evidence indicates this to be true in patients undergoing radical gynecologic procedures as well. Nutritional assessment (Table 21-19), detection of deficits, and appropriate supplementation or hyperalimentation can reduce hospital stay and postoperative morbidity.

Prophylaxis is important; however, some women still develop postoperative infection. Following radical procedures, these infections may predispose the patient to additional complications, such as urinary fistulas. Aggressive treatment is usually indicated with parenteral antibiotic coverage for gram-negative, gram-positive, aerobic, and anaerobic organisms. Single-drug broad-spectrum coverage may be less expensive and appropriate, particularly if the patient is to receive cisplatin and the physician wishes to avoid the potential nephrotoxic effects of aminoglycosides.

Table 21-19 Nutritional Assessment

History	
Weight loss[a]	Unless rapid, losses of less than 10% of usual body weight do not increase risks.
Anthropometrics	
Tricep skin fold (TSF)	Measure of body fat stores: Standard is 16.5 mm; values less than 13.2 mm should prompt additional evaluation.
Mid-arm muscle circumference (MAMC)	Measure of muscle mass and protein stores: Standard is 23.2 cm; values less than 18.6 cm require investigation.
Laboratory	
Serum albumin[a]	Visceral protein with $t\frac{1}{2}$ = 20 days may not reflect acute changes. Lowered levels reflect increased perioperative risk of infection.
Serum transferrin	Short $t\frac{1}{2}$ (8 days) permits prediction of acute deficit. Levels less than 150 mEq/L should arouse suspicion.
Prealbumin	High-priority visceral protein with a very short $t\frac{1}{2}$ (2 days) not routine screening.
Retinol-binding protein	High-priority visceral protein with ultrashort $t\frac{1}{2}$ (10 hours); clinical investigation is required.
Vitamin levels	Unless specifically indicated, assessment is rarely beneficial.
Immunologic	
Delayed hypersensitivity testing[a]	Anergy correlates with postoperative risk. Reversal with alimentation improves these risks.
Total lymphocyte count[a]	Unprovoked levels of less than 1,500/mm³ should arouse suspicion.

[a] Standard assessment.
(Modified from Orr JR Jr, Shingleton HM: Importance of nutritional assessment and support in the surgical and cancer patients. J Reprod Med 29:635, 1984.)

In most instances, *Psuedomonas* or *Serratia* coverage is unnecessary; however, failure of clinical response might indicate the presence of unusual organisms.

NEUROLOGIC

Patients with cerebrovascular disease and tansient ischemic attacks may require specific preoperative treatment that might include extracranial carotid end-arterectomy, systemic anticoagulation, or medical platelet inhibition. While no prospective studies compare these treatment regimens, the risk of postoperative stroke after simultaneous carotid and noncarotid surgery may be as low as 2.4 percent. However, the risk of other thrombotic events remains high (15 percent).

Following a completed stroke, cerebral blood flow is unstable and brain metabolism depressed. Large cerebral infarcts may take 6 to 8 weeks to resolve, and elective operations should not be done during this critical recovery phase. An emergency procedure requires careful maintenance of adequate intravascular volume and normal or elevated blood pressure. Following a stroke, sequential cerebral computed tomography (CT) scanning may assist in determining the time of complete resolution of the cerebral clot and permit optimal timing for the surgical procedure.

Patients with vertebral basilar ischemic episodes appear to have a lower stroke risk than patients who demonstrate carotid ischemia. Primary therapy for these patients includes the administration of anti-platelet drugs. The value of surgical repair of the vertebral arteries has not been tested in a controlled study.

The presence of an asymptomatic cervical bruit serves as a general index of the presence of atherosclerotic disease; however, there is no good correlation between the location of an asymptomatic bruit and the risk or site of eventual brain infarction. In fact, cervical bruits have little influence on the neurologic morbidity following systemic surgical procedures. Investigation and surgical treatment of patients with an asymptomatic cervical bruit does not alter central nervous system morbidity following systemic surgery.

Thromboembolic events are more common in patients with thrombocytosis, with an increased risk in those patients with platelet counts exceeding 1,000,000/mm³. Depending on the etiology, counts can and should be lowered preoperatively by myelo-suppressive therapy or platelet pheresis.

HEMATOLOGIC

Postoperative hemorrhage is not uncommon, following cancer-related surgical procedures. In the absence of a specific coagulopathy, intraabdominal hemorrhage can often be localized by arteriographic means. Selective embolization with Gelfoam or steel coils is frequently successful and avoids the necessity of anesthesia. While complications can occur, this procedure has gained widespread acceptance. In each situation, surgical judgment is necessary to determine which patient is most suited for repeat operation or arteriographic embolization.

Patients with sickle cell anemia, autoimmune hemolytic anemias, thrombocytopenia, granulocytopenia, and congenital or acquired coagulation deficiencies have specific perioperative risks. Most hospitals in the United States require hemoglobin levels greater than 9 g/dl before proceeding with elective surgery. However, there is little evidence to support an increased surgical risk based solely on compromised oxygen-carrying capacity. Perhaps more important is the cause of altered hemoglobin levels. Chronic losses may relate to a second primary cancer or metastatic disease. A hemoglobin of 10 g/dl provides an adequate level of oxygen for most tissue metabolic needs. Associated problems may indicate a need for preoperative transfusion (Table 21-20). However, if transfusion is performed, a 24-hour delay permits equilibration, provides easier fluid management, and facilitates tissue delivery of oxygen by the repletion of RBC 2,3-DPG levels.

Patients with sickle cell disease are at increased risk of vaso-occlusive crisis during the perioperative pe-

Table 21-20 Preoperative Transfusion for Anemia

Probable Need For Higher Hemoglobin	Low Hemoglobin (More Acceptable)
Age > 50 years	Age < 30
Atherosclerosis	Chronic anemia
Cardiovascular disease	Religious convictions
Cerebral ischemia	
Significant estimated blood loss	
Reduced PaO_2	

riod. Helpful prophylactic methods include maintaining oxygenation, normal body temperature, and adequate hydration. Exchange transfusions may reduce the number of potentially sickling cells to less than 50 percent of the total RBC population, which may benefit some of these patients.

Autoimmune hemolytic anemia may be related to the presence of a cold or warm antibody. When hemolysis is complement mediated, cross-matching difficulties can occur. RBCs, if given, should be administered through a blood-warming device. Neither splenectomy nor corticosteroids are beneficial. Those patients with warm antibodies may benefit from preoperative corticosteroid therapy or splenectomy. Preoperative transfusion should be avoided, as it is usually ineffective in raising hemoglobin levels.

Thrombocytopenia increases the risk of bleeding. If thrombocytopenia is chronic, bleeding rarely occurs unless platelet counts are below 30,000 to 50,000/ mm^3. Drug-induced thrombocytopenia usually resolves within 1 to 3 weeks after stopping the offending drug, and perioperative steroid administration may prove beneficial. In patients with thrombocytopenia associated with other problems or in those requiring emergency procedure, it may be necessary to transfuse 1 unit per 10 kg body weight to elevate the platelet count to acceptable levels. Drug-induced platelet dysfunction can be a potential problem, and risks are prolonged. Aspirin, a potential offender, consistently exerts an adverse effect on platelet function for 7 to 10 days after discontinuation.

Granulocytopenia, particularly with counts of less than 500 mm^3, increases the risk of infection. These patients usually require intensive antibiotic therapy for febrile episodes. Multiple drug regimens have been proposed; however, no consistent benefit of any antibiotic or combination of antibiotics exists. Coverage must be directed to both the usual and unusual pathogens. There is no proven consistent benefit of granulocyte transfusion; however, they might be considered in those granulocytopenic patients who exhibit fever unresponsive to medical treatment.

Specific coagulation factor deficiencies suspected on the basis of clinical history or examination can be diagnosed with appropriate coagulation studies. After diagnosis, treatment with specific component therapy can decrease bleeding risk. Von Willebrand's disease, associated with platelet dysfunction and abnormal factor VIII, is inherited as an autosomal-dominant trait. The diagnosis is established by demonstrating prolonged bleeding time and abnormal platelet aggregation. Cryoprecipitate or fresh-frozen plasma contains adequate levels of factor VIII. Levels of this factor are rapidly depleted during the storage of blood.

PAIN

One of the most common postoperative problems or complications involves the management of patients who have significant pain. Preoperative discussions allay the fears and reassure patients that adequate medication will be available, as ambulation and pulmonary recovery will be improved in those patients receiving adequate postoperative analgesia. A number of medications are available and may be given by a parenteral or enteral route (Table 21-21). The physician may further decrease the need for medication by simple methods, such as the local injection of bupivacaine (0.5 percent). Alternative postoperative management of pain might include the use of patient-controlled analgesia, which offers a cost-effective method for providing continuous pain relief. In this situation, the patient is connected to an apparatus that permits self-induced medication by incremental dose or altering rate of injection of the incremental dose. A number of methods are currently available, and it would appear that the apparatus in general can be used without direct supervision. This method is relatively safe, if modest incremental doses are used, and the average patient will actually require less medication. Epidural anesthesia using morphine derivatives offers long-term (12 to 24 hours) postoperative analgesia with few side effects. This method may also be used with longer-term infusion pumps or percutaneous catheters for palliative or terminal care.

In those patients with chronic pain, a search for treatable causes should be undertaken with surgery or radiation used as needed. In this latter group of patients, some will have no reversible cause, and the physician must overcome any fears concerning patient addiction. Medications should be given on an hourly basis and avoid p.r.n. needs. Estimates indicate that at least 25 percent of cancer patients die without adequate pain relief. Neurologic ablative or stimulatory procedures should be considered in those patients with a short life expectancy. Unfortunately, pain re-

Table 21-21 Narcotic Analgesics

Analgesic	Equianalgesic Milligram Dose (Morphine 10 mg IM)		Onset of Analgesia (min)	Duration of Analgesia (hr)	Contrasted with Morphine
	IM	PO			
Morphine	10	60	30–60 (IM)	4–7	—
Oxymorphone (Numorphine)	1	6	10–15 (IM)	3–6	Rapid onset; available in rectal suppository
Hydromorphone (Dilaudid)	1.5	8	15–20 (IM or PO)	4–5	Short-acting; available as rectal suppository
Levorphanol (Leov-Dromovan)	2	4	60–90 (IM or PO)	6–8	Long-acting; high oral potency; may accumulate
Butorphanol (Stadol)	2	—	30–60 (IM)	4	Nalorphine-like antagonistic properties
Heroin	5	30	—	5	Short-acting; illegal in the United States
Methodone	10	20	30–60 (IM or PO)	4–6	High oral potency
Nalbuphine (Nubain)	10	—	15 (IM)	3–6	Rapid onset; nalorphine-like antagonistic properties
Oxycodone (Percodan, Percoset)	15	30	10–15 (PO)	3–6	Rapid onset; high oral potency
Alphaprodine (Nisentil)	45	—	1–2 (IV)	0.5–1	Rapid acting; short onset
Anileridine (Heritine)	30	50	15 (IM or PO)		Rapid onset; short-acting, high oral potency
Pentazocine (Tacwin)	60	180	20 (IM)	3	Shorter acting halorphine-like antagonistic properties; may precipitate withdrawal
Meperidine (Demerol)	75	300	30–50 (IM) 40–60 (PO)	2–4	Shorter-acting; metabolites may produce CNS excitation
Codeine	130	200	15–30 (IM or PO)	4–6	High oral potency; constipation

lief is often accompanied by the development of new pain on the contralateral side or at another site.

PREOPERATIVE EVALUATION

Estimating surgical risks or making therapeutic decisions involves weighing the risks and benefits of appropriate medical/surgical intervention against the known natural history of the disease process. While surgical risk is defined as the probability of morbidity or mortality resulting from the preoperative preparation, anesthesia, operation, and postoperative convalescence, data about the outcome of interventions remain incomplete. In this situation, experience, convention, and intuition may become important in decision making.

Appropriate patient factors that affect surgical risk have been outlined and include the nature and duration of the surgical illness, underlying medical illnesses, age, and nutritional status. Surgical factors include the type of anesthesia, type of operation, urgency of the operation, experience of the surgical team, and hospital resources. In each situation, the physician and patient must discuss and determine the relative rewards and risks of a given treatment.

For the determination of operative risk and factors requiring specific preoperative correction, a simple list should be made of each abnormality at physical examination. Personal and family history of any bleeding tendency with laboratory definition of its presence should be noted. Allergic responses to previous medications and current medications must be recorded with specific physician awareness that patients often forget to list drugs and fail to remember certain drugs including nonprescription items such as aspirin.

Any time a surgical procedure is contemplated, it is essential that the physician and patient form a bond of communication and personal responsibility; the patient's confidence is based on genuine understanding, permitting her appropriate participation in judgments affecting her risks, future lifestyle, and postoperative convalescence. The explanation concerning the operative procedure should include a frank and optimistic discussion of the possibilities of preoperative care of postoperative use of drainage devices and intubation as well as further plans; the approach should be open, so that the patient will learn to trust the physician to manage specific problems. Unlike general surgical procedures, gynecologic procedures are often performed in patients who are not newly referred but who have been patients or who know of the physician's skills and the treatment possibilities. The relationship evolving between the patient and physician should not convey a sense of hurry or inadequate time, and questions should be answered with matter-of-fact responses and "I don't know," if necessary.

It should not bother the physician if a patient desires a second opinion nor should it disturb the patient if the individual physician would like consultation. The surest perception of a true informed consent is obtained in a setting in which there is full and frank discussion with the patient, in the presence of a witness.

History

Obtaining an accurate patient history remains crucial. It may be taken by interview or by a patient-completed form. While self-filled forms may be appropriate for most answered questions, it is imperative that the physician personally review all the possibilities, including allergies and current medications. Any potential problems, such as bleeding, neurologic abnormalities, or pain, must be discussed in detail.

Physical Examination

The physical examination relates not only to the process for which the surgical procedure is performed but serves to alert the surgeon to other possible complicating factors, such as cardiovascular or pulmonary disease. In fact, the physical examination coupled with the history constitutes the best possible screening process and provides nearly all the clinical data necessary for the detection of most diseases that may adversely affect surgical outcome. The incidence of major asymptomatic medical problems is small (Table 21-22) and, with careful questioning and physical examination, many of these conditions can be discovered and the appropriate laboratory studies performed. In contrast to healthy asymptomatic patients, those with symptoms or signs require additional laboratory evaluation.

Table 21-22 Prevalence and Cost of Detecting Asymptomatic Conditions in 1,000 Women

Condition/Test	Estimated Asymptomatic Prevalence per 1,000	Estimated Asymptomatic Cases Detected	False-Positive Cases	Cost of Testing ($)	Cost per Case Detected ($)
Anemia/hematocrit	10	10	0	4,000	400
Ischemic heart disease					
ECG	5	1	189	20,000	20,000
Stress test	5	3	90	20,000	6,666
Arrhythmia					
24-hr monitoring	5	5	0	179,000	35,800
Obstructive pulmonary disease					
Spirometry	19	19	0	22,500	4,500
Diabetes					
2-hr PP sugar	2.9	2	439	8,000	4,000
Bleeding disorder					
PTT	0.01	0.01	280	11,000	1,100,000
Thrombocytopenia					
Platelet count	0.05	0.05	0	7,000	140,000
Interstitial lung disease					
Chest radiograph	0.1	0.1	0	50,000	500,000
Chronic renal disease					
Creatinine	0.3	0.3	0	9,000	30,000

(Modified from Robbins JA, Mushlin AI: Preoperative evaluation of the healthy patient. Md Clin North Am 63:1145, 1979. Reprinted with permission from WB Saunders Co.)

Laboratory Studies

Minimal recommended tests for otherwise healthy preoperative patients includes a hematocrit, as the cost is low and the predictive value high. Surgery results in the administration of medications and sometimes catheterization. In this situation, the detection of preexisting urinary infection should be assessed, as the urinalysis is a potential cost-effective method of detecting problems and potentially preventing postoperative difficulties. Women who are at risk, who have a history suggestive of being pregnant, or who are concerned about being pregnant should have a pregnancy test. In most instances, a urinary pregnancy test is sensitive and specific; however, a serum pregnancy test may be necessary. Although little is known about the specific effects of anesthetic gases on the fetus, there appears to be no increase in maternal morbidity or mortality if anesthesia is knowledgeably and carefully administered to a pregnant woman. Perioperatively, the goal includes avoiding maternal hypoxia and hypotension. Postoperatively, tocolytic agents might be considered.

Abnormal values in the screening clinical chemistry profile may be present in as many as 60 percent of all hospitalized patients. At a benign obstetrics and gynecology service, only 8 percent of patients demonstrate abnormalities; however, 19 percent of surgical patients and 55 percent of medical patients have abnormal studies. Abnormalities are infrequent (14 percent) in patients under 40 years of age as compared with patients over 70 years of age (43 percent).

Whitehead and Wootton (1974) studied the results of 31,434 chemistry profiles performed in England. Only 7 percent were unsuspectedly found to be abnormal that had or provided new diagnostic information. Importantly, the use of routine admission testing in asymptomatic patients does not shorten the hospital stay but increases the total cost of hospital care by as much as 5 percent.

Abnormalities in serum glucose are present in approximately 5.5 percent of patients and represent the most frequently detected abnormality in patients undergoing biochemical profiles. In general, the detection of glucose intolerance may lead to measures to prevent osmotic diuresis and nonketotic coma or may alter management to assist healing and combat impaired WBC function. While the value of measuring preoperative serum glucose is undecided, many clinicians obtain this study, particularly for older, obese, high-risk patients.

Serum calcium screening is not a useful study in asymptomatic women. Minimal evaluation has little effect on surgery, and the incidence of hyperparathyroidism is only 27 per 100,000. However, in preoperative patients with malignancy, this study becomes more appropriate, as hypercalcemia related to bone metastases or ectopic parathormone may be present.

Evaluation of liver function studies in asymptomatic patients may detect underlying hepatic disease that could influence metabolism or medication dosages. However, evaluation of their routine use indicates that these studies do not regularly affect care. While the actual incidence of abnormalities in serum alkaline phosphatase (5 percent), SGOT (14 percent), and lactate dehydrogenase (12 percent) is numerically significant, their clinical effect on outcome or care is rarely important. Evaluation in those patients with cancer is probably more important. While the incidence of liver metastases is small at initial presentation, their presence may drastically alter the therapeutic approach. Fortunately, these serum studies are rather specific and sensitive in the detection of liver metastases as compared with CT or ultrasound. Routine evaluation prior to any oncology procedure is appropriate.

Complete blood counts are traditionally performed and potentially important in preoperative patients. Asymptomatic thrombocytopenia in women is rare (0.005 percent); however, those with cancer are likely to undergo more radical procedures or may have been or will be subjected to marrow toxic drugs. Anemia may also be detected and in cancer patients may be a clue to the existence of other problems such as malnutrition or chronic GI blood loss. Patients with a history of anticoagulant use, a history of physical examination suggestive of liver dysfunction, active bleeding, a history or physical examination indicative of bleeding. In patients not at risk, less than 3 percent, have abnormal coagulation studies. By contrast, 18 percent of those patients who have a defined risk will have an abnormal study. In those women with abnormal studies and no defined risk, careful follow-up suggests that they rarely have bleeding complications and bleeding problems have occasionally developed despite normal studies. Because these patients have radical dissections and will often be exposed to additional therapies, preoperative evaluation should be considered essential.

While electrocardiograms (ECG) are considered a potentially beneficial screening test for cardiac disease, the sensitivity and specificity of an ECG for detecting cardiac disease have been reported to be only 27 percent and 81 percent, respectively. Because of the relatively low prevalence of cardiac disease in the asymptomatic population, the positive predictive value is also low. Since the ECG has only limited value as a screening test, its routine use adds little to history and physical examination; however, older patients are at increased risk.

Malnutrition poses a significant risk to patients undergoing gynecologic procedures. While the overall incidence in gynecology patients is thought to be small, nutritional deficits are common in patients with cancer and occur even in patients who appear to be obese. Appropriate evaluation might include anthropometric measurements, assessment of weight/height ratio, serum albumin, serum total iron binding capacity, and total lymphocyte count.

Radiologic Studies

Chest radiographs account for more than 50 percent of all radiography performed in the United States. The Royal College of Radiologists, in the review of 10,619 patients, found that preoperative radiographs do not alter the choice of anesthesia or the decision to operate. In a study of 607 patients, Rees (1976) found 126 significant abnormalities, 4 percent of which consisted of cardiomegaly and 19 percent which were due to chronic respiratory disease. Rees and others have found that unless there are predisposing factors, history, laboratory, and clinical examination are more sensitive detectors of disease than radiography, except in the presence of tuberculosis. Single-view films are less expensive, result in less radiation exposure, and are equally predictive.

The benefit of a chest radiograph in the asymptomatic patient is small; however, it is an essential part of preparation in patients with gynecologic malignancy. The detection of pulmonary metastatic disease at the initial examination is rare, but its presence can drastically effect patient management. Moreover, long radical operations are associated with more blood loss and postoperative pulmonary dysfunction. Chest tomograms or CT has been recommended in patients with pelvic sarcomas. While these studies are more sensitive, the patients usually require surgery to control pelvic symptoms. Since no therapy is available for distal disease, the CT findings add little to clinical care. However, these more sensitive studies might be indicated in those undergoing ultraradical salvage treatment for pelvic malignancy.

While CT of the pelvis and abdomen is a preoperative test used commonly in patients with gynecologic cancers, its routine use is not recommended. It should not serve as an extension of the pelvic examination, as it is helpful in approximately 50 percent of cases and may be misleading as frequently. It does not accurately identify intraabdominal metastasis. However, it may evaluate and identify enlarged retroperitoneal lymph nodes and permit percutaneous needle biopsy.

Intravenous pyelography is considered a part of cancer staging but is rarely indicated in patients with apparent localized gynecologic disease. Unless specific symptoms exist, the incidence of abnormalities is extremely low. In addition, there is a slight risk of toxicity or creating problems with its use. Barium studies of the GI tract may detect coexisting disease and are considered essential for those women with risk factors for other diseases.

Mammograms should be routinely obtained for all patients undergoing gynecologic procedures for malignancy. While the precise need and benefit of a yearly mammogram remains unknown, preoperative screening should be undertaken in all older patients.

Endoscopic Studies

Preoperative endoscopic evaluation of the bladder and rectum should be performed in patients who have apparent tumor spread or who are at risk of coexisting disease. Occasionally, evaluation may require endoscopic evaluation of the upper GI tract to detect or eliminate significant disease.

Preparation

The goal of any preoperative evaluation is to lower risk by detecting and correcting any abnormalities prior to the surgical procedure. Volume losses are not considered common in the gynecologic patient; however, many have been NPO and have had multiple diagnostic studies requiring bowel preparation. Many others have third-space losses from ascites, effusion or bowel obstruction. As many as 38 percent of these women entering the operating room have unrecognized volume defects. The correction of volume loss will depend on the tonicity and amount of the losses. Approximately 5 to 10 percent of body weight loss occurs before alterations in skin turgor are evident. These same alterations are necessary before vital sign changes are detectable. There is no "cookbook" method to preoperative volume replacement, but many patients will benefit from the placement of intravenous lines and slow hydration the night prior to surgery.

Nutritional defects should be corrected with enteral or parenteral calories and protein. At least 7 days of preoperative nutritional supplementation is necessary prior to affecting the surgical outcome of the malnourished patient. Daily replacement of 1,500 to 2,000 calories is generally sufficient. Higher metabolic needs are only rarely present. Attempts to use the GI with elemental or as special nutriments may be beneficial. However, these patients usually require total parenteral nutrition. Glucose and protein are required to decrease nitrogen losses. Regardless, postoperative supplementation should always be considered. In patients undergoing emergency procedures, the institution of nutritional support during the immediate postoperative period may be of potential benefit.

Surgery in patients with hepatic disease is fraught with major problems. Patients with liver impairment are at high risk and patients with childs C classification or cirrhosis have a 76 percent likelihood of postoperative death, as do 58 percent of patients who have ascites. Associated poor nutrition has a mortality rate of 62 percent, and an abnormality in bleeding studies is associated with mortality rates of 50 percent.

In addition to the correction of any abnormalities, the bowel and abdomen require preparation for most gynecologic surgical procedures. Any procedure that is thought to have the potential to interrupt the bowel should be preceded with a mechanical and antibiotic bowel preparation. Clear liquids with cathartics for 48 to 72 hours preoperatively or some other osmotic solution delivered orally or by nasogastric tube are efficacious. Parenteral antibiotics may be beneficial.

The abdominal preparation should be performed as close to the operative procedure as possible. Preoperative shaving should be avoided, as it increases the risk of infection. If hair removal is necessary, clipping is preferable to shaving and creates less microtissue injury. Preoperative showers with hexachlorophene or some form of antiseptic are inexpensive methods of decreasing the risk of wound infection. There is no rationale for preoperative antiseptic douching. Although douching may dilute or decrease the numbers of bacteria in the vagina, this effect is short-lived.

SUGGESTED READINGS

Agarwal N, Shibutani K, SanFilippo JA, Del Guercio LR: Hemodynamic and respiratory changes in surgery of the morbidly obese. Surgery 92:226, 1982

Aitkenhead AR: Anaesthesia for bowel surgery. Ann Chir Gynaecol 73:177, 1984

Andersen BL, Lachenbruch PA, Anderson B, DeProsse C: Sexual dysfunction and signs of gynecologic cancer. Cancer 57:1880, 1986

Aranha GV, Greenlee HB: Intra-abdominal surgery in patients with advanced cirrhosis. Arch Surg 121:275, 1986

Askanazi J, Hensle TW, Starker PM, et al: Effect of immediate postoperative nutritional support on length of hospitalization. Ann Surg 203:236, 1986

Blanchard CG, Ruckdeschel JC, Fletcher BA, Blanchard EB: The impact of oncologists' behaviors on patient satisfaction with morning rounds. Cancer 58:387, 1986

Bland R, Shoemaker WC, Shabot MM: Physiologic monitoring goals for the critically ill patient. Surg Gynecol Obstet 147:833, 1978

Burke GR, Gulyassy PF: Surgery in the patient with renal disease and related electrolyte disorders. Med Clin North Am 63:1191, 1979

Burke JF: The effective period of preventive antibiotic action in experimental incisions and dermal lesions. Surgery 50:161, 1961

Babu SC, Sharma PV, Raciti A, et al: Monitor-guided responses. Arch Surg 115:1384, 1980

Benigno BB, Evrard J, Faro S, et al: A comparison of piperacillin, cephalothin and cefoxitin in the prevention of postoperative infections in patients undergoing vaginal hysterectomy. Surg Gynecol Obstet 163:421, 1986

Charlson ME: The effects of anesthesia in patients with specific chronic illnesses. Infect Surg Dec:67, 1984

Chazan JA: Oliguria in the postoperative patient. Infect Surg Jan:909, 1983

Committee on Pre and Postoperative Care, American College of Surgeons. In Dudrick SJ, Baue AE, Eiseman B, et al (eds): Manual of Preoperative and Postoperative Care. WB Saunders, Philadelphia, 1983

Craig DB: Postoperative recovery of pulmonary function. Anesth Anal 60:46, 1981

Crapo RO, Kelly TM, Elliott CG, Jones SB: Spirometry as a preoperative screening test in morbidly obese patients. Surgery 99:763, 1986

Cunningham AJ, Donnelly M, Bourke A, Murphy JF: Cardiovascular and metabolic effects of cervical epinephrine infiltration. Obstet Gynecol 66:98, 1985

Czer LSC, Shoemaker WC: Optimal hematocrit value in critically ill postoperative patients. Surg Gynecol Obstet 147:363, 1978

Dagi TF, Chilton J, Caputy A, Won D: Long-term, intermittent percutaneous administration of epidural and intrathecal morphine for pain of malignant origin. Am Surg 52:155, 1986

Del Guercio LR, Cohn JD: Monitoring operative risk in the elderly. JAMA 243:1350, 1980

Del Guercio LR, Cohn JD: Monitoring: methods and significance. Surg Clin North Am 56:977, 1976

Detsky AS, Abrams HB, Forbath N, et al: Cardiac assessment for patients undergoing noncardiac surgery. Arch Intern Med 146:2131, 1986

Dicker RC, Greenspan JR, Strauss LT, et al: Complications of abdominal and vaginal hysterectomy among women of reproductive age in the United States. Am J Obstet Gynecol 144:841, 1982

Drucker WR, Gann DS, McCoy S: Response to surgery: Neuroendocrine and metabolic changes, convalescence, and rehabilitation. p. 3. In Handy JD (ed): Hardy's Textbook of Surgery. JB Lippincott, Philadelphia.

Eisenberg PR, Jaffe AS, Schuster DP: Clinical evaluation compared to pulmonary artery catheterization in the hemodynamic assessment of critically ill patients. Crit Care Med 12:549, 1984

England GT, Randall HW, Graves WL: Impairment of tissue defenses by vasoconstrictors in vaginal hysterectomies. Obstet Gynecol 61:271, 1983

Farnell MB, Worthington-Self S, Mucha P Jr, et al: Closure of abdominal incisions with subcutaneous catheters. Arch Surg 121:641, 1986

Faro S: Patient cost in the treatment of postsurgical female pelvic infection. Am J Med 78(suppl 6B):165, 1985

Farquharson DIM, Orr JW Jr: Prophylaxis against thromboembolism in gynecologic patients. Reprod Med 29:845, 1984

Feigal DW, Blaisdell FW: The estimation of surgical risk. Med Clin North Am 63:1131, 1979

Foley KM: The treatment of pain in the patient with cancer. CA 36:194, 1986

Forney JP, Morrow CP, Townsend DE, DiSaia PJ: Impact of cephalosporin prophylaxis on conization-vaginal hysterectomy morbidity. Am J Obstet Gynecol 125:100, 1976

Goldberg M: Computer-based instruction and diagnosis of acid-based disorders. JAMA 223(3):269, 1973

Goldman DR, Brown FH, Levy WK, et al: Medical Care of

the Surgical Patient. A Problem Oriented Approach to Management. JP Lippincott, Philadelphia, Penn., 1982

Goldman L: Cardiac risks and complications of noncardiac surgery. Ann Intern Med 98:504, 1983

Goldman L, Caldera DL, Nussbaum SR, et al: Multifactorial index of cardiac risk in noncardiac surgical procedures. N Engl J Med 297:845, 1977

Goldstein MB: Acute renal failure. Med Clin North Am 67:1325, 1983

Gould SA, Rosen AL, Sengal LR, et al: Fluosol-DA as a red-cell substitute in acute anemia. N Engl J Med 314:1653, 1986

Hammond GL: Acute respiratory failure. Surg Clin North Am 60:1133, 1980

Harman E, Lillington G: Pulmonary risk factors in surgery. Med Clin North Am 63:1289, 1979

Humphreys MH, Sheldon GF: Fluid and electrolyte management. Textbook of Surgery. WB Saunders, Philadelphia, 1981

Jewell ER, Persson AV: Preoperative evaluation of the high-risk patient. Surg Clin North Am 65:3, 1985

Kelly CS, Ligas JR, Smith CA, et al: Sepsis due to triple lumen central venous catheters. Surg Gynecol Obstet 163:14, 1986

Knighton DR, Halliday B, Hunt TK: Oxygen as an antibiotic. Arch Surg 121:191, 1986

Kohler T, Palder SB, Tilney NL: Evaluation of the patient with coronary artery disease for noncardiac surgery. Infect Surg June:427, 1984

Kram HB: Noninvasive tissue oxygen monitoring in surgical and critical care medicine. Surg Clin North Am 65:1005, 1985

Krames ES, Gershow J, Glassberg A, et al: Continuous infusion of spinally administered narcotics for the relief of pain due to malignant disorders. Cancer 56:696, 1985

Krebs HB, Goplerud DR: The role of intestinal intubation in obstruction of the small intestine due to carcinoma of the ovary. Surg Gynecol Obstet 158:467, 1984

Ledger WJ, Gee C, Lewis WP: Guidelines for antibiotic prophylaxis in gynecology. Am J Obstet Gynecol 121:1038, 1975

Lennard TW, Shenton BK, Borzotta A, et al: The influence of surgical operations on components of the human immune system. Br J Surg 72:771, 1985

Liedtke AJ: Clinical assessment of the surgical patient with heart disease. Surg Clin North Am 63:977, 1983

Lucas CE, Ledgerwood AM: The fluid problem in the critically ill. Surg Clin North Am 63:439, 1983

Lucas CE, Martin DJ, Ledgerwood AM, et al: Effect of fresh-frozen plasma resuscitation on cardiopulmonary function and serum protein flux. Arch Surg 121:559, 1986

McBride K, La Morte WW, Menzoian JO: Can ventilation-perfusion scans accurately diagnose acute pulmonary embolism? Arch Surg 121:754, 1986

McGowan L: Abdominal incisions and staging in ovarian cancer. Arch Surg 121:800, 1986

McIrvine AJ, Mannick JA: Lymphocyte function in the critically ill surgical patient. Surg Clin North Am 63:245, 1983

Mann WJ Jr, Jander HP, Orr JW Jr, et al: The use of percutaneous nephrostomy in gyn oncology. Gynecol Oncol 10:343, 1980

Mattox KL: Disorders of surgical bleeding and blood transfusion problems. Handy JD (ed): Handy's Textbook of Surgery. JB Lippincott, Philadelphia, 1983

Morrow CP, Hernandez WL, Townsend DE, Disaia PJ: Pelvic celiotomy in the obese patient. Am J Obstet Gynecol 127:335, 1977

Moss G, Regal ME, Lichtig L: Reducing postoperative pain, narcotics, and length of hospitalization. Surgery 99:206, 1986

Orr JW Jr: Sutures and closures: An update. Ala J Med Sci 23:36, 1986

Orr JW Jr, Shingleton HM: Importance of nutritional assessment and support in the surgical and cancer patients. J Reprod Med 29:635, 1984

Orr JW Jr, Taylor PT: Reducing postoperative infection in the patient with gynecologic cancer. Infect Surg 6:666, 1987

Orr JW Jr, Kilgore LC Shingleton HM: Guidelines for CV monitoring of the surgical patient. Contemp Obstet Gynecol 27:71, 1986

Orr JW Jr, Ball GC, et al: Surgical treatment of women found to have invasive cervix cancer at the time of total hysterectomy. Obstet Gynecol 68:353, 1986

Orr JW Jr, Barter JF, Kilgore LC, et al: Closed suction pelvic drainage following radical pelvic surgery. Am J Obstet Gynecol 155:867, 1986

Orr JW Jr, Cornwell A, Wilson K, et al: Nutritional status of patients with untreated cervical cancer. I. Biochemical and immunologic assessment. Am J Obstet Gynecol 151:625, 1985

Orr Jw Jr, Cornwell A, Wilson K: Nutritional status of patients with untreated cervical cancer. II. Vitamin assessment. Am J Obstet Gynecol 151:632, 1985

Orr JW Jr, Wilson KW, Bodiford C, et al: Pretreatment comparison of nutritional parameters in patients with cervix and corpus cancer. Trans Am Gynecol Obstet Soc 111:159, 1985

Orr JW Jr, Wilson K, Bodiford C, et al: Corpus and cervix cancer: A nutritional comparison. Am J Obstet Gynecol 153:775, 1985

Orr JW Jr, Shingleton HM, Soong SJ, et al: Hemodynamic parameters following pelvic exenteration. Am J Obstet Gynecol 146:882, 1983

Orr JW Jr, Hatch KD, Shingleton HM: Gastrointestinal

complications associated with pelvic exenteration. Am J Obstet Gynecol 145:325, 1983

Orr JW Jr, Shingleton HM, Soong SJ: Hemodynamic parameters following pelvic exenteration. Am J Obstet Gynecol 146:882, 1983

Orr JW Jr, Shingleton HM, Hatch KD, et al: Urinary diversion in patients undergoing pelvic exenteration. Am J Obstet Gynecol 142:883, 1982

Orr JR Jr, Shingleton HM, Hatch KD, et al: Correlation of perioperative morbidity and conization to radical hysterectomy interval. Obstet Gynecol 59:726, 1982

Orr JW Jr, Austin JM Jr, Hatch KD, et al: Acute pulmonary edema associated with molar pregnancies: A high risk factor for the development of persistent trophoblastic disease. Am J Obstet Gynecol 136:412, 1980

Pemberton LB, Lyman B, Lander V, Covinsky J: Sepsis from triple- vs single-lumen catheters during total parenteral nutrition in surgical or critically ill patients. Arch Surg 121:591, 1986

Penn I: Cancer is a complication of severe immunosuppression. Surg Gynecol Obstet 162:603, 1986

Pierson DJ, Hudson LD: Monitoring hemodynamics in the critically ill. Med Clin North Am 67:1343, 1983

Pitkin RM: Vaginal hysterectomy in obese women. Obstet Gynecol 49:567, 1977

Polk HC Jr: Principles of preoperative preparation of the surgical patient.

Prorok JJ, Trostle D: Operative risk of general surgical procedures in patients with previous myocardial revascularization. Surg Gynecol Obstet 159:214, 1984

Rees AM, Roberts CJ, Bligh AS, Evans KT: Routine preoperative chest radiography in noncardiopulmonary surgery. Br Med J 1(6021):1333, 1976

Robbins JA, Mushlin AI: Preoperative evaluation of the healthy patient. Med Clin North Am 63:1145, 1979

Rodeheaver GT, Nesbit WS, Edlich RF: Novafil, a dynamic suture for wound closure. Ann Surg 204:1983, 1986

Rose SD, Corman LC, Mason DT: Cardiac risk factors in patients undergoing noncardiac surgery. Med Clin North Am 63:1271, 1979

Schreve RH, Terpstra OT, Ausema L, et al: Detection of liver metastases. A prospective study comparing liver enzymes, scintigraphy, ultrasonography and computed tomography. Br J Surg 71:947, 1984

Shapiro M, Schoenbaum SC, Tager IB, et al: Benefit-cost analysis of antimicrobial prophylaxis in abdominal and vaginal hysterectomy. JAMA 249:1290, 1983

Shapiro M, Munoz A, Tager IB, et al: Risk factors for infection at the operative site after abdominal or vaginal hysterectomy. N Engl J Med 307:1661, 1982

Shennib H, Mulder DS, Chiu RC-J: Effects of pulmonary atelectasis and reexpansion on lung cellular immune defenses. Arch Surg 119:274, 1984

Shingleton HM, Orr JW Jr: Cancer of the Cervix. Current Reviews in Obstetrics and Gynecology. Churchill Livingstone, London, 1983

Shires GT, Canizaro PC: Fluid and electrolyte management of the surgical patient. p. 91. In Schwartz ST (ed): Principles of Surgery, 4th Ed. McGraw-Hill, New York, 1983

Shoemaker WC, Bland RD, Appel PL: Therapy of critically ill postoperative patients based on outcome prediction and prospective clinical trials. Surg Clin North Am 65:811, 1985

Simon NL, Orr JW Jr, Hatch KD, Shingleton HM: Lower extremity edema due to deep vein thrombosis in patients with recurrent cervix cancer. Gynecol Oncol 19(1):30, 1984

Smoller BR, Kruskall MS: Phlebotomy for diagnostic laboratory tests in adults. Pattern of use and effect on transfusion requirements. N Engl J Med 314:1233, 1986

Stone KI, von Fraunhofer JA, Masterson BJ: The biomechanical effects of tight suture closure upon fascia. Surg Gynecol Obstet 163:448, 1986

Strauss RJ, Wise L: Operative risks of obesity. Surg Gynecol Obstet 146:286, 1978

Tilney NL, Lazarus JM: Acute renal failure in surgical patients. Causes, clinical patterns and care. Surg Clin North Am 63:357, 1983

Tobin GR: Myocutaneous and muscle flaps: Refinements and new applications. Curr Probl Surg in press

Wallace LM: Psychological preparation as a method of reducing the stress of surgery. J Hum Stress 10:62, 1984

Watson-Williams EJ: Hematologic and hemostatic considerations before surgery. Med Clin North Am 63:1165, 1979

Waxman K, Lazrover S, Shoemaker WC: Physiologic responses to operation in high risk surgical patients. Surg Gynecol Obstet 152:633, 1981

White VA, Kumagai LF: Preoperative endocrine and metabolic considerations. Med Clin North Am 63:1321, 1979

Whitehead TP, Wootten ID: Biochemical profiles for hospital patients. Lancet 2(7894):1439, 1974

22

Radical Hysterectomy

Hugh M. Shingleton
S. B. Gusberg

Radical hysterectomy, combined with pelvic node dissection, is a major treatment modality for low-stage, small-volume invasive cervical cancer. During the 1890s, the German surgeon, Ries,[1] devised the radical operation in concept; it was first performed, however, by Clark[2] in 1895 at the Johns Hopkins Hospital. Wertheim performed his first such operation in 1898. By 1912 Wertheim[3] had accumulated a series of 500 cases, with an operative mortality of 30 percent in the first 100 cases. Radium and x-rays were first used for treatment of cervical cancer in 1903 and largely replaced radical surgery as treatment for several decades due to the lower morbidity and mortality.

In 1944, noting that radiation was not the ideal method of treatment, Meigs[4] cited its high incidence of severe morbidity as well as low salvage rates. For these reasons, he reintroduced radical surgery in 1945, reporting 65 consecutive operations without an operative death. Now, many pelvic surgeons prefer surgery for selected patients, although the cure rates for early-stage patients treated either by radiation therapy or surgery are equal.

Some differences in the techniques of Meigs and Wertheim should be mentioned. Wertheim's operation was less radical than the one performed by Meigs and was similar to what present-day gynecologic oncologists refer to as modified radical hysterectomy, type II operation[5] (Fig. 22-1). In addition, Wertheim did not perform node dissections in all instances. Meigs' operation involved extensive dissection of the pelvic nodes, the ureters, and the ureterosacral and cardinal ligaments. While Wertheim and the British surgeon, Bonney,[6] advocated exploratory operations to determine resectability and believed that parametrial induration was not a barrier to performing radical hysterectomy, Meigs advocated restricting the surgery to young healthy patients with early-stage disease, the ideal stage being stage IB. Gynecologic oncologists in the United States use Meigs' operation, the type III radical hysterectomy (Fig. 22-1) for clinical stage Ib and IIa cervical cancers, and many use the type II (modified) radical hysterectomy, Wertheim's operation, for more than microcarcinoma of the portio.

SELECTION OF PATIENTS

Radiation therapy as treatment for cancer of the cervix can be applied to all patients; the survival rate for early disease equals that of surgery. This technique has the disadvantage, however, of causing serious bladder or bowel damage in 2 to 6 percent of cases and vaginal stenosis with resultant sexual dysfunction in one-half of cases. Such radiation complications may be delayed in appearance and are often difficult to correct. By contrast, a surgical approach permits conservation of the ovaries (the adnexa are very rarely involved in early-stage disease), establishes the precise extent of the tumor, and leaves a more functional

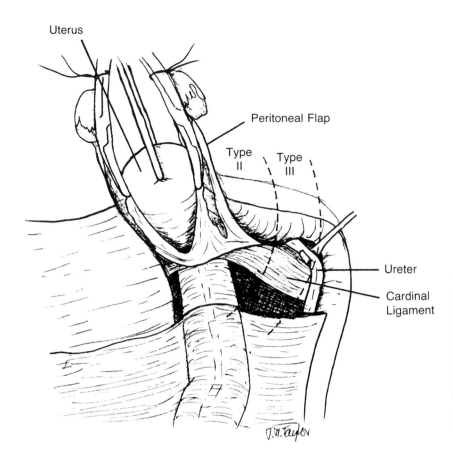

Uterus

Peritoneal Flap

Type II

Type III

Ureter

Cardinal Ligament

Fig. 22-1 The cardinal ligament is excised medially in women with microscopic lesions (type II operation) or laterally in those with larger volume lesions (type III operation). (Modified from Piver MS, Rutledge F, Smith JP: Five classes of extended hysterectomy for women with cervical cancer. Obstet Gynecol 44:265, 1974. Reprinted with permission from the American College of Obstetricians & Gynecologists.)

vagina; also, the major complications appear early and are more easily correctable. Surgical treatment has a psychological advantage to the woman in that it appears to be more decisive and has a shorter duration, and more prognostic information is made available.

The disadvantages of surgery are that thromboembolic phenomena, urologic injury or dysfunction, and occasional operative deaths occur. If the physician believes that discovery of metastatic disease to pelvic nodes requires postoperative whole-pelvis radiation therapy, the combination of the surgical dissection and the radiation therapy leads to more serious complications than does either modality alone. On the University of Alabama service, more than one-half of cervical cancer patients seen are diagnosed in stage IB and 60 to 70 percent of them are treated surgically. Usually excluded from surgical consideration are those over age 65; those who are morbidly obese (as this makes the procedure more difficult); and those with pulmonary, cardiovascular, or serious metabolic diseases. Those with stage IIB and III disease are excluded, not because they are unresectable (clinical stage III is approximately 50 percent inaccurate if one refers to the literature on surgical staging), but because high-volume lesions extending into the paracervical tissues are commonly associated with pelvic and extrapelvic node metastasis as well as close surgical margins. The major advantages of surgical treatment are lost if the disease is metastatic and adjunctive modalities are required thereafter.

THE OPERATION IN CONCEPT

In the ideal circumstance, radical hysterectomy is performed on the young slender woman in excellent general health and with small volume tumors. The uterus is resected en bloc with the paracervical lymphatics, vessels, and regional pelvic nodes; the pelvic lymph nodes are found to be negative for metastases, and an excellent margin is found around the primary tumor. With such a scenario, 5-year survival rates above 90 percent are expected. Under less than ideal circumstances (large lesions, nodal metastases, or poor surgical margins), the results are poorer. When nodal metastases or close margins are encountered, recurrence rates soar; such findings have often led many pelvic surgeons to advocate the use of adjunctive postoperative whole-pelvis radiotherapy. It is difficult, however, if not impossible, to show by literature review that radiotherapy used in this manner is effective and, indeed, salvages anyone.[7]

The completeness of the pelvic nodal dissections is a point in question. European surgeons appear to perform more extensive pelvic node dissections than do American surgeons, such operations being monitored by chlorophyll injected into the lymphatics (for better visualization) or under lymphangiographic control. Such meticulous and time-consuming node dissections may not be necessary, as they have not been shown to be associated with significantly higher salvage rates, while definitely associated with increased complications. For instance, Martimbeau et al.[8] reported lower extremity edema in 23 percent of women, 5 percent of whom had severe edema. The 5-year survival of Alabama patients with stage IB pelvic node metastases is 60 percent, equal to that reported by Martimbeau et al.[8] for the more extensive dissection, yet using the less meticulous node dissection technique, chronic leg edema occurred in less than 2 percent of cases.

Should a radical hysterectomy be abandoned if the patient has node metastases? In a recent informal survey of members of the Society of Gynecologic Oncologists, we found great variation in practice. A few stopped when any positive nodes were encountered and did not complete the hysterectomy; a considerable number of surgeons never stopped the procedure regardless of the number of positive nodes encountered or even in the presence of metastases to the aortic nodes. The question of whether the uterus should be removed in the presence of nodal metastasis is of interest. Bortolozzi et al.[9] and Heller et al.[10] reported increased 5-year survival in patients whose surgery was completed as compared with those patients in which the uterus was left in place as a receptacle for radium. Further studies are needed to answer these questions.

P.J. DiSaia (personal communication) posed the question of reevaluating the concept of en bloc dissections. He suggested that metastases to regional lymph nodes occur as embolic events, leaving the intervening normal tissue bridges at low risk. Certainly, the use of modified type II (Fig. 22-1) radical hysterectomy results in decreased morbidity from bladder dysfunction, so one might question the routine use of the type III Meigs operation for small lesions confined to the exocervix. Extirpation of the primary cervical tumor by total abdominal hysterectomy does not preclude pelvic node dissection; with proper patient selection, such a reduced operation might result in the same cure rate with better preservation of bladder function and resultant improved quality of life following the cancer treatment. Individualization of treatment for each patient seems in order.

PREOPERATIVE EVALUATION

The general history and physical examination should exclude those with the contraindications for surgery previously described. A chest radiograph and intravenous pyelogram are recommended to rule out pulmonary disease and urinary tract abnormalities, respectively. Postmenopausal women should have electrocardiograms (ECGs) performed to rule out subclinical cardiac disease. A blood chemistry profile focusing on hepatic and renal function is in order. Cystoscopic and proctoscopic examinations and barium enema studies are not essential in patients with small lesions, unless physical findings or symptoms suggest bladder or rectal invasion.

PROPHYLACTIC ANTIBIOTICS

While it is not clear that perioperative antibiotics reduce febrile morbidity in patients undergoing radical hysterectomy, the belief is that since they have proved effective in the treatment of women undergoing conservative hysterectomy, they should be effective in radical surgery as well. We have tended to use antibiotic coverage in radical hysterectomy patients and believe it decreases the risk of serious pelvic sepsis. This parallels experience of other authorities who believe that abscess formation is less likely in those treated by such regimens as single-dose doxycycline.[11]

The optimal number of doses for this purpose, and the appropriate drugs remain to be determined.

TECHNIQUE OF RADICAL HYSTERECTOMY AND BILATERAL PELVIC LYMPHADENECTOMY: SHINGLETON METHOD

We use the technique of Meigs for clinical stage IB and IIA lesions and a less radical technique for those with small-volume disease[12,13] (Fig. 22-1). Positioning of the patient is important, as is the availability of proper instruments (Figs. 22-2 and 22-3). A transverse incision of the Maylard type (muscle cutting) has been favored because of the lateral exposure for the pelvic lymphadenectomies, but it is true that a vertical midline incision permits better exposure for the periaortic node sampling, important in the patients with larger-volume lesions. Familiarity with the surgical anatomy is essential (Fig. 22-4). After manual exploration of the entire peritoneal cavity, particular attention is paid to the presence of suspicious lymph nodes either in the pelvis or along the aorta or common iliac vessels. A dissection of the aortic nodes between the bifurcation of the aorta and the renal vessels on the right side is carried out as well as dissections of nodes along both common iliac arteries

(Fig. 22-5). The left aortic nodes are not routinely sampled unless suspicious for metastases. These tissues are submitted for frozen section; if positive, we discontinue the surgical procedure and use the information gained in planning radiation therapy. Should the high nodes be negative, attention is turned to the pelvic nodes. After dividing the round ligament and ligating the infundibulopelvic ligaments bilaterally (in women over 40 whose ovaries are removed), the retroperitoneal space is widely opened and the pelvic vessels exposed. A careful dissection of nodal tissue by sharp and blunt dissection is carried out with separate specimens submitted from the common iliac, external iliac, and hypogastric and obturator areas (Fig. 22-6). While it is possible to dissect the nodes en bloc with the uterine specimen, it is more time-consuming to do so and offers no special advantage otherwise. We occasionally use small clips to close lymph vessels at the caudal portion of the pelvic node dissection, but make no serious attempt to ligate all open lymphatics. Careful attention is paid to avoiding damage to perforating vessels deep in the obturator fossa; venous bleeding in this area can be very troublesome and on occasion controlled only with packs. During this dissection, should matted nodes be found, or nodes attached to large vessels, one again might reconsider whether the surgery should proceed. We believe that if metastases are present bilaterally in the pelvic nodes or if nodes are densely attached to the major pelvic vessels, the

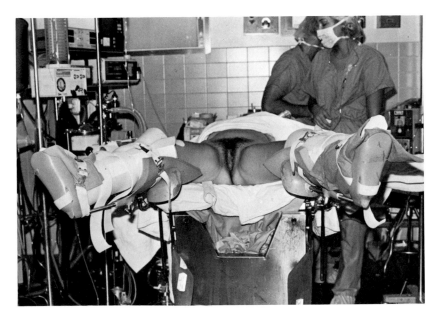

Fig. 22-2 Positioning of patient in stirrups (Crawford crutches) allows better access to the operative field for three surgeons.

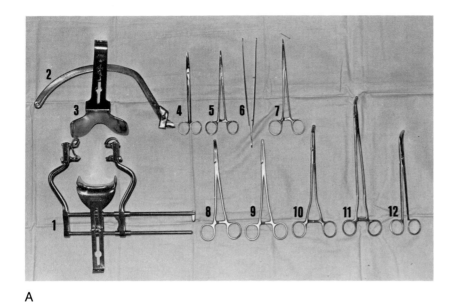

A

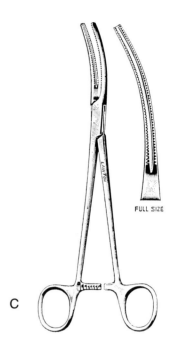

FULL SIZE

C

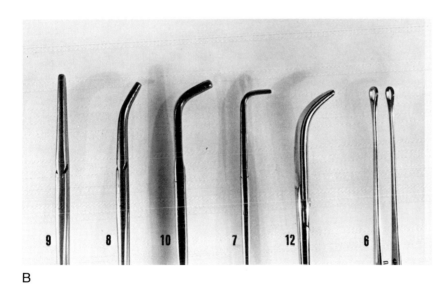

B

Fig. 22-3 Instruments for radical hysterectomy and node dissections. **(A)** Instruments, **(B)** Detail of selected instruments. 1. Balfour retractor. 2. Fourth blade extension arm. 3. Hammond winged retractor blade. 4. Potts-Smith scissors (sharp dissection). 5. Sawtell tonsil artery forcep (dissector). 6. Singley tissue forceps (for node dissections). 7. Mixter angular clamp forcep (right angle clamp). 8. Heaney-Ballentine curved hysterectomy forceps. 9. Heaney-Ballentine straight forceps. 10. Parametrium forceps. 11. Laing hysterectomy forcep. 12. Jorgenson scissors. **(C)** Gusberg hysterectomy clamp.

procedure should be terminated, leaving the uterus in place as a receptacle for intracavitary radioactive sources.

Should the decision be made to continue the operation after the node dissections, the uterine artery and vein are ligated at their junction with the hypogastric vessels laterally (Fig. 22-7A) and are reflected over the ureter (Fig. 22-7B). The ureter is separated from its peritoneal attachments in the deep pelvis and suspended on a penrose drain and by blunt dissection medial to the distal ureter, its entry into the cardinal ligament tunnel is identified. This tunnel is developed such that the further dissection of the vesicouterine ligament can be performed (Fig. 22-8). As part of this dissection, a peritoneal bladder flap is developed anterior to the cervix and the bladder dissected free from the vagina by sharp and blunt dissection. We have generally favored blunt (rather than sharp) dissection in the region of the tunnel and vesicouterine ligament and use a right-angle clamp (Fig. 22-8B) to develop

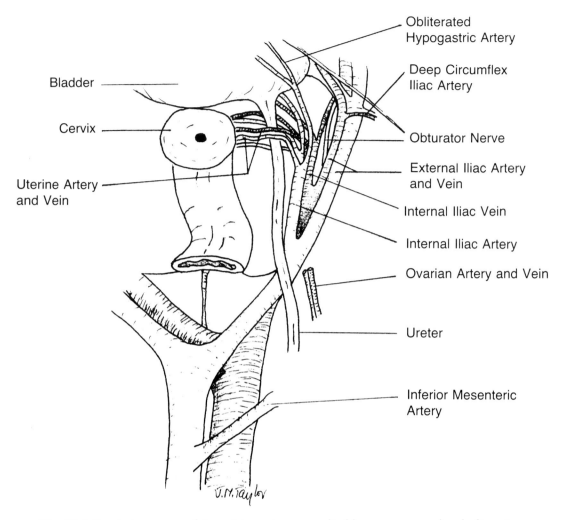

Bladder

Cervix

Uterine Artery
and Vein

Obliterated
Hypogastric Artery

Deep Circumflex
Iliac Artery

Obturator Nerve

External Iliac Artery
and Vein

Internal Iliac Vein

Internal Iliac Artery

Ovarian Artery and Vein

Ureter

Inferior Mesenteric
Artery

Fig. 22-4 Surgical anatomy of the pelvis pertinent to radical hysterectomy and node dissections.

the space beneath the ligament. Once the vesicouterine ligament is double-ligated and divided, further sharp dissection occurs to release the attachments of the ureter, especially posterior to the ureterovesical junction (Fig. 22-9). The bladder and ureterovesical junction can now be reflected away from the cardinal ligament, permitting that structure to be isolated, clamped, and divided (Fig. 22-10).

Dissection of the lower ureter and mobilization of the bladder angles are the most delicate and difficult part of this operation. Until this has been mastered, both in concept and in regard to the variation in anatomy from patient to patient, the operation may be associated with urologic injury and major bleeding.

Venous complexes beneath the ureterovesical junction and in the vicinity of the vesicouterine ligament are often prominent and must be handled with care. Most of the blood loss from the procedure (mean 1,900 ml) occurs at this stage of dissection and ends only with ligation of the cardinal ligaments and vaginal angles.

The cardinal ligament is further developed by dissecting the rectovaginal septum and the ligament is prepared for removal with the specimen. After bluntly separating the posterior vagina from the rectum in the open posterior cul-de-sac, we use gloved fingers to separate the medial portions of the uterosacral ligaments from the rectum as well. This permits

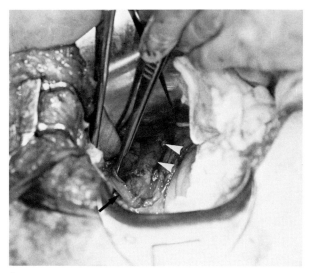
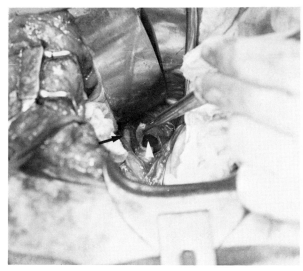

A

B

Fig. 22-5 Aortic node dissection. Fatty node-bearing tissue anterior to the vena cava in the area between the bifurcation of the aorta and the right renal artery is removed for frozen section, as are any other suspicious nodes on either side of the aorta. **(A)** The fat pad (white arrows) will be removed, exposing the underlying vena cava **(B)** (white arrow). In both views the right ureter is marked with a black arrow.

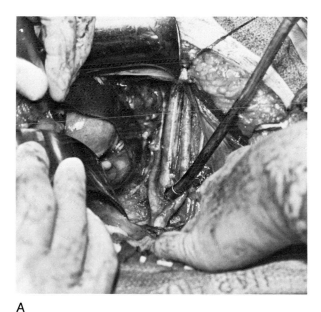
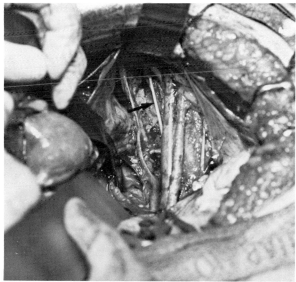

A

B

Fig. 22-6 Shingleton (HMS) technique: Pelvic node dissection. **(A)** Dissection of common iliac artery, external and internal iliac arteries, and veins in right pelvis. **(B)** Obturator fossa dissection with obturator nerve exposed (arrow).

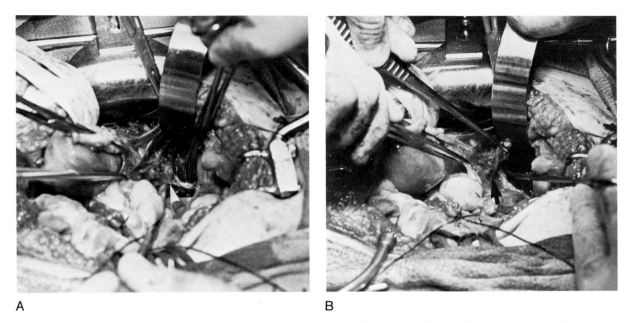

A   B

Fig. 22-7 HMS technique: Ligation of uterine vessels and initiation of ureteral dissection in right pelvis. **(A)** Uterine vessels exposed, crossing over the ureter (arrow). **(B)** After ligation, the uterine vessels are brought upward and the tunnel is developed medial to the ureter (arrow).

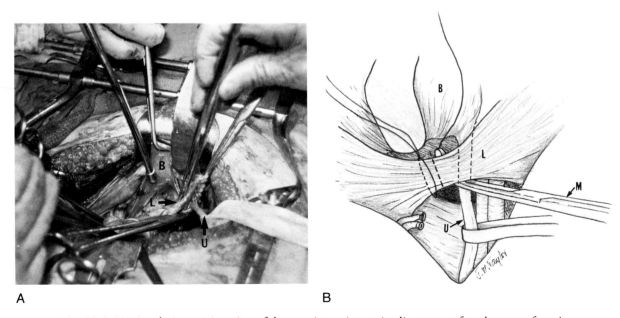

A   B

Fig. 22-8 HMS technique: Dissection of the anterior vesicouterine ligament to free the ureter from its tunnel. **(A)** The ureter passes below the anterior vesicouterine ligament as it enters the bladder. **(B)** A right angle clamp is passed medial to the ureter in the tunnel beneath the anterior portion of the vesicouterine ligament in order to pass ligatures around this tissue. B, bladder; U, ureter; L, vesicouterine ligament; M, Mixter right angle forcep.

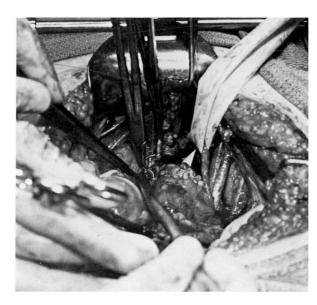

Fig. 22-9 HMS technique: Further dissection of the ureter involves its release from posterior attachments and mobilizing the ureterovesical function and bladder angle to allow isolation of the cardinal ligaments at the pelvic sidewall. Arrow, dissected bladder angle.

more distal excision of this ligament and prevents rectal injuries (Fig. 22-10). After excision of the uterosacral and cardinal ligaments, the vaginal angles can be clamped and the specimen excised (Fig. 22-11). The excised specimen (Fig. 22-12) has an ample vaginal margin; the wide lateral excision of the cardinal ligaments and uterine vessels is apparent. By varying the dissection of the bladder and ureterovesical junction, one can vary the length of upper vagina removed. Most or all of the vagina can be removed in this manner if the circumstances warrant, for example, as with vaginal extension of tumor.

After removal of the specimen, the vaginal cuff is managed with a running and locked absorbable suture along the cut edges (Fig. 22-13). The deep pelvis and node dissection areas can be drained by use of a Penrose drain brought out the vaginal cuff, while the dissection area can be closed off by reperitonealizing the pelvic floor with either running or interrupted sutures. Alternatively (and especially if hemostasis is excellent), one might elect to use suction drains brought out through a punch wound adjacent to the abdominal incision, after closing the vaginal cuff with hemostatic sutures. The abdominal incision is closed,

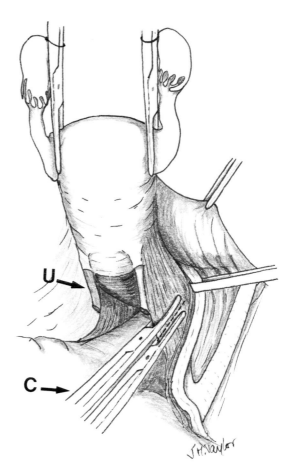

Fig. 22-10 HMS technique: After ligation of the uterosacral ligaments (U), Heaney-Ballentine clamps (C) (usually curved) are used for the first portion of the cardinal ligament. The rectum is carefully dissected away from the medial sides of the cardinal ligaments before these clamps are placed.

generally using a Smead-Jones en bloc technique, with staples used to close the skin. The average operation time for this operation is $3\frac{1}{2}$ hours on our service.

MODIFIED RADICAL HYSTERECTOMY

The operation proceeds as above, with the exception that the ureter can be unroofed by dividing the vesicouterine ligament superior to it. The ureter can be pushed aside without extensive detachment from the underlying tissues and peritoneum as described for

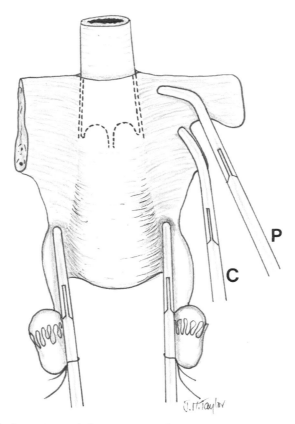

Fig. 22-11 HMS technique: An angled parametrium forcep (P) is used for the caudad portion of the cardinal ligament in order to guarantee excellent parametrial margins. The medial Heaney-Ballentine clamp (C) remains from the previous step. Curved Jorgensen scissors are used to excise the tissue at the medial side of the clamp. The cervix and upper vagina are shown diagramatically to denote the width of dissection.

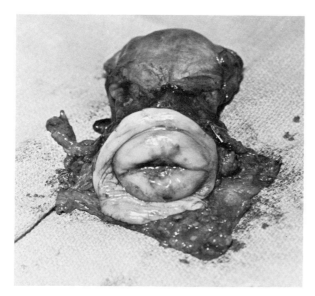

Fig. 22-12 HMS technique: Excised uterus with wide vaginal cuff and parauterine tissues. The ovaries were not removed in this patient.

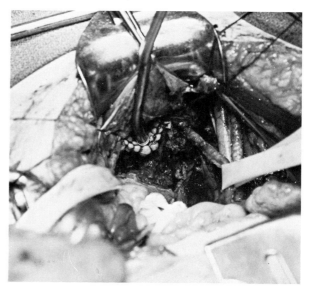

Fig. 22-13 HMS technique: Running locked sutures are used to secure the edges of the vaginal cuff or to close it. The ureters are held by Penrose drains for traction.

the type III operation. The cardinal ligament can be clamped and divided at the junction of the inner and middle thirds to assure some paracervical margin. This modification has the effect of decreasing chances of ureteral injury and bladder dysfunction associated with the more radical operation, to some degree because of less disturbance of bladder innervation.

TECHNIQUE OF RADICAL HYSTERECTOMY AND BILATERAL PELVIC LYMPHADENECTOMY: GUSBERG METHOD

The Gusberg operation incorporates the methods of Wertheim,[3] Meigs,[15] and Okabayashi[16] in its technical approach. It has been evolved by Gusberg over the years as the technique that will give the widest dissection compatible with the least pelvic disfiguration and the greatest surgical facility. The steps in this pelvic dissection may be outlined as follows:

1. Manual exploration is used for the pelvic side walls for operability, palpation of the paraortic regions for the presence of lumbar nodes, and careful palpation of the upper abdominal organs. Any palpable nodes of significance should be subjected to frozen section (Fig. 22-14A).

2. If operability is established, we begin by suture-ligating the infundibulopelvic and round ligaments close to the side wall. Following their division with scissors, the bladder flap is freed and blunt dissection permits the operator to free the bladder from the cervix and upper vagina in the central zone of the pelvis. The bladder pillars are allowed to remain laterally at this stage, although palpation lateral to them will usually permit definition of the lower ureters close to their entry into the bladder (Fig. 22-14B).

3. Sharp dissection with scissors will free the cul-de-sac now with care to avoid injury to the ureters laterally and the sigmoid colon centrally. As the uterosacral ligament is approached on each side, it must be clamped, suture-ligated, and divided close to the bowel. This will permit mobilization of the bowel and separation of the areolar tissue between it and the vagina to the depth of the dissection. This maneuver early in the operation affords greater facility in the later dissection of the parametria and ureteral tunnels. It will convert this later difficult area of dissection into a readily accessible tissue with great surgical freedom (Fig. 22-14C).

4. The lymphadenectomy is now carried out bilaterally. The peritoneum may need to be incised superior and medial to the infundibulopelvic ligature to attain the common iliac trunk after which the node-bearing fat over the external iliac vessels is cleared by blunt and sharp dissection down to the femoral canal with the careful dissection of the Cloquet's node region in its most inferior sweep. When its vessels are cleared of fat and areolar tissue, the psoas muscle and genitofemoral nerve are exposed. The operator should now return to the superior pole of the dissection and locate the bifurcation of the iliacs; the lymphatic chain here may then be ligated, the constant node dissected at the bifurcation, and then the node-bearing fat and areolar tissue freed along the hypogastric vessels, until the obturator fossa is reached. Gentle retraction of the external iliac vessels permits dissection of the obturator space until the obturator nerve and vessels are clean. As the dissection proceeds downward toward the paravesical fat and pelvic floor, the superior vesical-obliterated hypogastric artery and the uterine vessels are exposed. The former is preserved; the uterines are suture-ligated close to their hypogastric origin. The node-bearing fatty triangle is now separately excised unless its continuity with the specimen medially is firm enough to warrant preservation. In any case, the concept of en bloc dissection is not hampered (Fig. 22-14D). The pararectal and paravesical spaces are easily defined with the finger at this stage exposing the upper border of the parametrium, sometimes referred to as the web.

5. The ligature of the medial cut end of the uterine artery now points to the ureteral tunnel. The ureter may be freed from the roof of its tunnel by blunt dissection after which the tunnel is opened through its roof by sharp dissection with scissors. The ureter may now be freed completely from its attachment to the parametrium and to the cervix. Preservation of the delicate septum between the ureter and the superior vesical-obliterated hypogastric vessel and the small amount of loose tissue about the bladder entry will not restrict the radicality of the dissection but will aid in the prevention of later fistulae. Dissection of the bladder pillars will be necessary to reach the level of ureteral entry into the bladder and to free the bladder from the upper vagina (Fig. 22-14E).

6. With bladder, bowel, and ureters free, the poste-

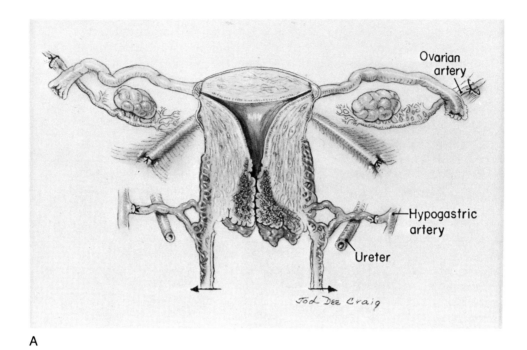

A

B

C

Fig. 22-14 Gusberg technique **(A)** Step 1, radical hysterectomy. **(B)** Step 2, radical hysterectomy. **(C)** Step 3, radical hysterectomy. (*Figure continues.*)

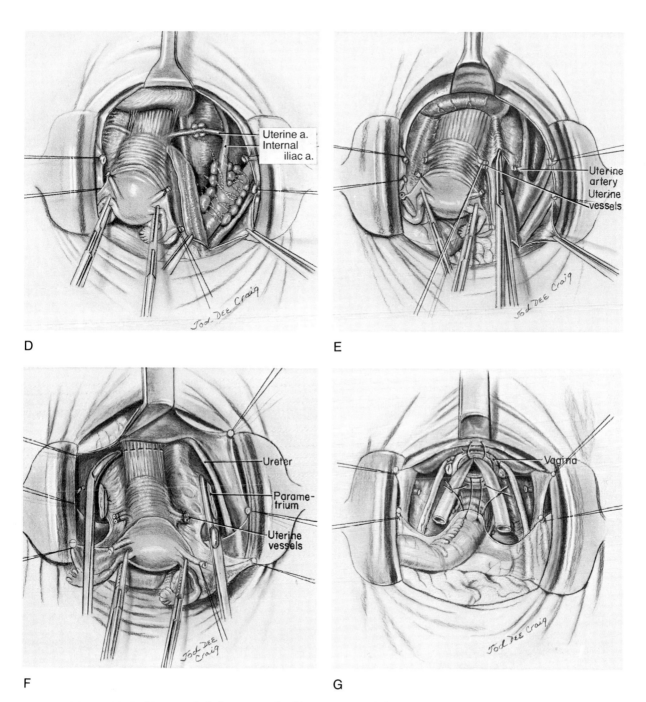

D

E

F

G

Figure 22-14 (*Continued*). (**D**) Step 4, radical hysterectomy. (**E**) Step 5, radical hysterectomy. (**F**) Step 6, radical hysterectomy. (**G**) Step 7, radical hysterectomy.

rior and lateral parametria may be clamped at the side walls, suture-ligated and freed. The paracolpos is also suture-ligated at the desired level, and the specimen is completely removed by incision through the vagina (Fig. 22-14F).

7. Peritonization is accomplished in the usual manner laterally, but the vaginal stump is used for central peritonization; that is, the bladder flap is sutured to the anterior vaginal wall and the sigmoid peritoneal flap to the posterior vaginal wall. With Penrose drains led into the vagina from each parametrial gutter, peritonization may be completed with a few stitches in the peritoneum over these drains (Fig. 22-14G).

RADICAL VAGINAL HYSTERECTOMY FOR CANCER OF THE CERVIX

As devised by Schauta[17] and carried forward by Mitra[18] and Adler,[19] this approach to cancer of the cervix is logical, except for the importance of removing the pelvic lymph nodes. This approach cannot be done efficiently from below. In order to overcome this objection, Mitra[20] devised a combined abdominal extraperitoneal lymphadenectomy and vaginal hysterectomy. Adler[19] improved the results of the operation by introducing radium into the tissues of the lateral pelvic wall after the vaginal removal of the uterus. Diaz-Bazan[21] reported the use of the Schauta[17] operation combined with lymphadenectomy in patients with carcinoma of the cervix associated with partial or complete procidentia. The technique and results of these studies are extremely interesting and worth studying. Partly from custom but more from the belief that the abdominal radical hysterectomy is more thorough, few surgeons have used this procedure in the modern era of safe abdominal surgery.

POSTOPERATIVE CARE

Drainage from the denuded pelvis and ileus and bladder care require the attention of the surgeon in the first few postoperative days. Accumulated lymph and serum in the retroperitoneal pelvic spaces is to be avoided. Many pelvic surgeons advocate the use of pelvic suction drains for a number of days until the drainage from each side decreases to 30 ml/day or less.

Others advocate leaving the vaginal cuff open and draining the retroperitoneal spaces using Penrose drains. The Penrose drains have been used successfully in hundreds of operations in Alabama and New York without contributing to infectious morbidity or to increased ureteral complications. We believe that either method of drainage is acceptable and have used both. In those patients who have copious drainage of serum, one should be wary of loss of serum albumin. Serum proteins should be checked postoperatively and replaced if the albumin falls below 2.5 g/dl. In regard to avoidance of ileus, we keep the patient nil per os (NPO) for 2 or 3 days, until such time as bowel function is apparent. We have never advocated the use of nasogastric tubes routinely following this operation, nor do we consider them beneficial. Ambulation is encouraged even on the first postoperative day. The bladder is drained in all instances using a suprapubic Foley catheter. Our habit is to discharge the patient within 7 to 10 days postoperatively without voiding trials and 2 to 3 weeks postoperatively to perform a residual urine determination and voiding trial. This is accomplished by filling the bladder to the point of urgency through the suprapubic tube and asking the patient to void. Once voiding is possible, the suprapubic tube is removed. This can be accomplished in more than 90 percent of patients by the twenty-first postoperative day. A few require more protracted catheter drainage, and only very rarely have we had to suggest intermittent self-catheterization as a method of bladder drainage. The high percentage of patients with bladder atony reported in former years was almost certainly the result of overdistention of the bladder secondary to use of transurethral catheters; atony as such is a very rare complication if suprapubic drainage is used.[22]

MORBIDITY AND COMPLICATIONS

The more serious complications include (infectious) morbidity, urologic injury, and thromboembolic phenomena. Other complications include development of lymphocysts, bladder dysfunction, ureteral strictures, and stress urinary incontinence.

Infections occur in significant numbers of patients following radical hysterectomy. In reporting 311 patients having surgery at the University of Alabama at Birmingham, Orr[23] found 33 percent of patients to have febrile morbidity. Early (days 1 to 2) fever ordinarily relates to pulmonary atalectasis, while later morbidity is attributable to urinary tract infections, wound infections, infected hematoma, pelvic cellulitis, pelvic or deep vein thrombophlebitis, or pelvic abscess. Pelvic cellulitis and abscess accounted for 10 percent of morbidity; such infections were thought to be especially ominous in that they may predispose patients to developing urinary fistulae due to the close proximity of pelvic infection, ureters, and bladder.

UROLOGIC INJURY

Ureteral fistulas, the scourge of pelvic surgeons of an earlier era (usual fistula rate: 12 to 15 percent), are now uncommon complications of radical hysterectomy. In a collected series of 4,860 patients,[13] the

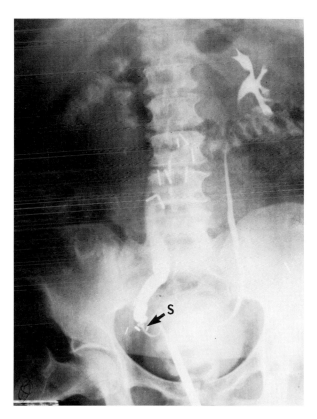

Fig. 22-15 Dilated ureter above a ureteral stricture (S) in a 54-year-old woman 2½ years following a radical hysterectomy for squamous cell carcinoma, as demonstrated by retrograde pyelogram. The stricture was managed by percutaneous placement of an internalized pigtail ureteral stent.

ureteral fistula rate was 2.3 percent and the vesicovaginal fistula rate 0.58 percent. The rates in these categories at Alabama are 1.4 percent and 0.23 percent, respectively. Ureteral strictures following radical surgery in the absence of pelvic radiotherapy are even less common than are fistulas. Ureteral fistulas and strictures are managed successfully in most instances by ureteral stenting using percutaneous techniques, even in patients in whom transvesical retrograde catheter replacement is unsuccessful. This recent advance in management reduces the necessity for repeat operations in most instances (Fig. 22-15).

BLADDER DYSFUNCTION AND URINARY INCONTINENCE

Voiding dysfunction related to partial bladder denervation resulting from the cardinal ligament excision presents more serious problems to more patients than do either fistulas or strictures. Following radical hysterectomy, diminished bladder sensation, voiding dysfunction, and stress incontinence are commonly encountered. In fact, many women complain of some degree of desensitization of the bladder, but this improves with time. Following surgery, a transient hypertonic bladder phase occurs, slowly returning to normal function over a few weeks. Stress urinary incontinence is more common following this surgery than previously appreciated or reported, occurring in 10 to 52 percent of women.[24] The precise mechanism of this incontinence is unclear due to paucity of well-designed, well-controlled studies including both preoperative and postoperative objective testing. Farquharson et al.[25] at Alabama demonstrated no evidence of loss of bladder neck support as a cause of postoperative incontinence in radical hysterectomy patients; Low et al[26] confirmed a reduction in urethral closure pressure previously reported. Farquharson and Orr[27] found that an appreciable number of patients had preexisting bladder dysfunction and theorized that those with borderline preoperative vesical neck function developed incontinence due to reduced urethral pressures occurring postoperatively. They observed that one-half of women following radical hysterectomy voided by abdominal straining compared with only 10 percent who were treated exclusively by radiotherapy. In other studies, Farquharson et al.[28] observed that in more than one-half of women who had radical hysterectomy followed by postoperative radiation therapy urinary incontinence developed; in this group, the severity of the incontinence was considerably greater as compared with those developing incontinence following the operation alone.

THROMBOEMBOLIC EVENTS: PROPHYLAXIS

The recent literature on the use of minidose heparin fails to demonstrate a decrease in pulmonary emboli when comparing those receiving low-dose heparin with control groups. The risk factors for thromboembolic phenomena are weight in excess of 85.5 kg, advanced stage of malignancy, and radiation therapy within 6 weeks of the operative procedure.[29] For a number of years at Alabama, we used minidose heparin (2,500 units SC on the morning of surgery). After documenting that the intraoperative blood loss was significantly higher in such patients and failing to be convinced that minidose heparin invariably prevented postoperative pulmonary emboli, we have more recently switched to the use of pneumatic calf compression by an externally applied device. Such calf compression has been shown to be effective in studies from this institution[27] as well as other centers.[30] The intermittent pressure is applied to the large calf muscles during surgery as well as in the first 1 to 2 postoperative days prior to full ambulation.

RARER COMPLICATIONS

Lymphocysts are uncommon findings following radical abdominal hysterectomy, perhaps related to better techniques of draining the retroperitoneal space used in recent years. We have seen only one symptomatic lymphocyst in the past 600 operations; in a collected series of almost 2,500 patients (including our own), the mean rate of lymphocysts was 2.1 percent.[31] Asymptomatic lymphocysts can be managed conservatively and often resolve over time. Percutaneous drainage under sonographic control might be tried if deemed necessary; if surgery is elected for treatment, opening and unroofing the lymphocyst from an abdominal approach has been suggested. We have not had occasion to treat any in this fashion.

Other complications include nerve injuries or vessel injuries during the course of the procedure. The obturator nerve may be damaged or divided and may result in a weakness in adduction of the thigh. Femoral neuropathies may occur if the blades of self-retaining retractors are used to compress the psoas muscles. Peroneal nerve damage may occur from pressure on the popliteal fossa when the patient's legs remain in stirrups during the operation. Such nerve damage may result in a foot drop that may last for weeks or months. Repair of lacerations of the vena cava or of large pelvic arteries and veins require skills in vascular surgery on the part of the pelvic surgeon, or consultation with those who possess such skills.

Operative deaths are rare. In a collected series consisting of 4,860 patients,[23] the mean operative death rate was 0.45 percent (range 0 to 1.4 percent). Currently, our operative mortality is one in 600 operations, or 0.17 percent.

TREATMENT RESULTS

The expected 5-year survival of surgically treated stage IB cervical cancer patients is 85 to 90 percent, depending on the volume of tumors in any given series. At the University of Alabama at Birmingham, we have achieved a 5-year survival rate of 92 percent, and 10-year survival of 79 percent. Survival after radical surgery can be related to lesion size, positivity of nodes, and the number and location of the positive lymph nodes. In regard to lesion size, we recently reported 181 patients with surgically treated stage IB cervical cancer, in whom those with lesions less or equal to 2 cm in diameter had a 5-year survival of 91.4 percent.[32] Patients whose lesions were over 2 cm had a 5-year survival of 63.9 percent. Recurrences can be related to lesion diameter and depth of stromal invasion (Fig. 22-16). These figures are similar to those reported by other recent authors. Reduced survival of women with stage IB lesions exceeding 2, 3, or 4 cm treated surgically has been used often as a justification for recommending radiotherapy as the primary treatment for all such women. At Alabama, using modern radiation therapy techniques, we have been unable to show an advantage in survival in the bulky stage IB lesions using radiotherapy as the sole therapy, yet concede that women with such bulky lesions are much more likely to have nodal metastases than are those with smaller lesions and thus are not routinely considered good operative candidates for that reason.

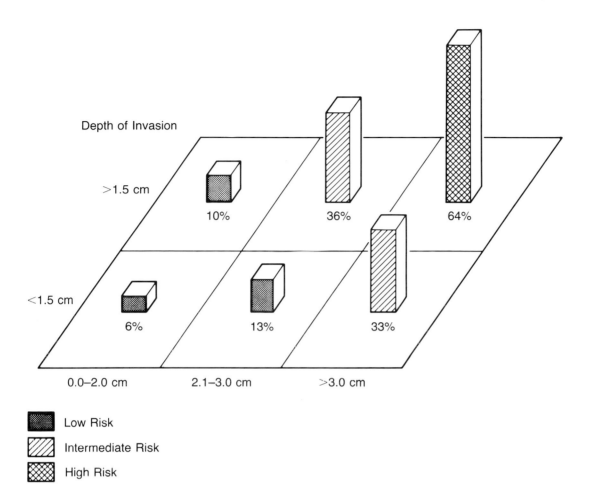

Depth of Invasion

>1.5 cm

10%   36%   64%

<1.5 cm

6%   13%   33%

0.0–2.0 cm   2.1–3.0 cm   >3.0 cm

Low Risk

Intermediate Risk

High Risk

Fig. 22-16 Stage IB squamous cell carcinoma of the cervix; recurrence rates in 100 patients by size of lesion and depth of stromal invasion. (Gauthier P, Gore I, Shingleton HM et al: Identification of histopathologic risk groups in stage 1B squamous cell carcinoma of the cervix. Obstet Gynecol 66: 569, 1985.)

One might make the argument, however, that the young patient (under age 35) with a large-volume stage IB tumor might be offered surgical exploration in any event (and resection if feasible) in an attempt to be aggressive in management and to guarantee that all disease is included in the treatment fields of subsequent radiotherapy. Selection of radiotherapy as sole therapy in this group of patients often fails to consider the significant number of women with extrapelvic nodal disease, much of which cannot be demonstrated by CT scanning or lymphangiography. The potential for gaining valuable information and altering therapy by surgically staging this group of women should be apparent.

REFERENCES

1. Ries E: Eine neue Operationsmethode des Uteruscarcinoms. Z Geburt Gynaekol 32:266, 1895
2. Clark JG: More radical method of performing hysterectomy for cancer of the uterus. Johns Hopkins Hosp. Bull 6:120, 1895
3. Wertheim E: The extended abdominal operation for carcinoma uteri: Based on 500 operated cases (Gradd H transl.) J Obstet Gynecol Dis Women Child 66:169, 1912
4. Meigs JV: Carcinoma of the cervix — The Wertheim operation. Surg Gynecol Obstet 78:195, 1944
5. Piver MS, Rutledge F, Smith JP: Five classes of ex-

tended hysterectomy for women with cervical cancer. Obstet Gynecol 44:265, 1974

6. Bonney V: The treatment of carcinoma of the cervix by Wertheim's operation. Am J Obstet Gynecol 30:815, 1935

7. Baltzer J, Kopcke W, Lohe KJ, et al: Surgical treatment of cervical carcinoma. Geburt Frauenheilkd 44:279, 1984

8. Martimbeau PW, Kjorstad KE, Iversen T: Stage IB carcinoma of the cervix, the Norwegian Radium hospital. II. Results when pelvic nodes are involved. Obstet Gynecol 60:315, 1982

9. Bortolozzi G, Rossi F, Mantioni C, Candiani GB: A contribution to the therapy of cervicocarcinoma: Remarks on 40 patients presenting paraaortic metastases (1970–1979). Eur J Gynaecol Oncol 4:9, 1983

10. Heller PB, Lee RB, Leman MH, Park RC: Lymph node positivity in cervical cancer. Gynecol Oncol 12:328, 1981

11. Rosenshein NB, Ruth JC, Villar J, et al: A prospective randomized study of doxycycline as a prophylactic antibiotic in patients undergoing radical hysterectomy. Gynecol Oncol 15:201, 1983

12. Shingleton HM, Palumbo L Jr: Ureteral complications of radical hysterectomy: Effects of preoperative radium and ureteral catheters. Surg Forum 19:410, 1968

13. Shingleton HM, Orr JW Jr: Cancer of the Cervix: Its Diagnosis and Treatment. 2nd Ed. Churchill Livingstone, Edinburgh, 1987

14. Gusberg SB, Frick HC II (eds): Corscaden's Gynecologic Cancer. 5th Ed. Williams & Wilkins, Baltimore, 1978

15. Meigs JV: Results of surgical treatment of cancer of the cervix uteri. AJR 65:698, 1951

16. Okabayashi H: Radical abdominal hysterectomy for cancer of the cervix uteri. Surg Gynecol Obstet 33:335, 1921

17. Schauta F: Die Berechtigung des vaginalen. Totalestirpation bei Gebarmutterkrebs. Monatsschr Geburt Gynakol Berl 19:475, 1904

18. Mitra S: A new approach to the extended radical vaginal hysterectomy for cancer of the cervix. Cancer 6:765, 1953

19. Adler L: Treatment of cervical cancer. Acta Radiol (Stockh) 28:474, 1947

20. Mitra S: Extraperitoneal lymphadenectomy and radical vaginal hysterectomy for cancer of the cervix (Mitra technique). Am J Obstet Gynecol 78:191, 1959

21. Diaz-Bazan N: Histerectomia radical vaginal (operation de Schauta) en cancer y prolapso. Arch Col Med Salv 21(3):156, 1968

22. Green TH Jr, Meigs JV, Ulfelder H, Curtin RR: Urologic complications of radical Wertheim hysterectomy: Incidence, etiology, management and prevention. Obstet Gynecol 20:293, 1962

23. Orr JW Jr, Shingleton HM, Hatch KD, et al: Correlation of perioperative morbidity and conization-radical hysterectomy interval. Obstet Gynecol 59:726, 1982

24. Petri E: Bladder after radical pelvic surgery. p. 220. In Stanton SL (ed): Clinical Gynecologic Urology. CV Mosby, St. Louis, 1984

25. Farquharson DIM, Varner RE, Orr JW, et al: Immediate and short term effects of abdominal and vaginal hysterectomy on bladder function and symptomatology. J Obstet Gynaecol 7:279, 1987

26. Low JA, Mauger GM, Carmichael JA: The effect of Wertheim hysterectomy upon bladder and urethral function. Am J Obstet Gynecol 139:826, 1981

27. Farquharson DIM, Orr JW Jr: Thromboembolic complications in gynecology. J Reprod Med 29:845, 1984

28. Farquharson DIM, Shingleton HM, Sanford SP, et al: The adverse effects of cervical cancer treatment on bladder function. Gynecol Oncol 27:15, 1987

29. Clarke-Pearson DL, Jelovsek FR, Creasman WT: Thromboembolism complicating surgery for cervical and uterine malignancy: Incidence, risk factors and prophylaxis. Obstet Gynecol 61:87, 1983

30. Clarke-Pearson DL, Synan IS, Hinshaw WM, et al: Prevention of postoperative venous thromboembolism by external pneumatic calf compression in patients with gynecologic malignancy. Obstet Gynecol 63:92, 1984

31. Orr JW Jr, Shingleton HM: Choosing the best urinary diversion in gynecology patients. Contemp Obstet-Gynecol 22:253, 1983

32. Gauthier P, Gore I, Shingleton HM, et al: Identification of histopathologic risk groups in Stage IB squamous cell carcinoma of the cervix. Obstet Gynecol 66:569, 1985

SUGGESTED READINGS

Kottmeier HC (ed): The Annual Report of the Results of Treatment in Gynecologic Cancer: Statement of Results Obtained in 1973 to 1975 Inclusive. Vol. 18. Stockholm, International Federation of Gynecology and Obstetrics, 1982

Masterson BJ: Manual of Gynecologic Surgery. 2nd Ed. Springer-Verlag, New York, 1986

Mattingly RF: Te Linde's Operative Gynecology. 5th Ed. JB Lippincott, Philadelphia, 1977

Meigs JV (ed): Surgical Treatment of Cancer of the Cervix: Radical Hysterectomy with Bilateral Dissection of the

Pelvic Lymph Nodes. Grune & Stratton, New York, 1954

Nelson JH Jr: Atlas of Radical Pelvic Surgery. Appleton-Century-Crofts, E. Norwalk, CT, 1985

Parsons L, Ulfelder H: An Atlas of Pelvic Operations. WB Saunders, Philadelphia, 1968

Simon NL, Orr JW Jr, Hatch KD, Shingleton HM: Lower extremity edema due to deep vein thrombosis in patients with recurrent cervix cancer. Gynecol Oncol 19:30, 1984

Wheeless CR: Atlas of Pelvic Surgery. Lea & Febiger, Philadelphia, 1981

23

Pelvic Exenteration

Hugh R. K. Barber

During the 1940s, pelvic exenteration was an operation whose time had come. By the 1950s, there were approximately 29,000 new cases of cancer of the cervix with 10,000 deaths, and 11,000 new cases of carcinoma of the endometrium with 4,000 deaths. Since approximately 50 percent of these cases would present as persistent or recurrent carcinomas, a new modality of therapy had to be employed. Since many of these had previously been treated by radiation therapy, additional therapy of this type would only increase the complication rate and would not improve the survival rate. Chemotherapy, hormonal therapy, and immunotherapy as employed today was in its infancy at that time.

The projected figures for 1987 are as follows[1]: cervical cancer, 12,800 new cases with 6,800 deaths; carcinoma of the endometrium, 35,000 new cases with 2,900 deaths; and cancer of the ovary, 19,000 new cases with 11,700 deaths. For other and unspecified genital female cancer, 4,600 new cases with 1,100 deaths. It is interesting to evaluate these figures; stage for stage, not a great deal of progress has been made, but in the overall evaluation the mortality has dropped, and survival rate has improved. This is due in no small measure to a better informed public and professional groups, translated into early diagnosis. The American Cancer Society (ACS) and the National Cancer Institute (NCI) have played a role in achieving these results.

During World War II and immediately after, there was increased interest in advancing the frontiers of surgery. Better trained surgeons with improved backup teams and ancillary services expanded the role of surgery, and the era of radical surgery was born.

Joe Vincent Meigs and Alexander Brunschwig were among the pioneers in advancing radical surgery for cancer of the pelvic organs. In 1939 Meigs combined the Wertheim procedure with the Taussig node dissection and introduced the radical hysterectomy with pelvic node dissection. Although he selected his cases for surgery during the early years of his program, it served to prove that surgery could be carried out with a low morbidity and very low mortality. Brunschwig, however, operated on all comers with selection held to a minimum and confirmed the possibility of low morbidity and mortality.

Approximately 40 years have passed since Brunschwig carried out the first one-stage pelvic exenteration for pelvic cancer. At that time, there were no guidelines, the operation was attempted in any and all cases in which the possibility existed that the disease could be cured and reasonable palliation achieved. The necessary surgical technique had to be established initially and then with greater experience had to be refined. Pitfalls of the operation were gradually elucidated, often by bitter experience, but in the end, Brunschwig and his students learned how to do the operation so that the patient would have the maximum chance for survival and possible cure. Brunschwig must be given the credit for planning, expediting, and producing an additional operative procedure for the treatment of advanced pelvic cancer.

At that time, there were few certified radiation therapists in the United States, and radiotherapy was lagging behind surgery. The lack of trained radiotherapists resulted in a great number of pelvic cancers that recurred locally or persisted. It was this group that responded best to a radical surgical approach. At the same time, basic research was expanding, and fluid and electrolyte therapy had been initiated during World War II. The use of blood transfusions, central venous monitoring, increased number of antibiotics helped advance the indications for pelvic exenteration. The question is rightfully asked as to why so many exenterations were carried out during the late 1940s, 1950s, and 1960s, with the current decrease in number. The answer is that with better trained radiotherapists there are very few central recurrences and other modalities can be employed, such as chemotherapy and hormonal therapy. The pelvic exenteration was born out of frustration resulting from inadequacy of therapy available to patients at that time who were condemned by the ravages of recurrent and persistent gynecologic cancer. Much of that has been eliminated today.

Having studied with and been associated with Alexander Brunschwig, I can give first-hand information on the evolution of the operation. Brunschwig reported that between 1935 and 1937 he made a few desultory attempts to excise the bladder, prostate, and colon for advanced cancer of the colon by a three-stage operation: (1) colostomy; (2) cutaneous ureterostomies or nephrostomies; and (3) excisions of pelvic organs; however, the results were disappointing, morbidity was high, and the technique was not pursued.

Brunschwig returned to this operation in December 1946 and carried out an en bloc one-stage excision of the bladder, vagina, uterus, lower ureters, and rectocolon, with thorough node dissection as well as the construction of a so-called wet colostomy wherein the ureters were put directly into the colostomy. Subsequently, he did two more pelvic exenterations in early 1947. Later, at the Memorial Hospital in New York City, the one-stage procedure was performed as frequently as patients presented with the proper indications, and the first clinical report was published in 1948.[2] A less radical procedure, the anterior pelvic exenteration, was devised and reported in 1950. Brunschwig considered the term exenteration more appropriate for the operation than the original term visceral evisceration. He pointed out that the exenteration is surgical removal of the inner organs commonly used to indicate radical excision of the contents of a body cavity as of the pelvis. Used in connection with the eye, it denotes removal of the entire contents of the orbit.

Some credit Appleby[3] with doing the first pelvic exenteration. In 1950, he reported on six patients who had a proctocystectomy with ureteral transplantation; four were followed for $4\frac{1}{2}$ to 7 years. However, Alexander Brunschwig is traditionally identified with pelvic exenteration for recurrent cervical cancer and is credited with planning, expediting, and producing an additional operative procedure for the treatment of advanced pelvic cancer. The greatest number of cases was carried out at the Memorial-James Ewing Hospital from 1947 until approximately 1970. During this time, there was an increasing realization of the need for teamwork by radiotherapists and surgically oriented gynecologists in exploring the potential of existing techniques, and possibly the development of new ones, giving promise for improving the survival rate. This new orientation has changed the emphasis from which is better — radiation or surgery — to a more enlightened attitude of which is better for a given patient; whether surgery or radiation or combinations of treatment. In turning from treating the cancer to treating the patient with cancer, the philosophy has swung from standardization to individualized therapy.

TYPES OF EXENTERATION

Essentially there are three types of exenteration: anterior, posterior, and total pelvic.[4] The total pelvic exenteration is a synthesis of four major procedures: (1) radical hysterectomy with pelvic lymph node dissection and excision and bilateral salpingo-oophorectomy, (2) total cystectomy, (3) combined abdominoperineal resection of the rectum, and (4) construction of a colostomy and a urinary conduit. An anterior pelvic exenteration is employed to encompass disease located in the region of the bladder; it is a fusion of radical cystectomy, radical hysterectomy, bilateral pelvic lymph node dissection, bilateral salpingo-oophorectomy, and vaginectomy with the construction of an ileo conduit.

In those instances in which the malignant disease

arises in the posterior wall of the fornix and involves the rectovaginal septum and the rectum, a posterior pelvic exenteration may be indicated to excise the disease en bloc. In a posterior exenteration, which is merely an extended form of abdominoperineal resection, a radical excision of the lower bowel and rectum is carried out along with radical hysterectomy, bilateral pelvic lymph node dissection, bilateral salpingo-oophorectomy, and vaginectomy with the construction of a colostomy. The posterior exenteration should not be employed except in extremely rare instances for the management of cancer of the cervix. In cancer of the cervix that is recurrent, persistent, or extensive, it is important to remove most of the vagina. This leaves the bladder denuded, and the slough and fistula rate is too high to be an acceptable method of management of cancer of the cervix.

THE ROLE OF PELVIC EXENTERATION

The number of articles appearing in the literature in the past 5 years indicates that fewer pelvic exenterations are being done. It is difficult to understand this when the patients with recurrent pelvic cancer have a 40 or 50 percent second chance to live when the indications are carefully followed. Chemotherapy and hormonal and immunotherapy have not been able to provide anywhere near these good results.[5] The ideal patient is one with recurrent or persistent carcinoma of the cervix with central recurrence. Ten major cancers have been subject to pelvic exenteration and in another 10 rare cancers pelvic exenteration has been employed to provide cure or palliation. Palliation as used in this presentation does not mean prolonging the patient's life, but rather prolonging the patient's life with the quality that provides dignity and with the patient able to carry out her usual lifestyle.

In the beginning of the exenteration project, the survival and the mortality approximately equalled each other. However, with better selection the survival rate has approached 50 percent with a mortality rate of less than 5 percent. It is important that the physician carrying out the procedure have knowledge of pelvic anatomy and the ability to carry out the procedure in less than 6 hours. The blood loss should be held to fewer than five bottles of blood and in very favorable cases one or no bottles of blood are required.

The team concept has taken hold in carrying out a pelvic exenteration. There may be many reasons for this: (1) for the urologist and the general surgeon to have enough cases to maintain their expertise, and (2) it may represent an effort on the part of the gynecologist to solicit their goodwill. Unfortunately, in my opinion, this approach decreases the expertise of the gynecologist and damages the aim of the division of gynecologic oncology of the American Board of Obstetrics and Gynecology. With time, the gynecologic oncologist will either be an interested spectator or a consultive observer. The two- and three-team approach is to be discouraged. The exenteration is most commonly carried out for gynecologic lesions and is therefore ideally performed by a surgically oriented gynecologist who will benefit the patient most.

PREOPERATIVE EVALUATION TO DETERMINE OPERABILITY AND RESECTABILITY

History

The overall general health of the patient is important in the outcome of management of patients with advanced or recurrent cancer of the pelvis.[6] The cardiopulmonary and renal systems must be carefully evaluated prior to surgery. Metabolic problems should be corrected.

The age of the patient at diagnosis is an important but highly variable factor. Chronologic age is not as important as physiologic age. However, at age 70 and older, the patient must be carefully evaluated. In this age group, when one complication occurs, it is usually followed by a series of complications that all too often result in a hospital mortality. In addition to the age of the patient, there are other considerations. The time that has elapsed from the initial treatment to the recurrence is important. If the interval is short, patients usually do not do well because of either the potency of the tumor or the decreased immunologic response of the patient. Patients with stages I and II disease with recurrence or persistence do infinitely better than those patients who have recurrence after stage III disease. Weight loss over a short period of time, anemia without obvious blood loss, and swelling of the leg with pain radiating down the back of the leg are all associated with decreased chance of removal of the tumor.

Physical Appearance

In general, the chronically ill, pale, emaciated patient who has difficulty ambulating is a poor candidate for pelvic exenteration. The extremely obese patient presents not only technical difficulties during the procedure but is a difficult patient to care for postoperatively. Many develop severe pulmonary complications. Any evidence of extrapelvic spread is a contraindication to surgery. In general, as the tumor spreads from the midline toward the pelvic wall, the incidence of complication increases and the survival decreases. A large infected cancer is often followed by a stormy course with sepsis despite the potent broad-spectrum antibiotics available today.

Laboratory Data

The usual metastatic work-up should be carried out. However, the backbone of the laboratory work-up consists of blood count, urinalysis, blood chemistry, intravenous pyelogram, chest radiograph, and electrocardiogram (ECG). A variety of other scans and tests are optional. However, the best and the most accurate evaluation can be carried out at exploratory surgery.

Ideally, the patient should be admitted to the hospital approximately 2 days before the scheduled surgery. However, with the current diagnosis related groups and peer review organizations programs, this is difficult to do and the bowel prep must be managed on the outside. However, by careful instruction, the patient will be able to do this fairly well. The bowel prep should be both mechanical and with antibiotics. The anesthesia should be supervised by an expert anesthesiologist who works carefully with the gynecologic surgeon in managing the patient during the procedure and during the immediate postoperative period. From the preoperative workup and evaluation, it can be determined whether the patient is a candidate for exploratory laparotomy.

Resectability

Having determined that there is no contraindication to surgery, the patient is taken to the operating room for exploratory laparotomy and anticipated pelvic exenteration. The patient's tumor is determined to be operable by the preoperative workup, but resectability will depend on the findings at exploratory laparotomy.

The patient is ideally prepared by being placed in the frog position with the legs flexed and the knees out to the side with the soles of the feet brought together. By careful preparation of the vagina and rectum, it is possible for the operating surgeon to palpate the lower pelvis and serve as a general guide during the procedure. The abdomen is ideally opened through a left paramedian incision extending up above the umbilicus. The pelvis and abdomen should be washed with fluid to detect any positive cytology. Ideally, this should be spun down and examined immediately. Visceral and paraaortic involvement has proved to be associated with very poor survival. However, there are a limited number of cases in which the small bowel has dropped against the tumor and can be resected en bloc with excision of all the tumor or a small local encroachment of the tumor on the large bowel, which can be resected with the potential for extended survival or marked palliation. However, if the mesentery of the bowel is involved, the procedure should be abandoned.

Pelvic Evaluation

Difficulty in establishing the planes of dissection often indicates extension of disease. These areas should be very carefully biopsied. The planes should be adequately opened to determine whether the disease has extended too far laterally or is attached to the levator (and would therefore be nonresectable). This should be done very early in the procedure and is described under Technique.

Patients with positive nodes at the periphery of the pelvis must be carefully evaluated before continuing with the pelvic exenteration.[7] The survival rate among these patients is very poor, and there is increased morbidity and mortality. Two nodes in the same chain is not nearly as bad as a single node in two separate chains; when there is contralateral involvement, the results achieved by the author have been dismal. The presence of positive pelvic nodes following radiation therapy for cure carries a poor survival. The question is often raised whether pelvic bone excision has any place in the management of pelvic exenteration. In patients in whom the bone is excised in order to get a wide margin, a small survival rate may be anticipated, but in the presence of positive bone histology the procedure should be abandoned. The question of bone excision usually has relevance only in those patients who have carcinoma of the vulva.

Other Considerations

The intravenous pyelogram has prognostic significance. It has been observed that if the obstruction occurs at the ureterovesical junction, the 5-year survival figures are similar to those patients in whom normal bilateral visualization is recorded. However, the survival rate falls progressively as the blockage occurs deeper in the pelvis, reaching practically zero when the obstruction is in the posterior lateral part of the pelvis.[8] Hydronephrosis is merely a stage in the progress to total obstruction and represents the extent of disease at that particular moment.

The question is raised whether untreated advanced cervical cancer should be treated initially by pelvic exenteration. Despite the good survival rate following radical surgery in the treatment of cancer of the cervix, stage III and IV, the loss of bladder and/or rectum with urinary and/or fecal diversion is a major complication, and therefore radiation therapy should be tried as an initial form of treatment. Million and associates[9] reported a 28 percent survival of patients with bladder invasion managed only by radiation therapy. This survival was equivalent to survival after exenteration, and no fistula developed in these patients. On the basis of this study, radiation therapy is the preferred method over primary exenteration in fresh cancer cases. In general, pelvic exenteration should be reserved for those patients in whom there is no chance of cure by any other modality.

Inflammatory carcinoma is a recognized syndrome in the breast, characterized by widespread lymphatic permeation. However, little attention has been given to this finding in the pelvis, possibly because observation is not as easy as in the breast. The pelvic peritoneum appears red and the vessels are dilated, presenting a picture not too dissimilar to that seen in early peritonitis. The clinical findings are not secondary to infection but rather extensive lymphatic permeation, carrying a poor prognosis and high morbidity. It is important to rule out widespread disease. In this clinical setting, pelvic exenteration is not indicated.

The traditional philosophy has been to tailor the procedure to fit the needs of the patient and the extent of disease. With limited disease, a procedure less than total pelvic exenteration should contribute a significant 5-year survival. This has been borne out in patients with anterior pelvic exenteration. Certain vulvar, vaginal, and colon recurrences are candidates for treatment by anterior pelvic exenteration. However, recurrent cervical cancer is probably best treated by total pelvic exenteration. Cancer of the cervix spreading posteriorly quickly becomes adherent to the pelvic floor and also invades the venous plexus in this area. In treating recurrent cancer of the cervix, it is most important to excise the vagina, leaving behind a denuded bladder and ureters; in patients treated by posterior pelvic exenteration, this results in a slough from lack of support and blood supply to the bladder. A high morbidity and mortality rate contraindicates posterior pelvic exenteration for the treatment of recurrent or persistent cancer of the cervix.

The question is raised as to whether pelvic exenteration should be carried out for palliation or only in the hope of a cure. It can be stated that pelvic exenteration should not be carried out if disease is left behind or even if disease is thought to be left behind. There will be no palliation, and the brief survival would be accompanied by high morbidity. Only when all disease is removed, and when the clinical setting indicates a good chance for long-term survival can resection be justified on the basis of palliation. Among those patients with known disease left at the time of surgery for recurrent cervical cancer, the average survival was little over 3 months and there was little, if any, palliation. It is a common observation that patients in whom disease is left behind at the time of pelvic exenteration or in whom it was not recognized that disease was left, do poorly postoperatively and have slow convalescence, characterized by ileus, low-grade temperature, and lethargy without any other clinical cause for the poor postoperative course following the procedure.

Technique

It is important to have a firm microscopic proof of recurrent cancer before starting the resection. There are guidelines to the operative technique for pelvic exenteration. However, the seasoned gynecologic oncologist will not approach the operation in a ster-

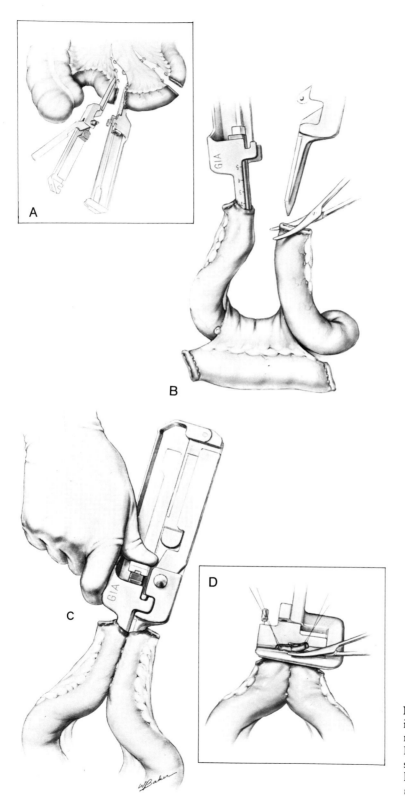

Fig. 23-1 **(A)** Ileal segment is identified and isolated with a GIA stapler. **(B)** Bowel continuity is reestablished using a GIA stapler. **(C)** Forks are inserted fully to ensure maximum stomal size. **(D)** Care must be taken to overlap the ends of the previous staple lines. *(Figure continues.)*

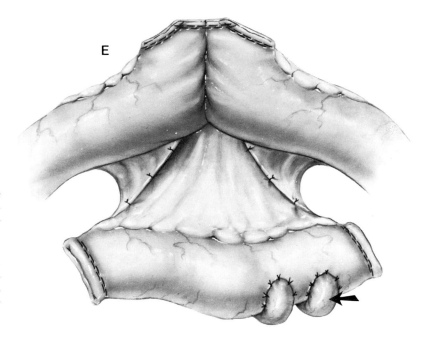

E

Fig. 23-1 *(Continued).* **(E)** The continuity of the ileum is reconstituted, and the ureters (arrows) are anastomosed to the ileal conduit. (This artwork was originally prepared for the United States Surgical Corporation's General Atlas and for publications by Professors Mark Ravitch, M.D., and Felicien Steichen, M.D., © 1981 USSC.)

eotyped manner but will have flexibility and make adjustments to the pathology. The use of hemoclips, stapling apparatuses, and suction apparatuses fitted with a light, with irrigating solution combined with suction all in one have helped speed up the time required for a pelvic exenteration. The steps in a total pelvic exenteration are listed as follows[10,11]:

1. The abdomen is opened through a left paramedian incision that can be extended as needed for better exposure.

2. Washings are taken from the pelvis and the upper abdomen for cytologic analysis.

3. The abdomen and pelvis are carefully explored, paying particular attention to the paraaortic area. If there is any question, the posterior peritoneum should be incised and nodes and lymphatic tissue removed for frozen-section analysis. If they are found to be positive, the pelvic exenteration operation should be abandoned, but any procedure needed to make the patient comfortable should be carried out. Patients with rectovaginal fistulas should have a colostomy, and for those with large vesical fistulas a urinary conduit should be constructed.

4. The self-retaining retractor is set in place, and the intestines are carefully packed out of the pelvis. In

pelvic exenteration, exposure is the keystone of success.

5. The planes are developed. The posterior peritoneum is picked up lateral to the infundibulopelvic ligament at the pelvic brim and is incised superficially, allowing the areolar tissue to fall away.

6. The peritoneum is incised to the round ligament.

7. The round ligament is clamped and tied, and the incision in the peritoneum is carried to the inguinal area. When the anatomy is greatly distorted, it is possible to find the round ligament especially when pelvic landmarks are obliterated by radiation fibrosis. It is then possible to start by ligating the round ligament near the internal abdominal ring.

8. The ureter is dissected medially with finger dissection, care being taken to keep the ureter attached to the peritoneum. The dissection is carried down to the pelvic floor.

9. The common and external iliac vessels are freed from the pelvic wall by incising the tissue between the vessels and the pelvic wall; then, by finger dissection, the tissue is separated from the pelvic wall down to the pelvic floor, thereby exposing the lateral edge of the sacroiliac nerve plexus (sciatic nerve). This is accomplished by

keeping the ureter medial and the hypogastric artery lateral and going down in a plane between these two areas.

10. By identifying the distal portion of the obliterated vessels along the lateral edge of the bladder, another relatively avascular plane is located, and the dissection is carried down to the pelvic floor; this approach facilitates identification and isolation of the obturator vessels and nerves. With the development of this plane and the one previously described, it is possible to determine whether the tumor is resectable.

11. The lymphatic fatty tissue and lymph nodes are dissected from the common and external iliac vessels by starting at the origin of the common iliac artery and continuing along the external artery to the inguinal ligament.

12. At the distal segment of the external iliac vein, the pelvic tissue is dissected from the vein and removed from the obturator and levator ani muscles by finger dissection. This, in combination with the previous dissection, mobilizes the entire area.

13. The distal dissection is carried along the proximal part of the vein to the level of the hypogastric vessels. As the dissection is carried higher, care must be employed to prevent damage to the hypogastric vein, as it joins the common iliac vein.

14. The obturator nerve is identified and protected from injury, while the obturator vessels are clamped, cut, and ligated at the obturator foramen.

15. The hypogastric artery is ligated either at its origin from the common iliac artery or wherever it can be mobilized easily, while the vein is ligated distally and then excised proximally. Since there is usually an increased amount of blood loss by taking the entire hypogastric vein, most gynecologic surgeons only take the branches rather than the entire vein.

16. The vessels over the sacroiliac plexus are ligated individually. The entire side is now mobilized, and a similar procedure is carried out on the contralateral side.

17. The colon is mobilized at the pelvic brim, clamped, and transected, the inferior mesenteric artery and vein having been ligated. Autosuture instruments such as GIA work very well and allow no spillage of bowel content.

18. The rectal colon is freed from the posterior pelvis down to the coccyx; injury to the middle sacral veins must be avoided. In mobilizing the specimen from the pelvic wall, large hemoclips provide good hemostasis and reduce the amount of blood loss.

19. The bladder is mobilized readily from the posterior part of the pubis and is retracted backward.

20. The mass of pelvic viscera is now freed from its attachments to the pelvic floor, and the dissection is carried to the perineum, including the vulva.

21. A pack may be placed in the pelvis and removed the following day, after which terramycin suppositories are placed in the pelvic cavity, or the omentum can be mobilized and brought down to cover the pelvic floor.

22. Urinary diversion is carried out, using a segment of the ileum or sigmoid. When the ileum[12] or sigmoid is used, the use of the GIA and TA55 speeds up the anastomosis and cuts down on the length of the operation (Fig. 23-1).

23. A colostomy stoma is placed on the left at a different level from that of the ileal stoma (for urinary diversion); the urinary conduit is usually brought out to the skin in the right lower quadrant.

24. A perineal phase may or may not be employed as the operator chooses.

25. The abdomen is closed in layers with interrupted retention sutures.

Although it is generally in the best interest of the patient to do a perineal phase, there are some patients whose pathology is located in the rectosigmoid; with new stapling instruments and by preserving a small area around the sphincter, the continuity of the bowel can be restored. This is carried out with autosuture instruments.

Result

Pelvic exenteration has been used to treat advanced and recurrent cancer of all pelvic organs.[13] A quick review of the generally accepted 5-year salvage rates for cancer involving the different pelvic structures shows that about 30 to 40 percent of vulvar, 60 to 70 percent of vaginal, 40 to 60 percent of cervical, 30 percent of corpus, and 80 percent of ovarian cancers recur and need further treatment.

CANCER OF THE VULVA

The cure rate for vulvar cancer is 60 to 70 percent; therefore, 30 to 40 percent of patients present with a recurrence. However, since many of these patients are in the geriatric age group, the number dying from an intercurrent disease will cut down the number that presents finally for definitive therapy. Carcinoma of the vulva is not a common cancer. It accounts for 0.3 percent of all female cancers at a rate of 1.5 per 100,000 females. It occurs most frequently after the ages of 60. There are about 500 deaths annually from cancer of the vulva in the United States and the death rate is about 0.5 per 100,000 females or about 0.3 percent of all female cancer deaths.

It has been reported that although all patients had a node dissection with the original radical vulvectomy, up to 33 percent of patients with recurrent vulvar cancer had positive nodes at the time of pelvic exenteration. This indicates that either nodes were missed at the time of the original procedure or that regeneration of lymph channels had occurred. Survival following treatment for cancer is related to the type of tumor and host resistance.

A well-differentiated tumor usually remains localized for a longer period than an anaplastic cancer. The lymphatics in the vulva course anteriorly, and the type of operation required to excise en bloc recurrence of vulvar cancer is directed toward eradication of this lymphatic distribution. Failure following initial therapy probably results in small cancer emboli present in the lymphatics draining the cancer-bearing area that were not excised with the original procedure. Most recurring cancers of the vulva can be managed with an anterior exenteration. The complication rate is high among these patients, and the survival rate ranges from 15 to 20 percent at 5 years or more.[14] However, there are others who with careful selection have achieved an absolute 5-year survival rate of 54 percent.[15]

CARCINOMA OF THE VAGINA

Carcinoma of the vagina is less common than carcinoma of the vulva. Cancer of the vagina accounts for 0.1 percent of all female cancers, or a rate of 0.6 per 100,000 females and usually occurs after the age of 65. There are about 350 deaths from cancer of the vagina annually at a rate of 0.3 per 100,000 females or about 0.2 percent of all female cancer deaths. The number of reported cases is increasing probably because of better diagnostic criteria. Cancer of the vagina often is well advanced when first diagnosed. The lesion may be concealed by the speculum, unless the speculum is rotated to expose the entire vagina at the time of its removal. These lesions are often large by the time signs and symptoms are evident. Vaginal lymphatics drain in three ways: the upper third of the vagina drains along the cervical lymphatics, the lower third along vulvar channels, and the middle third along either cervical or vulvar channels.

The difference in the type of operation required to excise vaginal disease is of some interest: with advanced vulvar cancer, most can be treated with an anterior pelvic exenteration while with advanced vaginal cancer most require a total pelvic exenteration to encompass their disease. This could reflect either the location of the disease or possibly a more virulent cancer. In a group of unselected patients, the 5-year survival was 15 percent.

CARCINOMA OF THE ENDOMETRIUM

The Annual Report on the Results of Treatment in Gynecologic Cancer (1976–1978) reports that 67.7 percent of the patients were alive at 5 years; 22.4 percent died of carcinoma of the corpus and could not be considered candidates for pelvic exenteration. Carcinoma of the cervix and carcinoma of the endometrium do not have similar or natural histories or method of spread. During an interval when several hundred exenterations were carried out for carcinoma of the cervix, only 36 pelvic exenterations were carried out for advanced or recurrent cancer of the endometrium.[16]

The finding of positive nodes at the time of the initial treatment for carcinoma of the endometrium carries a poor prognosis. Therefore, it follows that in patients with persistent or recurrent disease, positive nodes indicated an almost hopeless prognosis. Since there is an increased incidence of paraaortic node involvement in carcinoma of the endometrium, it is imperative that a special effort be made to rule out any possibility of paraaortic spread of disease before carrying out a pelvic exenteration.

Although there are fewer indications for pelvic exenteration in patients with carcinoma of the endometrium than in those with carcinoma of the cervix, there is a place for pelvic exenteration in the management of this malignancy. A survival rate of approximately 20 percent can be anticipated.

CARCINOMA OF THE OVARY

At laparotomy in patients with advanced ovarian carcinoma, a characteristic finding is wide dissemination of tumor over the peritoneal surfaces of the pelvis, upper abdomen, and omentum, as well as frequent involvement of both ovaries that either have spread from one primarily malignant or bilateral primary growths. There is also a high incidence of paraaortic node involvement in the presence of advanced ovarian carcinoma. In general, it can be stated that advanced and recurrent ovarian cancer is not amenable to surgical treatment except for a complication of the tumor, such as the relief of an obstruction or drainage of an abscess.

Theoretically, the natural history of ovarian carcinoma ordinarily would contraindicate pelvic exenteration. However, there are instances in which recurrence is late and limited entirely to the pelvis, and a more radical surgical procedure may be a reasonable approach to management of this patient. Endometrioid cancer may lend itself to radical surgical treatment, since it has been shown that only 30 percent of the cases were bilateral and 45 percent showed metastases to the upper abdomen. Endometrioid cancer of the ovary thus appears to be a less aggressive cancer than other ovarian cancers, especially in its potential for distant spread.

Patients with advanced recurrent ovarian cancer are an unfavorable group for pelvic exenteration, and except in rare instances the surgical procedure is not indicated for the management of carcinoma of the ovary. Less than 10 percent 5-year survival can be anticipated when pelvic exenteration is carried out as a definitive treatment for carcinoma of the ovary.[17]

CARCINOMA OF THE CERVIX

The Annual Report on the Results of Treatment in Gynecologic Cancer (1976–1978) reports that 55.0 percent of patients survive 5 or more years.[18] The Annual Report shows that 35.9 percent died of carcinoma of the cervix. Therefore, approximately one-third of cases of carcinoma of the cervix will have persistence or recurrence of their disease.

Carcinoma of the cervix in most instances remains confined to the pelvis for long period of time. Those patients are suitable for further treatment of their disease. Repeat irradiation therapy has little to offer in terms of cure and is accompanied by a high rate of complications and exacerbation of symptoms. The belief that if radiation has failed there is no further treatment affording cure is untenable today. The tendency for carcinoma of the cervix to remain localized to the pelvis provides an opportunity to encompass the disease by a surgical approach. It is apparent that operation can provide a very significant salvage rate for patients with recurrent carcinoma of the cervix (up to 50 percent), and no other equally curative form of therapy exists for this distressing condition. Although central recurrence of cervical carcinoma represents the most suitable lesion for exenterative operation, the procedure can provide salvage in some patients with lateral spread.

It is important to diagnose and treat recurrent carcinoma of the cervix soon after the recurrence is detected. The diagnosis of recurrence is often difficult. In early stages of recurrence the patient has no symptoms and few objective signs. A high index of suspicion is paramount in making the diagnosis. However, on pelvic examination any change from previous examinations should indicate that more aggressive diagnostic procedures be carried out. Intravenous pyelogram, ultrasound, and/or computed tomography (CT) scan contribute to making a diagnosis. Occasionally, by using a CT scan and the fine biopsy needle, it is possible to biopsy a paraaortic node and determine whether the patient should be explored. Unfortunately, exploratory surgery is usually indicated and required to make a definitive diagnosis. At the time of exploration, the survival rates reported indicate that the best results occur in the presence of a central lesion. The results fall off as the disease moves toward the pelvic wall; if there is no free space between the recurrence and pelvic wall, the chances for a 5-year survival are almost zero. In the favorable group of patients who have a central lesion, approximately 50 percent or higher 5-year survival can be anticipated. This can be achieved with a mortality rate of less than 5 percent.[19] However, if there is lateral spread or selection is held to a minimum, approximately 20 percent will survive 5 or more years.

The presence of positive pelvic lymph node involvement decreases the chance for survival. If more than one chain of nodes is involved, the results drop precipitously and when there is bilateral pelvic lymph node involvement the survival rate is about zero. The overall results from the presence of positive pelvic lymph nodes among patients with recurrent carcinoma is approximately 5 to 10 percent. There are some series reporting a survival rate of less than 5 percent.

EXTENSIVE RADIATION NECROSIS

The management of radiation necrosis presents a real challenge.[20] The clinical picture is complicated by severe pain, urinary and/or intestinal fistula, bleeding, copious foul discharge, and physical deterioration of the patient. It is difficult clinically to differentiate recurrent cancer from irradiation reaction and damage but, with proper selection of patients, pelvic exenteration is justified even though only radiation necrosis is found.

Among patients treated for extensive radiation necrosis with confirmation histologically following the operation, a few will die of cancer despite the fact that none was found at the time of pelvic exenteration. This confirms the natural history of cervical cancer and also reinforces the observation that it is difficult to differentiate clinically between persistent cancer and radiation necrosis even in the presence of a negative biopsy. Patients treated by pelvic exenteration for visceral necrosis are labile, and constant supervision is essential. Many develop complications, and most of these are small bowel fistulas. The results achieved in terms of physical welfare appear to justify the operation, since before surgery, existence is hardly bearable

in most instances. It appears that pelvic exenteration is indicated in selected patients for radiation necrosis and other damage producing severe symptoms.

However, before carrying out the pelvic exenteration the patient should be evaluated to see whether diversion of the urinary and fecal streams could possibly palliate the patient. If in the judgment of the gynecologic surgeon this can be achieved, there is a great deal less morbidity and no mortality as opposed to those receiving pelvic exenteration. However, this method of management will not control bleeding or the foul discharge or the pain that accompanies visceral necrosis.

EXENTERATION FOR OTHER CANCERS

Pelvic exenteration has been carried out for approximately 20 different disease entities. Aside from those already discussed, exenteration has been employed to control carcinoma of the rectum, embryonal carcinoma of the vagina, sarcoma of the uterus, cancer of the bladder, mixed mesodermal tumor of the uterus, granular cell myoblastoma, cancer of the urethra, adenocarcinoma of the tube, cancer of the perineum, lymphosarcoma, leiomyosarcoma of the bladder, leiomyosarcoma of the cervix, sarcoma of the prostate, fibrosarcoma, and reticulum cell sarcoma of the cervix.

In summary, it can be stated that the natural history of cancer of the cervix permits a radical surgical attack by pelvic exenteration, while all other malignant tumors listed lend themselves to radical surgical attack only if they do not have their usual method of spread.

SURGICAL-PATHOLOGIC CLASSIFICATION

The surgical-pathologic classification of cervical cancer[21] affords an opportunity for an accurate evaluation and at the same time serves to document the natural history of the tumor. The correlation of clinical and histopathologic findings permits a comparison of results among clinics carrying out a surgical program. This classification is not to be confused with the international classification. Classes of carcinoma of the cervix according to the surgical-pathologic classification are designated as shown below.

SURGICAL—PATHOLOGIC CLASSIFICATION OF CARCINOMA OF THE CERVIX

A	Limited to the cervix
B	Involves vagina and/or corpus
C	Parametrial extension
CN	Parametrial node
D	Peripheral node and parametrial extension
E	Bladder and/or rectum
EN	Same as E, plus node involvement
F	Pelvic wall—beyond pelvis
FN	Same as F, plus node involvement
AO	After positive biopsy specimen of infiltrating carcinoma, no tumor in the cervix in the surgical specimen
PR	Preoperative irradiation
R	Curative radiation followed by failure
S	Surgical attempt at cure prior to recurrence
RS	Irradiation and surgery employed for cure but requires further surgery for persistence or recurrence of disease

---

ROLE OF PELVIC EXENTERATION IN THE TREATMENT OF RECURRENCES FOLLOWING RADICAL SURGICAL EXCISION AS THE INITIAL TREATMENT

Of 222 patients presenting with recurrence following radical surgery, only 35 were treated by pelvic exenteration.[22] A comparison of the surgical-pathologic classification at the time of the initial surgery and at the time of treatment for recurrence reveals that there had been marked progression of the disease. Of the 35 patients, 8 survived 5 or more years. It is con-

cluded that fewer patients are suitable for pelvic exenteration after primary surgery than after primary irradiation. However, if it is technically possible to carry out pelvic exenteration, the results are about the same.

PELVIC EXENTERATION IN UNTREATED CANCER OF THE CERVIX

Since the patient loses bladder and/or rectum with pelvic exenteration, there is little enthusiasm for exenteration as a primary form of treatment. In general, pelvic exenteration should be reserved for patients who have no chance of cure by any other modality.

DISCHARGE FROM THE HOSPITAL

Criteria have been established for discharge from the hospital and have been formulated as shown below.

CRITERIA FOR DISCHARGING THE PATIENT WITH PELVIC EXENTERATION

1. Feels well physically and mentally
2. Tolerates a normal diet
3. Has no fever for at least 5 days
4. Walks without difficulty
5. Shows interest in being discharged from the hospital
6. Starts to resume interest in her previous work or hobbies
7. Demonstrates that she can take care of herself at home
8. Has skill and confidence in managing her ostomies
9. Has stable or increasing weight
10. Has minimal drug requirements
11. Understands the labile nature of her condition and accepts her responsibility for reporting any complications immediately

(Continues)

12. Understands the importance of continued follow-up examinations
13. Has immediate family members who understand the nature of the problem
14. Can return to home surroundings in which the problems presented by the patient are accepted

CRITERIA FOR ESTIMATING PROGNOSIS

The result of the treatment and the chances for long survival are difficult to predict. The operation is of considerable magnitude, and the patient has less resistance to any physical insult than has the nonexenterative patient, who is susceptible to the development of infection. A high percentage of patients require additional surgery, usually for complications of the bowel or urinary tract. The success of treatment may be evaluated by the following factors.

CRITERIA OUTLINED

1. At the time of operation, planes of dissection were developed with relative ease.
2. The recurrence was confined to the midline with minimal lateral spread.
3. There is relative certainty that all macroscopic disease was removed.
4. Technically, the urinary and bowel anastamoses were carried out with little trauma and no tension.
5. There was a reasonably uncomplicated postoperative course.
6. The hospital stay did not exceed 1 month.
7. Postoperative pyelograms were within normal limits.
8. There were no attacks of pyelonephritis.
9. No fever occurred beyond the first 5 or 6 postoperative days.

(Continues)

10. There has been subjective improvement in association with a marked decrease in requirements of analgesic or narcotic drugs.
11. The clinical appearance correlates with the laboratory findings, indicating progressive improvement.
12. There has been a leveling off or reversal of the downward weight curve.
13. The performance status of the patient has improved.
14. The patient has shown emotional adjustment to the operation.
15. Chemical and roentgenographic findings remain within normal limits.
16. All of the above are met and maintained for at least 12 months.

ROLE OF PELVIC EXENTERATION

Based on the experience at the Memorial-James Ewing Hospital, pelvic exenteration is established as a method of treatment of recurrent cancer of the cervix.[23] The increased complication rate and poor operative survival are anticipated and accepted, since the only hope for survival is offered by extended radical surgery. Surgical morbidity and mortality depend on the condition encountered in each patient, for example, extent of secondary infection, previous irradiation and tissue reaction, status of the urinary tract, and extent of disease. The following guidelines have been proposed and have been published by the author.[24]

ABSOLUTE CONTRAINDICATIONS TO SURGERY FOR CURE

1. Metastasis outside the pelvis (lung; supraclavicular, inguinal, or paraaortic nodes; and peritoneum) or malignant cells in peritoneal fluid
2. Visceral spread to the upper abdomen

(Continues)

3. Positive nodes above the periphery of the pelvis in the paraaortic area
4. Psychoses
5. Borderline cardiopulmonary reserve
6. "Skip" metastases to the bowel
7. Direct invasion or "skip" metastases to the mesentery
8. Skin metastases
9. Metastases beyond the introitus of the vagina, to the vulva, or fixed to the levator muscles
10. Bilateral ureteral obstruction secondary to disease
11. Bedridden from cancer or its complication for more than 1 month
12. Excessive weight loss secondary to cancer or its complications over a 1- or 2-month period
13. Markedly abnormal liver-function tests
14. Abnormalities of the clotting and bleeding mechanisms
15. Unilateral ureteral obstruction in the posterior lateral pelvis
16. Technical inability to remove all disease
17. For palliation, with known disease left behind
18. Permeation of disease to blood vessels at the periphery of the pelvis
19. Malignant disease involving bone
20. Positive pelvic nodes following radiation failure
21. Bilateral or multiple positive nodes in untreated cancer of the cervix
22. Sepsis
23. Cancer that has broken through the serosa of the uterus
24. Implants on the peritoneum within or beyond the confines of the pelvis
25. Reticulum cell sarcoma or lymphoma
26. Inadequate hospital facilities
27. Lack of ability and training of the physician to cope with all complications
28. Presence of multiple contraindications

RELATIVE CONTRAINDICATIONS TO SURGERY FOR CURE

1. Obesity
2. Over age 65
3. Low hemoglobin and hematocrit values not explained by evidence of active bleeding
4. Question of whether all disease can be completely excised
5. Microscopic evidence of blood vessel invasion at the primary site of the cancer
6. Indecision about the wisdom of completing the exenteration
7. Difficulty in mobilizing the specimen
8. Ovarian cancer
9. Radiation necrosis
10. Lack of a positive biopsy
11. Sarcoma
12. Active pulmonary tuberculosis

JUDGMENT DECISIONS

1. Big, bulky, infected tumor
2. Marked anaplasia of tumor
3. Small cell carcinoma
4. All malignant tumors, except cancer of the cervix
5. Localized abscess in pelvis
6. Lateral spread of tumor, especially that characterized by nodularity at the ischial spine
7. Excessive blood loss in attempting to mobilize the specimen
8. Persistence of disease after adequate initial treatment
9. Previously untreated cancer of the cervix
10. Marked emotional instability
11. Living alone with no one to take a general interest in giving help
12. Inflammatory cancer, characterized by lymphatic permeation

(Continues)

13. Spread of tumor posteriorly toward the pelvic and sacral areas
14. Inordinately difficult procedure
15. Physical disability limiting ability to care for ostomies
16. The hospital mortality surpasses the anticipated survival rate
17. Biologic spread equated against geographic spread

Obviously, there is only a limited place for pelvic exenteration. Since horrendous complications and relatively poor results follow pelvic exenteration in patients in whom the procedure is contraindicated, there must be strict observance of the indications and contraindications. In selected patients, pelvic exenteration may give years of additional useful life; under some circumstances there is a place for this ultraradical surgical operation.

PSYCHOSEXUAL ADJUSTMENT AND REHABILITATION

The rehabilitation of the patient who has had a pelvic exenteration should be well structured. It has been stated that patients who have survived for some time following pelvic exenteration are happy. Happiness probably means that they have become well adjusted. There are many reasons for the patient to become well adjusted.[25] After a period of time, the patient realizes that the cancer is being controlled. The patient's partner often can play a significant role in rehabilitating the patient. It is important to take a careful sexual history during the preoperative period. It is important to explain to the patient that it is possible to make a psychosexual adjustment following pelvic exenteration.

Sexual functioning, particularly under age 65, continues as the area of greatest disruption for these patients. It is important to construct a vagina for these patients. If a perineal phase is not required to encompass the entire disease, the vulva and clitoris can be left in place. This provides some psychologic uplift for the patient, particularly when they realize that a functioning vagina can be constructed.[26] These women are able to recapture some of their previous sexual activity and, although it may not be as complete and satisfying as it had been prior to the exenteration, it is usually satisfying for both the patient and her partner. Patients who have a fairly strong sex drive before the pelvic exenteration do better than those who have had a low sex drive.[27-29]

It is important to provide continuing support and regular counseling to the patient who has had a pelvic exenteration. Every gynecologic oncologist should enlist the aid of one or two patients who have had a pelvic exenteration and who have made a satisfactory physical, psychological, and sexual rehabilitation, to meet with the patient about to undergo a pelvic exenteration. In my experience, this has provided an important support mechanism, particularly when the patient who has survived a pelvic exenteration for a long period of time is available at any time to talk to the patient who is about to have an exenteration or who has recently recovered from a pelvic exenteration.[30] These patients should be encouraged to return to productive activity as soon as possible. They should be encouraged to engage in all their previous social functions, including golf, horseback riding, or whatever activities they had enjoyed. The aim is to bring about total rehabilitation and a satisfactory adjustment to their loss of bladder, rectum, and vagina.

SUMMARY

Pelvic exenteration was born out of frustration in managing recurrent cancer of the pelvis. During the 1940s, 1950s, and 1960s, a great deal of interest was shown, but a survey of the literature now indicates that interest is waning. It is difficult to know why this is so. It still plays an important role for treating patients with recurrent pelvic carcinoma.

It can be stated that the natural history of carcinoma of the cervix permits a radical surgical attack by pelvic exenteration, while other gynecologic cancers lend themselves to radical surgical attack if they violate the usual method of spread characteristic of their natural history. The ideal patient for pelvic exenteration is a patient under 60 who has central recurrence following adequate radiation therapy.

It is difficult, clinically, to differentiate recurrent cancer from radiation necrosis but with proper selection of cases and under individual circumstances, pelvic exenteration is justifiable even though only radiation necrosis is found. The current concept is to follow the principle of individualization of treatment rather than standardization of treatment.

The new and improved methods of treating patients with radiation therapy and the employment of combination therapies, such as radiation, surgery, chemotherapy, immunotherapy, and hyperthermia, reduce the number of patients requiring pelvic exenteration. However, rather than relegating patients with recurrent carcinoma to the scrap heap of repeated irradiation and chemotherapy, which are rarely curative, the physician in charge should consider pelvic exenteration, regardless of the origin or cell type of the tumor.

REFERENCES

1. Cancer Facts and Figures: American Cancer Society, New York, 1987
2. Brunschwig A: Complete excision of pelvic viscera for abdominal carcinoma. Cancer 1:177, 1948
3. Appleby LH: Proctocystectomy: The management of colostomy with ureteral transplants. Am J Surg 79:57, 1950
4. Barber HRK: Exenteration procedures in pelvic malignancy. Ch. 63. In Davis' Gynecology and Obstetrics. Vol. 3. Harper & Row, Hagerstown, MD, 1971
5. Symmonds RE, Webb MJ: Pelvic exenteration. In Coppleson M (ed): Gynecologic Oncology. Fundamental Principles and Clinical Practice. Churchill Livingstone, New York, 1981
6. Creasman WT, Rutledge FN: Preoperative evaluation of patients with recurrent carcinoma of the cervix. Gynecol Oncol 1:111, 1972
7. Barber HRK, Jones W: Lymphadenectomy in pelvic exenteration for recurrent cervix cancer. JAMA 215:1945, 1971
8. Barber HRK, Roberts S, Brunschwig A: Prognostic significance of the preoperative nonvisualizing kidney in patients receiving pelvic exenteration. Cancer 16:1614, 1963
9. Million RR, Rutledge F, Fletcher GH: Stage IV carcinoma of the cervix with bladder invasion. Am J Obstet Gynecol 113:239, 1972
10. Nelson JH Jr: Atlas of Radical Surgery. 2nd Ed. Appleton-Century-Crofts, New York, 1977
11. Parsons L, Ulfelder H: An Atlas of Pelvic Operations. 2nd Ed. WB Saunders Company, Philadelphia, 1968
12. Bricker EM: The technique of ileal segment bladder substitution. In Meigs JA (ed): Progress in Gynecology. Vol. 3. Grune & Stratton, New York, 1957
13. Averette HE, Lachtinger M, Sevin B, Girtanner RE: Pelvic exenteration: A 15 year experience in a general metropolitan hospital. Am J Obstet Gynecol 150:179, 1984
14. Barber HRK, Brunschwig A, Mangioni C: Advanced cancer of the vulva and vagina treated by anterior and total pelvic exenteration 1947–1962 at the Memorial-James Ewing Hospital. Estratto dalla Rivista, Annali di Ostetrica e Gynecologica, 1968
15. Morley GW: Infiltrative carcinoma of the vulva: Results of surgical treatment. Am J Obstet Gynecol 124:874, 1976
16. Barber HRK, Brunschwig A: Treatment and results of recurrent cancer of corpus uteri in patients receiving anterior and total exenteration 1947–1963. Cancer 22:949, 1968
17. Barber HRK, Brunschwig A: Pelvic exenteration for advanced and recurrent ovarian cancer. Surgery 58:935, 1965
18. Annual Report on Results of Treatment of Gynecological Cancer: Vol. 19. Statement of Results Obtained in 1976 to 1978 inclusive. International Federation of Gynecology and Obstetrics, Stockholm, 1986
19. Morley GW, Lindenauer SM: Pelvic exenterative therapy for gynecologic malignancy: An analysis of 70 cases. Cancer 38:581, 1976
20. Barber HRK, Brunschwig A: Definitive treatment of radiation necrosis. Five year results in 77 patients. Obstet Gynecol 35:344, 1970
21. Meigs JV, Brunschwig A: Proposed classification for cases of cancer of the cervix treated by surgery. Am J Obstet Gynecol 64:413, 1952
22. Barber HRK, O'Neil W: Recurrent cervical cancer after treatment by a primary surgical program. Obstet Gynecol 37:165, 1971
23. Brunschwig A: What are the indications and results of pelvic exenteration? JAMA 194:274, 1965
24. Barber, HRK: Relative prognostic significance of preoperative and operative findings in pelvic exenteration. Surg Clin North Am 49:431, 1969
25. Lamont JA, DePetrillo AD, Sargeant EJ: Psychosocial rehabilitation of exenterative surgery. Gynecol Oncol 6:236, 1978
26. Berek JS, Hacker NF, Lagasse LD: Vaginal reconstruction performed simultaneously with pelvic exenteration. Obstet Gynecol 63:318, 1984
27. Lagasse LD, Berman ML, Watring WG, et al: The gynecologic oncology patient: Restoration of function

and prevention of disability. p. 398. In McGowan L (ed): Gynecologic Oncology. Appleton-Century-Crofts, New York, 1978

28. Andersen BL, Hacker NF: Psychosocial adjustment following pelvic exenteration. Obstet Gynecol 61:331, 1983

29. Wabrek AJ, Gunn JL: Sexual and psychological implications of gynecologic malignancy. JOGN Nursing 13:371, 1984

30. Crosson K: A patient teaching aid for the pelvic exenteration patient. Oncol Nursing Forum 8(4):53, 1981

24

Urinary Diversion

Vicki V. Baker
Hugh M. Shingleton

Urinary diversion for the patient with gynecologic cancer has become an integral procedure in the surgical armamentarium of the gynecologic oncologist. With the advent of improved surgical technique and advances in postoperative care, the attendant morbidity and mortality associated with urinary diversion have substantially decreased. The technical aspects of the more commonly used operative methods of urinary diversion, the relative advantages and disadvantages of each, and the recognition and management of postoperative complications are reviewed.

INDICATIONS

The classic indications for urinary diversion include correction of severe congenital anomalies, relief of ureteral obstruction, and as a component of anterior or total exenterative procedures. There are numerous other indications in which urinary diversion might be considered when medical management or less extensive surgical procedures fail. These situations include incontinence, severe cystitis, vesicovaginal fistula, and urinary tract complications following radiation therapy, to name a few.

Most patients evaluated by the gynecologic oncologist for a urinary diversion procedure have recurrent carcinoma of the cervix. Other less frequent indications include malignancy of the vagina, endometrium, and vulva or complications of therapy.

METHODS OF URINARY DIVERSION

The ideal method of urinary diversion is one which ensures continence and avoids damage to renal function with acceptable operative and postoperative morbidity. The first description of urinary diversion was published in 1852 by Simon[1]; since that report, a

---

METHODS OF URINARY DIVERSION

I. Vesical
II. Supravesical
  A. Nephrostomy
    1. Cutaneous
    2. Percutaneous
  B. Ureterocutaneous diversion
  C. Ureteroenteric diversion
    1. Small bowel
      a. Ileal conduit
      b. Jejunal conduit
      c. Kock reservoir
    2. Large bowel
      a. Sigmoid colon conduit
      b. Transverse colon conduit
      c. Rectal pouch

plethora of ingenious surgical procedures have been advocated. There is no universally acceptable or clearly superior method of urinary diversion. A rigorous comparison of one method over another is difficult because reported series exhibit variation in patient selection criteria, surgical technique, criteria for morbidity, and the duration and type of postdiversion follow-up.

The flow of urine may be diverted at the level of the bladder (vesical diversion) or more proximally (supravesical diversion). Because the gynecologic oncologist primarily performs diversion as part of an exenterative procedure in which the bladder and urethra are removed, only methods of supravesical diversion are considered.

Nephrostomy

Cutaneous nephrostomy entails an operative procedure to divert the flow of urine to the skin. It is difficult for the patient to manage and may pose unacceptable risks to the surgical candidate who is in poor general medical condition. Percutaneous nephrostomy is an excellent alternative to cutaneous nephrostomy in that it achieves the same end result, but with a lower morbidity and mortality. This method of supravesical diversion is performed by directly inserting catheters percutaneously into the renal pelvis using fluoroscopic guidance.

Favorable patient acceptance and the low incidence of immediate and long-term complications make it an attractive method of urinary diversion in a high-risk surgical patient. It is generally considered a method of palliative diversion in those patients suffering from ureteral obstruction in whom curative therapy is not available. Although percutaneous nephrostomy will prolong survival in these incurable cases, the marginal quality of life experienced by many of these patients must be kept in mind by the surgeon and carefully explained to the patient and her family.

Ureterocutaneous Diversion

The end cutaneous ureterostomy and transureteroureterostomy involve implantation of one or both distal ureters through the abdominal wall, where they drain into an external appliance. The ureter must be significantly dilated and well vascularized. Although electrolyte abnormalities do not occur and the occurrence of pyelonephritis is infrequent, both procedures have been largely abandoned because of the high incidence of ureteral and skin strictures, which ranges from 45 to 64 percent.

Ureterointestinal Diversion

In an effort to avoid the stomal complications associated with ureterocutaneous diversion, numerous ureterointestinal anastomoses have been proposed. Although the incidence of stomal complications is decreased by the use of ureterointestinal anastomoses, there is an increase in the likelihood of electrolyte imbalances. In addition to the influence of the patient's renal function on her postdiversion electrolyte balance, the risk of clinically significant electrolyte abnormalities is influenced by the segment of bowel used, the absorptive mucosal surface area available, and the duration of contact between the urine and bowel mucosa. As one proceeds in an aboral direction, the electrolyte resorption capacity of the bowel decreases. A distal colonic segment of bowel resorbs fewer electrolytes than does a segment of bowel from the proximal jejunum. Within each regional segment of bowel, electrolyte resorption occurs in proportion to the exposed mucosal surface area; thus, longer bowel segments pose a greater risk of the development of electrolyte abnormalities than do shorter bowel segments. In addition to the surface area available for electrolyte resorption, the duration of contact between urine and mucosa influences the amount of electrolytes resorbed. A conduit, which is an isolated segment of bowel that permits free passage of urine via a stoma to the exterior, results in minimal stasis of urine as compared with a reservoir, which is an isolated segment of bowel fashioned to store urine until it is conveniently drained by the patient. Largely because of the prolonged exposure of urine to intestinal mucosa, reservoirs are associated with a higher incidence of metabolic complications as compared with conduits, regardless of the bowel segment considered.

Ureterocolonic Diversion

The ureterosigmoidostomy, performed as part of an anterior exenteration, and the wet colostomy, performed as part of a total exenteration, both function as cloacae, collecting urine and fecal material in a common reservoir. These techniques have been largely abandoned because of the high incidence of recurrent pyelonephritis. In addition, as compared with the general population, there is a 280- to 550-fold increase in the incidence of adenocarcinoma arising at the ureterocolonic anastomosis, with an attendant mortality of approximately 50 percent. These tumors have been hypothesized to result from the exposure of metaplastic colonic mucosa to N-nitrosoamines, which are produced by the action of fecal bacteria on the urine.

Techniques for the creation of a rectal pouch or bladder were introduced during the mid-1950s. The rectal pouch is a variation of the ureterosigmoidostomy in that the bowel is transected proximal to the ureterocolonic anastomosis and exited as a colostomy and urine is drained into the rectosigmoid. The advantage of the rectal pouch as compared with the ureterosigmoidostomy is the separation of urinary and fecal streams, thereby decreasing the incidence of pyelonephritis. However, incontinence is a frequent problem, and the uncontrollable drainage of urine from the perineum is unacceptable to most patients.

Another problem shared by the ureterosigmoidostomy and rectal pouch is hyperchloremic metabolic acidosis. Colonic mucosa normally exhibits a differential absorption of choride. The urinary stasis associated with these methods of diversion result in the excessive absorption of chloride with a secondary loss of bicarbonate. The resulting metabolic acidosis may be further exacerbated by renal tubular dysfunction and hepatic dysfunction.

Jejunal Conduit

A conduit fashioned from an isolated segment of jejunum carries a considerable risk of electrolyte disturbances because of the normal absorptive capability of this portion of the small bowel. Because of the frequent metabolic complications, which can include hyperchloremic acidosis, hyponatremia, hyperkalemia, and azotemia, this method of diversion should be undertaken only when other more distal segments of bowel cannot be used.

Kock Continent Ileal Reservoir

The Kock ileal reservoir[2] has been introduced as a method of continent supravesical diversion. The procedure requires a 60- to 70-cm segment of bowel,

40 cm of which is folded on itself and then divided to create a continent pouch. Although this method is theoretically attractive, it has not gained widespread acceptance among gynecologic oncologists, primarily because of the length of bowel required.

Ileal Conduit

The ileal conduit, popularized by Bricker in 1950,[3] has been the method of supravesical urinary diversion most frequently chosen by gynecologic oncologists during the past two decades. This method of diversion uses an isolated segment of distal ileum as the conduit segment. Immediate postoperative complications include urosepsis, urinary leak, ureteral fistula, bowel anastomotic leak, and bowel obstruction. The incidence of these complications ranges from 6.2 to 14.1 percent. When the data are analyzed with respect to prior therapy, it is evident that the incidence of these complications is greater in those patients who have been previously irradiated. Apart from an increase in complications attributable to prior radiation therapy, it has become clear that the ileal conduit also suffers from a notable delayed complication: the deterioration of renal function. Patients who have undergone ileal conduit diversion and survived at least 5 years exhibit a progessive deterioration in renal function, regardless of the indication for diversion or history of prior irradiation therapy.

The increased incidence of complications in previously irradiated patients and the loss of renal function with time have led to the suggestion that colonic conduits should be considered as superior alternatives to the ileal conduit. The colon offers certain intrinsic advantages for the creation of a conduit: (1) a thick muscular wall, which makes it easier to create a nonrefluxing ureteral anastomosis; and (2) a relatively large lumen, which minimizes the occurrence of stomal strictures.

A sigmoid conduit with a descending colostomy avoids the potential problems of a bowel reanastomosis. However, if the patient has received prior radiation therapy, there is an increased incidence of ureterointestinal anastomotic leaks. In previously irradiated patients, who constitute the majority of patients evaluated for a diversion procedure by the gynecologic oncologist, the transverse colon conduit is the method of choice, since this segment of bowel is generally out of the field of irradiation.

GENERAL CONSIDERATIONS

Several factors will influence the type of diversion undertaken. However, certain considerations are common to virtually any method of urinary diversion.

CONSIDERATIONS GERMANE TO URINARY DIVERSION

Curative versus palliative indications

Simple versus staged procedure

Prior radiation therapy

Operative time required and technical simplicity of the procedure

Patient considerations
    Age
    Medical condition
    Comprehension of the proposed procedure
    Ability for self-care
    Psychological status
Technical considerations
    Associated bowel injury
    Selection of stomal site(s)
    Method of ureteral anastomosis

Advanced age as an isolated criterion should not be a deterrent in considering a patient for urinary diversion. However, even in the young and otherwise healthy patient, urinary diversion alone or as part of an exenterative procedure is a major operation associated with significant morbidity and mortality. A careful and complete preoperative evaluation is mandatory.

In the patient previously treated for a gynecologic malignancy, the intent and type of diversion will be influenced by the presence and extent of disease. Temporizing intervention, as provided by percutaneous nephrostomy, might be appropriate for the poor-prognosis patient for whom curative therapy is not available, whereas a more permanent type of diversion would be attempted in the patient treated with curative intent. A history of prior radiotherapy should also influence the decision concerning the type of urinary diversion undertaken, since surgery on radiation-damaged tissue is associated with a higher complication rate as compared with nonirradiated tissue.

Radiographic studies of the genitourinary and gastrointestinal (GI) systems are recommended. An intravenous pyelogram is necessary to establish the number of ureters on each side and to identify hydroureter or hydronephrosis. In addition, a preoperative intravenous pyelogram is a useful baseline study against which subsequent studies may be compared. A barium enema followed by an upper GI series with a small bowel follow through study should be obtained to identify any areas of stricture or internal fistulization and to diagnosis coexisting intrinsic bowel disease.

One of the most important yet occasionally neglected items in the preoperative assessment is the evaluation of the patient by an enterostomal therapist. Potential ostomy sites should be chosen and marked preoperatively. The patient should be observed in several positions, so that skin creases and bulges are avoided. The ostomy should be placed at a site that can easily be seen and managed by the patient. In general, ileal conduits are brought out in the right lower quadrant. A transverse colon conduit can be placed in any abdominal quadrant within reach of its mesentery. When both a conduit and colostomy are planned, special consideration should be given to their placement. Some patients experience difficulty managing the stomal appliances when the ostomies are placed on the same side of the midline or at the same level on opposite sides of the midline.

Regardless of the specific technique chosen to create the ostomy, it should result in an everted stoma. A particularly important point in the construction of the stoma is to secure it adequately at the peritoneal, fascial, and skin levels. This will minimize the risks of parastomal herniation and stomal retraction or prolapse. Among its other advantages, an everted stoma will facilitate secure application of the appliance and protect against urinary leakage as compared to a flush stoma.

Certain technical considerations germane to urinary diversion are basic to any surgical procedure involving bowel transection and subsequent reanastomosis. A mechanical bowel preparation will reduce the risk of intraoperative fecal contamination and will ensure that all the barium has been evacuated from the GI tract. The standard bowel preparation includes a clear liquid diet for 2 or 3 days preoperatively, followed by magnesium citrate and cleansing enemas. An equally efficacious and less time-consuming bowel preparation that avoids any fluid or electrolyte disturbance can be achieved using colonic lavage solutions. Regardless of how the bowel is prepared, prophylactic antibiotics should be administered preoperatively. Various regimens may be used, including oral erythromycin and neomycin, intravenous metronidazole, or an intravenous cephalosporin.

The use of automatic stapling devices in the creation of urinary conduits has been well established since its introduction in 1972 by Johnson and Fuerst.[4] The advantages of these devices for the construction of GI anastomoses as compared to hand-sewn anastomoses include decreased operative time, decreased tissue trauma and improved blood supply to the anastomosis. The safety and decreased postoperative morbidity associated with the use of these instruments in gynecologic oncologic surgery have been reported. However, it is important to recognize the potential complications associated with the use of automatic stapling devices, including anastomotic leakage, enteric stenosis, and bleeding from the staple line.

A purported disadvantage of the automatic stapling device is the risk of calculus formation around the metal staples. There is little doubt that exposed wire staples can serve as a nidus for calculus formation, although its clinical significance is subject to question, since the stones generally pass through the stoma without difficulty. The incidence of staple-induced urolithiasis appears to be less than 5 percent. Theoretically, these stones could serve as a nidus for infection. However, the occurrence of pyelonephritis and persistent bacteriuria is so much more frequent than staple-induced stones that it is difficult to evaluate the influence of staple-induced stones on the risk of infection.

To minimize the occurrence of staple-induced urolithiasis, several techniques have been proposed to prevent contact of the staple line with urine. Costello and Johnson[5] suggested that the bowel be manually transected to isolate the conduit segment. Bowel continuity is then restored as a side-to-side open-lumen enteroenteric anastomosis using the automatic stapling instruments. The proximal end of the conduit is oversewn with a double layer of running chronic sutures reinforced with a layer of interrupted seromuscular sutures. Alternatively, Delgado[6] has advocated the placement of a running suture in front of the GIA staple line so that the urine cannot contact the staples.

To retain the general advantages of the staple device and avoid the potential problems associated with stone formation, two applications of the TA 55 automatic staple device loaded with absorbable staples (i.e., Polysorb, manufactured by Autosuture) may be used in place of the single application of the GIA instrument to divide the proximal end of the conduit. In the absence of data demonstrating a significant clinical problem secondary to staple-induced urolithiasis, most surgeons simply transect the bowel with the GIA instruments.

One of the more controversial issues that must be considered by the surgeon is whether the freely refluxing versus antirefluxing ureterointestinal anastomosis is the better method to preserve long-term renal function. A significant number of patients with freely refluxing ileal conduits followed for a minimum of 5 years exhibit a decline in renal function based on a rise in serum creatinine or radiographic evidence of progressive hydronephrosis. This progressive deterioration in renal function has been attributed to reflux-associated nephropathy. However, the role of reflux as the primary etiologic factor is subject to question. Neal[7] performed follow-up studies of refluxing and antirefluxing ureteroileal anastomoses for a minimum of 5 years and demonstrated no difference in the incidence of upper tract dilation or radiographically demonstrable reflux between the two types of anastomoses. Other long-term follow-up studies have demonstrated little or no evidence of renal deterioration in the absence of reflux in colon conduits, in which it is technically easier to create an antirefluxing ureterointestinal anastomosis. Although this might suggest an advantage with the use of colonic conduits, Sullivan et al[8] could not document any significant differences between freely refluxing ileal and antirefluxing colonic conduits with respect to long-term preservation of renal function in patients followed for a minimum of 5 years. These observations indicate that the adverse effects of conduit diversion observed in some patients may not be solely attributable to reflux.

There is little debate concerning the risk of renal damage when the kidney is exposed to increased ureteral back pressure for prolonged periods of time. In a patient diverted by a conduit, an increase in backpressure can obviously occur with outflow obstruction secondary to stomal narrowing of a conduit with a freely-refluxing ureterointestinal anastomosis or as a consequence of ureterointestinal anastomotic stricture. In addition, a urinary conduit without evidence of stomal narrowing and a freely refluxing ureteral anastomosis can also subject the kidney to increased backpressures if the intraluminal pressure of the conduit is elevated. Daniel and Singh[9] have documented unusually high intestinal pressures in some patients diverted by conduit and noted that these pressures were similar to the intravesical pressures recorded in patients with chronic urinary retention associated with bilateral hydronephrosis and hydroureter.

Numerous techniques are described in the literature for the creation of freely refluxing and antirefluxing ureterointestinal anastomoses. Regardless of the method chosen, ureteral intubation is recommended. The use of Silastic ureteral stents prevents immediate postoperative obstruction secondary to edema of the anastomosis, permits small leaks to heal without additional intervention and has not been associated with any complications attributable to their insertion.

SURGICAL CONSIDERATIONS

The gynecologic oncologist generally chooses among the ileal, sigmoid, and transverse colon con-duits to accomplish supravesical diversion (Fig. 24-1). Detailed descriptions of the techniques for manual transection of the bowel and hand-sewn GI anastomoses may be found in general surgical textbooks and should be familiar to any surgeon performing these operations. We favor the use of automatic staple devices because of the decreased operative time, ease of use and satisfactory results observed with their use.

Ileal Conduit

A segment of distal ileum, 10 to 15 cm proximal to the ileocecal valve and out of the field of previous irradiation, is chosen for the conduit. This segment of bowel must be of sufficient length to extend from the sacral promontory to a position 1 to 2 cm above the skin. However, the bowel segment should be as short as possible to minimize urine solute resorption. Trans-illumination and palpation of the bowel mesentery assist in the identification of a well-developed vascular arcade. Preservation of the last branch of the superior mesenteric artery or a segment of the ileocolic artery will provide an adequate vascular pedicle. The mesentery is incised so that the distal margin is longer than the proximal one. This asymmetric mesenteric incision provides adequate length without tension for the distal end of the conduit, which must

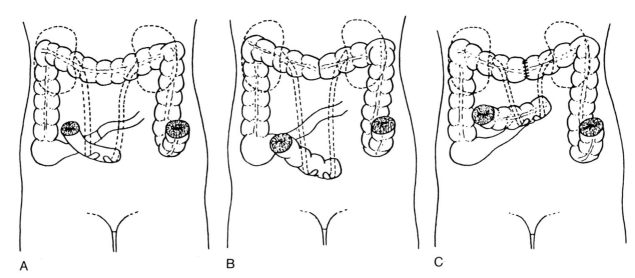

A   B   C

Fig. 24-1 The most commonly used methods of supravesical urinary diversion in gynecologic oncology: **(A)** ileal conduit, **(B)** sigmoid conduit, and **(C)** the transverse colon conduit.

reach above the skin surface. The bowel is transected using the GIA and the isolated ileal segment brought below the bowel mesentery. Small bowel continuity is reestablished by an end-to-end ileoileostomy or an end-to-end ileo-ascending colonostomy. The closed method of enteric anastomosis as described by Ravich and Steichen[10] using the GIA and TA 55 automatic stapling devices avoids any spillage of bowel contents. The mesenteric defect is closed with interrupted sutures to prevent internal herniation.

Isoperistaltic orientation of a small bowel conduit must be conserved. The proximal end of the isolated segment remains closed, and the distal end is used to create an everted stoma.

The ureters are transected at the pelvic brim and mobilized beneath the peritoneum, taking care to preserve the periureteral tissue and a flap of peritoneum attached to the distal ureter. The right ureter is easily isolated where it crosses the bifurcation of the common iliac artery. The left ureter is isolated beneath the sigmoid mesocolon and mobilized for a sufficient distance to carry it across the midline via a tunnel created in the retroperitoneal space by blunt dissection below the level of the inferior mesenteric artery. The free end of the ureter may be spatulated to facilitate the creation of the anastomosis and to decrease the incidence of stenosis although the authors do not routinely find that this is necessary. A freely refluxing simple end-to-side ureteroileal anastomosis is the most frequently utilized method of implantation.

A 5- to 6-mm ellipse of ileal serosa and mucosa is sharply excised approximately 2 cm from the closed proximal end of the conduit between the antimesenteric and mesenteric margins. A Silastic stent is placed in the ureter and brought out through the conduit stoma. The authors place a resorbable suture through the ureter to hold the stent in place (Fig. 24-2). The ureter is then sutured to the conduit using through and through interrupted sutures of 4-0 absorbable suture with the knots tied on the outside. A similar procedure is followed for anastomosis of the contralateral ureter, placing it approximately 3 cm from the closed proximal end of the conduit. The peritoneal flap left attached to the distal ureter is sutured over the anastomosis to relieve any tension on the ureteroileal anastomosis.

Following completion of the ureteroileal anasto-

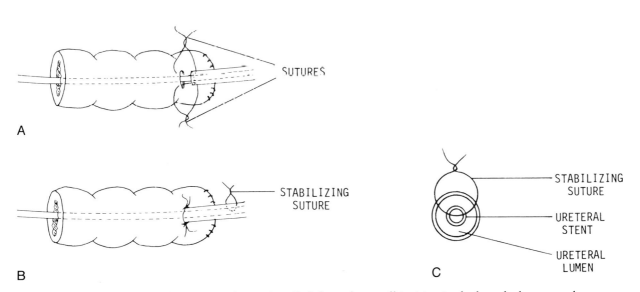

Fig. 24-2 (A) A Silastic ureteral stent is pulled through a small incision in the bowel; the mucosal surfaces are sutured together. **(B)** The stent is then fixed to the ureter (to prevent peristaltic expulsion) with a loosely tied 4-0 absorbable suture. **(C)** This stabilizing suture is passed through the walls of the ureter and stent.

mosis, the proximal end of the conduit is sutured to the posterior peritoneum at the level of the sacral promontory. The distal end of the conduit is used to create an everted stoma. The muscular, fascial and peritoneal layers of the incision are approximated and grasped with Kocher clamps. An ellipse of skin approximately 2.5 cm is excised. A cruciate incision that easily admits two fingers is made through the fascia and peritoneum. The conduit is gently brought through the anterior abdominal wall opening paying particular attention not to twist the mesentery. The seromuscular layer of the conduit is sutured to the abdominal wall peritoneum and fascia, which minimizes the risk of stomal retraction and parastomal herniation.

The ileal stoma is everted using the modified Brooke technique. Sutures are placed through the subcuticular tissue at the cutaneous margin and through the seromuscular layer of the conduit at the skin level. This suture is tied, and the free end is passed through the full thickness of the ileum at the top of the loop. When these sutures are tied, the stoma turns down on itself creating a rosebud (Fig. 24-3).

An end-loop ileostomy as described by Turnbull and Hewitt[11] is favored by some surgeons. This technique is less likely to produce tension on the mesentery but is technically more difficult because of the amount of bowel that must be brought to the exterior abdominal wall. A Penrose drain is placed through the most mobile part of the distal ileal loop mesentery immediately beneath the bowel. The loop is delivered through the anterior abdominal wall to permit several centimeters of bowel to protrude above the level of the skin. The functional limb of the loop is oriented caudad to the nonfunctioning limb of the loop. Near the junction of the defunctionalized end, the loop is opened transversely, and the mucosa is sutured to the subcutaneous tissue with interrupted 4-0 suture. The superiority of the end-ileostomy as compared with the loop ileostomy has not been established. As discussed by Emmott et al.[12] contradictions among reported series result from varying definitions and the criteria for diagnosis of stomal stenosis.

Sigmoid Conduit

A sigmoid conduit, performed as part of a total exenteration, is an excellent method of supravesical diversion in the patient who has not been previously irradiated. Given this qualification, this method of supravesical diversion is not routinely used by the gynecologic oncologist. A 20- to 25-cm segment of sigmoid colon is chosen and transected using the GIA instrument. One should isolate a segment that is longer than appears necessary because of the shortening secondary to spasm of the longitudinal muscles that occurs intraoperatively.

The creation of a descending end-colostomy will avoid the attendant complications of a bowel anastomosis. If sufficient mobility of the colon is achieved after the splenic and hepatic flexures are taken down, an end-to-end colonic reanastomosis may be created using the EEA stapling device in the previously non-irradiated patient. The proximal end of the conduit segment is left with the closure created with the GIA stapler.

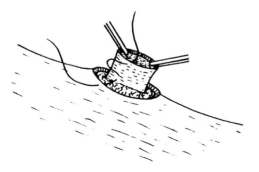 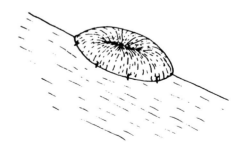

Fig. 24-3 The creation of an everted stoma requires that the bowel protrude above the skin surface for approximately 3 to 4 cm. Placement of absorbable sutures as illustrated folds the bowel upon itself, resulting in a rosebud stoma. (Shingleton HM, Orr JW: Cancer of the Cervix: Its Diagnosis and Treatment, 2nd Ed. Churchill Livingstone, Edinburgh, 1981)

A freely refluxing end-to-end ureterointestinal anastomosis may be performed as described for an ileal conduit. Alternatively, antirefluxing ureteral tunnels may be prepared. Staggered incisions through the taenia coli are made to avoid compromise of the blood supply to the bowel wall between the two sites of ureteral anastomosis. From the incision in the taenia, an oblique incision directed toward the mesenteric side of the bowel is then made through the seromuscular layer for a distance of approximately 5 cm. Development of the seromuscular flap is facilitated by infiltrating the wall of the colon with saline. Following sharp incision of the bowel mucosa, the ureter is sutured to the conduit mucosa with interrupted 4-0 suture with the knots tied on the outside. Insertion of a silastic ureteral catheter facilitates the creation of this anastomosis. Following completion of the anastomosis, the seromuscular layer of the tunnel is closed over the ureter, using interrupted 4-0 suture. The distal end of the conduit is used to fashion an everted stoma as described for the ileal conduit.

Transverse Colon Conduit

Use of the transverse colon for conduit diversion was first introduced by Nelson[13] and is probably the most versatile and generally applicable type of urinary conduit. Apart from its anatomic isolation from the field of pelvic radiotherapy, the transverse colon exhibits a generous blood supply, is easy to work with, and is a relatively mobile segment of bowel because of its lengthy mesentery.

Technically, a transverse colon conduit is constructed in a manner similar to that described for a sigmoid or an ileal conduit. A segment of transverse colon approximately 15 to 20 cm in length, supplied by the middle colic artery, is chosen as the conduit segment.

The greater omentum is dissected from the anterior wall of the transverse colon and the gastrocolic ligament divided. Although the hepatic and splenic flexure attachments may be taken down to facilitate the colonic reanastomosis, this is usually unnecessary.

The segment of transverse colon to be used as the conduit is isolated with two applications of the GIA. The bowel conduit mesentery is divided, taking care to make the distal incision approximately 2 to 3 cm longer than the proximal one to permit adequate mobility of the distal end of the conduit.

Using the automatic stapling device, the colon is reanastomosed as an end-to-end colocolonostomy. The mesenteric defect is closed with interrupted permanent suture to prevent internal herniation.

The conduit segment is placed below the colocolonostomy. Orientation of the conduit is influenced by the potential stomal sites, the length of ureters, and the end of segment closed with absorbable staples or oversewn with suture, if applicable. Orientation of the conduit with respect to peristalsis is not important since the colon empties by mass action.

The ureters are mobilized retroperitoneally as described for an ileal conduit. Following insertion of ureteral stents, the ureters are anastomosed within 3 to 5 cm of the occluded end of the conduit. A freely refluxing end-to-side ureterocolonic anastomosis can be constructed by placing interrupted 4-0 sutures through the wall of the ureter and through the wall of the colon, tying the knots on the outside (Fig. 24-4). Alternatively, an antirefluxing anastomosis can be constructed exactly as described for the ureterosigmoid anastomosis.

POSTOPERATIVE MANAGEMENT

Successful postoperative management of the patient who has undergone urinary diversion depends on a thorough understanding of the potential complications associated with the procedure. The operative mortality of urinary diversion alone ranges from 4 to 15 percent. When performed as part of an exenterative procedure, the operative mortality is reported to range from 7 to 37 percent. In most series, the risk of postoperative death is increased by advanced patient age, the presence of cancer and the performance of a total pelvic exenteration. The most common causes of operative mortality are sepsis, thromboembolic events and hemorrhage. The recognized risks of thromboembolic events, wound breakdown, wound infection, prolonged ileus, and bowel anastomotic leaks have led to certain general suggestions regarding the postoperative care of patients who have undergone urinary diversion. GI decompression, thromboembolic prophylaxis and empirical broad-spectrum antibiotic coverage are recommended. The administration of total parenteral nutrition is beneficial to most patients who are unable to eat for 7 to 10 days postoperatively.

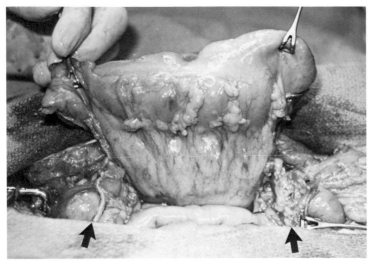

A

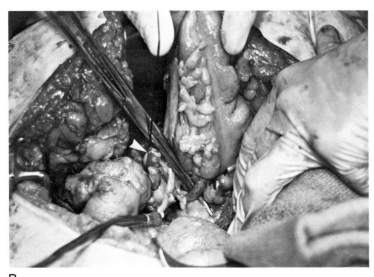

B

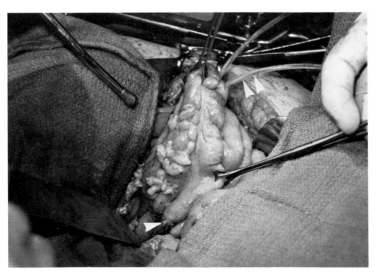

C

Fig. 24-4 The transverse colon conduit is technically straightforward and is associated with a low incidence of immediate and delayed postoperative complications. **(A)** The conduit segment is isolated using the GIA stapler device. The arrows indicate the colon segments to be reanastomosed behind the conduit segment. **(B)** One ureter has been anastomosed as described (indicated by the Kelly clamp). The contralateral ureter (white arrow), suspended by a silk suture, will be similarly anastomosed to the bowel. **(C)** The single white arrow indicates the completed uretcrointestinal anastomosis. The double white arrows show the Silastic stents exiting through the open end of the conduit.

A salutory effect of hyperalimentation upon postoperative mortality in gynecologic oncology patients who have undergone urinary diversion has been suggested by Hancock et al.[14]

The early postoperative complications of supravesical urinary diversion are largely referrable to conduit or bowel anastomotic leaks and stenosis and to urosepsis. The incidence of these various complications following supravesical urinary diversion varies greatly among reported series. Included among the factors that may directly or indirectly affect postoperative morbidity and mortality are the type of conduit created, the indication for the procedure, whether the patient received prior radiotherapy, the patient's general medical condition, and the presence or absence of cancer.

Urinary leakage following ureterointestinal anastomosis has been reported to occur in 1.7 to 16 percent of patients. The variation among reported series is due in part to the diagnostic criteria used. The routine use of retroperitoneal drains, as reported by Bagley et al.,[15] permits the recognition of small leaks that may or may not cause prolonged ileus and fever but that heal spontaneously. In contradistinction, the diagnosis of anastomotic leaks based on a rise in blood urea nitrogen and a stable creatinine, as reported by Hensle et al.,[16] may result in an underestimation of its true frequency. Although the median incidence of urinary leakage appears to be low (i.e., 3.2 percent), roughly one-fourth of patients in whom a leak develops will die. Although the cumulative number of transverse colon conduits from reported series is much smaller, the occurrence of a ureterointestinal leak or fistula is significantly less likely with a transverse colon conduit as compared with the ileal conduit. Presumably, this observation reflects the inherent advantage associated with the use of nonirradiated as compared to irradiated tissue.

If a ureteral leak is diagnosed, percutaneous nephrostomy with the antegrade passage of a ureteral catheter through the anastomosis and into the intestinal conduit will permit small leaks to heal spontaneously. Ureteral intubation intraoperatively will obviate the need for this intervention.

Bowel Complications

Gastrointestinal complications remain a major cause of early and delayed postoperative morbidity and mortality. Obstruction occurs in approximately 13 percent of diversion patients and is attributed to adhesions in approximately 50 percent of cases. Almost one-half of these bowel obstructions will occur during the early postoperative period and the remainder will necessitate a subsequent hospital admission. Other causes of bowel obstruction in patients who have undergone supravesical urinary diversion include the presence of metastatic disease, herniation, and volvulus.

Other GI complications include early postoperative anastomoic leaks and fistula formation. The risk of these complications increases when previously irradiated bowel is used. On the basis of the occurrence of bowel fistulae, Lichtinger et al.[17] have recommended the creation of an ileocolonostomy rather than an ileoileostomy in the previously irradiated patient undergoing ileal conduit diversion. However, the creation of a transverse colon conduit provides the most logical way to decrease early GI postoperative morbidity attributable to the use of irradiated tissue.

Stomal Complications

Stomal complications continue to be a major problem associated with conduit urinary diversion. The most common early stomal complications are attributable to an impaired blood supply. The management of these complications is dependent upon the extent of the damage. Although a mucosal slough may be followed closely, major necrosis of the stoma to or beyond the fascia requires prompt surgical revision.

Stomal retraction may result in a flush stoma (Fig. 24-5). As a result, the patient may experience considerable difficulty in attaching the appliance and maintaining a watertight seal. The resulting leakage of urine from the appliance will cause painful skin excoriation. Excessive retraction can also result in stomal stenosis, as will an impaired blood supply, persistently alkaline urine, and/or peristomal dermatitis. Peristomal dermatitis often results from the cutaneous aggregation of ammonia crystals produced by the action of urea-splitting bacteria on chronically alkaline urine. Suppressant antimicrobial therapy and acidification of the urine using methenamine mandelate with ascorbic acid and avoidance of urinary stasis will minimize these problems. Stomal stenosis will require surgical revision to avoid renal damage secondary to outflow obstruction.

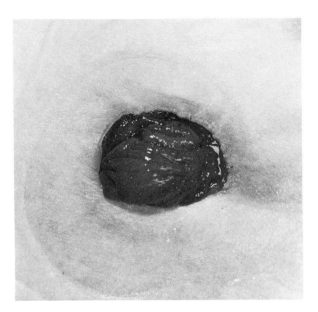

Fig. 24-5 An everted stoma should be created because it is easier for the patient to manage. It is difficult to achieve a watertight seal of an appliance with a flush stoma as pictured.

Metabolic Complications

Hyperchloremic metabolic acidosis is a potential problem with any type of urinary diversion through an intestinal segment. A clinically significant problem is most likely to develop in the colon conduit patient with impaired renal function.

Prolonged acidosis causes mobilization of the body's buffer stores and results in hypocalcemia and hypomagnesemia. Traditional therapy has included the empiric titration of the acidosis with sodium bicarbonate and a restriction of dietary chloride. Not only is this treatment frequently unsuccessful in the patient with preexisting renal dysfunction, but it also involves the administration of large salt loads. Koch and McDougal[18] recommended the administration of chlorpromazine (5 mg/kg/day) as a useful adjunct in the management of this complex metabolic disorder. Chlorpromazine nonspecifically retards intestinal absorptive and secretory processes by inhibiting the adenylate cyclase-cyclic adenosine monophosphate (cAMP) system.

Renal Function

The potential deterioration of renal function with time in the patient who has undergone conduit urinary diversion has been reviewed. To minimize the risk of subsequent renal damage, one type of conduit as compared to another cannot be recommended nor does the available data strongly support the use of an antirefluxing versus a freely refluxing ureterointestinal anastomosis in the adult patient. Because of the potential loss of renal function, any patient with a conduit must be followed at frequent intervals for an indefinite period of time.

Radionuclide scans are the best monitor of renal function but are not as available as other tests for many physicians. For this reason, it is recommended that the serum blood urea nitrogen and creatinine be measured frequently. An increase in these values signals the

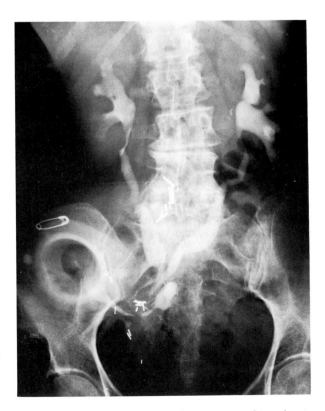

Fig. 24-6 Conduit stenosis results in increased intraluminal pressure, which may adversely affect renal function over time. This complication occasionally occurs in ileal conduits, but it is only rarely diagnosed in colon conduits.

need for a thorough assessment of renal function. It is important to recognize the limitations of the serum blood urea nitrogen and creatinine as indirect indicators of renal function in patients who have urinary conduits. Factitious elevations of both substances may occur in the event of urinary stasis.

An intravenous pyelogram should be obtained preoperatively, prior to discharge from the hospital and then at periodic intervals for an indefinite period of time. Conduit stenosis, which impedes the free low-pressure outflow of urine, is easily diagnosed radiographically (Fig. 24-6). Conduit stenosis requires surgical correction, since the prolonged exposure of the kidney to elevated ureteral pressures will adversely affect renal function. Similarly, the diagnosis of ureterointestinal obstruction also rquires prompt intervention to avoid irreversible renal damage. The man-

agement of partial obstruction involves percutaneous nephrostomy with the antegrade placement of a ureteral stent (Fig. 24-7). Because conduits are invariably colonized, patients who undergo stent insertion should be placed on some type of suppressant antimicrobial therapy to minimize the risk of pyelonephritis and subsequent urosepsis. Complete ureterointestinal obstruction is probably best managed by surgical revision or percutaneous nephrostomy alone.

SUMMARY

Many methods of supravesical urinary diversion have been described. The gynecologic oncologist generally relies upon the ileal conduit, transverse colon conduit or sigmoid conduit. The choice among

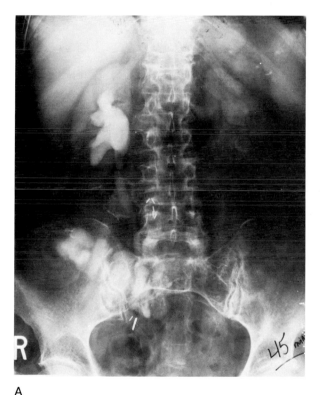
A

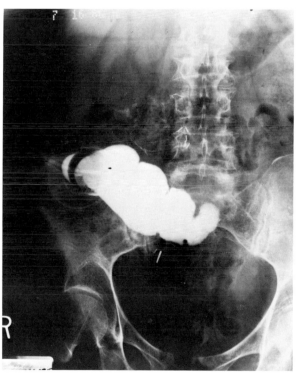
B

Fig. 24-7 The management of ureteral stenosis has changed dramatically with developments in interventional radiology. **(A)** A delayed intravenous pyelogram (IVP) illustrates a persistent nephrogram on the right and minimal renal function on the left. **(B)** The conduitogram demonstrates no reflux in this freely refluxing ureterointestinal anastomosis, underscoring the misleading interpretations that may occur, because spasm of the conduit or failure to provide sufficient intraluminal pressure may result in false-negative results. *(Figure continues.)*

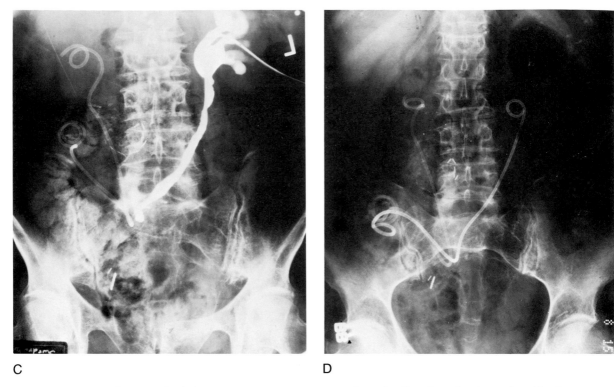

C   D

Fig. 24-7 *(Continued)*. **(C)** Using a percutaneous approach, a pigtail catheter has been placed in the right kidney and the instillation of dye through a catheter threaded down the left ureter clearly demonstrates the site of obstruction at the ureterointestinal anastomosos. **(D)** Double J pigtail catheters have been inserted in antegrade fashion.

the three is tempered by the indication for surgery, prior radiation therapy to the pelvis and personal experience. Functionally, there are no significant differences among the three types of conduits. There are no studies that demonstrate any advantage of colon conduits as compared with the ileal conduit in terms of the long-term preservation of renal function. However, the incidence of stomal complications is less for colonic conduits as compared with the ileal conduit. Of the three types of conduits most commonly used by the gynecologic oncologist, the transverse colon conduit offers several advantages. Apart from the stomal benefits shared with the sigmoid conduit, the transverse colon conduit is not affected by pelvic radiotherapy. As a consequence, the incidence of ureterointestinal fistulae, obstruction, and delayed stenosis is much lower as compared with sigmoid or ileal conduits.

REFERENCES

1. Simon J: Ectopia vesica: (Absence of the anterior walls of the bladder and pubic abdominal partietes): Operation for directing the orifices of the ureters into the rectum; temporary success; subsequent death; autospy. Lancet 2:568, 1852
2. Kock NG, Nilson AE, Nilsson LO, et al: Urinary diversion via a continent ileal reservoir: Clinical results in 12 patients. J Urol 128:469, 1982
3. Bricker EM: Bladder substitution after pelvic evisceration. Surg Clin North Am 30:1511, 1950
4. Johnson DE, Fuerst DE: Use of autosuture for construction of ileal conduit. J Urol 109:821, 1973
5. Costello AJ, Johnson DE: Modified autosuture technique for ileal conduit construction in urinary diversion. Aust NZ J Surg 54:477, 1984
6. Delgado G: Use of the automatic stapler in urinary

conduit diversions and pelvic exenterations. Gynecol Oncol 10:93, 1980

7. Neal DE: Complications of ileal conduit diversion in adults with cancer followed up for at least five years. Br Med J 290:1695, 1985

8. Sullivan JW, Grabstald H, Whitmore WF: Complications of uretero-ileal conduit with radical cystectomy: Review of 336 cases. J Urol 124:797, 1980

9. Daniel O, Singh ML: Measurement and control of bowel pressure in uretero-colic anastomosis. Br J Urol 41:32, 1969

10. Ravitch NM, Steichen FM: Techniques of staple suturing in the gastrointestinal tract. Ann Surg 175:815, 1972

11. Turnbull RB Jr, Hewitt CR: Loop-end myotomy ileostomy in the obese patient. Urol Clin N Am 5:423, 1978

12. Emmott D, Noble MJ, Mebust WK: A comparison of end versus loop stomas for ileal conduit urinary diversion. J Urol 133:588, 1985

13. Nelson JH Jr: Atlas of Radical Pelvic Surgery. Appleton-Century-Crofts, New York, 1969

14. Hancock KC, Copeland LJ, Gershenson DM, et al: Urinary conduits in gynecologic oncology. Obstet Gynecol 67:680, 1986

15. Bagley DH, Glazier W, Osias M, Lytton B: Retroperitoneal drainage of ureterointestinal conduits. J Urol 121:271, 1979

16. Hensle TW, Bredin HC, Dretler SP: Diagnosis and treatment of a urinary leak after ureteroileal conduit for diversion. J Urol 116:29, 1976

17. Lichtinger M, Averette H, Girtanner R, et al: Small bowel complications after supravesical diversion in pelvic exenteration. Gynecol Oncol 24:137, 1986

18. Koch MO, McDougal WS: Chlorpromazine: Adjuvant therapy for the metabolic derangement created by urinary diversion through intestinal segments. J Urol 134:165, 1985

SUGGESTED READINGS

Alfert HJ, Gillenwater JY: The consequences of ureteral irradiation with special reference to subsequent ureteral injury. J Urol 107:369, 1972

Baker VV, Dudzinski MR, Fowler WC, et al: Percutaneous nephrostomy in gynecologic oncology. Am J Obstet Gynecol 149:772, 1984

Bisson JM, Vinson RK, Leadbetter GW. Urolithiasis from stapler anastomosis. Am J Surg 137:280, 1974

Brochner-Mortensen J, Jensen S, Rodbro P: Assessment of renal function from plasma creatinine in adult patients. Scand J Urol Nephrol 11:263, 1977

Burstein JD, Furlit CF: Complications of cutaneous ureterostomy and other cutaneous diversion. Urol Clin North Am 10:433, 1983

Dagen JE, Sanford EJ, Rohner TJ Jr: Complications of the nonrefluxing colon conduit. J Urol 123:585, 1980

Ernstoff JJ, Degrasia AH, Marshall JB, et al: A randomized blinded clinical trial of a rapid colonic lavage solution (GoLytely) compared with standard preparation for colonoscopy and barium enema. Gastroenterology 84:1512, 1985

Golimbu M, Morales P: Jejunal conduits: Technique and complications. J Urol 113:787, 1975

Gonzales ET, Baum NH, Friedman A, Carlton Ce: Sigmoid conduit: Review and description of technique. Urology 10:579, 1977

Hill MJ, Hudson MJ, Stewart T: The urinary bacterial flora in patients with three types of urinary tract diversion. J Med Microbiol 16:221, 1983

Jeter KF: The flush versus the protuding urinary stoma. J Urol 116:424, 1976

Koch MO, McDougal WS: determination of renal function following urinary diversion through intestinal segments. J Urol 133:517, 1985

Mansson W, Colleen S, Stigsson L: Four methods of ureterointestinal anastomosis in urinary conduit diversion. A comparative study of early and late complications and the influence of radiotherapy. Scand J Urol Nephrol 13:191, 1979

Orr JW, Shingleton HM, Hatch KD, et al: Urinary diversion in patients undergoing pelvic exenteration. Am J Obstet Gynecol 142:883, 1982

Orr JW, Shingleton HM, Hatch KD, et al: Gastrointestinal complications associated with pelvic exenterations. Am J Obstet Gynecol 145:325, 1983

Rivard JY, Bedard A, Dionne L: Colonic neoplasms following ureterosigmoidostomy. J Urol 113:781, 1975

Schlesinger RE, Berman ML, Ballon SC, et al: The choice of an intestinal segment for a urinary conduit. Surg Gynecol Obstet 148:45, 1979

Stanley P, Craven JD, Skinner DG, Richie JP: The natural history of the upper renal tracts in adults following uretro-ileal diversion (Bricker procedure). 125:804, 1975

25

Intestinal Resection and Ostomy Care

Karl C. Podratz
Richard E. Symmonds
John V. Hagen

Whereas the surgical expertise for extended radical extirpation of malignant tumors of the pelvis, including segments of the adjacent gastrointestinal (GI) or urinary (or both) tract, was readily available at the turn of the century, the associated operative mortality predominantly attributable to postoperative sepsis tempered enthusiasm for such exercises. However, with the subsequent technologic advances in anesthesia, blood replacement, and antimicrobial therapy, followed more recently by developments in pharmaceuticals, electronic monitoring, and nutritional support, the experienced pelvic surgeon is seldom limited by the technical or physiologic constraints but rather by the biologic nature of the neoplasm and the effectiveness (or ineffectiveness) of adjunctive therapeutic modalities. Therefore, because of the intraperitoneal patterns of metastatic dissemination of several types of pelvic malignant lesions, as well as the proximity of the distal GI tract to the primary cancer of the internal female genitalia, intestinal resection with restoration of bowel continuity or ostomy formation frequently is necessary in the surgical management of these oncologic processes.

INDICATIONS FOR INTESTINAL RESECTION

Definitive Primary or Salvage Therapy

Definitive primary and more frequently salvage surgical management of cervical, vaginal, and vulvar malignant lesions require the concomitant resection of the adjacent distal large bowel to obtain adequate clearance. Local growth and direct extension, with invasion of the juxtaposition structures, are characteristics of the squamous cell carcinomas commonly associated with the distal internal and the external female genitalia. When the distal sigmoid, rectum, or anus is encroached upon by these neoplasms, a wide en bloc surgical resection of these structures is preferred. Extended radical hysterectomy or partial vaginectomy to include segmental resection of the involved bowel is an option in selected patients who have primary or recurrent cervical carcinoma with limited involvement of the rectum.[1] However, in the presence of extensive pelvic irradiation, radionecrosis, or significant central tumor volumes, an exenterative procedure should be contemplated, with the creation of an ileal, sigmoid, or transverse colon conduit.[2-7] In addition, extended radical vulvectomy, including partial resection of the rectum and anus, must be considered when extension is limited to the central portion of the vulva in patients with carcinoma of the vulva.[8] More extensive anal and rectal involvement or spread to two or more central vulvar structures requires ultraradical surgical management, combining radical vulvectomy with abdominoperineal resection or an exenterative procedure.[8-10]

Tumor-Reductive Surgery

Primary tumor reductive surgery has been advocated in the overall treatment schemata for malignant lesions of the more proximal portion of the müllerian system. Tumors originating in the ovaries, fallopian tubes, and endometrium are commonly adenocarcinomas with a propensity for cellular exfoliation and intraperitoneal dissemination. The resulting implantation and proliferation of the tumor on the intraabdominal serosa and peritoneal surfaces, particularly of the distal ileum and sigmoid, frequently requires resection of segments of bowel during the tumor reductive procedures. The theoretical merits of these procedures include optimization for adjunctive therapeutic modalities, reversal of immunologic processes, and positive psychological effects.[11] Surgical reduction of advanced disease to microscopic or minimal residual disease has been related to enhanced longevity after adjuvant therapy for ovarian, fallopian tube, and endometrial carcinoma.[12-19] In a recent report by Heintz et al.,[20] 70 percent of patients presenting with advanced ovarian cancer had their tumors reduced to a diameter of 15 mm or less. Bowel surgery, that is, invariably resection with or without stoma formation, was required in 23 percent of patients. Postoperative morbidity was relatively low and independent of whether intestinal resection was incorporated.

Complications of Surgery and Radiotherapy

Inherent in the radical or ultraradical surgical management of female genital cancers is an associated postoperative morbidity from compromise of the intestinal tract. Early postoperative complications, including obstruction, anastomotic dehiscence, vascular occlusion, infarction, and enterocolitis as well as delayed surgical-related sequelae such as fistula, obstruction, symptomatic blind loop, volvulus, intussusception, and herniations, frequently require prompt reoperation and resection of the involved segment(s) of bowel. The subsequent morbidity is acceptably low when the surgeon secures a technically sound, tension-free anastomosis of two well-vascularized bowel margins. By contrast, the surgical treatment of intestinal injuries after either pelvic or abdominal irradiation, or both, is more complex and is associated with significant perioperative morbidity. While technologic advances in instrumentation, dosimetry, fractionation, and radiobiology would predict enhanced treatment results, the ability to deliver high midplane doses of radiation, frequently in the presence of chemotherapeutic agents such as doxorubicin and cisplatin, have increased intestinal toxicity and morbidity.[21-23] Major treatment-related sequelae, including persistent obstruction, necrosis, perforation, hemorrhage, and fistula formation, will require surgical intervention. Whether the compromised bowel segment is bypassed or resected and the primary anastomosis or stoma formation is achieved, successful management is a challenge for even the most experienced surgeon.[24-27]

Surgical Palliation

Neither past surgical experience nor knowledge of the sparse literature addressing this subject facilitates the decision-making processes appreciably when a palliative procedure is contemplated for advanced malignant lesions of the pelvis. The consideration for surgical intervention is frequently precipitated by the clinical presentation of complete or partial bowel obstruction, which occurs with various frequencies in end-stage ovarian, fallopian tube, endometrial, and cervical carcinomas, as well as genital sarcomas. Progressive encasement of the bowel and its mesentery by tumor will lead to either mechanical obstruction or extended adynamic segments that are devoid of peristaltic function. Generally, management consists of either an attempt at long-tube decompression and holistic support or reexploration with bowel resection and frequent stoma formation with the incorporation of secondary tumor reduction when justifiable. Patient age, estimated patient longevity, tumor burden, prior chemotherapy or radiotherapy or both, and available second-line therapy are variables that influence the usual surgical criteria for management of such bowel obstruction. While the major operative morbidity (31 to 49 percent) and mortality (12 to 15 percent) are high for the surgical management of intestinal obstruction in advanced ovarian cancer, the median survival (10 to 20 weeks) and 1-year survival rates (14 to 17 percent) suggest that palliation is enhanced in a select minority of patients.[28–32] The existing clinical enigma is the inability to make an adequate prediction—on the basis of examination, imaging, and laboratory evaluation—those patients with post-treatment-related bowel obstruction who will benefit from additional surgical manipulation.

Management of Extragenital Entities During Pelvic Surgery

Finally, the detection of a secondary intestinal disease process during surgical management of (or what was presumed to be) a genital malignancy may require resection of a portion of the intestine. The most frequent extragenital entity that pelvic surgeons encounter is a diverticular process associated with acute or chronic diverticulitis of the distal descending colon or sigmoid, or both. If preoperative bowel preparations were performed, we suggest resection with anastomosis and adequate drainage, unless a paracolic, mesenteric, or diverticular abscess is encountered, requiring formation of a colonic stoma. A stoma is more frequently needed when either there is a free or concealed perforation or the bowel is not properly prepared. When a colostomy is mandatory, consideration should include reanastomosis with a proximal stoma, closure of the rectal stump (Hartmann procedure), or creation of an adjacent mucous fistula. If the patient's physical status will not permit more definitive surgery, adequate drainage with a proximal diverting colostomy is a reasonable alternative.

The incidental detection of an associated secondary malignant lesion in the GI tract is not a rare occurrence. Because 10 percent of ovarian cancers are metastatic and the colon is the second most frequent site of neoplasm (with an increasing prevalence) in females, the frequency with which pelvic surgeons will be involved in the primary treatment of colonic carcinomas will also increase. On the basis of our collective impressions, gynecologic surgeons must be prepared to manage the following unexpected surgical settings: (1) clinical ovarian lesions noted to be pathologically metastatic, with the most common extragenital site of origin being the right colon; (2) left adnexal mass lesions suspected to be ovarian in origin surgically identified as colonic carcinomas; and (3) incidental surgical detection of isolated neoplasms of either the small or the large bowel during pelvic surgery. Therefore, the gynecologic oncologist should keep up with state-of-the-art practices regarding the treatment of small bowel and colorectal cancers.

PREOPERATIVE PREPARATION AND STOMA SITE SELECTION

The preoperative assessment and preparation of an oncologic surgical candidate requires effective planning and management in order to (1) optimize the patient's tolerance for the intraoperative and postoperative stresses that result from physiologic and anatomic alterations, and (2) reduce postoperative morbidity. Even patients with relative contraindications to surgery, including age and significant medical problems, can be sufficiently rehabilitated medically to withstand the modest anesthetic and surgically induced stresses. Anticipation of the extent of surgical intervention, including the possible need for intestinal resection and ostomy formation, is generally based on the history, physical examination, and supplementary laboratory and diagnostic testing. The supplementary testing routinely includes electrocardiography, chest radiography, hematologic studies, serum chemistry studies, urinalysis, and a coagulation profile. Detectable deviations from the normal physiologic values or functions require expeditious clinical investigation and prompt correction. Because the cardiovascular and pulmonary systems are at greatest risk during the perioperative interval, the preanesthetic medical evaluation is intended to assess, stress, and enhance cardiopulmonary function to maximize the patient's cardiac index and oxygen-carrying capacities. Radiologic imaging of the GI tract, as well as excretory urography, endoscopic visualization of the distal urinary or intestinal tracts, computed tomography (CT), or sonography may be employed occasionally on a selective basis to provide additional information regarding the extent of disease and the anticipated degree of surgical radicality.

The nutritional status of the patient, which can adversely affect morbidity, must be carefully evaluated during the preanesthetic medical evaluation. Several of the disease processes in gynecologic oncology that require surgical intervention and bowel resection have pathologic lesions that contribute to a suboptimal nutritional state. Furthermore, intervals of relative starvation imposed before and after surgery further compound the situation. At presentation, the patient's recent dietary intake and associated weight changes as well as physical signs of a catabolic state, including edema or subcutaneous fat loss, or both, should be carefully assessed. Evaluation of the biochemical parameters of catabolism, including the blood urea nitrogen (BUN) and total protein and serum albumin levels, is useful, particularly for subsequent monitoring. Preoperative correction or reversal of the malnutrition generally requires parenteral hyperalimentation. Implicit in such therapy is the delivery of a quantity of carbohydrates, protein equivalents, and fat emulsions in excess of the basal nitrogen and caloric requirements needed to achieve an anabolic state. Fundamental to such therapy is adequate hydration and supplementation with electrolytes, minerals, and vitamins.

Bowel Preparation

The morbidity associated with resection of the distal GI tract is a reflection of the extent of soiling and size of the bacterial inoculum. Undoubtedly, the size of the inoculum is related to the intraluminal concentration of organisms, an index of the effectiveness of the preoperative bowel preparation. The frequency with which the gynecologic oncologist regrets not having requested a bowel preparation should diminish. On the basis of the patient's history and physical findings, most patients requiring intestinal resection can be identified and properly prepared. In patients without definable evidence of bowel involvement but at some risk of such according to the natural history of their disease, a modified preparation is suggested, thereby avoiding potential compromise of optimal therapy.

Controversy exists regarding the merits of mechanical, antibiotic, and combination preparations for adequately reducing the microbial count within the bowel. We favor the use of both mechanical cleansing and oral antimicrobial agents but emphasize the importance of the mechanical component. Reduction of the fecal content and lumen residue, which harbor and foster microbial growth, will sufficiently decrease intraluminal bacterial counts. Although antibiotics alone are of minimal value, their effectiveness in concert with mechanical purging is well recognized. Oral antibiotics are selected on the basis of demonstrated efficacy against intestinal organisms (preferably a broad-spectrum agent), minimal absorption, nonirritating to the intestinal tract, and lack of promotion of overgrowth of resistant organisms. While *Escherichia coli* is the most common organism associated with postoperative sepsis, *Enterococcus* and *Bacteroides* species are occasionally encountered in gynecologic surgery. We prefer the oral use of a combination of neomycin and tetracycline, erythromycin, or metronidazole. Either a 2-day or a single-day bowel preparation is used on our gynecologic surgical services (Table 25-1). With postoperative febrile morbidity, as well as wound and intraabdominal sepsis, used as a basis for comparison, the preliminary results of a prospectively randomized evaluation of the standard 2-day preparation versus the single-day intestinal lavage suggest that there are no significant differences among patients subjected to colorectal surgery at our institution (Wolff BG, personal communication).

Also, prophylactic antibiotics are administered systemically to all patients at our institution in whom the probability of bowel resection exists. The value of initiating antimicrobial therapy before operation for gastric, biliary, or colon surgery was demonstrated by Stone et al.,[33] who witnessed a significant reduction in wound sepsis. Furthermore, these workers showed that extension of perioperative antimicrobial coverage for several days after the operation was not beneficial.[34] Recent reports addressing the efficacy of perioperative antibiotics in radical pelvic surgery in the absence of bowel resection also demonstrated decreased febrile and infectious morbidity.[35,36]

Ostomy Education and Stoma Site Selection

The basis for favorable postoperative and extended ostomy function and care is formulated during preoperative counseling, preferably with an enterostomal therapist. Each patient requires individual

Table 25-1 Preoperative Bowel Preparation for Patients Undergoing Intestinal Resection

Time	Standard Preparation	GoLYTELY Lavage[a]
Two days before operation		
Mechanical		
AM	Phosphate of soda (15 ml)	
PM	Phosphate of soda (15 ml)	
	Water enemas (2)	
Antibiotic: qid	Neomycin (1.5 g) plus	
	tetracycline (250 mg)	
	or erythromycin (250 mg)	
	or metronidazole (250 mg)	
Diet	Clear liquids	
One day before operation		
Mechanical		
AM	Phosphate of soda (1)	12 to 6 PM: 4–6 L GoLYTELY preparation PO[b]
	Water enemas (3)	
PM	Water enemas (3)	
Antibiotic: qid	Same as previous day	6 and 11 PM: Neomycin (2 g)
		Metronidazole (2 g)
Diet	Clear liquids	Clear liquids
Day of operation	NPO after midnight	NPO after midnight
	Weigh at 6 AM	Weigh at 6 AM

[a] A polyethylene glycol-containing electrolyte solution.
[b] A feeding tube (Keofeed) may be needed.

rehabilitation, a process that commences with preoperative information regarding the anticipated surgical procedure and the postoperative convalescence, introduction to ostomy-related materials, and emotional support including, if possible, reassurance from a well-adjusted ostomate. The postoperative transition includes discussion of operative findings and prognosis, progressive direction in self-care skills, and building of the patient's confidence via continued reassurance and discussions. The patient's apprehensions are slowly supplanted by maturing independence with increasing knowledge in utilization of community resources and the recognition of the ready availability of the enterostomal therapist or physician with medical advice pertaining to stoma-related issues.

The emotional and physical problems resulting from leakage and appliance insecurity generally can be minimized or avoided by the proper selection of the preoperative site. The enterostomal therapist, with advice from the surgeon regarding anticipated operative management, should identify the preferred site(s) before the procedure. Generally, the more

functional locations avoid incisions, scars, skin folds, skin irregularities, and bony prominences such as the iliac crest and costal margins. Ideally, the stoma should be positioned below the waist line and at the crest of the infraumbilical fat roll. The site selection should be evaluated while the patient is lying, sitting, and standing; if uncertainty exists, the appliance should be secured and the exercise repeated.

SURGICAL TECHNIQUES

The need for resection of the GI tract during the treatment of oncologic or related diseases is generally anticipated before operation from the patient's history and clinical presentation. Therefore, the surgeon's choice of the primary or secondary incision should facilitate accessibility to the neoplastic process, as well as to optimize exposure for mobilization, resection, and reconstruction of the GI tract. We prefer a lower midline incision, skirting the umbilicus, which can be extended cephalad with ease when indicated. Furthermore, in patients previously subjected to multiple surgical procedures or high-dose irradiation, or both, access to the peritoneal cavity through the old scar or the irradiated fields, or both, may be difficult because of viscera adherent to the undersurface of the anterior abdominal wall. Hence, entry into the abdominal cavity is preferably gained at a less vulnerable point—generally more cephalad. After the initial entry into the abdominal cavity, placement of Kocher clamps on the fascial edges for anterior traction and posterior displacement of the adherent viscera will permit sharp dissection in the avascular plane, thereby minimizing visceral trauma and bleeding.

Inadvertent trauma to the small bowel during mobilization and exposure procedures, as well as deliberate serosal sampling and partial or complete resection during the surgical management of pelvic malignancies, requires familiarity with appropriate reparative approaches. Limited serosal tears or defects seldom require debridement and only seroserosal reapproximation employing interrupted 3-0 or 4-0 nonabsorbable sutures (Fig. 25-1). Preferably, the suture line is directed in a plane perpendicular to the long axis of the bowel, thereby minimizing potential compromise of the lumen. With enterotomies or wedge resections

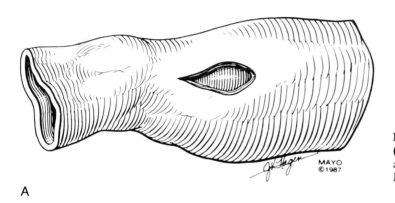

A

Fig. 25-1 Operative closure of serosal tear **(A)** employing interrupted 3-0 nonabsorbable sutures **(B, C).** (By permission of Mayo Foundation.)

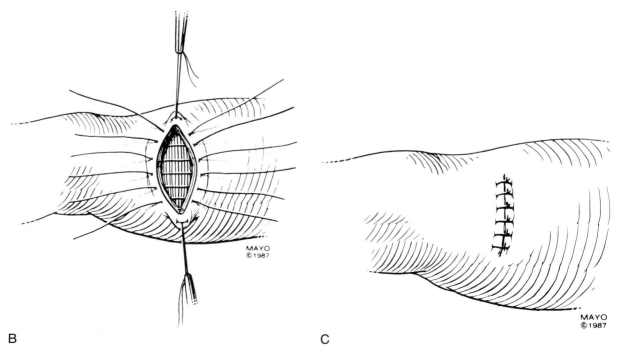

B

C

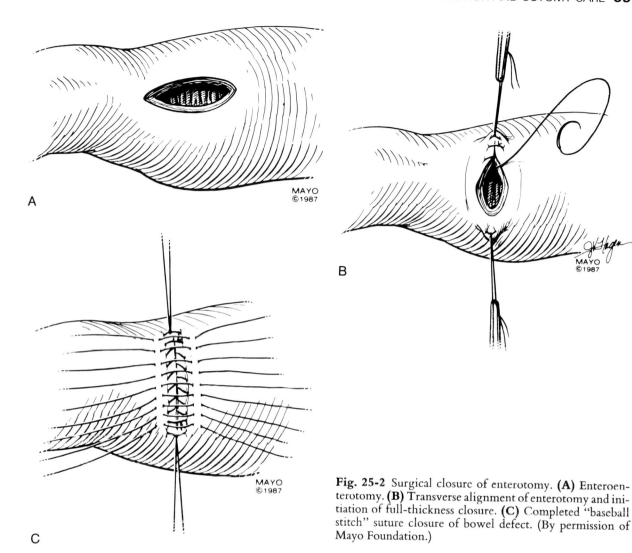

A

B

C

MAYO
©1987

Fig. 25-2 Surgical closure of enterotomy. **(A)** Enteroenterotomy. **(B)** Transverse alignment of enterotomy and initiation of full-thickness closure. **(C)** Completed "baseball" stitch" suture closure of bowel defect. (By permission of Mayo Foundation.)

for localized lesions or devitalization, the adjacent bowel is carefully assessed for viability, liberally debrided when necessary, and closed in a two-layer fashion, closure again being perpendicular to the long axis of the bowel lumen (Fig. 25-2). The mucosal margins are expeditiously approximated employing 2-0 or 3-0 absorbable sutures in a continuous "baseball" (outside-to-inside, outside-to-inside) or a simple through-and-through (outside-to-inside, inside-to-outside) manner, incorporating all layers of the bowel wall. Repair is completed with a second seroserosal layer, employing interrupted 3-0 nonabsorbable suture material.

Because the small intestine is near the pelvic viscera and is frequently involved metastatically when there is pelvic malignancy, partial resection of the small intestine, particularly the terminal ileum, is frequently required in the treatment of primary and recurrent genital neoplasms, as well as of complications resulting from primary or adjuvant radiotherapy. The more liberal incorporation of small bowel resection as part of tumor-reductive surgery and the management of treatment-related sequelae, at least in part, reflect the limited acute and chronic morbidity associated with this procedure. The morbidity is predominantly predicated on the facility with which anatomic and physiologic restoration of bowel continuity can be accomplished after resection. If there is no impairment in fibroblast activity, functional and leakage-free anastomoses are dependent on the preservation of an adequate circumferential blood supply and the accurate reapproximation of the gut wall. Operative exposure, as well as assessment of bowel viability, may be suboptimal in the presence of an excessively distended intestinal tract. Decompression can be readily secured by use of one of several methods. Because subsequent transnasal upper intestinal tract aspiration is frequently needed, we prefer transnasal long-tube decompression (ideally using a Tucker tube) with interoperative guidance through the more proximal GI tract. Occasionally, transmural decompression is required and effectively performed by using an initial pursestring placement in the bowel wall, through which a catheter (Angiocath or Intercath), Hemovac drain, or gallbladder-aspirating trocar can be inserted.

Rapid anastomotic union requires delivery of sufficient levels of nutrients, as well as tissue and blood constitutents, to the site of resection. Generous margins of clearance adjacent to the compromised intestinal segment will result in favorable blood flow to the resected margins. Furthermore, transecting the bowel at an angle of 45 to 60 degrees to the mesenteric border and avoiding excessive undermining (cleaning off) of the mesenteric border will further ensure satisfactory capillary flow, thereby promoting optimal primary healing. Meticulous ligation of the mesenteric vessels during bowel resection is important, particularly at the mesenteric-bowel serosal interface, thereby avoiding hematoma formation, which can produce significant perianastomotic venous stasis and occasional arteriolar occlusion, with subsequent compromise of the normal tissue reparative processes.

Generally, the functional integrity after segmental

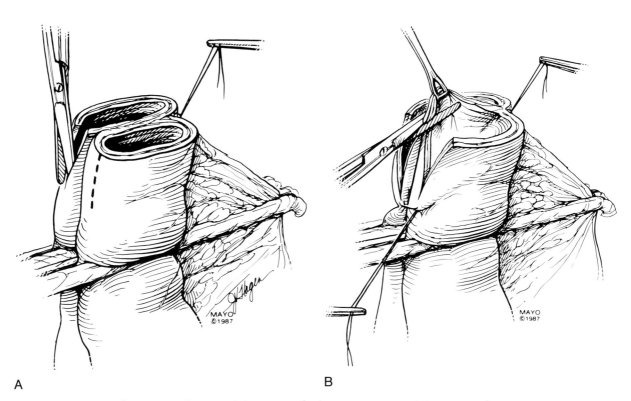

A   B

Fig. 25-3 Enlargement of intestinal diameter to facilitate anastomosis. **(A)** Incision of antimesenteric border. **(B)** Excision of intervening antimesenteric septum. (By permission of Mayo Foundation.)

small bowel resection is a reflection of the precision with which the anastomosis was originally performed. While various intraoperative presentations may dictate the use of any of three anastomoses (i.e., end-to-end, end-to-side, or side-to-side), we prefer, when the surgical setting permits, an open end-to-end anastomosis. This technique is theoretically the most physiologic approach for reestablishing continuity and, from a practical standpoint, can be most expeditiously performed. However, caution must be exercised when the opposing bowel lumina either are of small caliber or show a great disparity in diameter. The small luminal caliber is at risk of early obstruction from inversion of excessive tissue and the accompanying edema and for delayed obstruction from cicatricial contractures, resulting in stricture formation. Careful preanastomotic inspection will alert the surgeon to this potential complication, which can be readily circumvented without resorting to an alternative approach. Incising the antimesenteric borders of both opposing ends and obliquely excising a portion of the resulting antimesenteric septum will dramatically increase the anastomotic circumference in a noncircular fashion (Fig. 25-3). The luminal disparity is similarly approached by incising the antimesenteric border of the bowel with the smaller luminal diameter to approximate that of the opposed larger lumen. Additional minor discrepancies can be corrected by decreasing the distance between suture placement on the disparagingly smaller side while maintaining standard distances between sutures on the larger side.

After adequate mobilization and determination of the length of intestine requiring resection, the predetermined lines of excision on the mesentery are outlined by serosal incisions, exposing the underlying adipose tissue to be excised and vessels to be ligated (Fig. 25-4). The mesenteric borders are freed of adipose tissue for several millimeters, avoiding excessive undermining. Atraumatic intestinal clamps (linenshod clamp) are obliquely (45- to 60-degree angles) applied to ensure an optimal blood supply and lumen diameter. Crushing clamps are subsequently applied on the side of the lesion 2 to 3 cm from the atraumatic clamps, and the bowel is transected and cleansed with 70 percent ethanol and water. Although single mesenteric and antimesenteric nonabsorbable seroserosal bowel sutures are used for stabilization and proper

alignment of the lumen, we prefer to delay additional seroserosal approximation until completion of the initial layer. Mucosal closure is initiated by employing 2-0 or 3-0 absorbable sutures with placement of a four-bite coaptation suture in the corner nearest the surgeon. A continuous through-and-through (inside-to-outside, outside-to-inside) full-thickness suturing technique is used on the posterior margins and is converted to a baseball-type stitch (outside-to-inside, outside-to-inside) at the opposite corner for closure of the anterior edges. This approach adequately approximates all tissue layers but avoids excessive circumferential inversion of the tissue margin during the placement of the initial layer.

After removal of the bowel clamps, interrupted 3-0 nonabsorbable seroserosal sutures are placed anteriorly; after the bowel is rotated 180 degrees, the seroserosal layer is completed circumferentially. Palpation of the anastomotic site by use of the surgeon's thumb and index finger will document appropriate patency. The mesenteric defect is closed, with appropriate care being taken to avoid compromising the vascular supply.

An alternative to the two-layer, hand-sewn GI anastomosis is the restoration of bowel continuity, employing an automatic stapling device. Although staplers permit rapid and clean resections and anastomoses of the GI tract, we favor delaying the introduction of such mechanical union until sufficient expertise is demonstrable in the more traditional techniques, thereby preparing the resident surgeon for managing potential sequalae of technical failures or complications associated with stapling and bowel surgery in general. Successful GI stapling requires strict attention to details so as to avoid common pitfalls, including excessive or insufficient tightening of the instrument, failure to include the entire bowel width within the stapling lines, and withdrawing the device before adequately opening the limbs. Although decreased operating time is frequently mentioned as the main reason for using staplers, the cogent advantages derived from employing staplers are related more to the accuracy with which resections can be performed and the minimal probability of soiling and ease of managing disparities in bowel size. Furthermore, because type-B staples permit more favorable capillary flow to the stapled margins and stapling requires less bowel manipulation or reaction to the

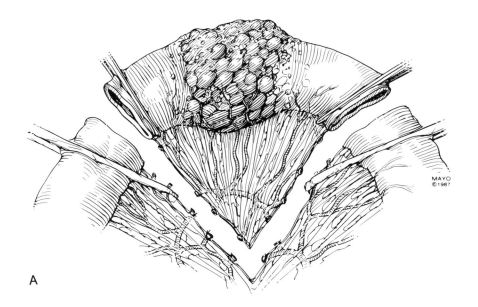

A

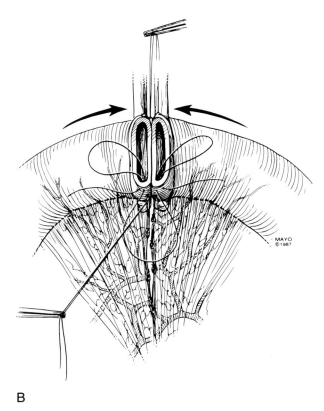

B

Fig. 25-4 Resection and hand-sewn end-to-end anastomosis of small bowel. **(A)** Intestinal and mesenteric resection. **(B)** Alignment and immobilization of intestinal margins. *(Figure continues.)*

materials, thereby reducing tissue trauma, the overall healing process at the site of union should begin earlier and progress more rapidly.

The stapled anastomosis most frequently employed for enteroenterostomies and other intestinal reapproximation is the functional end-to-end technique (Fig. 25-5). A mesenteric serosal incision is made and the vasculature interrupted in the fashion previously outlined. Two rows of type-B staples are automatically inserted along both margins of the line of transection during firing of the GIA stapler. The everted stapled margins are inspected for bleeding points, and hemostasis is secured with electrocautery. Linen-shod intestinal clamps are applied at equal distances from the stapled margins to minimize the efflux of the bowel content and to aid in approximation of the antimesenteric borders. The antimesenteric stapled corners are excised to permit insertion of the two limbs of the GIA stapler. After proper alignment of the bowel and instrument, the stapler is activated to form the anastomosis, and again the margins are inspected for hemostasis. The defect is closed, using a TA-55 stapler. To avoid closure apposition of the intraluminal anastomotic margins and to minimize the number of transecting staple lines, stab wounds are made in the opposing antimesenteric borders of the bowel 1.5 cm from the stapled lines, into which the limbs of the GIA stapler are placed, closed, and activated. The GIA staple lines are held apart, and the

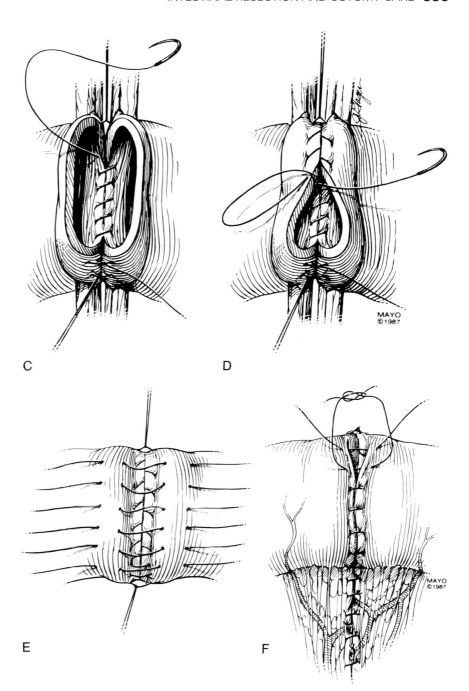

C   D

E   F

Fig. 25-4 *(Continued).* **(C)** Posterior continuous approximation. **(D)** Anterior "baseball stitch" approximation. **(E)** Placement of second-layer, inverting, reinforcing nonabsorbable sutures. **(F)** Second-layer closure. (By permission of Mayo Foundation.)

defect is closed with the TA stapler, resulting in a more favorable triangular anastomosis (Fig. 25-6).

Resection of the distal ileum proximal to the ascending colon is frequently required during primary tumor reductive surgery and for surgical management of radiation-related intestinal injuries. We believe that, except under unusual circumstances, surgical or pathologic processes resulting from pelvic malignancies or because of treatment causing intestinal dysfunction are preferably resected rather than bypassed.

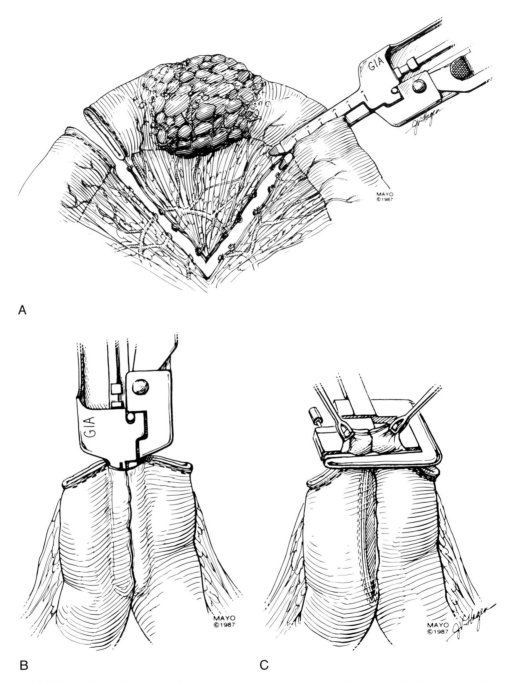

A

B   C

Fig. 25-5 Resection and functional end-to-end anastomosis of small bowel, employing stapling device. **(A)** Resection of small bowel. **(B)** Bowel alignment and proper placement of GIA stapler limbs. **(C)** Closure of defect with TA stapler after activation and removal of GIA stapler. (By permission of Mayo Foundation.)

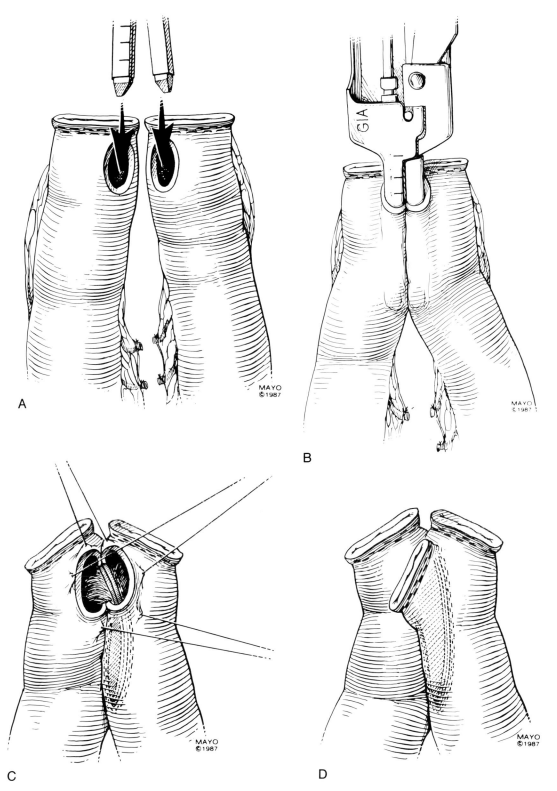

Fig. 25-6 Functional end-to-end ileoileostomy. **(A)** Direction of stapling limbs into enterotomies. **(B)** Alignment of bowel and stapler. **(C)** Anastomosis after activation of stapler. **(D)** Closure of common enterotomy. (By permission of Mayo Foundation.)

The technical advantages in postoperative monitoring, as well as medical, nutritional, and chemotherapeutic support have permitted greater liberalization in managing these problems. Therefore, when the adjacent small bowel is involved in a primary pelvic malignancy or is secondarily dysfunctional because of recurrent disease or postradiation-induced pelvic adhesions or obstructions, mobilization and resection, frequently including the resection of a portion of ascending colon, should be considered. Resection of the cecum and several centimeters of proximal colon affords (1) more adequate margins of clearance from the compromising process; (2) a more favorable blood supply, which enhances union, particularly in postirradiation settings; and (3) a more generous diameter at the anastomotic site.

After mobilization of the ileum from the peritoneal or serosal surfaces in the pelvis, the peritoneum lateral to the cecum and ascending colon is incised from the pelvic brim to an appropriate level. The hepatocolic ligament is divided if a right colectomy is anticipated. Medial mobilization will permit identification of the right ureter, ovarian vessels, perinephric fat of the inferior pole of the kidney, the second and third portions of the duodenum, and the inferior vena cava. If the tumor involves the colic gutter surfaces, the peritoneum lateral to the colon should be widely excised during colonic mobilization. The serosa of the mesentery is incised from the designated points of transection of the ileum and colon, with caution being used to avoid trauma to the superior mesenteric vessels. The right colic and ileocolic arteries and occasionally the right branch of the middle colic artery are divided, together with the corresponding venous network. Because the ileocolic artery supplies the distal segment of ileum, a minimum of 12 to 15 cm of terminal ileum is sacrificed with the cecum and proximal colon. The principles governing the mechanics of GI resection to minimize potential morbidity are equally applicable under these circumstances. An end-to-end enterocolostomy is performed in a similar fashion, as described, for the hand-sewn or stapled enteroenterostomy. Discrepancies in sizes of bowel lumen are occasionally encountered, but with a lesser frequency than might be anticipated because distention of the proximal small bowel generally accompanies the intestinal dysfunction caused by the offending pelvic process. Nevertheless, differences in lumen diameters are readily minimized by incising the antimesenteric border of the small bowel segment as described (see Fig. 25-3). Conversely, discrepancies in lumen sizes are of minimal concern when the anastomosis is accomplished by stapling—a distinct advantage of this mechanized approach.

In debilitated patients presenting with advanced primary or recurrent neoplasia or radiation-related intestinal injury, the surgeon may elect to forego mobilization and resection of the compromised intestinal segment(s). The selection of the palliative procedure to correct or minimize the resulting symptoms will require appropriate individualization on the basis of the urgency for intervention and the patient's perioperative status, the cause and natural history of the intestinal dysfunction, and the patient's anticipated longevity. A simple bypass, wherein the intestinal contents are shunted from a point proximal to the compromised segment to a more distal uninvolved portion of the bowel, can be accomplished with facility by either conventional hand-sewn or stapling techniques. The antimesenteric borders of the proximal small bowel and invariably the ascending or transverse colon are aligned employing linen-shod clamps, which also prevent efflux of intestinal contents. Stab wounds are made on the adjacent antimesenteric surfaces, and a limb of the GIA stapler is inserted into each enterotomy (Fig. 25-7). After proper closure and activation of the stapler, the two staple lines of the anastomosis are inspected for hemostasis and elevated and separated, permitting closure of the common enterotomy with a TA stapler. The mesenteric serosal surfaces are cautiously approximated to prevent internal herniation.

Complete exclusion of a compromised segment of intestine by exteriorizing a distal mucosal fistula (and also occasionally a proximal mucosal fistula) in addition to performing an ileocolostomy may be the treatment of choice, particularly in the postirradiation pelvis that harbors enteric fistulae. After transection of the ileum, both proximal and distal to the dysfunctional intestinal segment, the distal limb of the isolated segment is exteriorized, securing a mucous fistula, while the proximal limb is either doubly oversewn or likewise exteriorized as a second mucous fistula. An end-to-side ileocolostomy is secured employing a two-layered anastomosis (Fig. 25-8). After placement of the posterior interrupted seroserosal nonabsorbable sutures, a stoma is created in the colon; the posterior continuous full-thickness absorbable su-

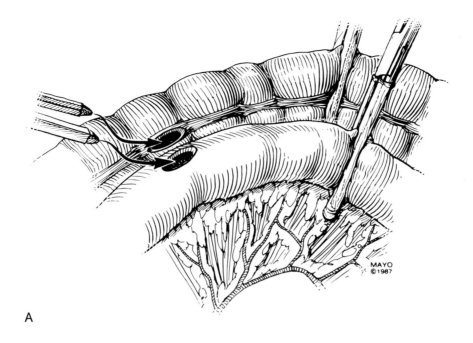

A

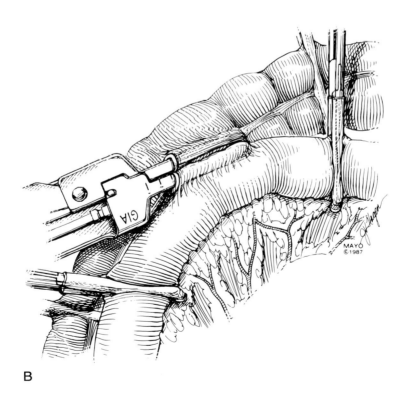

B

Fig. 25-7 Side-to-side ileocolostomy, employing GIA stapling device. **(A)** Detection of GIA stapler limbs into free-formed intestinal defects. **(B)** Alignment of GIA stapler *(Figure continues.)*

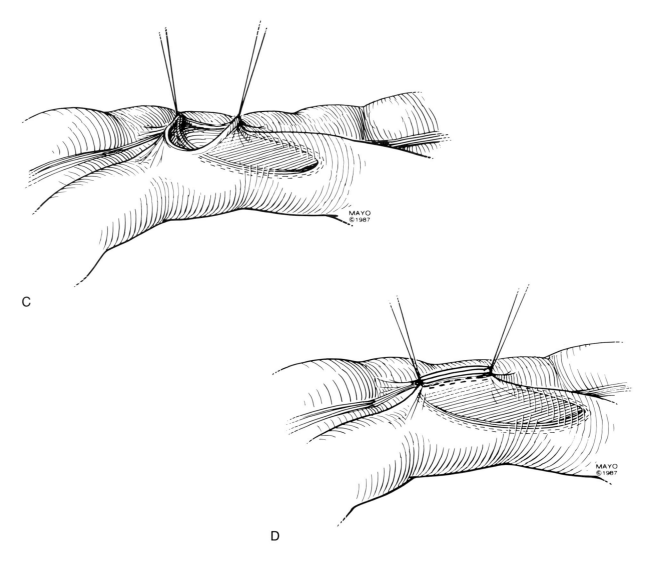

C

D

Fig. 25-7 *(Continued).* **(C)** Anastomosis after stapler activation. **(D)** Closed intestinal defect (TA stapler closure). (By permission of Mayo Foundation.)

ture layer is inserted; and the closure is continued anteriorly employing a "baseball stitch" approximation, after which the anterior seroserosal layer of nonabsorbable sutures is secured.

In the presence of postirradiation bowel necrosis with perforation and peritonitis, the experienced surgeon recognizes the morbidity associated with attempts at primary anastomosis. While the advisability of resecting the necrotic perforated segment continues to be debated (we endorse such resection when possible), consensus predicated on the associated de-

hiscence rates with immediate restoration of bowel continuity favors performing an end-ileostomy (see under Stoma Care). When it is elected to forego resection of the necrotic segment, creation of a mucous fistula is a necessary supplement to the diverting procedure. An alternative consideration would entail a primary anastomosis protected by a more proximal double-barrel or loop ileostomy.

Resection of the sigmoid colon, together with various lengths of rectum or descending colon, or both, is frequently required in the treatment of female genital

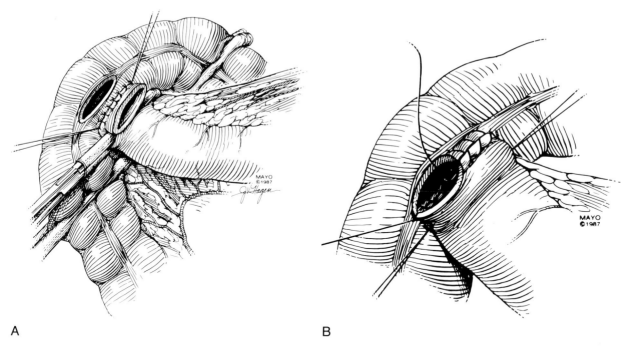

A   B

Fig. 25-8 End-to-side hand-sewn ileocolostomy. **(A)** Alignment and placement of posterior seroserosal nonabsorbable interrupted sutures. **(B)** Completion of posterior continuous second layer and conversion to anterior "baseball stitch." (By permission of Mayo Foundation.)

cancer. The inclusion of the distal large bowel in the extirpation of pelvic tumor burdens encountered with ovarian cancer or central recurrences observed with cervical cancer after radiation treatment affords the opportunity for optimal tumor reduction and adequate margins of clearance, respectively. With the uncommon penetration of the pelvic peritoneum by ovarian cancer, sufficient rectum is retained after the usual en bloc sigmoid resection to permit adequate mobilization and restoration of continuity with ease. A permanent end-sigmoid colostomy is seldom required in these settings. By contrast, postradiated surgical salvage of centrally located recurrent disease generally includes resection of both the distal sigmoid and a significant portion of rectum. Therefore, the surgeon must be familiar with several techniques to adequately accomplish a low sigmoidal rectostomy, including either a single-layered hand-sewn or a stapled end-to-end anastomosis, or both. An end-sigmoid colostomy may be selected, depending on the patient's prognosis, extent of resection and dose of radiation, anal sphincter function, and concurrent surgical procedures.

When an en bloc resection of the internal genitalia and the rectosigmoid is warranted, the round ligament is transected (if obliterated, entry into the retroperitoneal space is secured at the pelvic brim or higher), the peritoneum is incised, and the pararectal spaces are developed. After litigation of the infundibular pelvic ligaments and reflection of the bladder from the uterus and vagina, the uterine vessels are divided for lateral ureteral displacement. To facilitate mobilization, the superior hemorrhoidal vessels are identified and ligated and, with anterior and superior traction on the proximal sigmoid, the surgeon can readily free the rectum posteriorly from the presacral space by gentle but progressive elevation until the pelvic floor is reached. The lateral ligamentous supports are ligated in order to complete the mobilization process. Because the cul-de-sac is generally obliterated, the vagina is transected, the rectovaginal septum developed, and the rectum divided between properly placed Pemberton and linen Foss bowel clamps (Fig. 25-9). Thereafter, the proximal sigmoid is divided and the descending colon sufficiently mobilized to ensure a tension-free anastomosis. After two angle

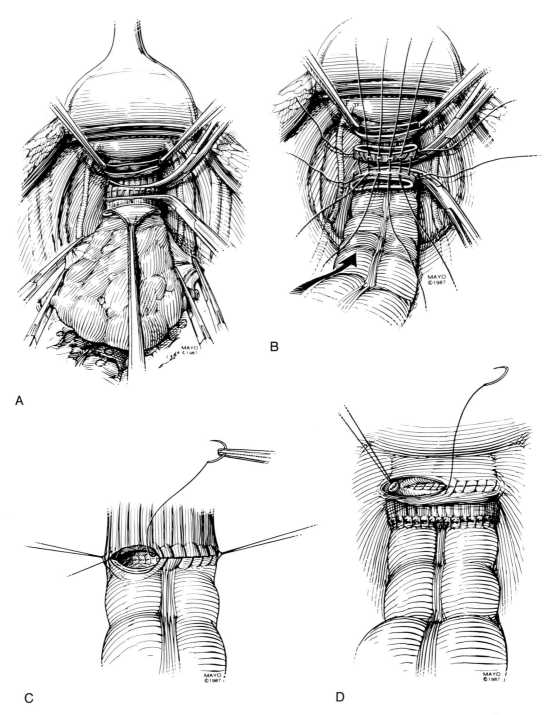

A

B

C

D

Fig. 25-9 En bloc hysterectomy/anterior resection. **(A)** Transection of vagina and circumferential mobilization of rectosigmoid. **(B)** Transection of rectum and placement of posterior interrupted nonabsorbable suture layer. **(C)** Completion of second posterior continuous suture layer and conversion to "baseball stitch" anteriorly. **(D)** Completion of sigmoidorectostomy and initial vaginal submucosal closure with initiation of the reapproximation of the fascial layers. (By permission of Mayo Foundation.)

sutures are placed for alignment, the posterior layer of the interrupted nonabsorbable seromuscular sutures are completed, followed by a continuous through-and-through second posterior layer, which is converted to a "baseball stitch" anteriorly. The anastomosis is completed by the anterior seromuscular layer. After a routine double-layer vaginal closure, fenestrated drains are placed adjacent to the anastomotic site for evacuation of blood, lymphatic fluid, and debris.

As more effective salvage management is realized, the indications for low anterior resections with immediate restoration of bowel continuity are usually considered. Familiarity with techniques to accomplish low anastomoses will occasionally circumvent the need for a permanent colostomy. The single-layer hand-sewn low anastomosis employing nonabsorbable sutures with the posterior row tied on the mucosal side has been used successfully at our institution. Critical to primary circumferential union is the assurance of a water-tight tension-free suture line between the two healthy segments of bowel harboring good vascular supplies. In addition, dilation of the anal sphincter before or after operation will minimize anal resistance.

An alternative approach to the hand-sewn low anastomosis is the use of the EEA stapling instrument. After completion of the low rectosigmoid resection and appropriate sizing of the opposing bowel lumina, either a pursestring or a full-thickness whipstitch suture is placed around the margins of both ends of the bowel. The EEA stapler is inserted transanally until the anvil cone is visualized. The instrument is opened, permitting the suture on the rectal margin to be secured about the central shaft. The sigmoid margin is delivered over the cone, and its pursestring suture is likewise fastened about the shaft (Fig. 25-10). The stapling device is properly closed, gently rotated in both directions to assess apposition, and activated. For removal, the stapler is opened and rotated, and the anvil is carefully withdrawn through the anastomosis. To ensure proper hemostasis and adequate circumferential approximation, the anastomotic site is inspected transanally by proctoscopy, and the double doughnuts within the cartridge are carefully inspected.

In certain surgical settings, particularly when advanced recurrent pelvic malignancies are treated, the creation of an intestinal stoma will be unavoidable.

We consider three broad indications for stoma formations, including (1) requirement for anal substitution; (2) surgical decompression of intestinal obstructions, specifically during end-stage palliation; and (3) fecal stream diversion of a more distal dysfunctional intestinal segment, particularly if perforation has occurred. The type of stoma best suited to the clinical circumstances will be dictated by the urgency for stoma formation, etiologic factors necessitating its creation, patient prognosis, and the temporary and permanent nature of the stoma. While a loop colostomy or ileostomy is frequently used under emergency surgical conditions or when temporary diversion is indicated, the end-on ostomy, matured according to anticipated effluent collection needs, is superior. The complications associated with stomas can be minimized by meticulous attention to detail, which commences with the proper selection of the stoma site before operation.

While the need for an ileostomy is infrequently required in gynecologic oncology, its proper maturation, when indicated, may circumvent many stomal- and peristomal-related problems after operation. These basic techniques are likewise applicable in the construction of the urinary conduit when suprapubic diversion is indicated. After transection of the ileum at a level that affords a generous vascular supply to the proximally transected margin, the mesentery is carefully skeletonized parallel to and 5 to 10 mm from the bowel wall for a distance of 2 to 4 cm. At the previously selected ileostomy site, a 2- to 2.5-cm disc of skin and underlying subcutaneous fat is excised and the anterior rectus sheath is incised both vertically and horizontally. A long hemostat is carefully inserted through the rectus muscle, posterior sheath, and peritoneum and then opened, splitting the tissue layers to permit placement of two fingers through the defect created. The diameter may need adjustment based on the depth of the abdominal wall and the amount of adipose tissue within the small bowel mesentery.

Formation of a Brooke-type stoma is readily accomplished by incorporating a portion of subcuticular tissue, the full-thickness edge of the ileum, and a seromuscular layer 2.5 to 3 cm from the intestinal margin within four equally spaced 3-0 absorbable sutures (preferably placed 45 and 135 degrees on both sides of the mesentery attachment) (Fig. 25-11). Additional subcuticular full-thickness anchoring sutures are employed, interspersed between the initial everting sutures.

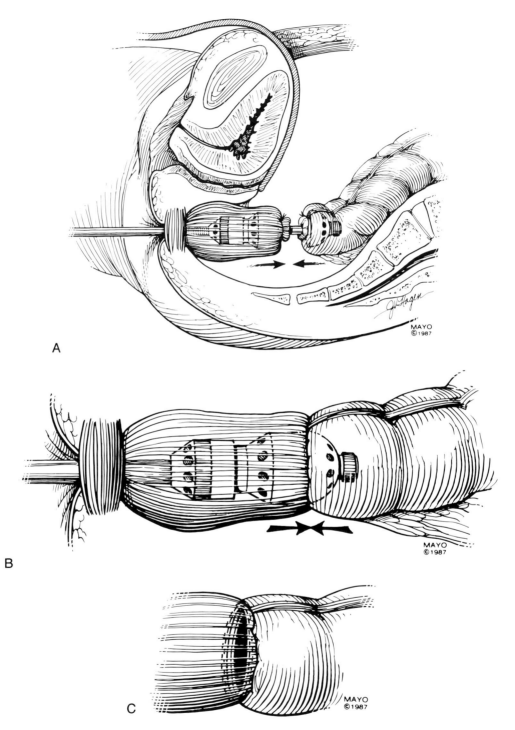

Fig. 25-10 Sigmoidorectostomy by use of mechanical stapling. **(A)** Proper alignment of rectal and sigmoid margins around shaft of stapler. **(B)** Activation of stapling device. **(C)** Completion of anastomosis, demonstrating double ring of staples. (By permission of Mayo Foundation.)

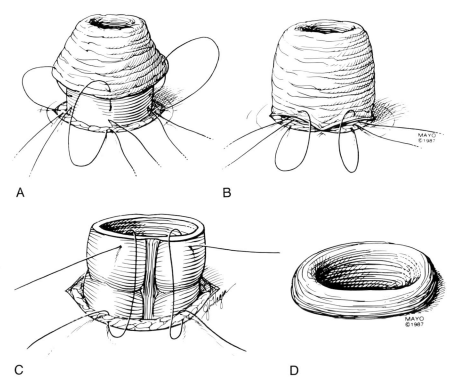

Fig. 25-11 Stoma maturation. **(A)** Subcutaneous-distal transmural-to-serosal suture approximation for inversion of small intestine. **(B)** Interval subcutaneous-distal transmural suture placement for completion of Brooke-type small bowel stoma. **(C)** Transmural to subcutaneous approximation for end colostomy. **(D)** Maturation of end colostomy. (By permission of Mayo Foundation.)

A

B

C

D

The principles of creating a colonic stoma are similar to those described for the ileostomy. The disc of skin and underlying subcutaneous fat and the deeper musculoaponeurotic defect must be enlarged to accept the increased bowel and mesenteric bulk. The descending colon and proximal sigmoid should be appropriately mobilized by incising the peritoneum along the left colic gutter and may also require mobilization of the splenic flexure, thereby avoiding subsequent stomal retraction.

After delivery of the colonic margin through the ostomy site defect, the left colic gutter is readily obliterated by suture approximation of the posterior sheath at the stoma site, the posterior lateral abdominal and gutter peritoneum, and the margin of the mesosigmoid to prevent lateral small bowel migration (and possible strangulation) and minimize postoperative retraction. The stoma is immediately matured using 3-0 absorbable sutures placed through the full thickness of the bowel edge and the subcutaneous tissue (see Fig. 25-11). When a significant length of colon

has been excised, therapy decreasing the absorptive surface sufficiently to anticipate a moderately active colostomy, we prefer creating a "rosebud end," employing a modification of the Brooke-type ileostomy, thereby allowing more ideal collection of bowel effluent.

A loop ileostomy or colostomy is generally employed as a temporizing procedure, with the intent of subsequently reestablishing bowel continuity or as part of symptomatic palliative therapy for advanced cancer. Selection of the ostomy site or sites is again of importance and dependent on the location of the process that dictates diversion. While the ileum and distal descending colon are readily adaptable, the transverse colon is the most commonly accepted site for diversion for several reasons, including (1) obstructive site or dysfunctional process frequently located in sigmoid or rectum, (2) generally excluded from previous local treatment modalities for pelvic malignancies, and (3) more optimal surgical accessibility.

A transverse incision is made superior and slightly

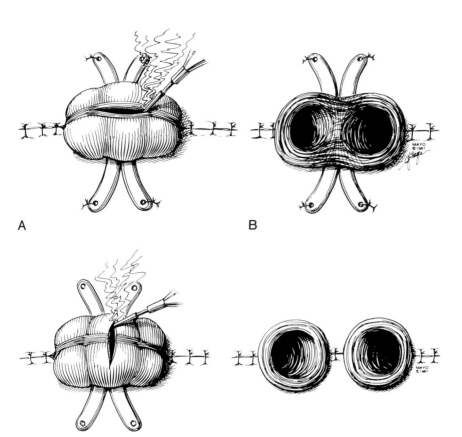

A

B

C

D

Fig. 25-12 Loop colostomy maturation. **(A)** Longitudinal colotomy, employing electrocautery. **(B)** Incision and eversion of matured loop colostomy with underlying Hollister bridge. **(C)** Transverse transection of loop colostomy. **(D)** Complete separation (defunctionalization) of loop colostomy stomas with intervening skin bridge. (By permission of Mayo Foundation.)

to the right of the umbilicus down through the anterior sheath. The rectus-abdominus muscle, as well as the posterior sheath, is incised sufficiently to deliver a loop of transverse colon. Identification of the middle colic vessels is essential to avoid trauma. The avascular attachment of the omentum to the colon is incised, a defect created in the transverse mesocolon near the bowel margin, a Hollister bridge inserted, and the abdominal incision closed. If the need for decompression or diversion is urgent, the bowel can be incised immediately; otherwise, a delay of 24 hours is preferred to minimize the possibility of peristomal soiling and subsequent infection (Fig. 25-12). We prefer electrocautery for incising the bowel wall, and the axis of the incision is usually dependent on the temporary nature of the ostomy and the requirement for complete defunctionalization. If there is a need for either a permanent or a totally defunctionalized os-

tomy, the bowel is opened transversely, and preferably the proximal ostomy and distal mucus fistula are separated at the time of abdominal wall closure by a skin bridge.

Colostomy closure is generally accomplished in an extraperitoneal fashion for the loop colostomy and for the end-colostomy with adjacent mucus fistula. Conversely, the isolated end-colostomy requires a laparotomy and intraperitoneal anastomosis. For extraperitoneal closure, an elliptical incision is made around the stoma(s), and with anterior traction (the index finger in the bowel lumen and a clamp on the cutaneous margin) and adequate counter traction, the bowel is circumferentially mobilized (Fig. 25-13). The cutaneous margin, together with a border of bowel mucosa, is excised and closed in the usual two-layer fashion, followed by a layered abdominal wall closure.

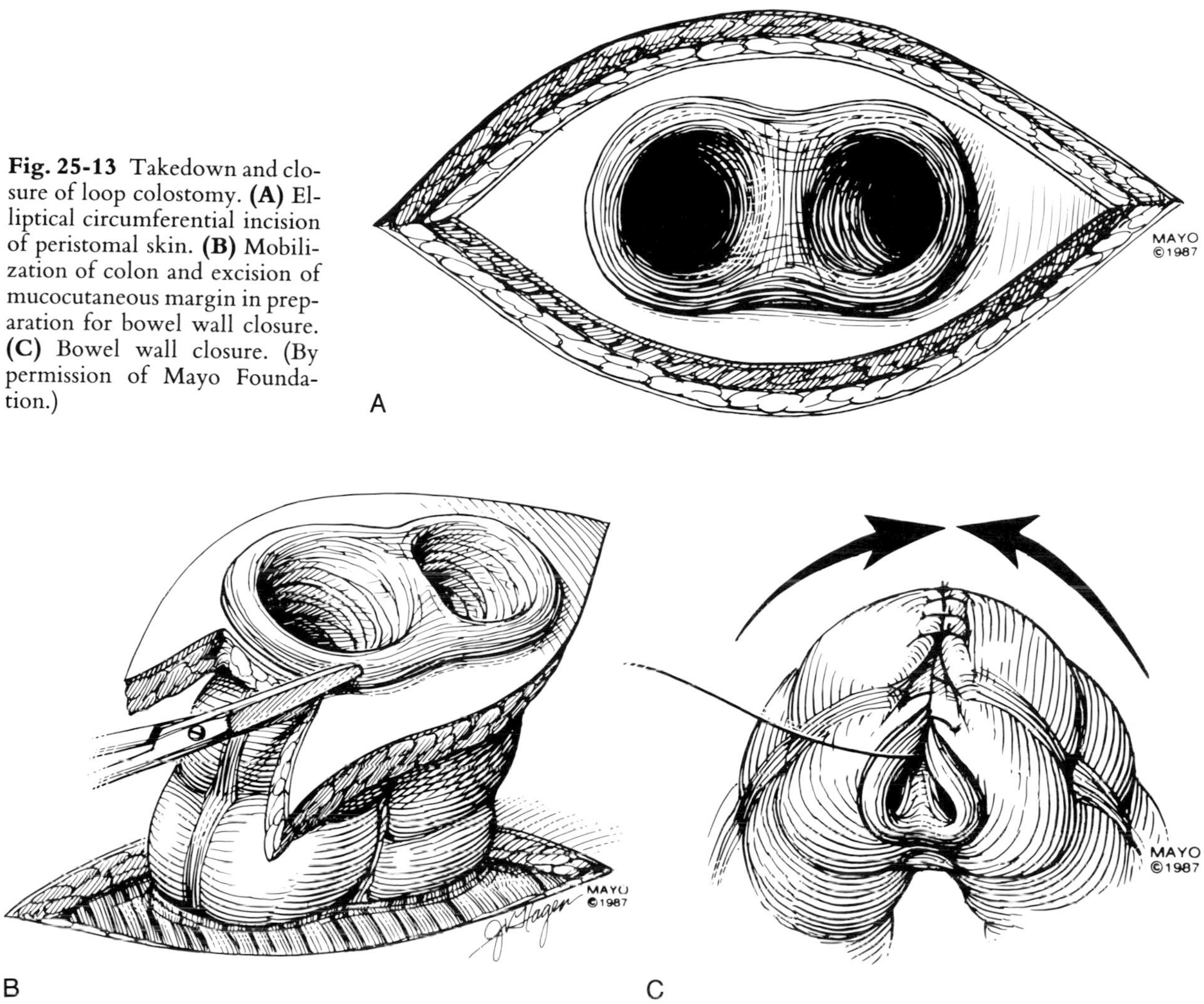

Fig. 25-13 Takedown and closure of loop colostomy. **(A)** Elliptical circumferential incision of peristomal skin. **(B)** Mobilization of colon and excision of mucocutaneous margin in preparation for bowel wall closure. **(C)** Bowel wall closure. (By permission of Mayo Foundation.)

POSTOPERATIVE MORBIDITY AND COMPLICATIONS

Wound Sepsis

While preoperative mechanical cleansing of the GI tract as well as liberal perioperative use of antimicrobials have decreased the frequency of postoperative wound infections, the presence of wound erythema and the subsequent development of purulent drainage continue to be encountered after abdominal procedures that include GI tract resections. The initiation and propagation of an infectious process require a sufficient inoculum of bacteria and the presence of a proper culture medium. Although either an exogenous or endogenous source may contribute to the infectious agents, the contamination probably occurred during the transection of the hollow viscus, because of the type of organisms that are usually identified on culturing of the septic wound. In addition, blood, serum, and tissue debris occasionally collect in the subcutaneous space, providing an ideal culture medium for microbes from the GI tract. Anticipatory preoperative bowel preparation, attention to details intraoperatively, meticulous hemostasis, and copious irrigation will reduce the frequency of wound sepsis. In addition, we have further minimized the incidence of wound infection in this high-risk population (having GI resections) by routinely incorporating, in the abdominal incision closure, a subcutaneous catheter for postoperative suction evacuation of serosanguineous debris for 3 to 4 days, as described by McIlrath et al.[37] The incidence of wound infection after primary closure of contaminated or dirty incisions was 1.4 percent with this technique, which presumably eliminates deadspace and the natural culture media of blood and other tissue fluids. However, once wound sepsis is suspected, prompt therapy is instituted, which should include opening the incision beyond the margins of inflammation and generally down to the fascia and obtaining appropriate specimens for microbial culturing in the process. Subsequent generous debridement, irrigation with water, saline, half-strength Dakin's solution (sodium hypochlorite), or diluted povidone-iodine solution, and open packing will secure a granulation base suitable for either secondary surgical or passive closure.

Paralytic Ileus

Although patients customarily experience some adynamic ileus after most major abdominal surgical procedures, the adynamic ileus is generally considered a temporary annoyance rather than a complication of surgery, usually resolving spontaneously within 3 to 5 days after surgery. The pathophysiology of paralytic ileus is undoubtedly multifactorial, including neural and humoral components. Whatever the cause, the clinical presentation of GI distention with air-fluid levels and absent bowel sounds (with occasional associated tachycardia) in an otherwise normal postoperative patient is generally a reflection of intraoperative manipulation and an extended time interval of either packing or exposure, or both, of the GI tract. Cautious observation, with monitoring and correction (when indicated) of serum electrolytes, is sufficient management with only an occasional requirement for long-tube (Tucker) decompression.

By contrast, prolonged ileus in the nonirradiated patient occasionally connotes the presence of a more subtle but significant underlying process. The presence of early wound sepsis, anastomotic leakage, prior or impending peritonitis, electrolyte imbalances, retroperitoneal hematoma formation, ureteral distention or retroperitoneal urinoma formation, and prolonged intestinal distention or ischemia, or both, must receive consideration under such circumstances. While conservative management is again indicated with adequate hydration, electrolyte replacement, and long-tube (Tucker) decompression, the definitive therapeutic approach entails identification and treatment of the causative phenomenon.

Mechanical Bowel Obstruction

The clinical presentation of mechanical bowel obstruction is characterized by abdominal distention, abdominal pain (typically colic in nature), vomiting, and absence of flatus. The abdominal distention is a reflection of nonabsorbable gases (mainly nitrogen from swallowed air and organic gases from fermentation) and intestinal fluids (distention enhances intestinal secretion, further increasing distention), which is readily visualized in most cases on radiologic evaluation of the abdomen. Patients with small bowel obstruction generally have a notable absence of colonic gas, while pronounced colonic distention is associated with large bowel obstruction, particularly in the presence of a competent ileocecal valve. Excessive distention (more than 9 cm) is associated with (1) an increased risk of vascular compromise, leading to strangulation, with its untoward sequelae; and (2) intestinal perforation, with the distended cecum being particularly vulnerable. The frequency of vomiting is greater with more proximal obstructions but is more feculent in nature with more distal or longstanding obstructions. After either GI resection or ostomy formation, or both, postoperative mechanical obstruction is preferably evaluated and managed based on the interval separating surgery and the presentation of symptoms.

Because of the gynecologic diseases or entities that require GI surgery, the etiologic factors for partial or complete intestinal obstruction are more divergent when they occur during the immediate postoperative time frame than when they occur at a time more distant from surgery. When they become clinically apparent during the initial hospital convalescence, the following recognized complications of intestinal resection should receive consideration as potential causes of bowel obstruction:

Excessive tissue inversion and subsequent edema at the anastomotic site

Injudicious use of a mechanical stapling device for anastomotic closures, internal hernias through mesentery defects or around colostomy loops or into retroperitoneal defects overlying retroperitoneal spaces under suction drainage

Adhesions

By contrast, the mechanical causes for delayed obstruction are varied:

Adhesions
Intrinsic strictures
Internal or external hernias
Extrinsic compression
Volvulus

Nevertheless, whatever the precise mechanism for luminal compromise, the recurrence, persistence, or progression of the primary insulting process that dictated the initial operative procedure remains the most frequent reason for subsequent mechanical obstruction; maintaining a high index of suspicion for either malignant or radiation-induced antecedents, or both, is recommended.

Management is likewise determined by the interval since the operation and the finding of the suggested cause. Generally, we favor prompt intervention for intestinal obstruction, with operative treatment commencing after adequate electrolyte, blood product, and fluid replacement; initiation of antimicrobial therapy; and placement of a long decompression tube (i.e., Tucker). Surgical management may range from simple lysis of adhesions or correction of internal or external hernia to the more frequently required segmental resection of compromised bowel and the associated recurrent disease or proximal diversion, with mucous fistula formation for palliative purposes, as described under Surgical Techniques.

Exceptions to prompt surgical intervention include situations in which obstructive symptoms occur during the immediate postoperative convalescence and when patients harbor advanced disseminated cancer. Under these circumstances, a trial of conservative management is recommended, with recognition of the associated risk of either strangulation or perforation or both, when there is prolonged or excessive intestinal distention. Our choice of management includes (1) direction of a long decompression tube (i.e., Tucker) through the pylorus under radiologic guidance to evacuate distending gas and fluid and reverse intraluminal fluid sequestration; (2) fluid, blood product, and electrolyte replacement; (3) parenteral alimentation; and (4) microbial therapy, when indicated.

Anastomotic Dehiscence

The reported incidence rates for anastomotic leakage are variable and dependent on the disease that originally mandated the GI resection, its relative location and associated environmental factors, and the methods employed for documenting the dehiscence. For instance, Goligher et al.[38] noted a leakage rate of 69 percent for low rectosigmoidostomy when detailed evaluation was obtained by digital, direct vision, and imaging procedures.

While the actual number of anastomotic leaks that escape recognition and detection is probably greater than appreciated, leaks that attain clinical significance in gynecologic oncology are infrequent and usually occur in patients who require intestinal resection for advanced disease or correction of adverse treatment sequelae. Nevertheless, if fibroblast activity is not impaired, functional and leakage-free anastomoses are dependent on the preservation of an adequate circumferential blood supply and an accurate tension-free reapproximation of the gut wall; both issues have been discussed. If the reapproximation is less than optimal, a diverting ostomy is preferred and, after subsequent assessment of anastomotic integrity, closure can be accomplished with substantially less risk than for an anastomotic leak. If vascularity and approximation are adequate, the primary union is enhanced by minimizing perianastomotic inflammation and infection by means of liberal suction drainage and use of antimicrobial agents, as well as by correcting any systemic metabolic or nutritional imbalances.

Abdominal distention, fever, and leukocytosis are clinical parameters associated with localized perianastomotic leaks, whereas the peritonitis and sepsis seen when soiling is more generalized is associated with anastomotic dehiscence or necrosis. Both clinical settings require prompt surgical drainage, decompression of the proximal bowel, and initiation of antimicrobial therapy. Surgical management of the anastomotic site is variable, depending on small or large bowel involvement, accessibility for drainage, abscess localization, and patient prognosis. Therefore, considerable individualization is necessary in planning effective therapy.

In the presence of peritoneal soiling from colonic

disruption, an end-on colostomy with a complementary mucous fistula (or Hartmann procedure) is generally the preferred approach. Rarely, consideration may be given to wide resection, reestablishment of local continuity, and more proximal diversion via loop colostomy. By contrast, locally confined enteroenterostomy dehiscences can be managed frequently with wide local resections, reanastomosis, long-tube decompression, and diversion of the more proximal small intestine. Regardless of environmental settings or variations in definitive intestinal management, copious irrigation and adequate suction drainage of the infected site(s) are imperative.

Enterocutaneous fistula formation after intestinal resection is suggestive of an unrecognized anastomotic dehiscence. Either an abdominal incision (or the perineal/vaginal suture line) or the adjacent stoma site may serve as the orifice for spontaneous drainage, which usually precedes the resolution of an indolent clinical course. A trial of conservative management is warranted; successful spontaneous closure can be anticipated in a significant percentage of patients, particularly those with low intestinal defects and no distal obstruction. More proximal fistulas are characteristically high-volume fistulas with their caustic intestinal contents causing cutaneous erosions. Continuous evacuation of the proximal bowel contents and total parenteral nutrition will afford conditions appropriate for spontaneous closure. If closure has not occurred by 6 weeks, surgical closure should be considered, occasionally requiring resection of the involved segment of intestine.

Vascular Compromise

Intestinal ischemia with subsequent necrosis is a rare complication of abdominal surgery, but every pelvic surgeon should be familiar with its clinical presentation. The sudden onset of abdominal pain, seemingly disproportionately severe to the patient's anticipated status, with progression to generalized peritonitis, rapid pulse, fever, metabolic acidosis, leukocytosis, and signs of shock are characteristic. While embolization or occlusion of a major mesenteric vessel, or both, will produce this surgical emergency, the most frequent cause in gynecology is generally mechanical bowel obstruction, that is, acute occlusion of the peripheral mesenteric vessels either by angulation or by twisting, as with volvulus or overdistention of the bowel lumen. The intramural pressure may exceed the vascular hydrostatic pressure and lead to strangulation and, when neglected, necrosis and death.

Optimal treatment is preventative management consisting of prompt effective correction of mechanical bowel obstruction, as outlined. If there is vascular compromise, effective and expeditious surgical management is mandatory. Isolation and resection of the compromised segment(s), with reestablishment of continuity, is customary in the absence of perforation. With extensive soiling of the peritoneal cavity, a proximal ostomy and distal mucous fistula are created after resection of the nonviable segment. Copious irrigation of the peritoneal cavity before closure and generous use of antimicrobial agents are essential to minimize subsequent morbidity.

Short Bowel Syndrome

Massive resection of the small bowel is generally accompanied by diarrhea and malabsorption, resulting in dramatic loss of weight from malnutrition. This clinical setting, referred to as short bowel syndrome, is characteristically seen after resection of more than 70 percent of the small intestine. Protracted sequelae are seldom observed in patients who have more than 100 cm of small intestine. However, the severity of the syndrome increases with decreasing length of preserved small bowel, particularly the ileum, and is further aggravated by concomitant colonic resection and loss of the ileocecal valve. While conservation of as much viable intestine as possible at the time of massive resection is paramount, improvements in medical and nutritional support systems have afforded enhanced survival with lower morbidity, thereby allowing for gradual intestinal adaptation.

Postoperative management includes maintenance of fluid and electrolytes, which is facilitated by controlling gastric hypersecretion, decreasing bowel motility, and avoiding dietary substances that have irritant or cathartic effects. Parenteral nutrition is preferably initiated early during the postoperative course, with subsequent gradual decreasing as intestinal adaptation permits progressive replacement with oral dietary management. Diets high in carbohydrates and proteins and low in fats and lactose are recommended and supplemented with readily absorbable triglycerides and essential vitamins and minerals.

Gastric hypersecretion can be controlled adequately by H$_2$-receptor antagonists, and bowel motility is further decreased with antidiarrheal agents.

We have no experience with the surgical correction of this syndrome and, because such massive resections constitute a treatment of neoplastic processes or sequelae of prior therapy, any anticipated benefits from antiperistaltic segments, colonic interposition, recirculating loops, or intestinal tapering, lengthening, pacing, or transplantation procedures would rarely indicate such secondary surgical manipulations.

Blind-Loop Syndrome

While the blind-loop syndrome is becoming less common, patients undergoing surgical bypass, isolation, or diversion of a segment of bowel rather than resection and who do not have adequate venting of the retained segment are susceptible to this condition. Typically, the procedure was used to correct or alleviate a postradiation intestinal injury. The clinical presentation commonly includes a history of abdominal pain, loss of weight, diarrhea, steatorrhea, and anemia. Bacterial action within the stagnant intestinal loop may alter the metabolism and absorption of certain vitamins and fats. Definitive treatment requires surgical resection of the blind loop; if such is not permissible or advisable, intermittent antimicrobial therapy may be beneficial and is generally warranted.

Pseudomembranous Colitis

Because of the routine inclusion of antimicrobial therapy in preoperative bowel preparations and the liberal utilization of perioperative systemic antimicrobial therapy in patients subjected to bowel resection, the oncologic surgeon should be familiar with the diagnosis and treatment of antimicrobial agent-induced diarrhea; this condition frequently presents as, or progresses to, pseudomembranous colitis. While pseudomembranous colitis historically was a diagnosis made by inspection and histologic sampling of the gut wall, the identification of *Clostridium difficile,* the most commonly associated cause, or its cytotoxin in a fecal specimen is believed to establish the diagnosis without requiring invasive techniques. The patient generally presents with watery or bloody diarrhea, fever, leukocytosis, and abdominal cramps or pain commencing after 5 to 10 days of therapy, al-

though symptoms may begin as early as 24 to 48 hours after the initiation of antimicrobial therapy or as late as 3 to 4 weeks after discontinuation of therapy. While most antimicrobial agents have been implicated, the agents most frequently associated with this entity in gynecology include cephalosporins, clindamycin, and ampicillin.[39] The normal bowel flora is believed to be altered sufficiently by the antimicrobial agents to permit an overgrowth of certain organisms, including *C. difficile.* However, the precise pathophysiologic mechanism of the diarrhea and colitis remains unknown. Nevertheless, *C. difficile* can be readily cultured and its cytotoxin assayed and, if culture is positive, the need for endoscopic evaluation is generally circumvented.

Regardless of the apparent insignificance of diarrhea during or after antimicrobial agent usage and bowel resection, a high index of suspicion for pseudomembranous colitis is warranted, and antidiarrheal agents should be avoided until completion of clinical investigations. Therapy commences with the discontinuation of the antimicrobial agent and initiation of oral vancomycin, bacitracin, or metronidazole and appropriate fluid and electrolyte replacement. While less effective than the use of vancomycin, an alternative approach is the administration of the ion-exchange resin, cholestyramine, which binds the cytotoxin. Continued follow-up evaluation is advised, because a significant number of patients subsequently will have relapse and require additional therapy.

Stoma-Associated Complications

The normal stoma is pink to red and moist during the immediate postoperative period, demonstrating a smooth, glistening surface from the associated surgically induced edema. Proper preoperative selection of the site, meticulous attention to detail intraoperatively during construction, and appropriate peristomal skin protection postoperatively will minimize the frequency of stoma-related problems.

Peristomal skin irritation is generally a reflection of either caustic irritation from the intestinal effluent or adverse reactions to the adhesive or plastic materials. Avoiding placement of stomas near skinfolds, scars, incisions, belt lines, or bony prominences will minimize leakage and extend the intervals between appliance replacement. Likewise, precise fitting of the skin barrier wafer around the stoma and the use of barrier paste will further minimize irritation from intestinal effluents. Dermatitis, excoriations, or ulcers related to sensitivities to the adhesives or pouches will require gentle skin care, as well as trials of alternative materials and possible skin testing if difficulties persist.

Stomal necrosis potentially represents the most serious early postoperative complication. The stoma will generally appear dusky to black within 24 hours to 3 days and represents compromise of the blood supply, possibly from excessive skeletonizing of fatty appendages or mesentery, or both. The dusky or poorly vascularized stoma frequently will regain its normal appearance as associated edema subsides. By contrast, the black stoma will slough and occasionally progress to either stenosis or retraction, or both, resulting in management problems for the patient. Revision may be required immediately if necrosis is complete, or revision may be delayed and considered later, as sequelae dictate.

Stomal retraction results from one or a combination of the following: inadequate mobilization of the more proximal bowel, radiation-induced shortening of the mesentery, shearing forces of the thick abdominal wall, or excessive weight gain after the operation. Persistent tension on the stoma causes progressive withdrawal of the stoma below the skin level, resulting in difficulty in maintaining a leakage-free seal and the related peristomal skin problems. Occasionally, revision of the stoma becomes mandatory.

Stomal stenosis can occur either superficially around the cutaneous margin or at the level of the fascia. Patients present with complaints of excessive pressure during stool passage, of constipation, or of small-caliber stools. Digital examination of a normal-appearing stoma may reveal a strictured fascial ring at various distances below the mucocutaneous junction. Although fascial stenosis may be related to inadequate fascial clearance at the primary operation, most stenotic ostomies result from postoperative vascular compromise of the stoma, which progresses to partial necrosis, retraction, and cicatricial scarification. Seldom is stomal dilation of long-term benefit, and surgical revision is the treatment of choice. However, stool softeners, irrigations, and dilations may temporize a critical setting sufficiently to avoid additional surgery in a terminally ill patient.

Stomal prolapse is a protrusion of bowel through the stomal opening, generally occurring as a delayed complication of surgery. While prolapse is relatively uncommon with end-colostomy, loop colostomy is at greater risk to lead to prolapse, specifically the nonfunctioning limb. Protrusion is generally gradual and progressive but is readily reducible. Nevertheless, definitive correction requires internal fixation of the bowel and occasional revision of the stoma.

Parastomal hernia occurring during the early postoperative period indicates that an overly generous fascial defect was created during stomal construction. More commonly, late herniation results from the progressive expansion of the fascial defect from increased intraabdominal pressure, resulting from obesity, chronic pulmonary disease, environmental factors, and constipation. The incidence is further enhanced if the stoma is constructed outside the rectus sheath. Most parastomal hernias are asymptomatic and are not recognized by the patient. Furthermore, the smaller symptomatic hernias are readily controlled by the use of special appliances. However, the larger parastomal hernias generally require surgical correction as the associated stomal management increases in complexity, irrigations frequently become unpredictable or undesirable, appliance accommodations become increasingly unsatisfactory as stomal topography changes, and the large hernia bulge becomes cosmetically more unacceptable. Nonoperative management consisting of individualized custom fitting of face plates and accompanying ostomy belts is preferable in patients with metastatic disease and chronic pulmonary disease, as well as in obese patients until sufficient weight is lost to justify the procedure.

Surgical repair entails either of two basic techniques. The first is creating a new site for the stoma. The original stoma is mobilized and moved to a new predetermined site, and the fascial defect is repaired. While accomplished with facility in patients harboring a single stoma, on a minimally altered abdominal wall, the making of a new stoma site can be difficult for even the most experienced surgeon in patients with two or more ostomies and an abdominal surface having multiple folds, incisions, or scars. The second is in situ parastomal herniorrhaphy.

While the techniques for preservation of the original stomal site are variable, the basic principles of hernia repair, including mobilization and high excision of the hernia sac as well as reapproximation of fresh fascial margins, remain constant. The reinforcing of the repair with synthetic mesh, the repositioning of the bowel through a new defect in the rectus sheath, the raising of skin flaps for repair, the selection of incisions for accessibility, and the type of stomal revision have all been debated.[40-44] We profess that the associated complexities with which this infrequent complication occurs in gynecologic oncology require careful individual assessment and familiarity with several alternative surgical approaches. For instance, if repair of a parastomal hernia associated with an ileal conduit cannot be accomplished without finding a new stoma site, the surgeon must be prepared to either extend the conduit with additional ileum or create a new conduit if finding a new stoma site mandates such.

STOMA CARE

The emotional and psychological impact of harboring a temporary or permanent ostomy is generally not fully appreciated before operation by patients with pelvic malignancies, in that significant energies are initially expended in fears and anxieties related to the discovery of their cancer. Nevertheless, proper stomal management entails early but appropriate professional counseling for the patient and her family. Ideally, it commences preoperatively with an educational visit from an enterostomal therapist, who discusses functional changes and the anticipated needs resulting from such alterations. The stoma site is likewise identified at that visit to ensure optimal appliance alignment. The planning of postoperative ostomy care must be individualized in that bowel activity varies from patient to patient, influenced by the patient's preoperative bowel habits, the surgical disease and procedure dictating the ostomy, and numerous environmental parameters, including diet, bowel activity, and medication. In addition, the choice of appliance, selection of adhesive agents and skin care, recommendations regarding dietary measures, and decisions regarding irrigation for regularity must be predicated on the patient's physical characteristics and personal desires.

Appliance

In addition to the patient's preference, the selection of an appliance will be determined by the stomal output, parastomal anatomy, and allergic tolerances. Disposable appliances are intended to be worn for several days and thereafter discarded. While one or two appliances can be employed daily for collection of colostomy effluents, drainable appliances are used with ileostomies and urinary conduits generally requiring replacement every 2 to 5 days. Appliance design favors a closed system; in the absence of leakage, recent advances have rendered them essentially odor free and noise free.

Skin Care

The effluents of both ileostomies and colostomies are irritants to exposed skin; appliances should therefore be secured with minimal exposure to the parastomal skin. Ostomy care includes gentle washing of the parastomal skin with warm water and mild soap. The surface is dried without rubbing; drying is frequently aided by a stream of warm or cool air from a hairdryer. A stencil simulating the topography of the stoma is made and used to aid in cutting the skin barrier wafer and pouch to the proper size to ensure a precise fit. The skin barrier minimizes the allergic reaction that occasionally develops to the plastics of the appliances. The barrier and appliance should fit within 1 to 3 mm of the mucocutaneous margin. Barrier paste can be employed to fill the space between the barrier plate and the stoma if necessary. Likewise, with a loop colostomy over a bridge, the barrier wafer and appliance are cut to the size of the stoma and barrier paste is applied around the bridge, permitting a sealed collection device. Reusable two-piece appliances are available with face plates, allowing the use of a belt to give additional support to the adhesive skin barrier. Regular drainage of the appliance will prevent distention, excessive pressure, and leakage.

Obviously, the ideal management of parastomal skin irritation is prevention. Routine cleansing and drying of the parastomal skin and prevention of leakage are of paramount importance. Should erythema develop, the skin is generally cleansed and allowed repeated intervals of exposure to air. Excoriations or ulcers are treated in a similar manner with the addition of a stomal adhesive or application of karaya powder before placement of a similar skin-barrier wafer. Skin sensitivity to the adhesives and plastics will require consideration of an alternative hypoallergenic skin barrier and a cotton cover for the appliance. Monilial infections, particularly in the diabetic patient, are readily suspected and treated with the appropriate antimicrobial powders. Parastomal hair should be removed at regular intervals, employing an electric shaver to minimize the frequency of associated folliculitis.

Dietary Measures

While dietary manipulation can regulate bowel activity, gaseous formation, and stool consistency to a certain extent, restrictive diets are generally not justifiable. The variability in eating habits and effects of certain foods are sufficient to warrant caution before suggesting dietary restrictions or alterations. Each patient will, by her own experience, identify specific food intolerances and selectively avoid foods that might result in unfavorable sequelae.

Irrigation

With the exception of elderly or handicapped patients (e.g., blind, arthritic), colostomy irrigation is discussed and encouraged for patients with distal descending or sigmoid colostomies. Before dismissal, each consenting patient is taught the irrigation technique by an enterostomal therapist. The irrigation system using a lubricated cone inserted into the stoma permits slow instillation of 700 to 1,200 ml water into the colon. If cramping becomes excessive, the volume of instillation is decreased or the instillation is stopped temporarily. After completion of return, which is variable from patient to patient, the stoma is cleansed and dried, and either a stomal cap or an appliance is secured.

In a recent report from our institution summarizing the irrigation practices of 72 women with end-sigmoid colostomies, Jao et al.[45] found that 71 percent were continent or experienced only minor leakage, while 15 percent and 14 percent were either incontinent with irrigation or had discontinued irrigation, respectively. The average irrigation volume was 1 L, and the average irrigation process required 45 minutes to complete. No colonic perforations occurred, and satisfactory results with irrigation were closely related to preoperative bowel habits. In addition to minimizing parastomal skin problems, flatus and odor are readily controllable with a stomal cap or appliance, permitting greater confidence to the physically and sexually active woman.

REFERENCES

1. Symmonds RE, Pratt JH, Welch JS: Extended Wertheim operation for primary, recurrent, or suspected recurrent carcinoma of the cervix. Obstet Gynecol 24:15, 1964
2. Spratt JS Jr, Butcher HR Jr, Bricker EM: Exenterative surgery of the pelvis. Major Prob Clin Surg 12:1, 1972
3. Barber HRK: Relative prognostic significance of preoperative and operative findings in pelvic exenteration. Surg Clin North Am 49:431, April 1969
4. Symmonds RE, Pratt JH, Webb MJ: Exenterative operations: Experience with 198 patients. Am J Obstet Gynecol 121:907, 1975
5. Rutledge FN, Smith JP, Wharton JT, O'Quinn AG: Pelvic exenteration: Analysis of 296 patients. Am J Obstet Gynecol 129:881, 1977
6. Orr JW Jr, Shingleton HM, Hatch KD, et al: Gastrointestinal complications associated with pelvic exenteration. Am J Obstet Gynecol 145:325, 1983
7. Averette HE, Lichtinger M, Sevin B-U, Girtanner RE: Pelvic exenteration: A 15-year experience in a general metropolitan hospital. Am J Obstet Gynecol 150:179, 1984
8. Podratz KC, Symmonds RE, Taylor WF, Williams TJ: Carcinoma of the vulva: Analysis of treatment and survival. Obstet Gynecol 61:63, 1983
9. Krupp PJ, Lee FYL, Bohm JW, et al: Therapy of advanced epidermoid carcinoma of vulva: Report of 13 patients, with review of recent literature. Obstet Gynecol 46:433, 1975
10. Podratz KC, Symmonds RE, Taylor WF: Carcinoma of the vulva: Analysis of treatment failures. Am J Obstet Gynecol 143:340, 1982
11. Barber HRK: Ovarian Carcinoma: Etiology, Diagnosis, and Treatment. Masson, New York, 1978
12. Griffiths CT: Surgical resection of tumor bulk in the primary treatment of ovarian carcinoma. Natl Cancer Inst Monog 42:101, 1975
13. Hanson MB, Powell DE, Donaldson ES, van Nagell JR Jr: Treatment of epithelial ovarian carcinoma by surgical debulking followed by single alkylating agent chemotherapy. Gynecol Oncol 10:337, 1980
14. Hacker NF, Berek JS, Lagasse LD, et al: Primary cytoreductive surgery for epithelial ovarian cancer. Obstet Gynecol 61:413, 1983
15. Edmonson JH, Fleming TR, Decker DG, et al: Different chemotherapeutic sensitivities and host factors affecting prognosis in advanced ovarian carcinoma versus minimal residual disease. Cancer Treat Rep 63:241, 1979
16. Dembo AJ, Bush RS, Beale FA, et al: Ovarian carcinoma: Improved survival following abdominopelvic

irradiation in patients with a completed pelvic operation. Am J Obstet Gynecol 134:793, 1979

17. Dembo AJ: Radiotherapeutic management of ovarian cancer. Semin Oncol 11:238, 1984
18. Podratz KC, Podczaski ES, Gaffey TA, et al: Primary carcinoma of the fallopian tube. Am J Obstet Gynecol 154:1319, 1986
19. Podratz KC, O'Brien PC, Malkasian GD Jr, et al: Effects of progestational agents in treatment of endometrial carcinoma. Obstet Gynecol 66:106, 1985
20. Heintz APM, Hacker NF, Berek JS, et al: Cytoreductive surgery in ovarian carcinoma: Feasibility and morbidity. Obstet Gynecol 67:783, 1986
21. Hoskins WJ, Lichter AS, Whittington R, et al: Whole abdominal and pelvic irradiation in patients with minimal disease at second-look surgical reassessment for ovarian carcinoma. Gynecol Oncol 20:271, 1985
22. Schray MF, Martinez A, Howes AE, et al: Advanced epithelial ovarian cancer: Toxicity of whole abdominal irradiation after operation, combination chemotherapy, and reoperation. Gynecol Oncol 24:68, 1986
23. Hainsworth JD, Malcolm A, Johnson DH, et al: Advanced minimal residual ovarian carcinoma: Abdominopelvic irradiation following combination chemotherapy. Obstet Gynecol 61:619, 1983
24. Wheeless CR Jr: Small bowel bypass for complications related to pelvic malignancy. Obstet Gynecol 42:661, 1973
25. Swan RW, Fowler WC Jr, Boronow RC: Surgical management of radiation injury to the small intestine. Surg Gynecol Obstet 142:325, 1976
26. Piver MS, Lele S: Enterovaginal and enterocutaneous fistulae in women with gynecologic malignancies. Obstet Gynecol 48:560, 1976
27. Schmitt EH III, Symmonds RE: Surgical treatment of radiation induced injuries of the intestine. Surg Gynecol Obstet 153:896, 1981
28. Castaldo TW, Petrilli ES, Ballon SC, Lagasse LD: Intestinal operations in patients with ovarian carcinoma. Am J Obstet Gynecol 139:80, 1981
29. Tunca JC, Buchler DA, Mack EA, et al: The management of ovarian-cancer-caused bowel obstruction. Gynecol Oncol 12:186, 1981
30. Piver MS, Barlow JJ, Lele SB, Frank A: Survival after ovarian cancer induced intestinal obstruction. Gynecol Oncol 13:44, 1982
31. Krebs H-B, Goplerud DR: Surgical management of bowel obstruction in advanced ovarian carcinoma. Obstet Gynecol 61:327, 1983
32. Clarke-Pearson DL, Chin NO, DeLong ER, et al: Surgical management of intestinal obstruction in ovarian cancer. I. Clinical features, postoperative complications, and survival. Gynecol Oncol 26:11, 1987
33. Stone HH, Hooper CA, Kolb LD, et al: Antibiotic prophylaxis in gastric, biliary and colonic surgery. Ann Surg 184:443, 1976
34. Stone HH, Haney BB, Kolb LD, et al: Prophylactic and preventive antibiotic therapy: Timing, duration and economics. Ann Surg 189:691, 1979
35. Rosenshein NB, Ruth JC, Villar J, et al: A prospective randomized study of doxycycline as a prophylactic antibiotic in patients undergoing radical hysterectomy. Gynecol Oncol 15:201, 1983
36. Sevin B-U, Ramos R, Lichtinger M, et al: Antibiotic prevention of infections complicating radical abdominal hysterectomy. Obstet Gynecol 64:539, 1984
37. McIlrath DC, van Heerden JA, Edis AJ, Dozois RR: Closure of abdominal incisions with subcutaneous catheters. Surgery 80:411, 1976
38. Goligher JC, Graham NG, de Dombal FT: Anastomotic dehiscence after anterior resection of rectum and sigmoid. Br J Surg 57:109, 1970
39. George WL, Rolfe RD, Finegold SM: *Clostridium difficile* and its cytotoxin in feces of patients with antimicrobial agent-associated diarrhea and miscellaneous conditions. J Clin Microbiol 15:1049, 1982
40. Thorlakson RH: Technique of repair of herniations associated with colonic stomas. Surg Gynecol Obstet 120:347, 1965
41. Rosin JD, Bonardi RA: Paracolostomy hernia repair with Marlex mesh: A new technique. Dis Colon Rectum 20:299, 1977
42. Leslie D: The parastomal hernia. Aust NZ J Surg 51:485, 1981
43. Todd IP: Mechanical complications of ileostomy. Clin Gastroenterol 11:268, May 1982
44. Abdu RA: Repair of paracolostomy hernias with Marlex mesh. Dis Colon Rectum 25:529, 1982
45. Jao S-W, Beart RW Jr, Wendorf LJ, Ilstrup DM: Irrigation management of sigmoid colostomy. Arch Surg 120:916, 1985

26

Reconstructive Surgery of the Vulva and Vagina

Kenneth D. Hatch
Hugh M. Shingleton

Techniques for reconstruction of the vagina and vulva in women undergoing radical pelvic surgery have been developed in recent years. Before the 1960s and 1970s, vulvar defects and pelvic cavities were permitted to epithelialize spontaneously, resulting in deformed pelvic structures, limited sexual function, and poor body image. Improved survival rates and increasing concern for sexual function of these women have led to the use of myocutaneous flaps, full-thickness transposition flaps, and split-thickness skin grafts as desirable techniques for rehabilitation following radical surgery of the vagina and vulva.

VAGINAL RECONSTRUCTION

A number of clinical situations require construction of a neovagina. The surgeon must be familiar with a variety of techniques in order to select the one most appropriate to the circumstance. It is essential, however, for the patient and her spouse to have thorough sexual counseling before the operation. The patient and her consort will require help in their adjustment to her new body image. Postoperatively, they will require considerable support.

Split-Thickness Skin Graft

The split-thickness skin graft is most successful when used to replace vaginal skin following skinning vaginectomy, but it can be used following more extensive surgery, such as radical vaginectomy, exenteration, or repair of vaginal strictures following radiotherapy.

TECHNIQUE

The donor site is chosen from the lateral thigh or the upper outer quadrant of the buttock, as these areas are usually covered by clothing and are subject to minimal irritation from daily activities. The skin is cleansed with acetone and alcohol. Mineral oil is placed over the donor site to ensure smooth passage of the dermatome over the skin. Several types of dermatome are available. The Brown dermatome is illustrated in Figure 26-1. The dermatome is set for a skin thickness of 0.014 inches and for a width of up to 8 cm. As the skin is harvested, an assistant picks up the skin with the thumb forceps and keeps it from rolling back into the dermatome blade (Fig. 26-1). The skin may then be placed on a 1.5-to-1 mesher in order to increase the size of the graft (Fig. 26-2). Meshing of the graft also makes for multiple drainage sites for

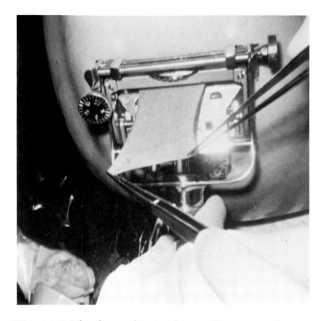

Fig. 26-1 The donor skin is taken with a Brown derma-tome.

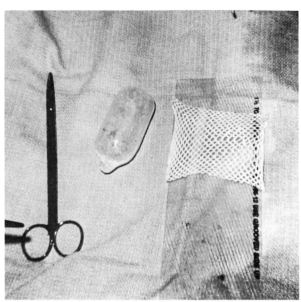

Fig. 26-2 The skin has been expanded by passing it through a 1.5-to-1 mesher.

serum and infection as well as easier attachment of the graft to the recipient site by permitting fibrin to form in the mesh holes.

The skin is sewn to a vaginal mold with dermal side out and inserted into the vaginal defect (Fig. 26-3). The edge of the donor skin is sewn to the vaginal edge, and the mold is fixed into the vagina with a suture. A urethral catheter is placed. The mold is re-moved on day 5, and the neovagina is irrigated gently with dilute iodine solution. The mold is replaced carefully to avoid avulsion of the new skin. The new vagina is irrigated daily with dilute iodine solution. The urethral catheter may be discontinued soon after the mold is first removed.

The patient may be discharged from the hospital as soon as she is comfortable removing, irrigating, and reinserting the mold herself. Estrogen vaginal cream is used to coat the vaginal mold to facilitate placement and increase the healing of the vagina. The patient is examined weekly in the clinic to monitor healing and to examine for strictures.

When the epithelium has completely regenerated and the vaginal size is adequate, the patient can begin coitus (Fig. 26-4). If the patient does not become sex-ually active, the mold should be inserted at night to

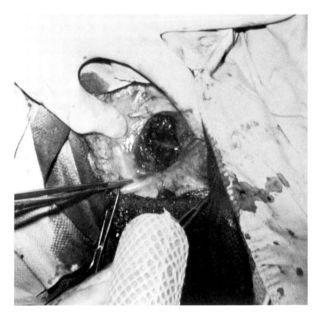

Fig. 26-3 The skin has been sewn around the vaginal stent and is being placed into the neovaginal cavity.

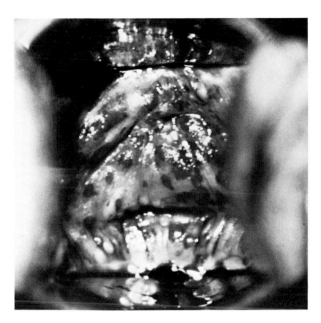

Fig. 26-4 Appearance of the neovagina at 4 months. The dark-stained islands are beginning glycogen formation.

prevent secondary strictures. This is a problem particularly with patients who have undergone previous radiation therapy. These patients will require regular dilation from coitus or vaginal mold insertion for several months in order to prevent fibrosis. This special care required by patients who do not have regular intercourse or who have had previous radiotherapy applies to all vaginal reconstructions using split-thickness skin grafts. Application of the split-thickness skin graft is described in the following operations; however, only special features of each operation is discussed.

SIMPLE VAGINECTOMY

The success of the split-thickness skin graft is dependent on the vascularity of the recipient site. The highest rate of success can be expected from those patients who undergo vaginectomy without previous radiotherapy. Here the skin take is high and the stricture rate low. The split-thickness skin graft undergoes an initial period of shrinkage for 2 to 3 weeks while the skin becomes vascularized. It is important for the patient to wear the mold until this period has passed. If regular coitus does not ensue, the mold should be

inserted nightly for an additional 3 to 4 weeks and then used two to three times weekly, until the skin has the appearance of normal vaginal skin with the production of glycogen and the risk of stricture has passed.

The fibrosis and lack of vascularity found in patients who have had radiotherapy significantly compromise the success of the graft. It is rare for such patients to demonstrate 100 percent take of the graft, and it will be necessary for them to continue to wear the mold while the skin that did survive spreads to cover the entire vagina. This process may require several months. Eventually, the vagina will become epithelialized, and regular coitus may ensue.

RADICAL VAGINECTOMY

The radical vaginectomy is most often performed as a part of radical hysterectomy for patients with disease extending into the vagina. Diethylstilbestrol (DES)-exposed patients with clear cell cancer often have cervix and upper vaginal involvement, and a number of them have undergone this treatment. The recipient site is composed of the bladder anteriorly and the rectum posteriorly. There will be little tissue laterally except for the paravaginal fat and areolar tissue. In the nonirradiated patient, the split-thickness skin graft has a high rate of success.

The patient should expect to wear the mold for up to 3 months while the operative site heals. Those patients with prior radiation have a high fistula rate and are better served by an exenterative operation.

EXENTERATION

In order to use the split-thickness skin graft following exenteration, a recipient site must be created. Following anterior exenteration, the rectum can provide the posterior surface for the split-thickness skin graft. If the omental pedicle is large enough, it is ideal to use as the remainder of the vagina. If the omental pedicle is not large enough, the bulbocavernosus flaps may be used. Berek et al.[1] used the redundant sigmoid successfully to help provide a recipient site.

In patients who have had a total exenteration with a low rectal anastomosis, it is preferable not to place the split-thickness skin graft directly on the suture line. In order to improve the rate of healing of the low rectal anastomosis, the suture line should be covered either with the omental pedicle, if it is large enough, or with the bulbocavernosus flap. In addition to providing a new blood supply, these two procedures provide a coital cushion that will decrease the tendency for future fistula formation as a result of coital trauma.

Following a total exenteration, which includes removal of the anus, it is difficult to prepare a recipient bed for the split-thickness skin graft, unless a large omental graft is available to serve as the entire recipient site. Morley et al.[2] successfully used a peritoneal patch onto which a split-thickness skin graft is placed after a granulation bed is established.

Postoperative management of the exenteration patient is similar to that of the patient with previous radiotherapy. The patient will use the vaginal mold until satisfactory epithelialization has taken place. As with the previously irradiated patient, this may take several months. Coitus is usually delayed by the extensiveness of the operation.

VAGINAL STENOSIS FOLLOWING RADIOTHERAPY

Reconstruction of a functioning vagina after radiotherapy obliteration requires careful dissection of the fibrotic skin away from the bladder and rectum and a new pocket in the pelvis is created for the split-thickness skin graft. Extreme care must be taken in dissecting this skin for damage to the rectum of bladder could result in a fistula. The lateral spaces should be developed first to gain entry into the pelvis. The vaginal epithelium overlying the rectum can be dissected with a protective finger in the rectum. The anterior dissection will begin at the site of vaginal obliteration. A urethral catheter can be inserted to help identify the bladder base. Postoperatively, the patients are manged similarly to the previously irradiated patients described above. The vaginal mold must be used for an extended period to prevent recurrence of the stricture.

Gracilis Myocutaneous Graft

The bilateral gracilis myocutaneous graft is ideally suited to reconstruction of the vagina following a total exenteration with a large perineal defect. The gracilis muscle is the most medial of the adductor muscle group and contains stable overlying skin and subcutaneous fat. The blood supply enters the muscle approximately 6 to 8 cm from the muscle origin at the pubic arch and is derived from both the profunda femoris and obturator vessels. For this reason, the obturator and the hypogastric arteries should not be ligated during the exenteration. The obturator nerve provides the innervation (Fig. 26-5).

TECHNIQUE

The patient is placed in the Lloyd Davis stirrups in the ski position with the thighs slightly externally rotated and the knees slightly flexed (Fig. 26-6). The gracilis can be palpated along the medial thigh as the most superficial of the adductor group. The skin island to be elevated with the graft is marked and can be 6 to 10 cm in width (Fig. 26-7). A width of 6 cm generally results in an appropriate-size vagina and reduces the risk of necrosis of the skin edge. It is important not to extend the flap distally onto the cutaneous area over the sartorius muscle in the lower third of the thigh, as the sartorius is dominant over the gracilis in this area. The length of the graft should be 12 to 20 cm. The incision at the tip of the graft should taper so as to aid in closure of the defect as well as reduce skin necrosis. Cephalad, the skin marks should end approximately 6 cm from the pubic arch. The posterior skin incision is made first; the anterior incision is then performed. The saphenous nerve and vein will be found near the anterior incision and should be conserved (Fig. 26-8).

The incision proceeds to the fascial investiture over the adductor muscle group. The crease between the gracilis and adductor longus is identified by blunt dissection, and the fascia is incised. The index and middle fingers are inserted behind the gracilis at about the mid-thigh, which will be caudad to the neurovascular bundle. In this area, there is an avascular plane, and the gracilis muscle can be elevated with a finger from the rest of the adductor group to its distal limits. By grasping the muscle and skin with the fingers behind and the thumb encircling the graft, the site of the incision in the fascia posterior to the muscle can be identified. This incision is carried distally by blunt dissection. The muscle should be mobilized 3 to 5 cm beyond the end of the skin incision to allow for contraction of the muscle after division. The muscle is divided, and a ligature is placed on both ends.

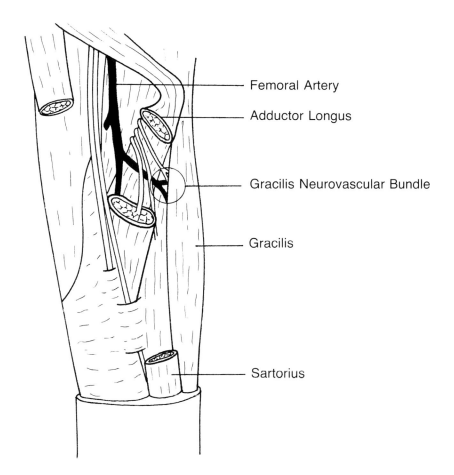

Fig. 26-5 Relationship of the gracilis muscle and its neurovascular bundle to the other structures in the thigh.

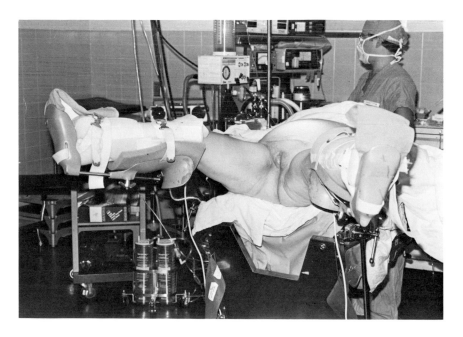

Fig. 26-6 The patient is positioned in the Lloyd-Davies stirrups prior to exenteration.

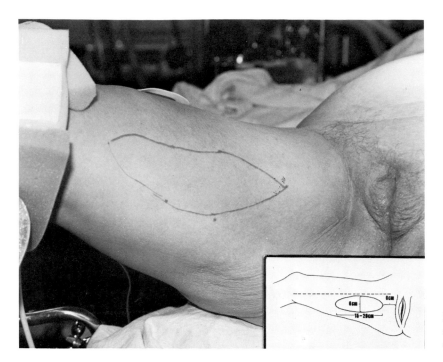

Fig. 26-7 The skin island to be elevated with the gracilis myocutaneous flap is outlined.

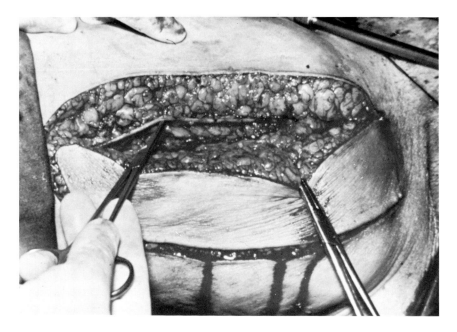

Fig. 26-8 The saphenous vein is identified at the upper edge of the myocutaneous flap.

The neurovascular bundle can now be localized by retracting the muscle medially (Fig. 26-9). The index finger is inserted ventral to the bundle under the fascia between the gracilis and adductor layers. The fascia is now incised cephalad using the index finger as a guide. This is repeated posteriorly. The tapered ends of the skin island are then trimmed to a more rounded appearance to reduce the tendency for skin necrosis at the tip. The fascial edges are sewn to the skin with 3-0 absorbable sutures to prevent shearing of the skin and

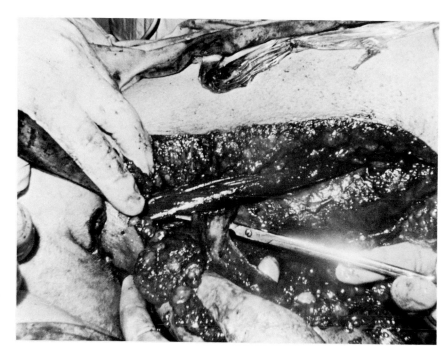

Fig. 26-9 The neurovascular bundle is isolated, and the flap is ready for placement in the vagina.

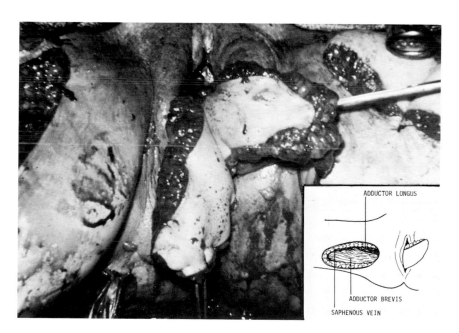

Fig. 26-10 Both flaps have been passed under the skin bridge and will be sewn together to form the vaginal pouch.

fat from the underlying muscle. The neurovascular bundle is carefully dissected from its fascia to allow for mobility during rotation. Since the blood supply to the graft enters the gracilis muscle approximately 6 to 8 cm from the pubic arch, the graft will be rotated around that point. The muscle is left attached to its origin at the pubic arch, but the fascia is incised to increase mobility. The graft is rotated posteriorly and brought under the skin bridge (Fig. 26-10). The skin bridge is established by sharp incision of the fibrous

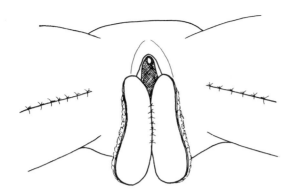

Fig. 26-11 The posterior edges of the two flaps have been sewn together. (Modified from Berek JS et al: Vaginal reconstruction performed simultaneously with pelvic exenteration. Obstet Gynecol 63:318, 1984)

attachments of Colle's fascia to the pubic arch. This tunnel should be large enough to permit easy passage of the graft so as to avoid pressure on the vascular pedicles.

To document skin viability, some authorities recommend the use of 1 g fluorescein IV, followed by exposure of the flaps to ultraviolet (UV) light in a dark room. Nonfluorescing skin areas are excised. If the entire flap does not show fluorescence, vascular spasm may be the cause; reinjection several minutes later should be performed. The bilateral flaps are joined in the midline with interrupted absorbable sutures performing the posterior line first (Fig. 26-11), then the anterior (Fig. 26-12). The neovagina is then inserted into the pelvic defect and sutured to the sacrum and remaining levator pedicles. To reduce the tension on the vascular pedicles, the thighs should be

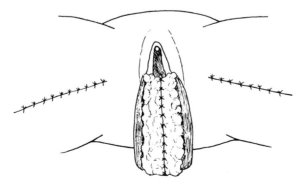

Fig. 26-12 The anterior edges of the grafts are sewn together. (Modified from Berek JS et al: Vaginal reconstruction performed simultaneously with pelvic exenteration. Obstet Gynecol 63:318, 1984)

adducted and rotated internally. The donor sites are closed with large, interrupted mattress sutures, and suction drains are placed. Suction drains are also placed in the dependent portion of the pelvis. The omentum is mobilized to cover the graft and prevent the small bowel from becoming adherent. A vaginal stent is unnecessary for the gracilis neovagina.

The patient must be ambulated as soon as she is able in an attempt to reduce the risk of pulmonary embolus. The skin edges of the graft should be inspected after 2 to 3 days. If significant discoloration is present, the graft should be inspected daily. Otherwise, a weekly inspection will suffice. Local debridement may be necessary if necrosis occurs. Even if significant skin loss occurs, the muscle often survives and a split-thickness skin graft can be applied when a healthy granulation bed is available. The patient should be seen frequently to monitor convalescence (Fig. 26-13).

Coitus may begin when overall recovery is satisfactory and the patient and her spouse have adjusted. Sensation during coitus will obviously be altered, and the patient and spouse should receive sexual couseling. Water-soluble lubricants may facilitate coitus, as vaginal secretions will be absent. If the patient is not sexually active, periodic irrigations may be helpful to reduce the vaginal odor associated with desquamation of keratinized epithelial cells and the sebaceous secretions.

RESULTS AND PRACTICAL OBSERVATIONS

Since McGraw et al.[3] published the first series of patients in 1976, the gracilis myocutaneous graft has become the favored method of neovaginal construction following total exenteration. This approach produces a neovagina with softness, pliability, and durability. The sensitivity to pressure is good, but tactile sensitivity is diminished. The donor tissue is expendable and can be transferred without significant patient morbidity. Although the gracilis muscle is somewhat bulky initially, it undergoes atrophy over several months and does not interfere with coitus. The neovagina rarely undergoes vault contraction unless the recipient pouch is not large enough or there has been significant skin loss due to necrosis. If skin loss occurs, a secondary split-thickness skin graft may be placed to prevent stricture. Prolapse of the neovagina is rare,

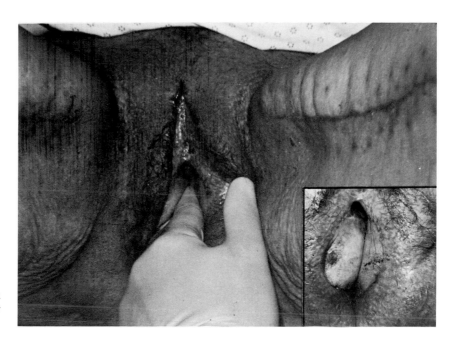

Fig. 26-13 Appearance of a gracilis neovagina 5 weeks after surgery is shown.

and herniation of abdominal contents has not been reported. If the skin in the lower vagina is somewhat redundant, it can be excised. Successful coitus can be anticipated in all those patients who have a sexual partner and who are so inclined following their convalescence. Orgasmic response has been reported even in patients who have undergone removal of a significant portion of their vulva as well as the clitoris.

The gracilis neovagina is most successful when performed at the time of exenteration. Most surgeons use a second surgical team, so that the operating time is not extended. The additional blood loss is approximately 250 ml. Attempting the procedure after the pelvic defect has healed leads to difficulty in preparing an adequate recipient bed, and prolapse or stenosis may result.

The obese patient presents special problems. The weight of the medial thigh fat will pull the skin posterior as well as obscure the landmarks for incision. The thigh skin should be rotated anteriorly 3 to 4 cm to compensate. In addition, the patient may have too much fat for bilateral myocutaneous grafts; a single graft can be placed in the pelvis with the omental carpet used as the remainder of the vaginal tube. It can then either receive a split-thickness skin graft or be allowed to undergo spontaneous epithelialization.

Patients who have undergone a supralevator exen-

teration often do not have enough room for a bilateral graft. A unilateral graft with omental carpet as described above may be used, or a vulvobulbocavernosus myocutaneous graft might be considered (Fig. 26-14).

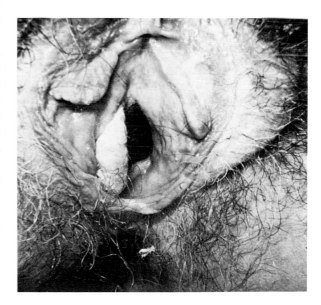

Fig. 26-14 A unilateral gracilis flap is shown 6 months postoperative. The left vaginal wall is formed by the omentum and undergoes spontaneous epithelialization.

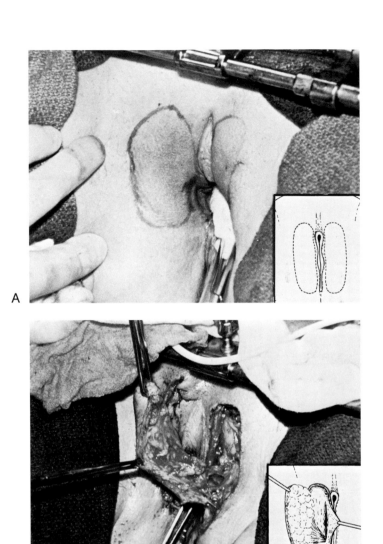

A

B

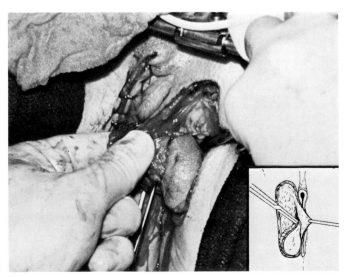

C

Fig. 26-15 (A) The marks for the vulvobulbocavernosus myocutaneous flaps are made. **(B)** The flap is clevated on its pedicle. **(C)** The flap is being passed under the skin bridge. *(Figure continues)*

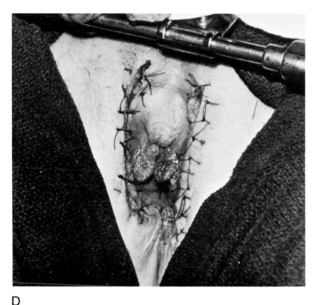
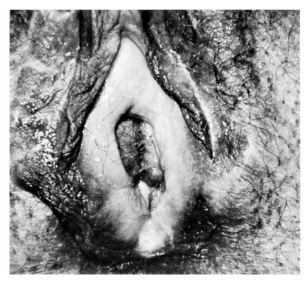

D   E

Fig. 26-15 *(Continued).* **(D)** The immediate postoperative appearance of the vulva. **(E)** The 6-month postoperative appearance of the neovagina and vulva. (Hatch KD: Construction of a neovagina after exenteration using the vulvobulbocavernosus myocutaneous graft. Obstet Gynecol 63:110, 1984)

Vulvobulbocavernosus Myocutaneous Graft

The vulvobulbocavernosus pedicle graft is best suited for the construction of a neovagina after supralevator pelvic exenteration. This includes the anterior exenteration and the total exenteration with low rectal anastomosis. The original description of the bulbocavernosus graft by Martius[4] did not include preservation of the overlying vulvar skin. The graft does, however, have a stable overlying skin that, together with the fat and rectal tissue, can be used as a pedicle to establish a successful graft. It brings both a new blood supply to aid in healing and a new epithelial surface into the pelvis. The blood supply is derived from the perineal branch of the pudendal artery, and the innervation is from the internal pudendal nerve.

TECHNIQUE

The bulbocavernosus muscle and fat pad are identified by grasping the labia between the thumb and fingers. The inner margin is the sulcus between the labia minora and labia majora. The outer margin is the lateral margin of the labia majora (Fig. 26-15A). The width varies, depending on the amount of fatty tissue,

but it may be up to 7 cm. The inferior pole is parallel with the perineal body, and the superior pole may extend above the base of the clitoris. The length may be up to 10 cm. The skin incisions are made, and the medial dissection is carried out first. A plane is developed between the bulbocavernosus pad and the skin of the introitus. The lateral incision is then performed and the dissection carried to the pubic arch. The blood supply enters at the inferior pole of the pedicle so the dissection should be in the mid- and upper portions first. The skin and subcutaneous tissue over the inferior pole are then incised, releasing the flap on its pedicle (Fig. 26-15B). A tunnel is developed by elevating the remaining introital skin away from the pubic arch. The graft is then passed through this tunnel and attached in the pelvis (Fig. 26-15C,D).

If a low rectal anastomosis has been performed, the grafts are sewn together posteriorly and placed over the anastomotic line. Laterally, the flaps are sewn to the levator muscle pedicles. The posterior and lateral walls of the vagina are thus formed by the vulvobulbocavernosus myocutaneous graft (Fig. 26-16A). The roof of the vagina is formed by the omental carpet (Fig. 26-16B), which is sutured to the pubic symphysis, the edge of the flap, and the rectosigmoid. The

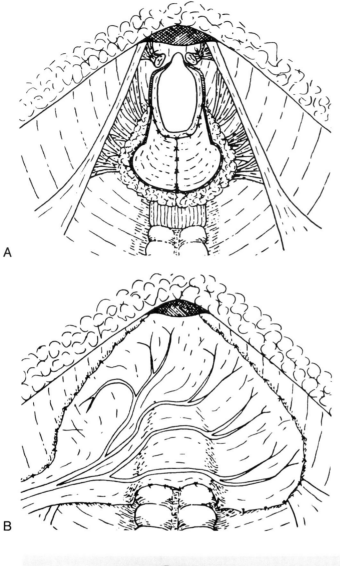

A

B

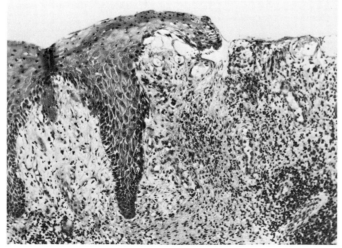

C

Fig. 26-16 (A) The vulvobulbocavernosus flaps are used to cover the rectum and lateral pelvic defect. (B) The omentum has been placed into the pelvis to complete the neovagina and to isolate the small bowel from the pelvic defect. (C) Spontaneous epithelialization of the omentum shown here at 3 months postoperative. (Hatch KD: Construction of a neovagina after exenteration using the vulvo-bulbocavernosus myocutaneous graft. Obstet Gynecol 63:110, 1984) omental carpet can be covered with a split-thickness skin graft, or spontaneous epithelialization can be allowed to take place (Fig. 26-16C). A vaginal stent is left in place. If the patient has undergone anterior exenteration with the preservation of a significant amount of posterior vaginal epithelium, the flaps may be sutured to the lateral margins of the posterior vagina and the grafts positioned laterally and superiorly. The omental carpet is placed in the pelvis as before and may provide the roof of the neovagina. Spontaneous epithelialization of the omentum occurs in approximately 3 months. The donor site is closed with interrupted 3-0 absorbable suture, and a Penrose drain is placed beneath the skin.

Approximately 1 week postoperatively, the patient is examined and the vagina irrigated. Subsequently, irrigation is carried out twice daily with a solution of hydrogen peroxide and saline (1:3). Upon discharge, the patient is instructed to continue irrigations with peroxide and tap water on a daily basis. Patients are examined periodically. Complete healing requires 4 to 6 months, with some need for cauterization of granulation tissue over the omental carpet. Vaginal obturators are unnecessary.

RESULTS AND PRACTICAL COMMENTS

The length of the vagina ranges from 6 to 10 cm and the diameter 3 to 6 cm. All the grafts have survived with virtually no loss of skin. In one patient, a significant hematoma occurred from the donor site, requiring removal of two sutures and evacuation of the hematoma, followed by compression dressing. Edema of the remaining labia minora has not been observed. The donor site incisions heal without chronic discomfort and have a near-normal appearance once hair has regrown (Fig. 26-15E).

The vulvar skin used to make the neovagina will grow normal vulvar hair. The amount of hair diminishes over time but has not disappeared in the longest-surviving patient at 5 years. The hair and sebaceous secretions may cause a significant vaginal odor requiring regular irrigation. One patient requested removal of the hair, and this was accomplished 4 months postexenteration by skin excision followed by split-thickness skin graft. This procedure resulted in a more normal-appearing and functioning vagina. In four patients, the skin was removed from the bulbocaver-

nosus flap at the time of reconstruction. A split-thickness skin graft was placed over the flap and omental carpet. This necessitated a vaginal obturator to prevent stricture and has resulted in a vagina that is shorter, smaller, more fibrotic, and in general less satisfactory than the myocutaneous graft technique. It is best to construct the neovagina with the myocutaneous graft. Should the hair remain a problem, it is excised after the neovaginal size has been well established.

RECONSTRUCTION OF THE VULVA

It is important to understand the relationships of the skin, subcutaneous fat, bulbocavernosus muscle, and pelvic diaphragm when considering vulva reconstruction. It should be noted that Scarpa's fascia merges into the inguinal ligament and extends for a short distance into the thigh as the cribriform fascia, which is penetrated by the saphenous vein and the other vessels exiting from the femoral artery and vein to the groin and vulva. It then merges with the fascia covering the thigh muscle. Over the mons pubis, Scarpa's fascia continues onto the labium majus, where it becomes Colle's fascia and lies just above the bulbocavernosus muscle. It merges with the superficial transverse perineal muscle inferiorly and laterally with the pubic arch. This attachment of Colle's fascia to the pubic arch produces the labial crural crease and severely limits the mobility of the skin at the lateral margin of the vulva. It also limits the lateral spread of any vulvar hematoma or abscess. The urogenital diaphragm forms the deep margin of the vulva. This is formed by the deep fascial investitures over the levator muscles as they pass from the pubic arch to the vaginal opening. These anatomic relationships must be kept in mind when considering reconstruction of the vulva.

Split-Thickness Skin Graft

Since its proposal by Rutledge and Sinclair,[5] this procedure has been employed by a number of oncologists for extensive areas of CIS or other chronic diseases of the vulva. Since only the skin is removed, the underlying Colle's fascia, subcutaneous fat, and bulbocavernosus muscle are preserved. For smaller areas of excision, the skin can be mobilized and the edges

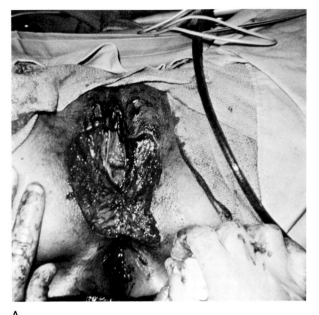

A

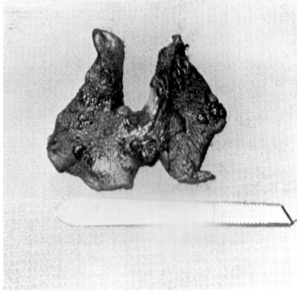

B

C

Fig. 26-17 (A) Vulvar defect following skinning vulvectomy. **(B)** Skin specimen from skinning vulvectomy. **(C)** Split-thickness skin graft applied to the defect. A fluff dressing will be applied. *(Figure continues)*

approximated. Occasionally, the edges are too far apart and a split-thickness skin graft is needed (Fig. 26-17). The donor site is selected, and the skin is harvested in the manner described in the section on vaginal reconstruction. The skin may be used either meshed or unmeshed. If a mesher is used, there will be more contraction of the skin as healing takes place.

The graft is sewn to the recipient site with 3-0 absorbable suture. A fluff dressing is applied; stay sutures are tied loosely over this dressing with just enough pressure for the skin to maintain contact with the underlying tissue and prevent collections of serum or small hematomas. The fluff dressing should be removed after 48 hours and examined for collection of

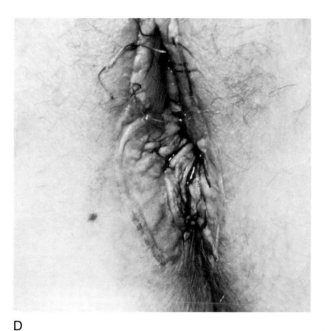

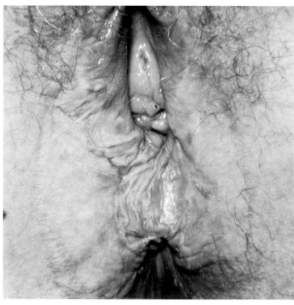

D   E

Fig. 26-17 *(Continued)*. **(D)** Appearance of the skin graft at 2 weeks showing the initial contracture. **(E)** Appearance of the graft at 6 months showing relaxation of the scar.

fluid beneath the graft. These should be drained using a scalpel to puncture the blebs, and the dressing is replaced. The graft is inspected daily and the dressing removed when no further fluid collections are noted. After the dressing is removed, a perineal squeeze bottle is used to irrigate the recipient site four times daily and after urination and defecation. A mixture of dilute betadine and saline is used.

Full-Thickness Rotational Flap

The split-thickness skin graft should not be used directly over bone and therefore cannot be used when the vulvectomy has removed tissue down to the pubic symphysis or pubic arch. When simple mobilization of the skin edges cannot be used to cover the defect, a full-thickness transposition flap should be used. These flaps are similar to that described by Limberg and Dufourmentel as a means to cover rhomboid shaped defects. Their use on the vulva was described by Barnhill et al.[6] as a means to cover perineal body defects after skinning procedures for carcinoma in situ. This technique can be used to cover large full-thickness defects on the vulva, particularly over the

posterior vulva. The adherence of Colle's fascia to the pubic arch laterally limits the applicability of this type of graft for the more anterior vulvar defects.

The skin over the buttock is ideal for mobilization and rotation over several centimeters to cover the large posterior defects (Fig. 26-18A). The defect to be covered is measured from the vaginal edge to the vulvar edge (points A and B). This distance is the width of the vertical incision of the donor graft (points C to B'). The distance from the anus to the vertical buttock incision should be the distance equal to the length of the vertical incision (points B to C). The horizontal incision for the donor graft is parallel to the defect to be covered and is of the same length as the vertical mark (B' C'). The full thickness of skin and underlying fat that infiltrates the subcutaneous fascia is mobilized from the underlying gluteal fat. A similar flap from the opposite side is mobilized, and they are brought together in the midline and attached to the vagina cephalad and anal margin caudad (Fig. 26-18B). The donor wound is closed by suturing A' to A', B' to B', and C' to C'. This leaves an inverted U (Fig. 26-19).

The anterior vulva may also be covered by full-

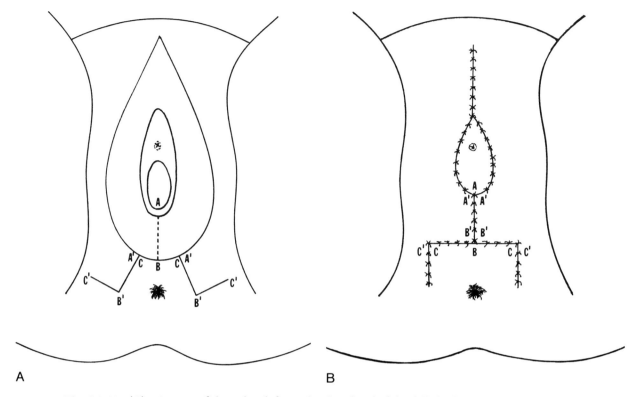

A   B

Fig. 26-18 **(A)** Diagram of the vulva defect to be closed and of the full-thickness transposition flaps marked for cutting. **(B)** The vulva defect is closed, and the flaps are sewn into place.

thickness transpositon flaps, however these will have to be based further out on the buttock or medial thigh and rotated over a 90-degree arc. The attachment of Colle's fascia to the pubic arch laterally limits the mobility of a flap based on the medial thigh (Fig. 26-20).

Postoperatively, the patient should have catheter drainage, and an ice pack should be placed. Ambulation may be started on the first postoperative day. Perineal hygiene using a squeeze bottle filled with dilute betadine solution can be started on the first postoperative day. Some minor separation, particularly at the corners, can be expected. This problem is managed by simple local irrigation. The results of this rotational flap closure are quite satisfactory. Nineteen patients have undergone radical vulvectomy and rotational flap reconstruction after radical vulvectomy with separate groin dissection incisions at the University of Alabama Medical Center. Their average hospital stay is 10 days, which is significantly less than the

stay of those treated by radical vulvectomy without reconstruction (23 days). No patient suffered a major separation, and no strictures of the introitus have occurred.

Full-Thickness Advancement Flaps

The lower abdominal skin can be mobilized and advanced to cover the pubic symphysis. This is aided by preserving some of the mons pubis and, in some cases, leaving a V in the midline (Figs. 26-5, 26-21, and 26-22).

The standard radical vulvectomy with en bloc bilateral groin dissection may be modified for selected patients with negative groin nodes.[7] The modifications include separate incisions for the vulvectomy and bilateral groin dissection. This modification enables the surgeon to conserve the skin bridge between the vulva and the groin dissection, which acts as a

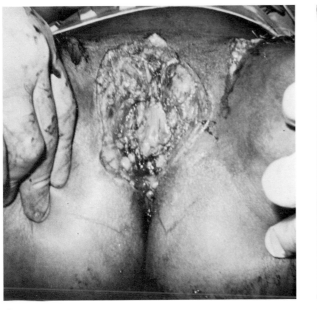

A

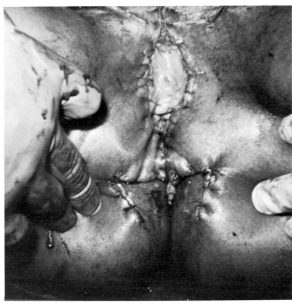

B

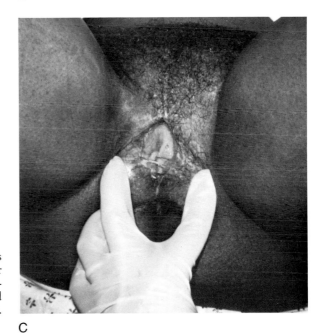

C

Fig. 26-19 (A) Clinical application of the full-thickness transposition flaps. The perineal body and 3 cm of lower vagina have been removed. **(B)** The flaps are used to provide a new perineal body and cover the anal sphincter and lower anal canal. **(C)** Appearance of the vulva at 6 months.

double pedicle advancement graft and facilitates the closure of the vulva by skin mobilization. In addition, more of the mons pubis is conserved, leading to a more normal appearing vulva with much needed coital cushion (Fig. 26-19C).

Myocutaneous Grafts

Myocutaneous grafts are required when very large defects need to be covered or when radiotherapy has been used and a new blood supply as well as unirra-

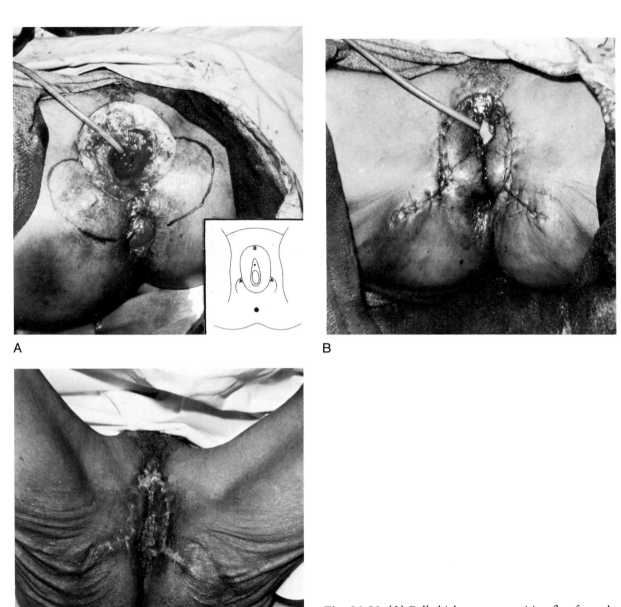

A

B

C

Fig. 26-20 **(A)** Full-thickness transposition flap from the buttock in a patient who has undergone excision of recurrent cancer of the vulva around the urethral meatus. **(B)** The flaps have been rotated up from the buttock onto the defect. **(C)** Appearance 4 months after surgery.

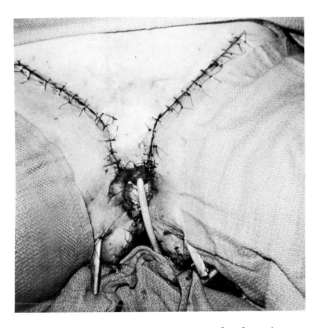

Fig. 26-21 Full-thickness advancement flap from the anterior abdomen used to cover the symphysis pubis.

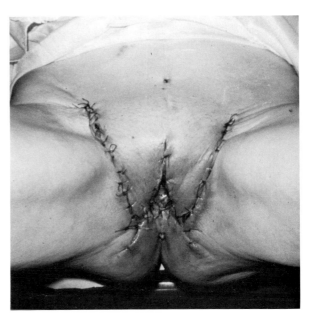

Fig. 26-22 Another full-thickness advancement flap from the abdomen.

diated skin are needed to cover defects of the vulva or groin. Three types of myocutaneous grafts have been reported useful in gynecologic oncology: gracilis, fascia lata, and gluteus.

Gracilis Myocutaneous Graft

The gracilis myocutaneous graft has gained the greatest acceptance and popularity. The patient is positioned as described earlier. This position gives access to the vulva, groins, and gracilis muscle; thus, the entire operation can be performed without further change in position. The gracilis muscle is identified by palpating the muscles on the medial aspect of the thigh. The marking of the graft to be harvested is different from that for vaginal reconstruction. Instead of an island of skin on the upper thigh, the entire skin from the tip of the graft to the pubic arch is often required. The skin can be tailored to fit the vulvar defect to be covered. If the vulvar defect is so wide that it extends to the upper thigh, the skin incision for the myocutaneous graft may extend to the vulvar defect, thereby leaving no skin bridge. If the vulvar incision did not extend completely to the thigh crease, a skin bridge will be left under which the myocutaneous

graft will be passed to reach the vulva. The graft may be used to cover the vulvar defect or it could extend over the mons and even into the groin. The graft is held in place by interrupted 2-0 absorbable sutures. A suction drain is left under the graft for 7 to 10 days. The graft is inspected each day to observe for skin edge necrosis. Some loss of skin may occur, particularly at the tips of the graft. This skin must be trimmed as necrosis occurs. The underlying muscle is often still quite viable even if the skin and subcutaneous fat are lost (Fig. 26-23).

The average operating time is extended by 2 hours over the usual time for a radical vulvectomy. Blood loss is 400 ml more, but the hospital stay is shorter than the standard radical vulvectomy and bilateral groin dissection performed without myocutaneous flap construction. Since these patients have defects that are too large for a primary closure, the alternative mechanism of healing would have been by granulation formation and secondary epithelialization. This results in extensive scarring of the vulva. In addition, patients typically have stricture of the vaginal introitus and become sexual cripples. The gracilis myocutaneous graft provides a soft, pliable skin surface that is very acceptable for coitus.

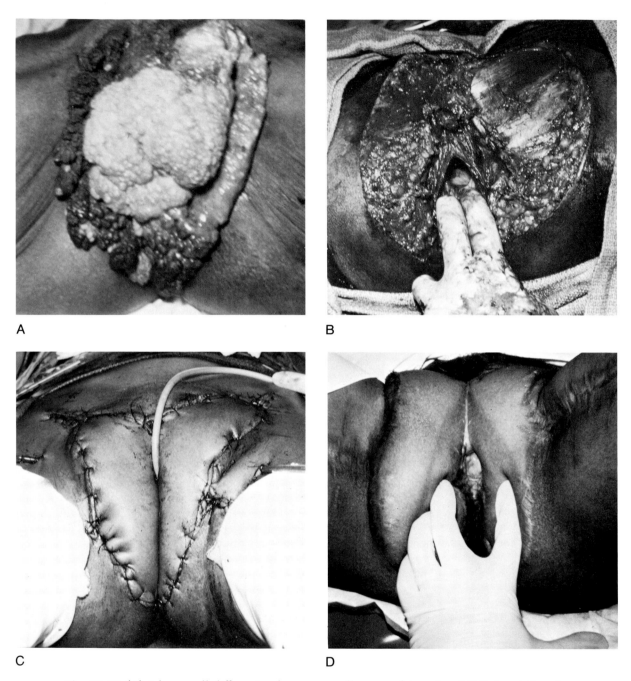

A

B

C

D

Fig. 26-23 **(A)** A large well-differentiated squamous cell cancer of the vulva. **(B)** Vulvar defect after excision. The fascia of the left medial thigh is exposed. **(C)** The gracilis myocutaneous flaps have been rotated into place. **(D)** Appearance at 6 months.

Tensor Fascia Lata Myocutaneous Flap

The tensor fascia lata myocutaneous flap is best used to cover large groin and anterior vulvar defects. It is a broad muscle that originates in the anterior portion of the lateral iliac crest and inserts into the fascia lata on the lateral thigh (Fig. 26-24). Its blood supply is from the transverse branch of the lateral femoral circumflex artery, and the innervation is from the lateral cutaneous nerve. The nerve enters the muscle posterior and deep to the vascular pedicle. The flap can be made as large as 25 × 40 cm, permitting coverage of the entire groin and perineum. The anterior border of the flap corresponds to a line drawn from the anterior superior iliac spine to the lateral condyle of the tibia. The distal border of the flap can extend to within 5 to 8 cm of the knee. The posterior border is marked by the greater trocanter. The incision is made through the fascia lata. The inferior end is elevated first to permit identification of the perforating vessels 8 to 10 cm below the anterior superior iliac spine. The flap can be rotated anteriorly to cover the groin, perineum, or lower abdominal wall. The flap can be brought directly to the defect or tunneled beneath a skin bridge. The flap may be rotated posteriorly to cover the sacrum or anus. The donor site may be closed primarily but occasionally requires skin grafting. Early ambulation is possible and desirable, in order to prevent pulmonary embolus. Patient acceptability has been excellent, with very few wound complications. Postoperative hospital stay is 10 to 12 days, and the chronic lymphedema often seen following vulvar and groin surgery has not been observed.

Gluteal Myocutaneous Thigh Flap

The gluteal myocutaneous flap is best suited for posterior pelvic, perineal, or buttock defects (Fig. 26-25). It is based on the inferior gluteal artery whose entry into the flap is 5 cm above the ischial tuberosity. The flap is approximately 12 cm wide, and its length may extend to the popliteal fossa. The dissection can be performed in the lithotomy position and is carried through gluteus muscle fibers. The fascia lata is tran-

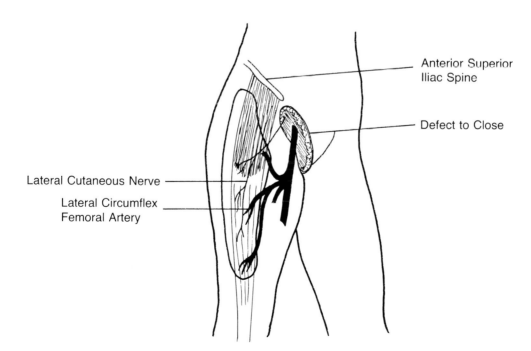

Fig. 26-24 Diagram showing the anatomy of the tensor fascia lata myocutaneous graft. (Modified from Goldberg MI, Rothfleish S: The tensor fascia lata myocutaneous flap in gynecologic oncology. Gynecol Oncol 12:41, 1981)

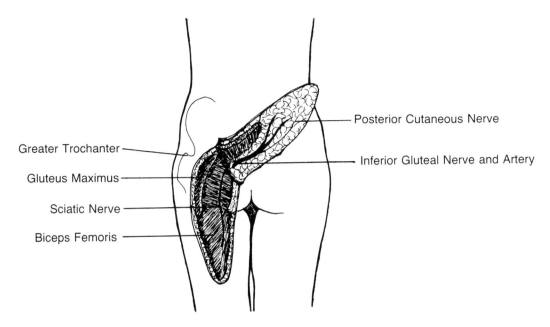

Greater Trochanter

Gluteus Maximus

Sciatic Nerve

Biceps Femoris

Posterior Cutaneous Nerve

Inferior Gluteal Nerve and Artery

Fig. 26-25 Diagram of the anatomy of the gluteal myocutaneous graft. (Modified from Achauer BM et al: Gluteal thigh flap in reconstruction of complex pelvic wounds. Arch Surg 11:18, 1983)

sected in the thigh, and dissection is carried out deep to its fascia, thereby including the inferior gluteal artery and the posterior cutaneous nerve of the thigh. The flap takes very well. It is accompanied by significant pain in the posterior thigh and causes disfigurement. Although the flap of choice for perineal and buttock wounds, it is not as satisfactory as the gracilis or bulbocavernosis flaps for neovaginal construction.

REFERENCES

1. Berek JS, Hacker NF, Lagasse LD: Vaginal reconstruction performed simultaneously with pelvic exenteration. Obstet Gynecol 63:318, 1984
2. Morley GW, Lindenauer SM, Youngs D: Vaginal reconstruction following pelvic exenteration: Surgical and psychological considerations. Am J Obstet Gynecol 116:996, 1973
3. McGraw JB, Massey FM, Shanklin KD, Horton CE: Vaginal reconstruction with gracilis myocutaneous flaps. Plast Reconstr Surg 58:176, 1976
4. Martius J: Operations for urinary incontinence. p. 327–329. In McCall M, Bolten, KA (eds): Operative Gynecology. Little, Brown, Boston, 1956
5. Rutledge E, Sinclair M: Treatment of intraepithelial carcinoma of the vulva by skin excision and graft. Am J Obstet Gynecol 102:806, 1968
6. Barnhill DR, Hoskins WJ, Metz P: Use of the rhomboid flap after partial vulvectomy. Obstet Gynecol 62:444, 1983
7. Hacker NF, Leuchter RS, Berek JS, et al: Radical vulvectomy and bilateral inguinal lymphadenectomy through separate groin incisions. Obstet Gynecol 58:574, 1981

SUGGESTED READINGS

Achauer BM, Turpin IM, Furnas DW: Gluteal thigh flap in reconstruction of complex pelvic wounds. Arch Surg 11:18, 1983

Andersen BL, Hacker NF: Psychosexual adjustment following pelvic exenteration. Obstet Gynecol 61:331, 1983

Becker DW, Massey FM, McCraw JB: Musculocutaneous flaps in reconstructive pelvic surgery. Obstet Gynecol 54:178, 1979

Berek JS, Hacker NF, Lagasse LD, Smith McL: Delayed vaginal reconstruction in the fibrotic pelvis following radiation or previous reconstruction. Obstet Gynecol 61:743, 1983

Chafe W, Fowler WC Jr, Walton LA, Currie JL: Radical vulvectomy with use of tensor fascia lata myocutaneous flap. Am J Obstet Gynecol 145: 207, 1983

Goldberg MI, Rothfleisch S: The tensor fascia lata myocutaneous flap in gynecologic oncology. Gynecol Oncol 12:412, 1981

Hatch KD: Construction of a neovagina after exenteration using the vulvobulbocavernosus myocutaneous graft. Obstet Gynecol 63:110, 1984

Heath PM, Woods JE, Podratz KC, et al: Gracilis myocutaneous vaginal reconstruction. Mayo Clin Proc 59:21, 1984

Jervis W, Salver KE, Busquets MAV, Atkins RW: Further applications of the Limberg and Dufourmental flaps. Plast Reconst Surg 54:335, 1974

Lister GD, Gibson T: Closure of rhomboid skin defects: The flaps of Limberg and Dufourmental. Br J Plast Surg 25:300, 1972

Magrina JF, Masterson BJ: Vaginal construction in gynecological oncology: A review of techniques. Obstet Gynecol Surv 36:1, 1981

Morrow CP, Lacey CG, Lucas WE: Reconstructive surgery in gynecologic cancer employing the gracilis myocutaneous pedicle graft. Gynecol Oncol 7:176, 1979

Pierce GW, Klabunde H, O'Connor GB, Long AH: Changes in skin flap of a constructed vagina due to environment. Am J Surg 92:4, 1956

Simmons RJ, Millard DR Jr: Reconstruction of a functioning vagina following radiation therapy for cancer of cervix. Surg Gynecol Obstet 112:761, 1961

Trelford JD, Silverton JS: Successful plastic procedures of the perineum. Gynecol Oncol 7:239, 1979

Wheeless CR Jr, McGibbon B, Dorsey JH, Maxwell GP: Gracilis myocutaneous flap in reconstruction of the vulva and female perineum. Obstet Gynecol 54:97, 1979

27
Endoscopy
Martin S. Goldstein

The early accurate diagnosis of adnexal masses is critical in the management and cure of ovarian malignancy. The imaging techniques of pelvic sonography, computed tomography (CT) scanning, and magnetic resonance imaging (MRI) are major advances in the differential diagnoses of a pelvic mass. These techniques are limited in their ability to separate solid ovarian neoplasms from uterine fibroids and in their inability to provide histologic confirmation of suspected findings. The application of laparoscopy as an adjunct to noninvasive imaging may be the only accurate method of differentiating an early malignancy from a benign process that requires no further surgical treatment. Laparoscopy as a first-look procedure in difficult differential diagnoses permits security of diagnosis prior to exploratory laparotomy and can permit an intelligent and secure selection of a more cosmetic incision site.

LAPAROSCOPY TECHNIQUE

Laparoscopy can be performed under local or general anesthesia. Local anesthesia eliminates the risks of general anesthesia and permits discussion of findings with the patient prior to laparotomy. The disadvantages of local anesthesia include patient anxiety, patient discomfort, inability to control respiration, and risks associated with patient movement if cautery or scissor techniques are used during the procedure. Laparoscopy under local anesthesia should not be used if there are previous incisions since large volumes of

CO_2 for abdominal distention cannot be used without causing discomfort to the patient. Laparoscopy under local anesthesia should not be used in lengthy procedures, for shallow and decreased respiration may lead to acidosis.[1,2] A standby anesthesiologist should be present with the ability to induce general anesthesia immediately if complications occur or laparoscopic findings confirm the need for exploratory laparotomy. In performing laparoscopy under local anesthesia, a diamond-shaped block is created by injecting a 0.5 percent solution of local anesthetic without epinephrine to minimize heart rate changes. The field block is carried through skin, subcutaneous tissue, fascia, and peritoneum. In operating under local anethesia, all movements must be explained to the patient, and gentle tissue handling is essential. The total amount of CO_2 used for abdominal distention must be limited to 1500 to 2000 cc CO_2. If larger volumes are used, general peritoneal and diaphragmatic irritation will prevent satisfactory visualization due to the patient's discomfort. In medically compromised patients, laparoscopy under local anesthesia without supplemental sedation may be the only chance of making a definitive diagnosis; in laparoscopy for the evaluation and diagnosis of malignancy, general endotracheal anesthesia permits a more complete diagnostic evaluation, including probe palpation of abdominal structures, diaphragmatic visualization, and biopsy if required.

Laparoscopy can be performed with the patient in the supine or lithotomy position. If the uterus is absent, inserting a vaginal packing will tent the cul-de-sac and permit better visualization of the pelvis and adnexa. The bladder should be drained by an indwelling catheter in laparoscopies for the evaluation of malignancy. A uterine elevator such as the Hulka tena-culum is helpful in moving the uterus and permitting better viewing of the adnexa. When a uterine elevator is required, the patient is in the lithotomy position; in other circumstances, the procedure can be performed with the patient supine. The choice of incision site for

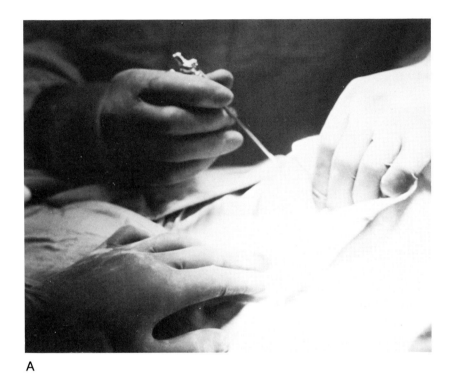

A

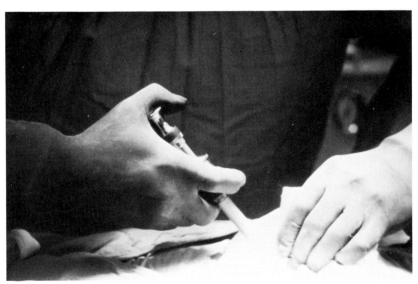

B

Fig. 27-1 Technique of manually elevating the anterior abdominal wall when inserting **(A)** a spring-loaded Veres insufflating needle and **(B)** a laparoscope trocar. By elevating the abdominal wall, all instruments are placed parallel to the spine, aorta, and vena cava.

laparoscopy is dictated by the presence of prior surgical incisions. In a patient who has not undergone previous surgery, an umbilical incision can be performed. A vertical or transverse incision is made either 5 or 10 mm wide to match the diameter of the laparoscope. The incision for laparoscopy can be lateral to the rectus muscle on either the right or left side if a midline scar extends to the umbilicus or if a supraumbilical paramedian incision is present. Careful selection of the incision site is of critical importance to prevent the complication of direct injury to abdominal organs. The spring-loaded Veres needle is placed while lifting the anterior abdominal wall. Repeat laparoscopies can be performed through the same incision site. In patients with prior abdominal surgery, the operative report should describe adhesions and their locations for future reference in performing repeat laparoscopy. The needle is inserted parallel to the spine to avoid damaging the aorta, illiac vessels, or vena cava. The abdominal wall is lifted, and the needle is inserted perpendicular to the fascia (Figs. 27-1 and 27-2). If local anesthesia is used, the patient must tighten her abdominal muscles to create resistance for the placement of the Veres needle and laparoscopic trocar. In extremely obese patients, the Veres needle can be placed transvaginally and a pneumoperitoneum introduced in this manner. The abdomen is usually filled with 1500 to 4000 cc CO_2. The smallest amount of gas that will permit safe placement of the laparoscopic instruments and adequate visualization will facilitate pulmonary gas exchange and diminish the possibility of acidosis. The abdomen contains an appropriate amount of gas for safe introduction of instruments and visualization when respiratory excursions can be identified in the insufflator flowmeter. In cases of prior surgery, increased gas insufflation will separate adhesions and increase the safety of performing the procedure. Thorough evaluation of the abdomen requires a second puncture for a 3- or 5-mm probe for manipulation and palpation. Laparoscopy without a second puncture is an incomplete procedure. At times, additional puncture sites are needed for scissors, graspers, biopsy instruments, aspirators, and cytology brushes. The laparoscopic trocar is inserted in a similar fashion by lifting the anterior abdominal wall. This technique permits trocar placement in a Z-type incision. When the laparoscope and trocar are withdrawn, the incisions made in skin, fascia, and peritoneum are staggered. This minimizes the chances of hernias in laparoscopic incisions.

Laparoscopy in patients with no previous surgery is accepted as a safe procedure when performed by an experienced surgeon under local or general anesthesia. The ability to lyse adhesions, perform biopsies,

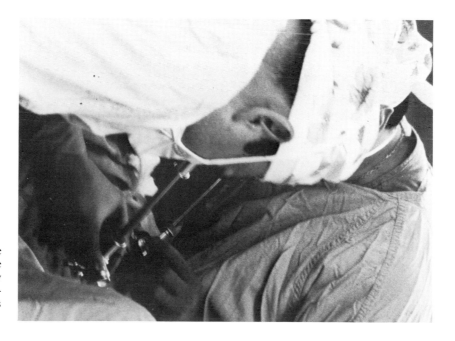

Fig. 27-2 A 5-mm laparoscope is placed in a second puncture incision to view the initial entry site to ensure that a transintestinal laparoscope placement has not occurred.

mobilize abdominal structures, and do cytologic washings requires training and experience in operative endoscopy. To perform an ovarian biospy, the ovary must be stabilized with a grasping instrument requiring a third puncture site. If a biospy is contemplated, bipolar and unipolar cautery should be available for hemostasis. Bleeding should be anticipated prior to biopsy or adhesiolysis, and blood vessels should be cauterized prior to dividing them. Bipolar cautery is safer than unipolar, since there is no risk of sparking or spread of the current and generated heat to adjacent tissues. This minimizes the risk of immediate or delayed tissue destruction.

In patients with prior surgery, the risks of laparoscopy are magnified. Some surgeons consider prior surgery a contraindication to laparoscopy. Most experienced laparoscopists are comfortable operating on people with prior incisions. To introduce a laparoscope in the previously scarred abdomen safely, areas of prior incisions should be avoided. Any infraumbilical area in the abdomen can be used as a site for the introduction of the Veres needle and laparoscope. Preliminary placement of a 14-gauge needlescope can identify adhesion-free sites for the placement of a 5- or 10-mm laparoscope.[3] To identify inadvertent damage to bowel by a transviscus puncture, a 5-mm scope

can be passed through a second puncture site and be used to visualize the initial puncture site (Fig. 27-2). Another method of viewing the initial scope entry site is by visualizing this area at the time the laparoscope sheath is removed, by leaving the scope within the trocar sheath as it is being withdrawn. This technique affords a view of the entry point of the laparoscope trocar in the peritoneum. If any inadvertent damage to bowel occurs, it will be identified and can be repaired. If prior surgery was extensive and the operator is uncomfortable with conventional laparoscopy, open laparoscopy can be used.

Open laparoscopy is the endoscopic method of visualizing the peritoneal cavity through a minilaparotomy incision.[4] Open laparoscopy offers the visual advantages of laparoscopy, including diaphragmatic evaluation with the security of open entry into the abdomen. The laparoscope can be used in any laparotomy for optimal visualization of the diaphragm and upper abdomen. In open laparoscopy, the abdomen is entered under direct vision by a small incision carried through skin, subcutaneous tissue, fascia, and peritoneum.[5] The wedge-shaped open laparoscopy trocar pictured (Figs. 27-3 through 27-7) is fixed into the incision by sutures. Carbon dioxide is then infused to create a pneumoperitoneum. The laparoscope is then

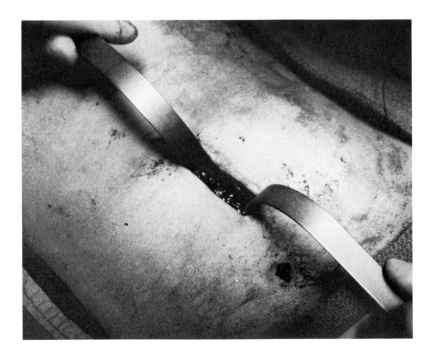

Fig. 27-3 Initial incision for the placement of the open laparoscope trocar sleeve.

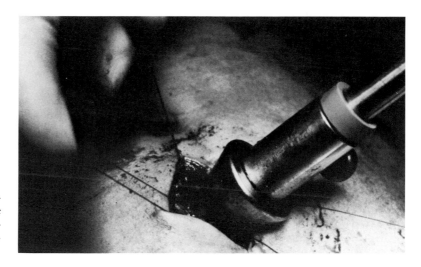

Fig. 27-4 Placement of an open laparoscope trocar sleeve. The wedge shape of the trocar sleeve permits creation and maintenance of a pneumoperitioneum.

inserted in the same manner as in closed laparoscopy. Additional puncture sites are placed as required for biopsy, manipulation, and cytologic sampling in patients who have undergone multiple prior surgical procedures. When we do not distend the abdomen with gas prior to the peritoneal incision, we may increase the risk of intraabdominal injuries. A CO_2 or N_2O pneumoperitoneum serves the function of separating adhesions and providing a large window for trocar placement in the closed technique. Modification of the open technique by prefilling the abdomen with gas prior to peritoneal penetration will increase the safety of this procedure.

The alternative to the total abdominal visualization afforded by the laparoscopic techniques is a large-incision exploratory laparotomy. The views of the dia-

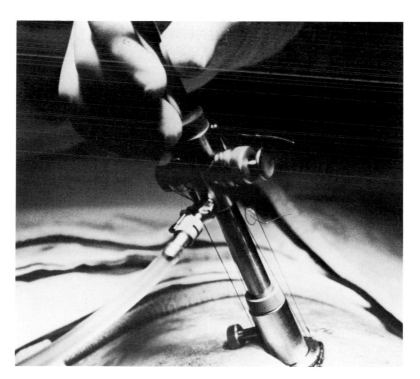

Fig. 27-5 Placement of the laparoscope in the sleeve and trocar of the open laparoscopy technique.

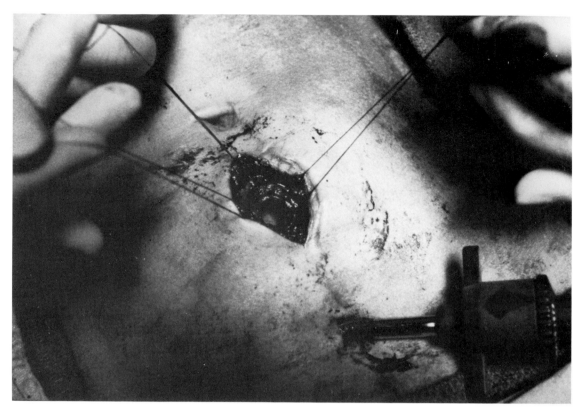

Fig. 27-6 Open laparoscopy incision after withdrawal of the laparoscope, trocar, and sleeve. This type of minilaparotomy incision is closed in layers.

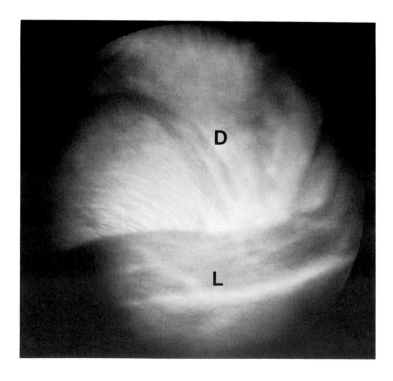

Fig. 27-7 Laparoscopic visualization of the liver (L) and diaphragm (D).

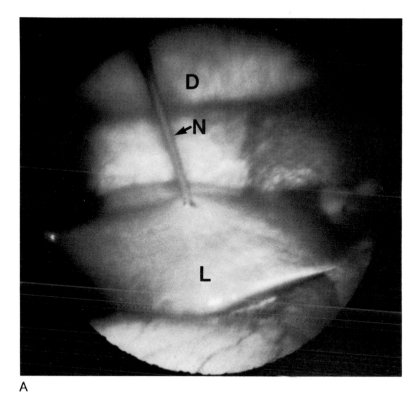

A

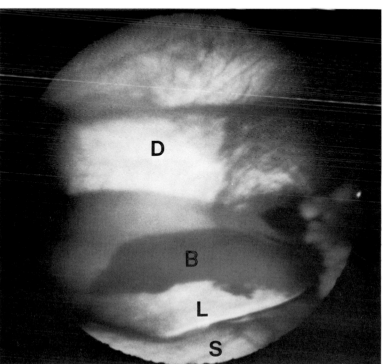

Fig. 27-8 (A, B) Laparoscopic visualizations of a liver biospy with a percutaneous biopsy needle directed to the liver parenchyma by direct vision. N, needle; L, liver; D, diaphragm; S, stomach; B, minimal bleeding at biopsy site.

B

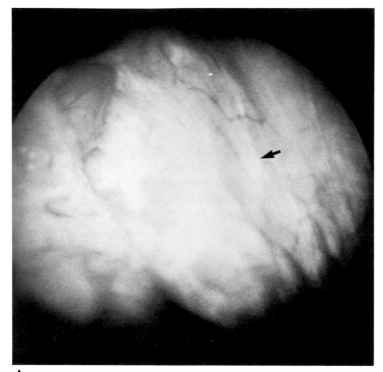

A

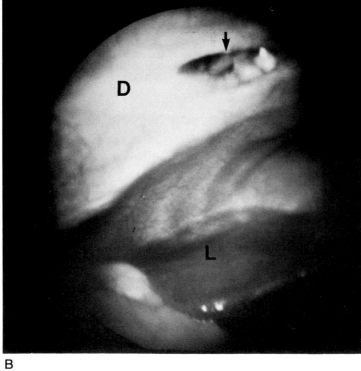

B

Fig. 27-9 (A) Visualization of possible metastatic site (arrow) for directed biopsy in a second-look laparoscopy. **(B)** Arrow shows biopsy site after the biopsy has been taken. D, Diaphragm; L, Liver.

phragm seen through the laparoscope (Fig. 27-7) are more complete than in an exploratory laparotomy.[6] Operative multiincisional laparoscopy can be performed on an ambulatory day-of-admission surgical basis. In all oncologic evaluations, the ability to perform immediate laparotomy to remedy complications or to complete diagnostic studies in laparoscopic negative second-look procedures must be readily available. Bowel preparation should be in place, and the patient should be prepared for the possibility of a formal laparotomy.

The objective of second-look surgical procedures is for diagnostic and therapeutic gain. Second-look laparoscopy may be considered as the initial step in the second-look procedure.[7,8] Laparoscopy has the limitation of not being definitive in the confirmation of a state of no evidence of disease since laparotomy with pelvic and periaortic node sampling is the definitive second-look procedure. Laparoscopy serves the valuable purpose of diagnosing residual disease that is too small for therapeutic debulking procedures and thus saves the patient an unnecessary exploratory laparotomy. The efficacy of laparoscopy may be improved when linked to CT scanning and MRI, which can be used to evaluate nodal enlargement and retroperitoneal structures.

Exploratory laparoscopy when performed as the initial stage of a second-look procedure requires a thorough aggressive approach by a skilled endoscopist. Cytologic washing of the lower and upper abdomen is performed first; 100 ml saline is infused into the lower abdomen by a 5-mm aspirating probe. The saline is then suctioned and studied cytologically and the diaphragm visualized. Then, 100 ml saline is infused in the right and left paracolic gutters and retrieved. Cytologic brushing can be used for cytologic screening, but washing appears to provide a more complete sampling technique. If pelvic adhesions prohibit complete cytologic sampling, the adhesions should be aggressively lysed. Cytologic results should be available prior to second-look laparoscopy. Piver et al.[9] advocated cytologic evaluation from the pelvis and right and left paracolic spaces. A 30-minute cytologic procedure can be performed by preparing the specimen with a cytocentrifuge and staining with a modified shortened technique of the classic Papanicolaou stain. The absence of visible tumor or malignant cells in the cytologic washings indicates the need for a second-look laparotomy while the patient is under a single anesthetic.

In addition to cytology, biopsies should be obtained from any suspicious areas on the liver, diaphragm, bowel or peritoneal surfaces (Figs. 27-8 through 27-10). Frozen sections will confirm persistent malignant disease. In the absence of biopsy-proven disease and cytologic evidence of malignancy, a laparotomy with node sampling should always be performed prior to the cessation of chemotherapy. If cytology is positive or frozen-section biopsy demonstrates persistent malignancy, formal laparotomy should be postponed until chemotherapy has achieved a laparoscopy-negative study. If significant gross disease is found on laparoscopy, debulking laparotomy is an option that must be considered by the oncologist.

The ability to visualize and explore the abdomen by laparoscopy is demonstrated in Figures 27-11 and 27-12. Figure 27-13 demonstrates two examples of the diagnoses of ovarian neoplasms by laparoscopy under local anesthesia. Both patients went on to exploratory laparotomy.

Documentation of laparoscopic findings can be made by articulating a 35-mm single-lens reflex camera to the laparoscope by an adapter. The laparoscopic light source provides adequate lighting when 1000 ASA film is used. A synchronized flash generator will provide superior-quality photographs. Videolaparoscopy is simple to perform by articulating a video camera to the laparoscope. It affords the advantage of a rapid complete method of documenting laparoscopic findings and demonstrates the location of adhesions increasing the safety margin of repeat laparoscopics.

HYSTEROSCOPY

Hysteroscopy is a simple atraumatic method of visualizing the endocervix and endometrial cavity. This nonincisional technique can be performed in an office or operating room setting. When used with colposcopy, it affords visualization of the squamocolumnar junction, when it is within the endocervical canal. Hysteroscopy can define and delineate endocervical involvement in endometrial cancer and permit accurate staging. In combination with aspiration curettage, hysteroscopy affords a definitive diagnostic way to define the etiology of abnormal vaginal bleeding in pre- and postmenopausal women.[10]

Hysteroscopy is performed by determining uterine position and size by a pelvic examination. The cervix

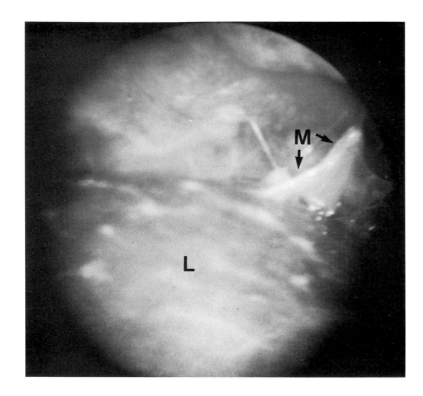

Fig. 27-10 Laparoscopic visualization of mucin (M) over the liver (L) and diaphragm in a pseudomyxoma peritonei recurrence after bilateral salpingooophorectomy.

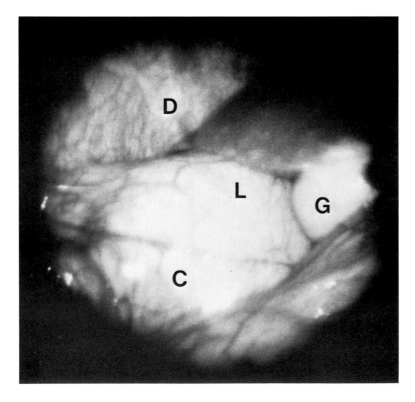

Fig. 27-11 Laparoscopic visualization of the liver (L), gallbladder (G), and a large renal cyst (C). D, diaphragm.

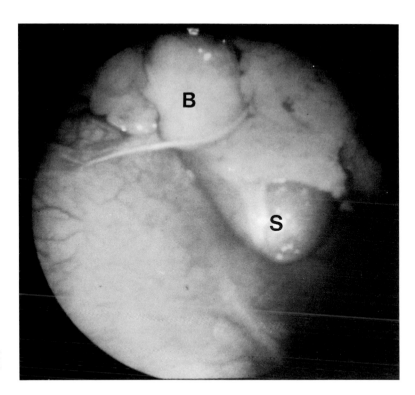

Fig. 27-12 Laparoscopic visualization of the spleen (S). B, loop of small bowel.

is grasped with a tenaculum, and a paracervical block is placed. The uterosacral ligaments are identified and a uterosacral block accomplished by injecting 3 cc of a 1 percent local anesthetic into each uterosacral ligament. The uterosacral block permits distention of the uterine cavity by CO_2, 32 percent dextran 70 (Hyskon Division, Pharmacia, Piscataway, NJ), or saline, with minimal patient discomfort. Adequate separation of the uterine walls to permit visualization of the endometrial lining can be obtained with uterine pressures under 150 mm Hg. If CO_2 is used as the distending medium, gasflow must be less than 100 m/min, and intrauterine pressure must be less than 200 mm Hg to prevent embolization. Saline hysteroscopy requires careful monitoring of the volumes used, to avoid fluid overload. Noncardiogenic pulmonary edema has been reported in hysteroscopy performed with 32 percent dextran 70.[11]

The choice of distending medium is dictated by surgeon's preference and bleeding circumstances. In the presence of uterine bleeding, only hyskon will afford continuous visualization. Operative hysteroscopy requires dextran or saline, since CO_2 causes bubbling and will obscure visualization if bleeding

occurs. Intrauterine YAG laser surgery is performed using saline. Carbon dioxide is simple to use in an office setting and will not clog the hysteroscopic channels, which can occur with dextran. The technique of hysteroscopic placement is simple, but visualization and interpretation of endometrial and endocervical anatomy require significant experience.

The hysteroscopist begins the study by viewing the endocervix and identifying the endocervical canal. The hysteroscope is slowly and carefully advanced under vision while the uterine cavity is being distended by hyskon, saline, or CO_2, which is infused through the hysteroscope. The lateral uterine surface is inspected until the uterine cornua and tubal ostium are visualized. The scope is then directed toward the fundus, and the opposite ostium is identified. This systematic approach affords a careful and complete anatomic evaluation of the uterine cavity. This study permits identification of uterine abnormalities, such as polyps, submucous myomas, scarring, congenital abnormalities, and malignancy. Polyps or small malignancies located at the apex of the uterine cornua may be seen; tubal carcinoma may be identified hysteroscopically if it involves the ostium. In contact

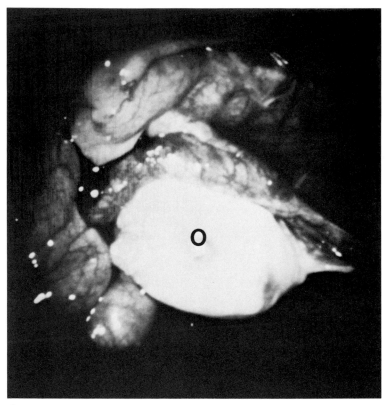

A

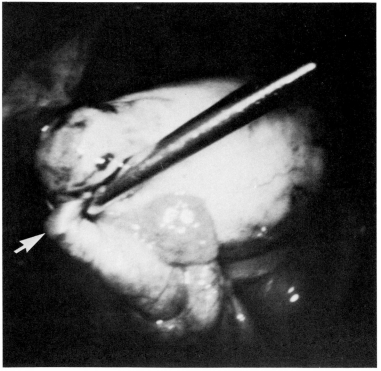

B

Fig. 27-13 (A, B) Laparoscopic visualizations of ovarian thecoma. Arrow indicates twisted infundibulopelvic ligament and fallopian tube. O, ovary.

hysteroscopy, the uterine cavity is not distended as it is in panoramic hysteroscopy. This eliminates the risks associated with distention of the uterine cavity with saline, hyskon, and CO_2, but the diagnostic advantages of panoramic hysteroscopy are lost. Uterine perforation is a rare complication that can be avoided by gentle, careful technique. In the unusual circumstance of uterine perforation, laparotomy is rarely required, as the perforation is under vision by a blunt instrument. The narrow diameter of the hysteroscope rarely evokes significant bleeding.

The Hamou colpomicrohysteroscope has a narrower diameter than the conventional panoramic hysteroscope. This permits its use in the office without anesthesia or analgesia. The magnification capability of the instrument of up to 150X gives it the versatility of being usable as either a panoramic or contact hysteroscope.[12,13] The colpomicrohysteroscope has been used to assess endocervical involvement in endometrial cancer and may prove useful in the clinical staging of endometrial carcinoma.[14,15]

Hysteroscopy has an important role in the differential diagnosis of uterine bleeding. The early evaluation of abnormal uterine bleeding coupled with directed hysteroscopic biopsies affords accurate diagnosis and staging of uterine malignancies. The application of hysteroscopy to oncology is important in the diagnosis, staging, and therapy of uterine cancer.

REFERENCES

1. Keith L, Silver A, Becker M: Anesthesia for laparoscopy. p. 91. In Phillips JM, Keith L (eds): Gynecological Laparoscopy. Symposia Specialists, Miami, 1974

2. Brown DR, Fishburne JI, Robertson VC: Ventilatory and blood gas changes during laparoscopy with local anesthesia. AM J Obstet Gynecol 124:741, 1976

3. Berek JS, Griffiths T, Leventhal JM: Laparoscopy for second look evaluation in ovarian cancer. Obstet Gynecol 58:192, 1981

4. Hasson HM: Open laparoscopy: A report of 150 cases. J Reprod Med 12:234, 1974

5. Hasson HM: Technique of Open Laparoscopy. Year Book Medical Publishers, Chicago, 1979

6. Mangioni C, Bolis G, Molteni P, Belloni C: Indications, Advantages, and limits of laparoscopy on ovarian cancer. Gynecol Oncol 7:53, 1979

7. Rosenoff SH, Young RC, Anderson T et al: Peritoneoscopy in the staging and follow-up of ovarian cancer. Ann Intern Med 83:37, 1975

8. Rosenoff SH, Young RC, Chabnaer B, et al: Use of peritoneoscopy for initial staging and posttherapy evaluation of patients with ovarian carcinoma. p. 81. In Symposium on Ovarian Carcinoma. NCI Monograph 42. 1975

9. Piver MS, Lele SB, Barlow JJ, Gamarra M: Second look laparoscopy prior to proposed second look laparotomy. Obstet Gynecol 55:572, 1980

10. Goldrath MH, Sherman AI: Office hysteroscopy and suction curettage: Can we eliminate the hospital diagnostic dilatation and curretage? Am J Obstet Gynecol 152:220, 1985

11. Zbelle EA, Moise J, Carson S: Noncardiogenic pulmonary edema secondary to intrauterine instillation of 32% dextran 70. Fertil Steril 43:479, 1985

12. Corson SL, Brooks PG: Experience with the Hamou colpomicrohysteroscope. J Reprod Med 10:654, 1983

13. Hamou JE: Microhysteroscopy. Obstet Gynecol 2:285, 1983

14. Savino L, Scarselli G, Branconi F, et al: Usefulness of hysteroscopy in endometrial adenocarcinoma staging. Eur J Gynaecol Oncol 3:210, 1982

15. Goldberg GL, Altaras MM, Levin W, Bloch B: Microhysteroscopy in evaluation of the endocervix in endometrial carcinoma. Gynecol Oncol 2:189, 1986

28

Staging Laparotomy and Lymphadenectomy in Gynecologic Cancer

Hervy E. Averette
Daniel M. Donato
John L. Lovecchio
Bernd-Uwe Sevin

Neoplasms of the genital tract have been routinely staged by clinical means, with the exception of ovarian carcinoma, in which a surgical-pathologic analysis is used to determine the extent of disease. In general, clinical staging facilitates comparative analysis of data between institutions but inherently lacks the ability to delineate disease extent precisely. As can be seen in Table 28-1, a substantial disparity between clinical and surgical disease extent has been consistently demonstrated in the literature.

Surgical staging is an attractive alternative to clinical staging in the planning of therapy for gynecologic tumors for the following reasons:

1. It is more accurate than clinical staging and provides precise histologic documentation of disease extent.
2. It permits individualization of therapy on the basis of specific patterns of disease spread.

Various diagnostic modalities have been employed as alternatives to surgical exploration, such as computed tomography (CT), lymphangiography, hysteroscopy, laparoscopy, and culdoscopy. However, all are limited in their ability to delineate disease extent and cannot compare with the accuracy of surgical staging.

Despite the appeal of surgical staging, we are obliged to demonstrate a distinct survival advantage to patients who undergo surgical staging and subsequent tailored therapy. It is also important to prove that the combined morbidity and mortality of surgical exploration and definitive therapy do not outweigh the benefits accrued by the precise definition of disease.

TECHNIQUE OF LYMPHADENECTOMY

The abdomen is generally opened through a longitudinal midline incision and carried approximately 5 cm above and to the left of the umbilicus. The in-

Table 28-1 Differences Between Clinical and Surgical Staging of Gynecologic Malignancies

Investigators	Site	% Difference
Way and Benedet (1973)[1]	Vulva	40
Homesley et al. (1986)[2]	Vulva	50
Knapp and Friedman (1974)[3]	Ovary	19
Piver et al. (1978)[4]	Ovary	28
Averette et al. (1985)[5]	Cervix	38
LaPolla et al. (1986)[6]	Cervix	42
Cowles et al. (1985)[7]	Endometrium	52
Morrow (1986)[8]	Endometrium	20

testines are packed into the upper abdomen in the usual fashion to expose the base of the mesentery. The right ureter is identified as it crosses the right common iliac artery, and the peritoneum medial to the ureter is gently elevated and incised with Metzenbaum scissors to expose the retroperitoneal space (Fig. 28-1). The incision is carried cephalad over the common iliac artery and descending aorta up to the crossing of the third portion of the duodenum. Care is

taken to identify the ureter and ovarian vessels throughout their course in the abdomen and pelvis, and these structures are retracted laterally with a Deaver retractor to expose the aorta and inferior vena cava. Once the posterior parietal peritoneum has been retracted, the right periaortic lymphatics are identified in the fat pad that lies adjacent to the aorta and superior to the vena cava.

The dissection is begun over the aorta, and a pedicle

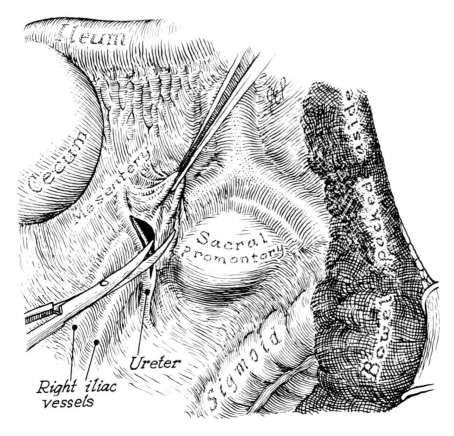

Fig. 28-1 Entering the retroperitoneum.

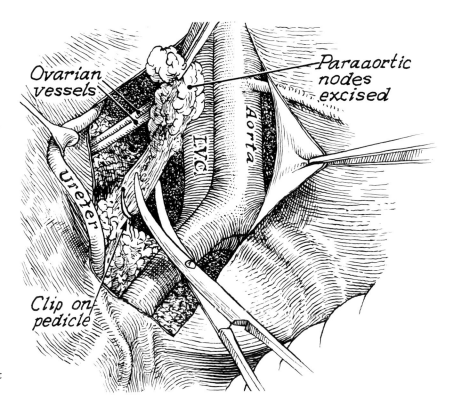

Fig. 28-2 Excision of the right periaortic nodes.

is formed by liberating the nodal group from the aorta medially, the vena cava inferiorly, and the psoas laterally. The pedicle, now free from the major vessels, is demarcated caudally with a hemoclip, and the nodal pedical is reflected cranially using hemoclips for hemostasis when necessary (Fig. 28-2). At all times, the surgeon must be cognizant of the ureter and ovarian vessels and must ensure that they are retracted laterally from the area of dissection. Once the third portion of the duodenum is reached, a hemoclip is applied cranially, and the nodal group is removed and sent for frozen-section evaluation.

Attention is then turned to the left periaortic area, which can be exposed through the same incision by reflection of the mesosigmoid laterally. The ureter and ovarian vessels are indentified once again and retracted out of the field of dissection. The inferior mesenteric artery is also palpated in the mesosigmoid and traced to its origin at the aorta, approximately 10 cm above the bifurcation. Continuing awareness of these structures is mandatory for performance of the left periaortic lymphadenectomy. The nodal group adjacent to the left common iliac artery is incised medially, and a pedicle is delineated caudally with a hemoclip. The periaortic and retroaortic nodes are swept cephalad with hemoclips up to and, if necessary, above the orgin of the inferior mesenteric artery (Fig. 28-3). A vein retractor assists in retracting the aorta, so that the retroaortic nodes can be seen and removed. These nodes are once again submitted for frozen-section evaluation.

If the periaortic nodes are tumor free on frozen section, and a pelvic lymphadenectomy is to be performed in conjunction with radical hysterectomy (early-stage cervical carcinoma or stage II endometrial carcinoma), attention is directed at exposing the paravesical and pararectal spaces. The anterior leaf of the broad ligament is opened just inferior to the round ligament to expose the paravesical space (Fig. 28-4). This avascular space is easily developed by sharp dissection posteriorly until the levator floor is reached. If one dissects too medially, injury to bladder or uterine vessels may occur, while too lateral a dissection may cause injury to the iliac vessels.

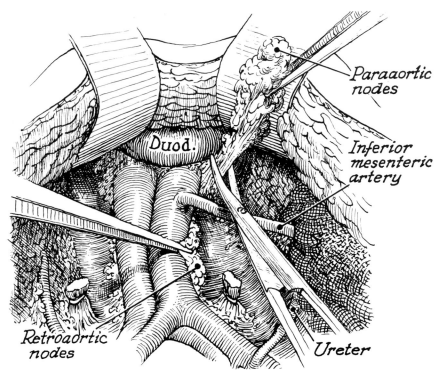

Fig. 28-3 Excision of left peri-aortic nodes above and below the inferior mesenteric vessels.

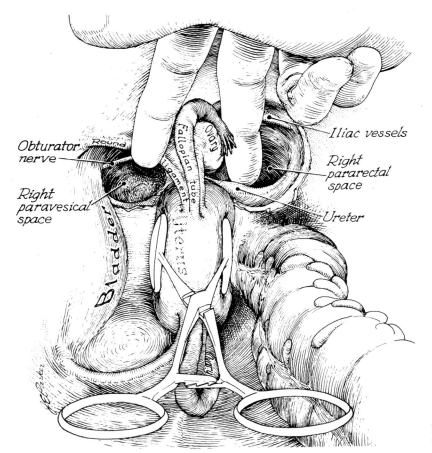

Fig. 28-4 Entering the para-vesical and pararectal spaces.

In a similar fashion, the pararectal space is entered by incising the posterior leaf of the broad ligament on the medial aspect of the uterosacral ligament. It is important to identify the path of the ureter in the pelvis and to retract it medially so that the avascular pararectal space may be visualized, inspected, and palpated.

When both paravesical and pararectal spaces have been opened, the cardinal ligament may be palpated by placing the index finger and middle finger into the paravesical and pararectal spaces, respectively, to evaluate for tumor extension. Once the spaces have been opened, any induration or suggestion of tumor extension may be studied by biopsy with an instrument such as Kervokian biospy forceps or by fine-needle aspiration of suspicious areas (Fig. 28-5).

After the parametrial areas have been explored, the pelvic lymphadenectomy may be accomplished in the usual fashion, submitting separate common iliac, hypogastric, external iliac, and obturator nodes for permanent section.

Ovary

The predilection for intraabdominal surface implantation as well as retroperitoneal lymphatic metastasis mandates that ovarian neoplasms be staged surgically. The lymphatic drainage of the ovary passes through collecting trunks in the broad ligament and coalesces in the infundibular pelvic ligament. From here the lymphatics enter the periaortic area between the bifurication of the aorta and the renal vessels. In view of this anatomic lymphatic network, it is not surprising that even "early-stage" ovarian cancers may have periaortic node involvement. The incidence of retroperitoneal node involvement by ovarian carcinoma can be found in Table 28-2. In fact, several sites of frequent subclinical involvement warrant close inspection and histologic sampling[9-13] (Table 28-3). Positive findings in any of these sites will upstage patients and alter subsequent therapeutic interventions.

Clearly, extensive surgical staging is an integral

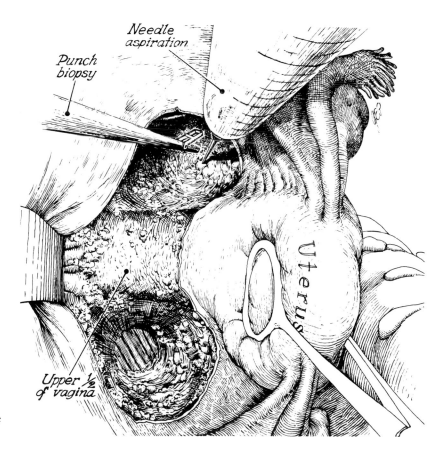

Fig. 28-5 Examination of the parametrium.

Table 28-2 Ovarian Cancer: Retroperitoneal Node Involvement for Each Stage

Stage	Positive Periaortic Nodes (%)	Positive Pelvic Nodes (%)
I	18	9
II	20	10
III	42	13
IV	67	33

(Data from Chen SS, Lee L: Incidence of positive periaortic and pelvic nodes in epithelial cancers of the ovary. Gynecol Oncol 16:95, 1983.)

part of the initial management of patients with ovarian malignancies, especially those with otherwise early-stage disease whose subsequent therapy will greatly depend on surgical extent of disease.

The importance of initial debulking for advanced disease (stage III/IV) has been consistently demonstrated in the literature.[13-18] Optimal cytoreduction is defined as a maximum debulking effort resulting in residual disease less than 1 to 2 cm in greatest diameter. Patients undergoing optimal initial cytoreduction have been shown to have a prolonged survival and augmented disease-free interval.[13,17,18] Based on the above findings, the FIGO committee on staging has proposed that patients with advanced disease be stratified into three subgroups based on residual disease remaining after initial maximal debulking effort.

The precise role of a surgical reassessment procedure (second-look) for ovarian cancer is still unclear. This procedure would have the following advantages:

Table 28-3 Ovarian Carcinoma: Sites of Subclinical Metastasis in Stage I and II Disease

Site of Involvement	Stage I (%)	Stage II (%)
Diaphragm	11	23
Periaortic nodes	12	10
Washings	31	12
Omentum	3	0

(Data from Piver MS: Ovarian malignancies: The clinical care of adults and adolescents. p. 74. In Current Reviews in Obstetrics and Gynecology. Vol. 4. Churchill Livingstone, New York, 1983.)

to restage patients not properly staged initially, to evaluate effects of chemotherapy and decide on further therapy, to evaluate patients who are clinically free of disease after chemotherapy, to define an end point of therapy, and to attempt a second debulking when initial debulking was not feasible. Multiple studies have demonstrated that the extent of residual disease after initial surgery was the most important predictor of findings at second laparotomy.[18-22] In a study by Piver et al.,[21] 95 percent of the patients who were optimally debulked initially had negative second look procedures after chemotherapy, whereas only 20 percent of patients who were suboptimally debulked had a negative secondary assessment.

The importance of an extensive exploration and lymphadenectomy after chemotherapy was demonstrated in a recent study.[22] It was found that 38 percent of patients who had no clinical evidence of disease after chemotherapy had negative findings at exploratory laparotomy. However, 14 percent of patients were found to have microscopic disease, and of these, most had pelvic and/or paraaortic lymph node involvement as the only site of persistance.

The role of secondary debulking at exploratory laparotomy is still unclear, although Berek et al.[23] demonstrated that in the small subset of patients who could be debulked, a significant improvement in median survival could be obtained. As secondary debulking in ovarian malignancy is not a universally accepted management practice, many investigators have attempted to use less invasive means to prove disease-persistence, such as CT scan, laparoscopy, culdoscopy, peritoneal lavage, and monitoring the CA 125 antigen.[21,22,24] These studies can be helpful when positive, however, when negative, a significant number of patients will be found to have disease persistence at laparotomy.[20,21,24,25]

Recently, a tumor marker (CA 125) has been isolated from more than 80 percent of patients with epithelial ovarian malignancies.[26] This marker has since been used to follow the clinical course of patients with ovarian malignancies undergoing therapy for their disease, and levels of this tumor marker seem to correlate with disease regression/progression in 93 percent of cases.[27] A recent study was performed correlating CA 125 levels just prior to secondary exploratory laparotomy with pathologic results found at surgery. Forty-three percent of patients with normal CA 125 levels prior to second-look procedures were found to have persistent disease, while all patients with a negative second look had normal CA 125 levels. The authors concluded that patients with normal CA 125 levels cannot be assumed to be disease free and should have further investigations to determine true disease status. Patients with elevated CA 125 levels almost assuredly have residual disease, especially if levels were previously normal.[25]

If the above methods fail to demonstrate disease, laparotomy must be performed before the patient can be declared disease free. An adequate second-look procedure requires a generous midline incision and, in the absence of ascites, cell washings are taken as usual. All peritoneal surfaces should be inspected and selective biopsies performed of the hemidiaphragm, both colonic gutters and pelvic peritoneum. Selective pelvic and pariaortic biopsies are performed as well. If not previously removed, the uterus, tubes and ovaries with the residual infracolic omentum are removed for pathologic analysis. Only when all the above biopsies and cell washings are negative is the patient declared free of disease.[21,22,24,28,29]

Despite negative surgical/pathologic findings after chemotherapy, 20 to 50 percent of patients will have recurrence of their disease.[22-24] Obviously the recurrence rate will depend on the adequacy of secondary exploration, and recurrences after a negative exploratory laparotomy performed adequately are probably lower than previously stated.[22] Because of the above recurrence rate, adjunctive modalities of therapy such as whole abdominal radiotherapy and chemotherapy have been employed. The success of these adjunctive measures has, in general, been limited.[30,31] Therefore, the precise role of adjunctive therapy in these patients needs further clarification.

The following conclusions can be drawn from the above data with respect to the surgical evaluation and treatment of patients with ovarian carcinoma. In patients with early stage (I to II) ovarian cancer, a meticulous pretherapy staging laparotomy, including omentectomy, pelvic and pariaortic lymphadenectomy, and multiple peritoneal and diaphragmatic biopsies, is performed. In young patients in whom conservative therapy is considered, removal of the involved adnexae is performed. In patients in whom child bearing is not being considered, a total abdominal hysterectomy/bilateral salpingo-oophorectomy is performed in addition to the above surgical staging. Further therapy is instituted on the basis of surgical/

pathologic findings. For patients with stage III to IV disease, optimal cytoreduction has been conclusively demonstrated to enhance survival. Total abdominal hysterectomy/bilateral salpingo-oophorectomy with the possible addition of radical peritoneal resection, small and/or large bowel resection is performed to reduce tumor bulk to less than 1 to 2 cm in maximum diameter.

After completion of chemotherapy, some evaluation of disease status is currently recommended to decide on the further management of patients who do not show gross evidence of disease persistance. Several diagnostic studies are available including the use of the CA 125 tumor marker, CT scan, or laparoscopy. However, when negative, one must proceed to a surgical reassessment procedure in order to histologically define disease status, as the above studies all have a significant false-negative rate.

The precise role of secondary tumor debulking in patients found to have persistent disease after chemotherapy is still not well defined. It is possible that secondary debulking may enhance survival in those patients who can be optimally cytoreduced after chemotherapy. However, further investigations are needed before conclusive statements can be made.

Patients who are shown to be disease free at surgical re-exploration may benefit from adjunctive therapy. However, the need for and the best modality of therapy for these patients is unclear.

ENDOMETRIUM

Although endometrial adenocarcinoma is currently staged clinically, several parameters that can only be reliably determined by surgical/histopathologic means have been demonstrated to influence patient survival (Table 28-4).

Unfortunately, the initial findings on examination and dilation and curettage (D & C) are often changed by definitive surgical/histopathologic examination. For example, while tumor differentiation has been known to influence overall survival for sometime,[32-34] it has repeatedly been demonstrated that both histologic type and grade were often changed after surgical/pathologic staging.[7,35,36]

Cervical involvement by endometrial cancer has generally been thought to confer a less favorable prognosis, however, multiple studies have demon-

Table 28-4 Prognostic Factors in Endometrial Cancer

Tumor grade/histology
Depth of myometrial penetration
Lymphovascular space involvement
Pathologic involvement of cervix/adnexae
Peritoneal cytology
Node status

(Data from Morrow CP: Tumors of the endometrium. p. 159. In Synopsis of Gynecologic Oncology. 3rd Ed. 1983.)

strated the inaccuracies of curettage in detecting endocervical involvement.[7,8,37] In Cowles's study, when the endocervical curettings were positive and the cervix was normal to palpation, 50 percent of patients were found not to have pathologic involvement of the cervix on final histology.[7] In addition, it seems that patients with gross cervical involvement have a worse prognosis than do those with only microscopic involvement (60 percent versus 75 percent 5-year survival).[8] Hysteroscopy has been used by some to attempt to improve the accuracy of endocervical curettage but this procedure does have the potential ability to disseminate tumor cells into the peritoneal cavity and vascular spaces.[8]

Obviously, the depth of myometrial penetration cannot be diagnosed by clinical means, and this has been found to be a significant predictor of lymphatic metastasis and overall survival.[37,38] Also, lymphatic and vascular space involvement by tumor seems to be an important risk factor for metastatic spread of this tumor.[37,39,40] Once again, this prognostic factor can only be determined at final pathological interpretation.

The significance of positive peritoneal washings in patients with early stage endometrial cancer remains controversial since first reported by Creasman and Rutledge.[41] While DiSaia and Creasman[42] reported a higher recurrence rate in stage I patients with positive washings, Yazigi et al.[43] found no significant difference in survival for patients with stage I disease, regardless of peritoneal cytologic findings.

Retroperitoneal nodal metastases have been documented even in early endometrial carcinoma, especially those with increasing grade or depth of myometrial invasion.[8,37,38,44] Table 28-5 demonstrates the incidence of positive nodes in stage I endometrial

Table 28-5 Endometrial Cancer: Node Metastasis by Maximum Invasion and Grade in FIGO Stage I Lesions

Depth	G_1 (%)	G_2 (%)	G_3 (%)
Pelvic node involvement			
Endometrium	1.7	3.7	0.0
Superficial	0.0	2.5	23.1
Intermediate	0.0	25.0	20.0
Deep	25.0	46.2	43.7
Periaortic node involvement			
Endometrium	2.1	0.0	0.0
Superficial	0.0	0.0	45.5
Intermediate	0.0	25.0	0.0
Deep	0.0	55.5	35.7

(Data from Boronow RC, Morrow CP, Creasman WT, et al: Surgical staging in endometrial cancer: Clinical-pathologic findings of a prospective study. Obstet Gynecol 63:825, 1984.)

cancer as found in the collaborative GOG study involving 222 patients.[37]

With the above-noted inaccuracies in clinical staging, multiple studies have compared clinical and surgical/pathologic staging for uterine cancer. Extrauterine spread has been documented in 18 to 20 percent of patients with stage I disease.[37,45–47] In Cowles's study, inaccurate clinical staging occurred in 52 percent of patients with stage I disease, 62 percent with stage II disease, and 60 percent of patients with stage III disease.[7]

Recent analysis by Morrow[8] demonstrated that isolated metastasis from endometrial cancer may influence recurrence rates (Table 28-6). When two or

Table 28-6 Two-Year Recurrence Rate of Endometrial Cancer for Isolated Metastasis

Site	Recurrence Rate (at 2 years) (%)
Aortic nodes	30
Lymph/vascular space	22
Adnexae	18
Cytology	14
Pelvic nodes	4

(Data from Morrow CP: Tumors of the endometrium. p. 159. In Synopsis of Gynecologic Oncology. 3rd Ed. 1983.)

more sites were involved, nearly 50 percent of cases recurred at 2-year follow-up. Based on the above data, an approach to patients with stage I endometrial cancer or patients with positive endocervical curettage in the absence of gross cervical involvement would include initial surgical staging, including cell washings, palpation of pelvic and paraaortic nodal areas, and simple extrafascial hysterectomy with bilateral salpingo oophorectomy. The uterus is bivalved intraoperatively and inspected for gross myometrial invasion or endocervical involvement. Selective pelvic and periaortic lymphadenectomy is performed if a serous, clear cell, or adenosquamous carcinoma cell type is present; if a grade 2 or 3 lesion is found; if a suspicion of at least 50 percent myometrial invasion exists; or if gross extension to cervix or adnexae is noted.

For patients who are found to be at risk of pelvic recurrence based on deep myometrial invasion, extension to the cervix or adnexae, and/or positive pelvic nodes, postoperative pelvic radiotherapy is employed. Patients without the above risk factors are not treated with additional pelvic radiotherapy, thus sparing the needless complications of this modality.

When gross cervical involvement is present in patients who are good operative candidates, a radical hysterectomy is performed. If all nodes and margins are free, no further therapy is used. In patients who are not good surgical candidates, preoperative radiotherapy is given followed with simple extrafascial hysterectomy and bilateral salpingo-oophorectomy.

In patients found to have positive periaortic nodes, a scalene node biopsy should be performed, as a positive scalene biopsy would contraindicate extended field radiation therapy. When scalene nodes are negative, and in the absence of other metastasis, extended field radiation therapy to the periaortic area is recommended. A 45 percent survival rate has recently been reported in this subset of patients.[48]

VAGINA/VULVA

As primary carcinomas of the vagina are rare, little has been written on surgical staging of these lesions. Also, the majority of these lesions are treated with primary radiotherapy, and the precise extent of disease is not usually established. An exception occurs with clear cell adenocarcinoma of the vagina, which

Table 28-7 FIGO Staging of Squamous Cell Carcinoma of the Vulva

Stage	TNM Status	Description
I	T1 N0 M0 T1 N1 M0	All lesions confined to vulva, with maximal diameter of 2 cm or less and no suspicious groin nodes
II	T2 N0 M0 T2 N1 M0	All lesions confined to vulva, with diameter greater than 2 cm and no suspicious groin nodes
III	T3 N0 M0 T3 N1 M0	Lesions extending beyond vulva but without grossly positive groin nodes
	T3 N2 M0 T1 N2 M0 T2 N2 M0	Lesions of any size confined to vulva, with suspicious groin nodes
IV	T3 N3 M0 T4 N3 M0	Lesions extending beyond vulva, with grossly positive nodes
	T4 N3 M0 T4 N0 M0 T4 N2 M0 T1 N3 M0 T2 N3 M0	Lesions involving mucosa of rectum, bladder, or urethra or involving bone
	M1A M1B	All cases with distant or palpable deep pelvic metastases

is commonly treated by surgical extirpation and lymphadenectomy. Further therapy may be instituted based on pathological disease extent. The approximate incidence of lymph node metastasis with adenocarcinoma of the vagina is 18 percent for stage I lesions and 30 percent for stage II lesions.[49]

The staging of squamous cell carcinoma of the vulva is based on the TNM system, which can be found in Table 28-7. Multiple studies have emphasized the importance of groin node metastasis in overall survival in patients with squamous cell carcinoma of the vulva.[2,50-52] The incidence of histologically positive groin nodes in relation to clinical stage can be seen in Table 28-8. Unfortunately, the clinical assessment of groin node status is unreliable in 25 to 50 percent of cases.[2,50,51] For example, a recent GOG collaborative study demonstrated that 49 percent of patients with clinical N0/N1 groin nodes were found to harbor metastasis.[2]

As the status of the groin nodes seems to be the single best predictor of survival, it would appear that

Table 28-8 Vulvar Cancer: Incidence of Positive Groin Nodes for Each FIGO Stage

FIGO Stage	No. of Patients	Positive Groin Nodes (%)
I	121	7
II	150	29
III	128	48
IV	26	58

(Data from Homesley HD: Carcinoma of the vulva. p. 98. In Conn HF (ed): Conn's Current Therapy. WB Saunders, Philadelphia, 1985.)

Table 28-9 Two-year Survival of Patients Based on Involved Groin Nodes

No. of Positive Nodes	No. of Patients	2-year Survival (%)
<1	42	80
2–3	44	66
≥4	27	27

(Data from Homesley HD, Bundy BN, Sedlis A, Adcock L: Radiation therapy versus pelvic node resection for patients with invasive squamous cell carcinoma of the vulva having positive groin nodes. Obstet Gynecol 68:732, 1986.)

the precise definition of node involvement by surgical/pathologic means would allow subsequent therapy to be directed appropriately and lead to an enhanced survival.

The GOG collaborative study randomized 114 patients with positive groin nodes to receive either pelvic node dissection or postoperative external groin and pelvic radiotherapy following radical vulvectomy and bilateral groin node dissection. Of 104 evaluable patients, the 2-year survival for the radiotherapy group was significantly improved (68 percent versus 50 percent). The progression-free interval for the radiotherapy group was also enhanced (68 percent versus 54 percent). The survival advantage was most significant for those patients with N2/N3 nodes or two or more histologically proven positive groin nodes. The relationship between survival and number of involved groin nodes can be found in Table 28-9. No significant morbidity was found when either of the above modalities were combined with radical vulvectomy and groin node dissection.[2]

Approximately 25 percent of patients with positive groin nodes will have positive ipsilateral pelvic nodes, and rarely are positive pelvic nodes found in the absence of involved groin nodes.[2,50,51] The survival of patients with positive pelvic nodes in most series is less than 25 percent.[2,50,51] It does not seem prudent to recommend the addition of pelvic node dissection to radical vulvectomy and bilateral groin dissection in patients with positive groin nodes, as adjunctive radiation therapy seems to be the best modality at this time.

Recent literature has focused on more conservative approaches to patients with superficially invasive (microinvasive) carcinoma of the vulva.[51-55] The major impetus for these studies was based on the significant morbidity (short- and long-term) with radical

vulvectomy and bilateral groin dissection. Unfortunately, no clear definition of microinvasive carcinoma of the vulva has been uniformly established. Controversy still exists as to the allowable depth of invasion, the point at which measurement of invasion is measured (e.g., basement membrane, surface epithelium), the maximum diameter of the primary lesion; the importance of lymphovascular space involvement, the importance of confluence, and the degree of tumor differentiation.

Recent studies indicate that unifocal lesions 2 cm or less in overall diameter with up to 1-mm stromal penetration (from basement membrane) are associated with a very low incidence of lymph node metastasis, whereas those lesions with up to 5-mm invasion may demonstrate lymph node metastasis in up to 34 percent of cases.[2,50,54,56-58] Table 28-10 demonstrates the relationship between depth of stromal penetration and incidence of groin node involvement for early-stage vulvar carcinoma.

Based on the above data, patients with small (up to

Table 28-10 Vulvar Cancer: Incidence of Positive Groin Nodes and Depth of Stromal Invasion

Depth (mm)	No. of Patients	Positive Groin Nodes (%)
1	19	0
2	47	9
3	50	16
4	49	22
5	41	34
>5	195	43

(Data from Homesley HD; Carcinoma of the vulva. p. 98. In Conn HF (ed): Conn's Current Therapy. WB Saunders, Philadelphia, 1985.)

2-cm) unifocal lesions that have up to 1-mm stromal invasion probably only require a wide excision with 2- to 3-cm margins. When an otherwise early vulvar carcinoma is found to have at least 1-mm but up to 5-mm stromal penetration, an evaluation of the ipsilateral inguinal nodes is required prior to conservative management. DiSaia's approach to patients with tumors up to 1 cm in diameter and up to 5-mm stromal invasion involves initial superficial lymphadenectomy. If, on frozen section, all nodes are negative, a wide excision with a 3-cm margin is performed. Eighteen patients have been studied with follow-up for up to 78 months without recurrence.[55] However, it is still unclear whether orderly lymphatic involvement of the sentinel groin nodes occurs in a reliable pattern (initial superficial involvement followed by deep nodal involvement). Until this controversy is resolved, we currently recommend en-bloc ipsilateral superficial and deep inguinal lymphadenectomy with wide excision of the primary lesion. If groin nodes are negative, no further therapy is indicated. If groin nodes are positive or multifocal areas of invasion are demonstrated, radical vulvectomy and contralateral groin node dissection is performed and subsequent therapy given based on final pathologic interpretation.

While local excision of small superficially invasive vulvar carcinoma appears to be a more desirable approach, one must be aware that multifocal sites of invasive carcinoma can occur on the vulva. For example, in a pathologic study of vulvectomy specimens by Gosling et al.,[59] 26 percent of specimens contained multifocal sites of invasion.

Vulvar melanomas are currently staged by the Clark or Breslow system employed for other skin melanomas. These staging techniques more closely

Table 28-11 Survival Based on Clark's Staging System for Malignant Melanoma of Vulva

Clark's Level	No. of Patients	10-Year Survival (%)
II	6	100
III	7	83
IV	11	65
V	23	23

(Data from Podratz KC, Gaffey TA, Symmonds RE, et al: Melanoma of the vulva: An update. Gynecol Oncol 16:153, 1983.)

Table 28-12 Survival Based on Breslow's Staging System for Malignant Melanoma of Vulva

Depth of Stromal Penetration (mm)	No. of Patients	Died of Disease (%)
<0.76	6	0
0.76–1.49	2	0
1.50–4.0	3	66
>4.0	4	75

(Data from Jaramillo BA, Ganjei P, Sevin BU, et al: Malignant melanoma of the vulva. Obstet Gynecol 66:398, 1985.

predict survival than the FIGO system used for squamous cell carcinoma of the vulva. Both systems are based on degree of stromal invasion. Clark's system describes depth of penetration relative to specific subepidermal layers, whereas Breslow utilizes a numerical value of disease extent, measured from the surface epithelium to the deepest tumor penetration in millimeters.

The survival of patients with vulvar melanoma based on the above staging strata is exemplified by the two studies quoted in Tables 28-11 and 28-12. In Jaramillo's series, 25 percent of patients were found to have positive groin nodes.[61] No patient in this report was found to have positive pelvic nodes. All patients with positive groin nodes had greater than 1.7-mm stromal invasion and all died of their disease. The overall 5-year survival in this series was 40 percent. The authors therefore did not recommend routine pelvic lymphadenectomy in patients with vulvar melanoma and suggested that patients with up to 0.76-mm stromal invasion could be managed with wide excision only.

In summary, with the exception of vulvar melanomas, a clinical staging system is employed for vulvovaginal neoplasms despite the inherent inaccuracies of the clinical evaluation of groin node involvement. Adjuvant radiation therapy based on surgical/pathologic involvement of groin nodes seems to improve survival in patients undergoing radical vulvectomy and bilateral groin dissection without increasing the morbidity. At this time, routine pelvic node dissection cannot be recommended for most patients with vulvar cancer (carcinoma or melanoma).

On the basis of currently available information, recommended therapy for patients with vulvar carcinoma can be stratified as follows:

1. For unilateral lesions up to 2 cm in diameter where less than 1-mm stromal invasion is noted, a wide excision into the deep subcutaneous tissue with 2- to 3-cm skin margins is performed. If final pathologic interpretation confirms the initial findings, no further therapy is indicated and close follow-up is instituted.

2. When early lesions are found to have at least 1-mm but less than 5-mm stromal invasion, we recommend wide excision (as above) combined with en bloc superficial and deep ipsilateral groin node dissection performed through a separate groin incision. If the groin nodes are not involved with metastasis and less than 5-mm invasion is confirmed microscopically, no further therapy is indicated. For patients found to have positive groin nodes, multicentric sites of invasion, or greater than 5-mm invasion on final histopathology, a radical vulvectomy with contralateral groin node dissection is performed. Subsequent therapy is then instituted based on final pathological findings.

3. For patients with greater than 5-mm invasion or multifocal invasion, a standard radical vulvectomy with en bloc bilateral groin node dissection is performed. When positive groin nodes are noted, groin and pelvic radiotherapy is employed. This form of adjunctive therapy seems to be superior to pelvic node dissection in the management of those patients with positive groin nodes.

4. For patients with vulvar melanoma, if up to 0.76 mm of stromal invasion is found, a wide local excision is probably all the therapy necessary; however, if 0.76-mm invasion or more is found, the procedure of choice would be a standard radical vulvectomy with bilateral groin node dissection. Routine pelvic lymphadenectomy does not seem to be indicated in the treatment of vulvar melanomas.

CERVIX

Cervical cancer is by international agreement staged by clinical criteria. Meigs[62] in 1954 documented the shortcomings of clinical staging in defining the true extent of cervical cancer and proposed a surgical/pathologic classification. Previously, Brunschwig and Pierce[63] and Henriksen[64,65] described the ultimate routes of metastases in cervical cancer utilizing autopsy material.

Subsequent to the above investigations, which primarily involved the evaluation of the pelvic spread of cervical carcinoma, renewed interest developed in the precise delineation of disease extent by exploratory laparotomy. Nelson[66] was the first to suggest routine surgical staging for the treatment planning of patients with advanced stage cervical carcinoma. During this time, Buchsbaum[67] and Uemakli and Bonney[68] reported discrepancies between surgical and clinical staging, and documented the frequent involvement of the periaortic lymphatics with metastatic disease. Many studies have reconfirmed the inadequacies of clinical staging in patients with cervical carcinoma.[5,6,67–77]

Of central importance, however, is not merely to demonstrate the inaccuracies of clinical staging, but to show that precise definition of disease extent will ultimately lead to alternatives in subsequent therapy and improved survival. In theory, pretreatment laparotomy can therefore be utilized to:

1. Identify extrapelvic sites of metastasis (retroperitoneal nodes, intraabdominal disease).

2. Remove inflamed adnexae or fibroids that may interfere with subsequent radiotherapy.

3. Downstage patients and allow more appropriate therapy to be instituted (radical hysterectomy, change in dosimetry planning).

Table 28-13 Cervical Cancer: Incidence of Positive Periaortic Nodes for Each Clinical Stage

Stage	No. of Patients	Positive Periaortic Nodes	
		%	N
IB	202	5.9	12
IIA	18	5.6	1
IIB	32	18.0	9
IIIA	3	0.0	0
IIIB	25	28.0	9
IVA	2	100.0	2

(Data from Averette HE, Sevin BU, Bell J, et al: Surgical staging of cervical cancer. p. 243. In Onnis A, Maggino P (eds): New Surgical Trends and Integrated Therapies in Endometrial, Vulva and Trophoblastic Neoplasia. Proceedings of the International Meeting of Gynecologic Oncology. Eur J Gynecol Oncol 1985.)

Table 28-14 Cervical Cancer: Modalities of Therapy Based on Surgical Staging

Treatment	No. of Patients	5-year Survival (%)
Radical hysterectomy and pelvic lymphadenectomy	158	89
Radical hysterectomy, pelvic lymphadenectomy combined with pelvic irradiation	26	58
Pelvic and paraaortic irradiation	27	25
Pelvic irradiation	62	46.7
Pelvic irradiation combined with surgical procedures to alter effectiveness of radiotherapy	3	100
Primary exenteration	1	100
Palliative radiotherapy combined with chemotherapy	1	100

(Data from Averette HE, Sevin BU, Bell J, et al: Surgical staging of cervical cancer. p. 243. In Onnis A, Maggino P (eds): New Surgical Trends and Integrated Therapies in Endometrial, Vulva and Trophoblastic Neoplasia. Proceedings of the International Meeting of Gynecologic Oncology. Eur J Gynecol Oncol 1985.)

In the University of Miami experience, a 38 percent discrepancy was found between the clinical and surgical staging of 282 patients undergoing pretreatment exploratory laparotomy and node dissection.[5] The incidence of positive periaortic lymph nodes for each clinical stage can be found in Table 28-13. Seven modalities of therapy resulted from the findings at staging laparotomy. These modalities, along with their corresponding 5-year survival can be found in Table 28-14.

Pretherapy staging laparotomy combined with subsequent extended-field radiation therapy has been associated with major intestinal complications in the past[69,77] (Table 28-15). A significant reduction in the gastrointestinal complication rate has been documented when the dose of radiotherapy was reduced to

Table 28-15 Cervical Cancer: Survival of Patients with Positive Periaortic Nodes and Complications Related to Surgery and Radiotherapy

Investigators	No. of Patients	Survival %	Survival Yr	Major GI Complications (%)	Procedure	RT Dosage (rad)
Wharton et al. (1977)[72]	24	17.0	3	NR[a]	T	5,500
Hughes et al. (1980)[79]	22	29.0	5	4.3	T	5,100
Ballon et al. (1981)[80]	18	23.0	5	0.0	E	5,500
Piver et al. (1981)[69]	67	11.9	2	62.0	T	6,000
Piver et al. (1981)[69]	31	9.6	5	10.0	T	4,500
Tewfik et al. (1982)[77]	23	21.0	5	60.0	T	5,500
Berman et al. (1984)[75]	98	15.0	3	N/R	T/E	4,400–5,500
Lovecchio et al. (1986)[78]	36	21.4	5	6.0	T	4,500
Lapolla et al. (1986)[6]	16	30.0	5	6.0[b]	T/E	4,000–5,000

[a] Complications for this subset of patients not reported.
[b] One of six patients who developed SBO explored transperitoneally.
T, transperitoneal; E, extraperitoneal.

4,500 to 5,000 rad.[69,75,78,79] The recent utilization of extraperitoneal staging may also favorably reduce the major GI complications of combined therapy.[6,75,80] Of the 282 patients staged by transperitoneal exploration and lymphadenectomy at the University of Miami, major GI complications occurred in only 6 percent of cases, and the maximum dose of external radiotherapy to the paraaortic area was limited to 4,500 R.[5]

In a follow-up study from the Miami series, by Lovecchio et al.,[78] 36 patients with positive periaortic nodes received extended field radiotherapy after pretherapy staging laparotomy. The 5-year survival was 21.4 percent. No difference in survival could be demonstrated based on the degree of nodal involvement (micro versus macro). These findings are concordant with other studies which demonstrate a 5-year survival of less than 30 percent for patients with positive periaortic nodes (see Table 28-16).[6,77,79,80] Despite the poor overall survival in these patients, numerous studies have shown that as many patients fail locally (intrapelvic persistence) as with distant metastasis.[6,74-76] Therefore, the subset of patients with positive nodes whose disease can be controlled in the pelvis appear to have the best overall survival after extended-field radiotherapy.

Patients may be downstaged as a result of pretherapy staging laparotomy when pelvic inflammatory disease and/or endometriosis gives the clinical impression of parametrial involvement.[5,6] Removal of diseased adnexae or large fibroids may improve dosimetry and reduce the possibility of interrupting radiation therapy because of inflammatory flareups.

Alternate approaches to pretherapy surgical staging have been proposed to enhance the accuracy of clinical staging and reduce the morbidity associated with surgery followed by radiotherapy. For example, computed tomography (CT) has been used to evaluate the extent of disease in patients with cervical cancer.[81-83] In a study by Vas et al.,[82] CT evaluation of intrapelvic disease extent was no more accurate than clinical evaluation. However, CT seems to be quite sensitive in the detection of periaortic lymph node involvement.[82-84] Fine-needle aspiration of suspicious periaortic nodes can be performed under CT guidance with minimum morbidity.[84] In Bandy's study, 67 percent of patients were adequately evaluated by a combination of the above methodologies.[84]

Lymphangiography has been employed for many years in the evaluation of patients with cancer of the cervix.[80,85-92] In Ballon's study, an 81 percent correlation was found between lymphangiographic results and surgical/pathological node involvement.[80] However, 27 percent of patients would have been overtreated, while 11 percent would have been undertreated, based solely on the results of the lymphangiogram. Most investigators believe that lymphangiography is too unreliable to use as a basis for therapeutic interventions.[87-92]

A retrospective analysis of 81 patients who recieved periaortic radiotherapy as part of the *primary* management of cervical cancer was undertaken by Potish et al.[93] All patients were staged by conventional clinical means with the addition of bipedal lymphangiography. The clinical justification for extended periaortic radiation was based on (1) abnormal lymphangiography (pelvic or periaortic); (2) abnormal IVP; or (3) extensive tumor volume. GI complications requiring laparotomy occurred in 5 percent of cases. The actuarial 5-year survival in this series was as follows: 80 percent stage IB; 100 percent, stage IIA; 40 percent, stage IIB; and 10 percent, stage IIIB. On closer inspection of the data, only 22 percent of all patients treated in this fashion (periaortic radiotherapy) actually had abnormal periaortic lymphangiography. In fact, most patients were treated on the basis of abnormal pelvic lymphangiograms only. If this interpretation is correct, many patients in this series may have been overtreated, as a significant number of patients with stage IIB to IV disease have been found to have negative periaortic nodes.[5] The 5-year survival in Potish's study was the same or lower than reported in other series where no extended-field radiotherapy was used.[5,94,95]

Table 28-16 Cervical Cancer: Survival of Patients with Positive Periaortic Nodes

Investigators	No. of Patients	Survival (%)
Wharton et al. (1977)[72]	24	17.0
Hughes et al. (1980)[79]	22	29.0
Ballon et al. (1981)[80]	18	23.0
Piver et al. (1981)[69]	67	11.9
Piver et al. (1981)[89]	31	9.6
Tewfik et al. (1982)[77]	23	21.0
Berman et al. (1984)[75]	98	15.0
Lovecchio et al. (1986)[78]	36	21.4
Lapolla et al. (1986)[6]	16	30.0

The issue of microinvasive carcinoma of the cervix (stage 1A) remains a controversial one since first described by Mestwerdt in 1947.[96] Numerous terms have been used to describe this entity, such as borderline microinvasion, early stromal invasion, microcarcinoma, carcinoma in situ with microinvasive foci, minimally invasive carcinoma, and confluent occult invasion carcinoma.[97-99] All these terminologies attempt to define the earliest stage in the transition of intraepithelial neoplasia to invasive carcinoma, where the incidence of lymphatic metastasis approaches nil. These lesions may therefore be treated by conservative measures with the expectation of complete cure.

Several histopathologic parameters have been used to help define this entity (depth of stromal penetration, width/volume of invading tongues, involvement of "capillary-like" spaces, and confluence of invasion). Although no international agreement exists as to precise definition of this entity, the Society of Gynecologic Oncologists proposed in 1974 that the term microinvasive carcinoma be restricted to lesions with 3 mm or less stromal penetration (measured from the base of the epithelium) without involvement of lymphovascular spaces.

Multiple studies have demonstrated that the risk of lymphatic spread is directly proportional to the depth of stromal penetration.[96,97,100-107] An example of this relationship may be seen in Table 28-17. Unfortunately, not all measurements are taken in the same manner, nor are all lymphadenectomies performed to the same degree. These discrepencies may account for the variability noted between studies with respect to the degree of lymphatic involvement for particular depths of stromal invasions. For instance, Roche and Norris[104] in 1975 reviewed the literature on 751 patients with less than 5-mm stromal invasions, and the overall incidence of positive nodes in reported cases was only 1.2 percent. However, a subsequent review by Van Nagell et al.[106] in 1983 demonstrated that the risk of lymphatic spread rose from 0.0 percent to 9 percent as the depth of invasion increased from 3 to 5 mm.

The area and volume of invasion have also been found to be associated with an increased risk of lymphatic spread.[97,101,103,108] In the GOG collaborative study involving 133 patients, both depth (more than 2 mm) and lateral extent (more than 4 mm) of invasion on cone-biopsy specimens were significantly correlated with the findings of residual invasive carcinoma on subsequent hysterectomy specimens. The lateral extent of the tumor was directly correlated with the depth of stromal invasion.[103] This relationship can be seen in Table 28-18.

Burghardt and Holzer[108] performed volumetric analysis of conization specimens and stated that the volume of invading tumor is the most important predictor of lymphatic spread. In their study, carcinomas with less than 400 mm³ invasion were not found to be associated with lymphatic metastasis.[108] These measurements, however, can be very difficult to obtain, and may often be inaccurate.[101]

The finding of tumor metastasis within endothelial-lined spaces (capillary-like spaces) has been said to impact a worst prognosis for patients with otherwise

Table 28-17 Cervical Cancer: Depth of Invasion and Pelvic Node Involvement

Depth (mm)	No. of Patients	Positive Pelvic Nodes (%)
3	59	0
4	87	4.6
5	68	4.4
6–10	330	15.8
11–20	247	25.9
>20	38	21.1

(Data from Delgado G, Stehman F, Zino R, et al: Surgical staging in IB cervical cancer: Clinical and pathologic findings of the Gynecologic Oncology Group (GOG). Annual Meeting, Soc Gynecol Oncol, Miami, FL. (SGO Abstracts 2, Feb 1985.)

Table 28-18 Cervical Cancer: Depth of Invasion Versus Extent of Lateral Spread

Depth (mm)	Lateral Extent					
	2 mm		2–6 mm		>6 mm	
	N	%	N	%	N	%
<1	40	80.0	8	16.0	2	4.0
1–3	11	18.0	27	43.5	24	38.5
>3	2	9.5	6	28.5	13	62.0

(Data from Sedlis A, Sell S, Tsukada Y, et al: Microinvasive carcinoma of the uterine cervix: A clinical-pathologic study. Am J Obstet Gynecol 133:64, 1979.)

early invasive carcinoma of the cervix.[99,103] Unfortunately, the identification of these spaces can vary depending on pathologic interpretation, and there is still some question whether these spaces truly represent lymphatic capillaries.[104] It has been demonstrated that, in general, as the depth of stromal penetration increases, more extensive involvement of capillary-like spaces occurs.[103,106,109] Therefore, the precise role of this parameter as an independent risk factor for lymphatic spread is still not precisely known. For example, in the study by Roche and Norris of 30 patients with microinvasive carcinoma of the cervix, 57 percent had involvement of capillary-like spaces, and none of these patients were found to have positive nodes.[104] However, a recent collaborative study involving more than evaluable patients with stage 1B-2A cervical cancer was completed and the findings suggest that involvement of capillary-like spaces does indeed seem to be an independent prognostic variable. The study demonstrated that 28 percent of patients with involvement of capillary-like spaces were found to have positive pelvic nodes, while only 8 percent of patients without capillary-like space involvement had positive pelvic nodes.[107]

The importance of confluence (coalescence of invasive tongues) as an independent variable in microinvasive disease of the cervix has also been imprecisely defined. It seems that confluence per se does not imply increased tumor virulence but serves as an indicator of tumor extent and, in this regard, may influence prognosis.[101,104,110]

On the basis of the available data, the following treatment schema is suggested for patients with cervical carcinoma. The diagnosis of microinvasive carcinoma of the cervix should be made only on an adequate cone biopsy specimen, where multiple sections have been reviewed. The depth of stromal penetration as well as the area (extent) of invasion seem to directly correlate with the risk of lymphatic spread. Tumors with up to 3-mm penetration and less than 4-mm width seem to be associated with a negligible incidence of lymphatic metastasis and may be managed conservatively. Invasion of capillary-like spaces by tumor does seem to be a significant independent variable for predicting lymphatic spread. Therefore, regardless of the depth of stromal penetration, when capillary-like space involvement is demonstrated histologically, we believe that radical hysterectomy and pelvic node dissection is the treatment of choice for

these patients. When lesions penetrate more than 3 mm into the stroma or extend at least 4 mm in width, a radical hysterectomy is indicated as the risk of lymphatic metastasis is significant.

For patients with early-stage (IB to IIA) cervical cancer who are good surgical candidates, staging laparotomy with initial periaortic lymphadenectomy is performed. If the periaortic nodes are negative, radical hysterectomy with pelvic lymphadenectomy is performed. If periaortic nodes are positive, scalene node biopsy is performed. If the scalene node biopsy is negative, patients receive pelvic and periaortic radiotherapy. For poor surgical candidates, pelvic radiotherapy alone is employed.

For patients with advanced-stage cervical cancer (IIB to IV), pelvic radiotherapy alone is used. It does not seem reasonable to employ extended-field radiotherapy in these patients without good evidence for periaortic nodal involvement. Routine pretherapy surgical staging does not seem justified unless patients are participating in prospective clinical trials investigating new treatment modalities, where it would be desirable to define disease extent outside the pelvic field of radiation prior to therapy.

SUMMARY

There is much controversy in the literature regarding the precise role of surgical staging for gynecologic neoplasms. It can undoubtedly be stated that surgical/pathologic investigations do lead to a more precise definition of disease. However, one must demonstrate that the patient will benefit from the information obtained at surgical exploration without incurring additional morbidity from the combination of surgical staging with primary of secondary modalities of therapy.

Ovarian carcinoma is conventionally staged surgically and surgical debulking remains an integral part of the initial treatment of this malignancy. It has been conclusively demonstrated that surgical delineation of tumor extent followed by appropriate adjunctive therapy will improve survival. Restaging laparotomy after chemotherapy remains as the most sensitive indicator of disease persistence, despite the introduction of less invasive techniques (CT scan, CA 125) that have been shown to possess a substantial false-negative rate. However, its precise role in the overall management of patients with stages III and IV disease has not been firmly established.

The staging of endometrial cancer seems more appropriately accomplished through surgical means based on our current knowledge of specific prognostic factors which cannot be precisely determined clinically. It is hoped that this modality will gain full acceptance in the near future.

In the evaluation of patients with squamous cell carcinoma of the vulva, the surgical definition of groin node status seems to more accurately predict survival. For those found to have positive groin nodes, the institution of groin and pelvic radiotherapy seems to enhance survival. The addition of pelvic node dissection does not seem to improve survival in patients with vulvar carcinoma.

The value of surgical staging for patients undergoing radical hysterectomy for early cervical cancer remains undisputed. However, its use in patients with advanced stage disease (IIB to IV) within a nonacademic setting, cannot be justified at this time. Until more effective means of treating these patients with advanced disease is found, the information obtained through pretherapy surgical exploration will not lead to improved survival in most patients.

ACKNOWLEDGMENT

We wish to thank Doris Hemingway and Gretchen Kroepil for their help in preparation of this manuscript.

REFERENCES

1. Way S, Benedet JL: Involvement of inguinal lymph nodes in carcinoma of the vulva: A comparison of clinical assessment with histologic examination. Gynecol Oncol 1:119, 1973
2. Homesley HD, Bundy BN, Sedlis A, Adcock L: Radiation therapy versus pelvic node resection for patients with invasive squamous cell carcinoma of the vulva having positive groin nodes. Obstet Gynecol 68:733, 1986
3. Knapp RC, Freidman EA: Aortic lymph node metastasis in early ovarian cancer. Am J Obstet Gynecol 109:1013, 1974
4. Piver MS, Barlow JJ, Lele SB: Incidence of subclinical metastasis in stages I and II ovarian carcinoma. Obstet Gynecol 52:1, 1978
5. Averette HE, Sevin BU, Bell J, et al: Surgical staging of cervical cancer. p. 243. In Onnis A, Maggino P (eds): New Surgical Trends and Integrated Therapies in Endometrial, Vulva and Trophoblastic Neoplasia. Proceedings of the International Meeting of Gynecologic Oncology. Eur J Gynecol Oncol 6:1985
6. LaPolla JP, Schlaerth JB, Gaddis O, Morrow CP: The influence of surgical staging on the evaluation and treatment of patients with cervical carcinoma. Gynecol Oncol 24:194, 1986
7. Cowles TA, Magrina JF, Masterson BJ, Capen CV: Comparison of clinical and surgical staging in patients with endometrial carcinoma. Obstet Gynecol 66:413, 1985
8. Morrow CP: Tumors of the endometrium. p. 159. In Synopsis of Gynecologic Oncology. 3rd Ed. 1986
9. Greer BE, Rutledge FN, Gallager HJ: Staging or restaging laparotomy in early stage epitheial cancers of the ovary. Clin Obstet Gynecol 23:293, 1980
10. Keettel WC, Elkins HB: Experience with radioactive colloidal gold in the treatment of ovarian cancer. Am J Obstet Gynecol 71:553, 1956
11. Rosenoff SH, DeVita VT, Hubbard S, Young RC: Peritoneoscopy in the staging and followup of ovarian cancer. Semin Oncol 2:233, 1975
12. Chen SS, Lee L: Incidence of positive periaortic and pelvic nodes in epithelial cancers of the ovary. Gynecol Oncol 16:95, 1983
13. Piver MS: Ovarian malignancies: The clinical care of adults and adolescents. p. 74. In Current Reviews in Obstetrics and Gynecology. Vol. 4. Churchill Livingstone, New York, 1983
14. Griffiths CT: Surgical resection of tumor bulk in the primary treatment of ovarian carcinoma. Symposium on Ovarian Carcinoma. Natl Cancer Inst Monogr 42:101, 1975
15. Young RC, Chabner NA, Hubbard SB: Advanced ovarian adenocarcinoma. N Engl J Med 299:1261, 1978
16. Parker LM, Griffiths CT, Yankee R, Canellos GP: Combination chemotherapy with adriamycin-cyclophosphamide for advanced ovarian carcinoma. Cancer 46:669, 1980
17. Aure JC, Hoeg K, Kolstad P: Clinical and histologic studies of ovarian carcinoma: Long-term followup of 990 cases. Obstet Gynecol 37:1, 1971
18. Griffiths CT, Parker LM, Fuller AF: Role of cytoreductive surgical treatment in the management of advanced ovarian cancer. Cancer Treatm Rep 63:235, 1979
19. Webb MJ, Snyder JA, Williams TJ, Decker DG: Second-look laparotomy in ovarian cancer. Gynecol Oncol 14:285, 1982

20. Roberts WS, Hodel K, Rich WM, DiSaia PJ: Second-look laparotomy in the management of gynecologic malignancies. Gynecol Oncol 13:345, 1982

21. Piver MS, Lele SB, Barlow JJ, Gamarra M: Second-look laparotomy prior to proposed second-look laparotomy. Obstet Gynecol 55:571, 1980

22. Berek JS, Hacker NF, Lagasse LD, et al: Second-look laparotomy in stage III epithelial ovarian cancer: Clinical variables associated with disease status. Obstet Gynecol 64:207, 1984

23. Berek JS, Hacker NF, Lagasse LD, et al: Survival of patients following secondary cytoreductive surgery in ovarian cancer. Obstet Gynecol 61:189, 1983

24. Mangiani C, Bolis G, Molteni P, Belloni C: Indications and advantages and limits of laparoscopy in ovarian cancer. Gynecol Oncol 7:47, 1979

25. Atack DB, Nisker JS, Allen HH, et al: CA-125 surveillance and second-look laparotomy in ovarian cancer. Am J Obstet Gynecol 154:287, 1986

26. Bast RC, Feeney M, Lazarus M, et al: Reactivity in a monoclonal antibody with human ovarian carcinoma. J Clin Invest 68:1331, 1981

27. Bast RC, Klug TL, St John E: Radioimmunoassay using a monoclonal antibody to monitor the course of epithelial ovarian cancer. N Engl J Med 309:883, 1983

28. Schwartz PE, Smith JP: Second-look operation in ovarian cancer. Am J Obstet Gynecol 138:1124, 1980

29. Raju KS, McKinna JA, Barker GH, et al: Second-look operations in the planned management of advanced ovarian carcinoma. Am J Obstet Gynecol 144:650, 1982

30. Menczer J, Modan M, Brenner J, et al: Abdominopelvic irradiation for stage II-IV ovarian carcinoma patients with limited or no residual disease at second-look laparotomy after completion of cisplatinum-based combination chemotherapy. Gynecol Oncol 24:149, 1986

31. Greiner R, Goldhirsch A, Nevenschwander H, et al: Whole abdominal radiation with advanced carcinoma after surgery, chemotherapy and second-look laparotomy. J Clin Res Oncol 107:94, 1984

32. Christopherson WM, Connelly PJ, Alberhasky RC: Carcinoma of the endometrium: An analysis of prognostic indicators in patients with favorable subtypes and stage I disease. Cancer 51:1705, 1983

33. Wallen TE, Malkasian GD, Gaffy TA, et al: Stage II carcinoma of the endometrium: A pathologic and clinical study. Gynecol Oncol 18:1, 1984

34. Silverberg SG, DeGiorgi LS: Histopathologic analysis of preoperative radiation therapy in endometrial carcinoma. Am J Obstet Gynecol 119:698, 1974

35. Macassaet M, Brigati D, Boyce J, et al: The significance of residual disease after radiotherapy in endometrial carcinoma: Clinicopathologic correlation. Am J Obstet Gynecol 151:1009, 1985

36. Piver MS, Lele SB, Barlow JJ, Blumenson L: Paraaortic lymph node evaluation in stage I endometrial carcinoma. Obstet Gynecol 59:97, 1982

37. Boronow RC, Morrow CP, Creasman WT, et al: Surgical staging in endometrial cancer: Clinical-pathologic findings of a prospective study. Obstet Gynecol 63:825, 1984

38. DiSaia PJ, Creasman WT, Boronow RC, Blessing JA: Risk factors and recurrent patterns in stage I endometrial cancer. Am J Obstet Gynecol 151:1009, 1985

39. Aalders JG: General discussion and conclusions. p. 96. In Prognostic Factors and Treatment of Endometrial Carcinoma: A Clinical and Histopathological Study. Drukkerji Dijkstra Neimeyer, BV, Groningen, 1982

40. Hanson MB, Van Nagell JR, Powell DE, et al: The prognostic significance of lymph-vascular space invasion in stage I endometrial cancer. Cancer 55:1753, 1985

41. Creasman WT, Rutledge FN: The prognostic value of peritoneal cytology in gynecologic malignant disease. Am J Obstet Gynecol 110:773, 1971

42. DiSaia PJ, Creasman WT: Adenocarcinoma of the uterus. p. 146. In DiSaia PJ, Creasman WT (eds): Clinical Gynecologic Oncology. 2nd Ed. CV Mosby, St. Louis, 1984

43. Yazigi R, Piver MS, Blumenson L: Malignant peritoneal cytology as prognostic indicator in stage I endometrial cancer. Obstet Gynecol 62:359, 1983

44. Creasman WT, Boronow RC, Morrow CP, et al: Adenocarcinoma of the endometrium: Its metastasis lymph node potential. Gynecol Oncol 4:239, 1976

45. Lewis BV, Stallworthy JA, Cowdell R: Adenocarcinoma of the body of the uterus. Obstet Gynaecol Br Commonw 77:343, 1970

46. Musemici R, DePalo G, Conti V, et al: Are retroperitoneal lymph node metastases a major problem in endometrial adenocarcinoma. Cancer 46:1887, 1980

47. Chen SS: Extrauterine spread in endometrial carcinoma clinically confined to the uterus. Gynecol Oncol 21:23, 1983

48. Potish RA, Twiggs LB, Adcock LL, et al: Paraaortic lymph node radiotherapy in cancer of the uterine corpus. Obstet Gynecol 65:251, 1985

49. DiSaia PJ, Creasman WT: Invasive Cancer of the Vagina and Urethra. p. 237. In DiSaia PJ, Creasman WT (eds): Clinical Gynecologic Oncology. 2nd Ed. CV Mosby, St. Louis, 1984

50. Podratz KC, Symmonds RE, Taylor WR, Williams TJ: Carcinoma of the vulva: Analysis of treatment and survival. Obstet Gynecol 61:63, 1983

51. Hoffman JS, Kumar NB, Morely GW: Prognostic significance of groin lymph nodes metastasis in squamous cell carcinoma of the vulva. Obstet Gynecol 66:402, 1985
52. Franklin EW, Rutledge FE: Prognostic factors in epidermoid carcinoma of the vulva. Obstet Gynecol, 37:892, 1971
53. Homesley HD: Carcinoma of the vulva. p. 98. In Conn HF (ed): Conn's Current Therapy. WB Saunders, Philadelphia, 1985
54. Hacker NF, Nieberg RK, Berek JS, et al: Superficially invasive vulvar carcinoma with nodal metastasis. Gynecology 15:65, 1983
55. DiSaia PJ, Creasman WT, Rich WM: An alternative approach to early carcinoma of the vulva. Am J Obstet Gynecol 133:825, 1979
56. Zucker PR, Berkowitz RS: The issue of microinvasive squamous cell carcinoma of the vulva: An evaluation of the criteria of diagnosis and methods of therapy. Obstet Gynecol Surv 40:136, 1985
57. Wharton JT, Gallager S, Rutledge FN: Microinvasive carcinoma of the vulva. Am J Obstet Gynecol 118:159, 1974
58. Donaldson ES, Powell DE, Hanson MB, Van Nagell JR: Prognostic parameters in invasive vulvar cancer. Gynecol Oncol 11:184, 1981
59. Gosling JR, Abell MR, Drolette BM, Loughrin TD: Infiltrative squamous cell carcinoma of the vulva. Cancer 14:330, 1961
60. Podratz KC, Gaffey TA, Symmonds RE, et al: Melanoma of the vulva: An update. Gynecol Oncol 16:153, 1983
61. Jaramillo BA, Ganjei P, Sevin BU, et al: Malignant melanoma of the vulva. Obstet Gynecol 66:398, 1985
62. Meigs JV: Surgical Treatment of Cancer of the Cervix. Grune & Stratton, New York, 1954
63. Brunschwig A, Pierce V: Necropsy findings in patients with carcinoma of the cervix. Am J Obstet Gynecol 56:1134, 1948
64. Henriksen E: The lymphatic spread of carcinoma of the cervix and body of the uterus. Am J Obstet Gynecol 58:924, 1949
65. Henriksen E: The dispension of cancer of the cervix. Radiology 54:812, 1950
66. Nelson JH: Pretreatment laparotomy in stages IIB-III carcinoma of the cervix. Presented at the Annual Meeting of the Society of Gynecologic Oncologists, January 1970 (abst)
67. Buchsbaum HJ: Paraaortic lymph node involvement in cervical carcinoma. Am J Obstet Gynecol 113:942, 1972
68. Uemakli A, Bonney WA: Exploratory laparotomy as routine pretreatment investigation of the cervix. Radiology 104:371, 1972
69. Piver MS, Barlow JJ, Krishnametty R: Five-year survival (with no evidence of disease) in patients with biopsy confirmed aortic node metastasis from cervix cancer. Am J Obstet Gynecol 139:575, 1981
70. Maggino T, Bonneto F, Catapano T, et al: Clinical staging versus operative staging in cervical cancer. Clin Exp Obstet Gynecol 10:201, 1983
71. Shah K, Olson MH, Dillard EA: Carcinoma of the cervix: Surgical staging and radiotherapy with 32 MeV Betatnon. Int J Radiat Oncol Biol Phys 8:1601, 1982
72. Wharton JT, Jones HW, Day TG, et al: Preirradiation celiotomy and extended field irradiation for invasive cancer of the cervix. Obstet Gynecol 49:333, 1981
73. Welander CE, Pierce VK, DattaReyudu N, et al: Pretreatment laparotomy in carcinoma of the cervix. Gynecol Oncol 12:336, 1981
74. Kademiam MT, Bosch A: Staging laparotomy and survival in carcinoma of the uterine cervix. Acta Radiol Ther Phys Biol 16:314, 1977
75. Berman ML, Keys H, Creasman W, et al: Survival patterns of recurrence in cervical cancer metastasis to paraaortic lymph nodes. Gynecol Oncol 19:8, 1984
76. Labasse LD, Creasman WT, Shingleton HM, et al: Results in the complications of operative staging in cervical cancer: Experience of the Gynecologic Oncology Group. Gynecol Oncol 9:90, 1980
77. Tewfik HH, Buchsbaum HJ, Latourette HB, et al: Paraaortic lymph node irradiation in carcinoma of the cervix after exploratory laparotomy and biopsy proven positive paraaortic nodes. Int J Radiat Oncol Biol Phys 8:13, 1982
78. Lovecchio JL, Averette HE, Donato DM: Five-year survival of patients with paraaortic nodal metastasis in clinical stage IB and IIA cervical carcinoma. Gynecol Oncol
79. Hughes RR, Brewington KC, HanJani, et al: Extended field irradiation for cervical cancer based on surgical staging. Gynecol Oncol 9:153, 1980
80. Ballon SC, Berman ML, Lagasse LD, et al: Survival after extraperitoneal pelvic and paraaortic lymphadenectomy and radiation therapy in cervical carcinoma. Obstet Gynecol 57:90, 1981
81. Whitley NO, Brenner DE, Francis A, et al: Computed tomographic evaluation of carcinoma of the cervix. Radiology 142:439, 1982
82. Vas W, Wolverson M, Freel J, et al: Computed tomography in the pretreatment assessment of carcinoma of the cervix. J Compt Tomog 9:359, 1985
83. Raber G, Potzschke B: Value of computerized tomog-

raphy for the assessment of the parametrium in cervical cancer. *ROFO* 143:544, 1985

84. Bandy LC, Clarke-Pearson DL, Silverman PM, Creasman WT: Computed tomography in evaluation of extrapelvic lymphadenopathy in carcinoma of the cervix. Obstet Gynecol 65:73, 1985

85. Averette HE, Hudson RC, Viamonte MI, et al: Lymphangioadenography in the study of female genital cancer. Cancer 15:769, 1962

86. Nelson JH, Masterson JG, Herman PG, Benninghoff DL: Anatomy of the female pelvic and aortic lymphatic systems demonstrated by lymphangiography. Am J Obstet Gynecol 88:460, 1964

87. Averette HE, LeMaire WJ, Lecart CJ, Ferguson JH: Lymphography in the preoperative detection of lymphatic metastasis. Obstet Gynecol 27:122, 1966

88. Jobson VW, Russell E, Girtanner RE, Averette HE: Predictive accuracy of lymphography in cervical cancer. Seventh Annual Meeting of the Western Association of Gynecologic Oncologists, Newport Beach, CAL, June 1979

89. Lagasse LD, Ballon SC, Berman JL, et al: Pretreatment lymphangiography and operative evaluation in carcinoma of the cervix. Am J Obstet Gynecol 134:219, 1979

90. Kolbenstredt A, Knudsen OS: A method for lymphographic and histologic correlation: Experience from 300 patients treated by pelvic lymphadenectomy. Gynecol Oncol 2:9, 1974

91. Ashraft M, Elyaderani MK, Gabriele OF, Krall JM: Value of lymphangiography in the diagnosis of paraaortic lymph node metastasis from carcinoma of the cervix. Gynecol Oncol 14:96, 1982

92. Brown RD, Buchsbaum HJ: Accuracy of lymphangiography in the diagnosis of paraaortic lymph node metastasis from carcinoma of the cervix. Obstet Gynecol 54:571, 1979

93. Potish RA, Ascock L, Jones J, et al: The morbidity and utility of paraaortic radiotherapy in cervical carcinoma. Gynecol Oncol 15:1, 1983

94. Currie DW: Operative treatment of carcinoma of the cervix. J Obstet Gynaecol Br Commonw 1978:385, 1971

95. Fletcher GH: External radiation therapy in cancer of the uterine cervix. p. 111. In Lewis GC, et al (eds): New Concepts in Gynecologic Oncology. FA Davis, Philadelphia, 1967

96. Mestwerdt G: Probeexzision and kolposkopie in der fruhdiagnose des portiokaszinomas. Zentralb. Gynaekol 4:326, 1947

97. Lohe KL: Early squamous cell carcinoma of the uterine cervix. Gynecol Oncol 6:10, 1978

98. Wilkinson EJ, Komorowski RA: Borderline microinvasive carcinoma of the cervix. Obstet Gynecol 51:472, 1970

99. Burghandt E: Microinvasive carcinoma. Obstet Gynecol Surv 34:836, 1979

100. Larsson G, Alm P, Gullberg B, Grundsell H: Prognostic factors in early invasive carcinoma of the uterine cervix. A clinical histopathologic and statistical analysis of 343 cases. Am J Obstet Gynecol 146:145, 1983

101. Coppelson M: The diagnosis and treatment of early (preclinical) invasive cervical cancer. Clin Obstet Gynecol 12:149, 1985

102. Burghardt E, Pickel H: Local spread and lymph node involvement in cervical cancer. Obstet Gynecol 52:138, 1978

103. Sedlis A, Sall S, Tsukada Y, et al: Microinvasive carcinoma of the uterine cervix: A clinical-pathologic study. Am J Obstet Gynecol 133:64, 1979

104. Roche WD, Norris HJ: Microinvasive carcinoma of the cervix: The significance of lymphatic invasion and confluent patterns of stromal growth. Cancer 36:180, 1975

105. Simon NL, Gore H, Shingleton HM, et al: Study of superficially invasive carcinoma of the cervix. Obstet Gynecol 68:19, 1986

106. VanNagel JR, Greenwell N, Powell DF, et al: Microinvasive carcinoma of the cervix. J Obstet Gynecol 145:981, 1983

107. Delgado G, Stehman F, Zino R, et al: Surgical staging in IB cervical cancer: Clinical and pathologic findings of the Gynecologic Oncology Group (GOG) SGO Abstracts #2, Feb, 1985. Annual Meeting of the Society of Gynecologic Oncologists, Miami, FL

108. Burghardt E, Holzer E: Diagnosis and treatment of microinvasive carcinoma of the cervix uteri. Obstet Gynecol 49:641, 1977

109. Lehman MH, Benson WL, Kurman RJ, Park RC: Microinvasive carcinoma of the cervix. Obstet Gynecol 48:571, 1976

110. Shingleton HM, Orr JW: Cancer of the cervix. Diagnosis and treatment. p. 917. In Singer A, Jordan J (eds): Current Reviews in Obstetrics and Gynecology. Vol. 5. Churchill Livingstone, New York, 1983

29

Second-Look Surgical Procedure

Vinay K. Malviya
Gunter Deppe

In 1948, Wangensteen introduced second-look surgical procedures to diagnose early recurrence in asymptomatic patients with colorectal cancer.[1,2] In 1966, Rutledge and Burns[3] used this concept of second-look surgery in assessing the disease status for ovarian cancer patients following cytotoxic chemotherapy.

A second-look operation is defined as a surgical re-exploration of patients who have completed a planned course of therapy after a definitive primary surgical procedure who, at present, have no clinical or radiographic evidence of disease. This operation is performed primarily to determine the status of a patient's tumor and to plan future treatment. The significant risk of developing acute leukemia, neurotoxicity, nephrotoxicity, cardiotoxicity, and other life-threatening complications with the use of cytotoxic chemotherapy mandates that patients who are clinically and radiologically free of disease be evaluated with the intent of discontinuing chemotherapy. Conversely, persistence of even a single small focus of tumor will ultimately result in recurrence of the disease and eventual death. Although few patients will benefit from extensive tumor reduction at second look, patients with minimal disease may benefit from additional treatment based on second-look findings.

Second-look laparotomy represents the basis on which curative second-line salvage therapy may be initiated. It has the potential to document a complete pathologic response to first-line chemotherapy and to identify those patients at risk of recurrence who may be candidates for additional adjunctive therapy.

DEFINITIONS AND TERMINOLOGY

Second-look surgery must be distinguished from re-exploration in other settings that have often been confused with second-look laparotomy:

Restaging: Used for a referred patient in whom the initial laparotomy findings are unclear and staging is incomplete

Reoperation: A patient with limited initial surgery who had significant tumor regression with postoperative therapy so that the patient now is operable

Re-exploration: Reoperation in patients who develop an isolated resectable recurrence

Re-evaluation: A surgical procedure performed on patients receiving chemotherapy to determine whether the nonpalpable disease is responding to chemotherapy or to detect early recurrence

Negative second-look: Findings at second-look laparotomy described as negative when no histologic or cytologic evidence of disease is found

Macroscopically positive second-look: Persistent tumor, identified grossly by the surgeon and confirmed by the pathologist, regarded as macroscopically positive

Microscopically positive second-look: When no tumor is identified by the surgeon, but cytologic washings or biopsies demonstrate persistent disease

Inadequate second-look: Incomplete surgical exploration due to surgical or anesthetic mishaps, the presence of extensive adhesions, or technical deficits of the surgeon

Sensitivity: The ability of a test to give a positive finding when the patient tested truly has persistent disease:

$$\text{Sensitivity} = \frac{\text{No. of true positive}}{\text{false negative} + \text{true positive}}$$

Specificity: the ability to give a negative finding when the person treated is free from disease:

$$\text{Specificity} = \frac{\text{true negative}}{\text{false positive} + \text{true negative}}$$

For patients with nonmeasurable disease, i.e., patients who have no clinical disease at the conclusion of their initial surgical exploration, second-look surgical reassessment is the usual method of evaluating response. In these cases, a patient is considered to have a pathologic complete response if there is no evidence of disease following laparotomy, which includes exploration of the entire abdomen from the pelvis to the undersurface of the diaphragm, biopsy of all suspicious areas, and random biopsy of the diaphragm and pelvic peritoneum.

TIMING OF SECOND-LOOK LAPAROTOMY

The optimal duration of chemotherapy and timing of second-look laparotomy is variable and must be individualized for each patient. Experience with single-agent chemotherapy melphalan at the M.D. Anderson Hospital supported the use of this alkylating agent for at least 12 cycles in advanced ovarian cancer.[4] The incidence of a negative second-look operation increased from 14.6 percent with less than 10 courses of Alkeran to 40 percent with 12 courses of Alkeran.

With the advent of combination chemotherapy and with a trend toward following chemotherapy with radiation therapy, fewer courses of chemotherapy are being administered prior to second-look surgery. Berek et al.[5] found no difference in the incidence of a negative second-look operation in patients treated with 6 to 9 cycles and those treated with 10 to 12 cycles of combination chemotherapy. Oldham and Greco and their co-workers reported negative second-look rates of 40 percent and 38 percent, respectively, after six courses of combination chemotherapy.[6,7]

Therapy should be planned on the basis of the stage of the disease at presentation and the volume of residual tumor at initial surgery. A reasonable approach may be to treat patients with early ovarian cancer optimally debulked at primary surgery, that is, residual tumor less than 2 cm, with six courses of combination chemotherapy. Conversely, the patient with advanced ovarian cancer and/or the patient who has residual tumor greater than 2 cm in diameter should receive at least eight courses of chemotherapy prior to second-look surgery.

There are no routinely available, diagnostic, clinical, radiographic, or serum biomarkers to monitor the cancer status of patients with common epithelial cancers of the ovary. Computed axial tomography and ultrasonography are less sensitive than serial pelvic examinations by an experienced gynecologist in determining early recurrence of gynecologic malignancies.[8] Serum biomarkers are available to monitor selected patients with germ cell ovarian malignancies. Recently, studies have been initiated to determine the sensitivity of CA 125 in determining disease status for recurrent epithelial nonmucinous ovarian cancers.[9-11]

COMPUTED TOMOGRAPHY

Computed tomography (CT) scan is the most accurate, noninvasive method currently available for detecting pelvic and abdominal masses, paraaortic lymph node involvement, pulmonary and hepatic metastases.[12] However, it does not detect small peritoneal or omental metastases less than 2 cm, diaphragmatic disease and bowel infiltration. Hepatic metastases may also be missed on CT scan especially when

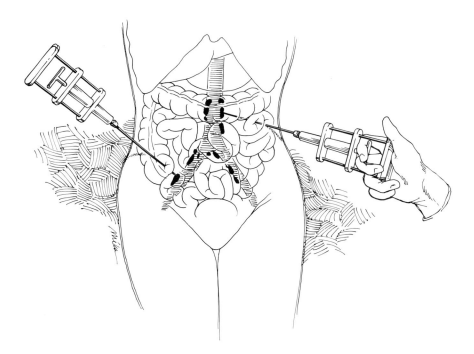

Fig. 29-1 (CT) scan directed aspiration biopsy of the enlarged paraaortic and pelvic lymph nodes prior to second-look laparotomy.

lesions are small or distorted due to streak artifacts produced by metal clips. Evaluation of retroperitoneal lymph nodes in hypoasthenic patients by CT scan is limited due to paucity of surrounding fat, since anatomic distortion from previous treatment may yield false-positive results.

CT scan directed fine needle aspiration may be used in selected cases to confirm positive cytologic findings prior to second-look laparotomy (Fig. 29-1). Attempts to replace second-look surgery with computed tomography in patients with ovarian cancer have been disappointing. Recently, Clarke-Pearson and colleagues studied 47 patients with no clinical evidence of disease following chemotherapy before second-look surgery and confirmed earlier findings that CT scan has a low sensitivity and a high false-negative rate.[13] Results of CT scans are inconclusive in patients who are most likely to benefit from an accurate definition of disease, those with minimal residual disease.

OTHER IMAGING TECHNIQUES

Ultrasound is helpful in detecting cystic hepatic metastases and fine-needle aspiration of these lesions; however, CT scan provides a clearer anatomic display and more reproducible images for assessment of disease and response to treatment when compared to ultrasound.[14]

The development of antibodies to ovarian cancer antigens and the conjugation of these antibodies to radioisotopes allows the radiographic imaging of primary, metastatic or recurrent disease. Using ^{131}I-labeled polyclonal heteroantisera to carcinoembryonic antigen, Goldenberg et al.[15] were able to image 10 of 10 primary and 11 of 14 metastatic ovarian cancer sites. The smallest tumor detectable by this technique measured approximately 2 cm in diameter. Van Nagell et al.[16] were able to image 13 of 13 primary ovarian cancers and 6 of 9 metastatic sites of disease. Tumors were successfully imaged in patients with both normal and elevated serum CEA levels. Epenetos et al.[17] used monoclonal antibodies directed against breast tissue components for radioimmunolocalization of epithelial ovarian cancers. The use of magnetic resonance imaging (MRI) in clinically undetectable cancer remains investigational but holds promise.

With further improvement in immunologic and imaging techniques, radioimmunolocalization of ovarian tumors offer great potential for clinical application.

Table 29-1 Summary of Primary Ovarian Cancer-Associated Antigens

Associated Antigen	Investigators
OCAA, OCAA-1	Bhattacharya and Barlow (1973, 1975, 1978, 1979)[20-25]
FRGP	Hamazaki and Hotta (1975)[26]
TA	Burton et al. (1976)[27]
OVC-1, OVC-2	Imamura et al. (1978)[28]
OCA	Knauf and Urbach (1978)[29]
IOTA	Stolbach et al. (1979)[30]
OCAA-2, -3, -4, -5	Bhattacharya and Chatterjee (1980)[31]
ID-3	Bhattacharya and Chatterjee (1980)[31]
Dawson-Ag	Dawson et al. (1980)[32]
NB/70K	Knauf and Urbach (1981)[18]
CA-125	Bast et al. (1983)[9]
90K/GP	Hanjani and Subba (1985)[19]

Table 29-3 Biomarkers in Ovarian Cancer

Carcinoplacental glycoproteins
  hCG
  HPL
  PAP
Oncofetal antigen
  α-Fetoprotein
  CEA
  Oncofetal antigent (BOFA)
  Ferritin
Abnormalities of glycosyltransferases and glycosidases
  Galactosyltransferase
  α_1-Fucosidase
Miscellaneous
  Serum lactic dehydrogenase
  Serum-mediated immunosuppression
  Serum ribonuclease

TUMOR MARKERS

A specific and sensitive serologic tumor marker would constitute an ideal monitoring device for evaluating the disease status of ovarian cancer patients. Although the perfect tumor marker is not available, progress has been made with CA 125 antigen.[9] Other tumor markers such as NB/70k and 90k-GP are also being studied.[18,19]

Presently, there are four major categories of potential tumor markers (Tables 29-1 through 29-3): (1) tumor-specific or tumor-associated antigens; (2) oncofetal antigens; (3) carcinoplacental glycoproteins; and (4) complex proteins or glycoproteins displaying enzymatic activity.

Table 29-2 Summary of Secondary Ovarian Cancer-Associated Antigens

Associated Antigen	Investigators
OV-1, OV-2	Order et al. (1975)[34]
FDP	Svanberg and Astedt (1975)[35]
A-1, A-4	Burton et al. (1977)[36]
M-1, M-4	Bara et al. (1977)[37]
CSAP	Pant et al. (1978)[38]
Pepsinogen	Hirsh-Marie et al. (1978)[39]
DUPAN-2	Metzgar et al. (1982)[40]
MOVI	Colnaghi et al. (1982)[41]

CA 125

CA 125, an antigenic determinant expressed by the majority of nonmucinous epithelial ovarian cancers, may be detected in serum with a solid-phase radioimmunoassay.

Several investigators have evaluated CA 125 as a tumor marker for epithelial ovarian cancer in patients undergoing second-look exploratory laparotomy. Antigen levels are reported to correlate with disease status in about 90 percent of patients. Elevation of CA 125 preceded the radiographic diagnosis of recurrence by 1 to 7 months.[11] It appears that a CA 125 titer greater than 35 U/ml predicts the presence of tumor. Berek found tumor at second-look operations in all 12 patients with an elevated CA 125 level greater than, or equal to, 35 U/ml.[10] Conversely, CA 125 levels less than 35U/ml were detected in 44 percent of patients with a positive second-look.

In Atack's series, 43 percent of patients with persistent disease had CA 125 values in the normal range; thus, normal CA 125 values do not obviate the need for second-look laparotomy in treatment planning.[42] An elevated level, however, will reliably predict the presence of tumor or future recurrence. Rising or falling trends reflect clinical disease progression or regression in 85 to 93 percent of cases. Furthermore, the absence of an elevated antigen level reliably indicates that, if intraperitoneal tumor is present, the largest tumor will probably not be greater than 1 cm in diameter. More experience is required before an elevated CA 125 level will be considered sufficient evidence of disease progression replacing the need for second-look surgery.

PREOPERATIVE EVALUATION

Prior to second-look laparotomy, all efforts should be made to rule out the presence of residual disease. In addition to a careful history and physical examination, the operative note from the initial surgery should be carefully reviewed with respect to the previous findings and sites of documented disease.

A significant correlation exists between positive biopsy sites at second-look laparatomy and sites of known initial residual cancer, particularly in patients with minimal disease at second-look (76 percent).

A complete blood count with differential and platelets, liver-function tests, serum lactic dehydrogenase, CA 125, and type and crossmatch for at least four units of packed cells should be ordered. Chest radiography, intravenous pyelogram, barium enema, and a CT scan of the abdomen and pelvis with contrast should be performed. Any abnormality is carefully assessed with appropriate studies.

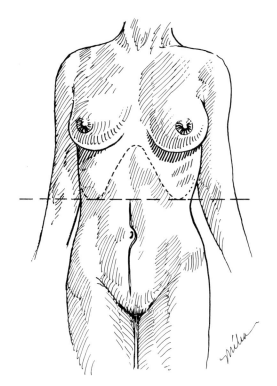

Fig. 29-2 Incision at the time of second-look exploratory laparotomy.

TECHNIQUE OF SECOND-LOOK OPERATION

Second-look laparotomy consists of a very methodical and meticulous search for persistent disease. It should be performed by the gynecologic oncologist who is familiar with the natural history, mode of spread of the cancer and the findings at initial surgery.

The operation should proceed in a fashion similar to the staging laparotomy for ovarian cancer. The patient is placed in a supine position and a midline vertical incision is made, extending approximately 6 cm above the umbilicus (Fig. 29-2). In the absence of ascites, cytologic washings are obtained from the pelvis, right and left paracolic spaces (Fig. 29-3), and the diaphragm (Fig. 29-4). Each site is washed with 100 ml saline solution. The fluid is withdrawn from each area separately and sent for cytology. The sample from the undersurface of the diaphragm is easily col-

lected with the use of a red rubber catheter. Adhesions are freed to permit adequate examination of all intra-abdominal surfaces and viscera, including the under-surface of the diaphragm, small and large bowel, liver, mesentery and residual omentum, gallbladder and spleen. Retroperitoneal lymph nodes are palpated.

Representative samples of the adhesions are sent for histopathologic examination. A laparoscope or sig-moidoscope may be used for examination of liver surface and diaphragm. Any suspicious appearing areas must be biopsied. Multiple random biopsies are obtained from the pelvic cul-de-sac, bladder dome, peritoneum of both pelvic side walls, paracolic gutters, diaphragm (Figs. 29-4 and 29-5), and known sites of residual disease recorded at the previous operation. Portions of both infundibulopelvic ligaments, round ligaments, and pelvic and paraaortic lymph nodes below the renal vessels are biopsied (Figs. 29-5 and 29-6). If present, the uterus, cervix, adnexae, and omentum are removed. If gross tumor is detected, secondary debulking is attempted provided optimal

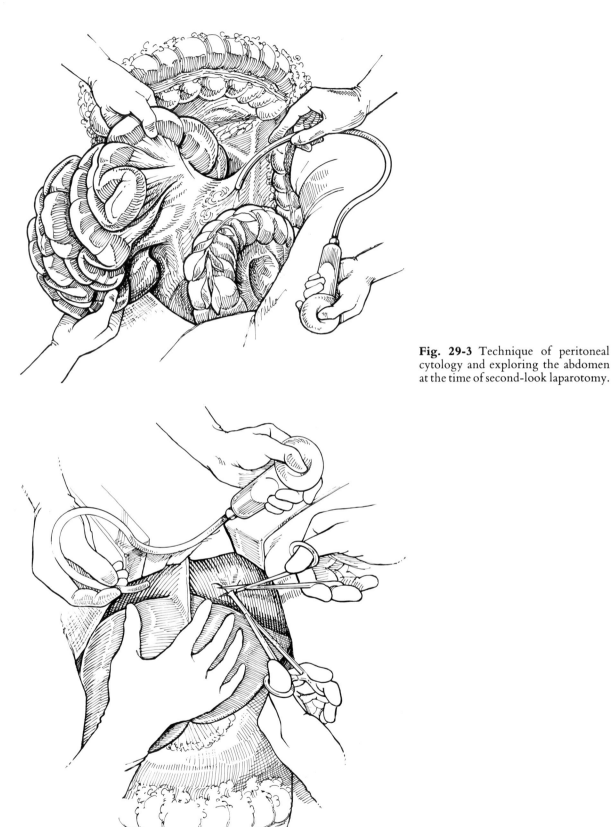

Fig. 29-3 Technique of peritoneal cytology and exploring the abdomen at the time of second-look laparotomy.

Fig. 29-4 Technique of subdiaphragmatic cytology and biopsy.

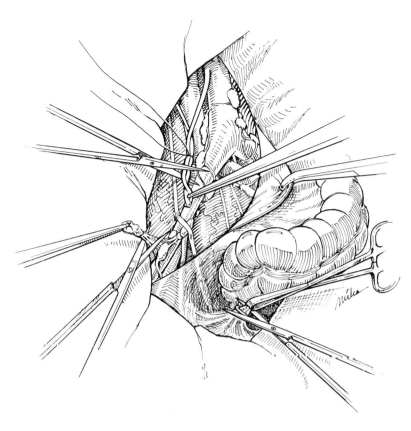

Fig. 29-5 Technique of biopsy of the infundibulopelvic ligament, pelvic lymph node and cul-de-sac peritoneum.

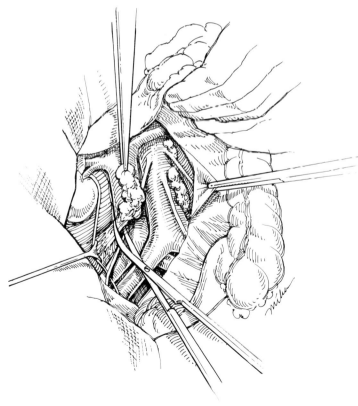

Fig. 29-6 Paraaortic lymph node biopsy.

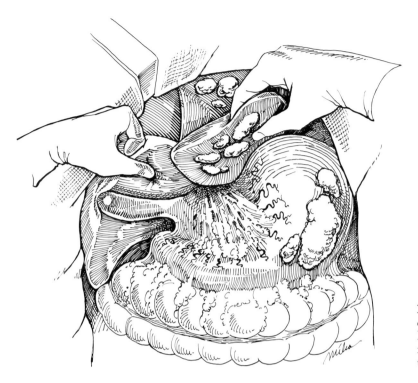

Fig. 29-7 Macroscopic disease encountered at the time of second-look laparotomy that cannot be satisfactorily debulked warrants termination of the procedure.

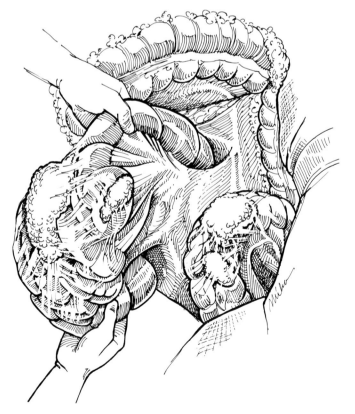

Fig. 29-8 Macroscopic intraperitoneal disease involving small and large bowel.

resection of all tumor appears to be feasible (Figs. 29-7 and 29-8). The aim should be to reduce the size of the largest residual tumor to less than 2 cm in diameter. Resection of the bowel and portions of the urinary tract may be necessary to accomplish this goal. The benefits and risks of urinary or fecal diversion, partial hepatectomy, and removal of other vital organs must be carefully individualized. Frozen section must be used liberally during the procedure and, unless debulking is planned, the procedure is terminated when histologic proof of persistent disease is obtained.

POSTOPERATIVE COMPLICATIONS

Second-look operations are performed in immunocompromised, elderly patients who are poor surgical risks due to their age and various other medical problems. The most common postoperative complications are related to the sampling of retroperitoneal lymph nodes and handling of the bowel. These may include prolonged ileus, intraoperative bleeding, pulmonary atelectasis and embolism or minor complications including wound and urinary tract infections, and deep venous thrombosis. Thrombocytopenia and leucopenia, secondary to chemotherapy and radiation therapy, may promote bleeding and infection. Thrombocytopenia may be exacerbated by prophylactic heparin. The hematocrit, white blood cell count, and platelets should be closely monitored during the perioperative period (Table 29-4). Most patients experience an uneventful postoperative course after second-look surgery, and the benefits appear to outweigh the risks.

SECOND-LOOK LAPAROSCOPY

Laparoscopy is helpful in the diagnosis, staging, and surveillance of various gynecologic neoplasms. It is not an alternative to second-look laparotomy but is a useful adjunct for determining the presence of resectable, unresectable, or diffuse disease following chemotherapy.

Second-look laparoscopy may be indicated (1) prior to second-look laparotomy in selected patients to obviate the need for extensive laparotomy in the event of unresectable disease; (2) for an interval evaluation of response during the course of chemotherapy; and (3) rarely to detect early recurrence in those patients who have undergone a thorough negative second-look laparotomy.

TECHNIQUE

The single-puncture technique is used in most patients. A second puncture for the insertion of ancillary instruments may be required in some patients (Fig. 29-9). The use of a needlescope and open laparoscopy has reduced the major complication rate significantly.[46,47]

Attempts are made to make a clockwise survey of the peritoneal cavity including the pelvis, paracolic gutters, omentum, if present, both hemidiaphragms, liver, stomach, anterior surface of the bowel, colon and their mesenteries. This is facilitated by altering the patient's position on the operating table and by probe manipulation. Lysis of intraperitoneal adhesions may be necessary in select cases. Peritoneal fluid,

Table 29-4 Complications of Second-Look Laparotomy

	Schwartz and Smith (1980)[43]	Curry et al. (1981)[44]	Roberts et al. (1982)[45]
Wound infection	18	1	6
Urinary tract infection	17	1	4
Hemorrhage > 500 cm³	16	—	5
Pulmonary	10	—	2
Other medical	8	1	5
Bowel injury-postoperative	5	—	1
Bowel injury at second-look	2	—	—
Postoperative intestinal obstruction	2	—	—
Other	9	—	—
None	124	24	NS
Total	211	27	23

NS, not specified.

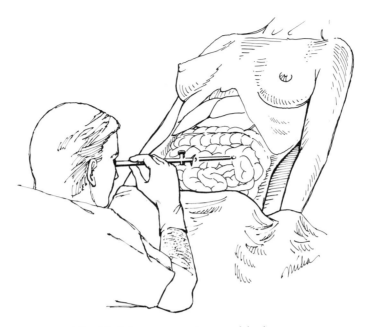

Fig. 29-9 Laparoscopy in second-look surgery.

if present in the cul-de-sac, is aspirated and submitted for cytology. If no fluid is present, approximately 150 ml normal saline is instilled through the puncture site and subsequently aspirated. Biopsy instruments inserted through the secondary puncture site are used to sample suspicious areas on the parietal or visceral peritoneum including the liver and diaphragm. The specimens obtained may be stained with a shortened modification of the classic Papanicolaou (Pap) stain.[48] The absence of tumor on frozen section and lack of malignant cells in the cytologic washings permits the surgeon to proceed with second-look laparotomy while the patient is still under anesthesia.

In the event of persistent disease, resectability is determined and sites of disease carefully documented. If the patient has extensive miliary unresectable disease, then she will not be explored. A Tenckhoff catheter or an infuse-a-port may be inserted at the same setting for intraperitoneal chemotherapy; however, in the event of finding resectable disease, the patient is explored and optimally debulked prior to further therapy. Patients with no laparoscopic evidence of disease are subjected to a second-look exploratory laparotomy.

The use of second-look laparoscopy is limited because of its high false-negative rate, ranging from 20 to 75 percent.[48] In addition, exploration of the peritoneal cavity is often suboptimal because of intraperitoneal adhesions from previous surgery. It is not possible to evaluate retroperitoneal structures, particularly the lymph nodes; thus, second-look laparoscopy should not be used routinely as a method of determining whether to discontinue therapy. It is contraindicated in patients who have received whole abdominal radiation therapy or intraperitoneal ^{32}P. Laparoscopy is of no value in patients who have obvious progressive disease on therapy and present with bowel obstruction.

COMPLICATIONS

The incidence of complications during second-look laparoscopy in various series have ranged from 2.5 to 14 percent. No mortalities have been reported. The complication with the greatest morbidity has been injury to the GI tract with bowel laceration requiring exploratory laparotomy. Other reported complications have included intraabdominal bleeding, injury to the inferior epigastric vessels, pneumothorax, subcutaneous emphysema, and incisional cellulitis.

Table 29-5 reviews the experience of various investigators with second-look laparoscopy in patients with ovarian cancer. In 32 percent of these patients

Table 29-5 Second-Look Laparoscopy in Ovarian Cancer

Investigators	No. of Patients	Persistent Tumor N	%
Rosenoff et al. (1975)[49]	13	5	30
Spinelli et al. (1976)[50]	47	11	23
Smith et al. (1977)[51]	24	14	58
Lacey et al. (1978)[52]	19	5	26
Mangioni et al. (1979)[53]	28	3	11
Quinn et al. (1980)[54]	58	10	17
Piver et al. (1980)[48]	22	8	36
Ozols et al. (1981)[55]	66	33	50
Berek et al. (1981)[46]	57	19	34
Qu et al. (1984)[56]	27	3	11
Xygakis et al. (1984)[57]	46	20	43
	407	131	32

(131 of 407), persistent tumor was found, and a laparoscopy was deemed unnecessary.

RESULTS

The findings at second-look surgery are related to the adequacy of the initial surgery. The three covariates that have been reported independently significant in predicting continued disease free status are the greatest diameter of the largest residual tumor remaining from primary surgery, histologic features of the tumor, and the diameter of the largest tumor aggregate found at initial surgery.[58] The use of cisplatin containing combination chemotherapy and patient under 50 years also were found to be significant variables in obtaining a complete response.

In 1976, Smith et al.[4] stated that the importance of removing all tumor masses larger than 2 cm was a more significant factor than reducing the total tumor volume by a fixed percentage such as 80 percent or even 95 percent, however, this group of patients was treated with single agent chemotherapy. Cohen et al.[59] demonstrated that the size of residual disease following initial cytoreductive surgery did not reduce the incidence of complete clinical remission in patients treated with cisplatin containing combination chemotherapy.[59] This study indicated that effective chemotherapy regimens may overcome the disadvantage of bulky residual disease.

Only approximately 20 to 30 percent of patients with bulky residual disease have a complete clinical response at second-look laparotomy. Of these, only one third are negative at second-look. The recurrence rates in these patients following negative second-look are 15 to 30 percent. Eighty percent of patients with less than 1 cm residual disease undergo second-look surgery. Sixty to 65 percent of these patients have complete pathologic response. Even if 10 to 15 percent of these patients have recurrences within the next 5 years, there is an improvement in 5-year survival in this group of patients.[60]

Second-look laparotomy affords the best diagnostic method available to determine future therapy. Table 29-6 summarizes the experiences in several institutions with second-look surgery for ovarian cancer. A cumulative review of the literature reveals that 23 percent of patients with negative second-look develop recurrence (Table 29-7). Since a negative second-look can no longer be equated with a high probability of cure, several investigators have suggested that patients with negative second-look results should be considered for consolidation therapy with intraperitoneal chemotherapy or whole abdominopelvic radiation therapy (Fig. 29-10).

Copeland et al.[80] studied 46 patients with stage III and IV ovarian cancer who had microscopic residual disease at second-look following combination chemotherapy. This study found that no patient with grade 1 disease and no patient who initially presented before the age of 40 died from disease. By contrast, the 5-year survival rates of patients with grade 3 disease was only 36 percent. Most of the patients had received 12 or more courses of chemotherapy. Several other workers have reiterated optimism with microscopic residual disease in patients with well differentiated cancer.[65,81] They have suggested that, of patients with microscopic residual disease, only those with poorly differentiated cancer were candidates for further therapy, that is either continuing intravenous or intraperitoneal chemotherapy, external radiation therapy, intraperitoneal instillation of radioactive ^{32}P, or perhaps immunotherapy.

Patients with persistent macroscopic disease found at second-look exploratory laparotomy should undergo secondary debulking. Berek et al.[82] found that optimal cytoreduction at second-look, the largest residual tumor less than 2 cm in diameter, significantly prolonged survival. Resection of either the GI or the

Table 29-6 Stage III and IV Ovarian Carcinoma Results of Second-Look Laparotomy

Investigators	No. of Patients	Negative Second-Look	
Wallach (1961)[61]	8	2	25
Mangioni et al. (1975)[62]	10	1	10
Phillips et al. (1979)[63]	21	19	83
Piver et al. (1980)[48]	11	5	45
Schwartz and Smith (1980)[43]	128	26	20
Curry et al. (1981)[44]	14	6	42
Greco et al. (1981)[7]	59	45	76
Park and Hoskins (1981)[64]	25	10	40
Webster and Ballard (1981)[65]	17	10	59
Wharton and Herson (1981)[66]	38	15	39
Roberts et al. (1982)[45]	27	8	29
Stuart et al. (1982)[67]	21	15	71
Webb et al. (1982)[68]	29	10	34
Cohen et al. (1983)[59]	73	29	40
Cohen et al. (1983)[59]	43	20	46
Ehrlich[69] (1983)	30	10	33
Copeland[70] (1983)	246	83	34
Onnis and Maggino (1984)[71]	48	25	52
Ballon et al. (1984)[72]	25	11	44
Barnhill et al. (1984)[73]	37	18	49
Berek et al. (1984)[5]	56	18	32
Rocereto et al. (1984)[74]	20	7	26
Luesley et al. (1984)[75]	50	12	24
Smirz et al. (1985)[76]	64	20	31
Miller et al. (1986)[58]	67	18	27
Dauplat et al. (1986)[77]	44	18	41
Cain et al. (1986)[78]	103	49	47
	1,314	510	39

Table 29-7 Recurrent Cancer Following Negative Second-Look Surgery

Investigators	No. of Recurrences/ No. of Second-Look Surgeries	Recurrence (%)
Mangioni et al. (1975)[62]	1/8	13
Phillips et al. (1979)[63]	1/21	5
Schwartz and Smith (1980)[43]	7/58	12
Curry et al. (1981)[44]	3/17	17
Greco et al. (1981)[7]	1/17	6
Roberts et al. (1982)[45]	6/36	16
Stuart et al. (1982)[67]	2/15	13
Berek and Hacker (1983)[46]	12/21	57
Gershenson et al. (1985)[79]	20/35	35
	53/228	23

urinary tract, or both, with colostomy is justified to achieve these goals. Our experience and the M.D. Anderson study support the favorable effect of optimal cytoreduction, while other investigators have reported unfavorable results.[43,83-85]

Patients with clinically insignificant ascites, less than 1000 ml, had a median survival of 18 months, significantly longer than the 5-month median in patients with clinically apparent ascites. In patients with symptoms of intestinal obstruction, even when sec-

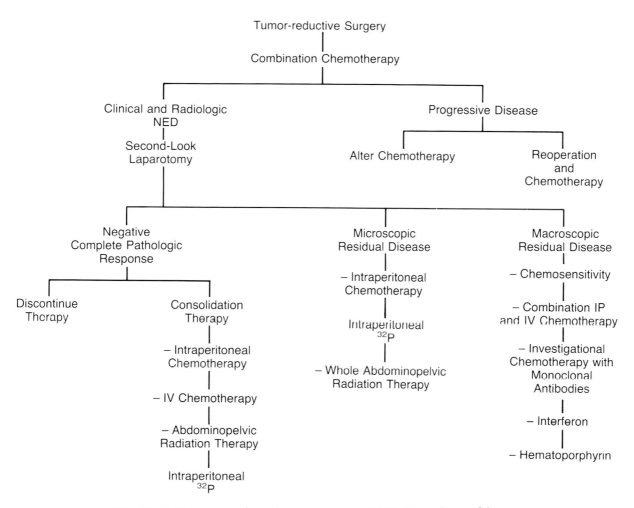

Fig. 29-10 Treatment schema in ovarian cancer. NED, No evidence of disease.

ondary debulking is not feasible, successful palliation was achieved in over 80 percent of the operations. Morbidity is high in this group and 1-year survival only 17 percent; however, in view of the palliation achieved, the morbidity is acceptable and justified.[82]

In conclusion, it appears that although second-look surgery to some extent identifies prognostic groups, it has little influence on survival. Some experts have questioned the value of second-look laparotomy because it does not directly benefit patients without gross tumor. Patients who have macroscopic disease at laparotomy rarely benefit from surgery, since no apparent effective second-line regimens are available for patients who have failed to respond to platinum containing combinations. With these objectives in mind,

alternatives to second-look laparotomy have been proposed. These might include indefinite treatment with cytotoxic chemotherapy, discontinuation of treatment without performing second-look surgery following a definite number of courses or until acceptable toxicity levels have been achieved. Less satisfactory options might include noninvasive radiologic or imaging methods to evaluate persistent tumor or serum markers to screen for the presence of tumor. Continuation of chemotherapy following a predetermined number of courses or discontinuation at the time of acceptable toxicity, may result in certain patients receiving insufficient treatment while others receive prolonged toxic chemotherapy. It is important, however, to delineate those who have persistent minimal disease because these patients may be resistant to further systemic chemotherapy, but responsive to other forms of treatment, such as radiation therapy, immunotherapy, or intraperitoneal chemotherapy.

OTHER GYNECOLOGIC MALIGNANCIES

Many ovarian germ cell tumors produce biologic markers that may be detected in the serum (Table 29-8). Serial measurements of the human chorionic gonadotropin (hCG) and α-fetoprotein (AFP) facilitate the diagnosis of these tumors, aid in detecting early subclinical recurrences, and monitor the response to treatment. Second-look operations are indicated only for those tumors that do not produce biologic markers.[86]

Since these tumors rarely involve the contralateral ovary or uterus, these organs are often preserved for future fertility at the primary surgery. Second-look surgery in these patients does not differ from that done for epithelial ovarian cancer except in the management of the remaining pelvic reproductive organs. The remaining ovary must be biopsied to detect occult cancer, and any ovarian cysts present must be removed intact if possible.

Experience with second-look surgery in patients with endodermal sinus tumor of the ovary is limited because of the availability of AFP as a biomarker. The largest series of patients is from the M.D. Anderson Hospital and Tumor Institute, where 13 of 41 patients with endodermal sinus tumor underwent second-look laparotomy.[87] Twelve of these 13 patients had

negative findings following 12 to 25 courses of vincristine–actinomycin–cytoxan. One patient who had stage III disease received only six courses of this triple-agent regimen and had positive second-look surgery but was negative at the third-look laparotomy after additional chemotherapy. Only one patient had a recurrence after a negative second-look procedure. Recently, two investigators reported negative second-look surgical procedures in patients with endodermal sinus tumor following the use of vinblastine–bleomycin–cisplatin.[88,89]

Anecdotal reports about second-look laparotomy in patients with sex cord stromal tumors have appeared, but the results and survival rates for these patients remain unclear.[90]

In a series of 106 patients with uterine sarcoma, 11 patients underwent re-exploration following chemotherapy and radiation therapy. Eight of these 11 patients had no evidence of disease and remained tumor free until the time of the report. Three patients had persistent disease, two are alive following local resection and continued chemotherapy, and one has died of progressive disease despite additional therapy.[91]

Two patients with stage I adenocarcinoma of the uterus had a second-look laparotomy and one was negative and free of disease after 6 months.[45] The patient with a positive laparotomy had a single focus of disease in the pelvis and is now free of disease after external pelvic irradiation. In 1980, Deppe et al.[92] performed second-look laparotomy in three patients with advanced endometrial carcinoma who had been in clinical remission after at least 1 year of chemotherapy. Two of these three patients had no evidence of residual tumor at second-look laparotomies.

Table 29-8 Clinically Useful Markers in Ovarian Cancer

Histologic Types	Marker
Choriocarcinoma	β-hCG
Dysgerminoma	β-hCG, LDH
Embryonal cell carcinoma	AFP, β-hCG
Endodermal sinus tumor	AFP
Mixed germ cell tumor	β-hCG, AFP, LDH
Immature teratoma	β-hCG, AFP, LDH
Polyembryoma	AFP, β-hCG
Serous cystadenocarcinoma	CA 125, OCA, OCAA
Mucinous cystadenocarcinoma	CEA, OCA, OCAA, CA 19-9

AFP, α-fetoprotein; CEA, carcinoembryonic antigen; β-hCG, β-human chorionic gonadotropin; LDH, lactic dehydrogenase.

THIRD-LOOK SURGERY

Patients with persistent cancer at second-look laparotomy who are placed on continued chemotherapy are at risk of developing potentially lethal drug toxicity. In some of these patients, it is impossible to assess accurately the tumor response to chemotherapy entirely on the basis of clinical findings. Copeland et al.[70] appraised the role of third-look surgery in the management of these patients. Twenty-seven patients with stage III epithelial ovarian cancer underwent third-look surgery. The findings at the third-look laparotomies were highly predictive; however, sufficient preoperative information, in most cases, was available to make the appropriate therapy decisions without the additional information obtained at third-look laparotomy. In Cain's series, 20 of 73 patients with persistent disease at second-look laparotomy and no clinical or radiographic evidence of disease on continued chemotherapy underwent third-look surgery. Nine of the 20 patients had no evidence of disease; however, two have recurred.[78]

In most cases, a careful appraisal of tumor grade, the findings at second-look surgery, and tumor reductive aspects should provide sufficient information to form the basis for discontinuation of chemotherapy; therefore, the role of third-look surgery is extremely limited.

CONCLUSION

Second-look exploratory laparotomy will remain the most reliable method of evaluating the disease status of ovarian cancer patients receiving chemotherapy until specific tumor markers or more sensitive radiographic techniques are developed. This surgery has a definite role in the management of epithelial ovarian malignancies; however, its role in the management of other gynecologic cancers remains ill-defined and limited. The benefits achieved by the ability to excise and delineate areas of residual cancer far outweigh and justify the risks of surgery. The findings at second-look surgery have tremendous prognostic impact on important therapeutic decisions, although its influence on survival mandates further study.

REFERENCES

1. Wangensteen OH: Cancer of the colon and rectum: With special reference to (1) earlier recognition of alimentary tract malignancy; (2) secondary delayed re-entry of the abdomen in patients exhibiting lymph node involvement; (3) subtotal primary excision of the colon; (4) operation in obstruction. Wisc Med J 48:591, 1949
2. Wangensteen OH, Lewis FJ, Arhelger SW, et al: An interim report upon the "second-look" procedure for cancer of the stomach, colon and rectum and for "limited intraperitoneal carcinosis." Surg Gynecol Obstet 99:257, 1954
3. Rutledge F, Burns B: Chemotherapy for advanced ovarian cancer. Am J Obstet Gynecol 96:761, 1966
4. Smith JP, Delgado G, Rutledge F: Second-look operation in ovarian carcinoma—Postchemotherapy. Cancer 38:1438, 1976
5. Berek JS, Hacker NF, Lagasse LD, et al: Second-look laparotomy in Stage III epithelial ovarian cancer. Clinical variables associated with disease status. Obstet Gynecol 64:207, 1984
6. Oldham RK, Julian CG, Johnson DH, et al: Combination chemotherapy and restaging of advanced ovarian carcinoma. p. 165. In Williams CJ, Whitehouse JMA (eds): Recent Advances in Clinical Oncology. Vol. I. Academic Press, London, 1982
7. Greco FA, Julian CG, Richardson RL, et al: Advanced ovarian cancer: Brief intensive combination chemotherapy and second-look operation. Obstet Gynecol 58:199, 1981
8. Sommer FG, Walsh JW, Schwartz PE, et al: Evaluation of gynecologic pelvic masses by ultrasound and computed tomography. J Reprod Med 27:45, 1982
9. Bast RC Jr, Klug TL, John E, et al: A radioimmunoassay using a monoclonal antibody to monitor the course of epithelial ovarian cancer. N Engl J Med 309:883, 1983
10. Berek JS, Knapp RC, Malkasian GD, et al: CA 125 Serum levels correlated with second-look operations among ovarian cancer patients. Obstet Gynecol 67:5, 1986
11. Niloff JM, Bast CC, Schaetzl EM, et al: Predictive value of CA 125 antigen levels in second-look procedures for ovarian cancer. Am J Obstet Gynecol 151:981, 1985
12. Brenner DE, Shaff MI, Jones HW, et al: Abdomino-pelvic computed tomography: Evaluation in patients undergoing second-look laparotomy for ovarian carcinoma. Obstet Gynecol 65:175, 1985
13. Clarke-Pearson DL, Bandy LC, Dudzinski M, et al:

Computed tomography in evaluation of patients with ovarian carcinoma in complete clinical remission. Correlation with surgical-pathologic findings. JAMA 225:627, 1986

14. Pussell SJ, Cosgrove DO, Hinton J, et al: Carcinoma of the ovary—Correlation of ultrasound with second-look laparotomy. Br J Obstet Gynaecol 87:1140, 1980

15. Goldenberg DM, DeLand F, Kim E, et al: Use of radio-labeled antibodies to carcinoembryonic antigen for the detection and localization of diverse cancers by external photoscanning. N Engl J Med 298:1384, 1978

16. Van Nagell JR, Kim E, Casper S, et al: Radioimmuno-detection of primary and metastatic ovarian cancer using radiolabeled antibodies to carcinoembryonic antigen. Cancer Res 40:502, 1980

17. Epenetos AA, Carr D, Johnson PM, et al: Antibody guided radiolocalization of tumors in patients with testicular or ovarian cancer using two radionated monoclonal antibodies to placental alkaline laparoscope phophatase. Br J Radio, 59:117, 1986

18. Knauf S, Urbach GI: Identification, purification and radioimmunoassay of NB/70K, a human ovarian tumor-associated antigen. Cancer 41:1351, 1981

19. Hanjani P, Subba RG: Identification of a 97 kilodalton glycoprotein (97K-GP)—An ovarian epithelial tumor marker. Gynecol Oncol 20:265, 1985 (abst)

20. Bhattacharya M, Barlow JJ: Immunologic studies of human serous cystadenocarcinoma of the ovary. Demonstration of tumor-associated antigens. Cancer 31:588, 1973

21. Bhattacharya M, Barlow JJ: An immunologic comparison between serous cystadenocarcinoma of ovary and other human gynecologic tumors. Am J Obstet Gynecol, 117:849, 1973

22. Bhattacharya M, Barlow JJ: A tumor-associated antigen from cystadenocarcinomas of the ovary. Natl Cancer Inst Monog 42:25, 1975

23. Bhattacharya M, Barlow JJ: Ovarian tumor antigens. Cancer 42:1616, 1978

24. Bhattacharya M, Barlow JJ: Tumor markers for ovarian cancer. Int Adv Surg Oncol 2:155, 1979

25. Bhattacharya M, Barlow JJ: Ovarian Cancer. p. 632. In Herberman RB, McIntire KR (eds): Immunodiagnosis of Cancer. Marcel Dekker, New York, 1979

26. Hamazaki MH, Hotta K: Ovarian cyst fluid specific antigens. Experientia 31:241, 1975

27. Burton RM, Hope NJ, Lubbers LM: A thermostable antigen associated with ovarian cancer. Am J Obstet Gynecol 125:472, 1976

28. Imamura N, Takahashi T, Lloyd KO, et al: Analysis of human ovarian tumor antigens using heterologous antisera. Detection of new antigenic systems. Int J Cancer 21:570, 1978

29. Knauf S, Urbach GI: The development of a double-antibody radioimmunoassay for detecting ovarian tumor-associated antigen fraction OCA in plasma. Am J Obstet Gynecol 131:780, 1978

30. Stolbach LL, Pitt A, Gandbhir L, et al: Ovarian cancer patient antibodies and their relationship to ovarian cancer associated markers. p. 553. In Herberman RB, McIntire KR (eds): Compendium of Assays for Immunodiagnosis of Human Cancer. Elsevier, New York, 1979

31. Bhattacharya M, Chatterjee SK: Antigen markers in ovarian cancer. Am Assoc Cancer Res 21:216, 1980 (abst).

32. Dawson JR, Kuttch WH, Whitesides DB, Gall SA: Identification of tumor-associated antigens and their purification from cyst fluids of ovarian epithelial neoplasma. Gynecol Oncol 10:6, 1980

33. Charpin C, Bhan AD, Zurawski VR Jr, Sculley RE: Carcinoembryonic antigen (CEA) and carbohydrate determinant 19-9 (CA 19-9) localization in 121 primary and metastatic ovarian tumors: An immunohistochemical study with the use of monoclonal antibodies. Int J Gynecol Pathol 1:231, 1982

34. Order SE, Thurston J, Knapp R: Ovarian tumor antigens: A new potential for therapy. Natl Cancer Inst Monog 42:33, 1975

35. Svanberg L, Astedt B: Coagulative and fibrinolytic properties of ascitic fluid associated with ovarian tumors. Cancer 35:1382, 1975

36. Burton RM, Hope NJ, Beyerle MP, Espinosa E: Tissue antigens in ovarian carcinoma. Oncology 34:146, 1977

37. Bara J, Malarewicz A, Loisillier F, Burtin P: Antigens common to human ovarian mucinous cyst fluid and gastric mucosa. Br J Cancer 36:49, 1977

38. Pant KD, Dahlman HL, Goldenberg DM: Further characterization of CSAP, and antigen associated with gastrointestinal and ovarian tumors. Cancer 42:1626, 1978

39. Hirsh-Marie H, Bara J, Loisillier F, Buyrtin P: Evidence of pepsinogen in ovarian tumors. Eur J Cancer 14:593, 1978

40. Metzgar RS, Gaillard MT, Levine SJ, et al: Antigens of human pancreatic adenocarcinoma cells defined by murine monoclonal antibodies. Cancer Res 42:601, 1982

41. Colnaghi MI, Canaveri S, Dellatorre G, et al: Monoclonal antibodies directed against human tumors. p. 55. In Proceedings of the Thirteenth International Cancer Congress, 1982

42. Atack DB, Nisker JA, Allen HH, et al: CA 125 surveillance and second-look laparotomy in ovarian carcinoma. Am J Obstet Gynecol 154:278, 1986

43. Schwartz PE, Smith JP: Second-look operations in ovarian cancer. Am J Obstet Gynecol 138:1124, 1980

44. Curry SL, Dembo MM, Nahhas WA, et al: Second-

look laparotomy for ovarian cancer. Cancer 11:114, 1981

45. Roberts WS, Hodel K, Rich WM, DiSaia PJ: Second-look laparotomy in the management of gynecologic malignancy. Gynecol Oncol 13:345, 1982
46. Berek JS, Hacker NF: Laparoscopy in the management of patients with ovarian carcinoma. Clin Obstet Gynecol 10:213, 1983
47. Hassan HM: A modified instrument and method for laparoscopy. Am J Obstet Gynecol 110:886, 1971
48. Piver MS, Shashikant BL, Barlow JJ, Gamarra M: Second-look laparoscopy prior to proposed second-look laparotomy. Obstet Gynecol 55:571, 1980
49. Rosenoff SH, Young RC, Anderson T, et al: Peritoneoscopy in the staging and follow-up of ovarian cancer. Semin Oncol 2:223, 1975
50. Spinelli P, Pilotti S, Suini A, et al: Laparoscopy combined with peritoneal cytology in staging and restaging ovarian carcinoma. Tumori 65:601, 1979
51. Smith WG, Day TG, Smith JP: The use of laparoscopy to determine the results of chemotherapy for ovarian cancer. J Reprod Med 18:257, 1977
52. Lacey CG, Morrow CP, DiSaia PJ, et al: Laparoscopy in the evaluation of gynecologic cancer. Obstet Gynecol 52:708, 1978
53. Mangioni C, Bolis G, Molteni P, Belloni C: Indications, advantages and limits of laparoscopy in ovarian cancer. Gynecol Oncol 7:47, 1979
54. Quinn, AM, Bishop GJ, Campbell JJ, et al: Laparoscopic follow up of patients with ovarian carcinoma. Br J Obstet Gynecol 87:1132, 1980
55. Ozols RF, Fisher RI, Anderson T, et al: Peritoneoscopy in the management of ovarian cancer. Am J Obstet Gynecol 140:611, 1981
56. Qu JY, Sun AD, Lien LC: Laparoscopy in the diagnosis and management of ovarian cancer. J Reprod Med 29:483, 1984
57. Xygakis AM, Politis GS, Michalas SP, Kaskarelis DB: Second-look laparotomy in ovarian cancer. J Reprod Med 29:583, 1984
58. Miller DS, Ballon SC, Teng NNH, et al: A critical reassessment of second-look laparotomy in epithelial ovarian carcinoma. Cancer 57:530, 1986
59. Cohen CJ, Goldberg JD, Holland JT, et al: Improved therapy with cisplatin regimens for patients with ovarian carcinoma (FIGO Stages III and IV) as measured by surgical end-staging (second-look operation). Am J Obstet Gynecol 145:955, 1983
60. Averette HJ, Cohen CJ, Hoskins W, Nelson JH: Ovarian CA: Optimal chemotherapy regimens. Contemp Obstet Gynecol 28:108, 1986
61. Wallach RC, Blinick G: The second-look operation for carcinoma of the ovary. Surg Gynecol Obstet 131:1, 1970

62. Mangioni C, Mattioli G, Natale N: The second-look operation in long-term therapy of ovarian malignancies. p. 15. In Excerpta/American Elsevier, New York, 1975
63. Phillips BD, Buchsbaum HJ, Lifshitz S: Re-exploration after treatment for ovarian carcinoma. Gynecol Oncol 8:339, 1979
64. Park RC, Hoskins WJ: Re-operating to assess ovarian cancer treatment. Contemp Obstet Gynecol 17:159, 1981
65. Webster KD, Ballard LA: Ovarian carcinoma. Second-look laparotomy postchemotherapy: preliminary report. Cleve Clin Q 48:365, 1981
66. Wharton JT, Herson J: Surgery for common epithelial tumors of the ovary. Cancer 48:582, 1981
67. Stuart GC, Jeffries M, Stuart JL, Anderson RJ: The changing role of second-look laparotomy in the management of epithelial carcinoma of the ovary. Am J Obstet Gynecol 142:612, 1982
68. Webb MJ, Snyder JA Jr, Williams TJ, Decker DG: Second-look laparotomy in ovarian cancer. Gynecol Oncol 14:285, 1982
69. Ehrlich CE, Einhorn LG, Stehman FB Response RL: "Second-look" status and survival in Stage III–IV epithelial ovarian cancer treated with cis-diamminedichloroplatinum (II) (cis-platinum, Adriamycin (ADR), and cyclophosphamide (CTX). Am Assoc Cancer Res 21:423, 1980 (abst)
70. Copeland LJ, Wharton JT, Rutledge FN, et al: Role of "third-look" laparotomy in the guidance of ovarian cancer treatment. Gynecol Oncol 15:145, 1983
71. Onnis A, Maggino T: Repetitive debulking surgery as adjuvant to chemotherapy in advanced epithelial ovarian cancer. Clin Exp Obstet Gynecol 11:21, 1984
72. Dallon SC, Portuff JC, Sikic BI, et al: Second-look laparotomy in epithelial ovarian carcinoma: Precise definition, sensitivity, and specificity of the operative procedure. Gynecol Oncol 17:154, 1984
73. Barnhill DR, Hoskins WJ, Heller PB, Park RC: The second-look surgical reassessment of epithelial ovarian carcinoma. Gynecol Oncol 19:148, 1984
74. Rocereto TF, Mangan CE, Guintoli RL, et al: The second-look celiotomy in ovarian cancer. Gynecol Oncol 19:34, 1984
75. Luesley DM, Chan KK, Fielding JWL, et al: Second-look laparotomy in the management of epithelial ovarian carcinoma: An evaluation of fifty cases. Obstet Gynecol 64:421, 1984
76. Smirz LR, Shehman FB, Ulbright TM, et al: Second-look laparotomy after chemotherapy in the management of ovarian malignancy. Am J Obstet Gynecol 152:661, 1985
77. Dauplat J, Ferriere J, Gorbinet M, et al: Second-look

laparotomy in managing epithelial ovarian carcinoma. Cancer 57:1627, 1986

78. Cain JM, Saigo PE, Pierce VK, et al: A review of second-look laparotomy for ovarian cancer. Gynecol Oncol 23:14, 1986

79. Gershenson DM, Copeland LJ, Wharton JT, et al: Prognosis of surgically determined complete responders in advanced ovarian cancer. Cancer 55:1129, 1985

80. Copeland LJ, Gershenson DM, Wharton JT, et al: Microscopic disease at second-look laparotomy in advanced ovarian cancer. Cancer 55:472, 1985

81. Nevin JE, Pinzon G, Baggerly TJ, et al: The use of intravenous phenylalanine mustard followed by supervoltage irradiation in the treatment of carcinoma of the ovary. Cancer 51:1273, 1983

82. Berek JS, Hacker NF, Lagasse LD, et al: Survival of patients following secondary cytoreductive surgery in ovarian cancer. Obstet Gynecol 61:189, 1983

83. Raju KS, McKinna JA, Barker GH, et al: Second-look laparotomy in the management of epithelial cell carcinoma of the ovary. Am J Obstet Gynecol 144:650, 1982

84. Mead GM, Williams CJ, MacBeth FR, et al: Second-look laparotomy in the management of epithelial cell carcinoma of the ovary. Br J Cancer 50:185, 1984

85. Malcolm W, Hainsworth JD, Johnson DH, et al: Advanced minimal residual ovarian carcinoma: Abdominopelvic irradiation following combination chemotherapy. Am Soc Clin Obstet 2:150, 1983 (abst)

86. Carlson RW, Sikic BI, Turbow MM, et al: Combination Cisplatin, Vinblastine and Bleomycin chemotherapy PVB) for malignant germ cell tumors of the ovary. J Clin Oncol 1:645, 1983

87. Gershenson DM, Junco GD, Herson J, et al: Endodermal sinus tumor of the ovary: The M.D. Anderson experience. Obstet Gynecol 61:194, 1983

88. Julian CG, Barrett JM, Richardson RL, et al: Bleomycin, vinblastine, and cisplatinum in the treatment of advanced endodermal sinus tumor. Obstet Gynecol 56:396, 1980

89. Lokey JL, Baker JJ, Price NA, et al: Cisplatin, Vinblastine and Bleomycin for endodermal sinus tumor of the ovary. Ann Intern Med 94:56, 1981

90. Schwartz PE: Current status of the second-look operation in ovarian cancer. Clins Obstet Gynecol 10:245, 1983

91. Hannigan EV, Freedman RS, Elder KS, Rutledge FN: Re-exploration after treatment of uterine sarcoma. Gynecol Oncol 16:1, 1983

92. Deppe G, Jacobs AJ, Cohen CJ: Second-look operation in endometrial cancer. Diagn Gynecol Obstet 2:193,1980

30

Surgical Management of Invasive Carcinoma of the Vulva

James H. Nelson, Jr.
Marcia C. Bowling

Radical surgery is almost unanimously accepted as the definitive treatment of choice for certain malignant lesions of the vulva: lesions greater than 2 cm in diameter or smaller lesions with evidence of lymph vascular space involvement by tumor emboli. This opinion reflects years of careful management of many vulvar cancer patients.

There have been several modifications of the original operation first described by Bassett[1] in 1912. The significance of Bassett's contribution stems from its rationale, namely, en bloc removal of the entire vulva along with the regional lymph nodes bilaterally. This procedure did not gain wide acceptance until much later, when it was introduced to the United States by Taussig[2] in 1941. He proved its superiority over other less extensive procedures (Table 30-1). Shortly thereafter, on the basis of Taussig's report, Bassett's[1] and Taussig's[2] philosophies, and Stoeckel's[3] suggestion of an extraperitoneal approach, Way[4] devised a more radical operation. His procedure resulted in the international adoption of radical surgery.

A detailed report by Green et al.[5,6] summarized characteristics of vulvar malignancy correlated to appropriate management. The conclusions deserve review here.

RADICAL VULVECTOMY

The localized lesion may be of multicentric origin and diffuse. Rutledge[7] found that 10 to 20 percent of patients with vulvar cancer had more than two grossly apparent sites of invasive disease. After evaluation 238 specimens by gross and histologic examinations, Green et al.[6] found that 20 percent had multiple independent foci of carcinoma. These workers suggested that the reported incidence of multicentric lesions was understated because of the difficulty of evaluating specimens in which the entire vulva was replaced by carcinoma. Both studies conclude that since one of five vulvar cancers have multicentric foci of origin, radical vulvectomy is the treatment of choice (Fig. 30-1).

BILATERAL GROIN LYMPH NODE DISSECTION

Cancer of the vulva has frequently metastasized to regional lymph nodes at the time of diagnosis and treatment[2,8-12] (Table 30-2). The incidence of positive nodes may reflect the acumen of the examiner. It

Table 30-1 Results of Radical Surgery for Malignant Lesions of the Vulva: Taussig's Modified Approach

Type of Treatment	No. of Cases	5-year Survival	Percent
Double-sided Bassett with vulvectomy	41	24	58.5
Superficial or one-sided adenectomy	21	6	28.6
Vulvectomy only	12	1	8.2
Radium (mostly advanced)	21	1	4.8
Palliative measures	6	0	0
Totals	101	32	33

(Taussig FJ: Results in treatment of lymph node metastasis in cancer of the cervix and the vulva. AJR 45:813, 1941. © American Roentgen Ray Society, 1941.)

is known that serial sections of lymph nodes will increase the frequency with which metastatic disease is found.

Green et al.[8] found that among those cases with lymph node metastases, 53 percent showed bilateral spread. Seven percent had metastases only to contralateral groin nodes. Collins and associates[11] reported that with a unilateral lesion, contralateral nodes were positive only when ipsilateral nodes were positive. Way's[4] findings agreed with those of Green and co-workers, with his report of 8 percent of lymph node metastases found in the contralateral groin only. For this reason, every patient with invasive vulvar cancer should undergo bilateral groin node dissection.

Preoperative clinical assessment is considered unreliable for predicting metastases. Way[10] found that of 81 patients with nonpalpable inguinal lymph nodes, 43 percent actually had metastatic disease.

Some tumors can be treated with less radical surgery. Rutledge et al.[11] identified patients with lesions less than 2 cm in diameter invading less than 5 mm deep as candidates for vulvectomy only, especially if complicated by poor medical status.

Extensive analysis of lymph node metastases demonstrate node status to be an important prognostic indicator. The indications for deep pelvic node (e.g., iliac, hypogastric) and paraaortic node dissections based on the findings in the groin nodes have been outlined by Green et al.[8] and Way[10] Green and associates did not find a single case of metastasis to the deep pelvic nodes, when the groin lymph nodes were negative for metastatic disease. Way found a 3 percent incidence of positive pelvic nodes in patients with negative groin nodes. Some workers suggest that in the case of grossly positive groin nodes, deep pelvic node dissection may be performed at the time of primary surgery. In the absence of grossly positive groin nodes, deep pelvic node dissection may be performed about 6 weeks later. The transperitoneal approach taken also permits paraaortic node sampling. The sig-

Table 30-2 Incidence of Lymph Node Metastases

Investigators	No. of Cases Reported	No. of Cases with Positive Nodes	Percent
Green et al.[8]	238	140	59
Taussig[2]	41	19	46.3
Boutselis[9]	60	24	40
Way[10]	84	44	52.3
Collins et al.[11]	98	31	31.6
Way[4]	81	45	61
Rutledge et al.[12]	86	33	38.4
JH Nelson Jr	70	27	38.5

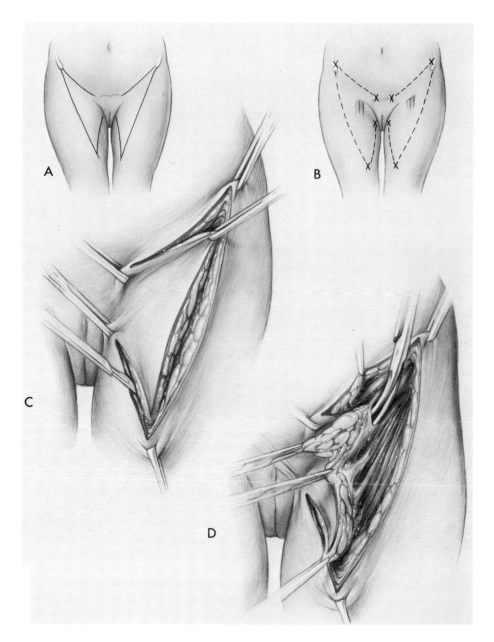

Fig. 30-1 Author's preferred procedure for radical vulvectomy and groin dissection. (**A**) Surface anatomy showing the skin and the subcutaneous tissues to be included in the resection. (**B**) Anatomic points, or landmarks, of the incisions. The incision above is made parallel and superior to the inguinal ligament. Then, the other two limbs of the incision attempt to follow the borders of the femoral triangle. (**C**) The three parts of the incision are made before any dissection is actually done. Otherwise, the skin retracts and distorts the area the surgeon intends to remove. (**D**) After the incisions have been made, dissection is begun and usually proceeds from lateral to medial, as it is being done here *(Figure continues.)*

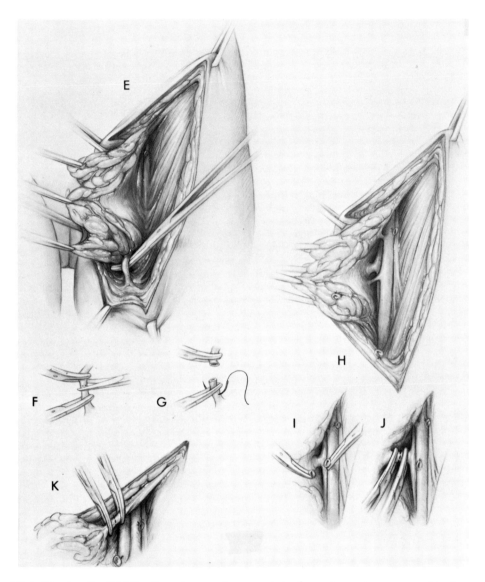

Fig. 30-1 *(Continued).* **(E)** The dissection continues, and the femoral vessels are exposed in the upper aspect of the dissection. Just medial to the apex of the inferior part of the incision the greater saphenous vein will be encountered. **(F)** This is clamped and transected, and the distal stump is transfixed with a 0 polypropylene suture ligature. **(G)** Ligation of the saphenous vein. **(H)** As the dissection progresses, the vessels in the femoral triangle are more fully exposed, and the junction of the greater saphenous vein and the femoral vein is dissected free. **(I)** The deep external pudendal artery is clamped, cut, and ligated at about this point. This artery is not always present in this location **(J)** Clamps are shown on the greater saphenous vein just before it joins the femoral vein. The stump is ligated with a 0 polyprophylene suture ligature. **(K)** The round ligament is encountered as it exits from the external ring. It is doubly clamped, cut, and ligated to permit the dissection to proceed en bloc *(Figure continues.)*

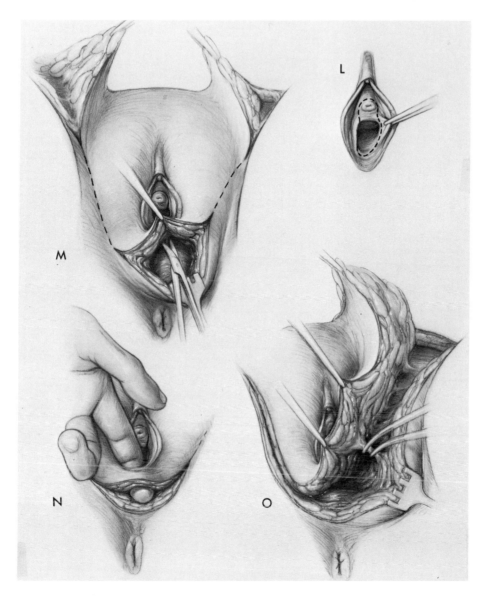

Fig. 30-1 *(Continued).* **(L)** The inner or vaginal incision is made along the dotted line, if the malignant lesion is out on the vulva. If the lesion is closer to the hymeneal ring or in the periurethral or perianal area, a very different incision may be necessary. It may require resection of the rectum with a colostomy. Partial resection of the urethra may have to be done. Each case must be individualized, according to the location of the lesion. Here, the most common incision is shown. It is used for the early lesion on the anterior half of the vulva, usually the labia majora. **(M)** The perineal incision is started just anterior to the anus, and the dissection is carried along the anterior rectal wall until the vaginal incision made in **(L)** is reached. **(N)** The incisions shown in **(L)** and **(M)** have been joined, and now the vulvectomy is begun. **(O)** The creases marking the lateral margins of the labia majora are used as guides for the vulvectomy incision, unless there is a bulky lesion spreading out toward this area. The internal pudendal vessels are exposed and clamped *(Figure continues.)*

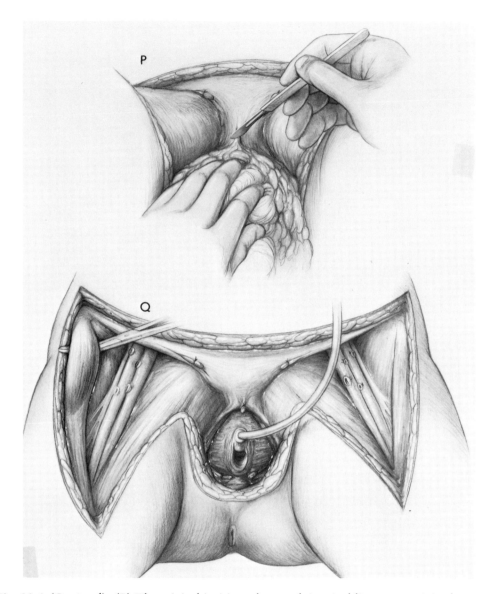

Fig. 30-1 *(Continued).* **(P)** The original incisions along each inguinal ligament are joined across the pubic symphysis. The dissection is then carried down over the symphysis. The stalks of the clitoris are transected and ligated in the process. **(Q)** Upon completion of the dissection, the sartorius muscles are mobilized (right side). The levator stumps are also tied into the vagina to build a structure more like a perineum *(Figure continues.)*

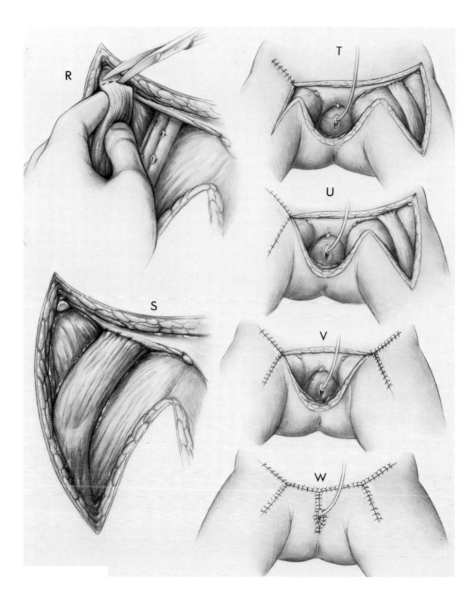

Fig. 30-1 *(Continued)*. (**R**) The sartorius is dissected to its origin. It can be transected at that point, and no bleeding will result (**S**) It is then swung medially to cover the femoral artery and vein. This step is extremely important. It is effective in preventing necrosis of the femoral artery. This complication was not uncommon before we adopted this step, but it has not occurred since. (**T**) Beginning closure of the incision. It is always started in the groin area using 3-0 chromic catgut sutures in the subcutaneous layer and 4-0 polyprophylene skin sutures. (**U**) Continuing the closure in the femoral triangle area. (**V**) Both groin areas have been closed. Drains are placed on each side up to the top of the inguinal incisions. The drains exit below the femoral triangle and are connected to continuous suction immediately. (**W**) Closure of the preineum and vaginal part is carried out with 2-0 chromic catgut. Suction drainage must be continued for 10 days, if it is to promote healing of the skin flaps. Pressure dressings, theoretically, are not sound as a means of promoting healing because of the risk of producing more severe ischemia in the skin by pressure *(Figure continues.)*

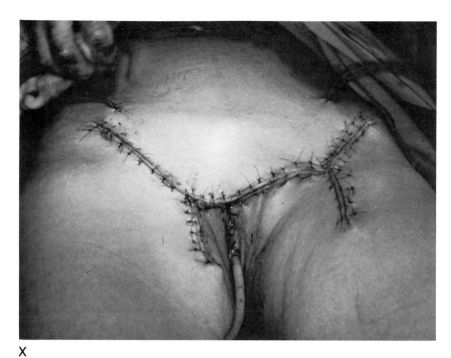

X

Fig. 30-1 *(Continued).* (**X**) Postoperative view of closing technique. (Figs. 30-1A–W from Nelson JH: Atlas of Radical Pelvic Surgery. 2nd Ed., Appleton-Century-Crofts, New York, 1977.)

nificance of lymph node involvement is shown in Table 30-3 (refs. 4, 8, 10, 11, 13). The influence of node status on 5-year survival rates at four institutions is listed. Numbers are corrected for deaths from intercurrent disease. In general, 5-year survival rates were reduced by about 50 percent with lymph node metastases, with about 40 percent surviving 5 years.

Green et al.[8] stressed the need for adequate therapy for vulvar cancer because of the high potential for cure. Before radical surgery was accepted, 5-year sur-

vival rates were 25 percent. Taussig[2] achieved a two-fold improvement by following Bassett's method of operation. This is particularly impressive because he worked before anesthesiology was a specialty and before the era of antibiotics and blood banking.

Further assessment of the results of adequate surgical therapy gives further insight about the curability of vulvar cancer. It is clear that in patients with lymph node metastases, prognosis was determined by the nodes involved. According to Green et al.,[8] if the

Table 30-3 Relative Survival Rates After Adequate Surgery With or Without Metastases to Lymph Nodes

		5-year Survival						Overall 5-year Survival (%)
		Negative Nodes			Positive Nodes			
Investigators	Total Cases	Total N[a]	(%)	Survivors[b]	Total N[a]	(%)	Survivors[b]	
Green et al.[8]	65	29	86	25	36	47.2	17	61[c]
Collins et al.[11]	51	32	68.7	22	19	21	4	51
McKelvey and Adcock[13]	106	75	74.6	56	31	29	9	61.3
Way[4,10]	134	75	88	66	59	49.1	29	70
	356	(211)	76.5	(169)	(145)	40.6	(59)	64

[a] Total number being considered.
[b] Number of patients alive after 5 years.
[c] Overall survival takes into account four operative deaths not shown in node groups.

metastases were limited to one groin, 86 percent of patients survived 5 years. This figure was similar to that for patients with negative nodes. With bilateral groin node involvement, 60 percent of patients were alive and well at 5 years. Metastases to deep pelvic nodes were associated with poor prognosis. If metastases were unilateral, 33 percent survived 5 years. If spread was bilateral, the prognosis was very grave, with only 12.5 percent surviving 5 years.

Collins et al.[14] described the influence of lesion size on curability. These investigators correlated the diameter of the vulvar cancer with the incidence of lymph node metastases. They found that as the greatest diameter of the lesion increased, the incidence of lymph node metastases increased as well. Way agreed that such a correlation exists, but Green did not find support. There are too many exceptions to generalize about lesion size and node metastasis, hence regarding lesion size and survival.

Extension of disease beyond the vulva seems to be an important determinant of survival. McKelvey and Adcock[13] reported 5-year survivals of 62.6 percent, regardless of lesion size, as long as there was no extension to the urethra, vagina, or anus. When there was involvement of any of these structures, only 22.7 percent survived 5 years. Green et al.[8] and Boutselis[9] found survival statistics to be even worse with extension to the urethra, vagina, or anus. As a result, pelvic exenteration is used more liberally as part of the primary therapy combined with radical vulvectomy and groin node dissections. Thornton and Flanagan[15] described 12 such operations done as primary therapy for vulvar cancer with involvement of the urethra, vagina, and/or anus. One-third survived more than 5 years. Similar findings have been described by Daily et al.[5] and others. Exenteration therefore has a role in the primary therapy of vulvar cancer in selected cases.

COMPLICATIONS OF SURGERY

Mortality

Operative mortality rates reported in the medical literature are shown in Table 30-4 (refs. 8, 10, 11, 13, 16). Reasons for the discrepancies are not entirely clear. One explanation may be that Way includes hospital deaths when calculating operative mortality. Many prefer this terminology because it includes death during surgery and during the hospitalization for that surgery, regardless of the number of intercurrent days. Operative mortality usually refers to deaths within 28 days of surgery. High hospital death rates are not unanticipated, since vulvar cancer is a disease of older women. Green et al.[8] found no increase in operative mortality when they compared a one step radical vulvectomy with groin and deep pelvic node dissection, to the operation done in two phases. The operative mortality was 6 percent. Twenty years later, Green's operative death rate was 3.5 percent with cardiac arrest and pulmonary embolism as causes of death.[16] More recently, Morley[17] found the overall operative mortality comparable at 3.9 percent, with a 1.8 percent surgical mortality and a 2.1 percent hospital mortality.

Postoperative Morbidity

The primary complication after radical vulvar surgery is wound infection that includes ischemic necrosis of the skin edges. Way[10] stated that one half the groin wounds healed by primary intention and that all vulvar wounds became infected to some extent. In their 1927 to 1950 series, Green and associates found that 80 percent of patients required subsequent secondary wound closure or skin grafts. At that time, the incision involved wide undermining of the upper and

Table 30-4 Operative Mortality

Investigators	No. of Cases Reported	No. of Operative Deaths	Percent
Way[10]	146	28	19.1
Collins et al.[11]	78	8	10.2
McKelvey and Adcock[13]	116	6	5.1
Green et al.[8]	131	8	6.0
Green[16]	142	5	3.5

lower skin flaps, which permitted excellent surgical exposure but was associated with high morbidity. In 1962, the surgical technique was modified with more limited undermining of the skin flaps.[16] This reduced the postoperative hospital stay by 50 percent and the need for secondary closure or skin grafts to 13 percent.

Thrombophlebitis is a potential complication after radical vulvectomy, seen in 7 percent of patients in Green's early series. Similar experiences are reported by others.

Late sequelae include edema and stress urinary incontinence. Some degree of edema of the lower extremities is consistently reported in all reviews. Green and associates[8] described transient edema in 14 percent, moderate persistent edema in 7 percent, and severe persistent edema in 5 percent of cases. McKelvey and Adcock[13] report persistent edema, frequently following radical vulvectomy and groin node dissection. Moderate edema usually begins 3 to 4 months postoperatively, resolving in about 2 years, as lymphatic channels regenerate.

Stress urinary incontinence may also be a late complication of radical vulvectomy, particularly with resection of more than 2 mm of the urethra. This issue is complicated by the age group under consideration, since this is a problem often seen with obesity or aging in women who have not undergone any operation.

The radical vulvectomy and groin node dissection technique is clearly improved with a two-team approach. Simultaneous vulvar and groin surgery can be performed, thereby shortening the operating time significantly, lessening the pulmonary complications and reducing the incidence of wound infection.

MANAGEMENT OF PREINVASIVE AND EARLY INVASIVE CARCINOMA OF THE VULVA

The problem of carcinoma of the vulva has changed dramatically over the past 25 years. This is best illustrated by an article published in the American literature by Woodruff some years ago, in which he demonstrated a marked shift from invasive carcinoma of the vulva to carcinoma in situ and microinvasive disease of the vulva.[18] Green had shown a somewhat similar shift in the stage of the disease, when he dem-

onstrated that in 25 years the incidence of lymph node involvement in the inguinal areas was 50 percent less than it had been 25 years earlier. Woodruff, on the other hand, demonstrated that whereas invasive carcinoma of the vulva in the early Hopkins series made up 3 of every 4 cases, their later studies, 20 years later, showed a reduction to the point where preinvasive carcinoma of the vulva made up 50 percent of cases. These experiences have been documented over and over again by oncologists around the country and the world. Of equal importance for the practicing gynecologist is the fact that as this shift is taking place the patients are younger and younger. This creates obvious problems for the gynecologist because it means that sexual function becomes a greater part of the problem of treatment. If one is dealing with a 75- or 80-year-old patient and has an invasive carcinoma of the vulva to deal with, that is relatively simple. On the other hand, if one is dealing with a 35-year-old woman with an extensive carcinoma in situ of the vulva or a microinvasive carcinoma of the vulva, the problem is quite different. As my former instructor might have said, deliver me from doing a vulvectomy on a sexually active woman.

The changes in the natural history and clinical manifestations of this disease may have come about by the medical education of the layman in this country. It is not clear from reports in the literature as to whether the same changes are occurring in other developed countries as well. Of major importance in the epidemiology of this disease is the clear-cut fact that virtually all these young women who develop extensive carcinoma in situ of the vulva and early invasive carcinoma of the vulva are heavy smokers. The logical explanation for this association has a two-part association. First, it is well known that certain excretion products from tobacco appear in the urine, the spilling of urine onto the vulva, as is inevitable may be the constant irritation that leads to neoplastic changes in the epithelium. Second, anyone who has been a heavy smoker is aware of the nicotine staining of the fingers used to hold the cigarette. This presents a problem similar to painting coal tars on the back of rats, which invariably produces a malignant lesion on the skin on the back of the rat. We hear almost daily of new associations between malignancies and tobacco; however, this one seems to have a logical explanation which make it difficult to refute an association between tobacco and vulvar carcinoma.

Materials

The main subject of this discussion consists of 24 cases of carcinoma in situ and microinvasive carcinoma of the vulva, which the author encountered in an 8-year period. The oldest patient in this group was 42 and the youngest 21 years of age. Most of these had extensive lesions requiring removal of the labia minora, but in all cases the clitoris could be salvaged and retained as a normal anatomic structure. In two cases, it was easy to do a local excision and primary repair, but in all other 22 cases, it was deemed necessary to take skin grafts and apply them in order to reconstruct the vulva and retain good anatomic appearance and function. Two patients with a microinvasive lesion had recurrence in the form of an in situ carcinoma at the edge of the skin graft. Three different clinical types of lesions were seen one showing a fiery-red but velvety lesion that was macular on gross examination. The second type was a warty papular lesion that could involve the entire vulva (at least in one case). The third had the classic appearance of lichen sclerosis, with marked white changes in the epithelium. In the two cases with this type of lesion, the white lesion was sharply demarcated from the surrounding vulvar epithelium.

Methods

The approach followed in treating these patients was that first reported by Dr. Rutledge from the M. D. Anderson Hospital. Dr. Rutledge described this as a skinning vulvectomy, although I prefer the term superficial vulvectomy with skin grafting where the lesions were extensive. In all these patients in whom skin grafting was done, a 100 percent take was achieved. All of the surgery was carried out by the author and his tumor fellows in training in gynecologic oncology. It is a very satisfactory operation that leaves the anatomic appearance of the vulva very close to normal and sexual function has been excellent in all of these patients. The skin graft was taken from the high gluteal region posteriorly and the graft donor site allowed to re-epithelialize. The graft was applied to the vulva using a pressure type of application with the skin graft sutures tied over cotton pledgets to apply pressure to the graft site.

REFERENCES

1. Bassett T: Traitement chirugical operatoire de l'epithelioma primitif du clitoris. Rev Chir Orthop 46:546, 1912
2. Taussig FJ: Results in treatment of lymph node metastasis in cancer of the cervix and the vulva. AJR 45:813, 1941
3. Stoeckel W: Zur. Therapie des Vulvakarzinomas. Zentralbe Gynaekol 54:47, 1930
4. Way S: The anatomy of the lymphatic drainage of the vulva and its influence on the radical operation for carcinoma. Ann R Coll Surg Engl 3:187, 1948
5. Daily LJ, Kaplan AL, Kaufman RH: Exenteration for advanced carcinoma of the vulva. Obstet Gynecol 36:845, 1970
6. Green TH Jr, Ulfelder H, Meigs JV: Epidermoid carcinoma of the vulva: An analysis of 238 cases. Part I. Etiology and diagnosis. Am J Obstet Gynecol 75:834, 1958
7. Rutledge FN: Cancer of the vulva and vagina. Clin Obstet Gynecol 8:1051, 1965
8. Green TH Ulfelder H, Meigs JV: Epidermoid carcinoma of the vulva: An analysis of 238 cases. Part II. Therapy and end results. Am J Obstet Gynecol 75:848, 1958
9. Boutselis JG: Radical vulvectomy for invasive squamous cell carcinoma of the vulva. Obstet Gynecol 39:827, 1972
10. Way S: Carcinoma of the vulva. Am J Obstet Gynecol 79:692, 1960
11. Collins CG, Collins JH, Barclay DL, Nelson EW: Cancer involving the vulva. A report on 109 consecutive cases. Am J Obstet Gynecol 87:62, 1963
12. Rutledge FN, Smith JP, Franklin EW: Carcinoma of the vulva. Am J Obstet Gynecol 106:1117, 1970
13. McKelvey JL, Adcock LL: Cancer of the vulva. Obstet Gynecol 26:455, 1965
14. Collins CG, Lee FYL, Roman-Lopez JJ: Invasive carcinoma of the vulva with lymph node metastasis. Am J Obstet Gynecol 109:446, 1971
15. Thornton WN, Flanagan WC: Pelvic exenteration in the treatment of advanced malignancy of the vulva. Am J Obstet Gynecol 117:774, 1973
16. Green TH Jr: Carcinoma of the vulva: A reassessment. Obstet Gynecol 52:462, 1978
17. Morley GW: Infiltrative carcinoma of the vulva: Results of surgical treatment. Am J Obstet Gynecol 124:874, 1976
18. Woodruff JD, Julian C, Puray T, et al: The contemporary challenge of carcinoma in situ of the vulva. Am J Obstet Gynecol 115:677, 1973

31

Breast Cancer: Treatment Options

Douglas J. Marchant

Controversy concerning the treatment of breast cancer has existed since the earliest descriptions by Celsus and Galen in the first and second centuries AD. It has long been realized that untreated breast cancer has a surprisingly predictable 5-year survival. In one series, 20 percent of patients were still alive at 5 years and 5 percent survived 10 years.[1] Thus, in discussing treatment, the surgeon must be aware of the natural history of breast cancer and the necessity for long-term (15 to 20 years) follow-up to determine the efficacy of treatment.

The American Cancer Society (ACS) predicts that in 1987 there will be 130,000 new cases of breast cancer and 41,000 deaths.[2] Breast cancer is a complex disease, and survival is influenced by several observations:

1. Divergent hypotheses of breast cancer biology
2. Curability
3. Multicentricity
4. Influence of local treatment
5. Biologic basis of systemic treatment

This chapter discusses each of these observations and provides recommendations for treatment based on a contemporary understanding of the disease.

HISTORY

Surgical removal of the breast was described in the first and second centuries. During the early nineteenth century, local excision was the custom, but cures were infrequent. In 1867, Moore[3] suggested that because of the pattern of spread and chest wall recurrence, the entire breast should be removed; by 1875, von Volkmann routinely removed the breast and the pectoralis fascia.[4] Halsted's mastectomy was first mentioned in the surgical literature in 1891, and by 1894 he had performed 50 so-called complete mastectomies.[5] This radical mastectomy, as the operation came to be known, was enthusiastically adopted both in the United States and abroad. Unfortunately, the Halsted operation was reserved for relatively advanced cases, and the early literature suggests that this operation was not associated with an increase in either cure rate or length of survival, although there was a dramatic reduction in chest wall recurrences. During the next several decades, the results of the radical mastectomy improved, principally due to the earlier diagnosis of breast cancer and the more selective use of this operation, through the efforts of Haagensen, who identified those cases in which it promised a cure.

Because the radical mastectomy did not take into

account the fact that the internal mammary lymph node chain constituted one of the primary routes of lymphatic drainage from the breast, especially from inner quadrant lesions, surgeons began to extend the classic operation to include a resection of the internal mammary nodes and even the chest wall. In 1951, Urban and others in the United States popularized the extended radical mastectomy that removed the internal mammary chain and an overlying portion of the chest wall en block with the radical specimen.[6]

With the increasing acceptance that cancer of the breast often is a systemic disease, previously held concepts for treatment have been reassessed and placed in proper perspective. The realization that most patients will not be cured with even the most extensive local treatment has resulted in a more conservative approach and the participation of the patient in treatment planning. Lesser surgical procedures, including the modified radical mastectomy and segmental resection combined with axillary dissection and radiotherapy, have largely replaced the classic Halsted radical mastectomy.

BIOLOGIC DETERMINANTS FOR BREAST CANCER TREATMENT OPTIONS

The classic nineteenth century Halstedian hypothesis that breast cancer spreads in an orderly fashion has been challenged by recent observations. A number of animal experiments and clinical trials have failed to demonstrate the superiority of the en bloc dissection. This suggests that lymph nodes are in fact not barriers to tumor cell dissemination but are possibly indicators of the biologic behavior of the disease. This alternative hypothesis stresses the importance of hematogenous spread and some have suggested that breast cancer is a systemic disease from its inception. In a recent article In the *Lancet*, Skrabanek[7] stated:

> The evidence that breast cancer is incurable is overwhelming. The philosophy of breast cancer screening is based on wishful thinking that early cancer is curable cancer. Unable to admit ignorance and defeat, cancer propagandists have now turned to blaming the victims. They consume too much fat, they do not practice breast self examination, they succumb to irrational fears and delay reporting the early symptoms. It would appear that no woman needs to die of breast cancer if she reads and heeds the leaflets of the Cancer Societies and has her breasts examined regularly. Adherence to these myths and avoidance of reality undermines the credibility of the medical profession with the public.

Obviously, a corollary to this hypothesis is that variations in local and regional treatment are unlikely to have any impact on survival.

MacDonald, like Skrabanek, suggested that human breast cancer is biologically predetermined from its onset. He failed to find any evidence that either early diagnosis, size of the lesion, or type of surgery had been of any influence on the outcome in this form of cancer.[8] The publication of Fisher's alternative hypothesis during the 1970s suggested that the only impact on survival would be the advent of effective systemic therapy.[9]

Contrary to the theory of biologic predeterminism, several pieces of data suggest that increasing tumor diameter is associated with decrement in survival. These data include findings from randomized screening trials. One reported by the Swedish National Board of Health, in essence confirming the findings from the Health Insurance Plan (HIP) of New York some years earlier, showed that the mortality of breast cancer could be reduced by approximately one-third in a population offered screening.[10] This finding appears to be independent of lead time and length time bias and suggests that there is a period between radiologic and clinical detection when the disease is more likely to become systemic. Other data relating to tumor diameter have suggested that there is a relationship between tumor volume and the probability of distant metastasis and that therefore breast cancer is not necessarily systemic from its inception.[11]

Another observation concerns the definition of curability. The definition of cure in a disease with a protracted time course has been much debated. For the patient, the most satisfactory definition of cure is freedom from cancer for the remainder of that patient's life. However, from a practical standpoint, clinicians generally measure survival over a fixed period of time, that is, the 5-year cure rate popularized by the ACS. When one is attempting to assess the benefits of cancer treatment, the forces of mortality must be taken into consideration, this definition of cure describes that proportion of the population treated whose mortality experience is the same as that of a matched unaffected population. A number of studies have addressed the forces of mortality; the results are conflicting, some showing that there is a perceptible inflection in the survival curve at approximately 10 years when the force of mortality begins to parallel that of the normal age-matched population.[12,13] However, others have found an exponential survival pattern in breast cancer and concluded that any form of treatment affected neither the time nor the cause of death.[14]

It is clear that with these divergent hypotheses of the natural history of breast cancer and questions concerning the curability of this disease, there can be no unified hypothesis; from a practical standpoint, the surgeon must accept that both could be true and not mutually exclusive. Obviously, screening discovers smaller cancers; whether they are early or not is debatable, but they certainly are more amenable to conservative and more cosmetic treatment options. Should the pessimists in the extreme be wrong, the patient will have benefited from appropriate and timely treatment.

Another determinant in selecting appropriate treatment is the assumption that multicentric disease in the breast is of clinical significance. Unfortunately, in spite of the findings from a number of studies, the extent of multicentric disease and its biologic significance are still debatable.[15] Whole-organ studies conducted by Gallager and Martin[16] reveal a 74 percent incidence of multicentric cancer. In these studies, the level of multicentricity was related to the tumor diameter and the histologic type. By contrast, the low level of multicentricity (13.4 percent) reported by Fisher et al.[15] is best explained by the limited extent of the examination of the residual breast tissue following mastectomy. There is considerable evidence that following wide local excision or quadrantectomy unassociated with radiotherapy, the local recurrence rate is 19 to 37 percent, a finding recently confirmed by the National Surgical Adjuvant Breast Project (NSABP) trial (B-06).[17] This study demonstrated a 28 percent local recurrence rate in those patients randomized to segmental resection and axillary dissection without radiation therapy. This protocol also studied the effect of multicentric disease in other quadrants of the breast and in the quadrant of the breast in which the primary tumor arose. Patients who had grossly positive margins were treated with mastectomy; however, even those with adequate macroscopic excision of the tumor apparently had multifocal disease that evolved into clinically invasive cancer at a later date.

Obviously, multicentricity is the central issue in the role of radiotherapy as part of the conservative treatment for breast cancer. A significant period of time must elapse before the results of this type of treatment can be properly assessed since local recurrence can occur many years following initial treatment. It would appear from current data that local control must be maximized, although the influence of such treatment on the natural history of the disease and survival is debatable.

A number of trials have demonstrated that only radical treatment can maximize local control. Whether this is to be done by surgical means such as mastectomy or a more limited surgical procedure and radiotherapy is a matter of some concern to surgeons treating this disease.[18,19]

The conflicting results of a number of trials concerning the efficacy of local regional treatment are difficult to explain. One thing is clear: long-term results of breast cancer treatment are critical and at least a 10-year period must elapse before any conclusion can be drawn concerning the efficacy of a treatment program. The NSABP protocol B-04 compared patients treated by radical mastectomy, by total mastectomy plus radiation, and by total mastectomy alone. There were no significant differences among the three groups of patients with clinically negative nodes or between the two groups with clinically positive nodes.[20] Contrary findings were reported in a trial from Southeastern Scotland, in which patients treated by total mastectomy and postoperative radiation therapy had a statistically worse survival when compared with those randomly allocated to the Halsted radical mastectomy.[21]

The recently reported NSABP B-06 trial compared patients with stage I and II breast cancer who were treated with total mastectomy and axillary dissection versus segmental mastectomy and axillary dissection without radiation therapy.[17] The latter group had high local recurrence rate over the mean follow-up period of 39 months. The group of pathologically negative lymph nodes undergoing segmental mastectomy and axillary dissection without radiation therapy had a significantly worse disease-free survival rate than did those treated by segmental mastectomy and radiation therapy. It is to be assumed that the increased distant disease rate will ultimately be reflected in decreased survival. These findings are in agreement with a trial conducted at Guy's Hospital in London, in which those randomized to partial mastectomy without axillary dissection and radiation therapy had a statistically significant higher local regional recurrence rate, lower distant disease-free rate, and increased death rate when compared with those randomized to radical mastectomy.[22] It should be noted that in this trial, low doses of radiation were used, which could explain the high local recurrence rate.

As stated initially, conflicting results of these trials are difficult to explain. However, the surgeon treating breast cancer should be optimistic simply because on balance the current evidence does not support the concept that breast cancer is necessarily a systemic disease from its inception, and the possibility that local regional recurrence resulting from inadequate local treatment can act as a source of tertiary spread must be considered a possibility.

Finally, it is important to discuss the biologic basis for systemic treatment. It is assumed that some patients have systemic disease and that there are certain major predictors of systemic recurrence, which are the basis for recommending systemic (adjuvant) treatment. These predictors include tumor diameter and the number of involved lymph nodes; the latter apparently are the most important. A number of less well-defined predictors, including tumor grade, nuclear grade, DNA synthesis, and estrogen receptors, have been described. Obviously, there is a need for more accurate predictors. In time, biochemical and immunopathologic methods may be of some value. Approximately 16 percent of patients with T1 N0 disease and 26 percent of patients with T2 N0 disease develop recurrence in 10 years. These patients are not treated with adjuvant therapy unless under protocol study. This raises the question of whether perhaps it is more of a matter of concern that adjuvant treatment is withheld from the patients rather than that some patients are overtreated who would not have developed systemic recurrence.

Theoretical and clinical considerations indicate that the best results with adjuvant therapy are obtained in patients with a low tumor burden. A number of reasons have been advanced for the failure of systemic adjuvant therapy. One hypothesis holds that spontaneous mutations result in drug resistance and therefore prevent chemotherapeutic cure.[23] Another hypothesis considers the growth rate of solid tumors, which follows a Gompertzian curve in which the rate of regression of the tumor decreases with shrinking

tumor size but a cure volume may never be reached.[24] Therefore, regardless of the treatment, tumors conforming to the Gompertzian type growth curve exhibit an increasing rate of regrowth as the tumor shrinks, and a level of therapy necessary to eradicate the disease completely cannot be achieved.

A number of strategies have been recommended to counter these hypotheses. One is to administer chemotherapy by what is called intensification. This takes into account the issue of biochemical resistance; the late intensification would use a crossover plan in which the drugs used would not be subject to resistance developed by the initial therapy. Another approach considers the use of adjuvant chemotherapy at the time of diagnosis or perioperatively, as was done in the initial trials of adjuvant therapy during the late 1970s.[25]

SCREENING

A number of methods for screening have been proposed, including thermography, ultrasonography, improved translumination, and mammography. Only the last need be considered in this presentation. Mammography is the only screening method that can provide a geographic presentation of the abnormality. With the use of dedicated mammography, safety is no longer an issue. The amount of ionizing radiation delivered by these units is negligible. The only issues are the guidelines to be used in recommending screening and the recommendations for treatment based on the mammographic findings. A number of committees are addressing the problem of guidelines. These include the American College of Obstetricians and Gynecologists, the American College of Radiology, and the American Cancer Society. There is agreement concerning the baseline mammogram that most experts agree should be obtained at approximately age 35. A difference of opinion concerns the frequency of screening between the ages of 40 and 49, and 50 and thereafter. There is some evidence based on the Swedish trials that yearly screening between the ages of 40 and 49 and then biannually thereafter makes more biologic sense than annual screening beginning at age 50 (Tabar L: personal communication). It is hoped that these issues will soon be resolved. The failure to do so presents a significant problem for the primary physician, who must recommend guidelines and who may be subject to litigation based on the failure to recommend appropriate diagnostic studies.

The major problem that has arisen with the frequent use of mammography, in particular, screening mammography, is the discovery of the occult lesion. This may represent an asymmetric density or geographic cluster of microcalcifications. In either event, a decision must be made whether to repeat the films to clarify the diagnosis, to repeat the films in several months to assess stability of these areas, or to recommend localization and biopsy. This requires considerable judgment on the part of the radiologist and the establishment of a dialogue among the radiologist, the physician, and the patient. In our experience at the Breast Health Center of the New England Medical Center, 80 percent of these lesions are benign; however, for the remaining 20 percent, the utmost judgment and skill are required to determine the diagnosis and provide for the conservative treatment of breast cancer.

At least three problems are associated with the discovery of the occult lesion:

1. The radiologist fails to define the lesion and make appropriate recommendations.
2. The surgeon fails to remove the lesion.
3. The lesion is removed but with inadequate margins and may be associated with postoperative induration, infection, and/or hematoma.

Consultation with the radiologist is essential regarding the patient who has an occult lesion. It must be determined with certainty that the lesion is in fact in the breast parenchyma. Occasional skin lesions may project as microcalcifications within the breast. Assuming that the lesion requires removal, a localization technique must be employed. We use a small needle with a hook placed in the vicinity of the occult lesion. This is inserted by the radiologist, with mammographic control.[26] It is essential that the surgeon and the mammographer confer to determine the precise location of the lesion relative to the needle in the lateral and the craniocaudad views. The patient is taken to the operating room and, usually under local anesthesia, the specimen is removed together with the needle. Specimen radiography is performed; if the occult lesion is present, the wound is closed. The pathologist determines whether a rapid section diagnosis is feasible, if the margins are adequate, and carefully inks the margins to permit determination of both microscopic and gross margins with the permanent sections. This is particularly important if wide local excision and radiotherapy are planned as the definitive treatment. With the increasing application of screening mammography more and more occult lesions are discovered and in many cases, the biopsy becomes part of the definitive treatment. It is therefore essential that the surgeon performing the biopsy be adequately informed about the technique of localization, the importance of the margins, the necessity for estrogen and progesterone receptor determinations, and the need for absolute asepsis and minimal induration and cosmetic deformity following the biopsy.

EVALUATION OF THE PATIENT

Treatment planning for breast cancer includes a multidisciplinary approach. Each patient should have her primary physician, but alternatives in treatment require the expertise not only of the surgeon, but of the radiotherapist and the medical oncologist as well. One approach has been developed by our Breast Health Center, which is a multidisciplinary clinic staffed by surgeons, radiotherapists, medical oncologists, pathologists, radiologists, and a full-time nurse. A key staff member of this clinic is the nurse coordinator, who acts as a liaison between the patient and the various medical disciplines. She coordinates the clinical appointments and arranges for appropriate follow-up. It is essential that each physician establish a protocol for the evaluation of the patient. This should include a rather elaborate checklist to be certain that patients are informed of their diagnostic studies and their follow-up appointments. Because of the increase in two-stage procedures for the diagnosis and treatment of breast cancer, a number of patients are referred for a second opinion. In some states, state law mandates that the physician discuss alternative treatment with patients; in California, this must be recorded in the patient's record.[27,28] Because of the legal implications, it is essential to evaluate all the pertinent material, including the biopsy material and the radiographs as well as the proposed treatment plan.

Once the diagnosis of breast cancer has been established, a number of preoperative studies should be obtained. Mammography is absolutely essential, even in the most obvious cases. Synchronous cancer is present in 4 to 5 percent of patients, and multicentric disease may be discovered in the involved breast. This, in fact, may preclude wide local excision and radiotherapy. Recently, we saw a patient at the Breast Health Center who demonstrates some of the problems associated with screening mammography, evaluation of the patient, and recommendations for treatment. This patient had a screening mammogram that demonstrated an occult lesion in the right breast. Localization and biopsy were performed, and a diagnosis of intraductal carcinoma was made. The margins indicated that not all of the disease had been removed. The patient sought a second opinion. She was seen 1 week following the biopsy, and the entire upper portion of her breast was indurated and ecchymotic. It was therefore impossible to determine the extent of a wide local excision, should this be the option chosen by the patient. We reviewed the slides, and indeed the lesion was an intraductal carcinoma extending to the margin of the biopsy. We recommended that she have a repeat mammogram in 2 weeks, because there was some question on the original mammogram of additional microcalcifications. It was clear that no additional surgery could be performed during this interval because of the induration and ecchymosis. A repeat mammogram in 2 weeks confirmed that the entire upper portion of the breast contained microcalcifications. It would therefore be impossible, on the basis of the original biopsy and these films, to determine which of these areas contained intraductal carcinoma or possibly invasive carcinoma; therefore, a modified mastectomy was recommended. At surgery, as expected, there was a wide area of intraductal carcinoma involving the entire upper portion of the right breast. All axillary nodes removed were negative for tumor.

Patients scheduled for treatment should have a pretreatment chest radiograph, routine blood studies, and liver-function tests. For invasive lesions, many surgeons recommend a bone scan; however, the yield is low for T1 lesions. By contrast, a number of medical oncologists prefer to have the studies as a baseline for later comparison with follow-up studies. Clinical staging using the TNM (primary *tumor*, regional lymph *nodes*, distant *metastasis*) system is recommended, although most students of breast disease recognize that this system does not adequately segregate patients, nor does it help select appropriate patients for surgical treatment.[29] The TNM system was designed so that patients could be categorized, thereby enabling centers to group patients similarly for intercenter comparison. It is well known that the clinical nodal status of the patient is apt to be incorrect. If a patient is thought to have clinically negative nodes, 40 percent of these patients will have histologically positive nodes, and 25 percent of these patients presumed to have clinically positive nodes are found to have negative nodes. In addition, it is difficult to get an accurate tumor size either from the pathologist or from the surgeon. At the moment, it is the best system available, and it does have some value in that it makes the physician record the patient and tumor information. Clearly, the future rests with some form of biologic staging.

Appropriate treatment planning requires formal consultation with radiotherapy and medical oncology. This should not be presented to the patient as a competition between the specialties. On the basis of the available information, a Tumor Board discussion should precede the recommendations to the patient. In most cases, this can be presented by the primary physician; however, in my opinion, it is essential that the patient have the benefit of a discussion with the radiotherapist concerning the effects and consequences of radiotherapy and with the medical oncologist concerning the potential need for adjuvant chemotherapy. This concept of pretreatment evaluation inevitably results in some delay of treatment, but there is no evidence that the delay of 2 to 3 weeks between the diagnosis and definitive treatment affects prognosis. Obviously, "shopping around" for treatment that suits the patient, that is, second, third, and fourth opinions, is to be discouraged. A number of treatment protocols are available, these should be appropriately discussed with the patient and her family.

SURGICAL OPTIONS FOR LOCAL TREATMENT

A number of factors influence the definitive surgical treatment for breast cancer. Important considerations include the size and histology of the lesion, the skill and experience of the multidisciplinary team, and the wishes of the patient. Beginning in 1979, a number of consensus development conferences have taken place on the treatment of primary breast cancer. The basic question asked has been: Which treatments provide the best chance for disease free survival of early breast cancer?[8,30] Specifically, these conferences dealt with the question of whether conservative surgery, including dissection of the axillary lymph nodes followed by irradiation to the breast, is as effective as either the modified or radical mastectomy. It is fair to say that dissention and contention continue. However, during the past 6 years, there has been increasing support for conservative surgery combined with radiotherapy as primary treatment for women with early (smaller) breast cancer. Since 1979, there have been a number of published reports from both retrospective studies and prospective randomized clinical trials, the latest of which concluded that segmental mastectomy followed by breast irradiation in all patients and adjuvant chemotherapy in women with positive nodes is appropriate therapy for stage I and stage II breast cancers, less than 4 cm, provided that the margins of the resected specimens are free of tumor.[17]

While the concept of conservative surgery has gained favor, there has been controversy concerning the technical details of the surgery and the radiotherapy employed. First, there must be agreement on the terms to be used. Conservative surgery implies wide local excision and resection of the tumor, with 1 to 2 cm of adjacent breast tissue designed to provide clear margins of resection. Quadrantectomy implies the resection of the tumor with the involved quadrant of the breast, including the overlying skin. The terms lumpectomy and segmental mastectomy are imprecise and their use is discouraged.

Axillary dissection implies the dissection of the axillary contents from the tail of the breast to the latissimus dorsi and the axillary vein superiorly and the lateral border of the pectoralis minor muscle medially. The use of the term axillary sampling is discouraged, again, because it is not a precise statement concerning the extent of the surgical procedure.

The use of conservative surgery and radiotherapy requires the consideration of four important criteria:

1. Patient selection
2. The surgery for the primary tumor
3. Radiotherapy for the primary tumor
4. The surgery for the axilla

The principal advantage of conservative treatment is cosmetic. Certainly, there are no data to indicate that the conservative approach provides improved survival as compared with the radical or modified radical mastectomy. Thus, the major criterion for patient selection is the ability to resect the primary tumor adequately without creating a cosmetic deformity. Patients who are poor candidates for breast-conserving treatment include patients with widely separated primary tumors in the same breast, those whose mammograms show diffuse disease in many quadrants, and those with large tumors in relatively small breasts. Patients with central lesions involving the nipple areolar complex can be successfully treated with the resection of the nipple areolar complex with careful attention to the final cosmetic result. Reconstruction of the nipple has been accomplished following radiotherapy. Other factors to be considered include patient age and the size of the breast. I have had patients in their middle 70s request conservative treatment for cosmetic reasons and younger patients request not only modified radical mastectomy but simple mastectomy of the opposite breast as well, in order to avoid future concern about the recurrence of the cancer in the treated breast and the development of a new cancer in the opposite breast. I therefore provide alternatives in treatment, when appropriate, to all patients, regardless of their age.

Adequate surgical resection implies grossly clear margins. The surgeon must appropriately mark the specimen for orientation by the pathologist. It is important to determine the distance of the tumor to the closest margin of resection. Tissue should be removed for estrogen and progesterone receptor studies without disturbing the evaluation of the resected margins. Microscopic involvement is best determined at the time of the evaluation of the permanent section. It is generally agreed that if the microscopic margins are positive after wide excision, further excision should be performed. This can be accomplished either at the time of the original biopsy or at the time of axillary dissection. Again, if a lesion is to be re-excised some weeks following the initial biopsy, it is absolutely essential that there be minimal induration and ecchymosis at the operative site; otherwise, it is impossible to define the lesion and provide a satisfactory cosmetic result. It must be re-emphasized that the biopsy may become part of the treatment and must be expertly and carefully performed.

Since the principal goal in conservative treatment is the final cosmetic result, I prefer to mark my incision with the patient in the sitting or the standing position. Frequently, a skinfold can be observed in the axilla that will disguise the incision and provide for unrestricted motion of the arm. The lines of Langer may not follow a circumareolar pattern when the patient is in the upright position; I therefore make the breast incision using the best cosmetic line. Many of our patients are admitted following the surgery and remain in the hospital for only 48 hours.

If meticulous axillary dissection is performed and adequate hemostasis obtained, drains are not employed. With careful closure of the surgical wound in the breast and adequate compression following the surgery, wound drains are not required. I prefer to place a small dressing over the axillary incision and then a large pressure dressing with fluffs held in place with a 6-inch Ace bandage. This can be applied before the patient is awakened. This provides stability for the operated breast and reduces discomfort. The dressings are removed before the patient is discharged. If the application of suction is required, it is important to avoid a hollow, and thus a cosmetic deformity. By employing intermittent suction, this deformity can be avoided. The sutures are removed in 4 or 5 days, and radiotherapy is started within 1 week to 10 days following surgery. Prior to discharge, the patient is seen by a physiotherapist, and appropriate range-of-motion exercises are given for the arm. The patient is also seen either in hospital or in the home environment by the Reach-to-Recovery team. Since the patient has been evaluated by a radiotherapist and medical oncologist, she is visited by these specialists while in the hospital; additional rapport is established for the continuation of treatment.

It is generally agreed that the breast should be treated with 180 to 200 rad/day, for a total of 4,500 to 5,000 rad. Doses in excess of 5,000 rad result in fibrosis and retraction and an unacceptable cosmetic result. For patients treated with a wide local excision and in whom the margins of resection are close on microscopic evaluation boost therapy may be recommended. There remains some controversy regarding the technique of this supplemental radiation; whichever technique is employed, it should not diminish the cosmetic result.

If the patient requires adjuvant chemotherapy for positive nodes, this treatment must be integrated with the radiotherapy. There is no agreement either concerning the concomitant use of chemotherapy and radiotherapy or a sequence in administering chemotherapy and radiotherapy. It has been our practice to initiate three cycles of chemotherapy, complete the radiotherapy, and then add three additional cycles of chemotherapy to complete the adjuvant therapy.

While the conservative approach is preferred by many patients, statistics clearly indicate that most patients are treated with the modified radical mastectomy. The Patient Care and Research Committee of the American College of Surgeons Commission on Cancer reported in their 1982 audit that 55 percent of patients treated in 1976 had undergone a modified radical mastectomy and that 28 percent had a Halsted radical operation. Comparable figures from the 1978 survey show that nearly 50 percent of women treated in 1972 had a Halsted mastectomy, and only 28 percent had a modified radical mastectomy.[31] It is estimated that at least 80 percent of patients now undergoing radical surgery for breast cancer have the modified operation. In this operation, the entire breast is removed without sacrificing the pectoralis major or minor muscles and an axillary dissection similar to that used in the conservative operation completes the procedure. The Halsted radical mastectomy is recommended only for those patients with lesions involving the pectoral fascia or muscle. In many of these patients, only a portion of the pectoralis muscle and its fascia may be removed and the patient treated with postoperative radiotherapy to this area.

Again, it should be emphasized that the modified mastectomy should be performed in a cosmetic manner, preferably with a transverse incision to permit a later cosmetic reconstruction. Meticulous dissection and accurate hemostasis is required and, as the term implies, the axillary dissection should be a dissection and not simply a sampling using blunt technique. Most authorities agree that at least 12 axillary nodes should be recovered. Obviously, this depends on the diligence of both the surgeon and the pathologist. The axillary dissection, in my opinion, can be facilitated by the elevation of the arm attached to a crossbar. This will relax the pectoralis muscles and permit a more extensive dissection of the axilla. Neither the thoracodorsal vessels nor the nerve should be sacrificed, and attention should be paid to the location of the long thoracic curve. It is impossible to determine the extent of axillary involvement, even at the operating table. Retrieval of a large number of obviously involved nodes often results in a negative report and what appears to be a clean axilla may be reported as showing significant nodal involvement. Therefore, except in rare instances, a careful and thorough axillary dissection should be performed removing all the adipose tissue, with constraints.

Postoperatively, these patients are managed similarly to patients having a wide local excision and axillary dissection. However, in the case of a modified mastectomy with the elevation of flaps, drainage is essential. The Hemovac is ideal. One is placed anteriorly and the other in the axilla. I prefer to have two separate reservoirs. This permits monitoring of the drainage from both areas. Neither Hemovac should be connected to suction until the wound is closed. Incomplete suction often results in the establishment of a clot in the tubing, preventing the full utilization of the drainage system postoperatively. I prefer to use fine nylon skin sutures that are removed on approximately the fifth postoperative day, depending on the healing of the wound. It is essential that these patients as well as those following wide local excision and axillary dissection be warned about overzealous use of the arm or untreated infection. Both might result in temporary edema and on occasion lymphangitis with more permanent swelling. Most patients are discharged on the fifth or sixth postoperative day, and some earlier if there is complete healing of the wound. Clearly, in these days of diagnostic-related groups (DRG), there is always the pressure to discharge the patient too early. The surgeon, in my opinion, must exercise his or her judgment. We must not succumb to treatment by a protocol or computer, given the very real possibility of a postoperative complication and the need to readmit the patient at a higher cost because of some avoidable complication.

There are advantages and disadvantages to the conservative and radical approaches. The main advantage of the conservative approach is the preservation of the breast. However, the price to be paid is the extended radiation treatments, and the real concern of some patients that future symptomatology in the retained breast is associated with recurrent tumor. In the more radical approach, treatment is accomplished in a few days, and obviously cancer cannot recur in the breast.

Many patients elect reconstructive procedures at a later date, and some surgeons are performing the reconstruction at the time of the modified radical mastectomy. We prefer to have the patient see the plastic surgeon prior to the surgical procedure, and we have established a support group that meets with the plastic surgeon at regular intervals to discuss reconstructive techniques and results. In some cases, following the mastectomy it is necessary to perform a reduction mammoplasty on the opposite side. This is a lengthy procedure, most appropriately accomplished at a second operative procedure. There is also the possibility that an unexpected finding will be discovered at the time of mastectomy that will adversely influence the constructive procedure. One of our patients required a mastectomy following a local recurrence after wide local excision and radiotherapy. She had been seen in consultation with the plastic surgeon and, after considerable discussion, it was decided that reconstruction would be performed at the time of the mastectomy. Unfortunately, the pathology report showed intradermal involvement of the cancer, that is, inflammatory carcinoma, seriously compromising the cosmetic result, as additional treatment was then required.

FOLLOW-UP

Our patients are seen during the immediate postoperative period by the Reach-to-Recovery team. Patients are matched to those who have undergone similar procedures, that is, the modified mastectomy or the conservative approach. Patients are also seen by the physical therapist and may return to our voluntary counseling sessions with the psychiatrist. Patients continue to be followed in the Breast Health Center for the first year, every 3 months, and for the second and third year, every 4 months. Yearly mammograms are obtained and, if indicated, repeat bone scan and other studies to detect metastatic disease.

Quality of life is of paramount concern, and patients are urged to discuss reconstructive procedures and psychosexual concerns. We are committed to the team approach in the treatment of breast cancer, but each patient has her own primary physician, in our case, the surgeon who initially saw the patient, and she is encouraged to call either this physician with any of her concerns or the nurse coordinator, who will then refer her to the appropriate physician for further discussion. We have found that about one-half of our patients request the mastectomy with a possibility of later reconstruction and about one-half request the conservative approach with wide local excision axillary dissection and radiotherapy. Properly performed, both approaches provide similar overall 10-year survival, approximately 60 percent for stage I and II lesions, with a local recurrence rate of 8 percent or less.

BREAST CANCERS WITH UNIQUE FEATURES

In Situ Carcinoma

IN SITU LOBULAR CARCINOMA AND LOBULAR NEOPLASIA

These lesions are almost always diagnosed as an incidental finding following biopsy of a dominant mass or an occult lesion. There are several key features of this lesion, when planning treatment:

1. Propensity for bilaterality
2. Multicentricity
3. Relatively low rate of the development of subsequent infiltrating carcinoma

Figures regarding the incidence of subsequent infiltrating carcinoma vary, but it is approximately 30 percent after a long follow-up and may involve the ipsilateral or contralateral breast.

Treatment options include surgery or a period of watchful waiting with appropriate follow-up diagnostic studies. If, following the initial biopsy, the margins are clear, a reasonable treatment plan includes reinforcement of breast self-examination, biannual physical examination and annual mammography. It must be said at the outset that some of these lesions do not produce calcium and therefore may actually be missed on the screening mammogram. The patient should be aware of this possibility; nevertheless, most patients choose this option. The alternative is to recommend mastectomy and, because bilaterality is common (50 percent), bilateral mastectomy as the treatment of choice. When presented with this option, few patients accept mastectomy. This seems reasonable, since in situ lobular carcinoma or lobular neoplasia is probably more widespread than generally appreciated, and many of these tumors never develop beyond the in situ stage.

IN SITU DUCTAL CARCINOMA

This is an entirely different lesion and of considerably more significance. Left untreated, infiltrating carcinoma will develop in the ipsilateral breast in up to 50 percent of cases. Again, many of the lesions are detected coincidentally. In one series, one-third presented as a mass, an additional one-third with nipple discharge, and the remaining one-third with suspicious mammographic findings. By contrast, intraductal carcinoma with microinvasion presents as a mass in two-thirds of patients.[32] A number of studies have indicated that several areas of the breast may be involved.[33] Because of this, there is considerable debate concerning appropriate treatment. Standard treatment has been total mastectomy with lower axillary sampling or a conventional axillary dissection. This should result in cure in nearly 100 percent of cases. Because of the advent of conservative techniques, for small invasive cancers, there has been considerable debate about the conservative treatment for the in situ ductal carcinoma. There are a number of trials in which the tumor is excised from the breast, and the retained breast is either left untreated or is treated with radiotherapy, much the same as one would treat an infiltrating lesion. Preliminary data suggest that the latter approach; that is, wide local excision and radiotherapy, is appropriate in the vast majority of cases.[34]

The widespread use of screening has led to the detection of more and more of these cases; to date, experience with the various treatment options is insufficient to make any definitive recommendations, particularly for lesions discovered only by mammography. There is some evidence that because of the multicentricity of this disease and the higher risk of local recurrence following standard radiation therapy, a strong case can be made for mastectomy and axillary dissection. Harris et al.[35] noted that with a marked intraductal component in the primary tumor and ductal carcinoma in situ in the adjacent tissue, these patients have a significantly lower 5-year local tumor-control rate (77 percent) than do patients with neither of these features (99 percent). Clearly, it is impossible to evaluate multicentricity in the breast unless a careful examination of the mastectomy specimen is performed; therefore, the intraductal cancer should not be down-graded. It is potentially a fatal disease if not treated adequately.

BREAST CANCER IN PREGNANCY

Breast cancer in pregnancy presents special problems. It is infrequent, comprising about 2.2 per 10,000 pregnancies, or 1.72 percent of all carcinomas of the breast. Seven percent of cancers are associated with pregnancy in premenopausal women. Several issues must be resolved:

1. Surgical curability
2. Appropriate therapeutic action
3. Dangers inherent in subsequent pregnancies

Numerous studies have indicated that the major problem of breast cancer discovered during pregnancy is delay in diagnosis.[36] If age and stage are comparable, pregnancy per se has little influence on prognosis. Therefore, pregnancy should not delay either prompt diagnosis or definitive treatment.

Breast examination should be part of every prenatal visit; if any abnormality is noted, appropriate diagnostic tests should be performed. Skinny-needle biopsy is as effective during pregnancy as in the nonpregnant patient, and certainly open biopsy can be performed under local anesthesia without adverse sequelae. It is absolutely essential to resolve a dominant mass.

A number of studies have indicated that many of these cancers are estrogen receptor negative; therapeutic abortion does not improve the chances for cure.[37] During the first trimester, once the diagnosis has been established, prompt treatment, including mastectomy and axillary dissection, should be performed. The chance of spontaneous abortion is very small. Patients presenting during the last trimester, depending on the maturity of the fetus, may be observed until delivery of a mature fetus is possible and then prompt therapy carried out. Patients with the diagnosis established during the middle trimester must be treated without delay, and observation to allow for maturity of the fetus is unjustified.

If regional involvement is discovered, a decision must be made concerning adjuvant therapy. Some studies have indicated that chemotherapy administered during the second and third trimesters has no adverse effects on the fetus.[38] It is probably wise to discuss these options with the patient, particularly if she is desirous of keeping the pregnancy. No long-term results are available regarding the effect of chemotherapy on the newborn.

As far as a future pregnancy is concerned, studies indicate that the vast majority of recurrences occur within 2 years following treatment.[39] It is therefore recommended that patients avoid pregnancy during this period; some form of barrier contraceptive is recommended. After 2 years, if the patient is clinically free of disease by appropriate studies, including chest radiography, bone scan, and liver-function tests, pregnancy need not be avoided. Some studies suggest that patients with positive nodes are not adversely affected by a future pregnancy.[39]

Another issue concerns the management of the patient who has been treated for breast cancer and who subsequently becomes pregnant. Each case must be considered on its merit, but no therapeutic benefit can be expected from abortion in these cases. As more and more data accumulate concerning the role of estrogen and progesterone receptors, certain subsets of patients may be discovered for whom these recommendations are not appropriate. However, at the present time, we simply do not have this information. The same situation applies to the recommendation for or against estrogen replacement therapy following the diagnosis of breast cancer. This is not recommended because of the possibility of exacerbation of the disease. On the other hand, when sufficient data have accumulated concerning the receptor status of these patients, again there may be certain subsets for whom estrogen replacement therapy is perfectly safe and appropriate.

ADJUVANT THERAPY

In 50 to 70 percent of patients with lymph node metastasis, systemic disease will develop. These patients will die from dissemination of these micrometastases. Theoretically, adjuvant chemotherapy should benefit patients at high risk of the development of these micrometastases that are not yet detectable. At least three variables are used to select chemotherapy. These include involvement of the axillary lymph nodes, the menstrual status and the hormone receptor activity. Premenopausal patients with axillary lymph node metastasis have a longer disease-free period and have a 25 percent relative reduction in early death after receiving adjuvant chemotherapy, in most cases cytoxan – methotrexate — 5-fluorouracil

(5-FU) compared with patients who have undergone a mastectomy without this form of adjuvant therapy. A number of trials have indicated that three-drug treatment is superior to single-agent treatment; however, further trials are indicated.[40]

In 1985, the National Institutes of Health Consensus Panel recommended tamoxifen adjuvant treatment for postmenopausal women who are estrogen receptor positive and who have positive nodes.[41] For postmenopausal women who are estrogen receptor protein negative, no treatment is recommended, since no benefit has been achieved from chemotherapy and the treatment produces appreciable toxicity.[42] Some studies have indicated that this is due to the level of treatment and that if adjuvant chemotherapy is given in appropriate dosages, there may be some benefit.[43] Adjuvant therapy, except in a trial or protocol setting, is not recommended for women whose nodes are negative, whether they are premenopausal or postmenopausal, since in these patients the prognosis is good and the attendant toxicity less acceptable.

Adjuvant radiotherapy is seldom given. Clearly, it can decrease the incidence of chest wall and lymph node recurrence; however, prospective randomized trials have shown that this is not associated with improved survival. Today adjuvant radiation therapy following mastectomy is used in patients with residual tumor or with surgical margins reported positive by the pathologist. This type of radiation therapy must be distinguished from curative use following wide local excision in the intact breast.

TREATMENT OF RECURRENT AND METASTATIC DISEASE

Metastatic disease is not curable; however, patients may be managed with a variety of palliative therapies and in some cases for many years, with excellent quality of life. It should be noted at the outset that local recurrence in a breast treated with wide local excision and primary radiotherapy is curable in many cases by mastectomy, and it is not necessarily representative of widespread metastatic disease. Nevertheless, in most cases, it indicates systemic metastasis and incurable disease.

A number of strategies are used to detect metastatic disease. Obviously, it is important to detect these cancers as early as possible. We obtain yearly liver-function tests, carcinoembryonic antigen (CEA) de-

terminations, and chest radiography. Biopsy is essential to document the recurrence and, if possible, to determine hormone receptor status. This is particularly true with lung lesions, which in fact may represent a new primary tumor. This may require needle biopsy, bronchoscopy, or media-stinoscopy or, in some cases, open biopsy. It is absolutely essential to know the complete picture of the extent of the metastasis and its hormonal receptor status before initiating any treatment. As might be expected, the treatment strategy depends on the extent of the disease, location of the disease, the menstrual status of the patient, and the disease-free interval.

Palliation may be achieved by using hormonal therapy; however, this should not be used in patients who need a rapid response, particularly those with visceral disease. Receptor status can be used in predicting this response. About 60 percent of women with estrogen receptor protein activity will respond to hormonal manipulation, and those who also have progesterone receptor protein activity have 80 percent or more chance of hormonal response. Patients who respond to hormonal maneuvers have a subsequent median survival of more than 4 years. Tamoxifen produces a response in about one-third of patients with metastatic disease and in two-thirds of those with estrogen receptor protein activity. It is of interest to note that for postmenopausal women, equivalent response rates can be achieved using tamoxifen or exogenous estrogen in pharmacologic doses. However, fewer side effects are seen with tamoxifen. It is important to monitor the patient's serum calcium during the first few days after the initiation of hormonal therapy. Transient exacerbation of the disease may occur with tamoxifen, estrogens, and androgens.

Oophorectomy may be used as an endocrine procedure for menopausal women. The expected response rate is in the range of 30 to 40 percent. Other surgical procedures such as adrenalectomy and hypophesectomy are seldom used. These have now been replaced with less toxic drug therapies, including tamoxifen and aminoglutethamide. Commonly used drugs include Adriamycin, cytoxan, prednisone, methotrexate, 5-FU, and vincristine. Combinations of these cytotoxic agents provide a response rate of 60 to 70 percent, but all these patients eventually die of their disease.

Patients with pathologic fractures may be stabilized by appropriate orthopedic procedures, and radiotherapy can be used to prevent pathologic fractures or control pain, soft tissue disease, and brain metastasis. Occasionally, an isolated metastasis can be resected with good palliation.

Because of the biology of this disease, metastatic cancer must be considered a chronic illness. Therefore, quality of life is of the utmost importance, and considerable psychosocial-sexual support is required of the treatment team. Continuity of the health care team and a positive attitude are essential in providing the support needed for these patients.

THE FUTURE

Recently, the American Board of Obstetrics and Gynecology indicated that it will require a knowledge of breast disease in its certification process.[44] A Consensus Meeting was held in May 1986 to define more clearly the role of the obstetrician gynecologist in the diagnosis and treatment of breast disease. This meeting was attended by obstetricians and gynecologists, general surgeons, pathologists, epidemiologists, radiotherapists, and psychiatrists together, with basic scientists discussing anatomy, physiology, and adjuvant and hormonal therapy. At this meeting, it was decided to develop a core curriculum and to define the requirements for residency programs to provide the necessary training for the diagnosis and treatment of breast disease.

It was recommended that the obstetrician-gynecologist, as the primary physician to women, should have a knowledge of the embryology, anatomy, and physiology of the breast. He or she should be able to provide adequate counseling in screening techniques, to perform appropriate diagnostic studies, including aspiration of cysts and skinny-needle biopsy, and to provide appropriate follow-up of patients referred for the treatment of breast cancer. Because the open biopsy often becomes part of the treatment, the Board stopped short of recommending that every obstetrician and gynecologist be prepared to perform the open biopsy. As the parameters for conservative treatment are more clearly defined, it is quite likely that some obstetrician-gynecologists will obtain the necessary additional training to participate as part of team treating of breast cancer. This will require a knowledge and proficiency in all the modalities, since it is impossible in a given patient to predict with certainty whether the patient is suitable for wide local excision or modified mastectomy, occasionally with resection of a portion of the pectoral muscle. This will require additional surgical training and close collaboration with the cytopathologist, the radiotherapist, and the medical oncologist, precisely the requirements for the certified gynecologic-oncologist.

REFERENCES

1. Bloom HJG, Richardson WW, Harries EJ: Natural history of untreated breast cancer (1805–1933). Comparison of untreated and treated cases according to a histological grade of malignancy. Br Med J 11:213, 1962
2. American Cancer Society: Cancer Facts and Figures. ACS, New York, 1987
3. Moore ZH: On the influence of inadequate operations on the theory of cancer. R Med Chir Soc (Lond) 1:245, 1867
4. von Volkmann R: Beitrage zur Chirgurie. Breitkoff and Hartel, Leipzig, 1875
5. Halsted WS: The results of operations for the cure of cancer of the breast performed at the Johns Hopkins Hospital. 4:297, 1894–1895
6. Urban JA, Marjani MA: Significance of internal mammary lymph node metastases in breast cancer. AJR, 111:130, 1971
7. Skrabanek P: False premises and false promises of breast cancer screening. Lancet 1:316, 1985
8. MacDonald I: The natural history of mammary carcinoma. Am J Surg 111:435, 1966
9. Fisher B, Redmond C, Fisher ER, and other participating NSABP investigators: The contribution of recent NSABP clinical trials of primary breast cancer therapy to an understanding of tumor biology. An overview of findings. Cancer 46:1009, 1980
10. Tabar L, Fagerberg CJC, Gad A, et al: Reduction in mortality from breast cancer after mass screening with mammography. Randomized trial from the breast cancer screening working group of the Swedish National Board of Health and Welfare. Lancet 1:829, 1985
11. Koscielny S, Tubiana M, Lea MG, et al: Breast cancer: Relationship between the size of the primary tumor and the probability of metastatic dissemination. Br J Cancer 49:709, 1984
12. Brinkley D, Haybrittle JL: The curability of breast cancer. Lancet 11:95, 1975
13. Brinkley D, Haybrittle JL: Long term survival of women with breast cancer. (Letter.) Lancet 1:1118, 1984
14. Mueller CB, Jeffries W: Cancer of the breast: Its outcome as measured by the rate of dying and causes of death. Ann Surg 182:334, 1975

15. Fisher ER, Gregorio R, Redmond C, et al: Pathologic findings from the National Surgical Adjuvant Breast Project (Protocol No. 4). 1. Observations concerning the multicentricity of mammary cancer. Cancer 35:247, 1975

16. Gallager HS, Martin JE: The study of mammary carcinoma by mammography and whole organ sectioning. Early observations. Cancer 23:855, 1969

17. Fisher B, Bauer M, Margolese R et al: Five-year results of a randomized clinical trial comparing total mastectomy and segmental mastectomy with or without radiation in the treatment of breast cancer. N Engl J Med 312:665, 1985

18. Harris JR, Hellman S: The results of primary radiation therapy for early breast cancer at the Joint Center for Radiation Therapy. p. 47. In Harris JR, Hellman S, Silen W (eds): Conservative Management of Breast Cancer. JB Lippincott, Philadelphia, 1983

19. Veronesi V, Zucali R, Luini A: Local control and survival in early breast cancer: The Milan trial. Int J Radiat Oncol 12:717, 1986

20. Fisher B, Redmond C, Fisher ER, et al: Ten-year results of a randomized clinical trial comparing radical mastectomy and total mastectomy with or without radiation. N Engl J Med 312:674, 1985

21. Langlands AO, Prescott J, Hamilton T: A clinical trial in the management of operable cancer of the breast. Br J Surg 67:170, 1980

22. Hayward J: The surgeon's role in primary breast cancer. Breast Cancer Res Treatm 1:27, 1981

23. Goldie JH, Coldman AJ, Gudauskas GA: Rationale for the use of alternating non-cross resistant chemotherapy. Cancer Treatm Rep 66:439, 1982

24. Norton L, Simon R: The Norton-Simon hypothesis revisited. Cancer Treatm Rep 70:163, 1986

25. Nissen-Meyer R, Kjellgren K, Malmio K, et al: Surgical adjuvant chemotherapy: Results with one short course with cyclophosphamide after mastectomy for breast cancer. Cancer 41:2088, 1978

26. Homer MJ: Non palpable breast lesion localization using a curved-end retractible wire. Radiology 157:259, 1985

27. General Laws of the Commonwealth of Massachusetts, an act providing certain rights to patients and residents in hospitals, clinic and certain other facilities, section H, 1979

28. Health and Safety Code, section 1704.5, State of California breast cancer informed consent law (SB 1893), 1981

29. Maguire WL (ed): Breast Cancer Research and Treatment. Vol. 6. Optimal surgical approaches to the local management of early breast cancer. A panel discussion. 1985

30. Harris JR, Hellman S, Kinne DW: Special report: Limited surgery and radiotherapy for early breast cancer. N Engl J Med 313:1365, 1985

31. Wilson RE: Progress in breast cancer treatment, today and tomorrow. Am Coll Surg Bull 68:2, 1983

32. Schuh ME, Nemoto T, Penetrante RB, et al: Intraductal carcinoma. Analysis of presentation, pathologic findings, and outcome of disease. Arch Surg 121:1303, 1986

33. Lagios MD, Westdahl PR, Margolin FR, et al: Duct carcinoma in situ, relationship of extent of non-invasive disease to the frequency of occult invasion, multicentricity, lymph node metastases, and short-term treatment failures. Cancer 50:1309, 1982

34. Fisher ER, Sass R, Fisher B, et al: Pathologic findings from the National Surgical Adjuvant Breast Project (protocol 6). 1. Intraductal carcinoma (DCIS). Cancer 57:197, 1986

35. Harris JR, Connolly JL, Schnitt SJ, et al: Clinical pathologic study of early breast cancer treated by primary radiation therapy. J Clin Oncol 1:184, 1983

36. King RM, Welch JS, Martin JK, et al: Carcinoma of the breast associated with pregnancy. Surg Gynecol Obstet 160:228, 1985

37. Nugent P, O'Connell TX: Breast cancer and pregnancy. Arch Surg 120:1221, 1985

38. Murray CL, Reichert JA, Anderson J, Twiggs LB: Multimodal cancer therapy for breast cancer in the first trimester of pregnancy. JAMA 252:2607, 1984

39. Harvey JC, Rosen PP, Ashikari R, et al: The effect of pregnancy on the prognosis of carcinoma of the breast following radical mastectomy. Surg Gynecol Obstet 153:723, 1981

40. Bonadonna G, Rossi A, Valagussa P: Adjuvant CMF chemotherapy in operable breast cancer: Ten years later. World J Surg 9:707, 1985

41. National Institutes of Health: Adjuvant chemotherapy for breast cancer. Consensus development conference statement, Sept. 9–11, 1985

42. Lippman ME (ed): Proceedings of the NIH Consensus Development Conference on Adjuvant Chemotherapy and Endocrine Therapy for Breast Cancer. Natl Cancer Inst Monog 1, 1986

43. Bonadonna G, Valagussa P: Dose response effect of adjuvant chemotherapy in breast cancer. N Engl J Med 304:10, 1981

44. Bulletin of the American Board of Obstetrics and Gynecology, Sept 1985

Section IV

SPECIAL PROBLEMS

32

Cancer in Pregnancy

Peter E. Schwartz

Invasive cancer occurring in pregnancy is, fortunately, an unusual event. It is highly emotionally charged, as there are two patients — the mother and the fetus, it occurs in young patients who are not psychologically prepared for a potentially devastating result, and it frequently evokes emotional responses from concerned physicians. Therapeutic recommendations are often based on scant support in the medical literature, and they may run counter to religious beliefs. As reported experience has increased, there appears to be no conclusive evidence that cancer in pregnancy is more virulent than cancer diagnosed in the nonpregnant woman. Delays in evaluating patient's symptoms are common in pregnancy, and this may lead to patients having more advanced cancer at diagnosis. Advances in the management of the premature infant have permitted earlier planned delivery of infants whose mothers have cancer and in whom earlier delivery will reduce fetal exposure to the untoward effects of therapeutic interventions.

This chapter reviews the effect of standard therapies (surgery, radiation, and chemotherapy) on the mother and developing fetus and reviews current management of cancer developing during pregnancy based on the site of origin of the malignancy. Gestational trophoblastic neoplasia is discussed in Chapter 18.

INCIDENCE

The actual incidence of cancer complicating pregnancy is unknown. It has been estimated that cancer may complicate 1 in every 1,000 pregnancies.[1] Table 32-1 summarizes the incidence of cancers occurring during pregnancy based on individual hospital statistics. The uterine cervix remains overall the most common site for neoplastic disorders (1 per 464 pregnancies) with cervical intraepithelial neoplasia occurring approximately once in 770 pregnancies and invasive cancer occurring once in 2,205 pregnancies. The breast is the next most common site for malignancy to be recognized in pregnancy, with a cancer frequency of 1 per 3,000 pregnancies. Less commonly occurring sites for malignancies to be found in pregnancy include the ovary, vulva, vagina, and skin (melanoma). Brain tumors, leukemias, lymphomas, and gastrointestinal (GI) tract cancers rarely complicate pregnancy.

In a population-based epidemiologic study of cancer occurring in the German Democratic Republic, Haas[2] was able to show a reduced incidence of cancer occurring in pregnancy as compared with the nonpregnant state, suggesting that patients with occult cancer have a reduced likelihood of conceiving, rather than there being an increase in cancer in the

Table 32-1 Cancer Diagnosed in Pregnancy

Site	Estimated Incidence	Investigators
Cervix		
Carcinoma in situ	1/767	Sokal and Lessmann[23]
Invasive	1/2,205	Sokal and Lessmann[23]
Breast	1/3,000	Benedet et al.[41]
Vulva	1/8,000	Nugent and O'Connell[62]
Ovary	1/9,000–1/25,000	Nugent and O'Connell[62]; Ribeiro and Palmer[63]
Vagina	1/37,000	Nugent and O'Connell[62]
Blood (leukemia)	<1/75,000	Applewhite et al.[51]
Colorectum	1/100,000	Fisher et al.[120]; Clark et al.[121]

gravid state due to the immunosuppression that normally occurs in pregnancy. This was an unexpected finding, as the pregnant women in this study were exposed to intense medical screening. The age-specific observed to expected ratios of pregnancy-associated cancers for all sites combined rose with each successive 5-year age group and ranged from 0.22 for women aged 15 to 19 years (1.9 cancers per 100,000 live births) to 1.40 (232.4 cancers per 100,000 live births) for those aged 40 to 44 years. In this population-based study, the cancer site, ranked in descending order, was cervix, breast, ovary, lymphoma, melanoma, brain, and leukemia. However, it is possible that one explanation for the low incidence of cancer reported in this series was due to incomplete reporting by physicians.

Metastases to the fetus are rare. In a literature review until 1970, seven of eight cancers reported to have spread from the mother to the fetus were melanomas.[1] The remaining lesion was a lymphosarcoma.[1] The occurrence of fetal metastases is so rare that its possibility does not influence management decisions. Metastases to the placenta have been reported in 24 cases until 1970, most often arising from malignant melanoma.

SURGERY AND PREGNANCY

Surgery may be required for the evaluation and treatment of cancer arising in pregnancy. Surgery, particularly intraabdominal surgery, should be avoided if possible until the second trimester, when the chance of spontaneous abortion is reduced. Ovarian resections may be safely accomplished in the sec-

ond trimester as the placental production of progesterone replaces the corpus luteum by 12 weeks gestation.[3] Anesthetic consequences of operating in pregnancy require that the patient be placed in a lateral position to avoid vena cava and aorta compression.[4] Alternatively, placing a 15-degree wedge under the right hip will produce left uterine displacement of the gravid uterus off the vena cava and will avoid the fetal complications of hypoxemia or hypotension.[5] In addition, gastric displacement by the gravid uterus results in a change in the angle of the gastroesophageal junction, relaxing the sphincter and its ability to control regurgitation. Progesterone also relaxes the gastroesophageal sphincter. Pyloric displacement by the gravid uterus impedes gastric emptying. Therefore, pregnant patients must always be considered by anesthesiologists to have a full stomach, no matter how long they fasted.[6]

RADIATION AND PREGNANCY

Radiation plays a prominent role in the management of common cancers that may complicate pregnancy. The deleterious effects of radiation on fetal development have been recognized for many years.[7,8] Muller[9] reported in 1927 that ionizing radiation is capable of producing genetic mutations experimentally that are identical to those that occur spontaneously. However, there are scant data directly applicable to humans.

Pregnancy may be divided into three general phases with regard to radiation damage.[10] The preimplantation phase between fertilization and the attachment of the blastocyst to the uterine wall lasts for approximately 7 to 10 days. It is likely that most embryos exposed to radiation during this phase will die, resulting in spontaneous abortion. Indeed, the pregnancy may not be clinically recognized.[11] The most sensitive time for the fetus with regard to radiation and chemical exposure is during the time of organogenesis from the first to the tenth week of gestation. Each of the developing organs has a specific time for maximum susceptibility to teratogenic agents, but the central nervous system (CNS), eye, and hematopoietic systems remain highly susceptible throughout pregnancy to the effects of ionizing radiation. In addition to the gestational age, the radiation dose and dose rate are also important to the common fetal effects of growth retardation, malformations, and death.

Dekaban[12] reported that one-half of children exposed in utero to 250 rad during the third to tenth gestational week had multiple congenital anomalies including low birth weight, microcephaly, mental retardation, retinal degeneration, cataracts, and skeletal and genital malformations. Similar irradiation administered prior to 2 to 3 weeks gestation was associated with an increased risk of spontaneous abortion but not with severe congenital anomalies. The incidence of anomalies significantly declined when exposure was between the eleventh and twentieth weeks. Effects of fetal radiation exposure after the twentieth week of gestation were limited to anemia, pigmentation changes and dermal erythema. Late fetal radiation increases the risk of growth retardation and eye and CNS abnormalities. In general, a fetal dose of less than 10 rad is not associated with gross fetal malformations or fetal growth retardation, but doses higher than 10 rad should lead to consideration of therapeutic abortion.[10]

Pregnant patients receiving radiation therapy directed to the pelvis for pelvic malignancies will suffer a fetal demise and will usually spontaneously abort. Patients receiving supradiaphragmatic irradiation will receive only minor exposure, due primarily to internal radiation scatter, and may safely carry an early pregnancy. However, supradiaphragmatic radiation later in pregnancy may expose the growing fetus to excessive radiation that will produce unacceptable fetal injury. It is necessary for the therapeutic radiologist to calculate the potential dose to the fetus before supradiaphragmatic radiation begins so that the mother understands the potential hazard to the fetus and alternative forms of therapy may be considered.

CHEMOTHERAPY AND PREGNANCY

Information on the effects of chemotherapy on the fetus remains incomplete. Cytotoxic chemotherapy should be routinely avoided during the first trimester, as experience with single agents has confirmed that many pregnancies will either result in spontaneous abortion after exposure to chemotherapy, or the fetus will experience teratogenic effects from these agents.[13,14] Avoidance of exposure to cytotoxic chemotherapy during organogenesis should be the rule, to be violated only under the most unusual circumstances. In turn, single-agent chemotherapy given during the second and third trimesters rarely causes congenital anomalies.[13,14] During the past decade, multiple case reports have appeared, indicating that combination chemotherapy may be successfully employed in the second and third trimesters of pregnancy for treatment of acute leukemia,[15,16] non-Hodgkin's lymphoma,[17-19] and ovarian endodermal sinus tumor.[20] Long-term consequences due to intrauterine exposure to cytotoxic chemotherapy remain unknown. It is possible that deleterious effects in the offspring of women exposed in utero to cytotoxic chemotherapy will occur; these patients require long-term monitoring.

A brief review of effects of single-agent treatment follows. It must be kept in mind that up to 3 percent of children have associated major congenital anomalies and 9 percent have minor anomalies in pregnancies not complicated by exposure to cytotoxic chemotherapeutic agents.[21]

Alkylating agents: Melphalan, chlorambucil, cyclophosphamide, triethylene thiophosphoramide, cis-diamminedichloroplatinum, streptozotocin, BCNU, CCNU, methyl CCNU, and busulfan are cell-cycle-nonspecific drugs that form crosslinkages with DNA, preventing DNA from dividing. In addition, by alkylating proteins, these agents interfere with normal intracellular mechanisms. Six of 39 patients exposed to alkylating agents during the first trimester had infants with congenital anomalies, but no congenital anomalies were noted in the offspring of patients treated in the second and third trimesters.[13] Chlorambucil exposure has been associated with a syndrome characterized by renal aplasia, cleft palate, and skeletal abnormalities.[22]

Vinca alkyloids: Vincristine, vinblastine, VP16, and VM-26 are cell-phase specific agents. They act predominantly in the M phase of the cell cycle on the microtubular protein involved in spindle formation during mitosis, causing a metaphase arrest. Only one of 15 pregnancies exposed during the first trimester resulted in a congenital anomaly and no anomalies were seen in 11 pregnancies treated later in pregnancy.[13,14]

Antimetabolites: Amethopterin (methotrexate), aminopterin, 5-fluorouracil (5-FU), cytosine arabinoside, 6-mercaptopurine, imidazole carboxamide, 6-thioguanine, 5-azacytodine, hydroxyurea, hexamethylmelamine, and L-asparaginase are cell-cycle-specific agents that interfere with the synthesis of DNA, RNA, and some coenzymes. These structural analogues of precursor purine and pyrimidine bases, when incorporated into DNA molecules, lead to nonfunctional DNA and cell death. Aminopterin and methotrexate can induce abortions when administered during the first trimester.[13,23] Aminopterin has been associated with congenital anomalies in 10 of 52 cases exposed during the first trimester. An aminopterin syndrome, characterized by cranial dysostosis, hypertelorism, anomalies of the external ears, micrognathia, and cleft palate, has been described.[24,25] Other antimetabolites appear safer in pregnancy, as only one congenital anomaly was observed in 56 patients exposed.[14] No congenital anomalies were observed in 37 fetuses treated with a variety of antimetabolites in the second and third trimester.

Antibiotics: Actinomycin D, doxorubicin, daunorubicin, bleomycin, mitomycin C, and mithramycin are cell-cycle-nonspecific agents that interfere with DNA-dependent RNA synthesis, leading to cell death due to a lack of RNA and an inability to produce cell proteins. Congenital anomalies are most likely to occur when exposure is during the period of organogenesis.

Steroids: Patients receiving steroids for the treatment of malignancies are exposed to corticosteroids as part of combination chemotherapy for lymphomas or Hodgkin's disease.[26] Cleft lips and palates were recorded in an extensive review by Sindu and Hawkins,[26] but it was not clear that this is statistically significant. These anomalies were most often observed during first-trimester exposure. Unrecognized hypoadrenalism due to exogeneous steroid administration in pregnancy may lead to infant death.

Barber[27] pointed out that there are effects in the fetus exposed to cytotoxic chemotherapy in addition to teratogenicity, death, and stunted growth. Hematopoietic suppression may occur in the fetus (anemia, leukopenia, thrombocytopenia) and infection secondary to leukopenia or immunosuppression has also been reported. The timing of chemotherapy in relationship to anticipated delivery must be carefully assessed, so that delivery does not occur when the patient is bone marrow suppressed from exposure to cytotoxic chemotherapy. Patients receiving cytotoxic chemotherapy are discouraged from breast-feeding, although the data to support this are weak.[27]

ASSESSING FETAL MATURITY

Numerous articles discuss the possibility of delaying treatment of cancer diagnosed during the third trimester of pregnancy until fetal viability or fetal maturity is ensured. Such statements assume that data are readily available to make intelligent recommendations for determining when to anticipate successful termination of pregnancy. Realistically, this is a highly individualized decision. Centers with newborn special care units are required to provide the best possible chance for survival of the premature baby. Table 32-2 presents the survival statistics for the Yale-New Haven Hospital newborn special care unit for 1984 to 1985. Those infants born after 30 weeks gestation had a definite survival advantage, compared with infants born earlier. These data are typical for newborn special care units in the United States (Gross, I : personal communication).

However, survival is not the ultimate goal. Quality of life is extremely important. The presence or absence of the respiratory distress syndrome is the single most important factor in determining the quality of a premature infant's life. Respiratory distress syndrome may be avoided if the lecithin to sphingomyelin (L/S) ratio in amniotic fluid is 2 or greater. Data support the use of corticosteroids to stimulate lung maturity immediately prior to delivery in patients between 30 and 34 weeks gestation. A recent collaborative group study on antenatal steroid therapy demonstrated that

Table 32-2 Survival Statistics: 1985-1986[a,b]

Gestation Age (Weeks)	Survivors/Total	%
<24	1/42	2.4
24	1/9	11.1
25	6/25	24.0
26	8/14	57.1
27	10/15	66.7
28	28/33	84.9
29	29/35	82.9
30	25/31	80.7
31	49/52	94.2
32	81/88	92.1
33	95/103	92.2
34	128/135	94.8
35	103/105	98.1
36	101/103	98.1
37	70/75	93.3
38	83/85	97.7
39	103/106	97.2
40	270/274	98.5
41	53/53	100.0
42	34/35	97.1
>42	9/10	90.1
Total	1,288/1,428	90.2

[a] Yale-New Haven Hospital Newborn Special Care Unit.
[b] Inborn.

dexamethasone phosphate administered at a dose of 5 mg IM q12 h for up to four doses statistically reduced the chance that a fetus would develop respiratory distress syndrome at birth, provided the fetus was at least 30 weeks gestation.[28] Specifically, female infants treated with dexamethasone had a statistically reduced incidence of respiratory distress syndrome compared with female infant controls and male infants. Overall, male infants showed no benefit from dexamethasone treatment. Black infants showed the most marked effect of treatment, whereas white infants showed only a moderate effect, but these trends were not statistically significant. The effects seen were all in singleton pregnancies, as infants in multiple births showed no benefit from treatment. The risk of respiratory distress syndrome is greatest in women who undergo cesarean section when not in labor. Steroid treatment could not completely overcome the apparent difference between cesarean and vaginal delivery. The infants most likely to benefit from corticosteroid therapy were in the group between 30 to 34 weeks gestational age delivered between 24 hours and 7 days after initiation of dexamethasone therapy.

CERVICAL CANCER

The cervix is the most common site in which malignant transformation occurs in pregnancy. A recent review reported that carcinoma in situ of the uterine cervix occurs in approximately 1 in 767 pregnancies and invasive cancer in 1 in 2,205 pregnancies.[29] In turn, pregnancy complicated 1 in every 34 cases of invasive cancer. The incidence of invasive cancer of the cervix presenting in pregnancy appears to be on the decline, perhaps due to more effective Papanicolaou (Pap) smear screening.[30,31] A similar trend has yet to be established for cervical carcinoma in situ. Women in whom carcinoma in situ and invasive cancer of the cervix develops in pregnancy as compared with nonpregnant women have been reported to be married at an earlier age (18 versus 20.8 years), have an earlier age of diagnosis of carcinoma in situ (22.9 versus 35 years) and invasive cancer (33.8 versus 48 years), and a higher parity (5.4 versus 2.2) compared with a control population.[32-34]

Squamous cell cancers are the most common histologic types of cervical cancer diagnosed in pregnancy (93.1 percent), followed by adenocarcinomas (3 percent), anaplastic cancers (2.6 percent), adenosquamous cancer (1.1 percent), adenoacanthomas (0.1 percent), and sarcoma (0.1 percent).[29] Neuroendocrine carcinoma of the uterine cervix in pregnancy has been the subject of our recent case reports.[35]

Cervical Intraepithelial Neoplasia

The diagnosis of cervical intraepithelial neoplasia is based on Pap smear screening, as this is an asymptomatic lesion. A Pap smear should routinely be performed at the time of the initial prenatal examination. Evaluation of an abnormal Pap smear should employ colposcopic examination of the cervix and colposcopically directed biopsies. The pregnant cervix is engorged with blood vessels precluding the utility of extensive random biopsies or cone biopsies for the routine evaluation of the abnormal Pap smear. The colposcope plays a major role in reducing the need for such biopsies. False-negative rates as high as 40 percent have been reported using Schiller stain directed biopsies in the evaluation of the gravid cervix.[36] Conization of the cervix has been associated most often with the complication of hemorrhage, but abortion or premature labor may also occur.[36]

For most pregnant patients, the endocervical eversion that normally occurs in pregnancy allows for successful colposcopic visualization of the transformation zone. If the transformation zone is not completely seen during the first trimester, it is safe to wait a few weeks and repeat the colposcopy examination as long as the Pap smear does not suggest invasive cancer. Colposcopically directed biopsies can often be limited to one biopsy of the worst-looking site on the cervix, thereby reducing the morbidity of the procedure. A false-negative rate of 0.5 percent and a complication rate of 0.6 percent has been reported when colposcopically directed biopsies have been used in the evaluation of the abnormal Pap smear in pregnancy.[29] I have recommended cone biopsies only twice in an 11-year period (1975 to 1986) for patients evaluated at Yale-New Haven Hospital. In each case, more extensive tissue was necessary because of the presence of microinvasive cervical cancer in the colposcopically directed biopsies.

Cervical intraepithelial neoplasia is a slowly progressive process. A spectrum of management recommendations have been suggested in the literature. Some investigators suggest that patients with biopsy-confirmed cervical intraepithlial neoplasia be followed on an every 4- to 6-week schedule, with cytology and colposcopy during the pregnancy,[37-39] whereas others suggest that further evaluation be deferred until after delivery.[40-43] At Yale-New Haven Hospital, patients with abnormal Pap smears in pregnancy are followed with repeat Pap smears every 3 months during the pregnancy, provided the initial Pap smear was consistent with the colposcopically directed biopsy. If subsequent Pap smears remain unchanged, the patient has a final Pap smear and colposcopy evaluation at 36 weeks; if no substantial change is present, a vaginal delivery is anticipated and re-evaluation of the cevix is recommended approximately 8 to 12 weeks postpartum and definitive treatment instituted.

It is unusual to see the development of rapidly progressing cancer from cervical intraepithlial neoplasia during pregnancy. Only one patient who delivered at Yale-New Haven Hospital between 1975 and 1986 had a diagnosis of cancer established after a Pap smear and colposcopically directed biopsy at 26 weeks gestation confirmed carcinoma in situ of the cervix. That patient was noted to have a small nodule in the posterior lip of the cervix at delivery. A subsequent biopsy confirmed the presence of invasive cancer that was then successfully managed with a type III radical hysterectomy and bilateral deep pelvic lymphadenectomy.

Patients found to have abnormal Pap smears that cannot be explained on the basis of colposcopically directed biopsies must undergo more extensive biopsies, usually in the operating room, using the colposcope to help limit the extent of the biopsy. The need for this approach is unusual. At Yale-New Haven Hospital, this has only been required twice during 1975 to 1986.

There is a limited role for cesarean section hysterectomies. This procedure has generally been limited to the management of patients who desire sterilization and are viewed as poor candidates to return for routine postpartum Pap smear follow-up or treatment and in whom there is a well-established obstetric indication for the cesarean section. Cesarean section hysterectomies are associated with significant morbidity, including hemorrhage and injury to normal viscera. It is best to limit this procedure to institutions with substantial experience performing this surgery.

Squamous cell carcinoma in situ of the cervix may infrequently be associated with an underlying adenocarcinoma or adenocarcinoma in situ of the endocervix.[44] In nonpregnant women, this can lead to inadequate management, unless an endocervical biopsy is performed. The eversion of the endocervical epithelium in pregnancy allows for more adequate inspection of this tissue. Figure 32-1 reveals the colposcopic findings in a 27-year-old gravida 2 para 1 patient who was 8 weeks pregnant. The patient's initially abnormal Pap smear was obtained 7 months earlier and showed dysplastic changes in squamous cells. The patient's next Pap smear was obtained in early pregnancy and revealed severe dysplasia of squamous epithelium and atypical endocervical cells. Coloposcopy revealed a bizarre overgrowth of endocervical tissue confirmed by biopsy to be invasive adenocarcinoma. The patient underwent a type III radical hysterectomy and bilateral deep pelvic lymphadenectomies; she remains alive and well 4 years later. Histologic evaluation of the cervix confirmed the presence of squamous

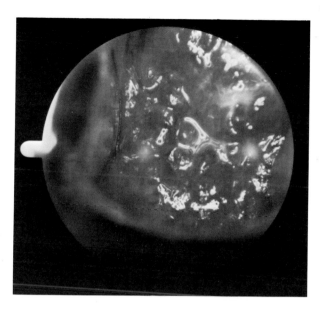

Fig. 32-1 Colposcopic view of adenocarcinoma of the endocervix presenting in an 8-week pregnant patient. This patient had a coexisting squamous cell carcinoma in situ of the exocervix, diagnosed on Pap smear. Note the luxuriant overgrowth of endocervical tissue.

cell carcinoma in situ of the exocervix with endocervical glandular involvement in association with invasive adenocarcinoma of the endocervix.

Microinvasive Cancer

The management of microinvasive cancer in pregnancy raises several issues. The establishment of this diagnosis requires a larger biopsy than that achieved with a colposcopically directed biopsy. Large wedges of the cervix, hemicone biopsy, or cone biopsy are necessary to secure sufficient tissue in order to confirm this diagnosis. Subsequent management must be based on the trimester of gestation. Insufficient data are available in the literature, in support of delaying definitive therapy for many months. An extrafascial hysterectomy is the routine recommendation for the management of microinvasive cervical cancer diagnosed during the first trimester of pregnancy. Management of microinvasive cervical cancer diagnosed during the second or third trimester is based on allowing the pregnancy to progress to near term and delivering the baby once fetal maturity is established. Delivery may be either by the vaginal route, in which

case an extrafascial hysterectomy would be performed postpartum, or by cesarean section and extrafascial hysterectomy.

The histologic criteria for the diagnosis of microinvasive cervical cancers vary among institutions, and the significance of lymphatic or vascular space involvement in the nonpregnant cervix remains debatable. Criteria for establishing the diagnosis of microinvasive cervical cancer in the gravid uterus are not clearly defined in the literature.[29] One must take into account the patient's desires as well as clinical judgment in deciding therapy. Anecdotal experience at Yale-New Haven Hospital suggests that a well-informed patient can be followed in pregnancy when focal microinvasive cancer is present and the pregnancy allowed to progress until fetal viability is established. Such patients are more likely to be seen now than in the past, as (1) the public has been informed of a need for Pap smears only once every 3 years if they have previously had negative annual Pap smears, and (2) many sexually active women are delaying childbearing until their mid-30s in order to pursue careers.

Invasive Cancer

The diagnosis of frankly invasive cervical cancer in pregnancy requires prompt management. Patients in the first or second trimester with International Federation of Gynecology nd Obstetrics (FIGO) stage IB or selected IIA disease who are suitable candidates for surgery should be treated by type III radical hysterectomies and bilateral deep pelvic lymphadenectomies. Patients found to have stage IB or selected IIA disease in the third trimester may be considered for carrying the pregnancy until fetal maturity is established, at which time a cesarean section and type III radical hysterectomy and bilateral deep pelvic lymphadenectomy is performed. A cesarean section will avoid the complication of bleeding and infection that may occur with a vaginal delivery. However, there is no evidence to support the contention that survival is compromised by having the patient deliver vaginally or that the cancer will be disseminated.[45]

The technique of radical hysterectomy and bilateral deep pelvic lymphadenectomy may be associated with significant morbidity, most often hemorrhage or injury to normal viscera. Thompson et al.[46] reported an increase in intraoperative blood loss and major postoperative complications when radical hysterectomies were performed in pregnancy. However, other investigators have reported no increase in fistulas or major complications with this approach.[31,33,47] The selection of cases in any surgical series can substantially influence complications. In my experience, the edema of pregnancy makes dissection planes easier to establish, such that radical hysterectomies and deep pelvic lymphadenectomies may be readily performed in pregnancy. Hysterotomy has been recommended to reduce the size of the gravid uterus when performing radical surgery. In general, I have not found this necessary when surgery is performed prior to 20 weeks gestation, as the uterus is mobile and may be lifted out of the incision in some patients to permit adequate exposure.

Radiation therapy may be employed for the management of all stages of cervical cancer in pregnancy. External beam radiation may be instituted first to induce an abortion, while treating the cancer during the first trimester. Prem et al.[48] reported an average time to abortion of 32.7 days (range 27 to 50 days), using this technique. Alternatively, abortion may be accomplished by suction dilation and curettage (D&C) prior to initiating radiation therapy. Radiation therapy in the second trimester requires a longer average time interval until abortion occurs (average time 43.9 days, range 33 to 60 days), suggesting to some that a hysterotomy may be the preferable initial method of management followed by external beam radiation.[48] At Yale-New Haven Hospital, external beam radiation is usually offered first rather than hysterotomy. The now rare patient found to have advanced-stage (IIB-IVA) cancer during the third trimester may be allowed to carry the pregnancy until fetal maturity is established prior to initiating radiation therapy. Excellent survival rates are now achieved in our New-Born Special Care nursery, particularly if the pregnancy can be maintained until at least 30 weeks gestation before terminating the pregnancy (Table 32-2).

The 5-year survival for patients treated for stage IB and II cancers of the cervix in pregnancy were 74.5 and 47.8 percent, respectively, as compared with 76.5 and 55.0 percent overall 5-year survival in the FIGO annual reports of the same era.[29] Survival for stage III and IV combined was 16.2 percent in the pregnant patient as compared with 27.9 percent overall 5-year survival in the FIGO annual reports.[29] The efficacy of treatment in advanced cervical cancer is unsatisfac-

tory. The clinician must routinely evaluate any abnormal bleeding in pregnancy by carefully performing a pelvic examination. Early diagnosis of invasive cervical cancer is essential to achieve a high cure rate. Avoiding pelvic examinations for fear of exacerbating a complication of pregnancy due to abnormal placentation may have a far more deleterious effect on the patient and fetus than careful, but active, investigation.

BREAST CANCER

Breast cancer is reported to occur once in every 3,000 pregnancies.[49] There is no conclusive evidence to support the contention that pregnancy influences the course of the cancer. Early diagnosis is critical for effective therapy. The enlargement of the breast in pregnancy and associated hyperemia may confuse the examiner and interfere with interpretation of mammograms. Mammograms may be employed in pregnancy, provided the abdomen is shielded. Clinicians must be alert to evaluate breast masses promptly in pregnancy. Delay in diagnosis of 2 to 7 months has often been related to the advanced stage of breast cancer in pregnant or lactating women.[50,51] Attention should be directed to the upper outer quadrants of breasts, as 50 percent of breast cancers arise there. A liberal use of the needle aspiration technique to separate cystic from solid masses may quickly resolve questions regarding the nature of breast masses in pregnancy.[52] Ninety percent of breast masses occurring in pregnancy are initially discovered by the patient.[53]

The diagnosis of breast cancer is best confirmed by excisional biopsy. Local anesthesia may be safely employed, as may general anesthesia. Only 1 of 134 patients undergoing a general anesthetic experienced a spontaneous abortion in one breast cancer series.[54] The histology of breast masses has the same distribution in pregnancy as in the nonpregnant state. Pregnancy does not select for any particular type of breast malignancy.[55] Occasionally, lactational mastitis or abscess may be confused with an inflammatory carcinoma. It has been suggested to biopsy all lactational abscesses at the time of incision and drainage in order to avoid missing an inflammatory carcinoma of the breast. A variety of neoplastic disorders can also present as breast masses including Hodgkin's disease,[50] Burkitt's lymphoma,[56,57] acute myelogenous leukemia,[58] and sarcoma.[59] If breast cancer is confirmed to be present, a piece of the cancer should be assayed for estrogen and progestin receptor content. Stage for stage, the prognosis for breast cancer patients initially diagnosed in pregnancy is almost the same as that in the nonpregnant state.[60] The best success is achieved in treating small cancers that have yet to spread to axillary lymph nodes.

It has been suggested that hormonal changes in pregnancy, that is, increased levels of estrogen, progesterone, corticosteroids, and prolactin, may stimulate the growth of breast cancer or indirectly decrease cellular and humoral immunity.[11] Peters[61] demonstrated considerable variation in the patterns of breast cancer growth first diagnosed in pregnancy, with some patients showing more rapid growth, others slower growth, and some no change in growth pattern. Nugent and O'Connell[62] reported on 176 patients with breast cancer in pregnancy. Poor survival was related to patients under 40 years of age and hormonally insensitive, as 71 percent had estrogen and progestin receptor-negative cancer specimens.

Ribeiro and Palmer[63] reported 5-year survival rates for patients with breast cancer diagnosed in pregnancy of 90 percent, 37 percent, 15 percent, and zero for clinical stages I, II, III, and IV, respectively, and no difference in survival, stage for stage, in each trimester of pregnancy or postpartum. An overall 5-year survival of 70 percent was reported. Breast cancer diagnosed late in pregnancy is often more advanced than is disease diagnosed early in pregnancy. This may have contributed to the erroneous impression in the past that breast cancers diagnosed in pregnancy have a uniformly poor prognosis.

Once the diagnosis of breast cancer is established, a limited evaluation for staging should be performed. A chest radiograph should be obtained, with the abdomen shielded. Radioisotope scanning must be avoided because of potential fetal injury.

Prior to definitive therapy, the patient and her family must be carefully counseled regarding therapeutic options. The emotional aspects of mastectomy in a young pregnant women cannot be overestimated, and the patient and her family must thoroughly understand the plan of management, the reasons for it, and the anticipated results of the therapy. A team approach involving the surgeon, obstetrician, therapeutic radiologist, medical oncologist, and medical social worker is extremely important, but the patient must have one physician who she can readily identify as being in charge of her overall care.

Modified radical mastectomy, removing the breast and axillary lymph nodes at levels I and II, is currently the standard treatment for early-stage breast cancer.[11] Axillary node removal is necessary to determine the need for additional chemotherapy or radiation therapy. Lumpectomy and radiation therapy would be inappropriate in a patient continuing her pregnancy, as the scatter to the fetus may be significant. It has been estimated that a fetus located 25 cm from a breast radiation field treated to 7,500 rad would be exposed to 30 rad[64] — an unacceptably high exposure rate to the fetus during organogenesis. The risks to the fetus from breast radiation therapy later in pregnancy would not be reduced, as fetal growth would bring the fetus closer to the radiation field. It is estimated that the chance of aborting as a result of mastectomy is approximately 1 percent.[54] There is no significant benefit to delaying surgery until fetal maturity is achieved.[60,63]

Women found to have locally advanced breast cancer without lymph node spread (T4 N0) will invariably develop massive recurrence at the mastectomy site if they have not received prior chemotherapy or radiation therapy. During the first trimester, these patients are best served by therapeutic abortion followed by radiation to the breast and regional nodes or chemotherapy. Mastectomy and regional node staging should be performed approximately 6 weeks later. During the second trimester, a hysterectomy is recommended first, to be followed by radiation or chemotherapy, and then mastectomy. Patients with massive local disease found in the third trimester may delay therapy until fetal viability is achieved.[65]

Women found to have metastases to axillary lymph nodes have a poor prognosis. Nonpregnant premenopausal women with axillary lymph node metastases benefit significantly from adjuvant cytotoxic chemotherapy.[66] This approach, if used in pregnancy, carries with it the possibility of teratogenic effects. Pregnant women must be counseled regarding the advisability of therapeutic abortion. Patients diagnosed in the third trimester may delay chemotherapy until after fetal maturity is achieved and the baby delivered. Anecdotal reports of successful pregnancy while the mother is receiving chemotherapy are available, but long-term effects on the children are not known.

Abortion is indicated if adjuvant cytotoxic chemotherapy is to be administered. However, there is no medical indication to justify the routine use of abortion in pregnant women with breast cancer. Indeed, several authorities have presented data showing no effect on survival with termination of pregnancy.[61,67,68] Prophylactic castration is not routinely recommended in the management of pregnant patients with breast cancer.[60] Its role may be limited to those few patients with disseminated disease whose cancers contain elevated levels of estrogen and progestin receptor protein. However, antiestrogen therapy would be an alternative choice.

Management of disseminated breast cancer usually requires systemic chemotherapy and possibly radiation or hormonal therapy. The deleterious effects on the fetus would be substantial, and a therapeutic abortion should be recommended in the first and second trimester under these circumstances. Disseminated disease presenting in the third trimester must be individualized, but delaying systemic treatment until fetal maturity is achieved is reasonable.

In the past, patients initially diagnosed as having breast cancer in pregnancy were advised not to become pregnant again, and many underwent prophylactic castration. Data now suggest that patients who appear to be successfully treated for breast cancer that initially presented during a pregnancy may subsequently be able to conceive again without endangering their lives.[69,70] It is possible that there is a natural selection of patients in the latter series for those patients who have been successfully treated, whereas those who were not rapidly succumbed to the disease and did not have the opportunity to become pregnant again. Patients who were first diagnosed to have breast cancer in pregnancy may be placed on birth control pills without incurring a risk of flareup of the cancer.[65]

OVARIAN CANCER

Ovarian cancer is the major health hazard for women in whom cancer develops in the female pelvic reproductive organs. More women (11,700) will die from ovarian cancer in the United States in 1987 than from cervical and uterine cancers combined (9,700).[71] Most patients diagnosed to have ovarian cancer are perimenopausal or postmenopausal, and overwhelm-

ingly they will have the common epithelial cancer. The incidence of ovarian cancer in women below age 35 is much lower; such patients often have histologically borderline malignant potential tumors or low-grade invasive epithelial cancers or the infrequently occurring germ cell or sex cord-stromal tumors. Overall, about 60 to 70 percent of the common epithelial cancers reported in any large series present as stage III or IV disease, as this disease usually remains silent until upper abdominal metastases occur, and even then symptoms are limited to vague nonspecific discomfort and bloating.[72]

Ovarian malignancies occurring in pregnancy are infrequent, with an estimated occurrence of 1 in 9,000 to 1 in 25,000 pregnancies.[73,74] Some asymptomatic lesions are recognized at the initial prenatal examination. However, ovarian malignancies represent only about 2 to 5 percent of ovarian neoplasms diagnosed in pregnancy as compared with 15 to 20 percent in nonpregnant women.[75,76] Ovarian neoplasms are usually followed until the second trimester, at which time many functional cysts will resolve; surgery, if necessary, may more safely be performed without endangering the fetus. Torsion appears to occur more frequently in ovarian malignancies presenting in pregnancy, perhaps due to the rapid enlargement of the uterus between the sixth to fourteenth weeks of gestation. Torsion is also a routine presentation of patients with ovarian germ cell malignancies in the nongravid state. Vague nonspecific abdominal discomfort is common during a normal pregnancy and may be confused with an intermittently torting ovarian neoplasm.

Ovarian malignancies are often silent during the second trimester and are difficult to identify by examination, as the expanding uterus lifts the ovaries out of the pelvis. Many ovarian malignancies do not become obvious until labor, when they can cause either obstructed labor or severe pain or are found as asymptomatic masses at cesarean section.

Diagnostic evaluation for patients found to have asymptomatic enlarged ovaries in the first trimester is limited. Patients clinically thought to have enlarging cysts should undergo an ultrasound examination. If simple cysts are identified, they may be followed with serial ultrasounds until they resolve. It has been suggested that unilateral mobile simple cysts up to 6 cm in diameter identified in the first trimester of pregnancy will be functional cysts in more than 99 percent of cases.[77] Complex cysts (i.e., cysts containing both solid and cystic elements) are more compatible with ovarian malignancies and require agressive therapeutic intervention. Solid tumors may present infrequently occurring ovarian malignancies, such as the dysgerminoma, and also require aggressive therapeutic intervention.

The role of magnetic resonance imaging is now being established.[78,79] Figure 32-2 demonstrates a fetus in the breech position. One can readily see fetal structures such as the fetal eyes, umbilical cord, thigh, amniotic fluid, and maternal spine. Figure 32-3 demonstrates a psoas abscess in the second trimester of pregnancy. Magnetic resonance imaging (MRI) is a safe technique for evaluating pelvic masses in pregnancy and gives clearer images than ultrasound. However, ultrasound is much more readily available. MRI in 16 pregnant patients with pelvic masses has been compared with ultrasound imaging. In seven patients, MRI contributed additional information, such as distinguishing leiomyomas, recognizing that a mass depicted by ultrasound was actually a loop of bowel and differentiating between a solid soft tissue mass and a hemorrhagic fluid-containing mass.[78] Other imaging

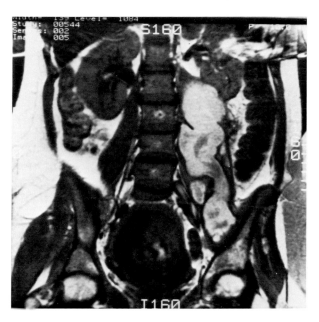

Fig. 32-3 Coronal magnetic resonance scan demonstrating a left psoas abscess in the second trimester of pregnancy. Note the gravid uterus in the pelvis. (Courtesy of Dr. E. Kanal.)

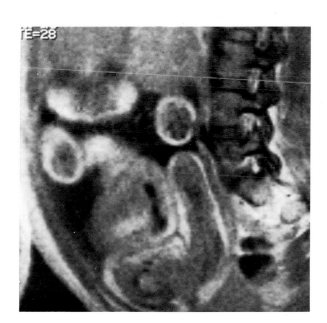

Fig. 32-2 Sagittal magnetic resonance scan through a 36-week gestation demonstrating a fetus in the breech position. Note the fetal eyes, umbilical cord, thigh, amniotic fluid, and maternal spine. (Courtesy of Dr. S. McCarthy.)

techniques that have been advocated include an intravenous urogram with only one exposure made to reduce fetal injury and the barium enema. In my experience, the latter two techniques add little to the evaluation of the asymptomatic adnexal mass in pregnancy and may be avoided.

Circulating tumor markers play a role in the diagnosis and management of ovarian germ cell malignancies in the nonpregnant state.[80] Endodermal sinus tumors secrete α-fetoprotein (AFP), embryonal carcinoma is associated with elevated levels of AFP and human chorionic gonadotropin (hCG), ovarian choriocarcinoma is associated with hCG, dysgerminomas may have dramatically elevated levels of lactic dehydrogenase (LDH), and mixed germ cell tumors may have elevations of any of the above markers. Unfortunately, each of the above markers is routinely elevated in pregnancy and, unless dramatically increased in patients being evaluated for an asymptomatic pelvic mass, their determination will be of little value. Indeed, one can wait until a histologic diagnosis is confirmed before using these markers for management of the malignancy. Preoperative values are of academic interest only and can be available by drawing an extra tube of blood and requesting the chemistry laboratory to store the serum until a histologic diagnosis is established.

The tumor antigen CA 125 has had a substantial impact in the monitoring of patients with ovarian cancer.[81,82] However, this antigen is also routinely elevated during the first trimester of normal pregnancy. It too will be of very limited value in the diagnosis of asymptomatic adnexal masses in pregnancy.[83]

Timing of surgery cannot always be controlled. Ovarian malignancies that twist on their vascular pedicle must be treated as surgical emergencies and should be rapidly removed. Spontaneous abortion following surgery for ovarian cancer is more likely to occur during the first trimester,[84] and premature labor will occur during the third trimester.[85] The second trimester is the safest time to operate on pregnant women. If it is possible to defer surgery from the first to the second trimester, the patient will be at reduced hazard for spontaneous abortion. Patients in the third trimester may be considered for conservative management until fetal maturity is established. Unfortunately, delaying surgery is inappropriate for patients with findings suspicious of an ovarian malignancy. If the preoperative evaluation suggests a high probability that an ovarian malignancy is present, surgery should be performed promptly.

Management of ovarian cancer is based on the histologic type of tumor as well as the grade, stage, and volume of residual disease. These factors have been well established based on ovarian malignancies treated in the nonpregnant patient.[72] The frequency of ovarian cancers presenting in pregnancy is low, but there is no evidence to suggest that ovarian cancers diagnosed in pregnancy are biologically different than those more commonly presenting in the nongravid state.

Surgical Staging

Surgical staging is based on an adequate incision that will permit inspection of the entire peritoneal cavity. Upon entering the abdomen through a vertical midline or paramedian incision, any peritoneal fluid present should be aspirated and sent for cytology and cell-block evaluation. If no free fluid is present, each of the paracolic spaces and the pelvis should be irrigated with 200 ml normal saline and the irrigant aspirated and sent for cytologic evaluation. The ad-

nexal mass should then be removed. It is in the patient's best interest to have the tumor sent for frozen-section histologic evaluation. If a malignancy is suspected clinically or by frozen-section evaluation, the contralateral ovary should be biopsied and biopsies obtained from multiple sites from the pelvic peritoneum, parcolic space peritoneum, omentum, pelvic and paraaortic lymph nodes, and diaphragm. Adhesions, if present, should be sampled and any intraperitoneal or retroperitoneal nodules removed. Patients who have visible involvement of both ovaries should have frozen-section analyses performed to determine the nature of the abnormality in each ovary. Epithelial ovarian cancers often involve both ovaries, but it is rare for an ovarian germ cell malignancy to be bilateral. However, ovarian germ cell malignancies may be associated with benign cystic teratomas in the contralateral ovary.[80] It is essential to establish a firm histologic diagnosis before subjecting a pregnant women to castration. It is far better to terminate the operation and await the final histologic diagnosis than prophylactically castrate a pregnant woman. Sex cord-stromal tumors, like ovarian germ cell malignancies, are usually unilateral, and the same caution applies. Removal of both ovaries in unusual circumstances can be performed in the second or third trimester, and the pregnancy can continue.

Epithelial Ovarian Cancers

Common epithelial cancers in young women are most often tumors of borderline malignant potential or early-stage low-grade tumors. Tumors of borderline malignant potential are the most common epithelial malignancies diagnosed in pregnancy in patients seen or consulted on at Yale-New Haven Hospital. Four of 100 consecutive patients with borderline malignant potential tumors seen between January 1978 and January 1986 presented in pregnancy.[86] Two tumors were first diagnosed at cesarean section; one patient underwent a unilateral oophorectomy at 22 weeks gestation and went on to complete a term gestation, and the remaining patient underwent a bilateral salpingo-oophorectomy at 16 weeks gestation and completed a term pregnancy (Fig. 32-4). In the latter patient, bilateral ovarian masses were recognized at 7 weeks gestation that on ultrasound imaging were suggestive or malignancy. The tumors were reevaluated at 11 and 15 weeks gestation. At 16 weeks

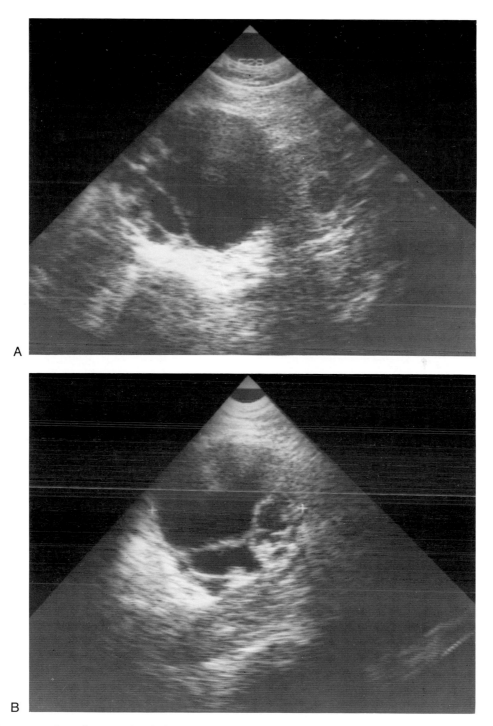

Fig. 32-4 Bilateral ovarian borderline malignant potential tumors of the ovaries arising in pregnancy. **(A)** Right ovary at 7 weeks gestation demonstrating multiple septa suspicious for malignancy. **(B)** Right ovary at 11 weeks gestation, unchanged in size. *(Figure continues.)*

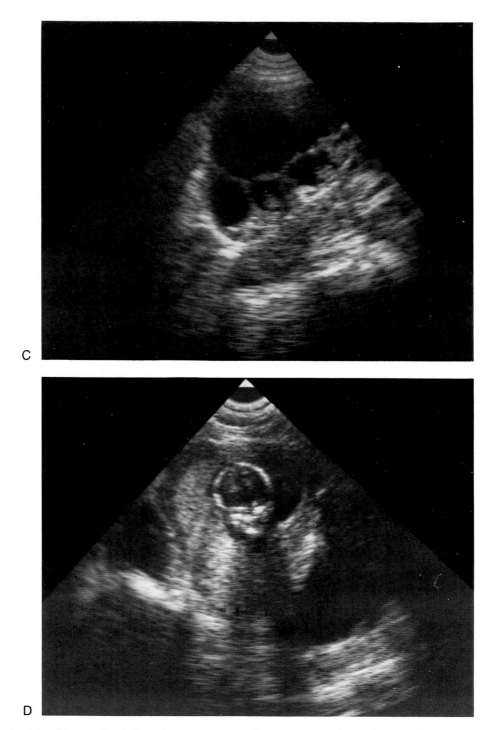

Fig. 32-4 *(Continued)*. **(C)** Right ovary at 15 weeks gestation, unchanged in size. **(D)** Fetal (midline) and bilateral ovarian neoplasms at 15 weeks gestation. (Courtesy of Dr. F. Malyska.)

gestation, the patient underwent an exploratory laparotomy and resection of each adnexal mass; she was found to have positive peritoneal cytology and an implant of tumor on the uterine serosa that was excised. At cesarean section, cytology was again positive, but at a subsequent reexploration no active disease was present.

A unilateral oophorectomy is adquate therapy for a stage IAi borderline malignant potential tumor. The role of adjuvant chemotherapy remains unclear for more advanced borderline malignant potential tumors.[86] Patients wishing to continue the pregnancy in the presence of borderline malignant potential tumors may, but should not receive adjuvant chemotherapy.

Patients found to have stage IAi invasive epithelial ovarian cancer may also be managed conservatively and permitted to continue their pregnancy. However, once the stage is more advanced, aggressive surgical debulking surgery should be performed, including a hysterectomy, salpingo-oophorectomy, omentectomy, and additional therapy with cis-diamminedichloroplatinum-based combination chemotherapy.[72]

GERM CELL MALIGNANCIES

Germ cell ovarian malignancies are infrequently occurring tumors that present most often in women in the second and third decades of life. As such, these malignancies may complicate pregnancy, but this is a very unusual event. These tumors are diagnosed at an early stage, as they tend to produce pain due to torsion of the vascular pedicle. Seventy percent present as stage I lesions and, with the exception of dysgerminoma, tend to be limited to one ovary. Karlen et al,[87] in 1979 reported that the dysgerminoma is the most commonly occurring germ cell malignancy in pregnancy and constitutes 25 to 35 percent of all ovarian cancer coexisting with pregnancy. Nevertheless, these workers were only able to obtain details on 27 such cases occurring in pregnancy and reported in the English literature between 1937 and 1978. Management of stage IA dysgerminomas tended to be conservative, with removal of the involved ovary in patients who wished to maintain the pregnancy and reproductive function. Patients with advanced disease or in whom the pregnancy was terminated usually underwent total abdominal hysterectomy, bilateral salpingo-oophorectomy, and postoperative radiation therapy. Surgical staging is extremely important. Cytologic washings may be positive in dysgerminoma visibly limited to one ovary, microscopic disease may be present in an otherwise unremarkable contralateral ovary, and metastases to paraaortic lymph nodes may occur as dysgerminomas have a tendency to spread via lymphatics. Data at Yale-New Haven Hospital in nonpregnant patients suggest that dysgerminoma is not only exquisitely sensitive to radiation therapy but is also extremely sensitive to chemotherapy.[80] Therefore, there is no reason to castrate a patient with a dysgerminoma to control the disease successfully. A recent report by Bianchi et al.[88] suggests that even when microscopic disease is present in the contralateral ovary, following intensive cytotoxic chemotherapy, fertility can be preserved.

Another type of germ cell ovarian malignancy is the endodermal sinus tumor, the most virulent of all germ cell tumors. In the era preceding modern combination chemotherapy, it had a 2-year survival of only 12 to 19 percent even though 70 percent present as stage IA disease. Other types include the immature teratoma, embryonal carcinoma, choriocarcinoma, and mixed germ cell tumors containing combinations of any germ cell malignances.[89,90] Experience at Yale-New Haven Hospital employing vincristine, actinomycin D, and cyclophosphamide combination chemotherapy has been uniformly successful in apparently curing all patients with stage I ovarian germ cell malignancies and patients with advanced-stage immature teratoma.[80] Patients with advanced-stage pure endodermal sinus tumors or mixed germ cell tumors containing endodermal sinus tumor are treated with a more toxic regimen, cis-diamminedichloroplatinum, vinblastine, and bleomycin; these patients are also routinely cured. Malone et al.[20] in 1986 reported on the first patient to be treated in pregnancy with the latter regimen for an endodermal sinus tumor with a successful outcome for both the mother and fetus. That patient was diagnosed at 25 weeks gestation to have an 18-cm mass associated with ascites, underwent a salpingo-oophorectomy, received two courses of combination chemotherapy postoperatively, underwent a planned cesarean section at 32 weeks gestation, delivering a healthy infant, and went on to receive three additional courses of combination chemotherapy postpartum. The patient and her infant were alive and well 10 months later, the child appearing to be developing normally.

Patients diagnosed to have a nondysgerminomatous ovarian germ cell malignancy would do best to undergo a termination of pregnancy when diagnosed in the first trimester and then to receive intensive cytotoxic chemotherapy. Patient diagnosed to have these lesions in the third trimester may undergo surgery followed by chemotherapy once fetal maturity is established and a cesarean section performed. Patients diagnosed to have a lesion in the second trimester may now be offered an option of cytotoxic chemotherapy. This latter approach must be viewed as experimental, as the long-term effects of the chemotherapy on the fetus remain unknown. Cytotoxic chemotherapy should not be given in the first trimester as the teratogenic effects are considerable when the fetus is undergoing organogenesis.

Sex Cord-Stromal Tumors

Sex cord-stromal tumors are infrequently occurring ovarian malignancies that include the granulosa-theca cell tumor, which is associated with estrogen production, and the Sertoli-Leydig cell tumors, which produce androgens. Rare forms of these tumors exist but are unlikely to complicate pregnancy. Seventy percent of these tumors present as stage I disease in young women, treatment for which is removal.[91] Each of the 36 sex cord-stromal tumors diagnosed in pregnancy and reported by Young et al.[92] were stage I disease. Thirteen of the 36 had ruptured at diagnosis, causing pain and, in two cases, shock. Only one patient in this series has had a recurrence. Advanced-stage disease, most often found in postmenopausal women, would be treated with aggressive debulking surgery followed by intense combination chemotherapy employing cis-diamminedichloroplatinum, vinblastine, and bleomycin.[93]

Nonspecific Mesenchyme Tumors

Nonspecific mesenchyme tumors are quite rare and should be treated as in the nonpregnant state with aggressive surgery and combination chemotherapy. Mixed mesodermal ovarian tumors invariably occur in perimenopausal or postmenopausal women and should not complicate pregnancy.

HODGKIN'S DISEASE

Hodgkin's disease has a peak incidence between ages 18 and 30.[94] It is extremely sensitive to therapy, with an 80 percent cure rate when localized and treated with radiation therapy. Advanced disease treated with chemotherapy is associated with prolonged disease survival in 65 percent of patients.[95,96] Failure to achieve complete remission is incompatible with cure. It has been estimated that one-third of premenopausal women with Hodgkin's disease are pregnant or have delivered within 1 year of diagnosis.[97,98] Pregnancy has not been reported to affect the course of Hodgkin's disease.[99,100] Ninety percent of Hodgkin's disease patients present with peripheral lymphadenopathy, 60 to 80 percent having cervical lymph nodes. Patients may be asymptomatic or present with variable histories of fever, night sweats, weight loss, malaise, and pruritis.[101]

A definitive diagnosis of Hodgkin's disease can only be made by histologic demonstration of the Reed-Sternberg cell, a dedifferentiated histiocyte.[101] Histologic appearance and patterns of spread of Hodgkin's disease are the most important prognostic factors. The four histologic subtypes of Hodgkin's disease are lymphocyte predominant, which carries the best prognosis, mixed cellularity, lymphocyte depleted, and nodular sclerosis, the latter being the most common type to occur in women and usually involves the neck and supraclavicular and anterior and superior mediastinal regions.[94,101] Staging (I to IV) is based on nodal or extranodal involvement. A reflects no systemic symptoms and B indicates systemic symptoms such as fever, sweats, and weight loss (Table 32-3). Staging allows one to determine whether the patient should receive local radiation or systemic chemotherapy. Once a decision is made for chemotherapy, no further diagnostic evaluations is necessary.

Minimal staging studies include a routine history and physical examination looking for systemic symptoms and identification of the clinical distribution of nodal disease, chest radiography, blood count, erythrocyte sedimentation rate, renal and liver-function studies, and a bone marrow aspirate and biopsy. These tests will identify patients with extranodal disease and, if positive, will eliminate the need for detailed nodal distribution studies. If these studies are negative, further evaluation of nodal distribution in the nonpregnant women would include a bipedal lym-

Table 32-3 Staging Classification for Hodgkin's Disease (Ann Arbor Classification)

Stage	Description Features
I	Involvement of a single lymph node region (I) or of a single extralymphatic organ or site (I_E)
II	Involvement of two or more lymph node regions on the same side of the diaphragm (II) or localized involvement of extralymphatic organ or site and of one or more lymph node regions on the same side of the diaphragm (IIE), optional recommendation: numbers of node regions involved indicated by a subscript (e.g., II3)
III	Involvement of lymph node regions on both sides of the diaphragm (III), which may also be accompanied by localized involvement of extralymphatic organ or site (IIIE) or by involvement of the spleen (IIIS), or both (IIISE)
IV	Diffuse or disseminated involvement of one or more extralymphatic organs or tissues with or without associated lymph node enlargement; reason for classifying the patient as stage IV should be identified further by defining site by symbols
	Lymphatic structures are defined as the lymph nodes, spleen, thymus, Waldeyer's ring, appendix, and Peyer's patches; liver involvement (H+) always considered diffuse, hence stage IV; bone marrow biopsies to be taken from a clinical or radiographically uninvolved area of bone
	Symptoms A or B
	Each stage will be subdivided into A and B categories: B for those with defined general symptoms, and A for those without. The B classification will be given to those patients with (1) unexplained weight loss of more than 10 percent of the body weight during 6 months previous to admission; (2) unexplained fever with temperatures about 38°C; and (3) night sweats.
	Note: Pruritus alone will no longer qualify for B classification; also a short, febrile illness in association with a known infection will not qualify for B classification.

(Report of the Committee on Hodgkin's Disease Staging Classification, 1971.)

phangiogram and an intravenous urogram or a computed tomogram (CT). If radiation is still planned, exploratory laparotomy, splenectomy, liver biopsy, and mapping of abdominal lymph node involvement are required.[102] Ultrasound or MRI of the liver, spleen, and retroperitoneal lymph nodes would be alternative imaging techniques for pregnant patients that would avoid the hazard of radiation exposure to the fetus.

Patients with stage I and II Hodgkin's disease are usually treated with radiation therapy; reported 5-year survival is 89 and 67 percent, respectively.[101] Most centers treat stage IIIA lymphocyte-predominant or nodular-sclerosing Hodgkin's disease with irradiation only, whereas stage IIIA disease with other histologic types is treated with combination chemotherapy and radiation. Stage IIIB and IV disease are predominantly treated with combination chemotherapy.[103]

Treating a mantle field employing a midline mediastinal dose of 4,000 rad yields an ovarian dose of approximately 65 rad.[104] Most ovarian radiation

comes from internal radiation scatter, which cannot be shielded. Whereas a fetal dose of greater than 10 rad has been suggested as the threshold for recommending therapeutic abortion in the first trimester of pregnancy, one should not recommend radiation in early pregnancy.[103] Patients with disease localized to the inguinal or abdominal region should undergo therapeutic abortion prior to receiving radiation therapy. Patients diagnosed as having Hodgkin's disease in the third trimester suitable for localized radiation therapy should have treatment withheld until fetal maturity is achieved. Similarly, chemotherapy should be avoided during the first trimester. Patients found to have rapidly progressing advanced disease should promptly receive chemotherapy, and decisions regarding continuation of the pregnancy should be based on the trimester of pregnancy and the patient's desires.

The MOPP regimen, consisting of Mustargen (nitrogen mustard), Oncovin (vincristine), procarbazine, and prednisone, has been extremely successful in achieving complete remissions and prolonged survival in previously untreated patients with stage III and IV Hodgkin's disease.[101] Eighty-one percent of patients in this category in the initial National Cancer Institute (NCI) series achieved these results with only 6 months treatment.[96] Side effects were considered tolerable. Other drugs active in Hodgkin's disease include cyclophosphamide, vinblastine, bleomycin, doxorubicin, and bischloroethylnitrosourea (BCNU).

Patients in remission from Hodgkin's disease should delay subsequent pregnancies for at least 2 years, as recurrence during the first 2 years following initial diagnosis is associated with a poor prognosis.[101]

NON-HODGKIN'S LYMPHOMA

Non-Hodgkin's lymphoma represents a spectrum of malignancies originating principally from lymphocytes and rarely reported to complicate pregnancy, as fewer than 20 cases have been published.[101] The two most important prognostic factors are the histology and stage of the disease. Histologically, the tumors may be divided into the nodular type, which tends to have a more indolent course with untreated median survivals of approximately 4 years, and the diffuse type, which is associated with a more rapid course and an untreated survival expectancy of months.[103] Non-Hodgkin's lymphomas tend to be much more widely disseminated at diagnosis than Hodgkin's disease, and staging evaluation is therefore less elaborate.

Management of non-Hodgkin's lymphoma is based on whether the disease is localized or disseminated. Localized disease regardless of histology is treated with radiation and has a 50 percent cure rate with radiation therapy. Data are available to suggest that localized disease might also be curable with chemotherapy.[105] Disseminated non-Hodgkin's lymphomas may be divided into favorable and unfavorable types. Disseminated nodular lymphoma and chronic lymphocytic leukemia are favorable types that are indolent.[103] Treatment is palliative in the favorable type, with survival about 5 years. Unfavorable types have a survival expectancy of 2 years. However, some patients may achieve complete remission and prolonged survival.[106]

Diffuse non-Hodgkin's lymphomas have a much more aggressive course than Hodgkin's disease and generally cannot wait for fetal maturity before initiating therapy. Two reports are available wherein com-

bination chemotherapy consisting of cyclophosphamide, vincristine, prednisone, and bleomycin was administered during pregnancy, resulting in normal infants and successfully treated mothers.[17,107] An additional patient was treated for diffuse histiocytic lymphoma with combination chemotherapy consisting of procarbazine and BCNU for 5 months prior to conception and during the first and second trimesters.[108] Streptozotocin was given throughout the third trimester. A normal male infant was then delivered. Rapid acceleration of non-Hodgkin's lymphoma postpartum is commonly observed.[109,110]

ACUTE LEUKEMIA

Acute leukemia rarely complicates pregnancy. Most pregnant acute leukemia patients are first recognized to have the disease during the second or third trimester.[111] The incidence is less than 1 case in 75,000 pregnancies.[112] The presenting symptoms usually reflect bone marrow failure and include easy fatigue, bleeding diathesis, and/or recurrent infection. Physical findings are nonspecific except for sternal tenderness, skin pallor, petechiae, ecchymoses, and hepatosplenomegaly. Laboratory examinations in the acute lymphocytic, myelocytic, or monocytic leukemias reveal a normocytic normochromic anemia, mild to marked thrombocytopenia, and leukocytosis.[101] At times, the leukocyte count may be low or normal. Auer rods in the cytoplasm of myeloblasts may help differentiate acute myeloblastic leukemias from acute lymphoblastic leukemias. Acute monoblastic leukemias may be identified by high serum and urine lysozyme levels. Bone marrow aspirates are used to confirm the clinical impression.[101] There is no evidence to suggest that pregnancy influences the natural history of acute leukemia.[13]

Survival of patients diagnosed to have acute leukemias in pregnancy has substantially improved with the use of chemotherapy, radiation therapy, and supportive care, including blood products and antibiotics. Modern therapy for patients with acute leukemia in pregnancy has now been associated with 100 percent maternal survival to delivery and 87 percent fetal survival.[101] Complications of therapy include severe infections secondary to bone marrow suppression and CNS leukemia, the latter being effectively treated with whole-brain irradiation and intrathecal methotrexate or cytosine arabinoside. Allopurinal should be administered to avoid the complications of hyperuricemia usually associated with organomegaly and high white blood cell counts.[113]

Acute lymphocytic leukemia in adults treated with combination chemotherapy has a complete response rate of 50 to 80 percent, the median duration of remission being 1 year. Agents used include prednisone, vincristine, asparaginase, daunorubicin, doxorubicin, 6-mercaptopurine, methotrexate, cyclophosphamide, and cytosine arabinoside. CNS prophylaxis with radiation therapy and intrathecal chemotherapy has yet to be proved effective.[101] Acute myelocytic leukemia has a poorer prognosis. While induced remission may be achieved in 50 to 80 percent of treated patients, the median survival is less than 1 year.[101] Whole-body radiation may be employed in preparing women to undergo bone marrow transplantation. Leukemic deposits in abdominal viscera may be irradiated palliatively. Such patients are unusual but should be recommended to undergo a termination of the pregnancy before being irradiated.

CHRONIC MYELOCYTIC LEUKEMIA

Chronic myelocytic leukemia presents with a history of progressive fatigability and a heaviness or ache in the left upper quadrant of the abdomen due to an enlarging spleen. Initial hematologic changes are limited to leukocytosis with basophilia or eosinophilia that may progress in time to several hundred thousand white cells per cubic millimeter.[101] Mature polymorphonuclear white cells, bands, metamyelocytes, and myelocytes predominate; platelets are normal or slightly increased and may be enlarged and functionally abnormal. Bone marrow examination reveals hypercellularity with mature forms predominating. Eighty-five percent of patients will have a Philadelphia chromosome, a 9:22 translocation.[101]

Chronic myelocytic leukemia represents 90 percent of chronic leukemias complicating pregnancy.[114,115] There is no indication that pregnancy adversely affects the natural history of chronic myelocytic leukemia.[13] Chronic myelocytic leukemia is most often diagnosed prior to pregnancy.[13] Treatment is palliative with a median survival from diagnosis of 45 months, but all patients eventually die,

most in acute blastic crisis that resembles acute myeloblastic leukemia, but has greater resistance to intensive therapy.[103] Median survival after acute blastic crisis is less than 1 year.[101] Poorer prognostic factors include absence of the Philadelphia chromosome, hyperdiploidy, chromosomal instability, presence of marked lymphadenopathy, basophilia, or gross soft tissue disease.[101]

Pregnant women with chronic myelocytic leukemia have a 96 percent chance of surviving to delivery, and fetal survival throughout the gestation is 84 percent.[101] Busulfan, hydroxyurea, dibromomannitol, and cyclophosphamide are the most useful drugs for this disease; radiation in nonpregnant patients is helpful in reducing the size of the spleen.

MELANOMA

Malignant melanoma is derived from pigment-producing melanocytes arising in the basal layer of the epidermis but is also found in the mucosa of the gastrointestinal (GI) tract and vagina and in the pigmented portion of the retina. Localized malignant melanoma that has not deeply invaded the dermis or spread to regional lymph nodes has a 50 to 80 percent cure rate, whereas those tumors that have invaded the lowest third of the dermis or metastasized to regional lymph nodes have a 20 percent cure rate.[101] Early recognition of malignant melanoma is essential for successful management. A pigmented nevus that becomes darker, irregular in outline, and elevated requires prompt biopsy. Bleeding and ulceration are late changes that may preclude surgical excision.[101] Pigmented nevi frequently darken in pregnancy, but a bluish or slate-gray appearance is cause for concern.[116] Malignant melanoma occurs most often in light-skinned caucasians exposed to prolonged ultraviolet or sunlight.[117] Its incidence increases the closer one lives to the equator.[118] There appears to be no convincing evidence that pregnancy changes the natural history of melanoma. Patients with malignant melanoma in pregnancy matched by site and stage have the same prognosis as nonpregnant patients.[119] Estrogen receptor protein has been demonstrated to be present in malignant melanoma,[120] but its clinical significance has yet to be established.[119] Clinical trials with pharmacologic doses of estrogen or antiestrogen therapy with tamoxifen, an estrogen agonist-antagonist, have not proved beneficial in the treatment of malignant melanoma.[101]

Treatment and prognosis for patients with malignant melanoma are based on the clinical and pathologic stage of the disease. Stage I disease is limited to a primary cutaneous lesion only. Stage II disease involves malignant melanoma demonstrated in regional lymph nodes or in lymphatic channels, leading to regional nodes. Stage III disease involves distant blood-borne metastases.[116] Most patients present with stage I disease, which may be pathologically staged according to the Clark level of deepest anatomic invasion[121] or the simpler Breslow system.[122] In the latter system, patients with disease invading to a maximum depth of less than 0.76 mm are at low risk, invasion of 0.76 to 1.5 mm are at intermediate risk, and invasion greater than 1.5 mm invasions are at high risk.

Ninety percent of melanomas originate in the skin, most arising in preexisting nevi.[116] Pregnant women found to have suspicious nevi should undergo complete excision of the nevi under local anesthesia. Lesions greater than 2 cm in diameter should undergo a full thickness punch biopsy through the darkest part of the lesion. Stage I lesions are treated surgically with wide local excision. Stage II lesions are treated surgically with complete regional lymph node resection. Stage III disease is treated with systemic chemotherapy with such agents as dimethyltriasenodimidazole carboxamide (DTIC) or nitrosoureas such as chloroethylcyclohexyl nitrosourea (CCNU). Response rates are low (20 to 25 percent), and the median duration of remission is only 8 to 10 months.[116] Adjuvant immunotherapy with bacillus Calmette-Guerin (BCG), *C. parvum,* and levamisole for completely resected stage I and II disease has shown no conclusive benefit.[116] Local injection of BCG intradermally may help control intradermal nodules.[101] Definitive surgery should be promptly performed in pregnant women with stage I and II disease. Patients with stage III disease can only be palliated. Salvaging the fetus is a very strong consideration in the presence of hematogenous dissemination. Early delivery of a mature fetus should be considered during the third trimester prior to administration of chemotherapy.

THYROID CANCER

Thyroid cancer may infrequently be diagnosed in pregnancy, as the peak age distribution for papillary adenocarcinoma of the thyroid is 30 to 34 years.[123]

The actual incidence of thyroid cancer in pregnancy is unknown due to the infrequency of its occurrence. Pregnancy changes do not routinely obscure the diagnosis of thyroid cancer in pregnancy, as most cancers present as solitary thyroid nodules. The most frequent cancers histologically are papillary, follicular, and anaplastic carcinomas. Medullary carcinomas account for fewer than 5 percent of primary thyroid malignancies.

Papillary carcinomas or mixed papillary follicular carcinomas are the most common malignancies of the thyroid, tend to occur most often in young women, and are the most common type of thyroid cancer to be diagnosed in pregnancy. Papillary thyroid cancers clinically present as solitary nodules in an otherwise normal gland, but on careful sectioning of the tissue, multifocal disease will be found in 30 to 40 percent of patients. Subclinical involvement of regional lymph nodes occurs in 50 to 70 percent of patients, but this does not affect prognosis. A 90 to 95 percent 15-year survival is expected in women under age 49.[124,125] A high risk factor for developing thyroid cancer is exposure to radiation therapy to the head, neck, or chest during childhood.[124,125] Follicular carcinoma occurs most often in women over age 40, presents as a hard mass, frequently spreads hematogenously, and has a slightly worse prognosis than that of the pure papillary tumor.[123] Anaplastic carcinomas most commonly present in patients over 50 years of age, have a fulminant course, and rarely complicate pregnancy. Medullary carcinomas occur in association with multiple endocrine neoplasia type II syndrome and are bilateral; only one case has been reported in pregnancy.[126] That patient died due to bilateral pheochromocytomas causing third-trimester hypertension.

Radionuclide scans are contraindicated in the evaluation of thyroid disease in pregnancy, as there is a theoretical risk of destroying the fetal thyroid. Fine-needle aspiration biopsies are the best way to diagnosis thyroid cancer in pregnancy.[127] The false-negative rate of thyroid fine-needle aspiration biopsies is only 6 percent.[128]

Pregnancy does not appear to alter the course of thyroid cancer,[60,129] and future pregnancies should not be avoided or therapeutic abortions recommended.[130] This recommendation is based on the overwhelming majority of thyroid cancers presenting in pregnancy being histologically well-differentiated lesions that can be readily treated with thyroid suppression until delivery regardless of the trimester of diagnosis.[123] Those few patients presenting with tumor fixed to surrounding tissue that then enlarges or in whom regional lymph node metastases develop despite suppression therapy should undergo surgery in the first two trimesters; surgery may be delayed in the third trimester until fetal maturity is accomplished. A subtotal thyroidectomy should be performed and ^{131}I administered postpartum. This approach avoids the surgical complication of permanent hypoparathyroidism.[131] A modified neck dissection should be performed if regional lymph nodes are involved,[124] but the chances of miscarriage occurring is high with extensive surgery.[132]

Medullary carcinoma of the thyroid gland requires total thyroidectomy and a prophylactic neck dissection. Patients diagnosed in the first two trimesters should undergo prompt surgery, whereas those diagnosed in the third trimester should be followed until fetal maturity is established. Concurrent pheochromocyomas must be treated promptly.

Undifferentiated cancers are associated with survival of less than 1 year.[123] Standard therapy is a radical total thyroidectomy followed by radiation therapy.[123] Chemotherapy, in particular doxorubicin, in combination with radiation therapy may play a role in prolonging survival.[134]

GASTROINTESTINAL CANCER

The incidence of GI cancer presenting in pregnancy ranges from 1 in 50,000 to 1 in 100,000 pregnancies. Most are carcinomas of the large bowel.[135,136] The distribution of colorectal cancer in pregnancy is similar to that of the nonpregnant state, with the majority of disease being located in the rectum and approximately 20 percent occurring in the sigmoid colon.[137] Delay in diagnosis is common, as early symptoms are easily attributable to the gravid state.[138,139] Severe constipation, abdominal pain, distention, or rectal bleeding require prompt evaluation; most diagnoses can be made by rectal examination. Unfortunately in many patients the diagnosis is not established until intussusception, obstruction, or perforation occurs.[60] The prognosis for carcinoma of the colon is poor but no different than in the nongravid state. Carcinoembryonic antigen (CEA) is of little value in diagnosing colorectal cancer in pregnancy because it is routinely elevated in pregnancy.[140] Digital rectal examination, testing stool for occult blood,

and proctoscopy or flexible colonscopy may be employed to establish the diagnosis, the latter being more difficult to perform late in pregnancy.

Pregnancy does not change the natural history of colorectal cancer.[141,142] Patients found to have early-stage colorectal cancer in the first two trimesters of pregnancy should undergo prompt surgery and the pregnancy allowed to proceed to term. Abortion is not necessary to perform the surgery.[60] Allen and Nisker[137] recommend that patients found to have large colorectal lesions with metastases suspected or present be allowed to carry the pregnancy until fetal maturity and then undergo a cesarean section and bowel resection. However, surgery may have to be performed earlier in the event of hemorrhage, threatened colon obstruction, or perforation.[60] A vaginal delivery should be avoided because large colorectal lesions may cause dystocia or hemorrhage in labor. Lesions diagnosed in the third trimester should be approached surgically once fetal maturity is established, at which time a cesarean section may be performed if the lesion is below the pelvic brim and the bowel is resected. Potentially curable lesions require either an anterior resection or abdominoperineal resection. Colon cancers diagnosed in pregnancy are almost invariably fatal, but 10 of 16 rectal cancer patients treated at the Mayo Clinic survived at least 5 years from initial diagnosis.[143]

UTERINE CANCER

Carcinoma of the endometrium is predominantly a disease of perimenopausal or postmenopausal women. Only 8 percent of endometrial cancers occur in women under age 40.[144] Women in whom endometrial cancers develop tend to be relatively infertile. Only seven patients with endometrial cancer diagnosed in pregnancy had been reported through 1979.[145] Two additional cases were reported in 1983 and 1984.[146,147] The reported patients ages ranged from 21 to 43 years. These cancers were usually associated with vaginal bleeding and were small well-differentiated adenoacanthomas. Only one death was noted, occurring in the only patient with cancer showing deep invasion into the myometrial unsuccessfully treated with irradiation and a hysterectomy. Hysterectomy remains the standard method of treating endometrial cancer, but one patient refused hysterectomy and subsequently had a normal pregnancy, suggesting that the diagnosis in the first pregnancy may not have been accurate.[145]

Malignant mixed mesodermal tumors of the uterus are infrequently occurring malignancies usually presenting in postmenopausal women and associated with a poor prognosis.[148] Figure 32-5 is an ultrasound image obtained from a 35-year-old woman at 22 weeks gestation in whom a diagnosis of a degenerating uterine leiomyoma associated with pain and vaginal spotting was observed. The patient was treated symptomatically but, because of severe progression of pain in association with intrauterine growth retardation, she underwent a primary cesarean section at 33 weeks gestation. The L/S ratio was 2.3, indicating fetal maturity. The patient delivered a viable infant but was found to have a mixed mesodermal tumor arising in the uterus and grossly infiltrating the rectovaginal septum and right pelvic sidewall. Postoperatively, the patient received intensive cytotoxic chemotherapy in combination with radiation therapy, failed to respond, and died 6 months after diagnosis.

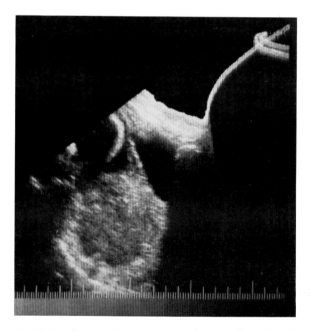

Fig. 32-5 Ultrasound examination of a mass thought to be a uterine leiomyoma undergoing degeneration in pregnancy that proven to be a uterine mixed mesodermal tumor. The gestational sac can be seen in the upper left side of the sonogram. (Courtesy of Dr. J. Copel.)

VULVAR CANCER

Carcinoma of the vulva is predominantly a disease of perimenopausal and postmenopausal women. Lutz et al.[73] reported that in 5 percent of women with vulva carcinoma seen at the Medical University of South Carolina, the diagnosis was made in pregnancy or within 2 to 6 months postpartum. A review of the world's literature through 1977 suggested that most patients with vulva malignancies have squamous cell cancer, but other histologies noted included sarcomas, melanoma, and adenocarcinoma of the Bartholin's gland.[73] While prolonged survival was noted in 3 of 5 patients treated by Lutz et al.,[73] the only cure was in the one patient with carcinoma in situ of the vulva. Two patients died of cancer 10 and 18 years following the original diagnosis, and Collins and Barclay reported a local recurrence 17 years after initial diagnosis.[149]

Carcinoma in situ of the vulva is increasing dramatically, based on Connecticut Tumor Registry data.[150] At least 40 percent of patients are under 40 years of age at diagnosis. It can be anticipated that many more cases presenting in pregnancy will be reported in the near future. Management in younger women has been a skinning vulvectomy with or without a skin graft.[73,151] Young women frequently have multifocal disease, whereas older women tend to have unifocal disease. The preferred treatment for carcinoma in situ of the vulva at Yale-New Haven Hospital in young women is laser vaporization, as this has a better cosmetic result than wide local exicision or skinning vulvectomy with or without skin graft. However, carcinoma in situ of the vulva can be managed by observation during pregnancy and can be treated by laser or excisional surgery postpartum.

Invasive vulva cancer is routinely treated surgically with a radical vulvectomy and bilateral superficial inguinal lymphadenectomies. At Yale-New Haven Hospital, patients with unilateral vuval lesions first undergo resection of the ipsilateral inguinal lymph nodes. If the lymph nodes are free of cancer by frozen-section evaluation, surgery is completed by performing a radical vulvectomy. If the ipsilateral inguinal lymph nodes contain metastatic vulva cancer, the contralateral inguinal lymph nodes are removed, as are the ipsilateral deep pelvic lymph nodes. A radical vulvectomy is performed once the lymphadenectomies are accomplished. Extensive surgery can be performed during surgery, but the risk of spontaneous abortion or premature labor may be substantially increased.

VAGINAL CANCER

Carcinoma of the vagina represents less than 1 percent of gynecologic malignancies, is a disease of older women, may be treated in early stages with either surgery or radiation therapy, and does quite poorly when presenting as advanced disease.[73] Histologically, most vaginal cancers are squamous cell.[152] The management of vaginal cancer is similar to that of cervical cancer. Cancer diagnosed during the first two trimesters should be treated promptly with either aggressive surgery, usually a radical hysterectomy and vaginectomy, or radiation therapy that will result in a termination of pregnancy. Patients diagnosed during the third trimester may maintain the pregnancy until fetal maturity and then undergo a cesarean section, followed by definitive therapy.

The largest report of vaginal cancer occurring in pregnancy is that of Senekjian et al.[153] reporting on women who were themselves exposed in utero to diethylstilbestrol (DES). Twenty of 24 patients in this series developed vaginal clear cell adenocarcinoma, and four had cervical clear cell adenocarcinomas diagnosed in pregnancy. Fifteen of the 24 patients had stage I disease, and all but one was successfully treated with either wide local excision (3) with or without radiation, radical hysterectomy (10) with or without radiation therapy, and radiation therapy alone (2). The more advanced stage cancers were treated with radiation and did poorly. Pregnancy did not appear to have adverse effects on clear cell cancers of the vagina and cervix.

MISCELLANEOUS CANCERS COMPLICATING PREGNANCY

Cancer is a disease predominantly of the very young and the elderly. This may in part be explained by the fact that the immune system is most competent in young adulthood through middle age.[101] Thus, women in the reproductive years would not be expected to have a high incidence of cancer. The immune tolerance demonstrated by the pregnant mother appears to be specific to the fetus, as an increase in cancer has not been demonstrated in pregnancy.[2,101] By contrast, patients intentionally receiving immunosuppressive drugs to promote renal allografts have a 100- to 1000-fold greater incidence of cancer than do age-matched controls.[154] Nevertheless, the literature is rich in case reports and small series of unfortunate patients in whom unusual malignancies develop during pregnancy. Overwhelmingly, there is no evidence to suggest that pregnancy influences the natural history of these diseases. A brief review of some of these malignancies follows.

Soft Tissue Sarcoma

Soft tissue sarcomas represent a diverse group of tumors that rarely complicate pregnancy. Delay in diagnosis is often responsible for the advanced stage and poor prognosis associated with this group of patients.[155,156] Overall survival is not different than for nonpregnancy patients, and subsequent pregnancies are not deleterious to the patient's health.[155]

Eighteen cases of osteogenic sarcoma diagnosed in pregnancy revealed no difference in survival when women were matched for skeletal tumor location, histologic appearance, and similar age with nonpregnant women.[157] Therapeutic abortion does not appear to be indicated except in first-trimester patients who require treatment with cytotoxic chemotherapy such as high-dose methotrexate. Early delivery is recommended in the third trimester.[158] Haerr and Pratt[159] reported a case of a large Ewing's sarcoma involving an iliac wing diagnosed at 25 weeks gestation and treated with multiagent chemotherapy before a cesarean section was performed at 34 weeks gestation. Mother and child were both alive and well 4 years later.

Endocrine Tumors

The most common tumor arising in the adrenal gland in pregnancy is the pheochromocytoma. This lesion requires prompt treatment, as it is associated with a high maternal mortality (58 percent) and fetal mortality (55 percent).[60] Antenatal diagnosis reduces the maternal mortality to 18 percent and fetal mortality to 15 percent. Donegan[60] reported on 128 patients with pheochromocytoma associated with pregnancy through early 1980. Forty-two were diagnosed antenatally. Only three of the 128 tumors were malignant. The characteristic symptoms experienced by patients with pheochromocytoma are episodic hypertension, headaches, anxiety, palpitations, sweating, and congestive heart failure. Supine hypertension with normal blood pressure in the sitting or standing position is characteristic of this tumor and may be secondary to pressure from the gravid uterus. The diagnosis is confirmed by elevated 24-hour urine collection levels of catecholamines, vanillylmandelic acid (VMA), and metanephrines.

Patients should undergo surgery to remove the tumor, but it is not necessary to terminate the pregnancy.[60] Preoperative α-adrenegic blockade with oral phenoxybenzamine effectively lowers the blood pressure; propranolol reduces the heart rate and prevents arrhythmias through β-adrenergic receptor blockade.[160,161] Stenstrom and Swolin[162] recommend that patients diagnosed as having a pheochromocytoma in the first trimester of pregnancy undergo prompt surgery but that patients first diagnosed later in pregnancy be treated with an α-receptor blocking agent until fetal maturity, at which time cesarean section and tumor resection is accomplished.

A single case of parathyroid carcinoma complicating pregnancy has been reported.[163] That patient presented with acute pancreatitis at 31 weeks gestation and underwent a left parathyroidectomy. She subsequently delivered a 1,750-g living infant and went on to have another pregnancy.

Gastrointestinal

Pancreatic cancer is rare in pregnancy.[164] It is a difficult diagnosis to make in the presence of pancreatitis.[165] Thoracoabdominal pain and GI symptoms are the presenting symptoms. Endoscopic retrograde pancreatography with cytologic examination of pancreatic secretions may be the most effective way of making the diagnosis of pancreatic cancer, short of surgery.[164] Each of the three cases of pancreatic cancer diagnosed in pregnancy resulted in a rapid maternal demise soon after delivery. Each of the infants of these mothers has survived. Biliary drainage and hyperalimentation may be necessary to maintain the pregnancy until fetal maturity is established.[164]

Gastrinomas rarely complicate pregnancy, present suddenly with symptoms of a severe ulcer diathesis postpartum, and are associated with elevated serum gastrin, peptic ulceration, and high secretion of gastric acid.[166,167] Management is surgical.

Gastric cancer is rare in pregnancy but is cited to have been reported in 44 Japanese patients between 1916 and 1980.[168] Only three cases are reported in the English literature.[168-170] Symptoms of gastric cancer are similar to those normally experienced in pregnancy and include GI discomfort, nausea, and vomiting. Gastroscopy avoids diagnostic radiation exposure in the patient suspect of having gastric cancer. In the nonpregnant state, only one-half of cases of gastric cancer are resectable, and the remainder are invariably fatal.

Hepatocellular carcinomas rarely occur in women, and the few that do usually present in postmenopausal women. A case report of hepatocellular carcinoma diagnosed at the fourth month of gestation resulted in a maternal death 12 weeks later. There was no evidence that the pregnancy enhanced the tumor evolution.[171] Hepatomas are treated by resection. One case of an extrahepatic biliary tract carcinoma complicating pregnancy has been reported.[172]

Urinary Tract Malignancies

Thirty-seven cases of renal tumors were reviewed by Tydings et al.[173] in 1978, 22 of which were renal cell carcinomas, the remaining being tubular adenomas, angioepitheliomas, hamartomas, or Wilm's tumors. Hematuria is the most common symptom for urinary tract malignancies, and nephrectomy with or without radiation therapy is standard treatment. Treatment should not be delayed in pregnancy except for third-trimester patients, for whom delay for a few weeks would lead to fetal maturity. The overall 5-year survival for renal cell carcinoma is 30 to 50 percent.[174] Renal cell carcinomas localized to the kidneys carry a 5-year survival of 60 percent. Anaplastic carcinomas have a poorer prognosis than that of well-differentiated cancers. Spontaneous regression of lung metastatses have been reported following nephrectomy, but this observation has not been consistently observed.[174]

Very few bladder cancers have been reported in pregnancy.[175-177] Most are transitional cell cancers, with 7 percent squamous cell and 1 percent adenocarcinoma, a distribution similar to that seen in the nonpregnant state. Superficial well-differentiated bladder cancers may be treated by fulguration, whereas deeply invasive cancers are managed with radiation therapy followed by partial or complete cystectomy. Patients requiring radiation therapy to the bladder should undergo a therapeutic abortion in early pregnancy, whereas therapy in late pregnancy may be delayed until fetal maturity is achieved. The 3-year survival for early cancer (stages 0, A, B1) is 54 percent, whereas those with deep invasion (stage B2, C) have a 3-year survival of 42 percent.[178] Bladder cancer most often metastasizes to bone, less frequently to liver, lung, or kidney.

Two cases of carcinoma of the urethra diagnosed in pregnancy have been reported.[179,180] The first was a squamous cell; the second was a low-grade adenocarcinoma diagnosed in the second trimester of pregnancy managed by allowing the patient to go to term, deliver vaginally, and then undergo definitive treatment consisting of radiation therapy and local excision. The latter patient was alive and disease free 7 years later.[180]

Central Nervous System Tumors

Central nervous system tumors rarely complicate pregnancy and are associated with a high (60 percent) maternal mortality.[181] Headaches and visual disturbances are the most common presenting symptoms. Evaluation by MRI avoids radiation exposure. Infratentorial lesions have a very poor prognosis. Therapeutic abortion has been recommended for patients discovered to have malignant brain tumors in the first trimester, because of the rapid course of such tumors. Surgical decompression should be performed in the presence of elevated cerebrospinal fluid (CSF) pressure, and patients should receive steroids to reduce cerebral edema.

Spinal cord tumors diagnosed in pregnancy are exceedingly rare. Neurologic symptoms developing in pregnancy deserve prompt evaluation. Magnetic resonance imaging may help in diagnosis and decompression procedures should be promptly performed.[182]

Kaposi's Sarcoma

The first case report of Kaposi's sarcoma in pregnancy occurring in a patient known to have acquired immune deficiency syndrome (AIDS) appeared in 1984.[183] The patient received doxorubicin, bleomycin, and vinblastine during pregnancy, and a growth-retarded infant was subsequently delivered vaginally. The frequency of this rare malignancy is undoubtedly on the rise and will present more often in pregnancy.

REFERENCES

1. Potter JF, Schoeneman M: Metastasis of maternal cancer to the placenta and fetus. Cancer 25:380, 1970
2. Haas JF: Pregnancy in association with a newly diagnosed cancer: A population based epidemiologic assessment. Int J Cancer 34:229, 1984
3. Csapo AI, Pulkkinen MD, Wiest WG: Effects of lutectomy and progesterone replacement in early pregnant patients. Am J Obstet Gynecol 115:759, 1973
4. Goodlin RC: Importance of the lateral position during labor. Obstet Gynecol 37:698, 1971
5. Eckstein K, Marx GF: Aortocaval compression and uterine displacement. Anesthesiology 40:92, 11974
6. Roberts RB, Shirley MA: Reducing the risk of acid aspiration during cesarean section. Anesth Analg 53:859, 1979
7. Bailey H, Bragg HJ: Effects of irradiation on fetal development. Am J Obstet Gynecol 5:461, 1923
8. Brill AB, Forgotson EH: Radiation and congenital malformations. Am J Obstet Gynecol 90:1149, 1964
9. Muller HJ: Artificial transmutation of the gene. Science 66:84, 1927.
10. Orr JW, Jr, Shingleton HM: Cancer in pregnancy. Curr Prob Cancer 8:1, 1983
11. Wallack MK, Wolf JA Jr, Bedwinek J, et al: Gestational carcinoma of the female breast. Curr Prob Cancer 9:1, 1983
12. Dekaban A: Abnormalities in children exposed to x-irradiation during various stages of gestation; tentative timetable of radiation injury to the human fetus. Part I. J Nucl Med 9:471, 1968
13. Nicholson HD: Cytotoxic drugs in pregnancy. J Obstet Gynaecol Br Commonw 75:307, 1968
14. Sweet DL, Kinzie J: Consequences of radiotherapy and antineoplastic therapy for the fetus. J Reprod Med 17:241, 1976
15. Durie BGM, Biles HR: Successful treatment of acute leukemia during pregnancy. Arch Intern Med 137:90, 1977
16. Krueger JA, Davies RB, Felal C: Multiple drug chemotherapy in the management of acute lymphocytic leukemia during pregnancy. Obstet Gynecol 48:324, 1976
17. Ortega J: Multiple agent chemotherapy including bleomycin for non-Hodgkin's lymphoma during pregnancy. Cancer 40:2829, 1977

18. Jones RT, Weinerman BH: MOPP (nitrogen mustard, vincristine, procarbazine and prednisone) given during pregnancy. Obstet Gynecol 54:477, 1979

19. Lowenthal RM, Funnell CF, Hope DM, et al: Normal infant after combination chemotherapy including teniposide for Burkitt's lymphoma in pregnancy. Med Pediatr Oncol 10:165, 1982

20. Malone JM, Gershenson DM, Creasy RK, et al: Endodermal sinus tumor of the ovary associated with pregnancy. Obstet Gynecol 68(suppl):86, 1986

21. Krepart GV, Lotocki RJ: Chemotherapy during pregnancy. p. 69. In Allen HH, Nisker JA (eds): Cancer in Pregnancy. Futura Publishing, Mt. Kisco, NY, 1986

22. Sieber SM, Adamson RH: Toxicity of antineoplastic agents in man: chromosomal aberrations, antifertility effects, congenital malformations, and carcinogenic potential. Adv Cancer Res 22:57, 1975

23. Sokal JE, Lessmann EM: Effects of cancer chemotherapeutic agents on the human fetus. JAMA 172:151, 1960

24. Milunsky A, Graef JW, Gaynor MF: Methotrexate-induced congenital malformation. J Pediatr 72:790, 1968

25. Warkany J: Aminopterin and methotrexate: Folic acid deficiency. Teratology 17:353, 1978

26. Sindu RK, Hawkins DF: Corticosteroids. Clin Obstet Gynecol 8:383, 1981

27. Barber HRK: Fetal and neonatal effects of cytotoxic agents. Obstet Gynecol 58(suppl):41, 1981

28. Collaborative Group on Antenatal Steroid Therapy: Effect of antenatal dexamethasone administration on the prevention of respiratory distress syndrome. Am J Obstet Gynecol 141:276, 1981

29. Hacker NF, Berek JS, LaGasse LD, et al: Carcinoma of the cervix associated with pregnancy. Obstet Gynecol 59:735, 1982

30. Stone ML, Weingold AB, Sall S: Cervical carcinoma in pregnancy. Am J Obstet Gynecol 93:479, 1965

31. Sall S, Rini S, Pineda A: Surgical management of invasive carcinoma of the cervix in pregnancy. Am J Obstet Gynecol 118:1, 1974

32. Kinch RA: Factors affecting the prognosis of cancer of the cervix in pregnancy. Am J Obstet Gynecol 82:43 1961

33. Creasman WT, Rutledge FN, Fletcher GH: Carcinoma of the cervix associated with pregnancy. Obstet Gynecol 36:495, 1970

34. Seltzer V, Sall S, Castadot M, et al: Glassy cell cervical carcinoma. Gynecol Oncol 8:141, 1979

35. Turner WA, Gallup DG, Talledo OE, et al: Neuroendocrine carcinoma of the uterine cervix complicated by pregnancy: Case report and review of the literature. Obstet Gynecol 67(suppl):80, 1986

36. Moore JG, Wells RG, Morton DG: Management of superficial cervical cancer in pregnancy. Obstet Gynecol 27:307, 1966

37. DePetrillo AD, Townsend DE, Morrow CP, et al: Colposcopic evaluation of the abnormal Papanicolaou test in pregnancy. Am J Obstet Gynecol 121:441, 1975

38. Ortiz R, Newton M: Colposcopy in the management of abnormal cervical smears in pregnancy. Am J Obstet Gynecol 109:46, 1971

39. Stafl A, Mattingly RF: Colposcopic diagnosis of cervical neoplasia. Obstet Gynecol 41:168, 1973

40. Boutselis JG: Intraepithelial carcinoma of the cervix associated with pregnancy. Obstet Gynecol 40:657, 1972

41. Benedet JL, Boyes DA, Nichols TM, et al: Colposcopic evaluation of pregnancy patients with abnormal cervical smears. Br J Obstet Gynaecol 84:517, 1977

42. Talebian F, Krumholz BA, Shayan A, et al: Colposcopic evaluation of patients with abnormal cytologic smears during pregnancy. Obstet Gynecol 47:693, 1976

43. Trombetta GC: Colposcopic evaluation of cervical neoplasia in pregnancy. J Reprod Med 16:243, 1976

44. Drew NC: Adenocarcinoma-in situ of the cervix uteri associated with cervical intraepithelial neoplasia in pregnancy. Case report. Br J Obstet Gynaecol 91:498, 1984

45. Lee RB, Neglia W, Park RC: Cervical carcinoma in pregnancy. Obstet Gynecol 58:584, 1981

46. Thompson JD, Caputo TA, Franklin EW, et al: The surgical management of invasive cancer of the cervix in pregnancy. Am J Obstet Gynecol 121:853, 1975

47. Dudan RC, Yon JF, Ford JR Jr, et al: Carcinoma of the cervix and pregnancy. Gynecol Oncol 1:283, 1973

48. Prem KA, Makowski EL, McKelvey JL: Carcinoma of the cervix associated with pregnancy. Am J Obstet Gynecol 95:99, 1966

49. Anderson JM: Mammary cancers and pregnancy. Br Med J 1:1124, 1979

50. Haagensen CD: Carcinoma of the breast in pregnancy. p. 660. In Haagensen CD (ed): Disease of the Breast. 2nd Ed. WB Saunders, Philadelphia, 1971

51. Applewhite RR, Smith LR, DiVincenti F: Carcinoma of the breast associated with pregnancy and lactation. Am Surg 39:101, 1973

52. Bottles K, Taylor RN: Diagnosis of breast masses in pregnant and lactating women by aspiration cytology. Obstet Gynecol 66(suppl):76, 1985

53. Zinn JS: The association of pregnancy and breast cancer. J Reprod Med 22:297, 1979

54. Byrd BF, Bayer DS, Robertson JC, et al: Treatment of breast tumors associated with pregnancy and lactation. Ann Surg 155:940, 1962

55. Donegan WL: Mammary carcinoma and pregnancy. Major Prob Clin Surg 5:170, 1967

56. Durodola JI: Burkitt's lymphoma presenting during lactation. Int J Gynaecol Obstet 14:225, 1976

57. Jones DED, d'Avignon MB, Lawrence R, et al: Burkitt's lymphoma: Obstetrics and gynecologic aspects. Obstet Gynecol 56:533, 1980

58. O'Donnell JR, Farrell MA: Acute myelogenous leukemia with bilateral mammary gland involvement. J Clin Pathol 33:547, 1980

59. Peters MV, Meakin JW: The influence of pregnancy in carcinoma of the breast. Prog Clin Cancer 1:471, 1965

60. Donegan WL: Cancer in pregnancy. CA 33:194, 1983

61. Peters MC: The effect of pregnancy in breast cancer. p. 65. In Forrest APM, Kunkler PB (eds): Prognostic Factors in Breast Cancer. Williams & Wilkins, Baltimore, 1968

62. Nugent P, O'Connell TX: Breast cancer and pregnancy. Arch Surg 120:1221, 1985

63. Ribeiro GG, Palmer MK: Breast carcinoma associated with pregnancy: A clinician's dilemma. Br Med J 2:1524, 1977

64. Denoix P: Treatment of malignant breast tumors. Rec Results Cancer Res 31:83, 1970

65. Bush H, McCredie JA: Carcinoma of the breast during pregnancy and lactation. p. 91. In Allen HH, Nisker JA (eds): Cancer in Pregnancy. Futura Publishing, Mt. Kisco, NY, 1986

66. Bonadonna G, Valagussa P: Dose-response effect of adjuvant chemotherapy in breast cancer. Engl J Med 304:10, 1981

67. Rosemond GP, Maier WP: p. 227. In Breast Cancer: Early and Late. Year Book Medical Publishers, Chicago, 1970

68. King RM, Welch JS, Martin JK, et al: Carcinoma of the breast associated with pregnancy. Surg Gynecol Obstet 160:228, 1985

69. Harvey JC, Rosen PP, Ashikari R, et al: The effect of pregnancy on the prognosis of carcinoma of the breast following radical mastectomy. Surg Gynecol Obstet 153:723, 1981

70. Cooper DR, Butterfield J: Pregnancy subsequent to mastectomy for cancer of the breast. Ann Surg 171:429, 1970

71. Silverberg E, Lubera C: Cancer statistics 1987. Ca 37:2, 1987

72. Schwartz PE: Gynecologic cancer. p. 1. In Spittell JA Jr (ed): Clinical Medicine. Harper & Row, Philadelphia, 1985

73. Lutz M, Underwood PB Jr, Rozier JC, et al: Genital malignancy in pregnancy. Am J Obstet Gynecol 129:536, 1977

74. Chung A, Birnbaum SJ: Ovarian cancer associated with pregnancy. Obstet Gynecol 41:211, 1973

75. Beischer NA, Buttery BW, Fortune DW, et al: Growth and malignancy of ovarian tumors in pregnancy. Aust NZ J Obstet Gynaecol 11:208, 1971

76. Munnell EW: Primary ovarian cancer associated with pregnancy. Clin Obstet Gynecol 6:983, 1963

77. Halmo SD, Nisker JA, Allen HH: Primary ovarian in pregnancy. p. 269. In Allen HH, Nisker JA (eds): Cancer in pregnancy. Futura Publishing, Mt. Kisco, NY, 1986

78. Weinreb JC, Brown CE, Lowe TW, et al: Pelvic masses in pregnant patients. MR and US imaging. Radiology 159:717, 1986

79. Weinreb JC, Lowe TW, Santo-Ramos R, et al: Magnetic resonance imaging in obstetric diagnosis. Radiology 154:157, 1985

80. Schwartz PE: Combination chemotherapy in the management of ovarian germ cell malignancies. Obstet Gynecol 64:564, 1984

81. Bast RC Jr, Klug TL, St John E, et al: A radioimmunoassay using a monoclonal antibody to monitor the course of epithelial ovarian cancer. N Engl J Med 309:883, 1983

82. Schwartz PE, Chambers SK, Chambers JT, et al: Circulating tumor markers in the monitoring of gynecologic malignancies. Cancer 60:353, 1987

83. Niloff JM, Knapp RC, Schaetzl E, et al: CA 125 antigen levels in obstetrics and gynecologic patients. Obstet Gynecol 64:703, 1985

84. Novak ER, Lambrose CD, Woodruff JD: Ovarian tumors in pregnancy. Obstet Gynecol 46:401, 1975

85. Jubb ED: Primary ovarian carcinoma in pregnancy. Am J Obstet Gynecol 85:345, 1963

86. Chambers JT, Kohorn EI, Schwartz PE: Borderline ovarian tumors. Am J Obstet Gynecol (in press)

87. Karlen JR, Akbari A, Cook WA: Dysgerminoma associated with pregnancy. Obstet Gynecol 53:330, 1979

88. Bianchi UA, Sartori E, Favall G, et al: New trends in treatment of ovarian dysgerminoma. Gynecol Oncol 23:246, 1986

89. Kurman RJ, Norris HJ: Endodermal sinus tumor of the ovary. A clinical and pathologic analysis of 71 cases. Cancer 38:2404, 1976

90. Jimerson G, Woodruff JD, Ovarian extra-embryonal teratoma. I. Endodermal sinus tumor. Am J Obstet Gynecol 127:73, 1977

91. Schwartz PE: Sex cord-stromal tumors of the ovary. p. 251. In Piver S (ed): Ovarian Cancer. Churchill Livingstone. London, 1986

92. Young RH, Dudley AG, Scully RF: Granulosa cell, Sertoli-Leydig cell and unclassified sex cord-stromal

tumors associated with pregnancy: A clinicopathological analysis of thirty-six cases. Gynecol Oncol 18:181, 1984

93. Colombo N, Sessa C, Landoni F, et al: Cisplatin, vinblastine and bleomycin combination chemotherapy in metastatic granulosa cell tumor of the ovary. Obstet Gynecol 67:265, 1986

94. Desforges JF, Rutherford CJ, Piro A: Hodgkin's disease. Engl J Med 301:1212, 1979

95. Sutcliffe SB, Wrigley PFM, Peto J, et al: MVPP chemotherapy regimen for advanced Hodgkin's disease. Br Med J 1:679, 1978

96. Devita VT, Simon RM, Hubbard SM, et al: Curability of advanced Hodgkin's disease with chemotherapy. Ann Intern Med 92:587, 1980

97. Chapman RM, Sutcliffe SV, Malpas JS: Cytotoxic-induced ovarian failure in women with Hodgkin's disease. I. Hormone function. JAMA 242:1877, 1979.

98. Smith RBW, Sheehy TW, Rothberg H: Hodgkin's disease and pregnancy. Arch Intern Med 102:777, 1958

99. Sweet DL, Jr: Malignant lymphoma: Implications during the reproductive years and pregnancy. J Reprod Med 17:198, 1976

100. Tawil E, Mercier JP, Dondavino A: Hodgkin's disease complicating pregnancy. J Can Assoc Radiol 36:133, 1985

101. Mitchell MS, Capizzi RL: Neoplastic diseases. p. 510. In Burrow GN, Ferris TF (eds): Medical Complications During Pregnancy. WB Saunders, Philadelphia, 1982

102. Timothy AR, Sutcliffe SBJ, Lister TA, et al: The management of stage IIIA Hodgkin's disease. Int J Radiat Oncol Biol Phys 6:135, 1980

103. Sutcliffe SB, Chapman RM: Lymphomas and leukemias. p. 135. In Allen HH, Nisker JA (eds): Cancer in Pregnancy. Futura Publishing, Mt. Kisco, NY, 1986

104. Meruk, ML, Green JP, Nussbaum H, et al: Phantom dosimetry study of shaped colbalt-60 fields in treatment of Hodgkin's disease. Radiology 91:554, 1968

105. Miller TP, Jones SE: Chemotherapy of localized histiocytic lymphoma. Lancet 1:358, 1979

106. DeVita VT, Jr, Chabner B, Hubbard SP, et al: Advanced diffuse histiocytic lymphoma, a potentially curable disease. Lancet 1:248, 1975

107. Falkson HC, Simson IW, Falkson G: Non-Hodgkin's lymphoma in pregnancy. Cancer 45:1679, 1980

108. Schapira DV, Chudley AE: Successful pregnancy following continuous treatment with combination chemotherapy before conception and throughout pregnancy. Cancer 54:800, 1984

109. Steiner-Salz D, Yahalom J, Samuelov A, et al: Non-Hodgkin's lymphoma associated with pregnancy. A report of six cases, with a review of the literature. Cancer 56:2087, 1985

110. Ioachim HL: Hodgkin's lymphoma in pregnancy. Three cases and review of the literature. Arch Pathol Lab Med 109:803, 1985

111. Hoover BA, Schumacher HR: Acute leukemia in pregnancy. Am J Obstet Gynecol 96:316, 1966

112. Yahia C, Hyman GA, Phillips LL: Acute leukemia and pregnancy. Obstet Gynecol Surv 13:1, 1958

113. Henderson, EJ: Acute leukemia: General considerations. p. 108. In Williams WJ, Beutler E, Erslev AJ, Rundles RW (eds): Hematology. 2nd Ed. McGraw-Hill, New York, 1977

114. McLain CR Jr: Leukemia in pregnancy. Clin Obstet Gynecol 17:185, 1974

115. Moloney WC: Management of leukemia in pregnancy. Ann NY Acad Sci 114:857, 1964

116. McCulloch PB, Dent PB: Melanoma. p. 205. In Allen AA, Nisker JA (eds): Cancer in Pregnancy. Futura Publishing, Mt. Kisco, NY, 1986

117. Movshovitz M, Modan B: Role of sun exposure in the etiology of malignant melanoma; an epidemiologic inference. J Natl Cancer Inst 51:777, 1973

118. Davis NC: Cutaneous melanoma, the Queensland experience. Curr Prob Surg 13:1, 1976

119. Houghton A, Flannery J, Viola MV: Malignant melanoma of the skin occurring during pregnancy. Cancer 48:407, 1981

120. Fisher RI, Neifeld JP, Lippman ME: Estrogen receptors in human malignant melanoma. Lancet 2:337, 1976

121. Clark WH, From L, Bernardino EA, et al: The histogensis and biologic behavior of primary malignant melanomas of skin. Cancer Res 29:705, 1969

122. Breslow AL: Tumor thickness, level of invasion and node dissection in stage I cutaneous melanoma. Ann Surg 182:572, 1975

123. Stuart GCE, Temple WJ: Thyroid cancer in pregnancy. p. 191. In Allen HH, Nisker JA (eds): Cancer in Pregnancy. Futura Publishing, Mt. Kisco, NY, 1986

124. Cady B, Sedgwick CE, Meissner WA: Changing clinical, pathologic, therapeutic and survival patterns in differentiated thyroid carcinoma. Ann Surg 184:541, 1976

125. Cady B, Sedgwick CE, Meissner WA: Risk factor analysis in differentiated thyroid cancer. Cancer 43:810, 1979

126. Chodanker CM, Abhyankar SC, Deodhar KP: Sipple's syndrome (multiple endocrine neoplasia) in pregnancy. (Case report.) Aust NZ J Obstet Gynecol 22:243, 1982

127. Goldman MH, Tisch B, Chattock AG: Fine needle

biopsy of a solitary nodule arising during pregnancy. J Med Soc NJ 80:525, 1983

128. Schwartz AE, Nieburgs HE, Davis TF: The place of fine needle biopsy in the diagnosis of nodules of the thyroid. Surg Gynecol Obstet 155:54, 1982

129. Hill CS, Clark RL, Wolf M: The effect of subsequent pregnancy in patients with thyroid carcinoma. Surg Gynecol Obstet 122:1219, 1966

130. Rosvoll RV, Winship T: Thyroid carcinoma and pregnancy. Surg Gynecol Obstet 121:1039, 1965

131. Farrar WB, Cooperman M, James AG: Surgical management of papillary and follicular carcinoma of the thyroid. Am Surg 192:701, 1980

132. Cunningham MP, Slaughter DP: Surgical treatment of diseases of the thyroid gland in pregnancy. Surg Gynecol Obstet 131:486, 1970

133. Thomas CG, Buckwalter JA: Poorly differentiated neoplasms of the thyroid gland. Ann Surg 177:632, 1973

134. Kim JH, Leeper RD: Treatment of analastic giant and spindle cell carcinoma of the thyroid gland with combination adriamycin and radiation therapy. Cancer 52:954, 1983

135. Byers T, Graham S, Swanson M: Parity and colorectal cancer risk in women. J Natl Cancer Inst 69:1059, 1982

136. Barber HRK, Brunschwig A: Carcinoma of the bowel. Am J Obstet Gynecol 100:926, 1968

137. Allen HH, Nisker JA: Colorectal cancer in pregnancy. p. 281. In Allen HH, Nisker JA (eds): Cancer in Pregnancy. Futura Publishing, Mt. Kisco, NY, 1986

138. Hill JA, Kassam SH, Talledo DE: Colonic cancer in pregnancy. South Med J 77:375, 1984

139. Nesbitt JC, Moise KJ, Sawyers JL: Colorectal carcinoma in pregnancy. Arch Surg 120:636, 1985

140. Lamerz R, Ruider H: Significance of CEA determinations in patients with cancer of the colon-rectum and the mammary glands in comparison to physiological states in connection with pregnancy. Bull Cancer 63:575, 1976

141. Zaridze DG: Environmental ethiology of large bowel cancer. J Natl Cancer Inst 70:389, 1983

142. Girard RM, Lamarche J, Baillot R: Carcinoma of the colon associated with pregnancy. Report of a case. Dis Colon Rectum 24:473, 1981

143. O'Leary JA, Pratt JH, Symmonds RE: Rectal carcinoma in pregnancy: A review of 17 cases. Obstet Gynecol 30:862, 1967

144. Kempson RL, Pokorny GE: Adenocarcinoma of the endometrium in women aged forty and younger. Cancer 21:650, 1968

145. Sandstrom RE, Welch WR, Green Th, Jr: Adenocar-

cinoma of the endometrium in pregnancy. Obstet Gynecol 53(suppl):73, 1979

146. Zirkin HJ, Krugliak L, Katz M: Endometrial adenocarcinoma coincident with intrauterine pregnancy. A case report. J Reprod Med 28:624, 1983

147. Suzuki A, Konishi I, Okamura H, et al: Adenocarcinoma of the endometrium associated with intrauterine pregnancy. Gynecol Oncol 18:261, 1984

148. Kohorn EI, Schwartz PE, Chambers JT, et al: Adjuvant therapy in mixed Mullerian tumors of the uterus. Gynecol Oncol 23:212, 1986

149. Collins CG, Barclay DL: Cancer of the vulva and cancer of the vagina in pregnancy. Clin Obstet Gynecol 6:927, 1973

150. Schwartz PE, Naftolin F: Type 2 herpes simplex virus and vulvar carcinoma in situ. N Engl J Med 305:517, 1981

151. Ruthledge F, Smith JF, Franklin E: Carcinoma of the vulva. Am J Obstet Gynecol 106:1117, 1970

152. Nori D, Hilaris BS, Stanimir G, et al: Radiation therapy of primary vaginal carcinoma. Int J Radiat Oncol Biol Phys 9:1471, 1983

153. Senekjian EK, Hubby M, Herbst AL: Clear cell adenocarcinoma (CCA) of the cervix and vagina associated with pregnancy. Gynecol Oncol 20:250, 1985

154. Pen I, Halgrimson CG, Starzl TE: De novo malignant tumors in organ transplant recipients. Transplant Proc 3:773, 1971

155. Cantin J, McNeer GP: The effect of pregnancy on the clinical course of sarcoma of the soft somatic tissues. Surg Gynecol Obstet 125:28, 1967

156. Lysyj A, Berquist JR: Pregnancy complicated by sarcoma. Report of two cases. Obstet Gynecol 21:506, 1963

157. Huvos AG, Bulter A, Bretsky SS: Osteogenic sarcoma in pregnancy women. Prognosis, therapeutic implications, and literature review. Cancer 56:2326, 1985

158. Simon MA, Phillips WA, Bonfiglio M: Pregnancy and aggressive or malignant bone tumors. Cancer 53:2564, 1984

159. Haerr RW, Pratt AT: Multiagent chemotheapy for sarcoma diagnosed during pregnancy. Cancer 56:1028, 1985

160. Fudge TL, McKinnon WMP, Geary WL: Current surgical management of pheochromocytoma during pregnancy. Arch Surg 115:1224, 1980

161. Leak D, Carroll JJ, Robinson DC, et al: Management of pheochromocytoma during pregnancy. Obstet Gynecol Surv 32:583, 1977

162. Stenstrom G, Swolin K: Pheochromocytoma in pregnancy. Experience of treatment with phenoxybenza-

mine in three patients. Acta Obstet Gynecol Scand 64:357, 1985

163. Hess HM, Dickson J, Fox HE: Hyperfunctioning parathyroid carcinoma presenting as acute pancreatitis in pregnancy. J Reprod Med 25:83, 1980

164. Gamberdella FR: Pancreatic carcinoma in pregnancy: A case report. Am J Obstet Gynecol 149:15, 1984

165. Boyle JM, McLeod ME: Pancreatic cancer presenting as pancreatitis of pregnancy. Case report. Am J Gastroenterol 70:371, 1979

166. Mentgen CN, Moeller DD, Klotz AP: Protection by pregnancy. Zollinger-Ellison syndrome. J Kansas Med Soc 75:37, 1974

167. Waddell WR, Leonsins AS, Zuidema GO: Gastric secretory and other laboratory studies on two patients with Zollinger-Ellison syndrome. N Engl J Med 260:56, 1979

168. Skokos CK, Lipshitz J: Adenocarcinoma of the stomach associated with pregnancy. J Tenn Med Assoc 75:103, 1982

169. Sims EH, Schlater TL, Sims M, et al: Obstructing gastric carcinoma complicating pregnancy. J Natl Med Assoc 72:21, 1980

170. Bowers RH, Walters W: Carcinoma of the stomach complicated by pregnancy: Report of an unusal case. Minn Med 41:30, 1958

171. Goncalves CS, Pereira FE, deVargas PR, et al: Hepatocellular carcinoma HBsA$_S$ positive in pregnancy. Arq Gastroenterol 21:75, 1984

172. Devoe LD, Moosa AR, Levin B: Pregnancy complicated by an extrahepatic biliary tract carcinoma. J Reprod Med 28:153, 1983

173. Tydings A, Weiss RR, Lin JH, et al: Renal cell carcinoma and mesangiocapillary glomerulonephritis. NY State J Med 78:1950, 1978

174. Abrams HL: Tumors and cysts of the kidney. p. 1043. In Hamburger J. Crosnier J, Grunfeld J-P (eds): Nephrology. Vol. 2. John Wiley & Sons, New York, 1979

175. Stanhope CR: Management of the obstetric patient with malignancy. p. 1. In Sciarra JJ (ed): Gynecology and Obstetrics. Vol. 2. Harper & Row, New York, 1984

176. Keegan GT, Forkowitz MJ: Transitional cell carcinoma of the bladder during pregnancy: A case report. Texas Med 78:44, 1982

177. Cruikshank SH, McNellis TM: Carcinoma of the bladder in pregnancy. Am J Obstet Gynecol 145:768, 1983

178. MacKenzie AR: Supervoltage x-ray therapy of bladder cancer. Cancer 18:1255, 1965

179. Smith FR: Effect of pregnancy on malignant tumors. Am J Obstet Gynecol 34:616, 1937

180. Severino LJ, Brockunier A, Davidian MM: Adenocarcinoma of the urethra during pregnancy: Report of a case. Obstet Gynecol 50(suppl):22, 1977

181. Carmel PN: Neurologic surgery in pregnancy. p. 203. In Barber HRK (ed): Surgical Disease in Pregnancy. WB Saunders, Philadelphia, 1974

182. Apuzzio J, Pelosi MA, Ganesh W, et al: Spinal cord tumors during pregnancy. Int J Gynaecol Obstet 17:608, 1980

183. Rawlinson KF, Zubrow AB, Harris MA, et al: Disseminated Kaposi's sarcoma in pregnancy: A manifestation of acquired immune deficiency syndrome. Obstet Gynecol 63(suppl):2, 1984

33

Cancer Pain

Arthur F. Battista
Joseph Ransohoff

The general incidence and intensity of cancer pain is not known, for no large-scale studies are available. Limited studies, however, have indicated as the disease progresses, pain usually increases in intensity and distribution. As the disease advances, significant pain has been reported in 60 to 90 percent of patients.[1] Global studies of the prevalence and intensity of pain in cancer patients worldwide have suggested that about 25 percent die in severe pain.[2]

The orientation of pain therapy in cancer patients being treated for their disease is therefore, to render relief of pain during the stage of treatment and in those with advanced disease to alleviate pain to a functional level and to maintain pain relief until death. Significant progress has been made in the treatment of cancer. In addition, great strides have been made in the investigation of the physiology and pharmacology of pain. This has resulted in renewed interest in the clinical treatment of pain in general and of cancer pain in particular. Thus, pain control is initiated at the onset of pain and continued when treatment is palliative and the disease progresses. At this stage, the main form of therapy in cancer patients is the alleviation of pain.

Because of the subjective qualities of pain, it cannot be defined satisfactorily. It is nevertheless known to us as a private experience, described by various descriptive terms: burning, shooting, cutting, aching, and others.

Pain is frequently associated with late gynecologic malignancy. The unremitting nature of this pain wears the patient down both physically and mentally. Since fully 50 percent of all gynecologic cancer when first seen can be treated only palliatively, pain frequently becomes the most urgent symptom demanding resolution. Gynecologic malignancy pain may take a variety of forms: mild lower abdominal discomfort by involvement of the uterus itself; dysuria, inguinal and lower flank pain by encroachment on the bladder neck or ureter with hydronephrosis; severe intense pain into the thighs, legs, and back by involvement of the lumbosacral plexus; and extension into the epidural space with invasion of the nerve roots. Many attempts have been made to classify pain on the basis of description and localization. Somatic pain may be superficial from the skin and of short duration; deep from muscle, joints, tendons, or fascia; and of intermediate duration. Visceral pain may be superficial or deep from thoracic, abdominal, or pelvic organs and of long duration. Superficial pain is usually described as cutting or pinching; deep pain as cramping, burning, or pulling and visceral pain as aching and nauseating.

Cancer pain may be classified according to the pathophysiology involved. Three categories result:

1. Damage by the pathologic process involving nerve fibers that may also result in deafferentation of the sequelae of anticancer therapy resulting in sensory or motor deficits associated or unassociated with dysesthesia or neuralgia

2. Compression of nerve elements resulting in a conduction block of large fibers decreasing their inhibitory action or the involvement of adjacent tissue producing hypersensitivity of nocioceptive nerve endings

3. Pain produced by multiple factors as the pathologic process spreads into various organs

Pain in cancer patients, as in patients with other illnesses, may be of two clinical types: acute and chronic. Acute pain is a common experience of the general population. It is well defined and has a special spatial and temporal pattern associated with a direct cause-and-effect situation. Both subjective and objective components are usually present and are usually easily recognized by the patients as well as the physician. The pain usually resolves when factors of pathologic etiology disappear. Acute pain has a short temporal duration. When pain lasts longer than 6 months, the spectrum changes, and it is generally classified as chronic pain. The objectivity of acute pain is usually absent. The physiologic and psychological reactions are different from those associated with acute pain.

Chronic pain affects most aspects of the patient's life and activity. It seems that the cause and effect in chronic pain have become one. In benign conditions, chronic pain usually stabilizes and is not life-threatening. By contrast, in cancer states, chronic pain usually increases in severity and represents progression of the disease process. This realization by the patient initiates a cascade, not only of physiologic but also of psychological changes, which must be considered in pain-therapeutic techniques.

Pain depends on signals transmitted from the peripheral site of stimulation along the nerves of the spinal cord and into tracts that ascend to the brain. These impulses do not pass into a static system but into a dynamic complex state affected by these inputs that can modulate the signal inputs from the periphery. Recent anatomic and physiologic studies have indicated that modulation of these peripheral inputs by the dynamic state of the nervous system occurs at each level of ascent. Such ascending sensory systems in the spinal cord of animals had been described by Galen in 150 AD.[3] During the early nineteenth century, the finding of Bell[4] and Magendie[5] that sensory fibers passed into the spinal cord only through the dorsal roots was a major advance in the study of sensory pathways. If the skin is stimulated by a noxious agent, potentials are generated in nerve endings, which at a certain intensity result in the axons developing action potentials that obey the all-or-none law. Impulses pass along nerve fibers into the dorsal root to their cells of origin in the dorsal ganglion, and their central projections pass into the spinal cord.

PAIN PATHWAYS

End Organs

The mechanism that initiates pain impulses passing into the spinal cord on noxious stimulation lies within the skin. Is there a specific end organ? This question has not been resolved. Although Goldscheider[76] in 1885 found specific points in the skin that produced pain on stimulation, identification of specific pain organs continues to be debated.

Von Frey[7,8] made extensive studies on pain spots using graded hairs. In his studies, he tried to correlate cold with Krause corpuscles, heat with Ruffini endings, and touch with Meissner's corpuscles. The classification has not been supported by other workers. Strughold[9] in 1924 produced evidence that correlated pain points with the unmyelinated nerve endings that branched profusely in the skin. These nerve fiber endings are found not only in the dermis but in the epidermis as well. They do not form a syncytium; each nerve fiber ending is quite distinct from the adacent one.

Nerve Fibers

Gasser and Erlanger[10,11] classified fiber size in peripheral nerves. The large myelinated A fibers could be divided into subgroups of fibers varying from 16 to 20 μm in diameter, conducting at 90 to 115 m/sec. At the other end of the spectrum were small unmyelinated C fibers, less than 2 μm in diameter, conducting at 0.6 to 2 m/sec. It is known from the work of Trotter and Davies[12] in 1909 that stimulating a peripheral nerve, which they did on themselves, produced pain. They also isolated the nerve stimulated and confirmed pain production on electrical stimulation. In patients undergoing operation, Foerster[13] in 1927 produced pain by electrical stimulation of their exposed nerve. Gasser[14] in 1943 had postulated that pain was probably carried by the fine unmyelinated slow-conducting C fibers in the peripheral nerves.

Posterior Roots

Both myelinated and unmyelinated fibers have their cell bodies in the dorsal root ganglion. The distal segments pass out to form the nerve fibers of the peripheral nerve, and the proximal segments pass through the posterior root into the spinal cord (Fig. 33-1). Gasser[15] in 1950 demonstrated that the fine unmyelinated C fibers divided before entering the dorsal horn, while the large myelinated A fibers divided only after the fibers reached the dorsal column. The afferent impulses entered the spinal cord through the dorsal roots, and efferent impulses left the cord through the ventral roots. This was observed by Bell[4] in 1811 and by Magendie[5] in 1882, when they sectioned the spinal cord roots and studied the response in animals.

Posterior Root Entry

Although studies conducted by Ranson[16-18] and collaborators (1913, 1916, 1931) indicated that the posterior rootlet fibers as they reached the tract of Lissauer in the spinal cord divided anatomically and physiologically into two groups—the lateral containing fine unmyelinated fibers and the medial large myelinated fibers—more recent studies by Earle[19] in 1952 have not substantiated their findings. Rather, he found that the fine fibers were mixed with large fibers as they passed into the spinal cord. No specific unmyelinated fiber group could be isolated at the root entry zone. The fine unmyelinated fibers pass into the spinal cord and, at the tip of the dorsal horn, bifurcate into ascending and descending fibers. These fibers then give off collaterals to the substantia gelatinosa and terminate either on cells of the substantia gelatinosa or on cells of the dorsal horn. Thus, Lissauer's tract extends throughout the spinal cord; each fiber traverses one to three segments superiorly or inferiorly. Experiments in the cat showed that only about 25 percent of the fibers of the Lissauer tract arose from the dorsal root ganglion cells; the remaining were short spinospinal fibers that formed a multisynaptic pathway for the transmission of impulses to higher levels.

Nociceptive impulses travel over A-delta and unmyelinated C nerve fibers evoked peripherally in the unmyelinated fine nerve endings pass into the dorsal root ganglion neurons and into the posterior root entry zone and then through proximal axons into the dorsal horn gray. Within the dorsal horn gray matter, a complex integration of incoming inputs from the periphery and descending inputs from the supraspinal centers take place. Within several laminae of the dorsal horn gray matter, synaptic connections are numerous, producing either excitatory or inhibitory activities. Based on cytoarchitectural studies, in 1952, Rexed[20] divided the spinal gray matter into a series of laminae identified by their cellular morphology. This consisted of 10 zones. In addition, axons of specific diameters terminated in certain laminae giving a restricted topography to these layers. Small delta fibers of the A group and C fibers converged mainly on cells in V and some in laminae IV and VI. The lateral spinothalamic tract fibers mainly arise from cells in lamina V.

Participating in the synaptic activities in these laminae are neurotransmitters that modulate the incoming information. Substance P serves as an excitatory transmitter of the primary pain afferents. Other peptides are present in high concentrations in the laminae of the dorsal horn gray matter: enkephalin and neurotensin. It has been found that morphine and enkephalin will block substance P release from primary afferent ends.

Descending System from Supraspinal Levels

From various regions in the brain stem, fibers pass down to the spinal cord, and many fibers end in the dorsal horn gray matter. They descend through the dorsolateral funiculus and are noradrenergic and serotoninergic. Lesions placed in the dorsolateral funiculus will reduce morphine analgesis.[21] This system modulates incoming impulses from the periphery prior to their ascent to supraspinal levels. Further research is required to define its role in pain control.

Lateral Spinothalamic Tract

From the cells of the substantia gelatinosa and from the dorsal funicular gray cells, fibers arise that form the lateral spinothalamic tract. These fibers carry deep

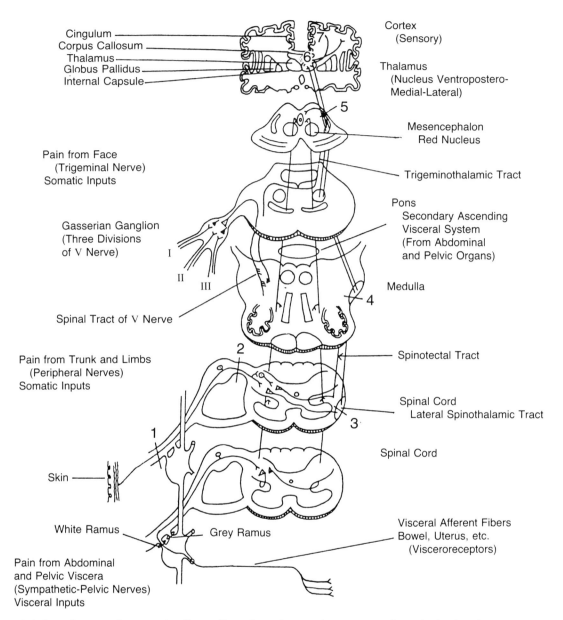

Fig. 33-1 Pain pathways. The somatic afferent fibers from the periphery passing through the dorsal root into the spinal cord are diagrammed. The lateral spinothalamic tract passes up through the spinal cord, medulla, pons, mesencephalon to end in the thalamic nucleus (ventroposterolateralis). The spinotectal tract follows along side the lateral spinothalamic tract; but ends in the superior colliculus area (related to head movements and pain). The trigeminal nerve fibers carry pain from the face and end in the spinal nucleus of the V nerve. The trigeminothalamic fibers cross and ascend to the thalamic nuclei (ventroposteromedialis). The visceral afferent fibers from the bowel, bladder, uterus, and other pelvic structures pass into the sympathetic chain and pelvic nerve and pass through the white communicating ramus into a peripheral nerve through the dorsal root to their neurons in the dorsal root ganglion. The central processes then pass to the dorsal horn gray region and end on cells, giving rise to ipsilateral and contralateral fibers, which pass superiorly as the secondary ascending visceral system: a multisynaptic pathway connecting with the reticular formation at higher levels. The following locations are sites of neurosurgical procedures for pain relief: (1) neurectomy, (2) rhizotomy, (3) cordotomy, (4) medullary tractomy, (5) mesencephalic tractomy, (6) thalamotomy, and (7) cingulotomy. (Battista AF, Ransohoff J: Pain in gynecologic malignancy. p. 407. In Gusberg SB, Frik HC (eds): Gynecologic Cancer. © 1978 The Williams & Wilkins Co., Baltimore)

and superficial pain to higher centers. In humans, the specific cells that give rise to the lateral spinothalamic tract have not been clearly identified. Most of the fibers pass to the opposite side through the central white commissure, which courses ventral to the central canal. The fibers then pass to the opposite anterolateral position in the spinal cord and ascend to higher centers. After the fibers cross and begin to ascend superiorly, collaterals are frequently given off, ending in the medial spinal gray area.

Within the lateral spinothalamic tract, a topographic arrangement of the fibers has been described. Fibers carrying inputs from sacral areas are located in the most dorsal and dorsolateral part of the tract, and fibers from the lumber, thoracic, and cervical areas in a ventral and ventromedial position. The lateral spinothalamic tract is joined by other ascending systems, as it passes up the spinal cord to the brain stem. The spinothalamic tract tends to maintain its lateral position. It proceeds to the posterolateral ventral nucleus of the dorsal thalamus (Fig. 33-1). Studies have shown that few fibers reach and end at the thalamic level.

At the medullary level, the spinothalamic tract is joined by crossed trigeminothalamic fibers from the spinal nucleus of the fifth nerve, which carry pain from the opposite side of the face. Together, both tracts end in the ventroposterolateral and the ventroposteromedial thalamic nuclei (VPL and VPW). Hassler[22,23] indicated that they end only on the basal part of the VPL-VPM complex. Fibers of the third order then pass from the thalamus to the somatic cortical arises S1 and S2 (Fig. 33-1).

Spinotectal Tract

In humans, the precise cells of origin of the spinotectal tract are unknown. They do, however, originate from cells in the substantia gelatinosa and the dorsal horn gray matter. Fibers pass to the opposite side of the spinal cord through the anterior commissure, which is ventral to the central canal. They ascend in close proximity with the spinothalamic tract (Fig. 33-1). However, in the mid-brain, the spinotectal fibers separate from the spinothalamic system and pass medially, ending in the deep layers of the superior colliculus and the lateral central gray regions.

Secondary Ascending Visceral System

Impulses from the viscera pass along thinly medullated axons. For the sake of clarity, a definition of the visceral system is necessary. It consists of both afferent and efferent components similar to those of the somatic system. Visceral afferent impulses are initiated by the stimulation of visceroceptors; their neurons are located on the dorsal root ganglion similar to somatic afferent fibers (Fig. 33-1). Visceral motor activity is exerted on smooth muscle and glands and tends to be automatic and unconscious. Although touch is sparsely distributed in the visceral system, distention of the walls of viscera or vessels usually produces severe pain. Langley[24] considered the autonomic system as mainly visceral efferent passing to tissue, except skeletal muscle, excluding the visceral afferent system.

The more recent attitude expressed by Hess[25] regarded the autonomic system as containing both afferent and efferent visceral components. The difference between the somatic and the visceral systems, however, is seen in the innervation of structures. For the somatic system, skeletal muscle is directly innervated by nerve fibers with their cell bodies within the nervous system (e.g., spinal cord). The visceral system differs in this respect: it involves two different neuronal groups. A preganglionic fiber is sent from the first cell within the brain or spinal cord, passing to an autonomic ganglion outside the brain or spinal cord. Here, the preganglionic fiber synapses with one or several postganglionic neurons. From the ganglion, unmyelinated fibers as postganglionic nerves pass to the viscera.

Basically, a simple visceral reflex will involve three cells: (1) the source afferent neuron forming the input from periphery to the central nervous system: (2) the preganglionic efferent visceral cell located within the brain or spinal cord; and (3) the postganglionic visceral motor cell located in the ganglion outside the central nervous system (CNS).

The visceral afferent fibers pass centrally through both sympathetic and parasympathetic systems. They pass from the thoracic, abdominal, and pelvic viscera through the sympathetic and splanchnic nerves, entering the sympathetic trunk. The fibers pass from the trunk through white communicating rami into peripheral nerves to their cells of origin in the dorsal root ganglia; their central processes pass into the Lissauer tract, into the substantia gelatinosa, and into the dorsal horn cell regions (Fig. 33-1).

Similarly, the parasympathetic system contains visceral afferent fibers. From the heart, lungs, and other viscera, afferent fibers pass through the vagus nerve to their cells of origin in the inferior (nodose) ganglion.

Likewise, visceral afferent fibers from the bladder, rectum, and accessory reproductive organs travel through the pelvic nerves into the spinal cord via the second, third, and fourth sacral dorsal roots to their cells of origin in the dorsal root ganglia. By cutting the dorsal root of S2, S3, S4, the sensation of a distended bladder is blocked. Visceral pain from the abdominal and pelvic organs is carried mainly through fibers in the sympathetic nerves. Thus, the peripheral visceral afferent fibers carrying pain pass to their cells of origin in the dorsal root ganglion; then their central processes continue, ending in the dorsal horn and in the secondary visceral gray areas. From these cells, crossed and uncrossed fibers pass to higher centers (Fig. 33-1).

The details of these pathways are unknown. Nevertheless, it has been demonstrated that fibers pass superiorly and inferiorly and ipsilaterally and contralaterally for a few segments, presumably connecting with cells in the visceral gray regions at these higher or lower spinal levels. New fibers probably arise and ascend for short distances and again end on cells in the visceral gray area. Thus a multisynaptic pathway is formed that conveys these visceral afferent impulses to higher levels (Fig. 33-1). It is not clear where this secondary ascending visceral system terminates, but physiologic evidence seems to indicate that this multisynaptic visceral system closely intermingles with the multisynaptic ascending reticular system.

PAIN THEORIES

The complexity of pain is well exemplified by the many theories proposed to explain it.

Specificity Theory

Muller[26,27] proposed the classic law of specific nerve energy, which implied the presence of specific receptors for pain. In 1882 Blix[28] detected what he described as cold spots in the skin. Von Frey[7,8] studied specific skin end organs, relating each to a specific sensory modality and presenting evidence that the free nerve endings were specific for pain sensations. Thus, the basis of the specificity theory of pain was formulated; pain resembled seeing and hearing. It was postulated that pain impulses generated in the free nerve endings pass along specific nerve fibers A delta and C fibers, into a specific tract in the spinal cord — the lateral spinothalamic tract — which then passes up the spinal cord, ending in a pain center in the thalamus.

The evidence presented to support the specificity theory of pain has been strongly disputed. Is there a specific pain ending? Is there a specific pain nerve fiber? Is there such an entity as a brain pain center? This has resulted in the claim that such a theory is untenable, and a pattern input concept to explain pain has been proposed.

Pattern Theory

Nafe[29] in 1934 proposed that cutaneous sensation depended not on specific inputs, but rather on a pattern of spatially and temporally oriented impulses from the periphery. Weddell[30] in 1955 and Sinclair[31] in 1955 proposed a more detailed pattern theory of pain. Temporal and spatial activity of peripheral inputs are coded into various nerve impulse patterns that are centrally interpreted as pain.

Other theories have been suggested to account for certain types of clinical pain. Livingston[32] in 1943 proposed that certain types of stimulation in some pathologic states would set up reverberating circuits at various levels of the spinal cord, especially in the internuncial pool, which would amplify non-noxious stimuli to be interpreted centrally as a pain experience. Similar suggestions with some variations have been made by other workers.[33,34]

Gate-Control Theory

A variation of the central summation theory to account for pain was the concept of input control by peripheral and central mechanisms. In the pain experience, impulses transmitted over the rapid conducting system were proposed by Noordenbos[35] in 1959 to modulate at the spinal cord and at central levels.

Pain inputs are carried by the slow conducting system. If the fast conducting system is defective, inputs that normally would produce no pain would now evoke pain.

Many variations of this concept have been suggested. Melzack and Wall[36] in 1965 critically reviewed both the specific and pattern pain theories and, as an alternative to both, proposed their gate-control theory of pain. They recognized the reality of physiologic specialization but maintained a wider concept to avoid the objections of the 1:1 relationship between input and pain sensations. They proposed that cutaneous sensory inputs are modulated in the spinal cord by a gating mechanism. Thus, impulses over the large fibers that pass into the spinal cord affect the dorsal horn cell, called the T or transmission cell and modulate the inputs of small fibers on the T cell. Thus, the number of impulses per unit time transmitted to the dorsal horn transmission T cell depends on the ratio of large (L) to small (S) fiber inputs as well as the ongoing CNS activity. When the input on the T cell exceeds a critical value, impulses discharge into the lateral spinothalamic tract fibers. These impulses, through collaterals, affect other adjacent ascending systems. This results in a sequence of sensation and behavior that characterizes a pain experience.

But pain comprises not only sensory but also an affective component. The affective constituent of pain has been recognized by many workers, including Head[37] in 1920 and Sherrington[38] in 1940. Within the concept of the gate-control theory, Casey and Melzack[39] in 1967 proposed that the sensory discriminative mechanism whereby stimuli are localized spatially and temporally is accomplished through the neospinothalamic system. The motivational drive for the action component of pain is effected through the old paramedial ascending system that activates the limbic and the reticular system.

The cognitive evaluation of pain and the integration with past experience are performed through higher-level brain structures, such as the cortex. Thus, the interplay of these three parameters results in the sensation of pain, as well as the psychological and physiologic reactions to pain. If the noxious inputs do not evoke activity in all three systems, there is no pain experience; anxiety or suffering that lack the direct peripheral inputs would not be pain. Although objections have been raised, this theory has stimulated pro-ductive pain research. It has also stimulated the physician to look at the complex picture of cancer pain in a different way.

PAIN THERAPY

Although there are no available objective methods to fractionate the various components of the pain experience, the physician must consider not only the sensory discriminative components directly related to the neoplastic process, but also the motivational and cognitive elements that are relegated, all too frequently, to a minor role in the pain experience. The physician must then use clinical judgment to quantitate the contribution of each of these three components to the patient's immediate complaints of pain and then to prescribe therapy.

Certain principles have been proposed for evaluating patients with pain due to cancer.[39a] Adherence to this scheme tends to prevent misdiagnosis and inadequate pain management. These directives are basic to medical practice in general: complete pain history, assessment of the social and psychological status, and through medical and neurologic evaluation with appropriate diagnostic tests. Patients with cancer pain require frequent re-evaluations regarding their pathologic process and the cause of their pain.

The management of patients with gynecologic cancer pain is complex. No single approach best serves as therapy for all such pain. At times, gynecologic pain may be due to various complications, including infection, pathologic fractures, and involvement of other viscera.

Radiographs, although used as a screening method for metastatic disease, are limited, since a 40 to 60 percent change in bone density is required for detectable changes by this modality. Pain can develop with minimal bone involvement. Bone scan requires 3 to 4 months before changes appear. The recent introduction of the computed tomography CT scan and magnetic resonance imaging (MRI) studies permit early detection of pathologic changes in retroperitoneal, pelvic, abdominal, paravertebral, and other areas. The pain due to gynecologic pathology may also result from the direct involvement of tissues and neutral elements in the lumbar and sacral areas. Aching pain of a dull quality localized to the lumbar area increased on lying or sitting may reflect such localization. Pain radiating anteriorly in a girdlelike fashion or into the inguinal area may indicate paraspinal lumbosacral encroachment. Pain radiating into the sacroiliac joint or referred to the anterior iliac crest region or into the perianal area associated with some sensory loss may reflect progression of the disease with manifestations of increased pain and a different localization.

Medical Therapy

Since pain is a heterogeneous entity, drugs may influence various components differently. Narcotics will decrease pain perception, while tranquilizers will alter pain reaction. Anxiety, fear, hope, cultural, and family elements, as well as ethnic and religious backgrounds, will affect pain perception and reaction. Some knowledge of the action of analgesics, narcotics, and tranquilizers is most helpful in the effective use of these medications for pain relief (Table 33-1).

Thus, the cause of the pain must be defined as early as possible; frequently associated symptoms may amplify the pain (e.g., generalized weakness, nausea, vomiting, or diarrhea). In addition, the patient's interpretation of the cause of her pain may be a most significant component; suffering and pain are frequently intermingled. In the early course of gynecologic neoplasms, it is usually the attending physician who directs pain therapy. Thus, we will consider the medical and then the surgical forms of pain control.

The treating physician has access to various therapeutic modalities for relieving cancer pain. Medical therapy consists of non-narcotic, narcotic, and other analgesic drugs. Each has its particular indications, advantages, and disadvantages. Effective pain therapy reflects the use of these drugs to their optimum activity.

CONSIDERATIONS IN MEDICAL THERAPY

Because the individual response to the same drug dose varies greatly, the management of pain with medication remains challenging. The difficulty is compounded frequently by the side effects of various analgesics. No one analgesic agent is the best in treating cancer pain; rather, determining the optimum analgesic for a particular patient seems the most effective therapeutic approach. A series of pain-relieving agents are available; knowledge of their action and the skill of their use will attain pain relief with minimal side effects. Guidelines are therefore most valuable.[44-47]

These reviews emphasize the need to relieve pain in advanced cancer patients with pain. In addition, the importance of well-informed physicians and supportive health personnel regarding the use of non-narcotic and narcotic medication is discussed in detail. For example, the half-lives of drugs vary: levorphanol (Levo-Dromoran) has a half-life of 12 to 16 hours and methadone (Dolophine) a half-life of 15 to 30 hours. Administration of either of these drugs provides analgesia for 4 to 6 hours.[48,49] These drugs, however, will accumulate with repeated administration, producing sedation and at times altering respirations.[50,51] Such awareness of drug action is essential for optimal scheduling of correct drug dosages.

At times, the combination of drugs will produce greater pain relief without increasing the amount of narcotic prescribed. For example, the addition of a non-narcotic such as aspirin or acetaminophen to a narcotic can effectively decrease pain without increasing the dosage of the narcotic.[52] Other medications, such as antihistamine, diazepam, and chlorpromazine, in conjunction with narcotics can also produce such beneficial effects.[53,54]

The Brompton cocktail, consisting of varying proportions of heroin (diacetylmorphine), phenothiazine, and cocaine, has been reported to be very effective in pain control in cancer pain. Studies have shown that heroin can be replaced by morphine with equivalent efficacy in pain relief.[1,55]

Prolonged use of narcotic medication usually leads to tolerance, for as the disease progresses and pain increases more narcotic analgesic is required to maintain pain relief. Changing to different narcotic agents, supplementing with non-narcotic drugs, and finally, where indicated, the use of destructive anesthetic or neurosurgical techniques to interrupt pain pathways may be required for relief of pain.

ADJUVANT DRUGS FOR PAIN RELIEF

Adjuvant drugs consist of a heterogeneous group of substances that have been used to relieve cancer pain.[56,57] They include tricyclic antidepressants,[58] phenothiazines,[59] antihistamines and steroids,[60,61] anticonvulsants,[62] and even L-Dopa.[63] The mechanisms

Table 33-1 Medical Treatment for Pain

Proprietary Name	Generic Name	Dosage mg/70-kg body weight		Clinical Use
		Oral	SC or IM	
Mild analgesics				
Aspirin	Acetylsalicylic acid	650 q 3–4 h		
Tylenol	Acetaminophen	650 q 3–4 h		
Strong analgesics				For mild to moderate pain
Butazolidin	Phenylbutazone	100 qid		
Indocin	Indomethacin	25 qid		
Dolobid	Diflunisal	500–1,000 q 12 h		
Clinoril	Sulindac	150–200 q 12 h		
Tolectin	Tolmetin	400 q 4–8 h		
Mild narcotic agents				For moderate to severe pain
Codeine		30–60 q 4–6 h	30–60 q 4–6 h	
Darvon	Proxylene hydrochloride	65 q 3–4 h		
Percodan	Oxycodone hydrochloride plus	5 q 4–6 h		
Talwin	Pentazocine	30–50 q 4–6 h	30 q 4–6 h	
Strong narcotics				For severe pain
Morphine			8–10 q 3–4 h	
Morphine — sustain release		30 q 8–12 h	8–10 q 3–4 h	
Demerol	Meperidine hydrochloride	50–100 q 3–4 h	50–100 q 3–4 h	
Methadone	Dolophine	5–10 q 3–4 h		
Tranquilizers				Nonanalgesics, adjuncts for relief of associated depression and/or anxiety
Valium	Diazepam	5–10 q 4–6 h	3–5 q 4–6 h	
Miltown	Meprobamate	200–400 qid		
Antidepressants				
Elavil	Amitriptyline hydrochloride	10–20 qid		
Tofranil	Imipramine	25 qid		
Phenothiazines				
Thorazine	Chloropromazine	10–20 qid	10 qid	
Phenergan	Promethazine hydrochloride	12.5 qid	25 h.s.	
Prolixin	Fluphenazine hydrochloride	2.5 qid	1.25 tid	

of pain relief obtained with these agents is not understood, but it is not a direct effect on the opiate receptors.

The effectiveness of anticonvulsant drugs in the treatment of certain benign chronic pain states, such as trigeminal neuralgia, postherpetic neuralgia, and other neuralgic disorders, has been known for many years. In 1962, Blum[64] introduced Tegretol (carbamazepine) for the relief of trigeminal neuralgia; this drug has been very beneficial.[65-67] Other anticonvulsant agents, such as Dilantin (phenytoin), Lioresal (baclofen), and Klonopin (clonazepam), have also

been reported to relieve pain in cancer patients.[62] The dosage of anticonvulsant drugs produces varied effects, and plasma levels differ from patient to patient. Since the relationship of dose to blood level is not linear, it is important to monitor plasma drug concentrations to ensure a therapeutic dosage.[68]

NON-NARCOTIC ANALGESICS

Non-narcotic agents may be effective in relieving mild to moderate cancer pain; therefore, they should be the first drugs used.[40,41] Additional evidence indicates that they can be effective in relieving certain types of bone metastatic pain.[42,43] The nonsteroidal noninflammatory drugs, aspirin, being the prototype, include acetaminophen and indomethacin; others (see Table 33-1) act at the periphery, inhibiting the pain system at its origin. They prevent prostaglandin production by inhibiting cyclooxygenase, the enzyme essential for the transformation of arachidonic acid to prostaglandin. By contrast, narcotics act on central pain-processing regions of the nervous system.

MILD ANALGESICS

Aspirin (Acetylsalicylic Acid)

Aspirin is the most widely used mild analgesic. It exhibits antipyretic, as well as analgesic actions. The mechanism of action is not well understood. Not only are peripheral mechanisms such as nerve conduction and chemoreceptors affected, but subcortical central activities as well.[69,70] Side effects include dizziness, gastrointestinal (GI) disturbances, and skin reactions. In susceptible patients, the prothrombin time may be altered, producing hemorrhage; in some asthmatic patients, exacerbation of symptoms may result. The dosage for an adult is 600 mg PO, every 4 to 6 hours. Some patients may obtain relief and tolerate higher doses up to 1 g every 4 hours.[71]

Tylenol (Acetaminophen)

Tylenol is both analgesic and antipyretic. By elevating the pain threshold, it produces analgesia and, by an action through the hypothalamic heat-regulating center, it produces antipyresis. It is well suited as a substitute for aspirin when the latter produces an allergic response. It has minimal side effects. The dosage for an adult is one to two tablets PO every 3 to 4 hours (one tablet contains 325 mg acetaminophen).

STRONG ANALGESICS

Butazolidin (Phenylbutazone)

Butazolidin is not a simple analgesic and should be administered with care. Detailed medical evaluation with close supervision of administration are indicated. Since it is related chemically, including its toxic action, to pyrazoline, it has antiinflammatory, antipyretic, and analgesic actions. The side effects are fre-

quently unpredictable, and close supervision to detect early adverse reactions is essential. Hematologic evaluation should be obtained every 1 to 2 weeks; any new symptoms should immediately be reported by the patient and evaluated by a physician. Usually within several days the effectiveness of the drug can be determined. If ineffectual, it should be stopped; if effectual, the dosage should be increased if possible. The dosage for an adult is 100 mg PO administered every 6 hours. The maintenance dose should not exceed 500 mg/day. For short-term pain relief in acute conditions, it can be very effective. Frequently a lower dosage of 100 to 200 mg/day will be effective.

Indocin (Indomethacin)

Indocin is an effective antiinflammatory nonsteroid drug. The antiinflammatory action is greater than that of aspirin. It has also antipyretic and analgesic actions. Indocin should be administered with great care and close supervision. Side effects, however, may develop in 50 percent of patients, and most patients cannot tolerate a dose greater than 100 mg/day. Patients with GI lesions should not recieve this drug. Its side effects are very diverse. The patient should be instructed to notify the physician of any new symptoms. Medical and hematologic evaluation at intervals should be part of the close supervision. The dosage for an adult is 25 mg PO, four times a day.

Dolobid (Diflunisal)

Dolobid is a nonsteroidal antiinflammatory analgesic drug. The analgesic effect of this salicylic acid derivative may persist up to 8 hours and may be as beneficial as aspirin or acetaminophen. Gastrointestinal side effects are less frequent than with aspirin. Like aspirin, it inhibits platelet aggregation. The dosage is 500 to 1,000 mg PO, every 12 hours.

Clinoril (Sulindac)

It is also an indole similar to indomethacin and tolmetin. Sulindac itself is inactive; however, in the liver it is metabolized to a sulfide that inhibits prostaglandin synthesis. Its analgesic and antiinflammatory action is similar to that of aspirin. The side effects involving the GI or CNS are usually mild. The dosage is 150 to 200 mg PO, every 12 hours.

Tolectin (Tolmetin)

Like indomethacin, Tolectin is an indole, useful as an analgesic agent, and has an antiinflammatory action greater than that of aspirin. It has a short half-life of about 1 to 1½ hours. The dosage is 400 mg every 4 to 8 hours.

NARCOTIC ANALGESICS

The earliest recorded medicinal use of the poppy was the Ebers Papyrus (600 to 1,500 BC) Hippocrates (463 to 377 BC) described various preparations using the poppy in the treatment of various medical conditions. Specific efficacy for pain relief was noted by Galen.[72] Modern use resulted from the isolation from opium of meconid acid, the precursor of morphine.

Narcotic agents are generally classified into three main categories: (1) natural opium, (2) semisynthetic opiate compounds, and (3) synthetic opiate substances. In a discussion of opiate compounds, morphine is considered the prototype. When administered orally, subcutaneously, or intravenously, it accumulates in free or bound form in various tissue, particularly, in the lung, kidney, liver, adrenals, spleen, and thyroid. Although morphine crosses the placental barrier, its permeability into brain across the blood-brain interface is very low.[73]

The effect of opiate compounds on CNS activity is complex. Opiate receptors have been identified throughout most regions of the brain as well as in the spinal cord. It is particularly high in the trigeminal nucleus, the intralaminar thalamic regions, and the periaqueductal gray.[74,75] Opiates in humans produce analgesia associated with different degrees of euphoria, drowsiness, and frequently, depending on dosage, a slowing in motor and intellectual activities. Many other side effects alter various biologic systems, including the respiratory, cardiovascular, and GI systems.

MILD NARCOTIC ANALGESICS

(Codeine)

Codeine is one of the alkaloids in opium; its action is similar to that of morphine. It has about one-eighth the analgesic action of morphine. Codeine suppresses the cough reflex but has little effect on respiration. As a mild narcotic, tolerance and dependence can de-

velop. It has been proposed that its analgesic action is due to demethylation in the liver, which converts it partly into morphine. Often used in combination with mild analgesic such as aspirin and phenacetin, it can be very effective for moderate to severe pain. Reactions are limited, consisting mainly of constipation or urticaria. The dosage for an adult is 30 to 60 mg PO every 4 to 6 hours; 30 to 60 mg SC or IM every 4 to 6 hours.

Darvon (Propoxyphene Hydrochloride)

Darvon is chemically related to methadone. Studies have shown that Darvon with aspirin produced greater analgesia than either compound alone. Its abuse can result in some drug dependence, more frequently of a psychic than a physical nature. Since it causes CNS depression, it may be additive to other depressive drugs. Although side effects are infrequent, dizziness, sedation, nausea, and vomiting have been reported. If chronic intake exceeds 800 mg/day, toxic psychosis or convulsions may be produced. The dosage for an adult is 65 mg PO every 4 to 6 hours.

Percodan (Proxylene Hydrochloride)

Percodan consists of a combination of drugs: oxycodine hydrochloride, oxycodone tetrephthalate, aspirin, phenacetin, and caffeine. Oxycodone is a semisynthetic narcotic. It has actions similar to morphine and affects the CNS and smooth muscle. Tolerance, physical dependence, as well as psychic dependence, may develop with chronic use. Thus, caution should be used in its administration. It may interact with other CNS depressants. Physicians unaware of the marked dependency possibilities of Percodan prescribe it too frequently. The dosage for an adult is one tablet PO every 4 to 6 hours.

Talwin (Pentazocine)

Talwin is a member of the benzazocine group. It is a weak narcotic antagonist (1/50 the antagonistic activity of nalorphine). It can be effective in the relief of severe pain due to neoplasm. Care must be exercised in replacing a strong narcotic with Talwin. Although it is a weak narcotic antagonist, it can evoke withdrawal symptoms if it suddenly replaces potent narcotics with moderate degrees of physical potent dependence. It can produce hallucinations and dysphoria. Since it has possible psychological and physical dependence, care should be used in its administration. The dosage for an adult is one tablet (50 mg) PO, every 3 to 4 hours, for a total daily dose of up to 600 mg.

STRONG NARCOTIC ANALGESICS

Morphine

Morphine is an alkaloid obtained from opium. It is the oldest known analgesic. Its action on the nervous system is uneven; some centers are depressed and others are activated. Morphine elevates the pain threshold. Its maximum analgesic action develops about 90 minutes after injection and remains for about 4 hours. It affects mood in addition to pain control. This dulling of attention, relaxation, and decreased anxiety are all additive effects in pain control. It affects visceral pain as well as somatic pain. The respiratory center is depressed; although it slows respiration, it increases the depth of respiration. It depresses the cough center and produces pupillary constriction. Morphine is excreted mostly through the kidneys in a conjugated form. Chronic use of morphine, as little as 60 mg/day for 2 days, will result in tolerance. As tolerance develops, so does physical dependency. The former is a signal of developing dependence. The dosage for an adult is 10 mg SC or IM, every 3 to 4 hours.

Demerol (Meperidine Hydrochloride)

Demerol is a narcotic analgesic with multiple actions similar to morphine. Its chemical structure resembles that of atropine. It is a central depressant with analgesic qualities similar to morphine, but of shorter duration. Morphine is about 10 times more potent than Demerol for an equal analgesic effect. Because of its antispasmodic action, it can be effective in relieving visceral pain. Similar to morphine, side effects such as sweating, nausea, vomiting, and confusion may develop. It is contraindicated if monoamine oxidase (MAO) inhibitors have been used. Chronic use over a few weeks leads to tolerance as well as physical dependency. Thus, it should be administered with great care. Such a narcotic should not be used until the late stages of the illness. The dosage for an adult is 50 to 100 mg PO, every 3 to 4 hours; 50 to 100 mg SC or IM, every 3 to 4 hours.

Dolophine (Methadone)

Dolophine is a narcotic analgesic with actions similar to morphine. It has the advantage of being active orally and is equal to 10 mg of morphine in analgesic effectiveness. It may be given subcutaneously or intramuscularly but not intravenously. Although tolerance and physical dependence can develop, these are less marked than with other potent narcotics. It has only slight euphoric sedative properties. The adverse reactions are similar to other narcotics, which include respiratory and cirulatory depression. Dizziness, nausea, vomiting, and sweating are the most frequently noted adverse effects. The dosage for an adult is 5 to 10 mg PO, every 3 to 4 hours; 2.5 to 10 mg IM or SC, every 3 to 4 hours.

Brompton Cocktail

Snow[77] in 1896 suggested the use of a narcotic and a stimulant combination for pain relief in cancer patients. He combined morphine and cocaine and reported significant benefit in relieving cancer pain.[76] The Brompton cocktail was finalized by its use and acceptance at the Brompton Hospital in 1952 for pain relief.[77] It consists of varying amounts of heroin (diacetylmorphine) or morphine, cocaine, alcohol, chloroform water, and phenathiazine. Studies have shown that either mixtures with heroin or morphine yield about an 85 percent pain relief.[78] In addition, it has been reported that cocaine is not necessary and little difference results from the use of heroin or morphine in the mixture in affording pain relief.[79] Thus, morphine can replace heroin in the mixture, and morphine in doses of 5 to 100 mg every 4 hours can produce effective analgesia in cancer pain.[1,55]

MINOR TRANQUILIZERS

Minor tranquilizers have little or no analgesic action but are used to allay anxiety and depression.

Valium (Diazepam)

Valium is a benzodiazepine derivative. Animal studies have indicated its action on the limbic system as well as on the thalamus and hypothalamus, producing a calming effect. In pain patients, it has value in the symptomatic relief of tension and anxiety states resulting from stress. It is also effective in the relief of skeletal muscle spasm. The dosage for an adult is 5 to 10 mg PO, three to five times a day; 2 to 10 mg IM or SC, three to five times a day.

Miltown (Meprobamate)

Miltown is a carbamate derivative. It acts at multiple sites in the CNS, including the thalamus and limbic system. It is effective in the relief of anxiety and tension. The side effects are mild, usually consisting of headache, anorexia, nausea, and occasionally diarrhea. Its chronic use exposes the patient to drug dependence. The dosage for an adult is 200 to 400 mg PO, three to four times a day.

ANTIDEPRESSANTS

Elavil (Amitriptyline Hydrochloride)

Elavil is a dibenzocycloheptadiene derivative. It acts as an antidepressant having an anxiety-relieving component as well as a sedative one. It acts by inhibiting the membrane pump responsible for the reuptake of norepinephrine into the adrenergic cells. Thus, it prolongs sympathetic activity. It should not be given concomitantly with MAO inhibitors. It may also block the antihypertensive action of quanethidine or similarly acting drugs. Care should be taken in the administration to patients with hyperthyroidism or taking thyroid medication. The dosage for an adult is 10 mg PO, four to five times a day, 75 to 100 mg at night.

Tofranil (Imipramine Hydrochloride)

Tofranil is a tricyclic antidepressant that does not primarily stimulate the CNS, but rather blocks the uptake of norepinephrine at nerve endings, potentiating adrenergic synaptic activity. It should not be administered to patients receiving MAO inhibitor drugs. Tofranil may block the action of such drugs as quanethidine or similar agents. The dosage for an adult is 25 mg PO, four times daily.

PHENOTHIAZINES

Thorazine (Chloropromazine)

Thorazine is a dimethylamine derivative of phenothiazine. It exerts a sedative and an antiemetic effect as well as a psychotropic action. It acts at all levels of the CNS but primarily on subcortical centers. It has a strong adrenergic and a weak peripheral anticholinergic action. It may counteract the action of quanethidine and related compounds. It also depresses the CNS. The dosage for an adult is 10 to 20 mg PO, three to four times daily; 10 mg IM, four times daily.

Phenergan (Promethazine Hydrochloride)

Phenergan has an antihistamine, an antiemetic, and a sedative action. The dosage for an adult is 12.5 mg PO, three to four times daily; 12.5 to 25 mg IM, before sleep.

Prolixin (Fluphenazine Hydrochloride)

Prolixin is a trifluoromethyl phenothiazine derivative. The precise mechanism of action is not understood. The dosage for an adult is 2.5 mg PO, four to five times daily; 1.25 mg IM, two to three times daily.

Surgical Therapy

Although the physiology of pain is poorly understood, the anatomic pathways related to pain have been described in detail. One must evaluate what specific neurosurgical procedure will be most effective for the relief of gynecologic malignancy pain.

The neoplasm usually spreads by direct extension or by the lymphatics. The lymph nodes about the internal iliac arteries lead to direct tumor spread into the lumbosacral nerve trunks, producing pain in the lower back, with radiation into one or both legs. Tumor spread through the nodes of the lumbar trunk to involve the upper lumbar nerve roots or adjacent bone produces pain in the lower lumbar area and abdomen. The external and common iliac lymphatic group affects a more anterior spread, invading the femoral, genitofemoral, or obturator nerves and evokes pain in the area of innervation.

In the evaluation of surgical therapy for gynecologic malignancy pain, the medical and neurologic conditions as well as the prognosis of the patient are most important. There are also many other significant considerations: Is the disease a local process? Does it involve adjacent structures? Are there metastases? The surgical interruption of pain pathways at the periphery and at various higher levels of the neural axis, by neurectomy, rhizotomy, cordotomy, tractomy, thalamotomy, frontal lobotomy, and cingulotomy, can result in pain relief. Each procedure has its indications, its limits, and its complications.

NEURECTOMY

Because gynecologic malignant processes rarely involve only one nerve, nerve resection for pain is seldom performed.

RHIZOTOMY

Rhizotomy consists of exposing the dorsal roots through a laminectomy and cutting the rootlets intradurally central to the ganglion. Because of the overlap of nerve root innervation, one to two roots above and below the level of pain are usually sectioned. Since dorsal rhizotomy eliminates all sensation to the innervated part, denervation of a hand, for example, produces marked functional loss, even if muscle strength is excellent. Thoracic rhizotomy does not produce significant incapacitation, whereas a bilateral S2 rhizotomy produces impotence and decreased sensation. If the S3 root is included, loss of bladder and rectal sphincter control also results. In addition to these considerations, posterior rhizotomy in malignant disease has an immediate success rate for pain relief of only 50 percent, and about one-half of these patients will have recurrence of their pain before death.[80]

Sindou[81,82] in 1972 made a thorough anatomic study of the distribution of fine and large fibers as they enter the spinal cord at the dorsal root entry zone in an attempt to develop a precise method of sectioning the posterior rootlets. Using magnification, he performed selective posterior rhizotomies. In 1986, he reported 12 hemiplegic patients with a painful upper limb; nine were relieved of their pain completely and three were partially improved with a follow-up of 1 to 12 years. Nashold and Ostdahl[83] in 1979 reported a series of patients with spinal cord pain syndromes who had thermolytic lesions placed in the dorsal root entry zone. Friedman and Nashold[84] in 1986 reviewed their results with this procedure in 56 patients with spinal cord pain followed for 6 months to 5 years: 50 percent had good pain relief, 8.9 percent had fair pain relief, and 41 percent had no pain relief. Further clinical studies are required to assess the effectiveness of this procedure to relieve pain in gynecologic cancer patients, since the innervation is from the lower lumbar and sacral cord regions.

CORDOTOMY

Clinical observations led to this important surgical procedure for pain. In 1905, Spiller[85] reported the autopsy findings of paired tuberculomas compressing the anterior quadrants of the lower thoracic spinal cord. This had produced the loss of pain and temperature over the lower trunk and extremities. The observation was made by Edinger[86] in 1889 and by Wallenberg[87] in 1895, that pain and temperature in humans were carried over the spinothalamic tract.

In 1911, Martin at the suggestion of Spiller[88] performed the first spinothalamic tract section in a human subject. Thus began one of the most effective surgical procedures for pain relief. It also introduced the surgical concept of interrupting pain pathways at various levels of the neural axis. Open surgical cordotomy can be very effective in pain relief, particularly in unilateral pain of gynecologic malignancy with no distant metastasis. Pain in the pelvis, low abdomen, perineum, and lower extremities responds well to thoracic cordotomy at the T2 and T4 levels, and neurologic complications have been markedly reduced since the advent of the operative microscope. Although postcordotomy analgesia usually drops several segments, adequate level of pain relief is usually maintained. Pain relief from cordotomy is obtained in about 70 to 80 percent of patients with gynecologic malignancy until their death.[89] When the pain becomes bilateral with progression of the disease, however, even bilateral thoracic cordotomy may not sustain pain relief.

In an attempt to diminish the risk and complication of open cordotomy so that the procedure could be done in medically poor-risk patients with intractable pain, Mullan et al.[90] in 1963 introduced the percutaneous needle approach to cervical cordotomy. A strontium needle was used that emitted β-particles, accomplishing a percutaneous chordotomy at the C1 to C2 vertebral level. Rosomoff et al.[91] in 1965 modified the Mullan technique using a radiofrequency (RF) current instead of β-radiation to produce a lesion. This made the technique generally applicable and set the basis for the introduction of percutaneous cordotomy as an acceptable method. It has replaced open cordotomy at many institutions. Although percutaneous cordotomy is performed at cervical C1 to C2, the level of analgesia can be controlled by the size and placement of the lesion. It has been widely used in controlling malignant pain.

Rosomoff[92] in 1969 reported a series of 100 patients who underwent bilateral percutaneous cervical cordotomy, 71 percent of whom had malignant disease. The abdomen, perineum, lumbar area, and lower extremities were involved in 73 percent of cases. An analgesic thoracic level was adequate for pain relief; 80 percent had immediate pain relief. Postoperative paresis was present in 10 percent, 3 percent being permanent. Bladder dysfunction resulted in 2 percent of cases. In this series, the Ondine syndrome (sleep-producing apnea) was present in four patients and appeared 24 to 72 hours after cordotomy. This complication, however, developed only in those patients with a high C3 analgesic level. Such a level for gynecologic malignancy pain is seldom required. Lipton[93] in 1968 reported in their Liverpool series that 90 percent of patients with malignant disease pain were relieved of pain by percutaneous cervical cordotomy until death. The sectioning of pain pathways at higher levels in the neural axis is performed in order to obtain a higher level of analgesia. Sectioning the spinothalamic tract at the medulla (medullary tractomy) produces a level as high as C1 to C2; at the mesencephalon (a mesencephalic tractomy), a level of analgesia of the face and scalp results.

THALAMOTOMY

Lesions for pain relief are placed in various nuclei of the thalamus using a stereotactic technique. It is used for pain arising from almost any body region, particularly when other surgical procedures have been ineffective or have produced painful dysthesias. Clinical evaluations have been correlated with histologic findings at autopsy, and the most effective regions in the thalamus have been determined.[94-96]

LOBOTOMY

Moniz[97,98] in 1936, based on the work of Fulton and Jacobsen[99] in 1935 on primates, persuaded Lima to perform a prefrontal lobotomy for psychiatric illness. The patient had a marked alleviation of anxiety. Since that time, many such procedures have been done for psychiatric illness and pain relief. Because of associated mental changes, prefrontal lobotomy has become markedly restricted in its use to relieve pain in cancer patients. Although suffering may be relieved by lobotomy, the associated personality alterations detract from this pain-relieving surgical procedure.

In order to decrease the serious side effects of lobotomy in patients with intractable pain, lesions have been placed in other brain areas, particularly the cingulum.[100,101] Unfortunately, with cingulotomy, mental alterations develop as well. Thus, only if the emotional suffering of a patient with gynecologic malignancy pain becomes the primary pain component would one consider an operation involving higher brain regions.

Intrathecal Injection

Another means of altering inputs that may afford pain relief is by destructive chemicals, such as alcohol or phenol instilled into the spinal subarachnoid space. Gynecologic malignancy rarely involves specific nerves; therefore, local nerve injections have a very limited application. To be able to affect many roots which are usually involved in pelvic malignancy, an intrathecal injection is required.

Dogliotti[102] in 1931 first introduced the use of intrathecal alcohol for pain relief. Absolute alcohol is lighter than cerebrospinal fluid (CSF); it will therefore float as a layer on CSF. By careful patient positioning, it is possible to affect first the dorsal roots. This is a difficult and unpredictable method. Complications include numbness, bladder dysfunction, and motor paresis. Usually more than one alcohol intrathecal injection is required for pain relief. In some patients, maximal pain relief may be delayed for several days after the injection, and the average duration of pain relief is about 3 months, ranging from weeks to years. Phenol and glycerine can also be used.[103] The mixture is heavier than CSF and will seek a more dependent level.

Thus, control can be easier than with alcohol. It has similar postinjection complications to those of alcohol, including bladder and motor dysfunction. Relief from pain by phenol in glycerin injection may be temporary or permanent. For unilateral limited root involvement by gynecologic malignancy, careful intrathecal phenol in glycerin injections may be effective for pain relief.[104,105]

In an attempt to obviate the direct destructive aspects of neurolytic agents on all neural elements, Hitchcock[106] in 1967 described hypothermic subarachnoid saline irrigation for pain relief. This consisted of performing a lumbar puncture, removing CSF, and then injecting saline at 2° to 4°C. Injections of 10 ml were repeated up to a total of 60 ml in some cases. Various modifications of this method for pain relief have been reported; hypertonicity or isotonicity with hypothermia or normothermia, as well as simple barbotage of the CSF. Reports indicate immediate significant pain relief, but also the return of pain within weeks to months.[107-110] Battista[111] in 1974 reported a series of 70 patients with intractable pain treated by hypothermic isotonic subarachnoid injections; 37 patients had neoplastic disease pain. Of the 37 patients, 75 percent had excellent to fair pain relief up to the time of death.

The mechanism of pain relief by this procedure is not understood, and various theories have been proposed. The complication rate is low, although severe muscle weakness and cardiac arrhythmias have been reported.[112-114] Myelography is recommended prior to the procedure, especially in the presence of any neurologic deficit.

Recent findings have confirmed the presence of opiate receptors in the dorsal horn region of the spinal cord. In addition, the local application of morphine to the dorsal horn cells suppresses the firing of spinothalamic neurons to noxious stimulation. On the basis of these findings, epidural and intrathecal administration of morphine has been used clinically to relieve cancer pain.[115-117] Technical developments have permitted the continuous infusion of narcotics by means of the infusaid pump. Marked analgesia results from small doses of morphine; however, epidural or intrathecal narcotic infusions over time will result in tolerance. The intraventricular route for narcotic administration using an Ommaya reservoir also produces marked pain relief with small doses.[118] Although tolerance does develop with continued use, increasing the dosage of the narcotic will maintain analgesia up to the limit determined by the severity of side effects. Changing the narcotic may restore some analgesia, but cross-tolerance will limit its efficacy.

Dorsal Column and Transcutaneous Nerve Stimulation

Another method by which inputs that produce pain can be altered is by nerve stimulation. Wall and Sweet[119] in 1967, based on the gate-control theory, experimented on themselves. They found that electrical stimulation of their own infraorbital nerves through needle electrodes produced paresthesias in the innervated skin regions as well as hypoalgesia in

the area to pinprick. This principle of pain relief was then applied directly to peripheral nerves as well as to the spinal dorsal column. A variety of stimulation units using the most recent electronic technology have been developed.

Sweet and Wepsic[120] in 1973 critically reviewed their results of dorsal column stimulation for pain relief over a period of several years. Their findings were similar to those reported by other workers.[121-126] Over time, the effectiveness of dorsal column stimulation decreased, ranging from 35 to 73 percent of excellent to good results immediately after implant to a decrease of 40 percent to 25 percent excellent to good results over a period of 6 months to 1 year. These results indicate the need for caution in the use of dorsal column implants for pain relief. The reason for this significant falloff in pain relief is not clear.

Alteration of pain inputs can also be produced by electrical stimulation of neural elements through the skin. This noninvasive transcutaneous electrical stimulation technique, although very simple, avoids the complication of dorsal column stimulation. Reports have indicated the use of transcutaneous electrical nerve stimulation in a variety of intractable pain conditions including gynecologic malignancy pain. In chronic pain, excellent to partial pain relief has been achieved in about 40 to 60 percent of cases.[124,125,127,128] The long-term effectiveness of this form of pain therapy is not yet known.

Within the past few years, pain has come of age. Pain, being one of the main symptom of disease in humans, at times becomes the disease itself. Physicians particularly interested in pain — its physiology and its therapy — have become knowledgeable in medical and surgical techniques for pain relief. This development brings hope for an effective form of therapy against pain as a disease.

REFERENCES

1. Twycross RG, Lack SA: Symptom Control in Far Advanced Cancer Pain Relief. Pitman, London, 1984
2. Daut RL, Cleeland CS: The prevalence and severity of pain in cancer. Cancer 50:1913, 1982
3. Keele KD: Anatomies of Pain. Charles C Thomas, Springfield, IL, 1957
4. Bell C: Idea of a new anatomy of the brain submitted for the observation of his friends. Strahan and Preston, London, 1811

5. Magendie F: Experiences sur les functions des racines des nerfs rachidiens. J Physiol Exp Pathol 2:276, 1822

6. Goldscheider A: Neue tatsachen uber die hautsinnesnerven. Pfuegers Arch Ges Physiol 1(suppl):1, 1885

7. von Frey M: Beitrage zur Physiologie des Schmerzsinns. Berlin Sachs Gesamte Wiss Math Phys Klin 46:283, 1894

8. von Frey M: Beitrage zur sinnesphysiologie der haut. Berlin Sachs Gesamte Wiss Math Phys Klin 47:166, 1895

9. Strughold H: Uber die dichte und schwellen der schmerzpunkte der epidermis in den verschiedenen korperregionen. Z Biol 80:367, 1924

10. Gasser HS, Erlanger J: The role of fiber size in the establishment of a nerve block by pressure or cocaine. Am J Physiol 88:581, 1929

11. Gasser HS: Mammalian nerve fibers, Nobel Lecture given December 12, 1945. Included in Les Prix Nobel en 1940–44, p. 128. PA Norstedt, Stockholm, 1946

12. Trotter W, Davis HM: Experimental studies in the innervation of the skin. J Physiol (Lond) 38:134, 1909

13. Foerster O: Ueber die vorderseitenstrang-durchschneidung. Arch Psychiatry Nervenkr 81:707, 1927

14. Gasser HS: Pain-producing impulses in peripheral nerves. Res Publ Assoc Res Nerv Ment Dis 23:44, 1943

15. Gasser HS: Unmedullated fibers originating in dorsal root ganglia. J Gen Physiol 33:651, 1950

16. Ranson SW: The course within the spinal cord of the non-medullated fibers of the dorsal roots; a study of Lissauer's tract in the cat. J Comp Neurol 23:259, 1913

17. Ranson SW, Billingsley PR: The conduction of painful afferent impulses in the spinal nerves. Am J Physiol 40:571, 1916

18. Ranson SW: Cutaneous sensory fibers and sensory conduction. Arch Neurol Psychiatry 26:1122, 1931

19. Earle KM: The tract of Lissauer and its possible relation to the pain pathway. J Comp Neurol 96:93, 1952

20. Rexed B: The cytoarchitectonic organization of the spinal cord in the cat. J Comp Neurol 96:415, 1952

21. Fields HL, Basbaum AI, Clanton CH, Anderson SD: Nucleus raphe magnus inhibition of spinal cord dorsal horn neurons. Brain Res 126:441, 1977

22. Hassler R: Trigeminal Neuralgia. Pathogenesis and Pathophysiology. Thieme, Stuttgart, 1970

23. Hassler R: Afferent system. p. 98. In Payne JP, Burt RAP (eds): Pain. Basic Principles — Pharmacology — Therapy. Thieme, Stuttgart, 1972

24. Langley JN: The Autonomic Nervous System. Vol. 1. W. Heffer, Cambridge, 1921

25. Hess WR: Die funktionelle Orginisation des vegetativen Nervensystems. Benno Schwabe, Basel, 1948

26. Muller J: Zur vergleichenden Physiologie des Gesichtssinnes des Menschen und der Augen und uber den menschlichen Blick. Knobloch, 1826

27. Muller J: Elements of Physiology. Vol. 2. Taylor & Walton, London, 1842

28. Blix M: Experminentela bidrag til losning affragan om hundnerveras specifika energies. Uppsala Lakforen Forh, 1 Ser, 18:427, 1882

29. Nafe JP: The pressure, pain, and temperature senses. p. 1037. In Murchison C (ed) Handbook of General Experimental Psychology. Clark University Press, Worcester, 1934

30. Weddell G: Somesthesis and the chemical senses. Annu Rev Psychol 6:119, 1955

31. Sinclair DC: Cutaneous sensation and the doctrine of specific nerve energies. Brain 78:584, 1955

32. Livingston WK: Pain Mechanisms. Macmillan, New York, 1943

33. Gerard MW: Afferent impulses of the trigeminal nerve. Arch Neurol Psychiatry 9:306, 1923

34. Hebb DO: The Organization of Behavior. John Wiley & Sons, New York, 1949

35. Noordenbos W: Pain. American Elsevier, New York, 1959

36. Melzack R, Wall PD: Pain mechanisms: A new theory. Science 150:971, 1965

37. Head H: Studies in Neurology. 2 Vols. Oxford University Press, London, 1920

38. Sherrington CS: p. 31. On the distribution of the sensory nerve-roots. In Denny-Brown D (ed): Selected Writings of Sir Charles Sherrington. Paul B Hoeber, New York, 1940

39. Casey KL, Melzack R: Neural mechanisms of pain: A conceptual model. p. 13. In Way EL (ed): New Concepts in Pain and Its Clinical Management. Davis, Philadelphia, 1967

39a. Foley KM: Clinical assessment of cancer pain. Acta Anesthesiol Scand 74(suppl):91, 1982

40. Twycross RG: Ventafridda V (eds): The Continuing Care of Terminal Cancer Patients. Pergamon Press, Oxford, 1980

41. Kantor TG: Control of pain by nonsteroidal anti-inflammatory drugs. Med Clin North Am 66:1053, 1982

42. Brereton HD, Halushka PV, Alexander RW, et al: Indomethacin-responsive hypercalcemia in a patient with renal-cell adenocarcinoma. N Engl J Med 291:83, 1974

43. Galasko CSB: Mechanisms of bone destruction in the development of skeletal metastases. Nature (Lond) 263:507, 1976

44. McGivney WT, Crooks GM (eds): The care of patients with severe chronic pain in terminal illness. JAMA 251:1182, 1984

45. Beaver WT: Management of cancer pain with parenteral medication. JAMA 244:2653, 1980

46. Inturrisi CE, Foley KM: Narcotic analgesics in the management of pain. p. 257. In Kuhar M, Pasternak G (eds): Analgesics: Neurochemical, Behavioral and Clinical Perspectives. Raven Press, New York, 1984

47. Foley KM: The practical use of narcotic analgesics. Med Clin North Am 66:1091, 1982

48. Inturrisi CE, Verebely K: Disposition of methadone in man after a single oral dose. Clin Pharmacol Ther 13:923, 1972

49. Dixon R, Crews T, Mohacsi C, et al: Levorphanol: Radioimmunoassay and plasma concentration profiles in dog and man. Res Commun Chem Pathol Pharmacol 29:535, 1980

50. Ettinger DS, Vitale PJ, Trump DL: Important clinical pharmacologic considerations in the use of methadone in cancer patients. Cancer Treatm Rep 63:457, 1979

51. Symonds P: Methadone and the elderly. Br Med J 1:512, 1977

52. Houde RW, Wallenstein SL, Beaver WT: Evaluation of analgesics in patients with cancer pain. p. 59. In Lasagna L (ed): International Encyclopedia of Pharmacology and Therapeutics. Section 6. Vol. 1: Clinical Pharmacology. Pergamon Press, New York, 1966

53. Twycross R: Value of cocaine in opiate-containing elixirs. Br Med J 2:1348, 1977

54. Singh PN, Sharma P, Gupta PK, et al: Chemical evaluation of diazepam for relief of postoperative pain. Br J Anaesth 53:831, 1981

55. Twycross RG: Clinical experience with diamorphine in advanced malignant disease. Int J Clin Pharmacol Ther Toxicol 9:184, 1974

56. Halpern LW: Psychotropics, ataractics and related drugs. p. 275. In Bonica JJ, Ventafridda V (eds): Advances in Pain Research and Therapy. Vol. 2. Raven Press, New York, 1979

57. Hanks GW: Psychotropic drugs. Clin Oncol 3:135, 1984

58. Watson CP, Evans RJ, Reed K, et al: Amitriptyline versus placebo in postherpetic neuroalgia. Neurology (NY) 32:671, 1982

59. Beaver WT, Wallenstein SL, Houde RW, et al: A comparison of the analgesic effect of methotrimeprazine and morphine in patients with cancer. Clin Pharmacol Ther 7:436, 1966

60. Schell HW: The risk of adrenal corticosteroid therapy with far-advanced cancer. Am J Med Sci. 252:641, 1966

61. Schell HW: Adrenat corticosteroid therapy in far-advanced cancer. Geriatrics 27:131, 1972

62. Swerdlow M: Anticonvulsant drugs and chronic pain. Clin Neuropharmacol 7:51, 1984

63. Minton JP: The response of breast cancer patients with bone pain to L-dopa. Cancer 33:358, 1974

64. Blom S: Trigeminal neuralgia: Its treatment with a new anticonvulsant drug. (G-32883). Lancet 1:839, 1962

65. Campbell FG, Graham JG, Zikha KL: Clinical trial of carbamazepine (Tegretol) in trigeminal neuralgia. J Neurol Neurosurg Psychiatry 29:265, 1966

66. Rockliff BW, Davis EH: Controlled sequential trials of carbamazepine in trigeminal neuralgia. Arch Neurol 15:129, 1966

67. Nicol CF, A four year double blind study of Tegretol in facial pain. Headache 9:54, 1969

68. Eadie MJ: Blood levels of anticonvulsants. In Winto RR (ed): Geigy Symposium on Epilepsy. Australasian Medical Publishing, Glebe, NSW, 1971

69. Lim RKS: Neuropharmacology of pain and analgesia. p. 169. In Lim RKS, Armstrong D, Pardo EG (eds): Pharmacology of Pain. Proceedings of the Third International Pharmacology Meeting. Vol. 9. Pergamon Press, New York, 1968

70. Woodbury DM: Analgesic-antipyretics. Anti-inflammatory agents and inhibitors of uric acid synthesis. p. 316. In Goodman LS, Gilman A (eds): Pharmacologic Basis of Therapeutics. Macmillan, New York, 1970

71. Twycross RG: Principles and practice of the relief of pain in terminal cancer. Update 5:115, 1972

72. Oeuvres complètes of Hippocrate. Paris, Littre, 1840–1849

73. Way EL, Kemp JW, Young JM, et al: The pharmacological effects of heroin in relation to its rate of biotransformation. J Pharmacol Exp Ther 129:144, 1960

74. Bunney WE Jr, Pert CB, Klee W, et al: Basic and clinical studies of endorphins. Ann Intern Med 91:239, 1979

75. Synder SH: Opiate receptors and internal opiates. Sci Am 236:44, 1977

76. Editorial: The Brompton cocktail. Lancet 1:1220, 1979

77. British National Formulary: London, 1976

78. Melzack R, Mount BM, Gordon JM: The Brompton mixture versus morphine solution given orally: Effects on pain. Can Med Assoc J 120:435, 1979

79. Twycross RG: Effect of cocaine in the Brompton cocktail. p. 927. In Bonica JJ, Liebeskind JC, Albe-Fessard DG (eds): Advances in Pain Research and Therapy. Vol. 3. Raven Press, New York, 1979

80. White JC, Sweet WH: Pain and the Neurosurgeon: A Forty-Year Experience. Charles C Thomas, Springfield, IL, 1969

81. Sindou M: Etude de la jonction radiculo-medullaire

postérieure: La radicellotomie postérieure selective dans la chirurgie de la douleur. These Med, Lyon, 1972

82. Sindou M, Mifsud JJ, Boisson D, Goutelle A: Selective posterior rhizotomy in the dorsal root entry zone for treatment of hyperspasticity and pain in the hemiplegic upper limb. Neurosurgery 18:587, 1986

83. Nashold B, Ostdahl PH: Dorsal rool entry zone lesions for pain relief. J Neurosurg 51:59, 1979

84. Friedman AH, Nashold BS: DREZ lesions for relief of pain related to spinal cord injury. J Neurosurg 65:465, 1986

85. Spiller WG: The location within the spinal cord of the fibers for temperature and pain sensation. J Nerv Ment Dis 32:318, 1905

86. Edinger L: Vorlesungen uber den bau der nervosen Centralorgane des Menschen und der Tiere fur Aerzie und Studirende. 2 Vols. FCW Wogel, Leipzig, 1904

87. Wallenberg A: Acute Bulbaraffection (Embolie dei Art. cerebellar post. inf. sinistra). Arch Psychiatry Nervenkr 27:504, 1895

88. Spiller WG, Martin E: The treatment of persistent pain of organic origin in the lower part of the body by division of the anterolateral column of the spinal cord. JAMA 58:1489, 1912

89. White JC: Cordotomy: Assessment of its effectiveness and suggestions for its improvement. Clin Neurosurg 13:1, 1966

90. Mullan S, Harper PV, Hekmatpanah J, et al: Percutaneous interruption of spinal pain tracts by means of a strontium-90 needle. J Neurosurg 20:931, 1963

91. Rosomoff HL, Carroll F, Brown J, Sheptak P: Percutaneous radiofrequency cervical cordotomy: Technique. J Neurosurg 23:639, 1965

92. Rosomoff HL: Bilateral percutaneous cervical radiofrequency cordotomy. J Neurosurg 31:41, 1969

93. Lipton S: Percutaneous electrical cordotomy in relief of intractable pain. Br Med J 2:210, 1968

94. Hecaen H, Talairach J, David M, Dell MB: Coagulations limitées du thalamus dans les algies du syndrome thalamique. Résultats thérapeutiques et physiologiques. Rev Neurol 81:917, 1949

95. Mark VH, Ervin FR, Yakovlev PI: Stereotactic thala motomy. III. The verification of anatomical lesion sites in the human thalamus. Arch Neurol 8:528, 1963

96. Spiegel EA, Wycis HT, Szekley EG, Glidenberg PL: Medial and basal thalamotomy in so-called intractable pain. p. 503. In Pain, Henry Ford Hospital International Symposium. Knighton RS, Dumke PR (eds): Little, Brown, Boston, 1966

97. Moniz E: Les prémières tentatives operatoires dans les traitement de certaines psychoses. Encephale 31:1, 1936

98. Moniz E: Essai d'un traitement chirurgical de certaines psychoses. Bull Acad Med Paris 115:385, 1936

99. Fulton JF, Jacobsen CF: Fonctions des lobes frontaux; étude comparée chez l'homme, les singes et les chimpanzes. Rev Neurol 64:552, 1935

100. Foltz EL, White LE Jr: Experimental cingulomotomy and modification of morphine withdrawal. J Neurosurg 14:655, 1957

101. Foltz EL, White LE Jr: Modification of morphine withdrawal by frontal lobe cingulum lesions. p. 163. In van Bogaert L, Radermeeker J (eds): First International Congress of Neurological Sciences. Pergamon Press, London, 1959

102. Doghotti AM: Traitement des syndromes douloureus de la peripherie par l'alcoolisation sub-arachnoidienne des racines postérieures à leur émergence de la moelle epinierro. Presse Med 39:1249, 1931

103. Maher RM: Relief of pain in incurable cancer. Lancet 1:18, 1955

104. Nathan PW, Scott TG: Intrathecal phenol for intractable pain; safety and danger of the method. Lancet 1:76, 1958

105. Nathan PW, Sears TA, Smith MC: Effects of phenol solutions on the nerve roots of the cat; an electrophysiological and histological study. J Neurol Sci 2:7, 1965

106. Hitchcock E: Hypothermic subarachnoid irrigation for intractable pain. Lancet 1:1133, 1967

107. Collins JR, Juras EP, Van Houten RJ, Spruell L: Intrathecal cold saline solution: A new approach to pain (evaluation). Anesth Analg 48:816, 1969

108. Mathews GJ, Ambruso VT, Osterholm JL: Hypothermic, hyperosmolar saline irrigation of cisterna magna: A new method for the relief of pain. Surg Forum 21:445, 1970

109. Savitz MH, Malis LI: Intrathecal injection of isotonic iced saline for intractable pain. Mt Sinai J Med NY 39:134, 1972

110. Lloyd JW, Hughes JT, Davies-Jones GAB: Relief of severe intractable pain by barbotage of cerebrospinal fluid. Lancet 1:354, 1972

111. Battista AF: Pain relief by subarachnoid hypothermic saline injection. Am J Surg 128:662, 1974

112. Nicholson MF, Roberts FW: Relief of pain by intrathecal injection of hypothermic saline. Med J Aust 1:61, 1968

113. McKean MC, Hitchcock E: Electrocardiographic changes after intrathecal hypertonic saline solution. Lancet 2:1083, 1968

114. Hitchcock E: Hypothermic saline subarachnoid injection. Lancet 1:843, 1970

115. Coombs DW, Saunders RT, Gaylor MS, et al: Relief of continuous chronic pain by intraspinal narcotics infusion via an implanted reservoir. JAMA 250:2336, 1983

116. Poletti CE, Cohen AM, Todd DP: et al: Cancer pain relieved by long-term epidural morphine with permanent indwelling systems for self-administration. J Neurosurg 55:581, 1981

117. Yaksh TL: Spinal opiate analgesia: Characteristics and principles of action. Pain 11:293, 1981

118. Lobato RD, Madred JL, Fatela LV, et al: Intraventricular morphine for control of pain in terminal cancer patients. J Neurosurg 59:627, 1983

119. Wall PD, Sweet WH: Temporary aboliton of pain in man. Science 155:108, 1967

120. Sweet WH, Wepsic JG: Stimulation of the posterior columns of the spinal cord for pain control; indications, techniques, and results. Clin Neurosurg 21:278, 1973

121. Long DM: Data presented at the seminar on electrical stimulation of the human nervous system for the control of pain, Minneapolis, December 1973

122. Long DM: Electrical stimulation for relief of pain from chronic nerve injury. J Neurosurg 39:718, 1973

123. Burton C: Data presented at the seminar on electrical stimulation of the human nervous system for the control of pain, Minneapolis, December 1973

124. Shealy CN: Transcutaneous electrical stimulation for control of pain. Clin Neurosurg 21:269, 1973

125. Shealy CN: Pain suppression through posterior column stimulation. p. 251. In Fields WS (ed): Neural Organization and Its Relevance to Prosthetic. Intercontinental Medical Book, New York, 1973

126. Friedman H, Nashold BS Jr, Somjen G: Physiological effects of dorsal column stimulation. Adv Neurol 4:769, 1979

127. Hymes AC, Raab DE, Yonehiro EG, et al: Acute pain control by electrostimulation: A preliminary report. Adv Neurol 4:761, 1974

128. Long DM, Carolan MT: Cutaneous afferent stimulation in the treatment of chronic pain. Adv Neurol 4:775, 1974

SELECTED READINGS

Abbe R: A contribution to the surgery of the spine. Med Rec NY 35:152, 1889

Ballantine HT, Cassidy WL, Flanagan NB, Marino R: Stereotaxic anterior cingulotomy for neuropsychiatric illness and intractable pain. J Neurosurg 26:448, 1967

Bennett WH: A case in which acute spasmodic pain in the left lower extremity was completely relieved by subdural division of the posterior roots of certain spinal nerves. Med Chir Trans 72:329, 1889

Clara M: Die anatomie der sensibilitat unter besonderer berucksichigtung der vergetativen leitungsbahnen. Acta Neuroveg (Wien) 7:4, 1953

Collins WF, Nulsen FE, Randt CT: Relation of peripheral nerve fiber size and sensation in man. Arch Neurol 3:381, 1960

Crosby EC, Humphrey I, Lauer E: Correlative Anatomy of the Nervous System. Macmillan, New York, 1962

Delgado JMR: Cerebral structures involved in the transmission and elaboration of noxious stimulation. J Neurophysiol 18:261, 1955

Dilly PN, Wall PD, Webster KE: Cells of origin of the spinothalamic tract in cat and rat. Exp Neurol 21:550, 1968

Feindel WH, Weddell G, Sinclair DC: Pain sensibility in deep somatic structure. J Neurol Neurosurg Psychiatry 11:113, 1948

Foerster O: Die Leitungsbahnen des Schmerzgefuhls und die chirurgische Behandlung der Schmerzzustande, 360. Urban and Schwarzenberg, Berlin, 1927

Foerster O: The dermatomes in man. Brain 56:1, 1933

Foerster O: Symptomatologie der Erkrankungen des Ruckenmarks und seiner Wurzeen. p. 1. In Bumke O, Foerster O (eds): Handbuch der Neurologie. Vol. 5. Springer, Berlin, 1936

Gasser HS, Erlanger J: The role played by size of the constituent fibers of a nerve trunk in determining the form of its action potential wave. Am J Physiol 80:522, 1927

Gillman J: Pain relief and other effects following barbotage. Lancet 1:746, 1972

Hay RC, Yonezawa T, Derrick WS: Control of intractable pain in advanced cancer by subarachnoid alcohol block. JAMA 169:1315, 1959

Head H: The afferent nervous system from a new aspect. Brain 28:99, 1905

Hosobuchi Y, Adams J: Data presented at the seminar on electrical stimulation of the human nervous system for the control of pain. Minneapolis, December 1973

Iggo A, Walsh EG: Selective block of small fibers in the spinal roots by phenol. Brain 83:701, 1960

Lele PP, Weddell G: Sensory nerves in the cornea and cutaneous sensibility. Exp Neurol 1:334, 1959

Lipton S: Other measures (percutaneous cordotomy, dorsal column electrostimulation of pain relief). p. 194. In Sweralow M (ed): Relief of Intractable Pain. Elsevier, Amsterdam, 1974

Magoun HW, Atlas D, Ingersoll EH, et al: Associated facial, vocal, and respiratory components of emotional expression. J Neurol Psychopathol 17:241, 1937

Maher RM: Neuron selection in relief of pain. Further experiences with intrathecal injections. Lancet 1:16, 1957

Matsushita M: The axonal pathways of spinal neurons in the cat. J Comp Neurol 138:391, 1970

Mehler WR, Ferferman ME, Nauta WS: Ascending axon degeneration following anterolateral cordotomy. An experimental study in the monkey. Brain 83:718, 1960

Melzack R, Stotler WA, Livingston WK: Effects of discrete brain stem lesions in cats on perception of noxious stimulation. J Neurophysiol 21:353, 1958

Mullan S, Hekmatpanah J, Dobben G, Beckman F: Percutaneous intramedullary cordotomy utilizing the unipolar anodal electrolytic lesion. J Neurosurg 22:548, 1965

Nashold B: Data presented at the seminar on electrical stimulation of the human nervous system for the control of pain, Minneapolis, December 1973

Pearson AA: Role of gelatinous substance of spinal cord in conduction of pain. Arch Neurol Psychiatry 68:515, 1952

Pick J: The Autonomic Nervous System. JB Lippincott, Philadelphia, 1970

Poirier LJ, Bertrand C: Experimental and anatomical investigation of the lateral spino-thalamic and spino-tectal tracts. J Comp Neurol 102:745, 1955

Ray BS: The management of intractable pain by posterior rhizotomy. Res Publ Assoc Res Nerv Ment Dis 23:391, 1943

Scarff JE: Unilateral prefrontal lobotomy for the relief of intractable pain and termination of narcotic addiction. Surg Gynecol Obstet 89:385, 1949

Shealy CN, Taslitz N, Mortimer JT, Becker DP: Electrical inhibition of pain; experimental evaluation. Anesth Analg 46:299, 1967

Shealy CN, Mortimer JT, Reswick JB: Electrical inhibition of pain by stimulation of the dorsal columns: Preliminary clinical report. Anesth Analg 46:480, 1967

Sherrington CS: Cutaneous sensations. p. 720. In Schafer EA (ed): Textbook of Physiology. Vol. 2. Pentland, Edinburgh, 1900

Spiegel EA, Kletzkin M, Szekley EG: Pain reactions upon stimulation of the tectum mesencephali. J Neuropathol Exp Neurol 13:212, 1954

Spiller WG: The occasional clinical resemblance between caries of the vertebrae and lumbothoracic syringomyelia, and the location within the spinal cord of the fibers for the sensations of pain and temperature. Univ Press Med Bull 18:147, 1905

Stewart WA, Lourie H: An experimental evaluation of the effects of subarachnoid injection of phenol-pantopaque in cats. A histological study. J Neurosurg 20:64, 1963

Swanson AG, Buchan GC, Alvord EC: Anatomic changes in congenital insensitivy to pain. Arch Neurol 12:12, 1965

Sweet WH: Lessons on pain control from electrical stimulation. Trans Stud Coll Physicians 35:171, 1968

Sweet WH, Wepsic JG: Treatment of chronic pain by stimulation of fibers of primary afferent neurons. Trans Am Neurol Assoc 93:103, 1968

Sweet WH, Wepsic JG: Relation of fiber size in trigeminal posterior root to conduction of impulses for pain and touch; production of analgesia without anesthesia in the effective treatment of trigeminal neuralgia. Trans Am Neurol Assoc 95:134, 1970

Sweet WH, Wepsic JG: Electrical stimulation for suppression of pain in man. p. 219. In Fields WS (eds): Neural Organization and Its Relevance to Prosthetics. Intercontinental Medical Book Corp, New York, 1973

Sweet WH, Wepsic JG: Stimulation of pain suppressor mechanisms; a critique of some current methods. Adv Neurol 4:737, 1974

Trotter W, Davis HM: The peculiarities of sensibility found in cutaneous areas supplied by regenerating nerves. J Physiol Neurol Leipzig Erganz 20:102, 1913

Tucker WI: Results of lobotomy. J Neuropsychiatry 2:153, 1961

Watts JW, Freeman W: Frontal lobotomy in the treatment of unbearable pain. Res Publ Assoc Res Nerv Ment Dis 27:715, 1948

Weddell G, Miller S: Cutaneous sensibility. Annu Rev Physiol 24:199, 1962

Weddell G, Palmer E, Pallie W: Nerve endings in mammalian skin. Biol Rev 30:159, 1955

Woollard HH: Observations on the terminations of cutaneous nerves. Brain 58:352, 1935

Woollard HH, Weddell G, Hartman JA: Observations on the neurohistological basis of cutaneous pain. J Anat 74:413, 1940

34

Psychosocial Issues in the Care of Gynecologic Cancer Patients

Cheryl F. McCartney
Julie Johnson Knox

A woman with a gynecologic malignancy faces enormous emotional trials. In a process that is often long and arduous, she experiences not only a threat to her body, but a series of challenges to personal adaptability, each challenge presenting a new situation to be mastered. From first suspicion of the diagnosis, to the last moment of life — whether she dies of cancer or not — she must deal with the disease and its consequences.

What role does the oncologist play in the process of psychosocial adjustment? In each encounter between patient and disease, the outcome depends on her repertoire of resources, both physiologic and psychological, as well as on the human context in which the encounter takes place. Relationships in the patient's life will tend to span a range from depleting and destructive to helpful and sustaining, and her own system of coping will be mobilized within this broader, ever shifting environment. The gynecologic-oncologist is a key support figure, as a physician trained and committed to help people cope with illness, and also as a leader, the head of the treatment team.

Both functions will be greatly affected by the doctor's aspiration as a healer. To the extent that the oncologist aims to mitigate the harm cancer does to a woman's whole life, the doctor-patient relationship will reinforce her efforts to adapt. As leader of the multidisciplinary team, the oncologist determines who will be told about the patient's condition, which consultants will be called, whether their recommendations will be followed, and to what degree the patient, her family, and the staff will participate in decisions about care. As in all human social systems, many of these decisions are conveyed through subconscious attitudes rather than made through conscious planning. A sensitive awareness of the overall impact of the disease process is thus critical to the oncologist's functioning.

These physicianly attitudes and the capacity for effective leadership are acquired skills, improved by learning and practicing new ways of thinking. The purpose of this chapter is to provide oncologists with the most useful concepts about the impact of cancer —specifically genital cancer—on the totality of a woman's life. We begin with a discussion of current thinking about quality of life in cancer patients. Subsequent sections examine the experience of cancer over time, individual factors involved in psychosocial adjustment, sexual problems, psychiatric disorders, and available resources.

QUALITY OF LIFE

Changing Perspectives

In a familiar scenario from just a few decades ago, the doctor would say, "It's cancer," and the patient would ask, "How long, Doc? How long have I got?" If cancer is seen only as the untimely end of a life-span, then "how long?" is the natural focus of attention. People seek mastery over a threat of impending death through a number of avenues, including efforts to lengthen the remaining expanse of time.

Not surprisingly, the search for definitive cures (and thus longer life) has dominated research activity in gynecologic oncology. The subspecialty was founded and fostered by surgically oriented physicians during a period of increasing societal concern to "find a cure for cancer." From the 1930s through the 1970s, death rates from infectious disease were declining, and medicine was slowly gaining power in the face of other well-known killers such as cardiac disease. In this setting, cancer was seen as the new adversary of modern technology.

The surgical pioneers of oncology appreciated that tumors of the uterine corpus, cervix, and vulva exhibit slow growth and a predictable pattern of spread. These accessible cancers, sometimes apparent before metastasis, presented a challenge to the rapidly advancing field of gynecologic surgery. Improved techniques in the operating room included progress in anesthesiology and other supportive disciplines, so that greater volumes of malignant tissue could be removed without undue physical risk.

At the same time, progress in radiotherapy and chemotherapy was allowing oncologists to explore what Howard Ulfelder, professor emeritus of gynecology at the Harvard Medical School, has called "the ultimate perimeters of radicality." In his keynote address at the 1980 American Cancer Society's National Conference on Gynecologic Cancer, Ulfelder[1] said:

> Although it may not be entirely accurate to state that we were determined to cure cancer at almost any cost, the surgical effort in particular occasionally included very extensive resections and rearrangements of function.

John Morris,[2] speaking at the same conference, also reflected on changing goals for gynecologic oncology. While optimistic about modern curative treatments, he urged physicians to accept the limitations of their technology:

> Do not take those who can be cured and injure or even kill them by overtreatment. Do not take those destined to die and make their death more undignified, prolonged, or painful. We all have fatal diseases.

Thus arose an ironic situation. Substanial progress in the rate of cure for female genital cancer[3] had set the stage for a question of whether a longer lifespan is worth the price.

This era in gynecologic oncology coincided with societal change in the direction of increased involvement of patients in making decisions about their care. Physicians and patients both began to assess therapy regimens not only by 5-year survival figures but also by cost, length of hospital stay, degree of disability, and interference with usual activities. Successful cancer cures contributed to further awareness of these issues, as a growing population of survivors challenged oncologists to redirect their therapeutic energy toward improving patients' overall lives. For example, the surgical creation of a neovagina (for women who had undergone pelvic exenteration) reflected an intuitive desire to restore sexual function. Increasingly, clinicians urged that considerations of quality of life—not just quantity—be included in efficacy studies.

Research Findings

During the past decade, several groups of researchers have looked at cancer treatment in light of these broader issues. A report on stage III ovarian carcinoma patients, for example, found that debulking surgery, while not curative, improved quality of life. Patients reported better ability to eat a regular diet, avoid confinement to bed, keep up normal activity, work at a job, and enjoy life. Quality-of-life improvement after debulking coincided with more traditional criteria, such as a reduced number of procedures per patient-survival month.[4] Another study described postoperative care after radical vulvectomy and groin node dissection for vulvar carcinoma, looking at the use of a myocutaneous graft from the tensor fascia lata for resurfacing the surgical deficit. The advantage of this procedure included not only improved cosmetic appearance but also fewer wound complications and shorter hospital stay.[5]

Other reports have examined the effect on quality of life of various palliative techniques for end-stage gynecologic cancer. One study, for example, questioned the use of percutaneous nephrostomy in cases of recurrent incurable disease: a group of nephrostomy patients spent 27 percent of their remaining life in the hospital and suffered more pain and weight loss than did controls.[6]

As this line of research develops, we can already see instances where the urge to preserve quality of life has spurred the development of better treatment options, in a positive feedback fashion. The newer approach to breast cancer, with a trend toward less radical, equally effective, treatment is a prominent example. When mastectomy is compared with lumpectomy plus radiation (for stage I and II cancer), there is no difference in efficacy, as measured by survival, but there is a significant difference in quality of life. Steinberg et al.[7] found that lumpectomy patients showed better overall adaptation to their surgery and less functional change — as assessed by better sense of attractiveness and femininity, less self-consciousness about their appearance, more emotional support from friends and more openness about the surgery and about sexuality.

Quality of life research does not always support the obvious or intuitive choice. Careful studies may disprove commonly held notions about which treatment would be preferable in the long run. Sugarbaker et al.[8] suspected that limb-sparing surgery with radiation and chemotherapy, for patients with soft tissue sarcoma of the leg, would be preferred to amputation with chemotherapy. Surprisingly, they showed very little difference between the groups on measures of physical and emotional function and some advantage to the amputation group on measures of sexual function.

Individuality of patient response adds yet another layer of complexity, again with often counterintuitive results. A physician cannot presume to know, in advance, how any given effect of illness will enter into a patient's assessment of life quality. For a description of quality of life to be meaningful, it must include both the objective event and the subjective reaction. In a follow-up study of women treated for breast cancer with mastectomy and chemotherapy, for example, some of the women who reported a reduction in sexual activity (objective loss) were in fact pleased with that change (subjective gain).[9] Good information about patients' life goals and needs can help tailor the treatment approach to the individual.

Personal values of physicians also play a role in what they seek for their patients. In the absence of good data to the contrary, well-intentioned doctors may impose their personal priorities on patients' lives. The following case history is an example:

> A 28 year-old divorced woman with carcinoma in situ of the cervix was the mother of one child. She was engaged to be married to a divorced man, who also had one child. Without asking, the doctor assumed that the patient would want another pregnancy. He advised her to go ahead and have a child with her new husband and then obtain the prescribed hysterectomy.

An important goal of quality-of-life research is to enable doctors to factor out these personal considerations through increased awareness of the complex issues involved. We will briefly review current thinking in this area, and then discuss its practical import for clinical decisions.

What Is Quality of Life?

All modern societies attach a positive value — either tacitly, or explicitly, as in "life, liberty, and the pursuit of happiness" — to the aim of maximizing individual quality of life. Various authorities have described quality of life as a sense of well-being, contentment, fulfillment, flourishing, or as a subjective index of satisfaction with present life circumstances.[10-12] As it is used in assessing the effect of disease, the concept implies a thorough overview of all potential areas of fulfillment. What we usually call psychological well-being, for example, is only one of several domains within which people seek to optimize their lives.

Some authorities define quality of life with respect to the perceived gap, at a single time, between the hopes and expectations of a person and what they are actually experiencing. Thus, efforts to improve quality of life can be directed either toward ameliorating problems (e.g., pain, loss of sexual function), or toward adjusting expectations to conform more closely to actuality (e.g., acceptance of loss, giving up hope for cure).[13]

How Do We Measure Quality of Life?

The earliest measures of quality of life in cancer patients focused almost entirely on physical function, using such measures as the Karnofsky Performance Status Scale, which assigns a grade to a patient's level of physical activity (e.g., bedridden, walks with assistance).[14] As social science researchers have attempted to characterize quality of life in a broader (biopsychosocial) context, they have developed a wide variety of both objective and subjective rating scales. There is no single "gold standard" for assessment of quality of life.

Some measures assess quality of life as a global construct (how the patient is doing overall), but many divide quality of life into specific domains, four of which are commonly addressed: psychological, physical, social, and economic.

Psychological status in cancer includes desired states of mind (e.g., feeling happy, relaxed, hopeful, and loved) as well as states of distress (depression or anxiety). Mental health, in other words, is an equation with both positive and negative terms. Change in psychological status has a strong interaction with changes in the other three domains. For example, Bukberg et al.[15] showed an association between physical performance status and clinical depression in hospitalized cancer patients. Similarly, depressed patients have been shown to interpret pain as more disruptive to activity, than nondepressed patients.[16]

Physical status encompasses both positive functions and negative symptoms. Functional areas include activity level (at work and in general), level of self-care, cognition (clear thinking, attention, memory), sexuality, and fertility. Symptoms of particular interest in cancer are pain, nausea, and vomiting.

Social interactions include quality of relationships with, and support from, people important to the patient (partner, family members, friends, co-workers).

Economic status must take into account not only lost income and expense of treatment but also the ancillary costs incurred by patients and family members, such as travel, meals in restaurants, babysitters, and other services. Even when patients have adequate insurance, the extended social context of their care includes many of these nonreimbursable expenses, especially high during terminal illness.[17]

An individual may be doing well in one domain and not so well in another. The most important step, in translating quality of life to the clinical setting, is in systematic attention to all facets of a patient's function:

A 70-year-old woman had a recurrence of cervical cancer. She puzzled her physician by refusing a second course of treatment, even though the first course had not been especially arduous, and her overall quality of life was good. Only after a psychiatric consult was called was it discovered that the woman's concern was in the area of economics: She did not know that she qualified for Medicaid, and when the first treatment exhausted her private insurance, she assumed that she couldn't afford a second round.

In this case, an initial review of systems, addressing separate domains of quality of life, would have smoothed the course for both patient and doctor.

The subjective/objective distinction must also be incorporated in assessment of quality of life. Patients' perception of how well they are doing, in any of the four domains, will not necessarily correspond to the external circumstances. One method of obtaining a subjective rating is to ask the patient to indicate where she stands along a continuum from "extremely satisfied" to "extremely dissatisfied." Whatever outside parameters are taken into account (e.g., the elderly patient's actual ability to obtain funds for her care), the physician must provide a forum for the patient to express her own sense of how she is doing.

Difficult Decisions

Although it is tempting to insist on quantitative measures, the final assessment emerges in discussion between patient and physician. Even without definitive measurement, clinical judgment is improved by clearer, more thorough, consideration of quality-of-life concepts.

When the chance for cure is high, and treatment is easily tolerated, decisions about therapy are straightforward. But what of the many cases in which doctor and patient must choose among a variety of evils?

Many physicians guide their thinking, and that of their patients, with the model of a risk-benefit analysis, with the data for the physical-health part of the equation drawn from a reasonably objective pool of shared information. The progressive deterioration of health, the pain and loss of function, and the ever-present threat of death are well-known consequences of an untreated malignancy. Also well documented are the unpleasant side effects and changes in body functions from some presently available treatments. Those risk-benefit factors not in the category of physical health, however, are not as well understood. In this area, physicians usually rely on a less codified, more subjective part of their clinical knowledge — their understanding of individual patients, and their personal attitudes toward different options.

Ultimately, the doctor must sit together with the patient, outline the alternatives in as balanced a manner as possible, and then ask "which do you want?" The patient's freedom of choice in this situation — her ability to make a decision in accordance with her own values — will depend critically on the accuracy of the doctor's portrayal of alternatives.

Even in the best of worlds, patients will differ widely in their handling of the risk–benefit equation. As in the game of poker, there is a continuum from people who will bet all their resources on a long shot, to those for whom no odds are favorable enough to take the risk. Some will opt for severe and possibly permanent effects of treatment, for example, if the likelihood of cure is great. Some will choose any treatment over no treatment, even if only palliation is possible. On the other hand, a regimen with lesser survival advantage may be selected for its more tolerable spectrum of predicted deficits and side effects: refusal of exenteration for recurrent cervical carcinoma or of second-line chemotherapy for ovarian cancer are examples of such choices.[18] In each case, patient and doctor both must attach a subjective weight to the importance of various life values, and a semi-quantitative weight to the effects of various treatments on each domain of life quality.

A 52-year-old woman decided to "gamble" for aggressive treatment (in this case, pelvic exenteration). The treatment was successful, in the sense of ensuring continued survival. Her marriage, though, had been held together by sex, and it fell apart in the aftermath of treatment. She turned to pain medications and alcohol for comfort and eventually suffered death from an overdose.

The challenge of quality-of-life research, and for each individual oncologist, is to make such decisions as fully informed as possible.[19]

THE TIME COURSE OF CANCER

As we move from an overview of quality of life issues, to a picture of the individual woman with genital malignancy, we must first examine the experience of cancer over time. Cancer is not a single stress, nor is it a homogeneous process: A series of adaptive tasks unfolds from diagnosis to treatment alternatives, through fluctuations of stress along the way as patient and family go through various stages of response, through repeated treatments and possible recurrence, and finally to an acceptance either of death, or of the price of survival. Dramatic changes take place in several spheres of function, so that each new phase brings overlapping and even conflicting emotional demands. Superimposed on all these events are the reactions of the woman's family and close friends — who may, at any one time, be "out of synch" with her phase of adjustment, and thus pose additional stresses.

The clinical course of cancer has been conceptualized as a series of nodal points.[20] Every patient goes through the stages of pre-diagnosis and diagnosis, but after these initial steps, the clinical course and thus, the spectrum of psychological challenge, is quite variable.

Before Diagnosis

Anyone who has ever worried about carcinogens in their diet or environment or fussed over a suspicious pain in the abdomen knows that the fear of cancer, and psychological adjustment to the threat of cancer, is not limited to those with a positive pathology report. The woman who eventually develops a genital malignancy will have formulated, long before diagnosis, a highly personalized set of notions about cancer.

Many of these beliefs will be colored by her individual life history, whether she has known people who died of cancer, for example. Other ideas will derive from cultural commonalities we are all exposed to: Cancer is not only a disease, but an allegory of a disease. Beliefs and meanings surrounding cancer, and the folklore that arises even in the most technologic of societies, cluster around the unknown origins and the potential lethality of the disease.

Susan Sontag, in *Illness as Metaphor,* has suggested that cancer is the modern symbol for the mystery of death — like bubonic plague or tuberculosis in times past.[21] Obscurity of onset of cancer, combined with the awareness of links between people's actions (diet, smoking, promiscuity) and the chance of disease, contributes an overlay of meaning about individual culpability. The Judeo-Christian tradition, in particular, emphasizes deterministic thinking as a way of accounting for the unknown: when something bad happens, the woman must have brought it upon herself. For the individual patient who fears that she has cancer, this thinking leads to both internal (sense of personal sin) and external (being shunned by others) stigmatization.

Many people believe there is something vaguely "dirty" about cancer, even apart from the implications of wrong doing. Cancer is one's own body destroying itself — it arises apparently from nowhere, starting very small and then growing indiscriminantly. Cancer conveys, for many, an image of messiness, of lack of control. Female genital cancer, in particular, implies a lack of control in the area of sexuality and procreation. Popular writer Stephen King, whose mother died of cancer, describes this horror in evocative terms in his novel *The Stand:* "The womb of his young wife had borne a single dark and malignant child."

The significance of these ideas, for the woman with a genital malignancy, is in the individual pattern of her adjustment to cancer, and in the lag time, the time from initial onset of symptoms to the seeking of medical care.[20] Psychological factors involved in lag time include dread of mutilation and death, fatalistic outlook, use of denial as a prominent defense, and excessive modesty.[22,23]

Diagnosis

Once the patient has presented with symptoms and data collection is under way, the doctor begins to play a role in her adjustment. The first step should be an acknowledgment of anxiety during the waiting period, and plans for how to convey the diagnosis. It is best not to give preliminary results, because they may need to be altered later, causing confusion. The physician should ask the patient to bring her husband, close friend, or trusted relative to the consultation when the findings and their implications will be discussed. With a family member present, the patient

feels less of a burden to memorize stressful information and has the assurance of immediate support.

Medical practice has changed from the days when, as in a 1961 study by Oken,[24] most physicians believed it was harmful to tell patients the truth about cancer. This study was repeated in 1979, and the trend had changed toward open communication.

The danger in withholding information is that patients feel isolated while the secret is being kept, depriving them of essential social support from the doctor and others[25]:

> A 57-year-old housewife with metastatic breast cancer had not been told directly of her condition. She noted feeling nervous because "I have lost 60 pounds in a year, my priest comes to see me twice a week, which he never did before, and my mother-in-law is nicer to me, even though I am meaner to her."

Patients in this situation figure out the gravity of their condition and then privately worry about why it is "unspeakable."

One recommended way to tell the truth includes three steps: (1) acknowledge the malignancy, (2) describe plans for treatment, and (3) assure the patient of the availability of medical attention throughout the course of the illness.

Common reactions to hearing the diagnosis include shock and denial, with patients making such statements as "I was too numb to hear any more," or "I just couldn't believe it." The human mind is slow to respond: a doctor who leaps in too quickly to express a hope for cure, may inadvertently convey an unwillingness to hear and share the patient's emotions. Oncologists should expect that information about prognosis and treatment will need to be repeated.

After the initial period of shock, other reactions include anxiety, sadness, guilt, and anger (in order of prevalence). These are typical of responses to severe stress of any kind, and are felt to comprise a sequence of emotions that signify successful coping. However, about one third of newly diagnosed gynecologic cancer patients exhibit clinical depression.[26]

Special meaning of gynecologic cancer may add to the woman's distress. Investigations of the psychological meaning of the uterus and its functions indicate that many women perceive their womb as a source of attractiveness and inner strength and also as a cyclic organizer of their lives. Threatened loss of this organ may convey fragility and vulnerability, and for some premenopausal women, a concern about how their bodies will be cleansed of the monthly buildup of "bad blood."[27,28] Ovaries, as well, may be seen as a source of femininity, the loss of which would suggest they are no longer "proper women."[29]

Avery Weisman, in his work on "psychosocial phasing" in cancer, calls the period following diagnosis the time of "existential plight," which may last as long as 4 months, but is usually briefer. Following this initial phase of free-floating anxiety and denial alternating with sadness, the patient begins to accommodate to the fact of cancer and shifts to a greater degree of engagement with the physician and with the process of cancer treatment.[30] Once the transition to this second phase has been made, the patient is more interested in obtaining information about her care, which then becomes her particular struggle, rather than a global assault. Multiple avenues of treatment open up, and the patient's adaptive challenges include not only her disease and the threat of death, but the specific impact from cancer therapy.

Surgery

Many patients experience a sense of relief when surgery is prescribed, because they can fantasize that all of the tumor will be removed. Reactions of anxiety beforehand, and discomfort afterward, are similar to those experienced with any major operation. In genital cancer, concern over mutilation is common. The gynecologist, whose work entails a sensitive awareness of a woman's personal valuation of her pelvic organs, may also experience stress from being in the role of mutilator.

Moderate levels of preoperative anxiety have been found to correlate with better psychological outcome than have very low or very high levels. A patient with high anxiety is presumably impervious to reassurance, whereas a patient whose preoperative anxiety is low is unrealistic about the stresses involved.[31]

Throughout the process of active treatment, of which surgery is often the first step, the patient's adaptive task includes mourning the loss of previous wholeness and autonomy and allowing enough dependency to rely on a physician's help. The emotional work of the postdiagnosis period will continue to occupy her energy. The cancer will become more "real" as she faces the changes in body parts and body func-tions involved in aggressive therapy. At the same time, she must also work through the impact of cancer on her nonphysical function. If the hospitalization for surgery represents the first extended absence from home or work, for example, the loss of familiar sources of satisfaction may be just as immediate, and devastating, as the operation itself.

Radiotherapy

The psychological consequence of external beam radiation includes fear of radiation and of physical side effects of treatment. Fatigue and nausea are common. Potential stresses induced by the treatment setting include loud intimidating machines and being left alone in a place that is "dangerous" for others.

Patients receiving intracavitary radiation frequently experience a characteristic pattern of agitation and anxiety, escalating over the 2 days prior to treatment, and then persisting and even increasing in the 2 or 3 days following, when it is often accompanied by fatigue and depressed mood.[32,33] The second and any subsequent courses of treatment are believed to be equally difficult. This anxiety may signal a pretreatment "work of worry" period, which includes attending to information geared to reducing the overall stress of treatment, accepting reassurance from others, and warding off feelings of helplessness.[34]

Even productive anxiety is an uncomfortable experience, and selective use of psychotherapy can help channel the patient's emotions into the ongoing work of accommodating to cancer treatment. Forester and others[35] describe a model of ten weekly sessions focusing on support, education, catharsis, and labeling of defenses. Patients receiving this therapy had a significant reduction in both emotional and physical symptoms, compared to controls.

Chemotherapy

Chemotherapy is a difficult project for both doctor and patient. It requires a high level of commitment, because it involves an extended and stressful regimen with multiple courses over months of time, with regular anticipated periods of illness following each treatment. The disruption of work, home, and school routines is considerable and takes a toll on perceived quality of life. Even between courses of treatment, overall social and work activity is reduced.[9]

Nausea and vomiting are a major psychological stressor in chemotherapy. Initially, these symptoms are induced only in the setting of direct stimulation by an emetogenic drug of chemoreceptor trigger zones in the brain. Many patients also develop an anticipatory nausea triggered by reminders of the treatment experience, such as foods the patient happened to eat beforehand or any smells, sights, and sounds associated with the treatment room. The development and maintenance of these symptoms appears to follow the patterns associated with classic conditioning to aversive stimuli. As many as 50 percent of patients report continued problems with nausea for 2 years after completion of treatment. Oncologists should advise their patients to avoid novel or strong-tasting foods on treatment days and should seek to minimize any distinctive smells (perfumes, cleaning fluids, deodorizers) presented in the treatment situation.[36] Hypnosis and relaxation techniques may also be helpful in the management of anticipatory nausea.[37,38]

Direct neurotoxic effects of chemotherapy agents should be considered in any patient who presents with mental status changes, however psychiatric they may at first appear.

Loss of hair is distressing for all women and especially for those patients for whom appearance is a significant component of their self-esteem. Adolescents, who depend critically on acceptance by their peer group, are especially vulnerable, but the oncologist should not assume that this loss is taken lightly by a woman of any age. Psychoanalytic investigators have described intense personal meanings associated with the cutting or the loss of women's hair.[39] Even with reassurance that hair loss is temporary, patients will experience a disturbance in body image that contributes to their sense of being diminished or altered by cancer.

Generalized weakness and fatigue, which occur with some chemotherapy regimens, further undermine the patient's function in such areas as work, school, family, and social life.

In discussing plans for chemotherapy with a patient, the oncologist should describe not only the treatment and its desired effects but also the many possible side effects that must be tolerated. Patients who are reluctant should be encouraged to try the treatment, since side effects vary widely between individuals. The notion that one may suggest side effects, by predicting them, is fallacious: patients do better if

they know in advance the worst-case version of what may happen, so they may develop an adaptive level of anxiety and avoid the helpless demoralizing situation of unexpected trauma.

As patients grow accustomed to the pattern of nausea and other symptoms, they should be encouraged to suggest modifications in the scheduling of treatment, so that symptomatic periods will coincide with weekends or planned absences from work or school. The more that patients can take an active role in making these decisions, the more they will feel empowered and engaged in the struggle against illness.

Experience of the Patient's Family

As we follow the woman with gynecologic cancer through various phases along the time course of the illness, we must keep in mind the extended family/ social context in which she carries out her work of adjustment. The family of a cancer patient tends to go through an initial crisis period immediately after the diagnosis, during which traditional role assignments may be either reinforced or changed dramatically. If the patient is a middle-aged woman who has always been the mainstay and support of her husband and children, for example, her adjustment to cancer will depend critically on the pattern of relationships that emerges on the other side of this initial crisis. When placed in the situation of being needy toward others, she may be reluctant to surrender her role of helper. Her adaptive resources may suffer unless she can either assume a new role or develop a new version of the old one.

Even after the initial crisis resolves and the family returns to previous rhythms, relationships continue to shift and change. The time course of the cancer treatment itself interacts with the developmental and adaptive timelines of various individuals in the family.

A psychiatric consultant was called to see the sister of a patient who had undergone pelvic exenteration. The sister's 4-year-old son had expressed great interest in his aunt's colostomy bag, and she was concerned about his vivid nightmares and fantasies about the patient's physical deficits. The boy had asked, "Will that happen to me, too?" The consulting psychiatrist was able to explain the relationship of these intense body concerns to the normal developmental tasks of a 4-year-old child.

Even in the healthiest of families, these shifting patterns of response cause waxing and waning of psychologic energies and repeated stresses in relationships. As the cancer patient goes through various phases of treatment, repeated and often unpredictable crises induce fatigue. Over time, family members may begin to hope, on a conscious or unconscious level, that the patient will die. They are faced, then, with either feeling guilty for the wish or with adopting any number of defensive maneuvers to avoid feeling guilty. Withdrawal of support, numbing of emotion, and immersion in outside activites are common responses at such times.

An awareness of the stresses on the patient's family and of the ups and downs in their level of adaptation over the course of illness can help the oncologist understand what might appear to be unexpected changes in the patient's degree of cooperation with treatment. Cancer caregivers must do their most active work and make many of the most critical treatment decisions, at times when the patient's social system is disrupted. To the extent that they are willing and able to do so, the family should be included at all stages of care. A patient whose social system is coping well with the multiple stresses of cancer has a good chance to be coping well herself.[40]

Recurrence

If we continue to track the patient and family through nodal points along the time course of gynecologic cancer, an important branch point is recurrence versus extended survival. The crisis of recurrence is considered by many authorities to be the most difficult phase of adjustment — more disappointing than the phase of decline toward death, when recovery is not expected, and more disillusioning than diagnosis. In Weisman's concept of psychosocial phasing, the period of recurrence and relapse is thought to be a second round on the existential plight — without the hope for cure that lent optimism during the initial postdiagnosis phase. Even in the face of a probable remission, a woman who is discouraged by failure may find it hard to rise, once again, to the challenges of further treatment and further tough decisions. In the best of circumstances, patients find reserves of quiet resignation and make a transition to limited horizons, seeking respite and reprieve rather than ultimate cure. Patients who were originally resistant to the need for follow-up (having assumed

they were cured), may become more cooperative at this time.[30]

When palliative therapy is contemplated, the patient's quality of life should be reassessed in all domains of function. Even patients who have hope for extended remission may believe they have reached the point of diminishing returns from further treatment. This is an important treatment decision, which merits careful and balanced consideration of the impact of both the disease and anticipated treatment. Oncologists should state explicitly, at the outset of the decision-making process, that their commitment to caring for the patient will be unaffected by the particular choice that is made. Patients may fear that if they do not choose aggressive treatment, their doctor will abandon them.

Death and Dying

The woman with terminal cancer experiences her imminent death within a context of the unfolding course of treatments and treatment failures: she may have several episodes of critical illness punctuated by periods of remission before she begins her tacit adaptation to impending death. The decision about when someone is a dying patient is not an easy one; it is unwise to discuss death too early, for if they do not die as predicted, adjustment to eventual death or unexpected recovery will be complicated by the false alarm.[41]

When curative treatment fails, patient and doctor both must make the transition to mourning her life and planning for her death. Common concerns expressed by dying patients include fear of pain, of dependency, of loss of control, of isolation, and of becoming repugnant to other people. In the well-known framework proposed by Kubler-Ross,[42] the process of dying involves a series of psychosocial phases:

1. *Denial:* usually adaptive and not to be challenged unless interfering with treatment
2. *Anger:* may be expressed as irritation toward caregivers or family members and as refusal to cooperate in care
3. *Bargaining:* a search for temporary reprieve
4. *Sadness:* not a clinical depression, but rather a grief over loss of self
5. *Acceptance*

These phases should not be viewed as taking place, like clockwork, in a definite order: denial and acceptance, in particular, will tend to alternate from day to day, or week to week, throughout the course of dying.[43] Kubler-Ross's contribution was in recognizing that dying patients need communication and support, and in giving caregivers a way of conceptualizing the often confusing and contradictory attitudes of patients in the final stage of life.

Cassem[44] described several essential features in psychosocial management of the dying patient:

1. *Competence:* caregivers skilled and effective in their work, so the patient can feel confident in those to whom she yields control
2. *Concern:* compassionate caregivers who can bear the burden of emotional involvement, which is very intense but also rewarding
3. *Comfort:* such as adequate pain medication
4. *Communication:* an open-ended dialogue with the patient about her unique achievements and her everyday thoughts and feelings
5. *Family members:* including young children
6. *Cheerfulness:* a "gentle and appropriate sense of humor"
7. *Consistency and perseverance:* to offset the fear of progressive isolation, a predictable schedule of visits, the quality and dependability of which are much more important than their length
8. *Equanimity:* the capacity to be comfortable around people who are dying

Compassion, attentive listening, unflinching commitment — these are heavy burdens. Oncologists, too, go through phases of denial, anger, bargaining, sadness, and acceptance, as they are slowly reconciled to the patient's death. In addition, they must absorb some of the patient's hostility and that of her family, which may be displaced from the death itself onto the doctor. Oncologists must also face their own mortality and memories of deaths of loved ones. Following are some comments of gynecology residents on this process:

"I feel like a failure when patients die."

"When patients die who are our age, it makes you think about yourself dying."

"I feel like I never go home from work, because at night I dream about my patients."

Cancer caregivers often worry that if they allow themselves to become emotionally involved with terminal patients, they will be in a constant state of bereavement. With experience, though, they discover that the process of helping patients to die well is a source of personal growth and energy.

Family members can also find rewards in the experience of helping dying patients. Patients, in turn, may find that their role of being supportive and strong for others, continues up until death.

A 42-year-old woman with ovarian cancer had recently found out she was terminally ill. When the doctor asked her husband, "What are your wishes for the time that is left?" he answered in terms of time remaining in the hospitalization. The dying woman gently corrected him, saying, "No, dear, the doctor means the time I have left to live."

Mismatch of timing between patients' and families' acceptance of death is not uncommon. If the patient accepts the inevitability of death, and the family does not, family members may press for additional uncomfortable treatments. If the family accepts the death, and the patient does not, they may withdraw and leave her feeling lonely and abandoned. It is important to intervene in such cases, so that remaining life tasks can be addressed with equal understanding on all sides.

Oncologists must distinguish between treatments that can reasonably be expected to prolong life and those that would only postpone death. Responding to the 1983 Presidential Commission Study on "deciding to forego life-sustaining treatment," a multidisciplinary group of experienced physicians suggested guidelines for the care of hopelessly ill patients. The doctor, they said, should discuss and choose with the patient from among several levels of care[41]:

1. Maximal life support, including emergency resuscitation
2. Intensive care and advanced life support
3. General medical care (including antibiotics, drugs, surgery, cancer chemotherapy, hydration, and nutrition)
4. General nursing care and comfort measures (pain relief, hydration, and nutrition in response to patients' requests)

Once doctor and patient have chosen a level of care, further decisions are easier. At the final (supportive only) level of care, chemotherapy is not an option, pain medications are used as needed without concern for addiction, and patients may prefer to move to a home or hospice setting.

Survival

Now that many patients with gynecologic cancer are cured, the psychosocial tasks faced by survivors are beginning to be described. Just as cancer has a mysterious origin, its demise is also mysterious, and survivors must cope, for the rest of their lives, with the uncertainty of possible recurrence. As one woman stated, "Every morning when I look in the mirror, I ask, 'Is the cancer back today.' " Survivors, as a group, report long-standing decreases in self-confidence, and an increased number of health worries.[45] Also important are the irreversible losses suffered as a result of cancer treatment: deficits from surgery, changes in sexual function, and sequelae of radiation and chemotherapy.

The family of a cancer survivor must adjust to yet another dramatic change in their social structure, as the patient re-establishes her position with respect to others. Some families experience the Lazarus syndrome ("and he that was dead, came forth"), in which the family has become so desensitized and uninvolved that they respond to the patient's recovery with hostility and displaced guilt.

Reports of life quality among survivors are often good, though. If the patient's psychological adaptation was successful, the experience of a close brush with death and the accompanying re-evaluation of life priorities may have a net positive impact. In one study, survivors of cancer were found to have better quality of life, on several different measures, than the general population.[46]

INDIVIDUAL FACTORS AFFECTING ADJUSTMENT TO CANCER

As a woman enters into the struggle with cancer, her chances for a successful response, both psychological and physical, depend on her individual set of adaptive capacities. In some areas of function, she will have reserves of strength and flexibility. In others, she

may have specific vulnerabilities to the stress of illness.

Physical Variables

If patients suffer from pain, disability, or any sort of central nervous system dysfunction, their adaptive resources will be reduced overall. The seriousness of the cancer and the extensiveness of cancer surgery and other treatment have been found to correlate negatively with measures of psychosocial adjustment.[47]

Stage of Life Cycle

The struggle with cancer occurs in the context of other psychological tasks, such as the series of life passages in adult development.

ADOLESCENCE

The adolescent patient, for example, is already engaged in a host of rapid changes: in body image, sexuality, mood stability, and personal identity. The conflicting emotions surrounding her budding efforts to become a woman make the adolescent girl vulnerable to the fear that genital cancer is a punishment. The threat of death stirs up intense fantasies about future achievement, evoking guilt and rage. Finally, increased dependency on family and cancer caregivers may seem like going backward to childish ways.

Typical coping behavior of adolescents draws on common fantasies of invulnerability and omnipotentiality. Defiance in the face of cancer is usually adaptive, but some may assert this position at the expense of their own best interests:

A 17-year-old girl with a germ cell tumor refused to undergo chemotherapy, and her mother was unable to persuade her. The Department of Social Services had to be brought in to enforce treatment.

The oncologist must strike a balance between insisting on potentially curative therapies and allowing the adolescent to carry out her developmental task of gaining independence and autonomy. Patients should be encouraged to establish boundaries in areas unrelated to the progress of cancer treatment. Many will engage more effectively with the doctor if they are able to play an active role in decisions.

Family members are an important source of information in evaluating the success of a patient's adjustment, since they will have a broader knowledge of multiple domains of quality of life:

> An 18-year-old girl with Sertoli-Leydig cell ovarian tumor appeared very depressed and withdrawn immediately after chemotherapy, but her mother reported that she was getting good grades and had been invited to her senior prom.

The patient's parents should be included in major treatment decisions, while being specifically warned against over-protectiveness, especially when the patient is striving to maintain normal behavior within her peer group.

YOUNG ADULTHOOD

The young adult patient with genital cancer will face a threat of unfulfilled potential in the areas of career and childbearing. Final separation from parents, the search for a partner, early marital adjustment, and plans for pregnancy are critical issues in this phase:

> A 27-year-old woman at 16 weeks gestation was noted to have a pelvic mass at her first prenatal visit. She was found to have cancer of the cervix and had to undergo not only radiation therapy but a spontaneous abortion, 2 weeks after the start of treatment.

Fertility is an important concern for patients who must lose their reproductive organs. Even a woman who has already decided not to have children will find that there is a difference between "I don't want to have kids" and "I'm not able to have kids." The inability to bear children may make a woman feel unattractive, and many of the feelings surrounding the uterus as a source of private satisfaction, womanliness and creativity will be especially acute in young adults:

> A 35-year-old woman was recently divorced, and childless, when her cancer was discovered. Despite her good prognosis, she was deeply concerned that her boyfriend would lose interest in her, if he could not anticipate fathering a child.

The impact of loss of fertility is variable from person to person. A woman may have so many children she feels overwhelmed, and yet want more anyway, because mothering is her only source of self-esteem. Another woman in the same situation might be relieved that she cannot get pregnant again. Other sources of self-worth can cushion the loss of childbearing capacity, and physicians must be careful not to make assumptions based on their own values about a patient's response.

MIDDLE AGE

The woman in her middle years may be engaged in any of a number of different developmental crises. Family structure may be in flux, as adolescent children leave home and elderly parents need additional care. The patient may be entering a phase of increasing self-definition, starting a new career or finding new sources of self-fulfillment. In midlife, the remaining time span seems finite, and patients are aware of limitations in the future remaining to them. The loss of fertility is less of a concern, although many of the personal meanings attached to the uterus and ovaries will continue to play a role in their adjustment.

OLD AGE

Older women will usually have begun to contemplate the ending of their lives and may respond to the diagnosis of cancer by saying, "At least now I know what I'll die of." In this phase of the life cycle, patients worry most about being abandoned by relatives and caretakers. The oncologist must help ease the patient's fear of loneliness and her fear of excessive suffering by describing plans for continued support.

Social Support

If an oncologist could choose a single variable to be tipped in the patient's favor, the one that consistently correlates with positive overall adjustment is the quality of the patient's social support.[48] In a review of nonmedical issues affecting survival, Weisman and Worden[49] found that "patients who live significantly longer than expected tend to maintain cooperative and usually sustaining relationships."

In working to optimize adjustment through the patient's social network, oncologists may find it helpful to conceptualize the family as falling on a spectrum between a closed system and an open system. A closed system is a tight unit with very defined, rigid relationships between members. Closed-system families tend to be more autonomous but less flexible, slow to incorporate new ideas, and only selectively responsive to what the physician says. An open system tends to be looser in structure, with more fluid boundaries with the outside environment. Open-system families are more vulnerable in the face of stress, because they have fewer internal resources, but they are more flexible and readily adopt the moods and attitudes of the cancer care team.[50]

Most women experience the stress of cancer within the context of a marriage or other partnership, where pre-existing role assignments may influence the course of adjustment.

> A 60-year-old woman suffered radiation damage to her bowel as a result of therapy for cervical cancer. She had always been the leader in her second marriage. Her husband had difficulty in empathizing, because of his own overwhelming need to depend on her.
>
> A strong-willed 40-year-old schizophrenic woman was found to have uterine cancer. Her upcoming hysterectomy was expected to be stressful within her long-standing lesbian relationship—her 36-year-old lover was a very dependent, borderline personality. Advance preparation of staff for psychological care of the patient allowed her to deal with the reversal of roles and prevented psychiatric complications.

In addition to family and friends, the patient's social network may include people she knows through work, community, or church activities. The oncologist should make an informal survey, at the outset of treatment, of the patient's psychosocial resources and should aim to work closely with significant helpers in the patient's life. These people will already be attuned to the patient's needs and eager to contribute to her care.

Personal Background

Preexisting personality plays a significant role in the patient's ability to recruit, and make use of, social support. Gynecologic cancer is experienced on a background of previous life history: past trauma, personality characteristics, and the special meaning she attaches to genitalia and sexuality.

The physician should pay attention to her history of previous life stresses. How has the patient coped, in the past, with losses? How does she respond in the face of impaired function? If she adapted successfully to the circumstances, a past psychological trauma may have given her practice in responding to stress. If she was overwhelmed and impotent, a past event may

predispose her to a fearful maladaptive response to genital cancer. A history of psychiatric illness, including alcoholism, indicates specific areas of vulnerability.

One line of research shows two individual coping styles employed in adaptation to stress: (1) monitoring, which involves constant scanning for information relevant to possible dangers; and (2) blunting, in which such information is actively screened out. Monitors are less anxious when they have detailed discussions with physicians, whereas blunters do better if they are allowed to distract themselves from the illness.[51]

Studies of personality attributes and adjustment to cancer suggest that people who display a fighting spirit and a zest for challenge suffer less psychological morbidity and may even live longer than do those who react with helplessness or passive acceptance.[52]

Religion is another factor that is protective of psychosocial adjustment. Patients who have strong religious beliefs and connections report lower levels of pain and better life satisfaction.[53]

SEXUAL PROBLEMS

Many of the experiences and factors discussed above are common to all types of cancer, but female genital cancer poses specific challenges in the area of sexuality.[54]

Somatic Effects

Sexual behavior consists of three dimensions—somatic, intrapsychic, and interpersonal—all of which are altered by the illness.[55]

Local treatments frequently cause loss, distortion, or dysfunction of the organs involved in sexual intercourse, changes affecting both physical and aesthetic aspects of sexual function. Radical hysterectomy may shorten and/or narrow the vagina; if ovaries are also removed, estrogen stimulation is lost.

Radiation therapy may weaken delicate connective tissues in the pelvis, causing vaginitis, proctitis, and cystitis. Veins and arteries surrounding the vagina are often damaged, further diminishing lubrication and elasticity.[56] Dyspareunia and postcoital bleeding are common, and complete obliteration of the vagina can result if intercourse or mechanical dilation are not encouraged.[57] Some patients, especially those who have had both surgery and radiation may suffer fistula formation: Communications between vagina and bowel or bladder lead to spillage of feces and urine into the vagina, which are both functionally and aesthetically disturbing.

Surgery for vulvar cancer usually includes removal of the clitoris, labia, and tissue adjacent to lymph nodes, resulting in lost sensitivity and occasional introital stenosis.[58,59] Pelvic exenteration is also extremely disfiguring, removing vagina, uterus, tubes, ovaries, rectum, and bladder and creating multiple ostomy sites. Surgical reconstruction of a neovagina may not be fully satisfactory, because of problems with pain and discharge.[60] In addition to local alterations of function, patients may also find their sexual fulfillment impaired by the physical debilitation of cancer and cancer treatments.

Intrapsychic Effects

All cancer patients are distressed by the threat of the illness to their life and health. Specific sources of anxiety in genital cancer include fears that sexual activity will cause spread, recurrence, or transmission of the cancer. Patients may also fear that sex will cause pain, bleeding, or disruption of postsurgical anatomy.[57,59,61]

The woman with genital cancer must mourn the loss of her sexual and reproductive organs, a process that often includes diminished libido and chronic anxiety. She may also suffer loss in her sense of personal attractiveness, femininity, and overall self-worth.[62,63] Alterations in the genital area have profound effects on the intrapsychic body image, a component of self-esteem that is closely tied to a woman's sense of herself as a sexual being.[64,65]

The individual impact of bodily change is further determined by personal meaning attached to the genitalia, which differs greatly between individuals. Sexual history is especially important. If she has residual guilt about past sexual activities, masturbation, premarital or extramarital sex, venereal disease, abortion, multiple partners, for example, genital cancer may seem like a retaliation for sin[59,65]:

A 32-year-old woman had become pregnant out of wedlock, 13 years earlier and, despite a successful experience of raising the child, had always felt deeply ashamed. She and her husband decided they were ready for another child, and she became pregnant. When she was discov-

ered to have choriocarcinoma, she viewed this as her punishment for the previous "sin."

Patients with a history of being sexually victimized (rape, incest, other abusive relationship) are also at particular risk. The trauma of genital cancer and treatment will reawaken earlier feelings of betrayal, helplessness, and self-blame.

Ideas associated with ostomies may be another source of shame and guilt. Control of one's sphincters is an achievement prized in childhood and is associated with parental love and personal autonomy.[66] In a study of pelvic exenteration patients, Vera[67] found that ostomies were considered to be the most difficult area of adjustment and were held responsible for decreased social and sexual activity. Ostomy stomas may become erotized, and thus an alternate source of sexual pleasure, but unless they are counseled about this change, patients may be too ashamed to benefit from it.[68]

A woman's perceptions of genital cancer are also influenced by beliefs about the function of sex, whether it is for pleasure, reproduction, and/or maintenance of emotional bonds. Other individual factors involved in sexual adaptation include (1) quality of premorbid sexual function, (2) nonspecific variables such as stage in life cycle and personal coping style, and (3) gender role definition.[62,64] Androgenous role definition is thought to provide a better platform for adjustment than a highly feminine role definition. Nongender sources of self-esteem are more flexible, permitting a woman to feel valued through work, hobbies, and relationships outside of sexual partner and children.

Interpersonal Effects

Women with cancer who are single, divorced, or widowed may be actively searching for companionship at the time of diagnosis. In some age groups, women outnumber men, further complicating their sense of being socially stigmatized by cancer:

A 70-year-old widow was one of several women courted by an attractive 75-year-old widower, who had recently lost his wife of 50 years to a long, painful illness. Shortly after they decided to marry, she discovered she had cancer. As soon as he heard this news, her fiancé canceled the engagement and left on a trip to visit his grandchildren. He never called her again and eventually married another elderly widow.

Even those who are content not to have a male partner may suffer limitations in other forms of sexual expression, such as masturbation or homosexuality.

Women who do have partners often fear deterioration, or termination, of their relationships as a result of sexual changes. These fears are well founded, according to many studies[59,69,70]:

> A 30-year-old woman with ovarian cancer was deteriorating rapidly. Her husband privately asked the doctor when she would die, because he had a new girlfriend and wanted to marry her.
>
> Another woman in her 30s was dying of ovarian cancer. Her husband told her he would not visit the next day, because he had to get his sexual needs met elsewhere.

Issues that may affect bonding include the man's fear of inducing injury, fear of contagion by the cancer, and feelings that the patient is now sexless or unacceptably disfigured. Unless open communication is established between the woman and her partner, the loss of intimate contact can demoralize her at a time when she is most in need of support.

Especially vulnerable are couples with preexisting marital problems or with emotional bonds highly dependent on sex:

> A 33-year-old woman with four children was discovered to have vulvar cancer at a postpartum visit. She was reluctant to undergo surgery because she thought her husband would leave her if sexuality was compromised.

Long-lasting relationships seem better able to tolerate the stresses of cancer than short-term ones.[69]

Societal attitudes also play a role in sexual adjustment. During the 1950s, sexuality was seen as only appropriate for healthy married women in the childbearing age group. Women who had undergone colostomy or other disfiguring surgery tended to disclaim any interest in sex.[71] During the 1980s, societal attitudes have shifted. Women with genital cancer are now more likely to complain about losses in sexual function and are better motivated for rehabilitation.[60,68]

Time Course of Sexual Problems

In a controlled prospective study of early-stage cervical and endometrial cancer patients, Andersen[72] found that changes in sexual function, along with such symptoms as fatigue, bleeding, pain, and vaginal discharge, were a stimulus for seeking medical attention. By 4 months after start of treatment, 30 to 40 percent of the sample reported sexual problems, in all phases of the response cycle (desire, arousal, orgasm). At 8 and 12 months, some improvement was reported.

Factors Related to Site or Type of Treatment

Severity of disease and radicality of procedure are the most important predictors of sexual dysfunction. In cervical cancer, for example, preinvasive disease treated by conization causes no reduction in sexual activity and may even improve function.[73] At the other extreme, central recurrence of disease (treated with pelvic exenteration) leads to complete cessation of sexual activity in 80 to 90 percent of patients. A similar spectrum of sexual dysfunction is described for vulvar cancer treatments, where sexual losses vary according to the radicality of surgery.[74]

The sexual costs of radical hysterectomy versus radiation therapy have been a matter of debate. It has long been thought that radiation is more damaging to sexuality.[73] A well-controlled study, however, found comparable changes for both interventions.[75]

Sexual Counseling

Decreased satisfaction in sexual relationships and reduced frequency of intercourse are common but not inevitable.[76,77] Some women are simply uninformed that sexual function can be preserved despite removal of genital organs. Dennerstein and Ryan[63] showed that the most significant determinant of posthysterectomy sexual dysfunction was a preoperative expectation (often incorrect) of change in ability to have, and enjoy, sex. Several reviews highlight the value of the oncologist's role in sexual counseling.[78-83]

The first step is to gather information on spoken or unspoken concepts that a woman may have about her sexuality within the context of a discussion of the effects of treatment. The physical examination, for example, should include an opportunity for the patient to view her genitals in a mirror during explanations of any visible changes and to ask questions about functions of organs being affected. Some patients may not be aware that treatments sparing the clitoris will preserve a greater range of sexual behavior or that orgasm is still possible after removal of the clitoris. Alternatives to vaginal intercourse, including those available after the most radical of procedures, should be described.

Essentials of sexual counseling include the following:

1. Privacy
2. Continuity (i.e., that the counselor is the same person and that the same issues are raised repeatedly for follow-up discussion)
3. Matter-of-fact tone
4. Scheduled time (patient should know both when, and how long, the meeting will be)
5. Permission to ask questions
6. Relevance of concerns to the patient's stage of illness

The timing of sexual counseling must match the readiness of patients. The first concern of a patient approaching surgery, for example, is the life-threatening nature of her problem. Once she has achieved some degree of emotional resolution on that issue, she can focus on sexuality.

> A 45-year-old woman with ovarian cancer was admitted to the hospital, where the cancer care team tried to counsel her about alternatives to intercourse. Her husband balked, saying, "All you people are interested in is sex. I love my wife. I can still hold her hand, give her a kiss. That is all we need right now."

This case also illustrates the point that patients and their partners can remain physically intimate, even with significant deficits. Couples may need encouragement to continue holding and touching, especially in the hospital setting.

Oncologists should be prepared for the wide range of psychological variables that may influence sexual rehabilitation:

> A 28-year-old single woman was referred for psychiatric evaluation when she refused to do vaginal dilation exercises, prescribed to retard scarring and constriction of her vagina. Two years prior to referral, she had broken up with her boyfriend and shortly thereafter had been diagnosed with leiomyosarcoma of the rectovaginal septum. She was angry over the timing of events, saying, "He went out and started dating and rebuilding his life, and I got cancer. It's not fair." Having already faced possible death and the loss of fertility, femininity, and sexuality,

she was frustrated at the long series of treatments that had been beyond her control. She considered the exercises as something the could control and therefore refused them.

In such a case, caregivers should support the patient's efforts to regain autonomy, counsel her about the risks and benefits of her refusal in short-term versus long-term gain, and then allow her freedom to make the decision. Sexual counseling and rehabilitation, as with other psychosocial interventions in cancer care, should be offered and then offered again. The patient should not feel she has missed her chance, if she is not ready to take advantage of it at any one point along the time course of disease.

PSYCHIATRIC PROBLEMS

While all women with gynecologic cancer experience, in varying degrees, the sequence of emotional reactions described above, some will also develop (or already suffer from) psychiatric illness.[15,84,85] An oft-cited study by Derogatis and others[86] found that about one-half of a population of cancer patients, both hospitalized and ambulatory, met criteria for a psychiatric disorder. Among that group, 85 percent had symptoms of anxiety and depression.[86] These symptoms appear most often at nodal points in timecourse, such as after diagnosis.[26] One study comparing women newly diagnosed with pelvic cancer with those with benign disease found both groups to have anxiety and fatigue, but the cancer patients were more likely to be depressed and confused as well.[87]

The risk of depression increases with advancing disease and physical deterioration. Cassileth et al.[40] showed that anxiety and mood disturbance were most severe during palliative therapy for incurable disease, next highest during active, curative treatment, and lowest during follow-up care.

The risk of psychiatric disorders in female genital cancer is roughly equivalent to that in heterogeneous cancer populations, for all sites except ovary. Ovarian cancer patients appear to have a disproportionately high prevalence of anxiety and depression throughout the course of illness. This is thought to reflect the greater severity of disease at time of diagnosis and the lesser hope for cure. Severe side effects from triple-agent chemotherapy also increase the risk of depression in this group.[26,88]

Depression

Common myths about depression in cancer are that all cancer patients are depressed and that cancer patients ought to be depressed, given the gravity of their illness. All cancer patients do have some degree of acute stress response after each crisis (e.g., diagnosis) with symptoms of shock, sadness, crying, anxiety, poor appetite, and disruption of sleep. It has been suggested that this response is adaptive, signaling a process of accommodation to the psychological injury. These symptoms are usually transient, lasting about 7 to 10 days, and are not of the severity seen in clinical depression.[89]

The diagnosis of depression in physically healthy patients depends heavily on somatic symptoms, such as anorexia, weight loss, pain, and fatigue. Since the woman with genital cancer may already have these symptoms as a direct result of her illness, the diagnosis must rest on emotional and cognitive criteria: sadness, anger, guilt, anxiety, difficulty in concentrating, loss of interest in usual activities, inability to experience pleasure, feelings of hopelessness or helplessness, and suicidal ideation.

In addition to the many psychosocial stressors associated with cancer, chemotherapeutic drugs should be considered as a possible etiology, especially when the temporal pattern of depression is closely linked to the administration of treatment:

A 15-year-old girl was receiving monthly courses of vinblastine. Each time she went for treatment, she became withdrawn, dysphoric, and suicidal. It was at first thought that a problematic relationship with her mother was the cause of her depression. On two separate occasions, though, she had a prompt recovery immediately after transfer to a psychiatric unit, which coincided with completion of chemotherapy. The pattern of recovery and relapse suggested vinblastine as the etiology.

Of drugs commonly used in gynecologic cancer, the vinca alkaloids can cause depression.[90] Other chemotherapy agents associated with mood disorders include steroids, L-asparaginase, and procarbazine.[89] Early investigations show that high doses of interferon may cause severe depression, with suicidal ideation.[91] The oncologist should be wary of possible CNS side effects from drugs that are still under investigation.

The first step in treatment of depression in cancer is emotional support given by the oncologist and the cancer care team. Psychiatric consultation should be considered when the patient has severe symptoms that last longer than a week, or any symptoms that are progressive or interfering with function, such as cooperation with treatment. Four treatment approaches are employed, often in combination: (1) short-term supportive psychotherapy, (2) antidepressant medications, (3) electroconvulsive therapy, and (4) relaxation techniques.

Depressive syndromes comprise a spectrum of neuroendocrine disturbances, any of which may respond to antidepressant medications.[92] There is rarely a contraindication to the use of these drugs. Some studies of antidepressants have suggested a decreased response rate (40 percent) in medically ill patients, as compared with physically healthy populations (60 percent). These figures may be misleading, though, because of the high rate of discontinuation (32 percent) due to the development of side effects.[93] Side effects such as delirium, urinary retention, and nausea more frequently become a limiting factor in patients who are medically ill, but they are reversible and should not preclude a trial of medication.

A depressed woman with genital cancer should be started on a very low dose of antidepressant, which the physician can describe to her as a test dose to determine her potential for side effects. A gradual approach to therapeutic range is more likely to be tolerated. In assessing the effect of antidepressants, the physician should look at behavioral symptoms, such as activity level and interest in family or hobbies, as well as mood. Patients may not report feeling better, even when they appear to be doing better overall.

It has been suggested that medically ill patients respond to lower doses of antidepressants. This is controversial,[94] though, and inadequate dosing is often cited as a reason for treatment failure.[95]

Tricyclic antidepressants are especially useful in patients who have pain: they act directly to relieve pain and also potentiate the action of other analgesics.[96] Studies of the syndrome of coexisting pain and depression, currently thought to be underdiagnosed, report an 80 percent response rate to antidepressants.[97,98]

Stimulant medications, such as dextroamphetamine and methylphenidate (Ritalin), are increasingly recommended for treatment of depression in the medically ill. They are fast acting and have minimal side effects that are usually correctible with adjustment of dose. A recent study showed three-fourths of depressed medically ill patients deriving benefit from stimulants, 93 percent of whom responded in the first 2 days. Stimulants may well be safer for patients with severe medical illness.[99]

Organic Brain Syndrome

The development of an acute mental disturbance in a patient with cancer suggests CNS dysfunction. An important distinction in organic brain disorder is between (1) delirium, characterized by clouding of consciousness, inability to sustain attention, sensory misperceptions, and a disordered stream of thought; and (2) dementia, characterized by loss of intellectual abilities, especially memory, judgment, and abstract thought, without alteration in consciousness. Delirium is more likely to be reversible.

Delirium is especially common in cancer patients, with prevalence rates up to 40 percent among those referred for psychiatric consultation, and 85 percent in the terminally ill.[100,101] Physicians unfamiliar with the dramatic disorganization of thought process and perception, including visual hallucinations, in delirium may misdiagnose it as functional psychosis, which is uncommon in patients without a prior history.

Causes of delirium in gynecologic cancer include, in approximate order of frequency:

1. Drugs, especially chemotherapeutic agents (methotrexate, vinca alkaloids, 5-fluorouracil, steroids)[102] and narcotic analgesics;
2. Metabolic derangement such as hypoxia, hypercalcemia, hyponatremia, hepatic/renal insufficiency, and hypoglycemia
3. Radiation therapy directed at brain
4. Anemia
5. Infection
6. Direct effect from metastasis to brain (rare in gynecologic cancer)
7. Other miscellaneous causes such as vitamin deficiency and coagulopathy

Delirium may occur prior to changes in physical exam or laboratory data to support one of these causes.

The primary treatment of delirium consists of careful work-up for etiology and correction of organic de-

rangement where possible. When pharmacotherapy is necessary for management of agitation and self-injurious behavior, agents commonly recommended are either haloperidol or an intermediate-acting benzodiazepine such as lorazepam, or both.[103]

RESOURCES

Gynecologic oncologists are fortunate to have access to a wide array of psychosocial resources: the doctor-patient relationship, multiple caregivers on the cancer team, and other people outside the hospital/clinic setting.

Doctor-Patient Relationship

In the overwhelming situation of life-threatening illness, the woman with genital cancer develops a complex and intense set of feelings toward her oncologist. She is dependent on the doctor for the basic needs of bodily care and preservation of life. She may revert to childlike ways of thinking and feeling, such as idealizing her doctor as a strong, protective parent figure. She also fears that if she expresses any anger or negative emotions, the doctor may withhold care from her. This simultaneous experience of the doctor as "good parent" and "bad parent" is a deep-seated response to the stress of illness, often coexisting with a rational awareness of limitations of the doctor's powers. Even in the healthiest of patients, unrealistic expectations are common. When no cure is realistically available, the patient may still believe in its possibility. She may also expect the process of being a cancer patient to be totally passive, requiring no effort on her part. All interactions between doctor and patient must be understood within the context of these unconscious fantasies.

The physician may be uncomfortable with being the object of so many strong feelings and may strive for more equality in the relationship. Consumerism and patient rights are frequently used as reasons for placing the patient in an active decision-making role. While patients should certainly be encouraged to maintain as much autonomy as they are ready for, the physician should be sensitive to the patient's needs. At some phases in the process of cancer care, it may be more adaptive for the patient to be childlike. Oncologists who seek a flexible balance between dependency and autonomy, taking cues from the patient about what she can handle, are most likely to create a doctor-patient relationship that serves as a source of strength.

The oncologist is also head of a treatment team: non-M.D. professionals help diffuse emotional burdens. The doctor must appreciate, though, how important he or she is, as an individual, to the patient:

> A 60-year-old woman recovering from radical vulvectomy was progressing well — more active each day, up and walking about — until the resident physician who was taking care of her went on a three-day trip. Suddenly she became whining, demanding, and much more passive. The resident had not told her he would be gone, having undervalued his own role in her postoperative care.

A structured approach to the clock (when you'll see the patient, and for how long) and the calendar (when you'll be gone, and for how long) is a way of gaining control over patients' emotional needs. A preset time length for meetings is especially important for very demanding patients: It guarantees to the patient that her doctor will not leave the room if she complains and helps the doctor avoid feelings of anger or guilt. The structure can be maintained with simple phrases, such as "We'll meet for 10 minutes each morning," and "Our time is up — I'll see you again tomorrow."

Another hint for effective use of doctor-patient time is to gather information in an open-ended fashion. The first step in good psychosocial management in cancer is the oncologist's assessment of how the patient is doing, through questions such as these:

What is your understanding of _____?
What were you thinking about just then?
What does _____ mean for you?
You have strong feelings about _____?
What are your thoughts about _____?

The doctor should not avoid questions that upset the patient or bring her to tears but should use these emotions as signals of areas that need further attention.

When enough information has been obtained to convince both doctor and patient that a topic merits more exploration, the oncologist should make a decision about who would be the best resource for the patient's needs. Just because the doctor often hears things first does not mean that he or she should necessarily provide therapy or counseling. The oncologist can be compared to an executive who assembles data, formulates plans, delegates projects, and then supervises their execution.

When other caregivers are asked to participate, they should be introduced to the patient as having special expertise in the area of depression, sexuality, and so forth. A careful introduction will serve to imbue the new relationship with some of the patient's positive feelings for the doctor. As long as this step is presented as another piece in the overall care plan, and the doctor continues to meet with the patient as usual, the patient will feel cared for, and not abandoned, by her physician.

Cancer Care Team

The ongoing relationship between doctor and patient is the focal point for information flow and the setting for critical treatment decisions, but much of cancer care is carried out by other professionals. Multiple disciplines work together, under the guidance of the team leader, to gather information and provide support in several domains of the patient's function.

NURSE

Patients are often more open with nurses and feel more on an equal footing with them. The oncologist should respect the nurse's unique awareness of the patient's day-to-day experiences and use them as an information source. Nurses can benefit, in turn, from hearing doctor's plans for meeting patients' overall physical and psychosocial needs.

SOCIAL WORKER

In addition to their work in gathering resources for transportation, financial aid, temporary housing, and disposition, social workers have training in psychosocial interventions. Depending on their degree of experience, social workers may be able to carry out family counseling, group therapy, and individual therapy. They are also skilled in finding mental health resources in the community. The oncologist should be receptive to their suggestions about when a psychiatric consultation is needed. Social workers often collaborate with psychiatrists, meeting regularly with the family, for example, while the psychiatrist is meeting with the patient.

CONSULTATION/LIAISON PSYCHIATRIST

Common reasons for consultation request include symptoms of excessive emotional reaction (depression, anxiety), grossly disturbed behavior, suicidal threat or attempt, refusal to cooperate, management of pain, and issues related to dying. In the ideal setting, the psychiatric consultant is available not only for specific consultation requests, but also functions as a liaison to the cancer team. This more informal collaborative function of the psychiatrist is thought to lower the diagnostic threshold of medical staff for recognition of psychiatric disorder.[88,104] In the absence of such a liaison, request rates for psychiatric consultations are quite low in the cancer population (2 to 5 percent).[100,105] Depression tends to be underdiagnosed and undertreated.[89]

CHAPLAIN

Religion has a protective effect on the patient's adjustment to cancer. The chaplain may intervene (1) by drawing church-affiliated people into the patient's social support system; and (2) by praying with the patient, soothing and renewing her, and helping her accept the realities of her illness.

RECREATION THERAPIST

Cancer patients often have idle time, when their movement is restricted. Recreation therapists can facilitate creative, satisfying use of this time (not just passive TV watching).

DIETICIAN

Because nutrition and enjoyment of food are often impaired in cancer, dieticians play an important supportive role. They can improve the quality — both subjective and objective — of a patient's diet.

OSTOMY THERAPIST

When ostomy therapists are doing their job, patients talk about difficulties they are experiencing and fears that they have. The physical intimacy of the relationship may allow the patient to talk more openly about sexual concerns.

FAMILY AND FRIENDS

Family members should be encouraged to feel that they are part of the team. They can help the patient control her environment and make it more reflective of her unique interests. In the hospital setting, they can bring in pictures, music, and other items that have special meaning for the patient. An audio tape machine can provide a link between patient and absent relatives, and enable a dying woman, for example, to make tapes of her voice for her children. The patient, in turn, derives satisfaction from providing support to family members, a respite from the role of being the dependent needy one.

STUDENTS

In the teaching hospital, medical students and so forth are another psychosocial resource, because they have time to spend listening to the patient, and are often more able to be empathic than overworked or sleep-deprived physicians. The oncologist should keep track of how many students are talking with the patient, though, because the disadvantage of so much attention is that a likeable verbal patient can grow weary of "pouring her heart out" again and again. The patient should be encouraged to decide for herself how much she wants to talk to students.

Cancer caregivers are unique people, just as patients are; a good fit between patient and therapist depends on personal characteristics as well as disciplinary affiliation. The oncologist should be flexible about working with the caregiver to whom the patient intuitively turns for support. If team members communicate freely with each other and their leader, multiple people can share the burden of psychosocial management. The patient will almost always view her doctor as the most important figure, however. The doctor is the "glue" that holds the treatment plan together.

Outside the Medical Setting

Many excellent self-help and other nonprofessional groups in the community provide support and assistance for cancer patients and their families. Oncologists should contact their local chapter of the American Cancer Society for information about these resources. Another suggestion is to keep a list of women who are veterans of various procedures and treatments who are willing to talk about their experiences with newly diagnosed cancer patients.

FUTURE DIRECTIONS

Because of the difficult treatment decisions posed in clinical practice, the field of psycho-oncology will be paying increasing attention, in years to come, to issues of quality of life. Another area of future development will be refinements in detection and treatment of psychiatric disorders in cancer patients.

A particularly intriguing area of active work is concerned with the mind-brain-body axis in cancer. Researchers in such fields as psychoneuroimmunology are finding increasing evidence for the role of psychological variables in the development of, and physical response to, malignancy.

The holistic approach to a woman with female genital cancer, not only the impact of cancer on her life, but also that of her life on cancer, is here to stay.

ACKNOWLEDGMENTS

We thank the following medical students whose literature review projects helped in the writing of this chapter: Ruth Dickinson, Allen Hamrick, James Lockwood, Deborah Russell, and Steve Shymansky.

REFERENCES

1. Ulfelder H: Gynecologic oncology: changing perspectives. Cancer 48:425, 1981
2. Morris JM: Risk/benefit ratios in the management of gynecologic cancer. Cancer 48:642, 1981
3. Cancer Facts and Figures 1987: American Cancer Society, New York, 1987
4. Blythe JG, Wahl TP: Debulking surgery. Gynecol Oncol 14:396, 1982
5. Chafe W, Fowler WC Jr, Walton LA, et al: Radical vulvectomy with use of tensor fascia lata myocutaneous flap. Am J Obstet Gynecol 145:207, 1983
6. Baker VV, Dudzinski MR, Fowler WC, et al: Percutaneous nephrostomy in gynecologic oncology. Am J Obstet Gynecol 149:772, 1984
7. Steinberg MD, Julianno MA, Wise L: Psychological outcome of lumpectomy versus mastectomy in the treatment of breast cancer. Am J Psychiatry 142:34, 1985
8. Sugarbaker PH, Barofsky I, Rosenberg SA, et al: Quality of life assessment of patients in extremity sarcoma clinical trials. Surgery 91:17, 1982
9. Meyerowitz BE, Watkins IK, Sparks FC: Psychosocial implications of adjuvant chemotherapy: A two year follow up. Cancer 52:1541, 1983
10. Andrews FM, Withey SB: Social Indicators of Well-Being: Americans' Perceptions of Life Quality. Plenum Press, New York, 1976
11. Cribb A: Quality of life: A response to KC Calman. J Med Ethics 11:142, 1985
12. Welch-McCaffrey D: Cancer, anxiety, and quality of life. Cancer Nursing 8:151, 1985
13. Calman KC: Quality of life in cancer patients: an hypothesis. J Med Ethics 10:124, 1984
14. Hutchinson TA, Boyd NF, Feinstein AR, et al: Scientific problems in clinical scales, as demonstrated in the Karnofsky index of performance status. J Chron Dis 32:661, 1979
15. Bukberg J, Penman D, Holland J: Depression in hospitalized cancer patients. Psychosomat Med 46:199, 1984
16. Cleeland CS: The impact of pain on the patient with cancer. Cancer 54:2635, 1984
17. Bloom BS, Knorr RS, Evans AE: The epidemiology of disease expenses. JAMA 253:2393, 1985
18. Newton M: Quality of life for the gynecologic oncology patient. Am J Obstet Gynecol 134:866, 1979
19. McCartney CF, Larson DB: Quality of life in gynecologic cancer. Cancer 60:2129, 1987
20. Holland JCB: Psychologic aspects of cancer. p. 1175. In Holland JF, Frei E (eds): Cancer Medicine. Lea & Febiger, Philadelphia, 1982
21. Sontag S: Illness as Metaphor. Farrar, Strauss and Giroux, New York, 1978
22. Henderson JG: Denial and repression as factors in the delay of patients with cancer presenting themselves to the physician. Ann NY Acad Sci 125:856, 1966
23. Lynch HT, Krush AJ: Attitude delay in cancer detection. Cancer 18:287, 1968
24. Oken D: What to tell cancer patients: A study of medical attitudes. JAMA 58:1120, 1961
25. Hackett TP, Weisman AD: The treatment of the dying. Curr Psychiatr Ther 2:121, 1962
26. Cain EN, Kohorn EI: Psychosocial reactions to the diagnosis of gynecologic cancer. Obstet Gynecol 62:635, 1983
27. Drellich MG, Bieber I, Sutherland A: The psycholog-

ical impact of cancer and cancer surgery: Adaptation to hysterectomy. Cancer 9:1120, 1958

28. Drellich MG, Bieber I: The psychological importance of the uterus and its function. J Nerv Ment Dis 126:322, 1958

29. Raphael B: The crisis of hysterectomy. Aust NZ J Psychiatry 6:106, 1972

30. Weisman AD: A model for psychosocial phasing in cancer. Gen Hosp Psychiatry 1:187, 1979

31. Janis IL: Psychological Stress: Psychoanalytic and Behavioral Studies of Surgical Patients. John Wiley & Sons, New York, 1958

32. Andersen BA, Karlsson JA, Anderson B: Anxiety and cancer treatment: response to stressful radiotherapy. Health Psychol 3:535, 1984

33. Peck A, Boland J: Emotional reactions to radiation treatment. Cancer 40:180, 1977

34. Andersen BL, Tewfik HH: Psychological reactions to radiation therapy: Reconsideration of the adaptive aspects of anxiety. J Pers Soc Psychol 48:1024, 1985

35. Forester B, Kornfeld DS: Psychotherapy during radiotherapy: Effects on emotional and physical distress. Am J Psychiatry 142:22, 1985

36. Cella DF, Pratt A, Holland JC: Persistent anticipatory nausea, vomiting, and anxiety in cured Hodgkin's disease patients after completion of chemotherapy. Am J Psychiatry 143:641, 1986

37. Redd WH, Andresen GV, Minagawa RY: Hypnotic control of anticipatory emesis in patients receiving cancer chemotherapy. J Consult Clin Psychol 50:14, 1982

38. Redd WH, Hendler CS: Behavioral medicine in comprehensive cancer treatment. J Psychosoc Oncol 1:3, 1983

39. Andresen JJ: Rapunzel: The symbolism of the cutting of hair. J Am Psychoanal Assoc 28:69, 1980

40. Cassileth BR, Lusk EJ, Strouse TB, et al: A psychological analysis of cancer patients and their next-of-kin. Cancer 55:72, 1985

41. Wanzer SH, Adelstein SJ, Cranford RE: The physician's responsibility toward hopelessly ill patients. N Engl J Med 310:955, 1984

42. Kubler-Ross E: On Death and Dying. Macmillan, New York, 1969

43. Raphael B, Maddison DC: Attitudes to dying. p. 1055. In Coppleson M (ed): Gynecologic Oncology. Vol. 2. Churchill Livingstone, New York, 1981

44. Cassem N: The dying patient. p. 300. In Hackett TP, Cassem NH (eds): Massachusetts General Hospital Handbook of General Hospital Psychiatry. CV Mosby, St. Louis, 1978

45. Schmale AH, Morrow GR, Schmitt MH, et al: Wellbeing of cancer survivors. Psychosomat Med 45:163, 1983

46. Danoff B, Kramer S, Irwin P, et al: Assessment of the quality of life in long-term survivors after definitive radiotherapy. Am J Clin Oncol 6:339, 1983

47. Andreson BL, Hacker NF: Treatment for gynecologic cancer: A review of the effects on female sexuality. Health Psychol 2:203, 1983

48. Goldberg RJ, Cullen LO: Factors important to psychosocial adjustment to cancer: A review of the evidence. Soc Sci Med 20:803, 1985

49. Weisman AD, Worden JW: Psychosocial analysis of cancer deaths. Omega 6:61, 1975

50. Hersh SP: Psychosocial aspects of patients with cancer. p. 264. In DeVita VT Jr, Hellmann S, et al (eds): Cancer: Principles and Practice of Oncology. 2nd Ed. JB Lippincott, Philadelphia, 1985

51. Miller SM: When is a little information a dangerous thing? Coping with stressful life events by monitoring vs. blunting. p. 145. In Levine S, Ursin H (ed): Coping and Health. Plenum Press, New York, 1980

52. Greer S, Morris T, Pettingale KW: Psychological response to breast cancer: effect on outcome. Lancet 2:785, 1979

53. Yates JW, Chalmer BJ, St. James P: Religion in patients with advanced cancer. Med Pediatr Oncol 9:121, 1981

54. McCartney CF: Sexual problems in women with pelvic cancer. Cancer (in press)

55. Greenberg DB: Measurement of sexual dysfunction in cancer patients. Cancer 53:2281, 1984

56. Abitbol MM, Davenport JH: Sexual dysfunction after therapy for cervical carcinoma. Am J Obstet Gynecol 119:181, 1974

57. Decker WH, Schwartman E: Sexual function following treatment for carcinoma of the cervix. Am J Obstet Gynecol 83:401, 1962

58. Moth I, Andreasson B, Jensen SB et al: Sexual function and somatopsychic reactions after vulvectomy. Dan Med Bull 30:27, 1983

59. Stellman R, Goodwin JM, Robinson J, et al: Psychological effects of vulvectomy. Psychosomatics 25:779, 1984

60. Andersen BL, Hacker NF: Psychosexual adjustment following pelvic exenteration. Obstet Gynecol 61:331, 1983

61. Bransfield DD, Horiot JC, Nabid A: Development of a scale for assessing sexual function after treatment for gynecologic cancer. J Psychosoc Oncol 2:3, 1984

62. Roeske NCA: Hysterectomy and other gynecological surgeries. p. 217. In Notman MT, Nadelson CC (eds): The Woman Patient. Plenum Press, New York, 1978

63. Dennerstein L, Ryan M: Psychosocial and emotional sequelae of hysterectomy. J Psychosomat Obstet Gynecol 2:81, 1982

64. Derogatis LR: Breast and gynecological cancers: their

unique impact on body-image and sexual identity in women. Front Radiat Ther Oncol 14:1, 1980

65. Schain WS: Sexual functioning, self-esteem and cancer care. Front Radiat Ther Oncol 14:12, 1980

66. Druss RG, O'Connor JF, Stern LO: Psychologic response to colectomy. Arch Gen Psychiatry 20:419, 1969

67. Vera MJ: Quality of life following pelvic exenteration. Gynecol Oncol 12:355, 1981

68. Lamont JA, DePetrillo AD, Sargeant EJ: Psychosexual rehabilitation and exenterative surgery. Gynecol Oncol 6:236, 1978

69. Sewell HH, Edwards DW: Pelvic genital cancer: Body image and sexuality. Front Radiat Ther Oncol 14:35, 1984

70. Dempsey GM, Buchsbaum HJ, Morrison J: Psychosocial adjustment to pelvic exenteration. Gynecol Oncol 3:325, 1975

71. Sutherland AM, Orbach CE, Duk RB et al: The psychological impact of cancer and cancer surgery. I. Adaptation to the dry colostomy: Preliminary report and summary of findings. Cancer 5:857, 1952

72. Andersen BL: Sexual functioning morbidity and the woman with gynecologic cancer: Outcomes and directions for prevention. Cancer 60:2137, 1987

73. Andersen BL: Sexual functioning morbidity among cancer survivors: Current status and future research directions. Cancer 55:1835, 1985

74. Andersen BL, Hacker NF: Psychosexual adjustment after vulvar surgery. Obstet Gynecol 62:457, 1983

75. Vincent CE, Vincent B, Greiss FC, et al: Some marital sexual concomitants of carcinoma of the cervix. South Med J 68:552, 1975

76. Capone MA, Good RS, Westie KS, et al: Psychosocial rehabilitation of gynecologic oncology patients. Arch Phys Med Rehabil 61:128, 1980

77. Cain EN, Kohorn EI, Quinlan DM, et al: Psychosocial benefits of a cancer support group. Cancer 57:183, 1986

78. Andersen BL: Sexual difficulties for women following cancer treatment. p. 257. In Andersen BL (ed): Women with Cancer: Psychological perspectives. Springer-Verlag, New York, 1986

79. Auchincloss S: Gynecological cancer: Psychological and sexual sequelae and management. p. 25. In Holland JC (ed): Current Concepts in Psycho-Oncology. Memorial Sloan-Kettering Cancer Center, New York, 1984

80. Capone MA, Good RS: Sex counseling for cancer patients. Contemp Obstet Gynecol 15:131, 1980

81. Donahue VC: Sexual rehabilitation of gynecologic cancer patients. p. 1050. In Coppleson M (ed): Gynecologic Oncology. Vol. 2. Churchill Livingstone, New York, 1981

82. Von Eschenbach AC, Schover L: The role of sexual rehabilitation in the treatment of patients with cancer. Cancer 54:2662, 1984

83. McCartney CF: Female sexual dysfunction. p. 331. In Dornbrand L, Hoole AJ, et al (eds): Manual of Clinical Problems in Adult Ambulatory Care. Little, Brown, Boston, 1985

84. Lansky SB, List MA, Herrmann C, et al: Absence of major depressive disorder in female cancer patients. J Clin Oncol 3:1553, 1985

85. Petty F, Noyes R Jr: Depression secondary to cancer. Biol Psychiatry 16:1203, 1981

86. Derogatis LR, Morrow GR, Fetting J, et al: The prevalence of psychiatric disorders among cancer patients. JAMA 249:751, 1983

87. Andersen BL: Psychological responses and sexual outcomes of gynecologic cancer. p. 1. In Sciarra JJ (ed): Gynecology and Obstetrics. Vol. IV. Harper & Row, Philadelphia, 1987

88. McCartney CF, Larson DB, Wada CY, et al: Effect of psychiatric liaison on consultation rates and reasons for consult in gynecologic oncology. J Psychosomat Obstet Gynecol 5:253, 1986

89. Massie MJ, Holland JC: Diagnosis and treatment of depression in the cancer patient. Clin Psychiatry 45:25, 1984

90. Holland J, Scharlau C, Gailane S, et al: Vincristine treatment of advanced cancer: A cooperative study of 392 cases. Cancer Res 33:1258, 1973

91. Adams F, Quesada JR, Gutterman JU: Neuropsychiatric manifestations of human leukocyte interferon therapy in patients with cancer. JAMA 252:938, 1984

92. Evans DL, McCartney CF, Nemeroff CB, et al: Depression in women treated for gynecologic cancer: Clinical and neuroendocrine assessment. Am J Psychiatry 143:447, 1986

93. Popkin MK, Callies AL, Mackenzie TB: The outcome of antidepressant use in the medically ill. Arch Gen Psychiatry 42:1160, 1985

94. Fava GA: Diagnosis and treatment of depression in the medically ill. Prog Neuropsychopharmacol Biol Psychiatry 10:1, 1986

95. Pollack MH, Rosenbaum JF: Management of antidepressant-induced side effects: A practical guide for the clinician. J Clin Psychiatry 48:3, 1987

96. Spiegel K, Kalb R, Pasternak GW: Analgesic activity of tricyclic antidepressants. Ann Neurol 13:462, 1983

97. Lindsay PG, Wyckoff M: The depression-pain syndrome and its response to antidepressants. Psychosomatics 22:571, 1981

98. Ward NG, Bloom VL, Friedel RO: Effectiveness of tricyclic antidepressants in the treatment of coexisting pain and depression. Pain 7:331, 1979

99. Woods SW, Tesar GE, Murray GB: Psychostimulant

treatment of depressive disorders secondary to medical illness. Clin Psychiatry 47:12, 1986

100. Levine PM, Silberfarb PM, Lipowski ZJ: Mental disorders in cancer patients. Cancer 42:1385, 1983

101. Massie MJ, Holland J, Glass E: Delirium in terminally ill cancer patients. Am J Psychiatry 140:1048, 1983

102. Silberfarb PM: Chemotherapy and cognitive defects in cancer patients. Annu Rev Med 34:35, 1983

103. Adams F, Fernandez F, Andersson B: Emergency pharmacotherapy of delirium in the critically ill cancer patient. Psychosomatics 27:33, 1986

104. Torem M, Saravay SM, Steinberg H: Psychiatric liaison: Benefits of an "active" approach. Psychosomatics 20:598, 1979

105. Massie MJ, Holland JC, Gorzynski GJ, et al: Psychiatric consultation in a cancer hospital. p. 67. In Syllabus and Scientific Proceedings. 133rd Annual Meeting of the American Psychiatry Association. American Psychiatric Press, Washington DC, 1980

35

Advances in Cancer Research

Frank J. Rauscher, Jr.

Much new and exploitable for the benefit of people is happening in cancer research, so much so that many in these fields believe that we may be in the golden age. True? The purpose of this chapter is to try to convey to the physician who may not have time to keep abreast of new technology in cancer research just what is going on, and especially what is happening that may help provide even better care of the patient and prospective patient (high-risk individual) now and within the next decade.

This chapter is presented as a synopsis of those areas of research that investigators in the mid-1980s would generally agree are most stimulating intellectually and concurrently the most promising for eventual translation to public health. Second, an attempt is made to summarize what we have learned from decades of research that can be used by patients and prospective patients now, particularly as to what can be done by personal choice to avoid advertent or inadvertent propensity to cancer. Throughout this chapter, when appropriate, emphasis is placed on research supported by the American Cancer Society (ACS) or on that recommended for support by hundreds of scientific advisors and participants in its peer review system. I have not summarized state-of-the-art technology with which the reader of this text is familiar, but rather have attempted to point out those research areas, especially in bench-biology, that you may wish to keep your eyes on.

PREVENTION

In all of cancer research, no series of findings is more important than the understanding that cancer is not an inherent fate of people because they are people. Cancer occurs for the most part because of something we do, eat, drink, or smoke and to a lesser extent because of where we work and live. Informed estimates by many investigators suggest that up to 85 percent of cancers are due to long-term environmental exposure to specific agents and/or to life-style. Of this estimate there is little disagreement that approximately 30 percent of all cancers (lung, head and neck, bladder, and probably cervical and pancreatic) are related to the use and amount of use of tobacco. In addition, 20 percent or more of cancers seem to be related to nutrition and diet. Interestingly, and contrary to public perception, relatively few of these diseases are proved to be induced by environmental chemicals. Each year for the past several decades more than 200,000 new chemicals have been developed in Western countries, with about 10,000 produced in quantities of 1 ton or more. Yet of those tested, fewer than 40 have been found to be carcinogenic in animals and humans. We must continue to be extraordinarily vigilant, and it is clear that programs to eliminate or reduce the impact of known carcinogens including public education and modification of life-styles are warranted.

Efforts must surely continue to "clean up the environment," but research into options for chemoprevention must be expanded as well. Are there effective ways in which we can protect people from the processes of carcinogenesis (reprogram genome?) despite onslaughts of life-style and inadvertent impact of an industrial society?

In any event, much of cancer research today has to do with diet and nutrition; vaccine development; oncogenic control; and the development, test, use, and evaluation of biologic response modifiers as immune stimulants as well as therapeutics.

Overview of Incidence and Survival Trends

In 1987 there will be an anticipated 965,000 new cases of cancer in the United States, with approximately 483,000 deaths. It is somewhat heartening that over the past decade the incidence of most cancers with the exception of lung has remained level or has decreased. Similarly the 5-year relative survival rate for all races and both sexes had improved to approximately 50 percent by 1982. Five-year survival is the probability of escaping death from cancer for 5 years following diagnosis.

The most disheartening trend, however, is that with the exception of white males, lung cancer incidence and deaths continue to increase at precipitous rates. As one of the least curable cancers, this phenomenon skews overall survival rates dramatically. For black males, incidence and mortality rates increased about 10 percent annually from 1973 through 1983 and 6 percent for women of both races. Lung cancer deaths have now surpassed breast cancer in 15 states despite the fact that 1 in 10 American women can be expected to develop breast cancer within a 75-year lifetime.

In summary, the following is excerpted from the National Cancer Institute's Surveillance, Epidemiology, and End Results (SEER) Program:

> The cancers with the highest 5-year relative survival rates, all races combined, for patients diagnosed between 1977 and 1982 are: thyroid cancer, 93 percent; testis, 88 percent; endometrium, 84 percent; melanoma, 80 percent; female breast, 74 percent; bladder 76 percent; Hodgkin's disease, 73 percent; prostate, 71 percent; larynx, 67 percent; and uterine cervix, 66 percent. Survival

continues to be poor for some cancers, such as pancreatic, lung, esophageal, and stomach cancer.

The 5-year relative survival rate was 61 percent for white children under 15 years of age diagnosed between 1977 and 1982, up from a rate of 54 percent for children diagnosed between 1973 and 1976. This is a statistically significant increase. A rate could not be calculated for black children because of the small number of patients in the SEER registries.

For the first time, 10-year relative survival rates by cancer site are now available from the SEER Program for patients diagnosed in 1973. This will allow researchers to determine better the long-term survival of cancer patients and their potential to be cured.

The annual number of newly diagnosed cancers per 100,000 population (incidence rate) has remained relatively constant from 1974 through 1983, increasing an average of 0.6 percent yearly. The number of people dying of cancer per 100,000 population (death rate) has remained fairly level from 1974 through 1983, with an average increase of only 0.4 percent yearly.

Death rates for some of the major cancers decreased substantially. Decreases, as measured by the percent of change in death rates between 1974–1975 and 1982–1983, occurred for cancers of the bladder, down 13 percent; testis, down 52 percent; colon and rectum, down 5 percent; stomach, down 20 percent; Hodgkin's disease, down 43 percent; cervix uteri, down 30 percent; ovary, down 8 percent; endometrium, down 11 percent; pancreas, down 1 percent; and leukemia, down 1 percent.

Death rates increased for some others: male lung cancer, up 15 percent; female lung cancer, up 72 percent; prostate, up 7 percent; and non-Hodgkin's lymphoma, up 12 percent.

Human Carcinogens and Processes

From time to time, my office is asked for a list of chemicals and other factors known to be carcinogenic for people. Table 35-1 includes those substances and processes that virtually all investigators in this field would agree are human carcinogens. This assessment is based on firm evidence from animal tests and from epidemiologic studies of human populations. This list was compiled principally by Myra Karstadt of Irving Selikoff's Environmental Sciences Laboratory, Mount Sinai, New York, funded by one of our Special Institutional Grants for Cancer Cause and Prevention Research.

Table 35-1 Substance/Process

Aflatoxins	Chlornaphazine	Melphalan
4-Aminobiphenyl	Conjugated estrogens	Mustard gas
Arsenic, arsenic compounds	Bis(chloromethyl) ether	2-Naphthylamine
Asbestos	Chlorambucil	Nickel refining
Azathioprine	Chromium, chromium compounds	Soots, tars, and mineral oils
Benzene	Coke oven emissions	Thorium dioxide
Benzidine	Cyclophosphamide	Thiotepa
Benzidine-based dyes	Diethylstilbestrol	Treosulfan
Chemotherapeutic regimens that include alkylating agents, vinca alkaloids, procarbazine hydrochloride, and prednisone	Estrogens generally	Vinyl chloride
	Underground hematite mining	Tobacco usage
	Iron-dextran	Ethyl alcohol with tobacco usage
	Isopropyl alcohol manufacture (strong acid process)	Marijuana
		x-rays and other sources of irradiation

Viruses (Probable Biologic Carcinogens)
Human t-cell leukemia viruses types I, II, III
Epstein-Barr virus
Hepatitis B virus
Herpes simplex virus type 2
Cytomegalovirus
Papillomaviruses, multiple types

The American Cancer Society Cancer Prevention Study II

One of the largest research studies ever carried out in the United States was launched in 1982. Cancer Prevention Study II (CPS II), a long-term prospective study, is examining the habits and exposures of more than one million Americans to learn how life-styles and environmental factors affect the development of cancer. Modeled after the first ACS Cancer Prevention Study (1959 to 1972), CPS II is similar in method but wider in scope and involves more participants.

More than 77,000 volunteers enrolled 1.2 million men and women in the study. These volunteer researchers distributed a four-page confidential questionnaire to participants who were asked about their exposure to certain environmental conditions, their history of disease, and their life-styles. The questionnaires were designed to elicit more than 500 pieces of information each, which was computerized for statistical analysis.

Many of the questions focus on health issues of current concern. These include risks of certain drugs, foods, and various occupational exposures; low-tar and nicotine cigarettes; consumer products; long-term exposure to low-level radiation; and the health effects associated with air and water pollution. For a period of 6 years, and possibly longer, the volunteers will keep track of the status and whereabouts of study participants. Various suspected relationships will be tested by comparing mortality rates of differently exposed groups.

The goal of the study is to identify those factors that increase a person's chances of developing cancer, those that carry little or no risk, and those that actually may help prevent cancer.

The first Cancer Prevention Study conducted by the ACS produced important findings about health and disease. Study data provided overwhelming evidence that cigarette smoking is the major cause of lung cancer and an important factor in other cancers. It also furnished information on risks of heart disease and other serious illnesses, and revealed a relationship between obesity and certain cancers.

Since the first study, new factors in our environment have been identified that may be related to cancer. The ACS decided to initiate a second study to respond to the concerns of the public and scientific community about suspected carcinogens. Inquiries may be addressed to Lawrence Garfinkel, ACS, overall director of CPS II.

Nutrition and Diet

As of 1986, there appears to be a reasonably close consensus as to what is good for us in terms of cancer and heart disease prevention among recommendations of the National Academy of Sciences, the American Cancer Society, and the American Heart Association. Principal among these are:

1. Eat more cruciferous vegetables (cabbage family)
2. Add more high-fiber foods
3. Choose foods, in a balanced diet, rich in vitamins A, E, and C
4. Reduce intake of total fat
5. Reduce alcohol consumption especially with use of tobacco
6. Reduce intake of salt-cured, smoked, and nitrite-cured foods
7. Reduce obesity by sensible monitored means to lower overall risk to many cancers.

More specifically, investigations continue on the protective action of the food preservative butylated hydroxyanisol (BHA) and on the identification of chemicals in foods that inhibit development of cancers, with brussels sprouts, cabbage, fruits, green coffee beans, and black tea among the interesting candidates.

Great interest centers on vitamin A, and its precursor, β-carotene, along with natural or synthetic analogues of vitamin A, the retinoids. Vitamin A appears critical for normal growth of epithelial cells of the skin and the linings of organs, including lungs, bladder, stomach, colon, esophagus, uterus, and kidneys. Vitamin A deficiencies are associated with abnormalities of these tissues. About one-half of all primary cancers begin in epithelial tissues, with many beyond effective treatment when they are diagnosed.

British researchers found lower levels of retinol in blood sera of men who later developed cancers of various kinds, compared with men having higher levels. Men developing lung cancers had the lowest levels of all. Might the risk of cancers be reduced therefore if blood levels of retinol could be increased? A long-term study of nearly 2,000 men in Chicago found less risk of lung cancer, even among smokers, among men who consumed large amounts of carrots, spinach, and other vegetables containing β-carotene. The seeming protective effect was against lung cancer

only, not other forms of cancer, or other penalties such as heart disease associated with cigarettes. Further studies are needed to confirm such a protective effect against lung cancers; in any case, foods rich in β-carotene are not a passport to "safe" cigarette smoking.

β-Carotene seems able to limit or prevent the growth of transplanted cells in animals and to prolong the animal's life-span even when the tumor burden is high or to make chemotherapy and radiation more effective, reports Dr. Eli Seifter of Albert Einstein College of Medicine. Similarly, Meyskens and associates of the University of Arizona report encouraging preliminary results from high doses of vitamin A to prevent the recurrence, after surgery, of melanoma.

Hundreds of retinoids have been synthesized in a search for toxicity lower than that of vitamin A. One of these, transretinoic acid, was found to be safe and able to reverse the precancerous lesions of the cervix when applied topically with a diaphram. The Arizona team finds that retinoids hold promise also in halting dysplasias of the bladder, oral cavities, and squamous dysplasia of the lung and bowel. Several institutions are pursuing such studies.

Michael Sporn of the NCI Laboratory of Chemoprevention reports substantial progress in arresting or reversing the development of premalignant cells with retinoids. Sporn and associates have shown that synthetic retinoids have prevented breast and bladder cancers in experimental animals. Retinoids given to human patients in trials aimed at preventing recurrent bladder cancers proved too toxic to continue. Safer trials are now appearing. Sporn and Meyskens emphatically warn against intake of high doses of vitamin A, or retinoids, to prevent cancer. Excess vitamin A is a hepatotoxin, and physicians using vitamin A experimentally do so with extreme caution.

The roles of vitamins C and E in health and cancer also remain puzzling. Both C and E are known as antioxidants, meaning they can prevent the conversion of many chemicals into active carcinogens after those chemicals have been eaten or inhaled. Studies on prevention of that conversion continue.

Talalay and Bueding of Johns Hopkins University have shown that BHA can increase the activity of enzymes that can detoxify chemicals capable of causing cell mutations, in particular the glutathione-S-transferases. Current studies by Wattenberg and associates, of the University of Minnesota, are exploring naturally occurring inhibitors in cruciferous vegetables, such as cabbages, brussels sprouts, cauliflower, and broccoli, as well as in green coffee beans and black tea. Specific compounds that cause these effects need to be identified and synthesized as potential food additives.

Finally, Lipkin et al., at the Memorial Sloan-Kettering Cancer Center, New York, have shown that up to 2 g calcium per day orally appears to diminish cellular changes in colon crypt cells generally associated with precancerous and neoplastic lesions. This finding could be very important, following extension and confirmation since calcium is also associated with diminished risk of hypertension and osteoporosis. Other considerations, however, have to do with the apparent contribution of calcium to higher cholesterol levels in some persons as well as risk of kidney stones and interference with copper and magnesium absorption.

Oncogenes

The human genome has the capacity to code for an estimated 50,000 to 100,000 things (e.g., characteristics, enzymes, growth factors). About 40 of the genes have been identified as being responsible for tissue or cell development in young life, largely embryonic. It now seems that when their task is completed, they turn off. We apparently do not need their early function any longer, but they are not lost —they are simply unexpressed. It seems also that mostly later in life they can turn on again, but in an aberrant uncontrolled way, to induce neoplastic lesions. Much remains to be learned of this phenomenon, but the following seem to pertain. These genes exist and can be characterized, the protein products of two or more are present frequently and in multiple copies in a high percentage of animal and human cancers, and cellular oncogenes often have a high degree of homology with gene sequences of known or suspect oncogenic viruses. The hope is that a major part of the molecular basis of cancer has been discovered and that further studies will determine what extrinsic influences turn these apparent common denominator switches on and how this is done. Can this activation be prevented, or can an active gene be rerepressed?

To give the reader a feel for the rapidity, quality, and promise of this effort, this morning (Oct. 16, 1986) a remarkable though expected but explosive finding was reported (Nature) by Robert Weinberg and his associates (Whitehead Institute, Cambridge, Massachusetts). They identified the first gene that functions to prevent cancer in humans, in effect an antioncogene. This finding will surely help clarify the fact of hereditary predisposition to some forms of cancer and may very well provide better means for individual risk assessment and therapy. This first gene discovered to restrain growth is directly associated with risk of retinoblastoma. In hereditary cases, both of two genes are absent or nonfunctional. While this lesion is rare, there is little doubt that other genes will be found that are linked to other familial cancers such as that of the breast; it may help explain why 90 percent of people who smoke do not develop tobacco-related cancers.

It is possible that no other area of cancer research has more potential for cancer prevention, determination of risk, and possibly also of therapy and prognostic evaluation than that of oncogenes and antioncogenes.

Early Specific Detection of Risk and Disease

The search for a $10 finger-prick blood test that would detect earliest cancers of any type has long been a dream of cancer research. Advantages for screening and prognostic evaluation as well as for detection of disease and perhaps even risk to disease are obvious. Within the past 15 years, some 20 such tumor-specific or cancer-specific antigens have been described and in most cases patented. The problem continues to be that no antigens have been found that are truly tumor or cancer specific. The most useful, such as α-fetoprotein (AFP), carcino-embryonic antigen (CEA), and human chorionic gonadotropin (hCG), are not uniquely expressed before or during disease. Rather they and others are tumor-associated antigens; that is, they are quantitatively more present in patients with various cancers than in the apparently noncancerous individual. Nonetheless, the rate of false-positive results, in particular, due to heavy smoking, chronic bronchitis, and a host of other conditions, is far more than acceptable. Monitoring for elevated CEA levels has proved effective in longitudinal evaluation of some patients with some cancers, but here too the rate of apparent false low or high values is problematic.

One of the most recent substance candidates to fill this hope is malignin or antimalignin antibody (AMA). Discovered and developed by a neurochemist, Dr. Samuel Bogach, in the 1970s, malignin is a small (10,000-M_r) peptide antigen detectable by an anti-AMA monoclonal against an antigen characteristic of malignancy (93 percent true-positives) rather than cancer cell type. Bogach et al. claim that tests (approved by FDA in 1976) with AMA pick up the antigen 1 to 19 months before clinical evidence of disease with obvious potential for screening of risk and disease. The authors further state that "This test is a prognostic indicator of how long you're going to live, the first antibody that relates to survival from cancer." My view is that we should keep an eye on this and especially confirmation studies yet to be published (as of September 1986).

A different approach to determination of risk and projected severity of induced disease is being taken by B. Weinstein and colleagues F. Perera and R. Santella, Columbia University, New York. In their studies on the molecular epidemiology of lung cancer, Weinstein and co-workers are exploring the possibility that lung cancer patients have higher levels of DNA and protein adducts in their lung tissue compared with autopsy controls, when exposure via cigarette smoking and other sources is generally the same. If so, one could speculate that, in addition to their exposure, efficiency in binding of carcinogens such as benzo-(α)-pyrene (BaP) to cellular DNA may have been a factor in their disease. They are also probing for activated oncogenes in the same lung tumor and normal (nontumor) lung tissue of lung cancer patients and autopsy controls, in an attempt to relate the different measures of binding to the presence of activated oncogenes. They ask whether these oncogenes are tumor specific and whether any pattern emerges between their presence and histologic or clinical features of cancer.

While data on this approach to molecular epidemiology are preliminary, these studies represent a promising example of a new effort to detect and quantitate risk of exposure to known human carcinogens and consequently may provide a more rational approach to behavioral modification and disease prevention.

The most recent (November 1986) promising blood test for symptomatic cancer and possibly for sequential prognostic evaluation is that of Eric T. Fossel et al., of Beth Israel Hospital and Harvard Med-

ical School, Boston. They reported that plasmas from more than 90 percent of 331 patients with cancers of the breast, ovary, lung, colon, and other organs had detectable changes in lipoproteins as determined by nuclear magnetic resonance (NMR) evaluation. With the exception of some pregnant women and patients with benign prostate hypertrophy, the test differentiated between those with cancer and those apparently without the disease, including patients with other proliferative diseases, such as psoriasis and ulcerative colitis. Furthermore, the test shows promise of correlation with clinical course of disease, being positive in active disease, negative in remission, and again positive in relapse. Much more needs to be done especially as to whether the test can detect very early (nonsymptomatic) cancer and even in those at highest risk of cancer.

Viruses and Vaccines

In 1986 we recognized the 75th anniversary of the beginning of the modern era of viral oncology and, therefore, of molecular biology. The science of viral oncology began around 1910, when a farmer walked into the relatively primitive laboratory of a young intern at Rockefeller Institute with a sick chicken. The doctor's name was Peyton Rous, and the chicken had a tumor. Rous cut the tumor out, ground it with saline and sand, passed its fluid through a diatomaceous filter capable of withholding intact cells, and induced the same kind of tumor in normal chickens inoculated with the brew. A filterable agent was present, similar perhaps to that peculiar phenomenon of Twort and d'Herelle and the lysis of bacteria in 1917 and perhaps even to that of Ellerman and Bang (Denmark) in 1908, who transmitted avian leucosis without cells. But Rous and Murphy, at the respected Rockefeller Institute, working with chickens and a reproducible neoplastic lesion, a fibrosarcoma, were frequently criticized with such comments as, "But it's infectious and, therefore, an inflammatory reaction, and in any event what does it have to do with mouse or human cancer?"

Next came the early seminal confirmations and contributions of scientists such as Andervont, Beard, Bittner, Bryan, Duran-Reynals, Gross, Groupe, Luke, Moore, Shimkin, Shope, and Syverton. Then it happened: the "sciences" became quantifiable, and the observations of Rous and Murphy were accepted, albeit with some reluctance. However, as late as about 1950, viral oncology people had to assemble in someone's hotel room to exchange information even at annual meetings of cancer research scientists.

Today we know of more than 100 different viruses that induce cancers in nearly all animals that have been carefully studied. Indeed, we can engineer new tumor viruses through the science of recombinant DNA technology, itself a product of research on viruses. We recognize four classes of viruses that cause or are an important component in the causation of cancers in people: HTLV-I and HTLV-III, hepatitis B, papilloma and EBV, and other herpes viruses. If these probabilities are true, up to 25 percent of the world's cancers may be virus induced or accountably related, especially hepatitis B virus and primary hepatoma.

During the 1950s to 1960s, investigators were looking for extractable viruses from human tissues that essentially had the same properties as the many viruses already isolated from animal cancers. For the most part, and for reasons not yet well understood, human cancer viruses were not there or did not behave predictably. Brave souls began talking about parasitism at the genetic level or the heritable and transmissible insertion by viruses of information into cellular genome. To virologists this was elegant but near heresy because it could have meant that the continued presence of the intact virus was not necessary for the continuation of the tumor as a tumor.

Then emerged the concept of the "hit-and-run" mechanism attributed largely to DNA viruses, such as polyomavirus, SV-40, and later other adenoviruses. (I can remember none who attributed this capacity to RNA viruses.) At least some of this RNA thinking had to do with many studies of their cousin RNA viruses of influenza, polio, measles, mumps, and the like. Also in particular, because of the concept and then proof, of vertical transmission. Mice born to carriers of AKR leukemia or C3H mammary tumor viruses developed these diseases because they were infected with intact and recoverable viruses in utero.

But then came the identification and biologic characterization of reverse transcriptase, by Baltimore and Temin, as a function of RNA tumor viruses. This work greatly enhanced the supposition that (1) the intact virus was not necessary for infection and disease inductions; (2) only a piece was necessary; (3) this piece might be a viral gene, and (4) this gene might be insertable into and transmissible in a heritable fashion by the cellular genome. Thus was born and extended the field of molecular virology/oncology. In a summary of virology the road ahead may not be straighter or quicker but the questions seem cleaner to ask and even possibly to answer:

To what extent can viruses pick up "normal" cellular genes required for normal growth and function? Are they changed in the pickup? Are their protein products changed or made in overabundance? How many oncogenes are there? Are two or more involved in initiation and promotion? Are they involved at all, or are relatively few etiologically involved as common denominators in the 100 or more diseases we call cancer?

If oncogenes become oncogenic somewhere along the chain of events that leads to clinical cancer, what can be done to prevent them from being turned on? And what can we do to turn them off? (Is cancer of adults so tied to the aging process that these questions are moot?)

The American Cancer Society has long supported research in virtually all areas discussed, most recently into the biology, including clinical and pharmacokinetic trial studies of the interferons, tumor necrosis factor, and lymphotoxin. Past support has contributed to the development of effective vaccines for cat leukemia and Marek's disease of chickens. Current virology support by the ACS includes further research into the cancer sequelae of acquired immunodeficiency syndrome (AIDS) and the development and preventive potential of vaccines, against the herpes and papillomaviruses that are probably causatively related to some cancers in people. Projections as to when these newer technologies will be usable for high-risk persons by the community physician are risky and, worse, smack of overpromise and overexpectation. But the hepatitis B vaccine (HBV) is here now, and some other newer technologies for prevention and treatment should be no longer than 2 to 5 years down the road. As virtually all clinician scientists well recognize, there is now a front-line body of information that may be exploitable for prevention and for new drug design, treatment, earlier detection of risk, and disease and prognostic evaluation.

And therein lies some of the new challenge—the obligatory opportunity for physicians who treat patients with cancer to test and use interferons, other cytokines, monoclonal antibodies, and antiviral agents (antisubcomponents?) for patient benefit. After 75 years, one can view with unabashed respect the efforts of those who argued steadfastly in the early years for support of a major research effort in this area.

The four principal candidate viruses as human oncogenes are (HBV), Epstein-Barr virus (EBV), papilloma virus (APV), and the family of human T-lymphotropic viruses (HTLV-I, II, and III). By and large, they are linked to cancers that affect relatively few Americans, although they are responsible for hundreds of thousands of deaths worldwide each year.

HEPATITIS B VIRUS

Spread from person to person by means of body fluids, such as blood, saliva, and mucus, hepatitis B infects the liver and can cause serious damage. Most patients get over an acute hepatitis attack and recover, carrying antibodies to the virus in their blood thereafter. But about 15 percent of these persons become carriers of the disease. Apparently well, they nevertheless continue to produce virus, which can be transmitted to other people through intimate contact, blood transfusions, or in the case of intravenous drug abusers, through shared needles. Hepatitis B carriers have chronic active hepatitis and stand at risk of developing cancer of the liver.

Hepatocellular carcinoma, is uncommon in the United States, but it is a major public health problem and the leading cause of death from cancer in many developing countries, particularly in Africa and the Orient.

Exactly how chronic active hepatitis infection leads to liver cancer is not known. One problem has been that until recently, there was no way to study the disease in animals. Recently, a few species other than humans were found to have their own forms of hepatitis B virus. Some of these animals become carriers and can develop liver cancers. Dr. William S. Robinson of Stanford University conducted pioneering studies of hepatitis in a colony of ground squirrels. The existence of animal models, which also include the common North American woodchuck and the domestic white duck, means that the events leading from the carrier state to the development of cancers can be studied. When that is known, perhaps ways can be found to interrupt the sequence and prevent the malignancy.

Meantime, even without specific understanding of

how liver cancer arises in hepatitis B carriers, an effective vaccine has been developed that prevents uninfected persons from infection. By removing this factor from the equation, physicians postulate that the vaccine will prevent liver cancers from developing. The hepatitis B vaccine made from viral surface antigen of infected plasma, now undergoing large-scale tests in Taiwan and in homosexuals in the United States appears to be the first true anticancer vaccine for humans. The recent production of surface antigen in yeast through recombinant DNA technology plasma should provide large quantities of an effective safe vaccine at a fraction of present cost, free of difficult dependence on human plasma.

On the other hand, the vaccine cannot help people who are already hepatitis B carriers, and at present there is no treatment that can terminate their chronic infection. They remain at risk of developing liver cancers later in life and of passing the virus on to other people who have not been vaccinated.

This points up one problem common to all the viruses associated with cancer and, indeed, with all viruses that affect humans and animals. With the exception of interferon, the natural antiviral factor, there are few other if any, effective drugs with which to treat viral infections that may lead to cancer. Some such as arabinoside a (ara-a), amantidine, and zovirin are under study, but so far none can stop viral infections as effectively as penicillin and other antibiotics do against bacterial infections. One of the great research challenges in cancer, then, is to develop compounds that can stop viral infections such as hepatitis B.

EPSTEIN-BARR VIRUS

Epstein-Barr virus, a member of the large family of herpes viruses, is ubiquitous. Few of us have not been exposed and infected. In most people, EBV causes a mild, sometimes barely noticeable infection. In some, particularly young adults, it causes infectious mononucleosis from which most patients recover completely.

Under certain circumstances, however, EBV is a factor in the development of two types of cancer: nasopharyngeal carcinoma and Burkitt's lymphoma (an extremely aggressive cancer of the B lymphocytes that mostly affects young children). Nasopharyngeal carcinoma is extremely rare in the United States, except among immigrants from southeastern China, where it is one of the commonest of cancers. Nasopharyngeal cancer cells have been found to contain active EBV. Burkitt's lymphoma is prevalent in certain parts of Africa, where it appears that EBV needs to interact with other endemic factors, including malaria.

Arnold J. Levine, of Princeton University, is using recombinant DNA methodology to analyze different parts of the very large EBV virus to discover what abnormal proteins are made by EBV-infected cells and whether these substances play a role in malignancy. Elliott Kieff, of the University of Chicago, is looking for differences in the nucleic acid fingerprints of different EBV strains. Viral infection, by hepatitis B in the case of liver cancer, and by EBV in Burkitt's lymphoma, appears to stimulate rapid proliferation of cells as the tissue tries to repair itself. During this proliferation, certain cells become immortalized; that is, they escape the restraints on growth that keep many normal cells from reproducing in vitro. When other factors, such as genetic predisposition or infection are present, neoplastic transformation can occur. This would be why some, but not all, hepatitis B carriers develop liver cancer and why the vast majority of people exposed to EBV develop neither Burkitt's lymphoma nor nasopharyngeal carcinoma.

A strong rational case has been made for further development and use of an EBV vaccine of a cellular membrane glycoprotein antigen (magp340) induced by the virus. This will probably be done initially for the prevention of infectious mononucleosis and then of Burkitt's lymphoma and nasopharyngeal carcinoma in high-risk individuals. The antigen is stable, safe, abundant, and assayable and induces 100 percent protection against malignant tumors induced by EBV in the cottontop tamirin, a rare Columbian monkey now bred in the laboratory.

More work needs to be done on this preventative approach, but it seems likely that recombinant DNA technology will provide a testable gp340 vaccine against EBV-induced diseases.

PAPILLOMAVIRUSES

There are many strains of papillomavirus, most of which cause unsightly but generally nonthreatening warts of one form or another. Warts are not malignant, they do not invade neighboring normal tissues as cancer cells do, nor do they metastasize. Their growth can be unpredictable, and they are often difficult to cure. A relatively rare type of wart, as juvenile laryngeal papilloma, can interfere with breathing or speech and, until it was found that interferon could stop the relentless growth of cells, this condition could not be treated with predictable success. Papillomaviruses transmitted sexually, and causing painful condyloma acuminatum or genital warts, can now be treated with interferon as well as with surgery.

It has recently been found that sexually transmitted papilloma viruses may play a role in the development of cancer of the cervix. In the United States, where Papanicolaou (Pap) smears detect this condition very early and where prompt treatment cures virtually all patients whose disease is detected early, cervical cancer is no longer the problem it used to be. It will nevertheless claim 6,500 lives in the United States in 1985 and is the leading cause of cancer death among women in Latin America.

Cervical cancer is most common among women who began sexual activity in their early teens and have multiple partners. It is thought that during this time, when the tissues of the cervix are still maturing and its squamous cells are proliferating rapidly, those viruses (HPV types 16 and 18 especially) integrate into the DNA of these cells as potential future oncogenes.

As with HBV and EBV, the relationship between papillomavirus infection and the development of cervical cancer may involve other factors. It is known, for example, that the mutation-causing chemicals in cigarette smoke travel quickly from the mouth throughout the body and concentrate in the mucous membranes elsewhere, including those in the vagina and cervix. Recently, a large study of women with cervical cancer in Czechoslovakia showed that while early sexual activity was a major risk factor, as expected, cigarette smoking increased the risk substantially. Possibly, chemicals in cigarette smoke that find their way to the cervix, where they act in concert with papillomavirus on the growing squamous cells to set the scene for cancer later in life.

Since squamous cells make up tissues in other parts of the body and are transformation targets in cancers of the bladder and some cancers of the skin and the lung, can papilloma viruses induce other cancers as well? Studies are now gearing up to investigate this possibility.

What continues to be badly needed since Shope

isolated the first tumor-associated papillomavirus of rabbits are cell culture systems in which to grow adequate quantities of virus for study, especially for gene mapping and function. An exciting experimental system used by Kreiden and Rapp, of the Hershey Medical School, involving the renal capsule of nude mice as a recipient chamber of cells from human papillomas, has permitted the recent demonstration of viral replication and of the transformation of human cells but apparently not yet to true malignancy.

Similarly, Lacy, Alpert, and Hanahan were able to transmit bovine papilloma virus-1 genome through a mouse germ line with resultant heritable incorporation in all cells of the mouse and induction of fibropapillomas of the skin.

Current data suggest that HPV 16 and 18 are the main candidates for cervical carcinoma and that types 5 and 8 are suspect in the etiology of epidermodysplasia verruciformis. Because many male partners of women with these diseases have similar lesions the hope (and current research emphasis) is that effective vaccines against the most prevalent strains can be developed, should this be warranted, as has already been done for cattle.

HUMAN T LYMPHOTROPIC VIRUS

Since many leukemias in animals are caused by viruses, scientists searched for decades to find an example of virally induced leukemia in humans. They were spurred on by reports of leukemia clusters — a number of cases of leukemia occurring in the same geographic area, at about the same time. Nowadays, statisticians view clustering skeptically, since it can be explained largely by chance, and no infectious agent, viral or otherwise, or chemical cause, has been pinpointed. It was impossible to ignore, however, the hard knowledge that viruses did cause cancer in animals other than humans. This was first discovered in 1911 by Dr. Peyton Rous of Rockefeller Institute, and over the years, scientists found that chickens, mice, monkeys, cats, cows, and virtually every animal they tested could develop some form of cancer as a consequence of viral infection. Was it likely that humans were exempt from so universal a pattern?

During the 1950s and 1960s, NCI scientists pursued a concerted effort to find a viral-cancer link in humans. But without monoclonal antibodies to detect and define viruses and their products, and without

recombinant DNA methods to analyze the sequences of nucleic acids in viruses and cells, they ran into many blind alleys. From 1974 through 1982, Myron T. Essex of the Harvard School of Public Health focused his research on a virus that caused leukemia in cats. His studies, supported by the American Cancer Society, paved the way for those that later established unquestionably that HTLV-I caused adult T-cell leukemia. Essex found that a cat infected with feline leukemia virus (FELV) had a 5 percent chance of later developing leukemia; in other words, the great majority of infected animals did not become leukemic. Unknowingly, he was working with an animal model that mirrored a virally-caused leukemia in humans.

In 1981, after 12 years of painstaking work, Robert C. Gallo of the National Cancer Institute proved that a virus was the cause of a human malignancy; one that paralleled the feline leukemia studied by Essex. The disease was a particularly aggressive form of leukemia in which the T cells, the soldiers of the immune system, become malignant and infiltrate everywhere in the body. Patients with this disease often have extensive and painful skin lesions, in addition to their symptoms of rapidly progressing leukemia; without a properly functioning immune system, each patient is at risk of severe infection.

The first patients in whom this leukemia was found were a group of eight black men from the southeastern United States; it was thought at first that this was an extremely rare form of leukemia.

As soon as the human T-cell leukemia virus (HTLV), as it was then called, was announced in the scientific literature, Japanese scientists at Kyoto University reported that in their part of southwestern Japan, very aggressive T-cell leukemia with the same clinical features as the rare American form was, in fact, very common. This leukemia, too, involved a virus, and in time it was known that the HTLV virus discovered at NCI and the virus associated with what the Japanese called adult T-cell leukemia were the same.

Extensive medical detective work has since demonstrated that viral-induced T-cell leukemia is not rare at all but worldwide. It is the leading malignancy of the blood-forming tissues in the Caribbean, and it has also been found in Latin America, Sicily, Africa, and elsewhere. The cases are nearly always from the same geographic area; patients who do not live in areas where the incidence is high generally turn out to have lived in such places in the past. Interestingly, in areas where there are many cases of this leukemia, there are also perfectly healthy people who have antibodies to the virus in their blood. This probably indicates that they too have been exposed to the virus in the past but that their bodies have fought it off, leaving them immune.

It would seem that the effects of HTLV differ among people, perhaps in a way that resembles the effects of the poliovirus. (Polio infection in the very young causes a minor illness that quickly passes; in older children and young adults, its effects can be devastating and may cause death.) Only about 1 in 80 people who have been infected with HTLV ever develops the leukemia. It also appears that HTLV is not "catching" in the ordinary sense, probably requiring long-term intimate contact in order to spread from one person to another. Family members of the leukemia patients are more likely to have antibodies to the virus, and at higher levels, than are people in the general population in the same area.

The form of the virus that causes the adult T-cell leukemia is now known as HTLV-I. A second strain was isolated from a patient with another type of leukemia and is known as HTLV-II. A third strain, HTLV-III, is now recognized as the cause of AIDS. Unlike HTLV-I, which turns T Cells into deadly leukemia cells, HTLV-III kills them outright. Instead of a flood of useless malignant T cells, HTLV-III leaves the patient with no appropriate T cells at all. So completely are the T cells eliminated that it was difficult to find the virus in AIDS patients, since they had no T cells left in which to harbor it. Stripped of disease-fighting T cells, AIDS patients are defenseless against infections. Within 2 years after diagnosis, 80 percent of AIDS patients are killed by infection. HTLV-I is probably spread through long-term close contact, within a family, for example. HTLV-III is spread through bodily fluids, which may contain infected T cells. Such fluids include blood, semen, and perhaps saliva; the virus is spread through sexual contact, through blood transfusions, from infected pregnant mother to newborn child, and from infected intravenous drug abusers to anyone sharing a contaminated needle. About 15,000 people in the United States have died with AIDS since the disease was first reported in 1981.

But of those who do not die of infections, well over one-third develop cancers of very specific kinds. Most closely associated with AIDS is Kaposi's sarcoma, a disease once found predominantly in elderly men of Italian or Jewish heritage. In them, this purplish cancer of the soft tissues near the skin grew indolently; most patients lived a normal span of years and died from some other cause.

In AIDS patients, however, Kaposi's sarcoma is a much more malignant disease, attacking much younger people. This form can be treated fairly successfully with interferon. In addition, patients with AIDS may also develop B-cell lymphomas in the brain, a very unusual type of cancer. Neither Kaposi's sarcoma nor the B-cell lymphomas seems to be caused directly by the HTLV-III virus, but although the mechanism is not understood, the link is clear.

Recently, William Haseltine, of Harvard Medical School found that all the viruses of the HTLV family produce gene-stimulating proteins that change the behavior of the infected cells. This phenomenon, known as transactivation, accounts for the ability of HTLV-I and -II to transform T cells into malignant cells. The process is much more pronounced in HTLV-III infected cells and apparently accounts for the devastation of the T cells.

FUTURE PROSPECTS

Although the idea that viruses can play a role in human cancer is sobering, much about this story is hopeful. Viruses can be prevented when vaccines are available to protect people. The worldwide use of vaccine against smallpox has wiped out this disease altogether. Polio, which killed and crippled thousands every year in the United States alone, is a shrinking public health problem. It is possible, at least in theory, to create vaccines against the viruses associated with human cancer, as seems to have been done with hepatitis B. Even when other factors associated with the development of the cancer remain, such as genetic predisposition, environmental conditions, and life-style, the elimination of the virus from the equation would mean that the other elements could not add up to cancer induction.

Work is proceeding on a vaccine against EBV, but because this is more than 20 times as large and complex as the other three viruses discussed here, progress is expected to be slow. Investigators are currently working on vaccines against the different strains of papilloma virus and the HTLV family of viruses, each of which involves special complications. The hepatitis B vaccine, however, does in fact prevent infection with this virus, after three properly timed injections. Vaccine research is slow, costly, and difficult and although promising, will not yield results immediately.

The down side of the strategy of preventing cancer by vaccinating against viruses is that it may take a long time for any impact on cancer incidence to be felt. Nor do most vaccines cure viral infections that have already occurred. For this reason, there is renewed effort to develop antiviral drugs, which could prevent cancer by cutting short the viral infections that precede them. So far, none is completely effective or free from serious side effects. Even the natural product interferon causes flulike symptoms and may have severe temporary psychological effects.

For the HTLV family of viruses, entirely different types of antiviral drugs may be needed. These are RNA viruses, or retroviruses; unlike others, which are DNA viruses, the retroviruses must go through an additional step in order to infect a cell. This step requires an enzyme called reverse transcriptase. Scientists believe that if they can create a drug to block this enzyme, they will be able to prevent infection.

Discovering that anything so specific as a virus is needed for a particular kind of cancer to develop is, for scientists, like finding a chink in that cancer's armor. It's a weak spot, an opportunity to attack, a chance to focus research, and possibly a place where, in the future, some kind of therapeutic intervention could be designed to prevent that cancer from developing. Another of the newer, still experimental, approaches to vaccine development is being pursued by Ariel Hollingshead, at George Washington University. Dr. Hollingshead isolates, purifies, and stabilizes quantitatively tumor-associated antigens (TAA) from surface membranes of lung cancer cells. In a cooperative study with Thomas H.M. Stewart, University of Ottawa, these proteins were given once a month for 3 months, following surgery, to 28 patients. Five years later, 80 percent were still alive, compared with 50 percent of 24 patients not receiving vaccine. Similar immunogens were also prepared against squamous cell, large cell, and small cell carcinomas, and adenomas of the lung, and are now being tested in cancer centers in the United States, Canada, England, and France in a larger long-term study of the efficacy of these materials involving more than 100 patients.

Tumor-associated antigens against melanoma, cancer of the colon, ovary, bladder, brain, and other sites are also being developed. This international collaboration could determine whether such vaccines might protect high-risk persons against cancer such as those of asbestos workers who smoke cigarettes.

A vaccine to permit cigarette smokers to indulge their habit is not in the offing. A single vaccine against all or even many cancers appears most improbable.

Not unlike these studies by Hollingshead are those of Michael Hanna, of the Litton Institute of Applied Biotechnology, Frederick Cancer Research Facility, Frederick, Maryland, on active specific immunotherapy (ASI). Vaccines or immunogenic substances are produced from tumor cells of an individual patient's colon resection which are then combined with bacillus Calmette-Guérin (bCG), a bacterial immunostimulant, and injected back into the same patient. Phase 3 trials through the Eastern Cooperative Oncology Group (ECOG) are showing a remarkable significant delay and a decrease in the incidence of tumor recurrence and mortality in patients treated with an autologous vaccine compared with those treated with surgery alone. Hanna and co-workers also demonstrated that peripheral lymphocytes of immunized patients produced large quantities of monoclonal antibodies (MAB) specific to their colon tumors. Human MAB therapy alone or combined with these vaccines with or without adjuvant chemotherapy is under way in patients with colon, lung, pancreas, and other cancers, through ECOG and Hanna's group.

OTHER NEW TREATMENT RESEARCH

Sidney Farber showed in the 1940s that the lives of some children with acute lymphocytic leukemia were extended significantly during and following treatment with the antifolate, aminopterin. An intensive program by the NCI followed through its Cancer Chemotherapy National Service Program that helped develop new drugs and drug combinations to extend further survival and cure of children with ALL and other cancers. The wisdom and success of this and other programs are reflected in Table 35-2, which compares the leading causes of death in children aged 1 to 14 in the United States, from 1959–1963 to 1979–1983. Note that the number and rates of mortality with childhood cancers declined by nearly one-

Table 35-2 Leading Causes of Death in Children Aged 1 to 14 Years: Number of Deaths and Death Rate per 1,000,000 Population in the United States, 1959–1963 to 1979–1983

Cause	1959–1963 Deaths/(Rate)	1964–1968 Deaths/(Rate)	1969–1973 Deaths/(Rate)	1974–1978 Deaths/(Rate)	1979–1983 Deaths/(Rate)
Accidents	59,656 (225.9)	64,580 (233.0)	62,674 (232.0)	50,319 (200.0)	40,542 (169.3)
Cancer	21,132 (80.0)	19,743 (71.2)	16,300 (60.3)	12,272 (48.8)	10,260 (42.8)
Congenital malformations	15,788 (59.8)	13,319 (48.1)	11,413 (42.2)	9,170 (36.5)	7,711 (32.2)
Pneumonia and influenza	16,168 (61.2)	12,344 (44.5)	7,854 (29.1)	4,214 (16.8)	2,066 (8.6)
Heart disease	2,287 (8.7)	2,465 (8.9)	3,043 (11.3)	2,918 (11.6)	3,215 (13.4)
Homicide	1,747 (6.6)	2,718 (9.8)	3,212 (11.9)	3,628 (14.4)	3,679 (15.4)

(U.S. National Center for Health Statistics.)

half during this 20-year period. This is especially impressive in view of incidence rates having remained virtually the same during that period. Most cancers of childhood are characterized as being rapidly growing wherein a large portion of their cells are in active DNA synthesis. So too virtually all drugs selected for use were picked up as active in animal systems with rapidly growing transplantable tumors. Within the past decade, major efforts have been launched to develop and use compounds (e.g., platinum, cytokines) against the preponderance of cancers that grow relatively slowly. Clearly, the further development of additional cytotoxic compounds and biologic response modifiers of lower general toxicity and their use as adjuvants to surgery and radiotherapy should herald the next quantum improvement in management of the cancer patient. Following Dr. Farber's seminal contributions to chemotherapy and ALL of children, many other technologies for meaningful life extension and cure are now used routinely, among which are (1) the studies of Pinkel et al. on total brain irradiation of ALL children with chemotherapy induced remission to kill protected reservoirs of leukemic cells; (2) improved use of single drugs and their analogues; (3) compilation, use, and improvement of combination chemotherapy; and (4) most recent reports of up to 50 percent induction of apparent complete second remissions by bone marrow transplantation of children resistant to chemotherapy. Other areas of intensive research considered most promising toward cure by most investigators include:

Antiangiogenesis

Tumors like any other tissue need a food supply to maintain viability and growth. This is most routinely accomplished by host vascularization into the tumor upon demand (angiogenesis factors) of the tumor. This is too often accomplished at the expense of normal host vitality, the familiar cachectic syndromes. Judah Folkman et al., of Harvard University, pioneered the development of animal models to test for factors that might inhibit angiogenesis. Their most recent studies show that heparin plus hydrocortisone (but not either alone) profoundly inhibit the growth of animal tumors or of human tumors transplanted to animals including embryonated eggs through processes of antiangiogenesis. This essentially nontoxic form of chemotherapy may well have value in the treatment of some human cancers. Other materials also known to inhibit angiogenesis include cartilage extracts, vitreous substance, aortic wall extracts, protamine sulfate and depletion of serum copper. Most recently (1986) Folkman and associates isolated and characterized a protein from human tumors, angiogenin, which enhances angiogenesis.

Hyperthermia

Attempts to exploit heat for selective toxicity of tumor tissue have been made for more than 100 years beginning with observations that fever associated with bacterial septicemia was sometimes associated with tumor regression.

More recent studies of heat as a therapeutic agent include the development of hardware for delivery and precise monitoring of energy to superficial and deep-seated lesions and its use in combination with radiotherapy and chemotherapy. Because 42°C is the upper limit for whole-body hyperthermia, its use as an adjuvant to radiotherapy or chemotherapy seems more feasible and promising than heat alone. Although more than 12,000 patients with different cancers have been treated with heat along or in combination with other modalities since 1977, much remains to be done in the design and evaluation of clinical trials before hyperthermia joins the armamentarium of cancer therapy.

Psychosocial Research

In 1984 the ACS began funding research into the other side of cancer: what the disease does to people psychologically and socially, in addition to physical impairment. Questions abound. How to induce people to seek early detection of cancers? How to induce cessation of smoking? How best to deal with family crises over cancer, especially when children are involved? How to handle fears, grief, despair? How to correct a misperception that cancer is always a sentence to lingering and painful death? How to inform people about the optimistic issues in cancer—the cured patients and their problems?

Psychosocial research in cancer is a new field, developing largely over the past 10 years. So keen is the interest among clinical investigators that 27 applications for grants were made to the ACS in the spring of 1983 before the formal announcement had been made that a support program was available; total support has reached approximately $4,169,100 million by 1986. Current projects include:

1. The effectiveness of methods used to teach breast self-examination
2. How attitude and behavior of physicians affect cancer patients both positively and negatively
3. The prevention of nausea when patients merely think about taking drugs
4. How to keep ex-smokers from succumbing again
5. The management of psychological and sexual concerns of men and women after treatment for certain cancers

6. How best to identify and screen high-risk people for colorectal cancer

Since approximately one-half of all patients now survive their cancer, a new issue is the care of the cured patient and the quality of life for long survivors and cured patients. Many people worry whether their cancer might recur. Too many learn they cannot get jobs or health insurance because they have had cancer. Most likely, they face a normal life but are victims of unreasoned prejudice. Their psychological hurts are real.

Another current objective is to make psychosocial research more scientifically sound by drawing on skills of various specialists and devising reliable research methods and tools specifically for use with cancer patients.

Some may need drugs to relieve depression and anxiety. Others need advice about colostomies and other ostomies. Cancer patients often have a sense of being damaged or impaired, not in control of themselves, of needing help in re-establishing healthy attitudes and normal functioning. Women often ask about breast reconstruction after cancer surgery, and many who have it report a significant improvement in their self-esteem and psychological sense of well-being.

Research is increasing toward understanding the interplay between the human body, mind and emotions, with provocative results. Grief over the death of wives seems to put some men at greater risk of dying in the next year, compared with matched, still-married men. The reason is not clear. It may involve altered life-style and health behavior or may involve some interaction of emotions with hormones and the immune reaction. Some cardiac researchers point to evidence for a personality prone to heart attacks, the so-called type A hard-driving, pushed-for-time man. While suggestive, data for a cancer-prone personality, similar to type A and heart disease, are incomplete.

Available evidence does not support the theory that techniques of reducing stress can change the risk of cancer or the length of survival. While there is need for research in this area, the use of clinical psychosocial interventions that claim to alter tumor growth cannot be recommended at this time. But stress and anxiety can influence physical well-being and behavior. The problem is that it can have both positive and negative effects, depending on the conditions of the experiment. The late Vernon T. Riley, a microbiologist at the Pacific Northwest Research Foundation in Seattle, sought to study this in experiments with mice susceptible to a virus-induced cancer. He proved that laboratory mice were being subjected to considerable stress, such as noise, odors, temperature changes, and handling. When he protected his mice against as much stress of this type as he could, only 7 percent of animals developed the virus-induced cancers after 13 months, compared with 60 percent that continued to live under the stress. The stressed mice showed more hormonal changes that might impair their immune defenses. Other investigations have shown that under certain circumstances, stress seems to *protect* animals from developing tumors.

Research in this area does not concern patients alone. Physicians, nurses, other caretakers, in families or hospitals, who must give people bad news, work many hours, see too many defeats, and often share the loss of patients with their families also need counseling and support.

Establishment of a clearinghouse for information on psychosocial research in cancer must be developed as an essential next step.

Biologic Response Modifiers

Beginning in about 1980, professional, lay, and media communities have heard much about immune enhancers probably associated with the unfortunate "hype" of interferon by the media, although not entirely by the media. This description is usually thought of as including essentially natural substances, less toxic than conventional cytotoxic chemotherapy that will prevent cancer or enhance the body's ability to live with cancer in a more pleasant way. Not at all surprising that patients are encouraged.

INTERFERON

Interferon as a modern prototype (BCG goes back further) holds the hope of allowing the physician the only available "nonchemotherapeutic" means of a systemic therapy adjuvant to surgery and radiation for immediate or maintenance therapy. As is well recognized, it used to be thought that the major reason cancer recurred was because of inefficient surgery or radiotherapy. We now know that for the most part cancer recurs because it was already metastasized in 60

percent of patients (United States: most cancers) at first presentation to the physician. As well and long recognized by oncologists, this can only mean that most patients must be treated systemically. Prior to biologic response modifiers (BRMs) the only way this could be done responsibly was by cytotoxic chemotherapy before, during, or after (and often long after) surgery or radiotherapy. BRMs may offer an additive or alternative means of systemic therapy. In keeping with the intent of this chapter, following are experimental areas that appear now (1986) to offer promise for application to people benefit.

A natural substance, later called interferon, was discovered by Issacs and Lindeman in England in 1957. It was produced in virus-infected cells that inhibited infection of adjacent cell by the same or other viruses.

This remained an interesting antiviral agent, one of the very few at that time, until the 1960s, when Gresser, in Paris, showed an apparent antimitotic anticancer effect in ACR mice with a high incidence of apparent virus-induced leukemia. The supposition followed that suspect virus-induced cancers (leukemia, lymphoma, breast) might be especially vulnerable to interferon therapy. But it was soon realized that interferon was species specific. That is, to treat chicken or mouse cancers with interferon, one had to make quantities of interferon in cells of chickens or mice, so too with human interferon for human cancers. Cantel, in Finland, developed a way to make more and better amounts of interferon in human leucocytes deliberately infected with an influenza virus, during the 1970s. Following that seminal contribution, Strander and others in Sweden published data suggesting that patients so treated, with osteogenic sarcoma, did better than historic controls with the same disease. Within a few years anecdotal observations on beneficial effects with a few patients with breast cancer and non-Hodgkins lymphoma became apparent. At that time, because of the stimulus of Gutterman at the M.D. Anderson Hospital and Tumor Institute, in Houston, and others, the ACS committed $2.8 million to purchase interferon from Finland for evaluation in American cancer patients.

Then and now, comparisons are as follows. In 1980 no American company produced interferon; it had to be purchased in Finland. Today interferon is produced by many companies in the United States. At that time, it was thought that only one form of interferon existed. Today we recognize at least 14 gene products of interferon. At that time, interferon was only one type with a purity of 1 part in 1,000. Today it is pure primarily through the sciences of recombinant technology. At that time, there was only enough of the impure natural product to treat no more than about 125 patients. Finally, at that time, that product alone cost about $30,000 to treat one patient. Today it costs about $200 to $300.

Interferon is not a magic bullet, but it has served as a prototype for the development of other BRMs and has in fact been approved (since August 1986) for use in wide treatment of hairy cell leukemia (90 percent remission response rate). Other uses for kidney cancer, Kaposi sarcoma, laryngeal papilloma, and cancer of bladder, bone marrow, and skin (melanoma) may join the list of approved for treatment-sensitive cancers.

As to the mechanism of action, an interesting and possibly important part of the biology of interferon is that in addition to being an immune modulator, it also has a capacity to be cytotoxic against "resting cells" or those not in active DNA synthesis. This is why newer protocols seek to determine whether interferon might work better in combination with traditional chemotherapeutic drugs — virtually all of which have been screened against and used against tumors which grow rapidly.

TUMOR NECROSIS FACTOR

Tumor necrosis factor (TNF) is a potent lymphokine produced by activated mononuclear phagocytes or lymphocytes with remarkable direct cytotoxic effects preferentially against cancer cells. Interestingly it is an extension of an observation made more than 100 years ago by Coley that some cancer patients with a bacterial septicemia underwent a spontaneous regression of tumor. For some time debate followed as to whether this was due to fever or to bacterial toxins. The technologies of bacteriology were not well advanced at that time, and Coley's toxins were neither quantitable nor reproducible. The advent of competent radiotherapy further made this approach to therapy less enduring. Years later, however, Lloyd Old, et al., at Memorial Sloan-Kettering, began to determine the scientific basis of this phenomenon. TNF is real and appears about ready to join those BRMs to be tested against human malignancies. Reportedly its genes (there seem to be two) produce anticancer prod-

ucts that, unlike interferon, are nonspecies specific but that may be almost identical to cachectin, a factor that appears to induce the wasting syndrome in many cancer patients, more needs to be done.

INTERLEUKINS

The interleukins were first described as growth factors for human T-leukocytes by Robert Gallo, of the NCI. This was the substance that allowed Gallo and others to propagate T-4 cells in culture for growth of what is now called the AIDS virus (HTLV-3). Recognizing that primed T-4 cells may be aggressively anticancer Rosenberg et al. of the NCI, developed a means to propagate and further sensitize these cells in tissue culture with IL-2 and then return the mix plus additional doses of IL-2 to the patient. Their results in inducing heretofor unseen remission rates in cancer patients were encouraging. Rosenberg and his colleagues, P. Spiess and R. Lafreniere, most recently have extended and refined these observations by isolating and propagating tumor-infiltrating lymphocytes (TIL) from murine tumors. When exposed to IL-2 and combined with cyclophosphamide in the treatment of murine tumors, this combination and procedure appears to be far more effective than the original lymphokine-activated killer (LAK) cell procedure with less than 10 percent of that procedure's toxicity. Application to human disease and especially micrometastases is imminent.

MONOCLONAL ANTIBODIES

The promise of monoclonal antibodies for detection, diagnosis, treatment, and prognostic evaluation remains extraordinarily high, but for the most part not yet realized. With few apparent exceptions, tumor-specific antigens have not yet been isolated, and monoclonal antibodies against tumor-associated antigens have not yet been developed that have specific activities for the above functions. It appears, however, to be a matter of time until this technology together with conjugated toxins, chemotherapeutic drugs, or radioisotopes will become a major or new means of therapy and prognostic evaluation.

One example of this promise was presented by Richard Miller, of Becton Dickson, Mountainview, California, at a recent M.D. Anderson conference. Using a hybridoma of mouse and human lymphoma cells, he made a monoclonal antibody against the idiotypic region of immunoglobulins secreted by a particular patient's B cells. Appropriate doses of this antibody had the effect of preventing tumor cells from producing circulating idiotype, lending hope that such antibodies may well selectively destroy these B cells.

DIFFERENTIATION-INDUCING FACTORS: MATURATIONAL THERAPY

Differentiation and maturational approaches to therapy are not new, but within the past several years seem to have gained impetus. Vitamin A and its analogues, the retinoids; polar solvents, including dimethylsulfoxide, dimethyformamide, and miromethyformamide; and butymic acid, among other compounds have the ability to drive immature cells through benign stages of maturation, function, and death. Much of this is derived from the original studies of Leo Sachs, at the Weizmann Institute of Science, Israel. Sachs showed that various types of calls make a myoloid protein called MGI1 that causes immature cells to multiply. Another related protein, MGI2, restricts multiplication but induces differentiation when MGI2 is added to leukemic mouse cells incapable of differentiation. This approach and others by Marks and Rifkind, Memorial Sloan-Kettering, New York, with other differentiation compounds are experimental, promising, but not yet well established in human cancers.

Nonetheless, Spremulli and Dexter suggest that polar solvents and other differentiation inducing factors may be useful as adjuvants to other treatment modalities. Compounds that induce maturation rather than kill tumor cells represent an important conceptual departure from standard cytotoxic chemotherapy.

SUMMARY

The primary purpose of this chapter is to give the physician overburdened by general and speciality literature a concise *smorgasbord* of what many believe to be the most promising areas of cancer research, and in particular those areas that may well provide improved means for patient care and for prevention. The commitment of the United States in 1971, and that of other countries, to an expanded attack on cancer was and continues to be the most important health program in the biomedical history of any nation. Cancer cost in this country alone is at least $40 billion per year, not including the humanitarian cost of patient and family suffering. An investment of less than $1 billion per year since that time has resulted in remarkable advances toward control of these diseases. Cancer is predominately a disease of older people; as the United States and other Western countries approach zero population growth together with increasing longevity, if present trends continue, we must anticipate much more neoplasia. Our job is to use existing and gain new information to prevent this.

COMMENT

Does the nation's cancer program have an appropriate balance between prevention and treatment in intellectual effort and use of finite funds? Money and scientists tend to go where there is research opportunity and promise of good science. I believe this is as it should be and that this marriage has served the public well. If this be so, might the current climate of politics, the economy, and public desire upset this balance? There is reason to believe, and to be concerned, that this is happening. Beginning about 1975, and now more strident than ever, the buzz word in Congress, and certainly in its relevant appropriation subcommittees, has been prevention. In turn this infers that we have not, and even are unwilling to get priorities in order. The NIH and the NCI in particular are being increasingly beseeched by Congress and public interest groups to get their thinking in line with what they perceive to be better priority for direct people benefit. Among other of their understandable concerns is that it is better to prevent than cure. The high cost of health care delivery (the cost of medical care increased by 12 to 14 percent in 1981), unequal access to quality medical care, and an aging American population with consequent more disease and also less federal and state commitment to Medicare, Medicaid, and so forth, remain concerns.

What new is being done in prevention and, most importantly, are there exploitable research opportunities not now being funded because of bias and turf protection by the scientific community?

Considerable emphasis as warranted by data and

apparent opportunity has been placed on the identification of risk factors (including occupational exposures and life-styles) than ever before. The ACS will spend $13 million over the next 6 years to enable 80,000 unpaid volunteers to query over 1 million of their neighbors as to life-style, occupation, diet, drugs, disease history, and so forth, to further identify and evaluate risk factors predisposing to cancer and other diseases. This will lead to better individual and group surveillance, early detection, and therefore prevention. The NCI as well as the ACS are supporting projects and programs in biologic response modifiers, the flagword of which is sometimes known as chemoprevention. There is nothing wrong with this descriptive term. In fact it is an excellent way to describe how we hope to exploit relatively natural products such as interferons, retinoic acids, and actual or potential vaccines against primary hepatoma, cervical carcinoma, and some lymphomas using antigens or the viruses of hepatitis B, herpes simplex virus type II, human papillomavirus, and Epstein-Barr, respectively.

Scientists will continue to pursue the antioxicative potential of vitamins C and E (and the controversies there surrounding) to prevent the formation of nitrosamines in the bowel, hence the possible prevention of colon and other cancers. Probable carcinogens have been identified and a data base for regulation of chemicals and protection of the worker at the workplace and of his family at home has been provided. Further research has confirmed Berenblum's hypothesis that carcinogenesis, for the most part, involves the processes of initiation and promotion, thus opening new strategies for intervention. Much new research is being supported in diet and nutrition not only as to what might cause cancer but what, including additives, might prevent it.

Despite the fact that the specific causes of about 50 percent of our cancers are well known, the incidence of some cancers continues to increase. This is because as the birthrate drops, we are becoming a nation of older people, and older people develop more cancer than the young. The increase is also attributable to the fact that people do not heed information available to them. Approximately 30 percent of our cancers are directly related to the usage of tobacco alone or together with excessive consumption of alcohol. In comparison, less than 5 percent of cancers are thought to be caused by occupational exposure of the worker at the work-place, by contacts with family members, or in general through environmental pollution and exposure of people in industrialized communities. Of our approximately 225 million Americans, a large majority are in or are coming into ages (and cumulative experiences) of high risk to more than 100 diseases that we call cancer. Exposures and processes that lead to cancer take 10 to 40 years. It appears most unlikely that current knowledge and exploitable technology for prevention will reverse this process now extant in most Americans and other peoples. We must therefore seek to balance our research and control efforts between prevention and treatment. Certainly prevention of disease must be our first priority. However, for the sake of one in four Americans living today, we must continue to seek ways to prevent morbidity and death from cancer through effective programs in education, detection, treatment, and rehabilitation.

SELECTED READINGS

Albert DM, Bernards R, Dryja TP, et al: A human DNA segment with properties of the gene that predisposes to retinoblastoma and osteosarcoma. Nature (Lond) 323:643, 1986

All cancers produce malignin; has potential for early detection. Oncol Times 17 Jan 1986

Alpert S; Hanahan D, Lacey M: Bovine papillomavirus genome elicits skin tumors in transgenic mice. Nature (Lond) 322:609, 1986

Dexter DL, Spremulli EN: Polar solvents: A novel class of antineoplastic agents. J Clin Oncol 2:227, 1984

Epstein NA: Vaccination against Epstein-Barr virus: Current progress and future strategies. Lancet 1:1425, 1986

Farber S, Diamond LK, Mercer RD, et al: Temporary remissions in acute leukemia in children prolonged by folic acid antagonist 4-aminoptrein glutamic acid. N Engl J Med, 1948

Folkman J: How is blood vessel growth regulated in normal neoplastic tissue? Proc AACER 26:384, 1985

Fossel ET, Carr M, McDonah J: Detection of malignant tumors, water-suppressed proton nuclear magnetic resonance spectroscopy of plasma. N Engl J Med 35 1986

Goldstein D, Laszlo J: Interferon therapy in cancer: From imaginon to interferon. Cancer Rcs 46:4315, 1986

Gori GB, Wynder EL: Contribution of the environment to cancer incidence: An epidemiologic exercise. J Natl Cancer Inst 58:825, 1977

Grady GF: The here and now of hepatitis B immunization. N Engl J Med 315:350, 1986

Henle W, Henle G: The relation between the Epstein-Barr virus and infectious mononucleosis, Burkitt's lymphoma and cancer of the postnasal space. E Afr Med J, 46:402, 1969

Holleb AI (ed): The American Cancer Society Cancer Book. Doubleday, Garden City, NY, 1986 (To know what your patients and their families may be reading, the reader may wish to consult this text.)

Lafreniere R, Rosenberg SA, Spiess P: A new approach to the adoptive immunotherapy of cancer with tumor-infiltrating lymphocytes. Science 233:1318, 1986

Marks PA, Rifkind RA: Differentiation modifiers. Cancer 54:2766, 1984

Index

Note: Page numbers followed by *f* denote figures; those followed by *t* denote tables.